Anatomy

A Regional Atlas of the Human Body

Carmine D. Clemente, A.B. M.S. Ph.D.

Professor of Anatomy and Cell Biology and
Professor of Neurobiology, Emeritus (Recalled)
University of California at Los Angeles School of Medicine

Professor of Surgery (Anatomy)
Charles R. Drew University of Medicine and Science
Los Angeles, California

5th Edition

(With More Than 150 Plates of Direct Clinical Importance)

Lippincott Williams & Wilkins
a Wolters Kluwer business
Philadelphia • Baltimore • New York • London
Buenos Aires • Hong Kong • Sydney • Tokyo

Acquisitions Editor: Crystal Taylor
Developmental Editor: Kathleen H. Scogna
Managing Editor: Cheryl W. Stringfellow
Marketing Manager: Valerie Shannahan
Production Editor: Laura Horowitz, Hearthside Publishing Services
Project Manager: Jennifer Glazer
Designer: Risa Clow
Compositor: Maryland Composition
Printer: RR Donnelley-Willard

351 West Camden Street
Baltimore, MD 212[illegible]
530 Walnut Street

Philadelphia, PA 19106

The publisher is not responsible (as a matter of product liability, negligence, or otherwise) for any injury resulting from any material contained herein. This publication contains information relating to general principles of medical care that should not be construed as specific instructions for individual patients. Manufacturers' product information and package inserts should be reviewed for current information, including contraindications, dosages, and precautions.

This 5th edition of *Anatomy: A Regional Atlas of the Human Body* is published by arrangement with Elsevier Germany GmbH, publisher and copyright holder of *Sobotta Atlas der Anatomie des Menschen, 22. Auflage, Band 1, Band 2; München: Elsevier/Urban & Fischer* ©2006. The English translation was undertaken by Lippincott Williams & Wilkins.

Illustrations in this atlas have been published previously in the following:
Clemente, Carmine D. *Anatomy: A Regional Atlas of the Human Body*, 4th Edition. Baltimore: Williams & Wilkins, 1997.
Sobotta. *Atlas of Human Anatomy*, 21st German Edition/13th English Edition, Volumes 1 and 2. Edited by R. Putz and R. Pabst. Munich: Urban & Fischer, 2000; Baltimore: Lippincott Williams & Wilkins, 2001.
Sobotta. *Atlas of Human Anatomy*, 11th English Edition, Volume 1. Edited by J. Staubesand. Baltimore, Munich: Urban & Schwarzenberg, 1990.
Sobotta. *Atlas der Anatomie des Menschen, 18. Auflage*, Band 2. Edited by H. Ferner. München: Urban & Schwarzenberg, 1982.
Wicke, L. *Atlas of Radiologic Anatomy*, 6th English Edition. Edited and translated by A.N. Taylor. Baltimore: Williams & Wilkins, 1998.

Printed in the United States of America

First Edition, 1975, Urban & Schwarzenberg; Lea & Febiger
Second Edition, 1981, Urban & Schwarzenberg
Third Edition, 1987, Lea & Febiger; Urban & Schwarzenberg
Fourth Edition, 1997, Williams & Wilkins

Library of Congress Cataloging-in-Publication Data has been applied for. ISBN: 0-7817-5103-9.

The publishers have made every effort to trace the copyright holders for borrowed material. If they have inadvertently overlooked any, they will be pleased to make the necessary arrangements at the first opportunity.

To purchase additional copies of this book, call our customer service department at **(800) 638-3030** or fax orders to **(301) 223-2320**. International customers should call **(301) 223-2300**.

Visit Lippincott Williams & Wilkins on the Internet: http://www.LWW.com. Lippincott Williams & Wilkins customer service representatives are available from 8:30 am to 6:00 pm, EST.

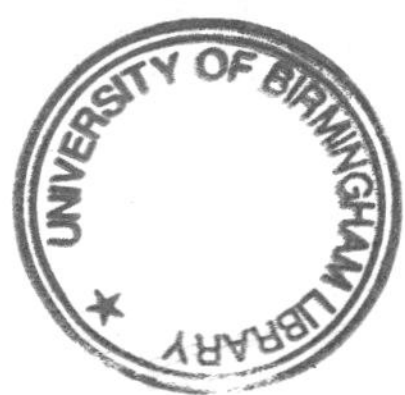
UNIVERSITY OF BIRMINGHAM LIBRARY

06 07 08 09 10
1 2 3 4 5 6 7 8 9 10

Preface to the Fifth Edition

I am most pleased that the broad-based acceptance of the 4th edition of this book has called for this new edition. I am equally happy to write that the publishers have allowed many changes and additions that, in my view, make this book an even better learning resource for all students in the health sciences and in the related professions. I continue to observe the use of this atlas in the anatomy classroom and laboratory here at the UCLA Center for the Health Sciences, and many suggestions I have received over the past 6 years from students and from friends around the world have been incorporated in this edition. Further, students have convinced me that a **special section on the cranial nerves** would be helpful to them. This has now been included and a series of diagrammatic drawings (patterned after Grant and other authors) along with a number of figures relevant to the cranial nerves have been collected in a group of **29 plates** at the end of the Neck and Head section. Most of the new cranial nerve drawings were done by Ms. Jill Penkhus several years ago when she was the resident artist in the Department of Anatomy here. In addition to these, several new pieces of art have been included in this atlas.

Among the new illustrations in this edition are modified replacements of the nine remaining illustrations in the 4th edition that originated from the controversial atlas *Topographical Human Anatomy* by Pernkopf. These new color illustrations were expertly rendered by the medical illustrators at Anatomical Chart Company (ACC) and David Rini. By far, however my deepest appreciation is extended to **Professors R. Putz** in Munich and **R. Pabst** in Hanover, Germany, for their exceedingly creative contributions for the 21st German and 13th English editions of the *Sobotta Atlas of Human Anatomy.* More than 325 figures in their most recent two-volume set are the principal new drawings on which this edition is based. The other figures are ones that were used in my 4th edition. I am responsible for all the notes that accompany all of the figures, and any mistakes that may be found in these are mine and those of no one else. I would be most grateful to any student or professor who may have suggestions or who may identify errors, if these were transmitted to me here in Los Angeles.

Many new clinically related plates have been added to those in the 4th edition. This atlas now contains more than 150 plates that are of direct clinical importance. These are listed in the front pages of the book and they include surface anatomy, radiographs (many of which come from the outstanding collection of Professor L. Wicke of Vienna), MRIs, CT scans, arteriograms, lymphangiograms, bronchograms, and even a series of arthroscopic images of the knee joint. These have been added because of the increased emphasis on the clinical relevance to the teaching of Anatomy that has become common in medical schools, not only in the United States but in many other countries as well. One plate (#146) is based on the work of Drs. R. Torrent-Guasp of Madrid and Gerald Buckberg of UCLA here in Los Angeles.

There are many who have helped to make this atlas possible. Among them are Ms. Betty Sun, Ms. Crystal Taylor, Ms. Kathleen Scogna, and Ms. Cheryl Stringfellow at Lippincott Williams & Wilkins in Baltimore and, of course, to many at the Elsevier Corporation, the publishers that acquired the Sobotta collection from Urban & Fischer. I am especially grateful to Dr. Constantine Karakousis, Professor of Surgery and Chief of Surgical Oncology at the University of Buffalo in Buffalo, New York, for his recommendations and comments on the clinical importance of several of the plates. Perhaps most of all, my continuing gratitude goes to Julie, my wife, who has helped me both at the computer and in being considerate for all the time it has taken me to do this manuscript, time that could have been given to some of her interests.

Carmine D. Clemente

Los Angeles, California — February 2006

Publisher's Acknowledgment

Lippincott Williams & Wilkins gratefully acknowledges the contribution of Thomas R. Gest, PhD, Associate Professor of Anatomical Sciences and Medical Education, University of Michigan Medical School, for his thorough review of nomenclature in the atlas.

From the Preface to the Fourth Edition

There are many changes in this edition. In fact, almost every plate and its accompanying notes have been altered. A larger type size and clearer leader lines, easier to follow, have replaced previous ones on most of the figures. Many of the notes have been rewritten and changes suggested by students here at UCLA and other students in the United States and abroad have been incorporated.

There are 135 more figures in this edition than in the third edition, representing an increase of nearly 17%. These have helped to make the various sections of the book more complete. About half of the additional figures (68) have been added to the sections on the Abdomen, Pelvis and Perineum, regions which students have asked for additional information. Most of these figures (44) were added to the section on the Pelvis and Perineum. The remainder of the new figures (67) have been distributed throughout other parts of the book, with the Lower Limb (additional 29 figures) and Neck and Head (additional 18 figures) sections receiving the most. More figures on Surface Anatomy and new Charts for each of the Muscle Groups have been included for the convenience of students. These figures and charts list simplified Origins, Insertions, Innervations, and Actions of the individual muscles. One additional feature in this edition is the detailed listing of the figures in front of each part of the Atlas. These can be used as a logical study guide sequentially consistent with the instruction in most Anatomy courses.

Most of the figures of this edition have come from the 3rd Edition of this Atlas or from the 20th German Edition of Sobotta, edited by Professor Reinhard Putz, Director of the Institute of Anatomy in Munich and Professor Reinhard Pabst from the University of Hannover in Germany. I am most grateful to them for their elegant anatomical figures. Also I am greatly indebted to Dr. Lothar Wicke for figures from his *Atlas of Radiographic Anatomy*. Additionally, a number of illustrations have been used from the classic Pernkopf textbook, *Atlas of Topographic and Applied Human Anatomy* and still others have come from the Benninghoff-Goerttler textbooks and from earlier editions of the Sobotta Atlas edited by Professors Helmut Ferner and Jochen Staubesand. I also wish to acknowledge with appreciation Professor Gene Colborn from the Medical College of Georgia in Augusta, Georgia, USA, for producing six line drawings.

Many of the drawings in this edition are new and many others are exact redrawings of figures used previously. I am especially grateful to the publishers both in Baltimore and Munich for allowing me to enlarge the Atlas, to enhance the clarity of the figures and to reset all of the plates and notes. Special thanks are extended to Dr. Michael Urban and Timothy S. Satterfield and to Renate Hausdorf, Dorle Matussek, Raymond Reter and Crystal Taylor for their enormous help in bringing this book to completion. I am also grateful to Deborah Tourtlotte for compiling the index. In Los Angeles, I thank Drs. Charles H. Sawyer and Anthony M. Adinolfi for their support and suggestions through the years. Finally, and most importantly, I dedicate this volume to my wife, Julie, for her love and unending kindness through the decades.

Carmine D. Clemente

Los Angeles, California — July, 1996

From the Preface to the First Edition

Twenty-five years ago, while a student at the University of Pennsylvania, I marvelled at the clarity, completeness, and boldness of the anatomical illustrations of the original German editions of Professor Johannes Sobotta's Atlas and their excellent three-volume, English counterparts, the recent editions of which were authored by the late Professor Frank H. J. Figge. It is a matter of record that before World War II these atlases were the most popular ones consulted by American medical students. In the United States, with the advent of other anatomical atlases, the shortening of courses of anatomy in the medical schools, and the increase in publishing cost, the excellent but larger editions of the Sobotta atlases have become virtually unknown to a full generation of students. During the past 20 years of teaching Gross Anatomy at the University of California at Los Angeles, I have found only a handful of students who are familiar with the beautiful and still unexcelled Sobotta illustration.

This volume introduces several departures from the former Sobotta atlases. It is the first English edition that represents the Sobotta plates in a regional sequence - the pectoral region and upper extremity, the thorax, the abdomen, the pelvis and perineum, the lower extremity, the back, vertebral column and spinal cord, and finally, the neck and head. This sequence is consistent with that followed in many courses presented in the United States and Canada and one which should be useful to students in other countries.

Many have contributed to bringing this Atlas to fruition. I thank Dr. David S. Maxwell, Professor and Vice Chairman for Gross Anatomy and my colleague at UCLA, for his encouragement and suggestions. I also wish to express my appreciation to Caroline Belz and Louise Campbell, who spent many hours proofreading and typing the original text. I especially wish to thank Mary Mansor for constructing the index—a most laborious task. I am grateful to Barbara Robins for her assistance in typing some of the early parts of the manuscript, and above all, to her sister Julie, who is my wife and who makes all of my efforts worthwhile through her encouragement and devotion.

Carmine D. Clemente

Los Angeles, California — January, 1975

Contents

5 Back, Vertebral Column, and Spinal Cord

6 Lower Extremity

7 Neck and Head

Index

Plates of Direct Clinical Importance

Plates of Direct Clinical Importance (Continued)

Plate 352	Intervertebral Discs
Plate 354, 355	Radiographs: Cervical, Thoracic and Lumbar Regions
Plates 364–367	Surface Anatomy of Lower Limb
Plates 388, 389	Sites for Intramuscular Injections: Lateral Thigh, Gluteal Region
Plate 397	Arteriogram of the Femoral, Popliteal, and Tibial Arteries Region
Plate 435	Radiograph of the Knee (A P Projection)
Plate 439, 442	MRIs of the Knee Joint
Plate 444	Arthrogram of the Knee Joint
Plate 445	Arthroscopic Images of the Knee Joint
Plates 448, 452	Radiograph of the Ankle Joint
Plate 456	Radiograph and MRI of Ankle, Subtalar, and Talocalcuneoventricular Joints
Plate 459	Longitudinal Arches of the Foot
Plates 460–465	Cross Sections and MRIs of the Thigh, Leg, and Foot
Plate 468, 469	Surface Anatomy of the Head and Neck
Plate 485	Scintiscan and Ultrasonogram of the Thyroid Gland
Plate 486, 487	Lymphatic Channels of the Head and Neck
Plate 505	Arthograph of the Temporomandibular Joint
Plate 527	Circle of Willis and its Variations
Plate 528	Internal Carotid Arteriogram
Plate 529	Vertebral Artery Arteriogram
Plate 538	Surface Anatomy of the Anterior Orbit
Plate 555	MRI through the Orbit
Plates 556, 557	The Retinal Vessels through an Ophthalmoscope and the Branches of the Vessels at the Optic Disc
Plate 564	Surface Projections of the Paranasal Sinuses
Plates 568, 569	Oral Cavity, Sublingual Region, Lower Teeth, and Dorsum of the Tongue
Plate 580	Innervation of the Teeth
Plate 584	The Permanent Teeth, Vestibular and Medial Aspects
Plate 601	Laryngoscopic Views of the Larynx
Plate 614–642	The Cranial Nerves I through XII

Plates Containing Muscle Charts

PECTORAL REGION, AXILLA, SHOULDER, AND UPPER LIMB

PLATES

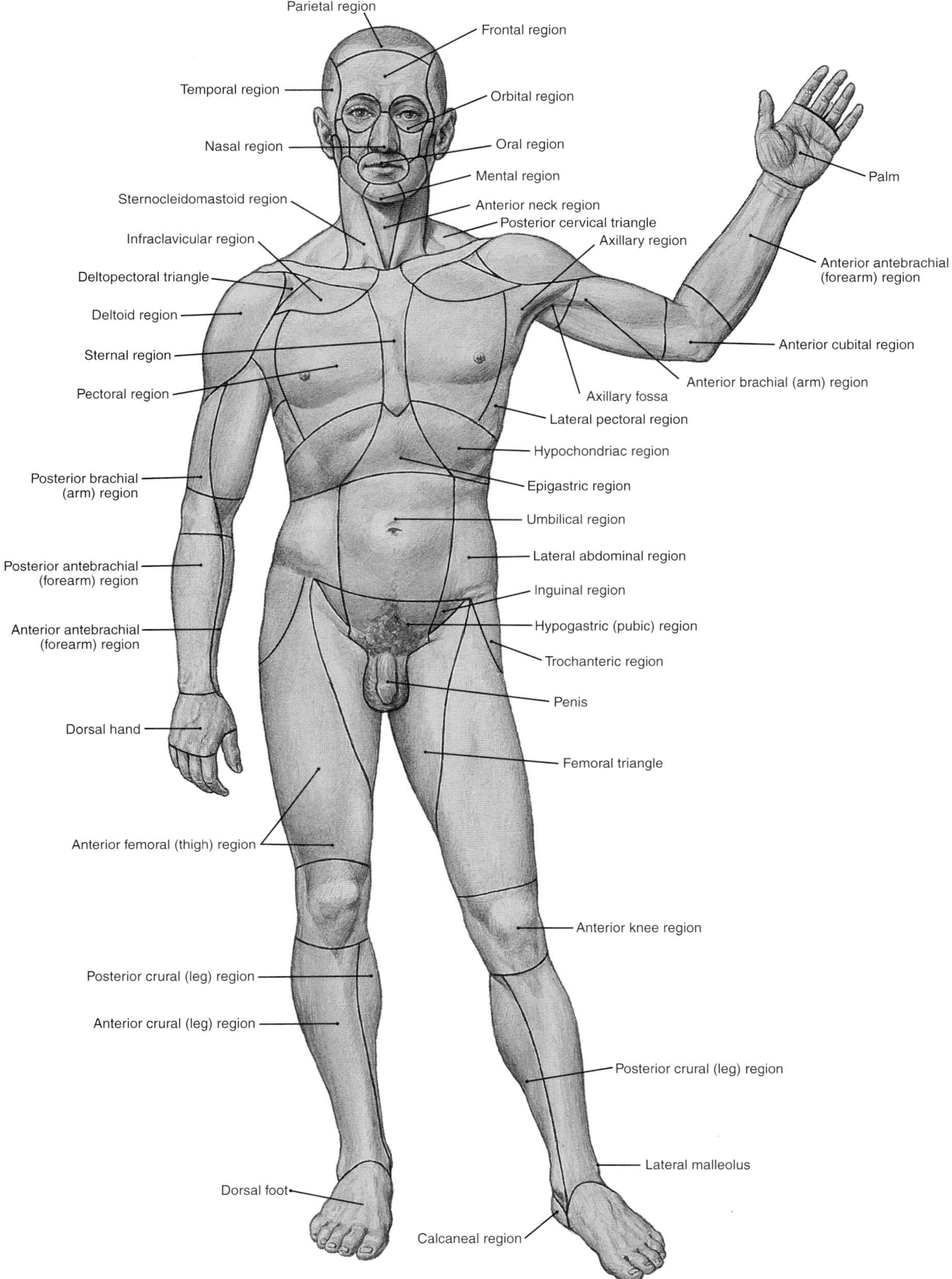
Parietal region
Frontal region
Temporal region
Orbital region
Nasal region
Oral region
Mental region
Sternocleidomastoid region
Anterior neck region
Posterior cervical triangle
Infraclavicular region
Axillary region
Palm
Anterior antebrachial (forearm) region
Deltopectoral triangle
Deltoid region
Sternal region
Anterior cubital region
Pectoral region
Anterior brachial (arm) region
Axillary fossa
Lateral pectoral region
Hypochondriac region
Posterior brachial (arm) region
Epigastric region
Umbilical region
Posterior antebrachial (forearm) region
Lateral abdominal region
Inguinal region
Anterior antebrachial (forearm) region
Hypogastric (pubic) region
Trochanteric region
Penis
Dorsal hand
Femoral triangle
Anterior femoral (thigh) region
Anterior knee region
Posterior crural (leg) region
Anterior crural (leg) region
Posterior crural (leg) region
Lateral malleolus
Dorsal foot
Calcaneal region

Figure 1 Regions of the Body: Anterior View

NOTE: (1) Surface areas are identified by specific names to describe the location of structures and symptoms precisely.

(2) Some regions are named after bones (sternal, parietal, infraclavicular, etc.), others for muscles (deltoid, pectoral, sternocleidomastoid), and still others for specialized anatomical structures (umbilical, oral, nasal, etc.).

(3) The principal regions of the body include the pectoral region and upper extremity, thorax, abdomen, pelvis and perineum, lower extremity, back and spinal column, and neck and head.

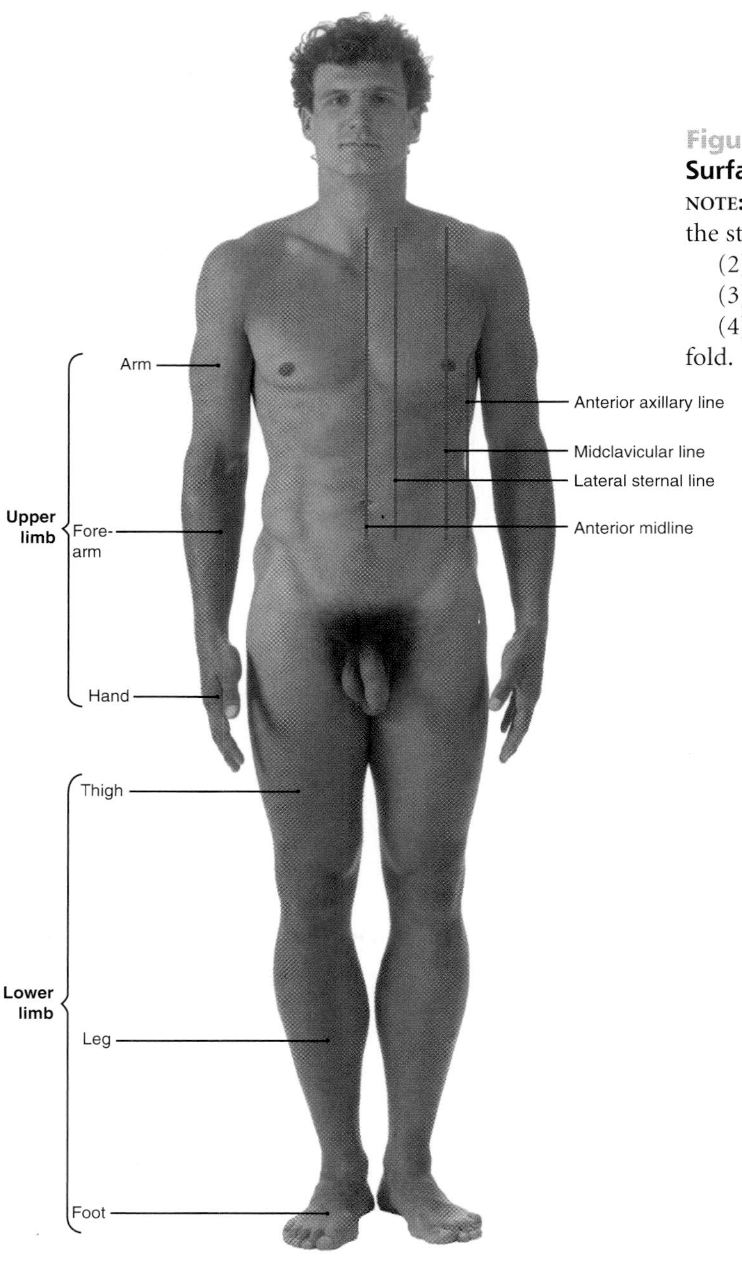
Arm
Upper limb
Fore-arm
Hand
Thigh
Lower limb
Leg
Foot
Anterior axillary line
Midclavicular line
Lateral sternal line
Anterior midline

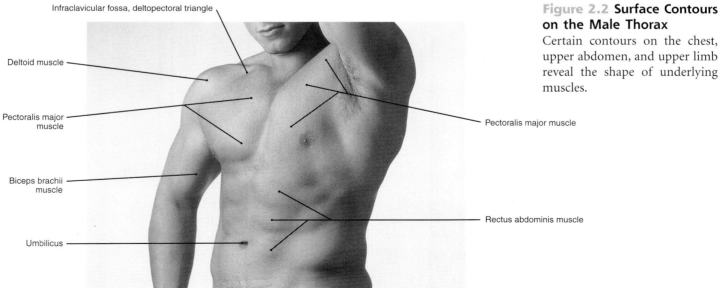

Figure 2.1 Regions and Longitudinal Lines on the Anterior Surface of the Male Body

NOTE: (1) The lateral sternal line descends along the lateral border of the sternum.

(2) Other lines parallel to this are called parasternal lines.

(3) The male nipple lies near the midclavicular line.

(4) The anterior axillary line descends from the anterior axillary fold.

Infraclavicular fossa, deltopectoral triangle
Deltoid muscle
Pectoralis major muscle
Biceps brachii muscle
Umbilicus
Pectoralis major muscle
Rectus abdominis muscle

Figure 2.2 Surface Contours on the Male Thorax

Certain contours on the chest, upper abdomen, and upper limb reveal the shape of underlying muscles.

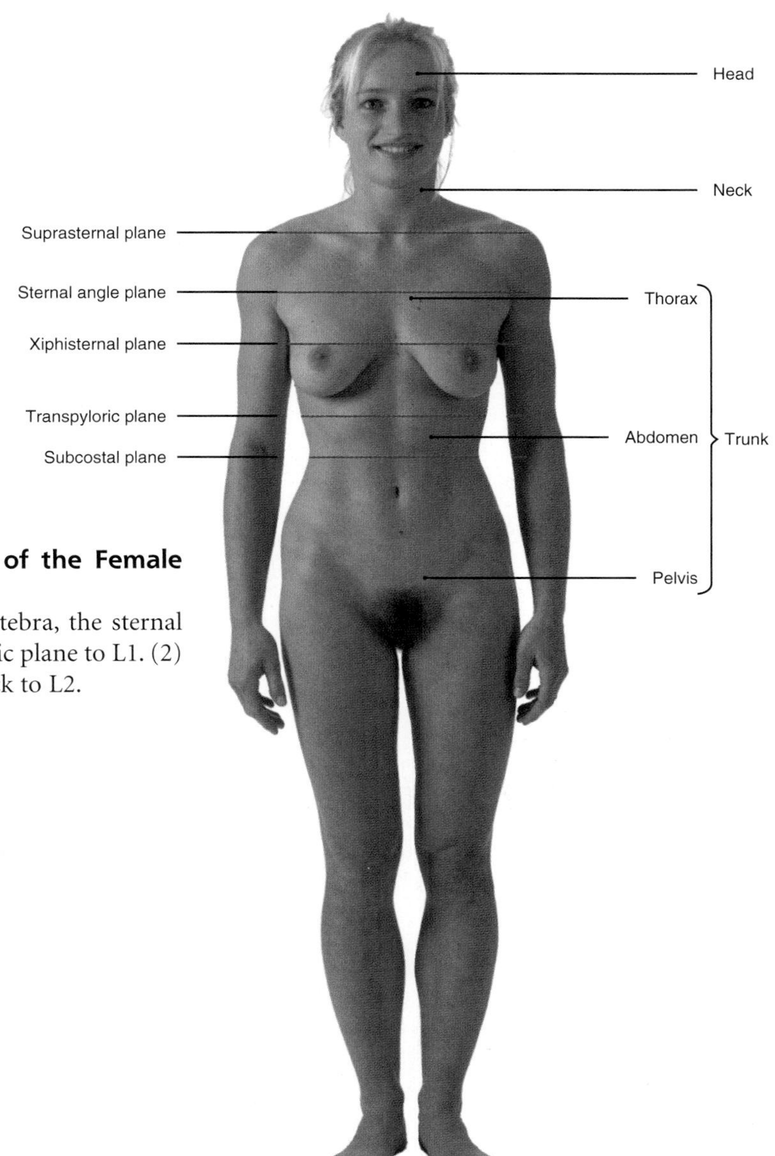
Head
Neck
Suprasternal plane
Sternal angle plane
Thorax
Xiphisternal plane
Transpyloric plane
Abdomen
Trunk
Subcostal plane
Pelvis

Figure 3.1 Transverse Planes Shown on the Surface of the Female Thorax

NOTE: (1) The suprasternal plane projects back to the T2 vertebra, the sternal angle to T4, the xiphisternal junction to T9, and the transpyloric plane to L1. (2) The subcostal plane, below the 10th rib anteriorly, projects back to L2.

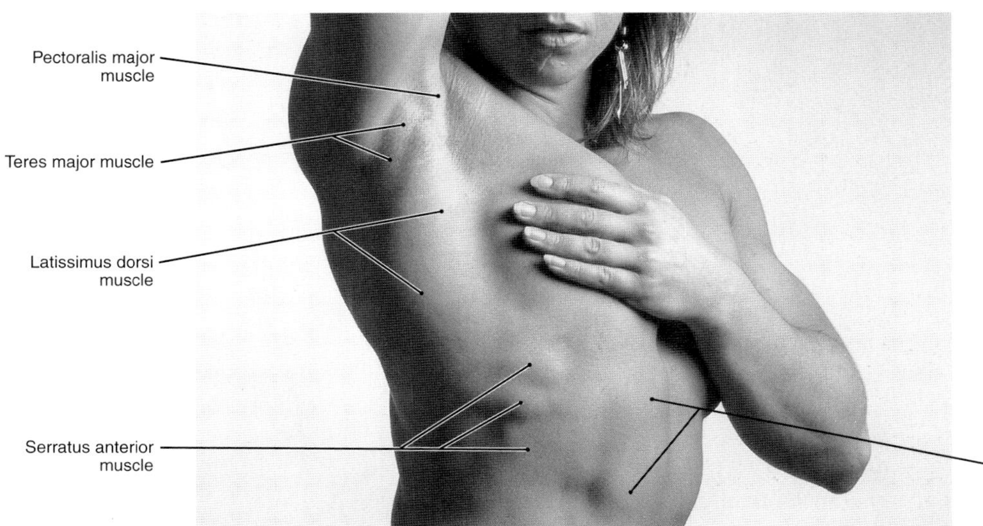
Pectoralis major muscle
Teres major muscle
Latissimus dorsi muscle
Serratus anterior muscle
Rectus abdominis muscle

Figure 3.2 Surface Contours on the Lateral Thorax of a Young Woman

Note the contours of well-developed latissimus dorsi, pectoralis major, teres major, and serratus anterior muscles.

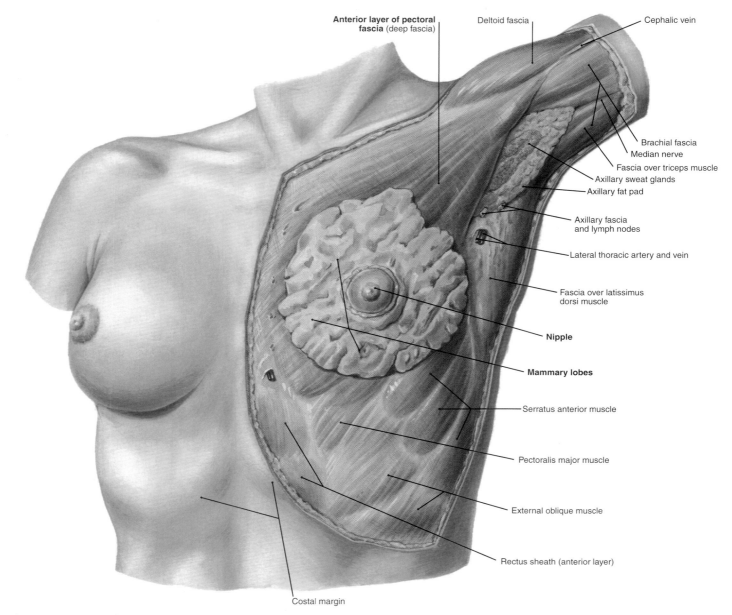

Anterior layer of pectoral fascia (deep fascia)
Deltoid fascia
Cephalic vein
Brachial fascia
Median nerve
Fascia over triceps muscle
Axillary sweat glands
Axillary fat pad
Axillary fascia and lymph nodes
Lateral thoracic artery and vein
Fascia over latissimus dorsi muscle
Nipple
Mammary lobes
Serratus anterior muscle
Pectoralis major muscle
External oblique muscle
Rectus sheath (anterior layer)
Costal margin

Figure 4.1 Anterior Pectoral Region and Female Breast ▲

NOTE: (1) The lobular nature of the breast.

(2) It extends from the lateral sternal line to the midaxillary line and from the second to the sixth rib.

(3) The breast is located in the superficial fascia anterior to the pectoral fascia.

(4) Shown are the superficial axillary lymph nodes and the axillary sweat glands.

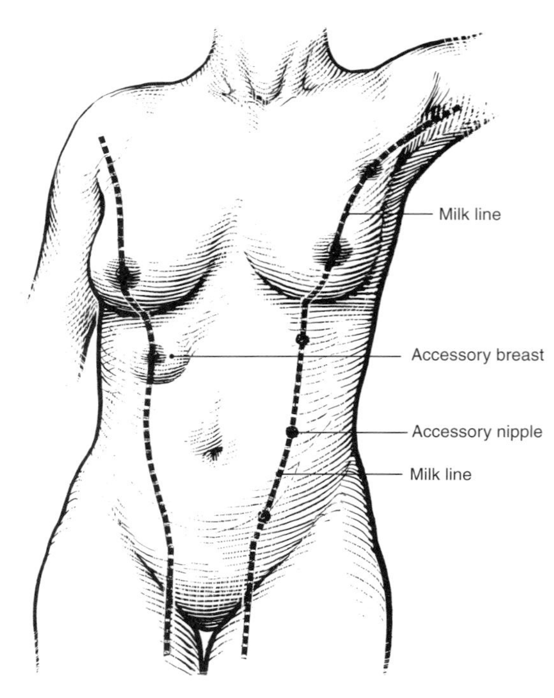
Milk line
Accessory breast
Accessory nipple
Milk line

Figure 4.2 Milk Line and Accessory Nipples and Breasts ▶

NOTE: (1) Supernumerary nipples (polythelia) and/or multiple breasts on the same side (polymastia) occur in about 1% of people.

(2) These are found along the curved milk line extending from the axillary fossa to the groin.

(3) This condition occurs slightly more frequently in males than in females and may easily be handled surgically.

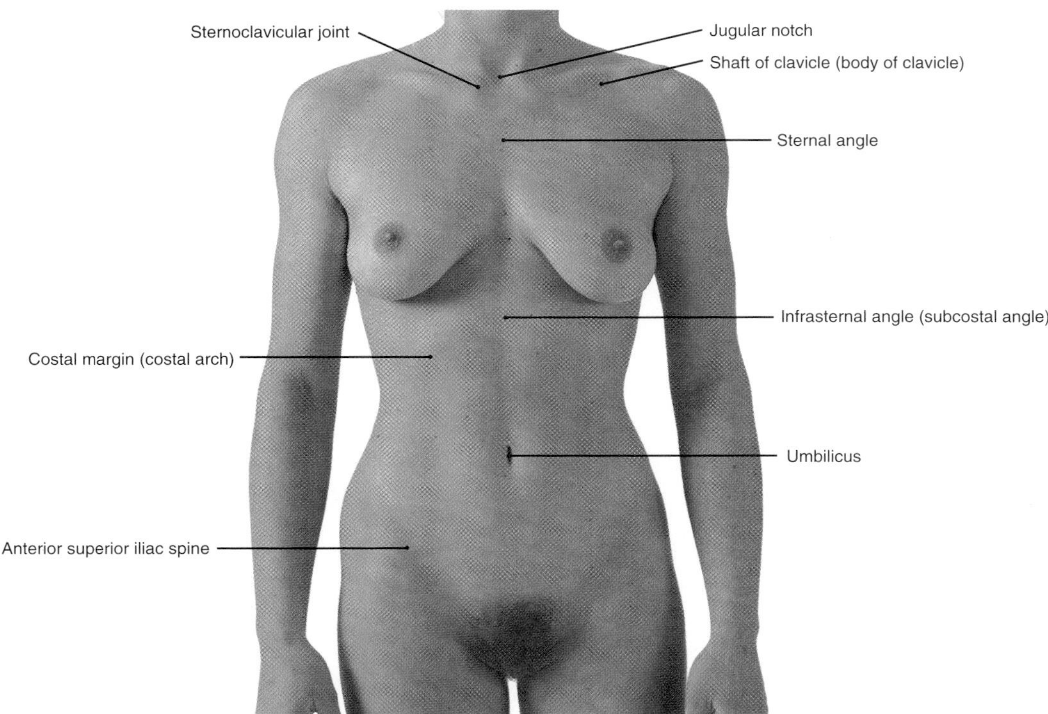
Sternoclavicular joint
Jugular notch
Shaft of clavicle (body of clavicle)
Sternal angle
Infrasternal angle (subcostal angle)
Costal margin (costal arch)
Umbilicus
Anterior superior iliac spine

Figure 5.1 Surface Anatomy of the Anterior Thoracic and Abdominal Walls of a Young Female
NOTE: Bony structures and the umbilicus are labeled.

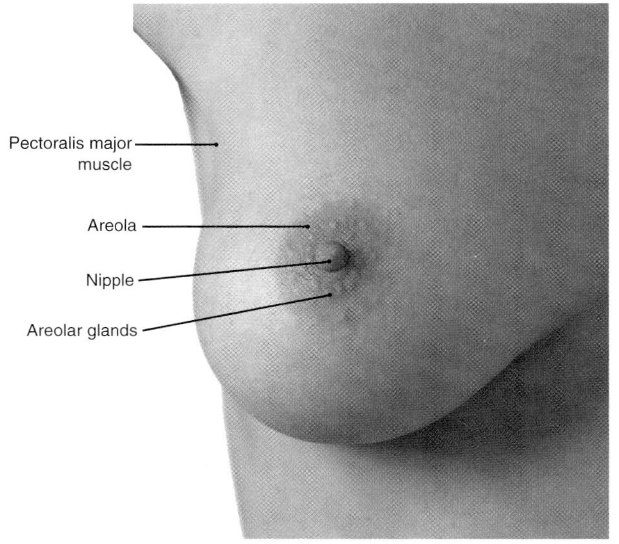
Pectoralis major muscle
Areola
Nipple
Areolar glands

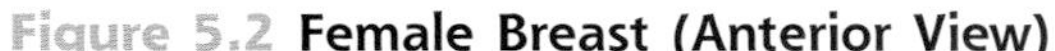

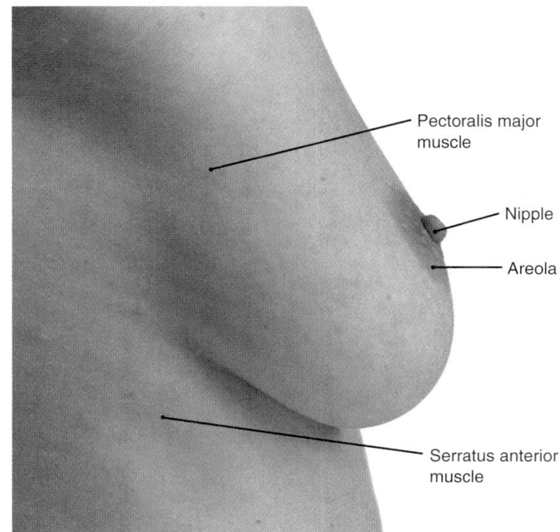
Pectoralis major muscle
Nipple
Areola
Serratus anterior muscle

Figure 5.2 Female Breast (Anterior View)

Figure 5.3 Female Breast (Lateral View)

NOTE: The nipple and areolar glands project from the surface of the pigmented areola. Also observe the muscular contours of the pectoralis major and serratus anterior muscles.

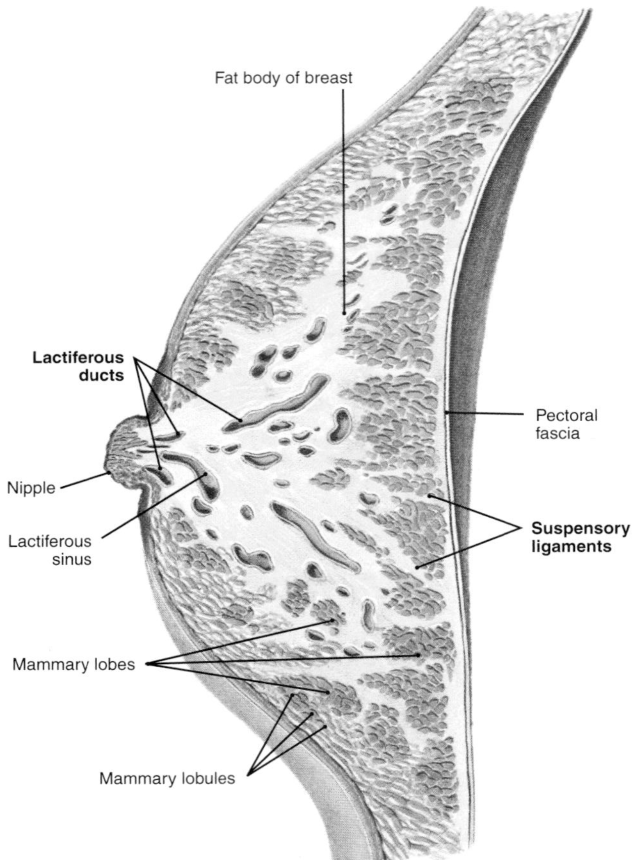
Fat body of breast
Lactiferous ducts
Nipple
Lactiferous sinus
Pectoral fascia
Suspensory ligaments
Mammary lobes
Mammary lobules

Figure 6.1 Sagittal Section through Mammary Gland of Gravid Female

NOTE: (1) The radial arrangement of the lobes, separated by connective tissue and fat.

(2) In the lactiferous duct system, each of the 15 to 20 lobes has its own duct.

(3) The pectoral fascia separates the breast from the pectoralis major muscle.

(4) The connective-tissue suspensory ligaments (of Cooper) extend to the pectoral fascia.

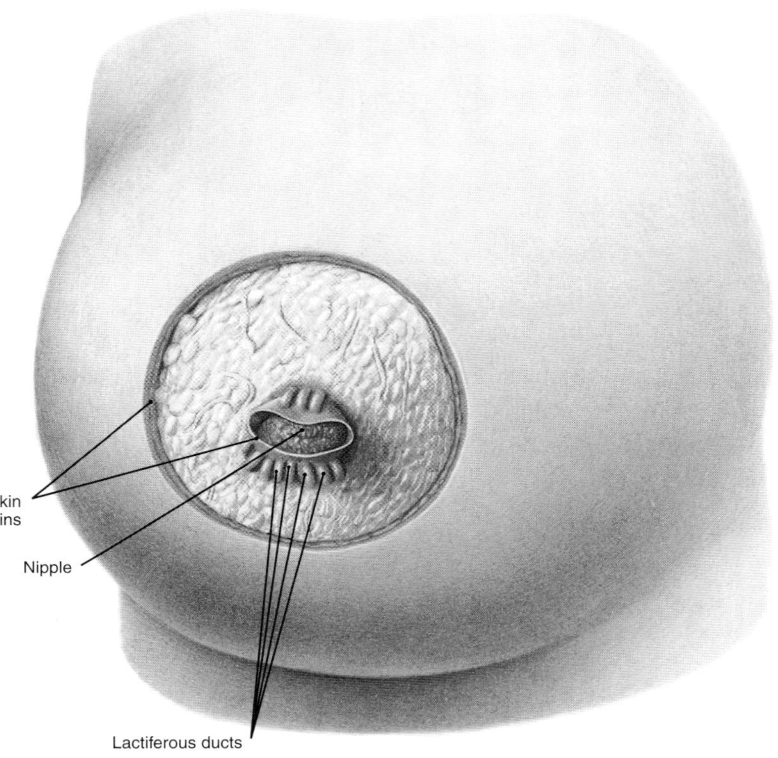
Cut skin margins
Nipple
Lactiferous ducts

Figure 6.2 Right Mammary Gland: Dissection of the Nipple ▶

NOTE: (1) A circular piece of skin has been incised from around the nipple.

(2) The 15 to 20 lactiferous ducts are arranged radially around the nipple and seen just deep to the skin.

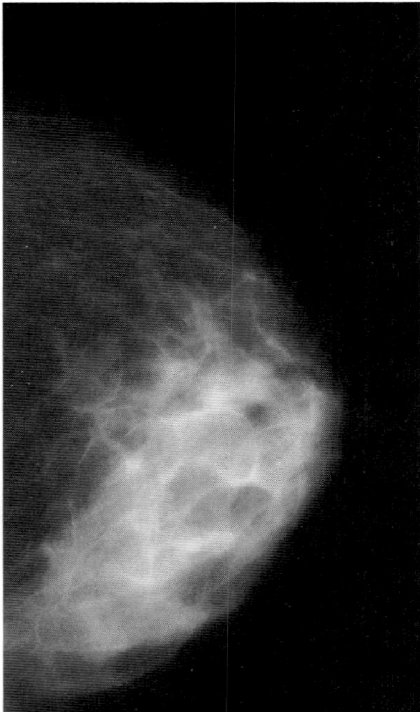

Figure 6.3 Radiograph of Normal Female Breast

Lateral mammograph of a 47-year-old woman.

Cancer of the Breast

Cancer of the breast usually develops in the epithelial cells that line the ducts of the glandular tissue. Often the initial clinical sign of breast cancer is a painless lump in the upper lateral quadrant of the organ. This may progress:

(1) to invade the connective tissue between the lobules (suspensory ligaments of Cooper) and cause a **retraction of the nipple**;

(2) to grow more deeply and **fix the breast to the pectoral fascia** overlying the pectoralis major muscle. This causes the breast to be **less movable** and it **tends to elevate** when the underlying pectoralis major contracts;

(3) to cause a **dimpling, a thickening, and a discoloration of the skin over the tumor**. The skin then assumes an appearance of an orange peel and hence has been called the **peau d'orange sign** of advanced breast carcinoma.

From the local primary tumor site, malignant cells spread by entering lymphatic capillaries and proceed to lymph nodes, where they may multiply to form metastatic secondary tumors. The most frequent routes of early metastatic spread involve the lateral thoracic and axillary lymph nodes as well as nodes that accompany the internal thoracic vessels lateral and parallel to the sternum. Spread of tumor cells also occurs by way of venous capillaries to larger veins and then to more widespread organs.

Lymphatic Drainage of the Breast; Lymphangiogram of Axilla

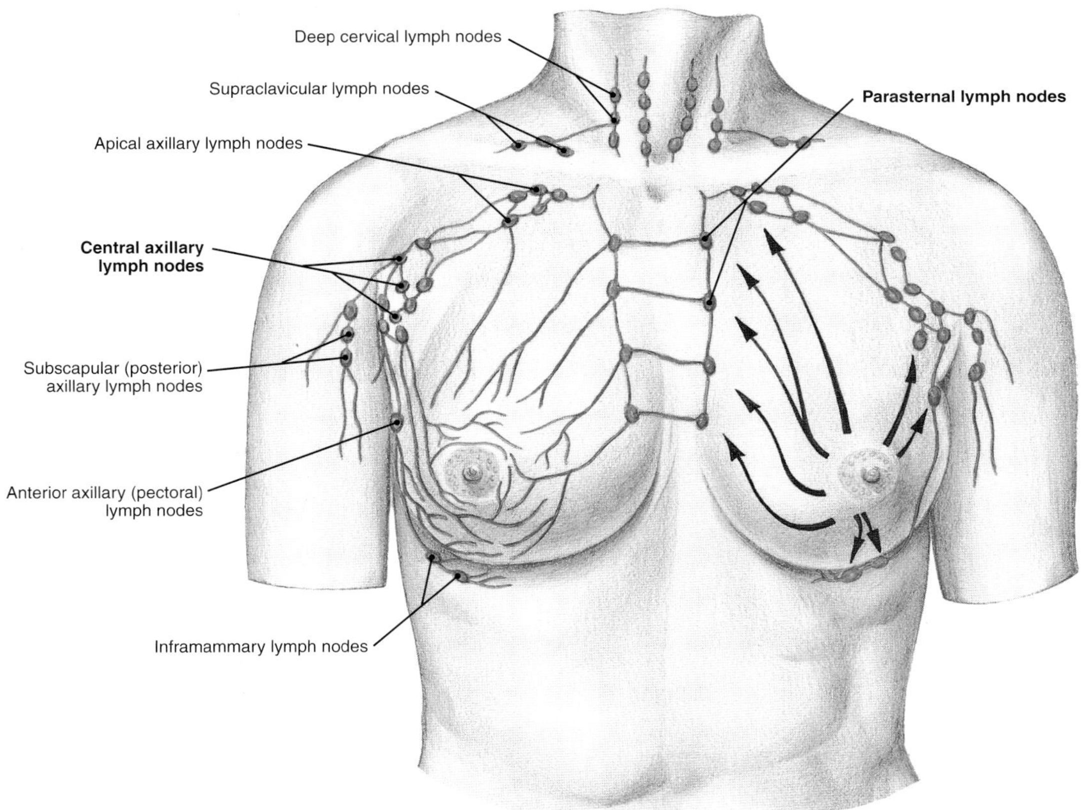
Deep cervical lymph nodes
Supraclavicular lymph nodes
Apical axillary lymph nodes
Central axillary lymph nodes
Subscapular (posterior) axillary lymph nodes
Anterior axillary (pectoral) lymph nodes
Inframammary lymph nodes
Parasternal lymph nodes

Figure 7.1 Lymphatic Drainage from the Adult Female Breast

NOTE: (1) Numerous lymph vessels in the breast communicate in a subareolar plexus deep to and around the nipple.
(2) About 85% of the lymph from the breast courses laterally and upward to axillary and infraclavicular nodes.
(3) Most of the remaining lymph passes medially to parasternal nodes along the internal thoracic vessels.
(4) Some lymph vessels drain downward to upper abdominal nodes and some go to the opposite breast.

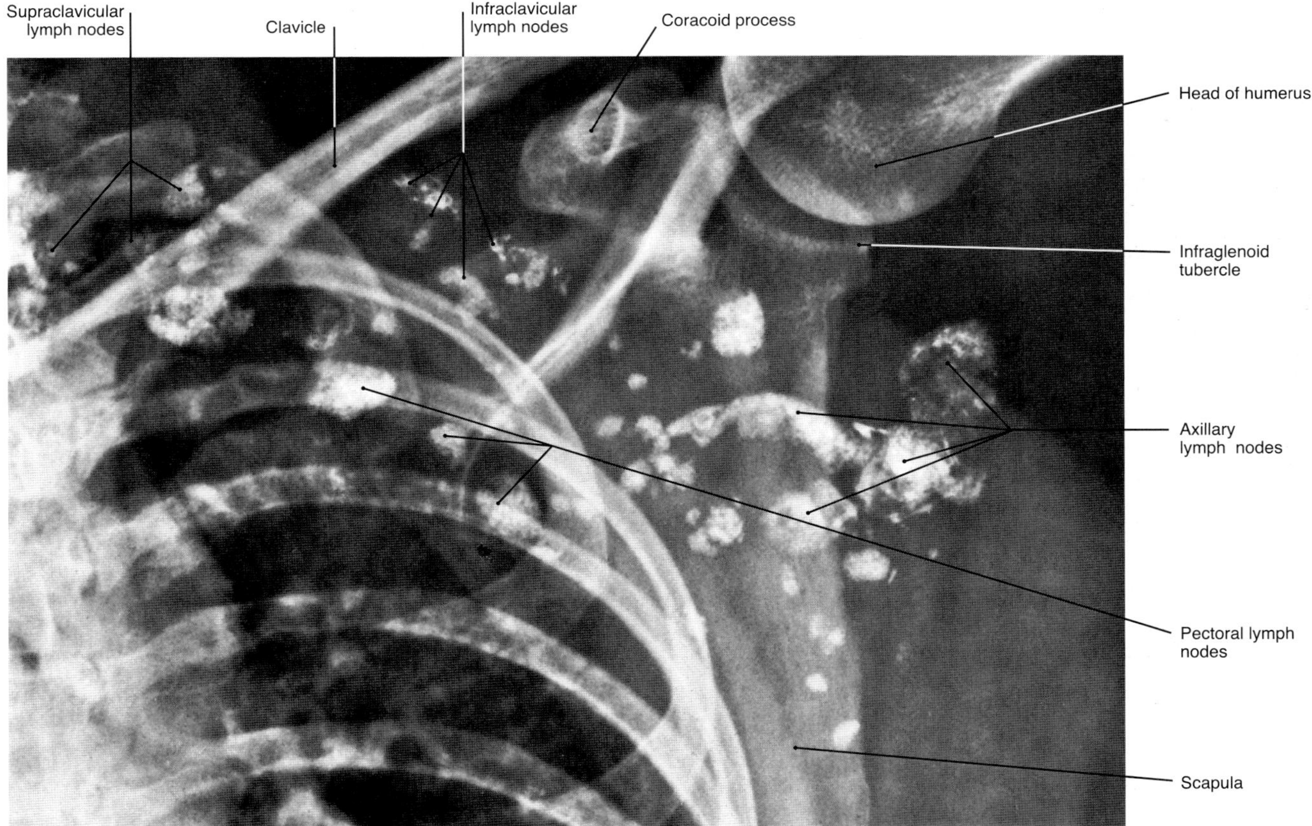
Supraclavicular lymph nodes
Clavicle
Infraclavicular lymph nodes
Coracoid process
Head of humerus
Infraglenoid tubercle
Axillary lymph nodes
Pectoral lymph nodes
Scapula

Figure 7.2 Lymphangiogram of the Pectoral and Axillary Lymph Nodes
(From Wicke, 6th ed.)

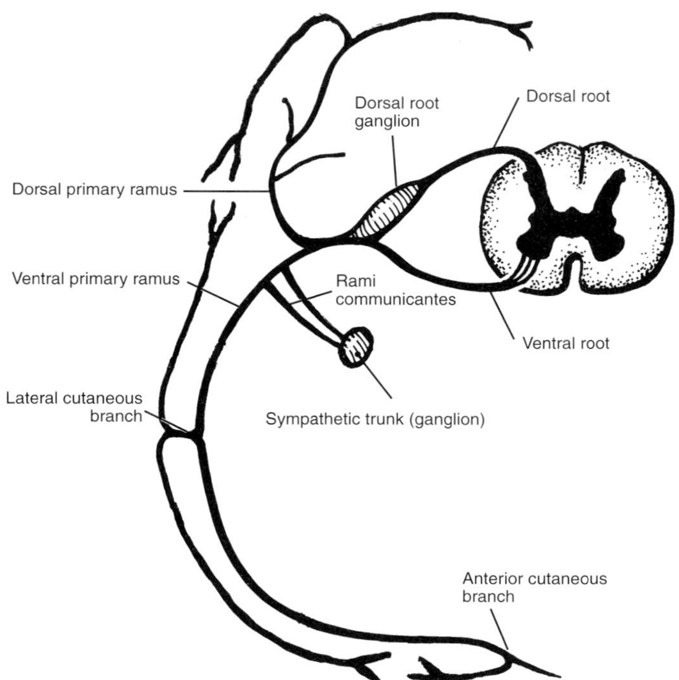
Dorsal root ganglion
Dorsal root
Dorsal primary ramus
Ventral primary ramus
Rami communicantes
Ventral root
Lateral cutaneous branch
Sympathetic trunk (ganglion)
Anterior cutaneous branch

Figure 8.1 Typical Spinal Nerve: Its Origin, Branches, and Connections to the Sympathetic Trunk

NOTE: (1) Each spinal nerve attaches to the spinal cord by a dorsal (sensory) root and a ventral (motor) root.

(2) Each dorsal root contains a spinal ganglion, where the cell bodies of sensory neurons are found.

(3) The dorsal and ventral roots of the same segment join to form a spinal nerve, which soon divides into dorsal and ventral primary rami.

(4) The dorsal primary ramus supplies the back; the ventral primary ramus supplies the lateral and anterior walls of the trunk.

(5) Spinal nerves communicate with the sympathetic trunk by way of rami communicantes.

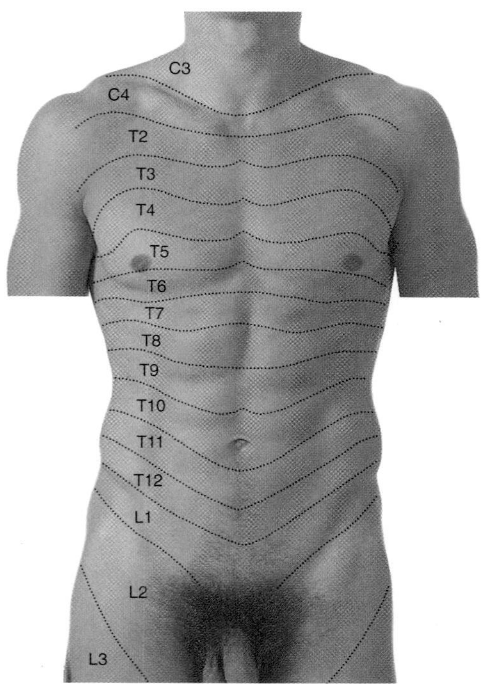
C3
C4
T2
T3
T4
T5
T6
T7
T8
T9
T10
T11
T12
L1
L2
L3

Figure 8.2 Segmental Sensory Innervation of Anterior Body Wall (Dermatomes)

NOTE: C5 to C8 and most of T1 do not supply the body wall, since they supply the upper limb.

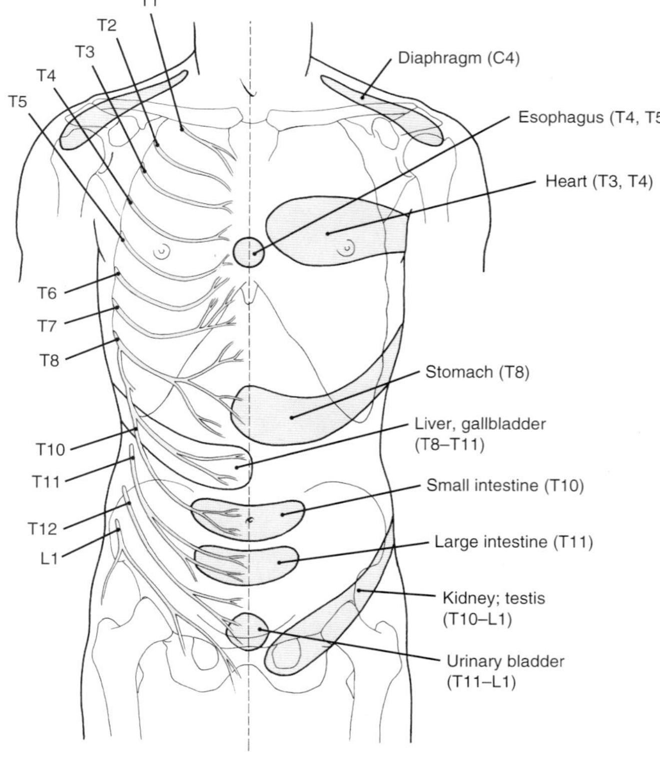
T1
T2
T3
T4
T5
T6
T7
T8
T10
T11
T12
L1
Diaphragm (C4)
Esophagus (T4, T5)
Heart (T3, T4)
Stomach (T8)
Liver, gallbladder (T8–T11)
Small intestine (T10)
Large intestine (T11)
Kidney; testis (T10–L1)
Urinary bladder (T11–L1)

Figure 8.3 Segmental Sensory Nerves (Right) and Pain Projection Regions (Left)

NOTE: (1) The sequential segmental sensory nerves from T1 to L1 supply the anterior body wall.

(2) The body wall regions to which pain from internal visceral organs is projected.

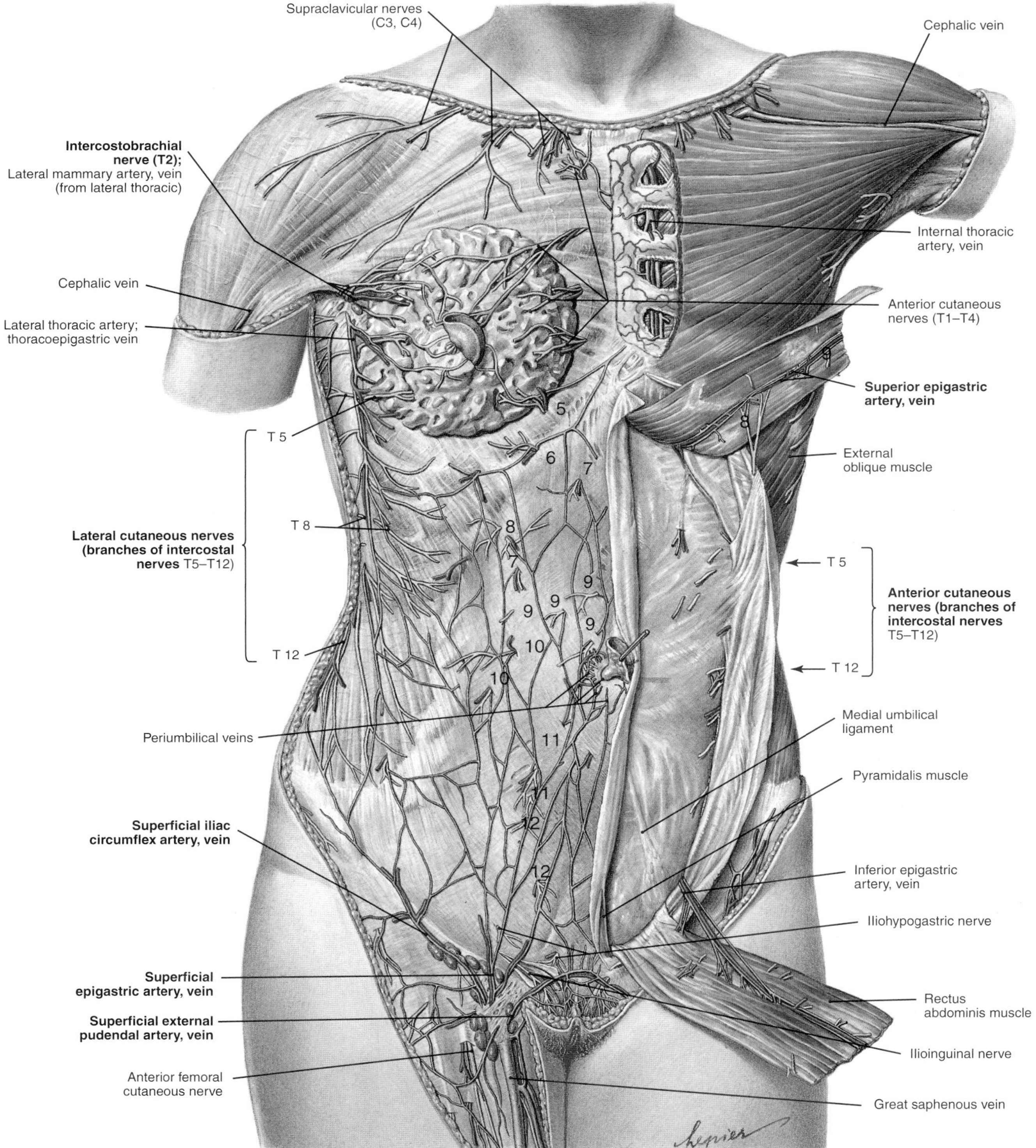
Supraclavicular nerves (C3, C4)
Cephalic vein
Intercostobrachial nerve (T2);
Lateral mammary artery, vein (from lateral thoracic)
Internal thoracic artery, vein
Cephalic vein
Anterior cutaneous nerves (T1–T4)
Lateral thoracic artery; thoracoepigastric vein
Superior epigastric artery, vein
T 5
External oblique muscle
T 8
Lateral cutaneous nerves (branches of intercostal nerves T5–T12)
T 5
Anterior cutaneous nerves (branches of intercostal nerves T5–T12)
T 12
T 12
Medial umbilical ligament
Periumbilical veins
Pyramidalis muscle
Superficial iliac circumflex artery, vein
Inferior epigastric artery, vein
Iliohypogastric nerve
Superficial epigastric artery, vein
Rectus abdominis muscle
Superficial external pudendal artery, vein
Ilioinguinal nerve
Anterior femoral cutaneous nerve
Great saphenous vein
5
6
7
8
7
9
9
9
9
10
10
11
11
12
12

Figure 9 Superficial Vessels and Nerves of the Anterior Trunk: Pectoral Region and Anterior Abdominal Wall

NOTE: (1) Cutaneous innervation of the trunk: supraclavicular nerves (C3, C4), intercostal nerves (T1–T12), and the ilioinguinal and iliohypogastric branches of L1.

(2) The intercostal nerves give off lateral and anterior cutaneous branches.

(3) Anastomoses between the thoracoepigastric vein above and the superficial iliac circumflex and inferior epigastric veins below.

(4) The breast, its innervation (T2 to T6 intercostal nerves) and its blood supply (internal thoracic artery, lateral thoracic artery, and intercostal arteries).

(5) The nipple at the level of T4 and the umbilicus at the level of T10.

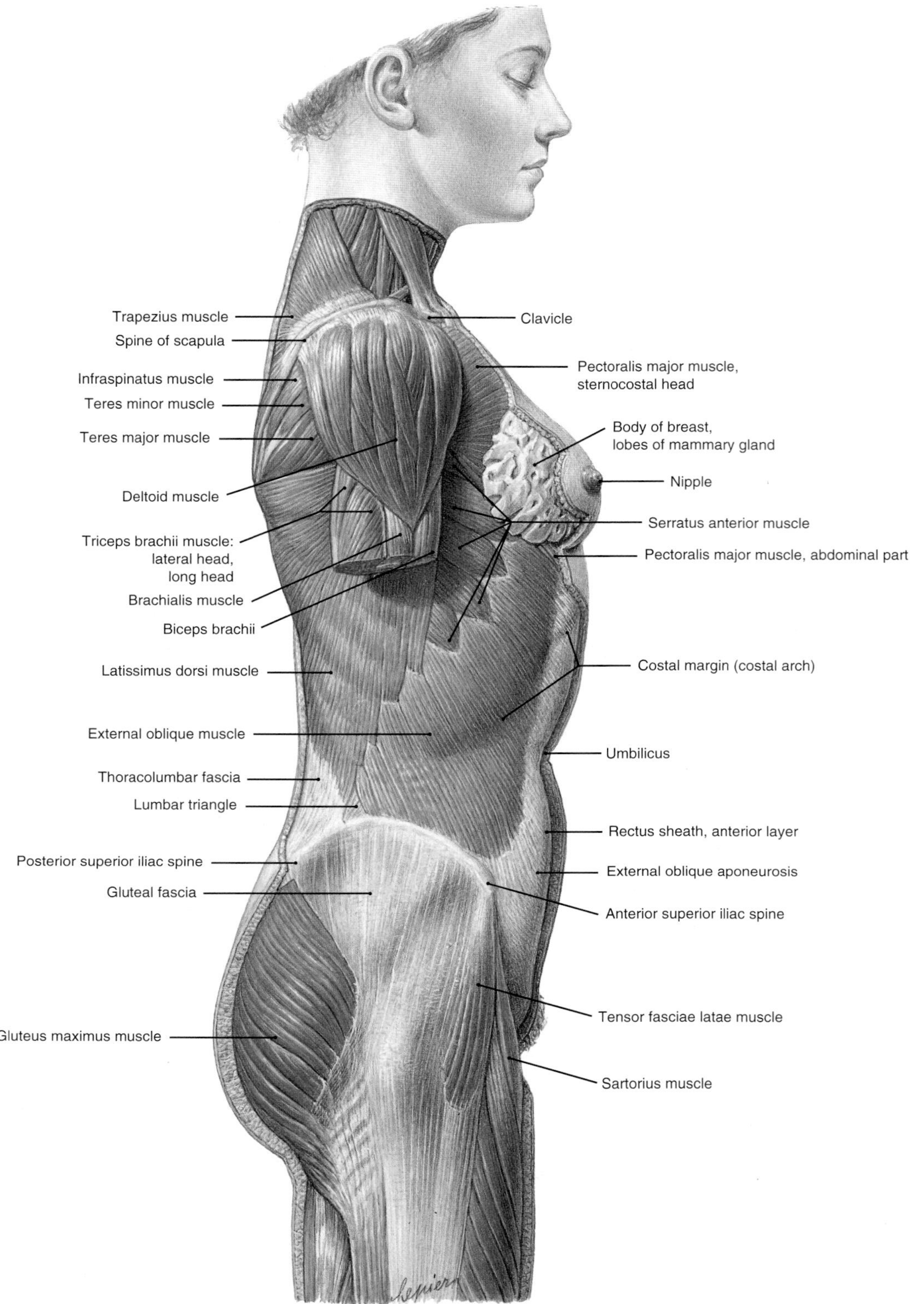
Trapezius muscle
Spine of scapula
Infraspinatus muscle
Teres minor muscle
Teres major muscle
Deltoid muscle
Triceps brachii muscle: lateral head, long head
Brachialis muscle
Biceps brachii
Latissimus dorsi muscle
External oblique muscle
Thoracolumbar fascia
Lumbar triangle
Posterior superior iliac spine
Gluteal fascia
Gluteus maximus muscle
Clavicle
Pectoralis major muscle, sternocostal head
Body of breast, lobes of mammary gland
Nipple
Serratus anterior muscle
Pectoralis major muscle, abdominal part
Costal margin (costal arch)
Umbilicus
Rectus sheath, anterior layer
External oblique aponeurosis
Anterior superior iliac spine
Tensor fasciae latae muscle
Sartorius muscle

Figure 10 Muscles of the Lateral Thoracic and Abdominal Wall

NOTE: (1) The interdigitations of the external oblique muscle with the serratus anterior muscle superiorly and the latissimus dorsal muscle inferiorly.

(2) The lumbar triangle. Its boundaries are the external oblique muscle (anteriorly), the latissimus dorsi muscle (posteriorly), and the crest of the ilium (inferiorly).

(3) The external oblique muscle ends in a broad and strong aponeurosis medially.

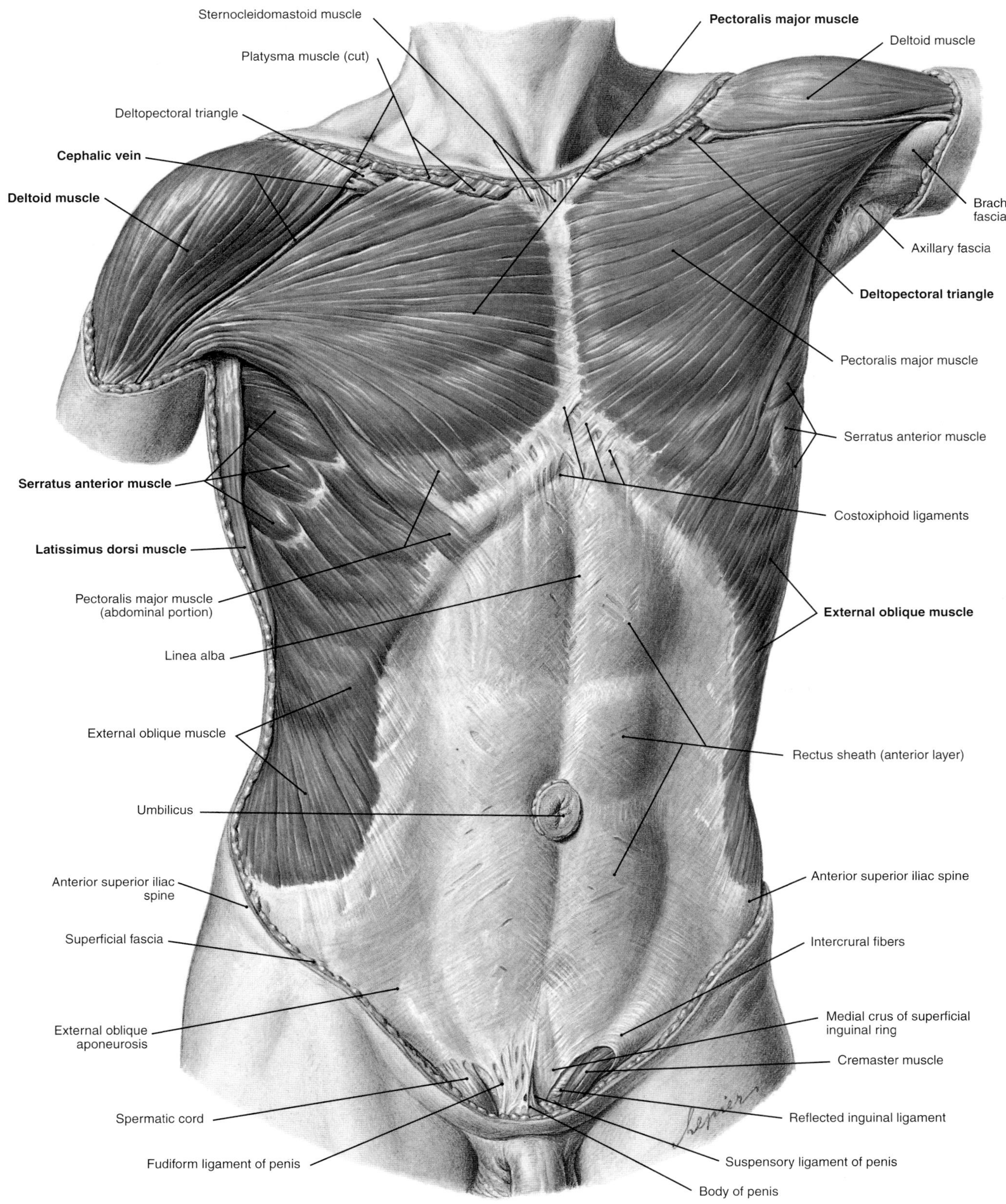
Sternocleidomastoid muscle
Platysma muscle (cut)
Deltopectoral triangle
Cephalic vein
Deltoid muscle
Pectoralis major muscle
Deltoid muscle
Brachial fascia
Axillary fascia
Deltopectoral triangle
Pectoralis major muscle
Serratus anterior muscle
Serratus anterior muscle
Costoxiphoid ligaments
Latissimus dorsi muscle
Pectoralis major muscle (abdominal portion)
External oblique muscle
Linea alba
External oblique muscle
Rectus sheath (anterior layer)
Umbilicus
Anterior superior iliac spine
Anterior superior iliac spine
Superficial fascia
Intercrural fibers
External oblique aponeurosis
Medial crus of superficial inguinal ring
Cremaster muscle
Spermatic cord
Reflected inguinal ligament
Fudiform ligament of penis
Suspensory ligament of penis
Body of penis

Figure 11 **Muscles of the Superficial Thoracic and Abdominal Walls**

Muscle	Origin	Insertion	Innervation	Action
Pectoralis major	Medial half of clavicle; second to sixth ribs; costal margin of sternum; aponeurosis of external oblique	Humerus, lateral lip of intertubercular sulcus	Lateral (C5, C6, C7) and medial (C8, T1) pectoral nerves	Adducts and rotates arm medially; **sternal part:** helps extend humerus; **clavicular part:** helps flex humerus

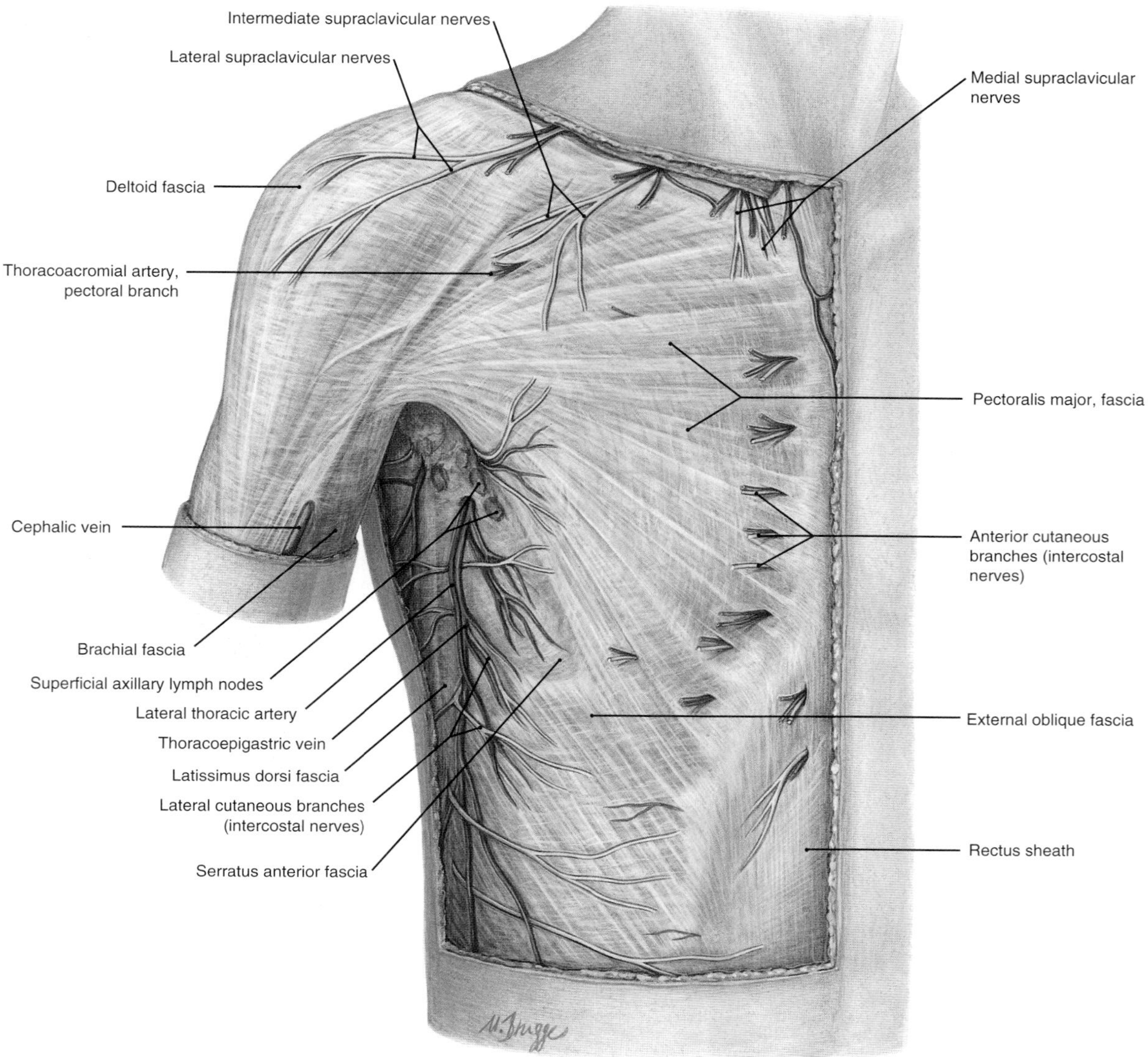
Intermediate supraclavicular nerves
Lateral supraclavicular nerves
Medial supraclavicular nerves
Deltoid fascia
Thoracoacromial artery, pectoral branch
Pectoralis major, fascia
Cephalic vein
Anterior cutaneous branches (intercostal nerves)
Brachial fascia
Superficial axillary lymph nodes
Lateral thoracic artery
External oblique fascia
Thoracoepigastric vein
Latissimus dorsi fascia
Lateral cutaneous branches (intercostal nerves)
Rectus sheath
Serratus anterior fascia

Figure 12 Anterior Thoracic Wall; Superficial Dissection in the Male

NOTE: (1) The skin and superficial fascia have been removed, but the cutaneous vessels and nerves have been retained.

(2) The cutaneous neurovascular structures penetrate through the deep fascia (pectoral fascia) to get to the superficial fascia and skin.

(3) Most of the cutaneous vessels and nerves are anterior and lateral cutaneous branches of the intercostal nerves.

(4) The supraclavicular nerves derived from C3 and C4.

(5) The intercostobrachial nerve (T2). It joins the medial brachial cutaneous nerve to supply the skin of the axillary fossa and upper medial arm.

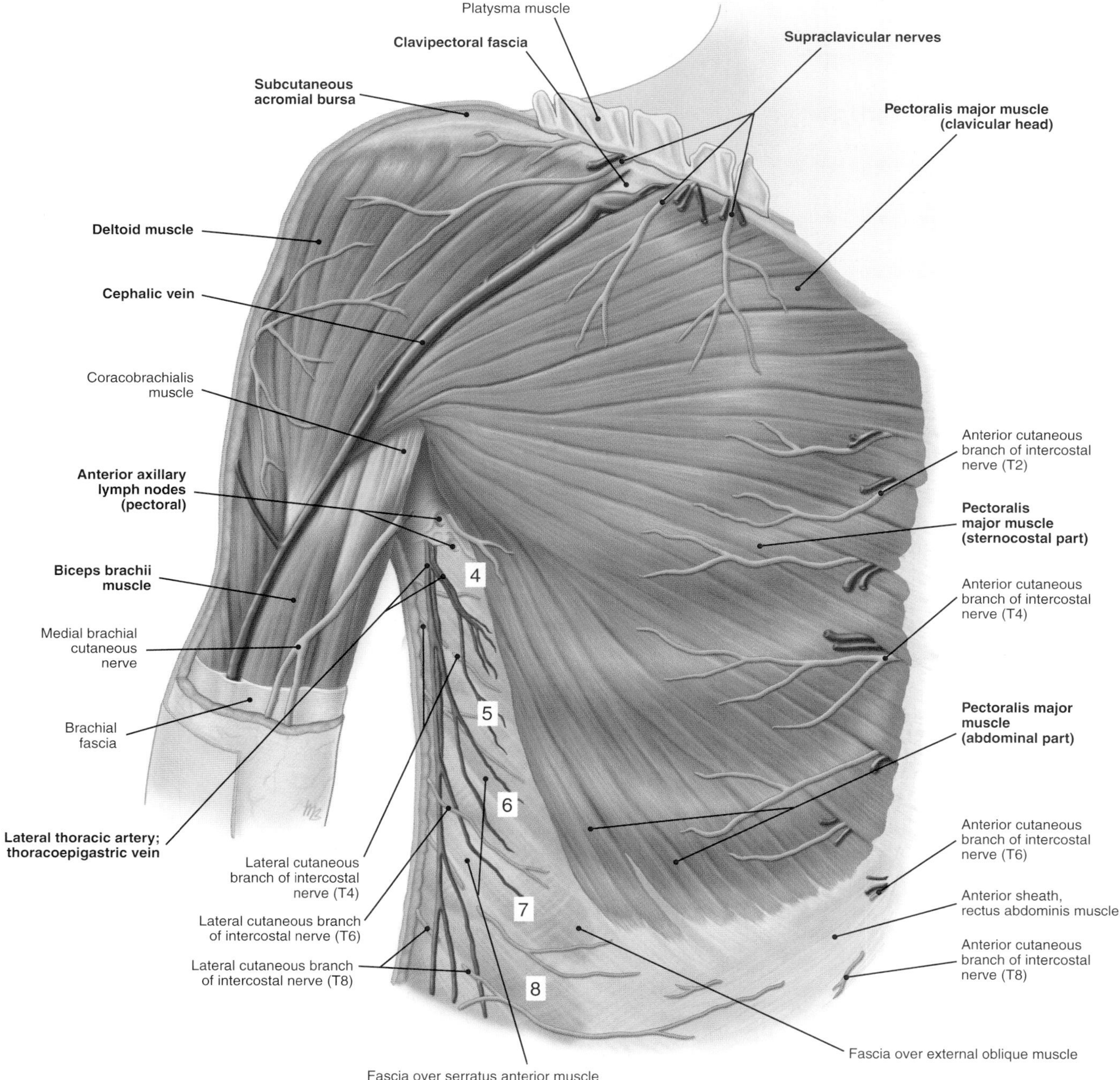
Platysma muscle
Clavipectoral fascia
Supraclavicular nerves
Subcutaneous acromial bursa
Pectoralis major muscle (clavicular head)
Deltoid muscle
Cephalic vein
Coracobrachialis muscle
Anterior cutaneous branch of intercostal nerve (T2)
Anterior axillary lymph nodes (pectoral)
Pectoralis major muscle (sternocostal part)
Biceps brachii muscle
4
Anterior cutaneous branch of intercostal nerve (T4)
Medial brachial cutaneous nerve
Brachial fascia
5
Pectoralis major muscle (abdominal part)
6
Lateral thoracic artery; thoracoepigastric vein
Lateral cutaneous branch of intercostal nerve (T4)
Anterior cutaneous branch of intercostal nerve (T6)
Lateral cutaneous branch of intercostal nerve (T6)
7
Anterior sheath, rectus abdominis muscle
Lateral cutaneous branch of intercostal nerve (T8)
8
Anterior cutaneous branch of intercostal nerve (T8)
Fascia over external oblique muscle
Fascia over serratus anterior muscle

Figure 13 Pectoralis Major and Deltoid Muscles (Anterior View)

NOTE: (1) The anterior layer of the pectoral fascia and the deltoid fascia as seen in Figure 12 have been removed.

(2) The lateral cutaneous vessels and nerves penetrating through the intercostal spaces in the midaxillary line.

(3) The anterior cutaneous vessels and nerves piercing the pectoralis major muscle along the lateral border of the sternum.

(4) The clavicular fibers of this muscle course obliquely downward, and laterally, the upper sternocostal fibers are directed nearly horizontally and the lower sternocostal and abdominal fibers ascend nearly vertically to the humerus.

(5) The natural cleft between the clavicular and sternocostal heads. Detaching the clavicular head uncovers some of the vessels and nerves that supply this muscle (see Figure 15.1).

(6) The fourth to the eighth ribs are numbered sequentially.

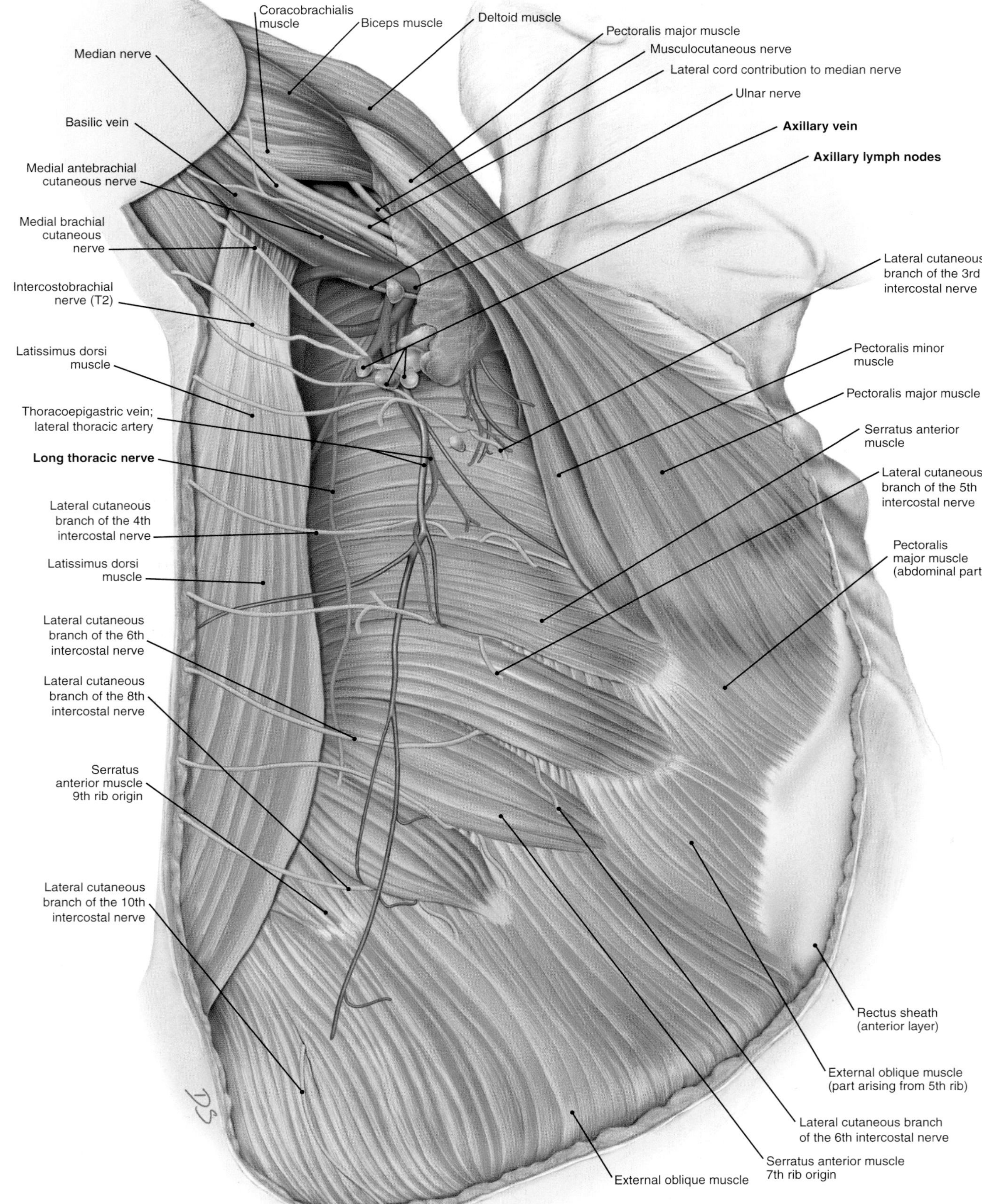
Coracobrachialis muscle
Biceps muscle
Deltoid muscle
Pectoralis major muscle
Musculocutaneous nerve
Lateral cord contribution to median nerve
Ulnar nerve
Axillary vein
Axillary lymph nodes
Median nerve
Basilic vein
Medial antebrachial cutaneous nerve
Medial brachial cutaneous nerve
Intercostobrachial nerve (T2)
Latissimus dorsi muscle
Thoracoepigastric vein; lateral thoracic artery
Long thoracic nerve
Lateral cutaneous branch of the 4th intercostal nerve
Latissimus dorsi muscle
Lateral cutaneous branch of the 6th intercostal nerve
Lateral cutaneous branch of the 8th intercostal nerve
Serratus anterior muscle 9th rib origin
Lateral cutaneous branch of the 10th intercostal nerve
Lateral cutaneous branch of the 3rd intercostal nerve
Pectoralis minor muscle
Pectoralis major muscle
Serratus anterior muscle
Lateral cutaneous branch of the 5th intercostal nerve
Pectoralis major muscle (abdominal part)
Rectus sheath (anterior layer)
External oblique muscle (part arising from 5th rib)
Lateral cutaneous branch of the 6th intercostal nerve
Serratus anterior muscle 7th rib origin
External oblique muscle

Figure 14 **Lateral Aspect of the Upper Right Thoracic Wall and the Superficial Axillary Structures**

Muscle	Origin	Insertion	Innervation	Action
Pectoralis minor	Coracoid process of scapula	Ribs 2 to 5	Medial pectoral nerve (C8, T1)	Protracts scapula; elevates ribs
Serratus anterior	Fleshy slips from upper nine ribs	Medial border of scapula	Long thoracic nerve (C5, C6, C7)	Protracts and rotates scapula; holds scapula close to thoracic wall

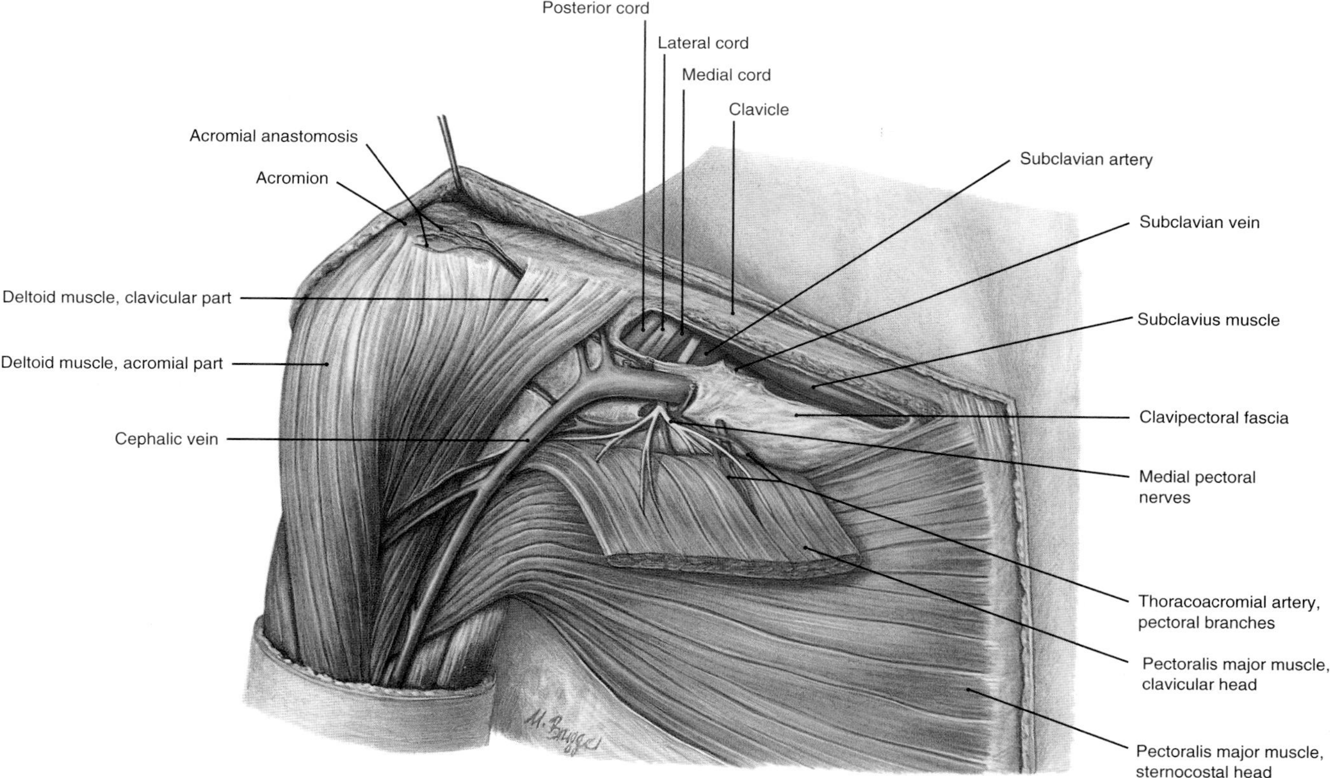
Posterior cord
Lateral cord
Medial cord
Clavicle
Acromial anastomosis
Acromion
Subclavian artery
Subclavian vein
Deltoid muscle, clavicular part
Subclavius muscle
Deltoid muscle, acromial part
Clavipectoral fascia
Cephalic vein
Medial pectoral nerves
Thoracoacromial artery, pectoral branches
Pectoralis major muscle, clavicular head
Pectoralis major muscle, sternocostal head

Figure 15.1 Deltopectoral Triangle (Right)

NOTE: (1) The clavicular head of the pectoralis major muscle has been severed and reflected downward.

(2) The investing layer of deep fascia covering the deep surface of the pectoralis major muscle and the clavipectoral fascia, which extends between the clavicle and the medial border of the pectoralis minor muscle, are exposed.

(3) The cephalic vein pierces the clavipectoral fascia to join the axillary vein.

(4) The thoracoacromial artery (from the axillary artery) and the lateral pectoral nerve (from the lateral cord of the brachial plexus) pierce the fascia from below to supply blood to the region and to innervate the pectoralis major muscle.

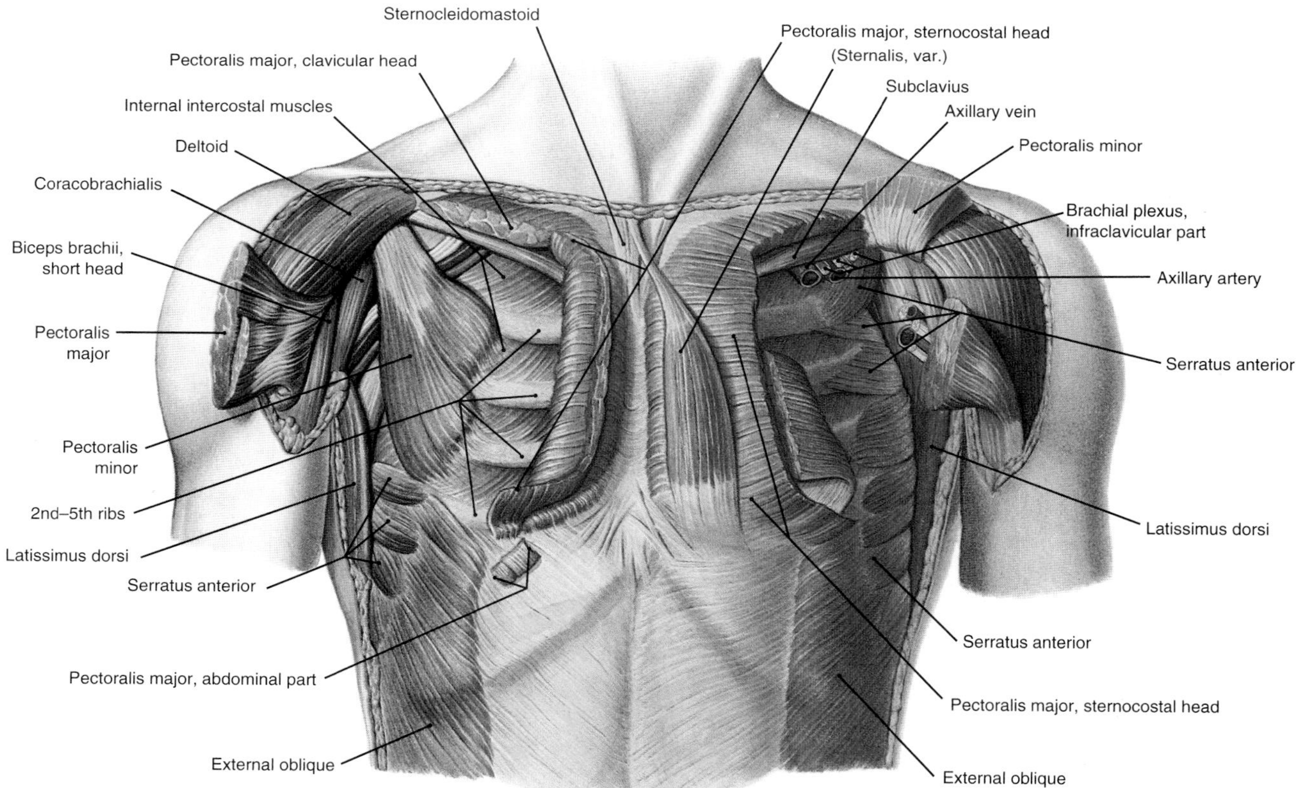
Sternocleidomastoid
Pectoralis major, sternocostal head
(Sternalis, var.)
Pectoralis major, clavicular head
Subclavius
Internal intercostal muscles
Axillary vein
Deltoid
Pectoralis minor
Coracobrachialis
Brachial plexus, infraclavicular part
Biceps brachii, short head
Axillary artery
Pectoralis major
Serratus anterior
Pectoralis minor
2nd–5th ribs
Latissimus dorsi
Latissimus dorsi
Serratus anterior
Serratus anterior
Pectoralis major, abdominal part
Pectoralis major, sternocostal head
External oblique
External oblique

Figure 15.2 Pectoralis Minor, Serratus Anterior, and Latissimus Dorsi Muscles (Right Lateral View)

NOTE that the pectoralis major muscle has been reflected, revealing the pectoralis minor muscle extending from the second to fifth ribs to the coracoid process. Also note that the serratus anterior muscle forms the medial wall of the axilla.

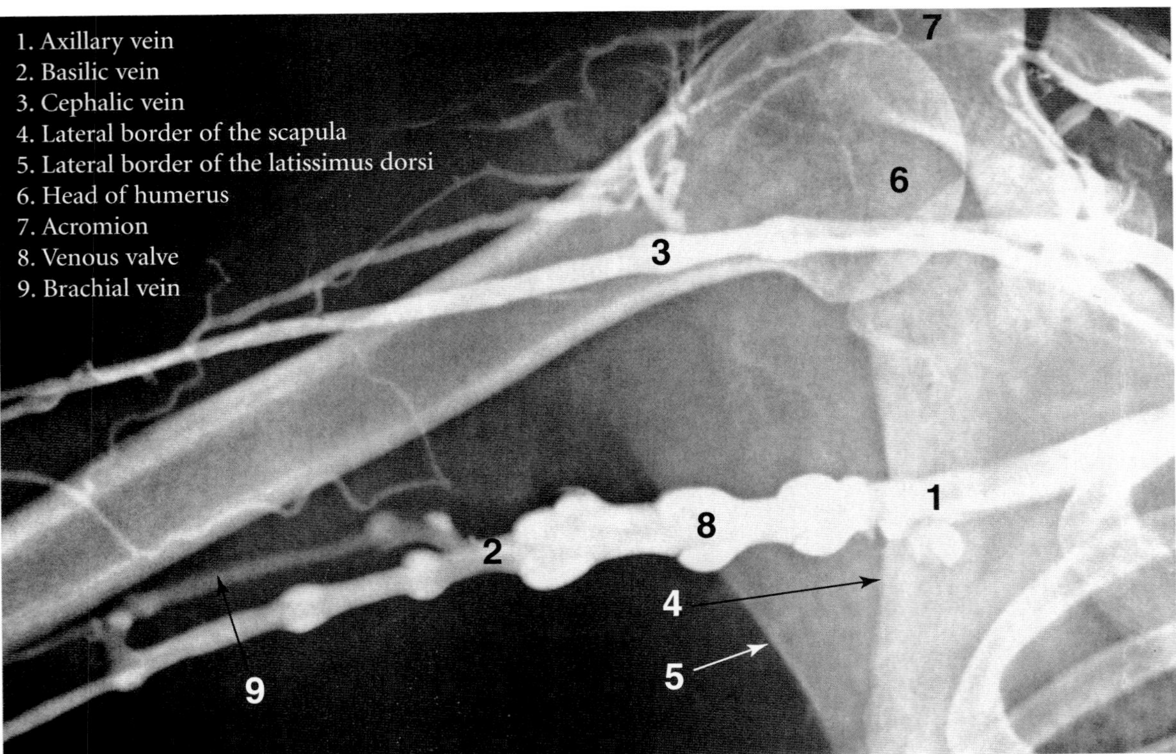
1. Axillary vein
2. Basilic vein
3. Cephalic vein
4. Lateral border of the scapula
5. Lateral border of the latissimus dorsi
6. Head of humerus
7. Acromion
8. Venous valve
9. Brachial vein
7
6
3
1
8
2
4
5
9

Figure 16.1 Radiograph of Veins in the Axillary Region

NOTE: (1) The basilic vein (2) becomes the axillary vein (1).

(2) One of the brachial veins (9) also flows into the axillary vein, as does the cephalic vein (3), the junction of which is medial to the field shown here.

(3) The venous valves (8) along the course of the axillary vein.

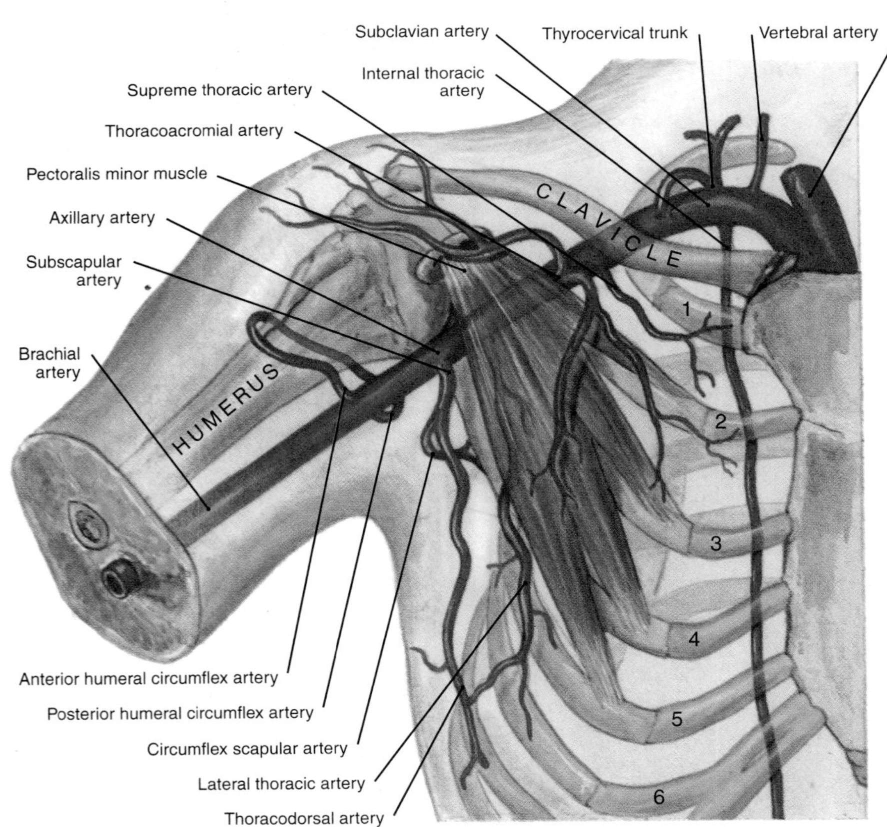
Subclavian artery
Thyrocervical trunk
Vertebral artery
Common carotid artery
Internal thoracic artery
Supreme thoracic artery
Thoracoacromial artery
Pectoralis minor muscle
Axillary artery
Subscapular artery
Brachial artery
CLAVICLE
HUMERUS
1
2
3
4
5
6
Anterior humeral circumflex artery
Posterior humeral circumflex artery
Circumflex scapular artery
Lateral thoracic artery
Thoracodorsal artery

Figure 16.2 Branches of the Axillary Artery

NOTE: (1) The subclavian artery becomes the axillary artery distal to the clavicle.

(2) Below the teres major, it becomes the brachial artery.

(3) The pectoralis minor crosses the axillary artery, dividing it into three parts:

(a) Medial to the muscle
(b) Beneath the muscle
(c) Lateral to the muscle

(4) From the first part there is one branch, the **supreme thoracic artery**.

(5) From the second part are derived two branches:

(a) **Thoracoacromial artery**
(b) **Lateral thoracic artery**

(6) From the third part come three branches:

(a) **Subscapular artery**
(b) **Anterior humeral circumflex artery**
(c) **Posterior humeral circumflex artery**

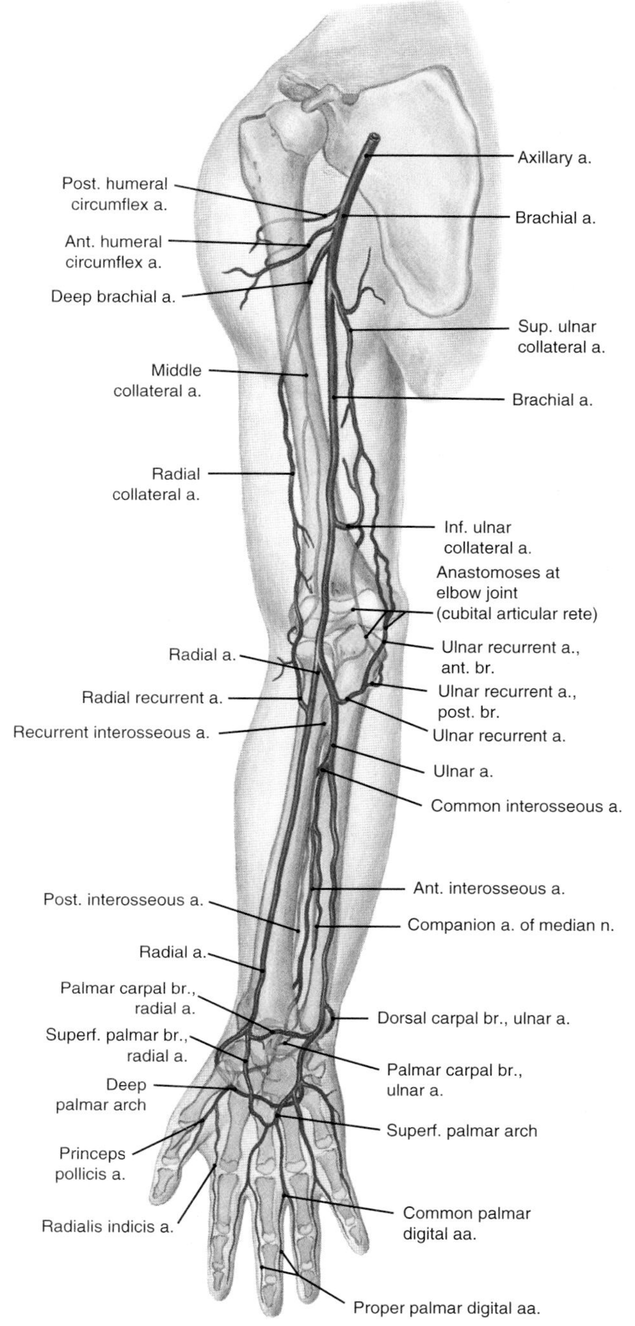
Axillary a.
Post. humeral circumflex a.
Brachial a.
Ant. humeral circumflex a.
Deep brachial a.
Sup. ulnar collateral a.
Middle collateral a.
Brachial a.
Radial collateral a.
Inf. ulnar collateral a.
Anastomoses at elbow joint (cubital articular rete)
Radial a.
Ulnar recurrent a., ant. br.
Radial recurrent a.
Ulnar recurrent a., post. br.
Recurrent interosseous a.
Ulnar recurrent a.
Ulnar a.
Common interosseous a.
Ant. interosseous a.
Post. interosseous a.
Companion a. of median n.
Radial a.
Palmar carpal br., radial a.
Dorsal carpal br., ulnar a.
Superf. palmar br., radial a.
Palmar carpal br., ulnar a.
Deep palmar arch
Superf. palmar arch
Princeps pollicis a.
Radialis indicis a.
Common palmar digital aa.
Proper palmar digital aa.

Figure 17.1 **Schematic View of the Arteries of the Upper Limb (Anterior View)**

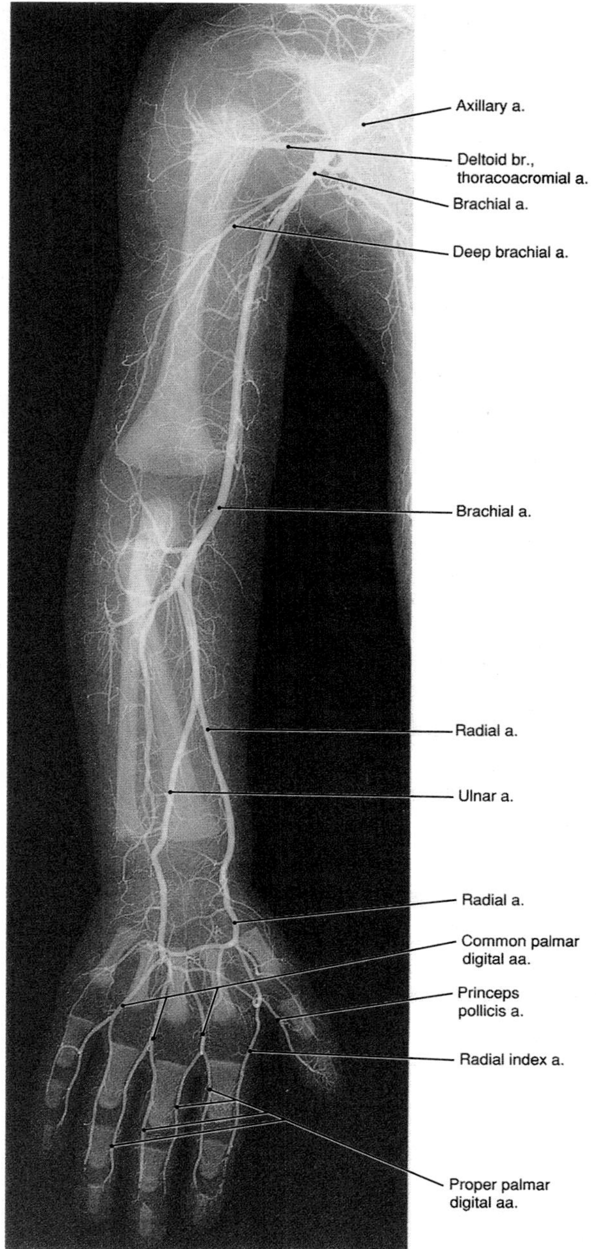
Axillary a.
Deltoid br., thoracoacromial a.
Brachial a.
Deep brachial a.
Brachial a.
Radial a.
Ulnar a.
Radial a.
Common palmar digital aa.
Princeps pollicis a.
Radial index a.
Proper palmar digital aa.

Figure 17.2 **Arteriogram of the Upper Limb in a Stillborn Infant**

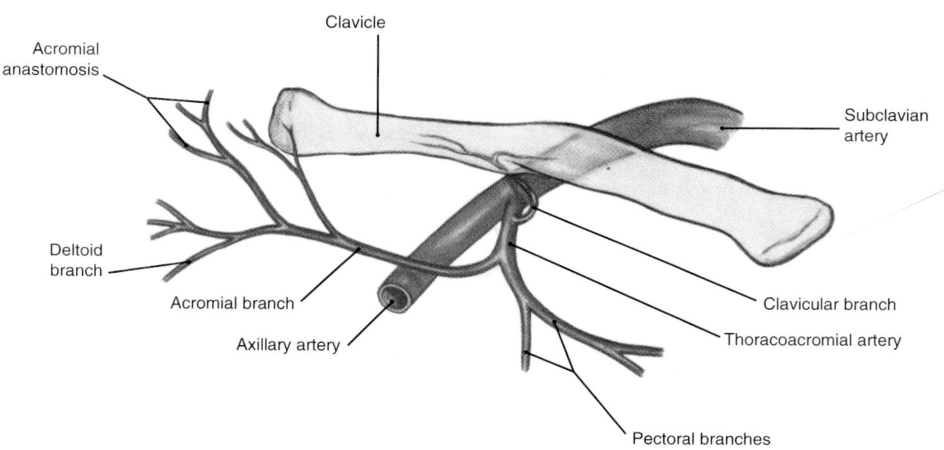
Clavicle
Acromial anastomosis
Subclavian artery
Deltoid branch
Acromial branch
Clavicular branch
Axillary artery
Thoracoacromial artery
Pectoral branches

Figure 17.3 **Thoracoacromial Artery and its Branches**

NOTE that the four branches of the thoracoacromial artery usually are the clavicular, pectoral, acromial, and deltoid.

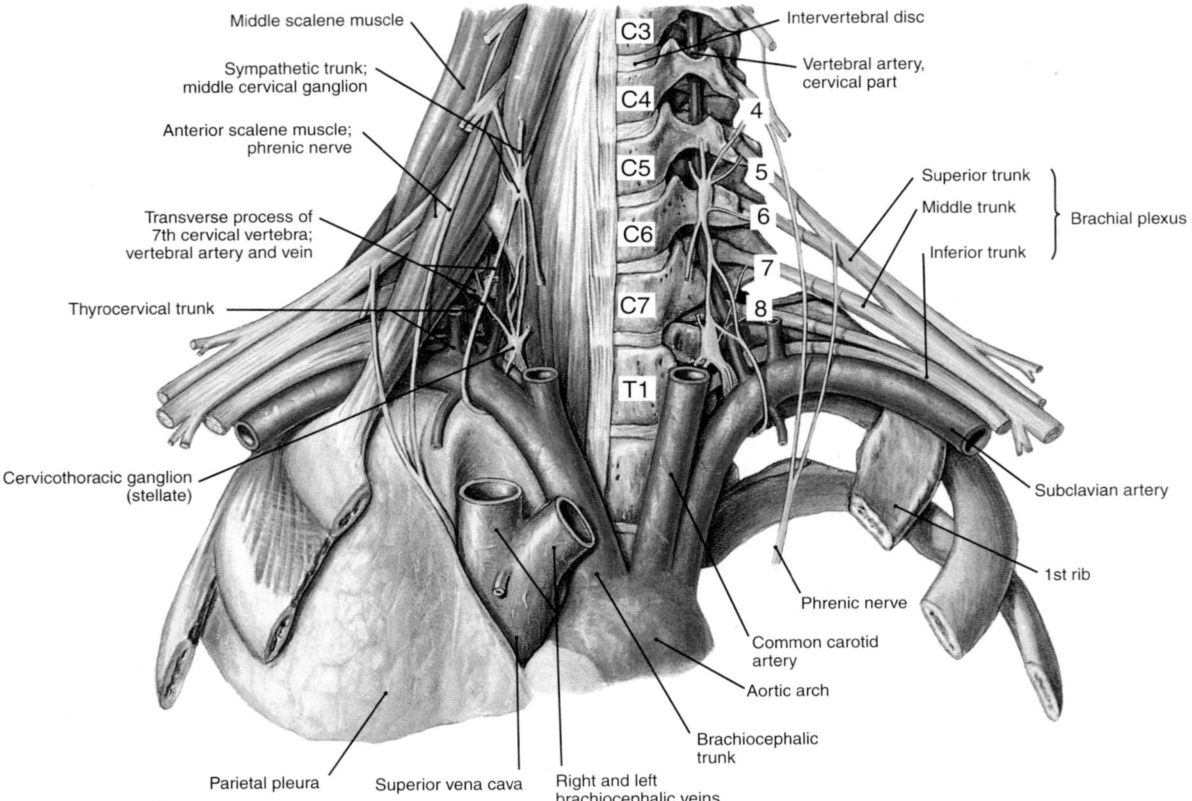
Middle scalene muscle
Sympathetic trunk; middle cervical ganglion
Anterior scalene muscle; phrenic nerve
Transverse process of 7th cervical vertebra; vertebral artery and vein
Thyrocervical trunk
Cervicothoracic ganglion (stellate)
Parietal pleura
Superior vena cava
Right and left brachiocephalic veins
Brachiocephalic trunk
Aortic arch
Common carotid artery
Phrenic nerve
1st rib
Subclavian artery
Superior trunk
Middle trunk
Inferior trunk
Brachial plexus
Intervertebral disc
Vertebral artery, cervical part
C3
C4
C5
C6
C7
T1
4
5
6
7
8

Figure 18.1 Roots of Origin of the Brachial Plexus in the Posterior Lateral Neck Region

NOTE: (1) The roots of C5, C6, C7, C8, and T1 emerge from the vertebral column and form the upper, middle, and lower trunks of the brachial plexus.

(2) C5 and C6 join to form the upper trunk, C7 forms the middle trunk, and C8 and T1 join to form the lower trunk.

(3) Crossing the first rib under the clavicle with the subclavian artery, each trunk splits into anterior and posterior divisions. The divisions then reassemble to form three cords: **lateral**, **medial**, and **posterior**. Now study Figure 18.2 and read its NOTE.

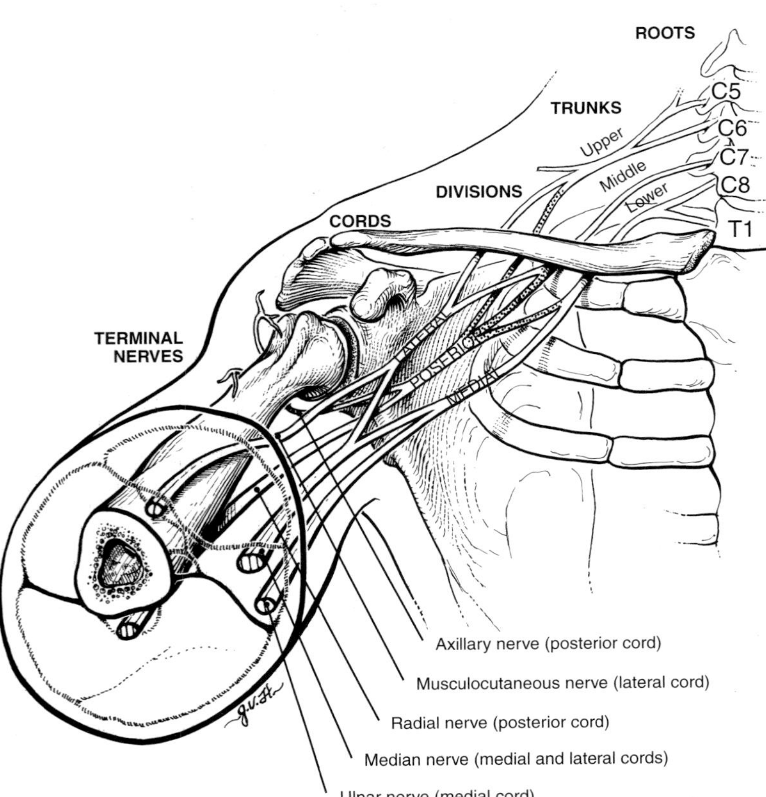
ROOTS
TRUNKS
DIVISIONS
CORDS
TERMINAL NERVES
C5
C6
C7
C8
T1
Upper
Middle
Lower
LATERAL
POSTERIOR
MEDIAL
Axillary nerve (posterior cord)
Musculocutaneous nerve (lateral cord)
Radial nerve (posterior cord)
Median nerve (medial and lateral cords)
Ulnar nerve (medial cord)

Figure 18.2 Diagram of the Brachial Plexus

NOTE: (1) Distal to the trunks and divisions the three cords form five terminal nerves.

(2) The posterior cord gives rise to **axillary** and **radial nerves**, the lateral cord gives off the **musculocutaneous nerve**, and from the medial cord arises the **ulnar nerve**. Both lateral and medial cords give branches to form the **median nerve**.

(3) The lateral, medial, and posterior cords course laterally, medially, and posteriorly to the axillary artery and are named according to this relationship.

ROOTS
TRUNKS
DIVISIONS
CORDS
TERMINAL NERVES
C4
C5
C6
C7
C8
T1
Dorsal scapular nerve (C5)
Long thoracic nerve (C5, 6, 7)
Upper trunk
Middle trunk
Lower trunk
Nerve to subclavius (C5, 6)
Suprascapular nerve (C5, 6)
Posterior division
Anterior division
Posterior division
Anterior division
Posterior division
Anterior division
Upper subscapular nerve (C5, 6)
Thoracodorsal nerve (C5, 6, 7)
Lower subscapular nerve (C5, 6)
Medial brachial cutaneous nerve (C8, T1)
Medial antebrachial cutaneous nerve (C8, T1)
Medial cord
Posterior cord
Lateral cord
Axillary nerve (C5, 6)
Medial cord root
Lateral cord root
Medial pectoral nerve (C8, T1)
Lateral pectoral nerve (C5, 6, 7)
Musculocutaneous nerve
Radial nerve
Median nerve
Ulnar nerve

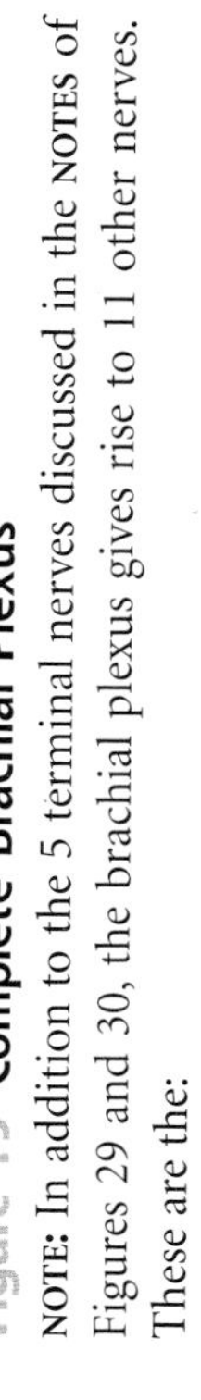

Figure 19 Complete Brachial Plexus

NOTE: In addition to the 5 terminal nerves discussed in the NOTES of Figures 29 and 30, the brachial plexus gives rise to 11 other nerves. These are the:

1. Long thoracic nerve (roots C5, 6, 7)
2. Dorsal scapular nerve (C5 root)
3. Nerve to subclavius muscle (upper trunk)
4. Suprascapular nerve (upper trunk)
5. Lateral pectoral nerve (lateral cord)
6. Medial pectoral nerve (medial cord)
7. Medial brachial cutaneous nerve (medial cord)
8. Medial antebrachial cutaneous nerve (medial cord)
9. Upper subscapular nerve (posterior cord)
10. Thoracodorsal nerve (posterior cord)
11. Lower subscapular nerve (posterior cord)

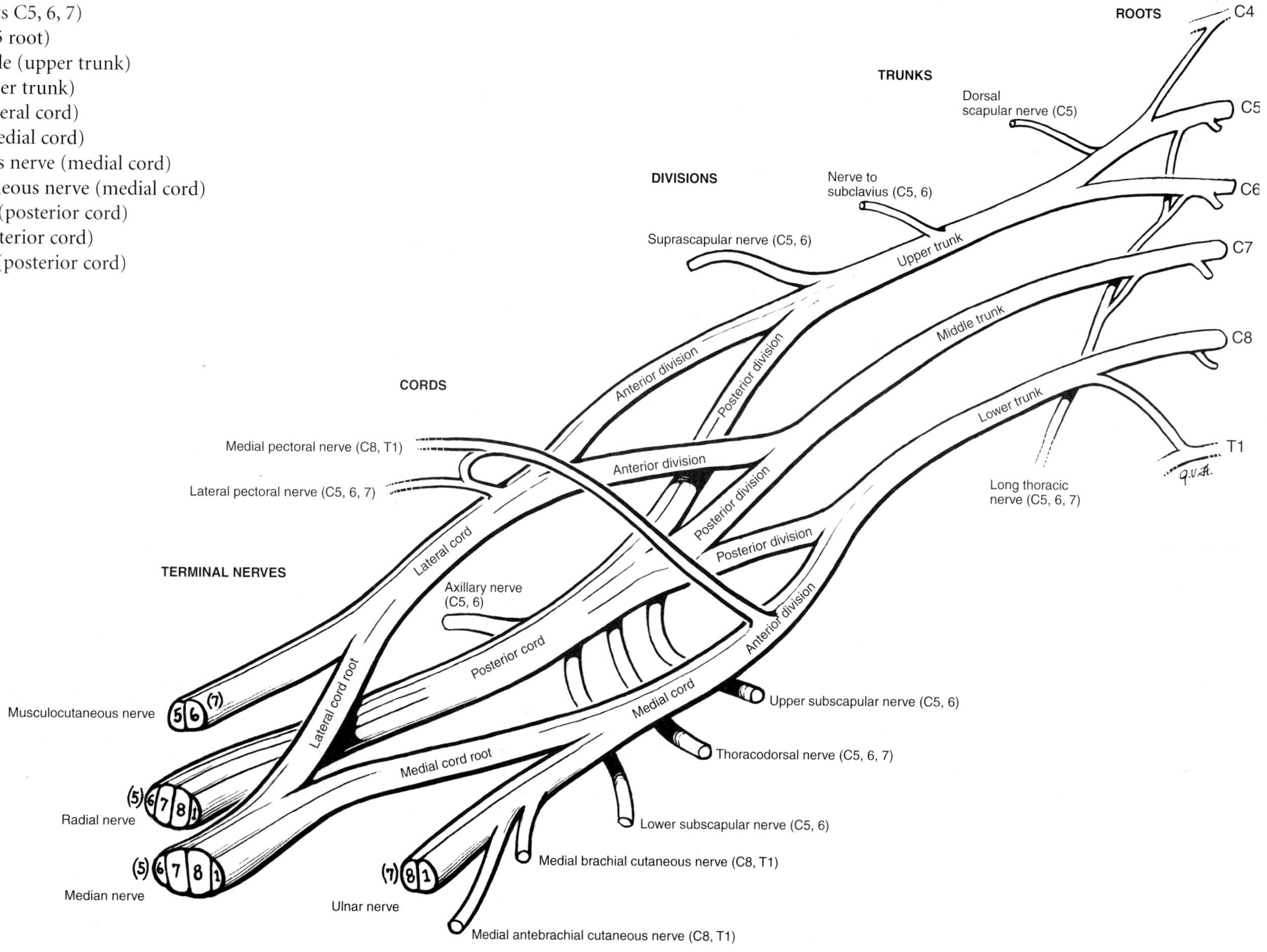

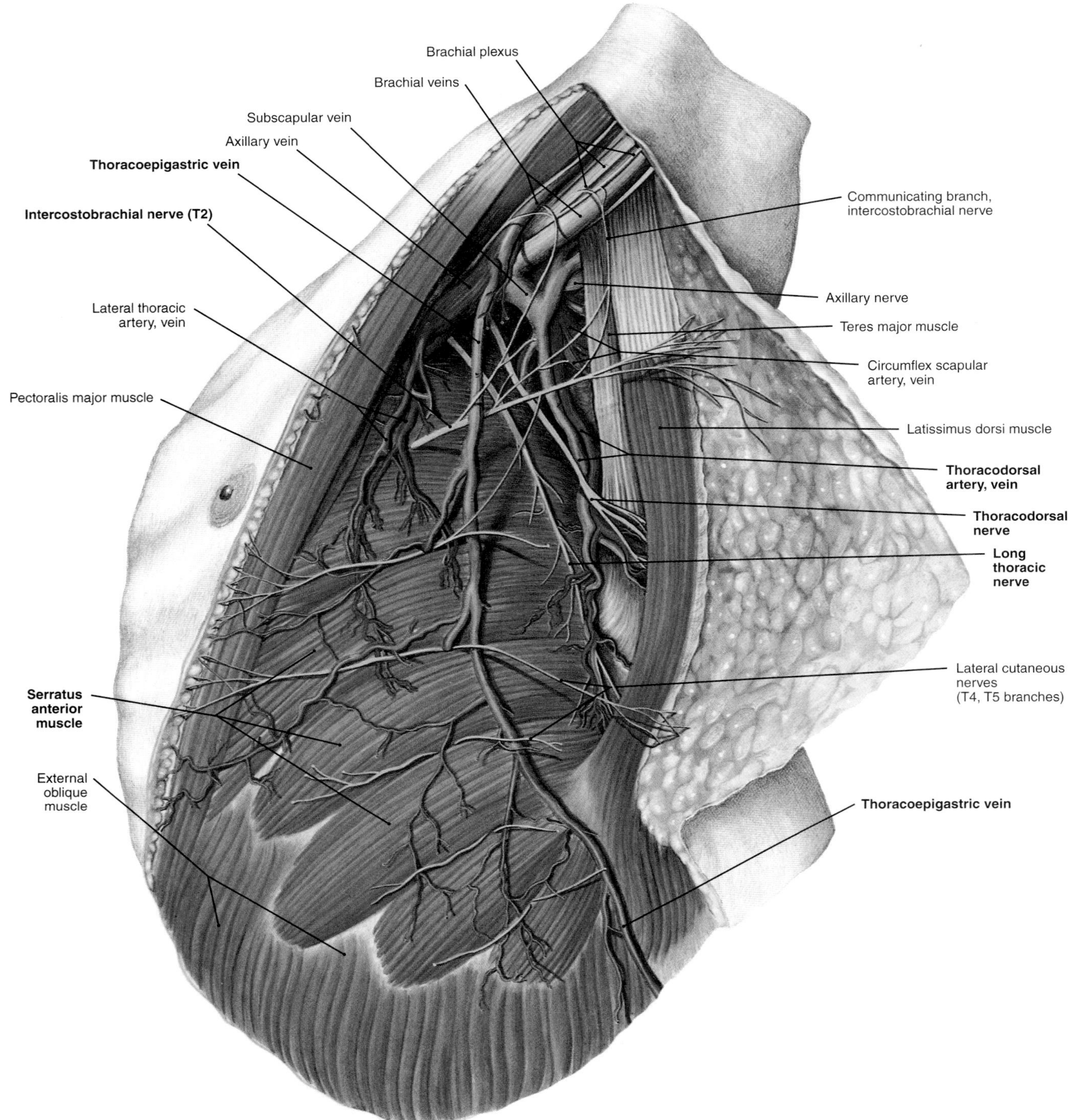
Brachial plexus
Brachial veins
Subscapular vein
Axillary vein
Thoracoepigastric vein
Intercostobrachial nerve (T2)
Lateral thoracic artery, vein
Pectoralis major muscle
Serratus anterior muscle
External oblique muscle
Communicating branch, intercostobrachial nerve
Axillary nerve
Teres major muscle
Circumflex scapular artery, vein
Latissimus dorsi muscle
Thoracodorsal artery, vein
Thoracodorsal nerve
Long thoracic nerve
Lateral cutaneous nerves (T4, T5 branches)
Thoracoepigastric vein

Figure 20 Axilla: Superficial Vessels and Nerves (Left)

NOTE: (1) The boundaries of the axilla are:

(a) **Anteriorly**, the pectoralis major muscle
(b) **Posteriorly**, the subscapularis, teres major, and latissimus dorsi muscles
(c) **Medially**, the serratus anterior muscle covering the second to the sixth ribs
(d) **Laterally**, the bicipital groove of the humerus.

(2) the lower part of the serratus anterior muscle arises from the lower ribs as fleshy interdigitations with the external oblique muscle.

(3) The serratus anterior is innervated by the long thoracic nerve, and the latissimus dorsi by the thoracodorsal nerve.

(4) The axillary vein lies medial to the axillary artery and the brachial plexus.

(5) The descending course of the thoracoepigastric vein and the lateral thoracic vessels.

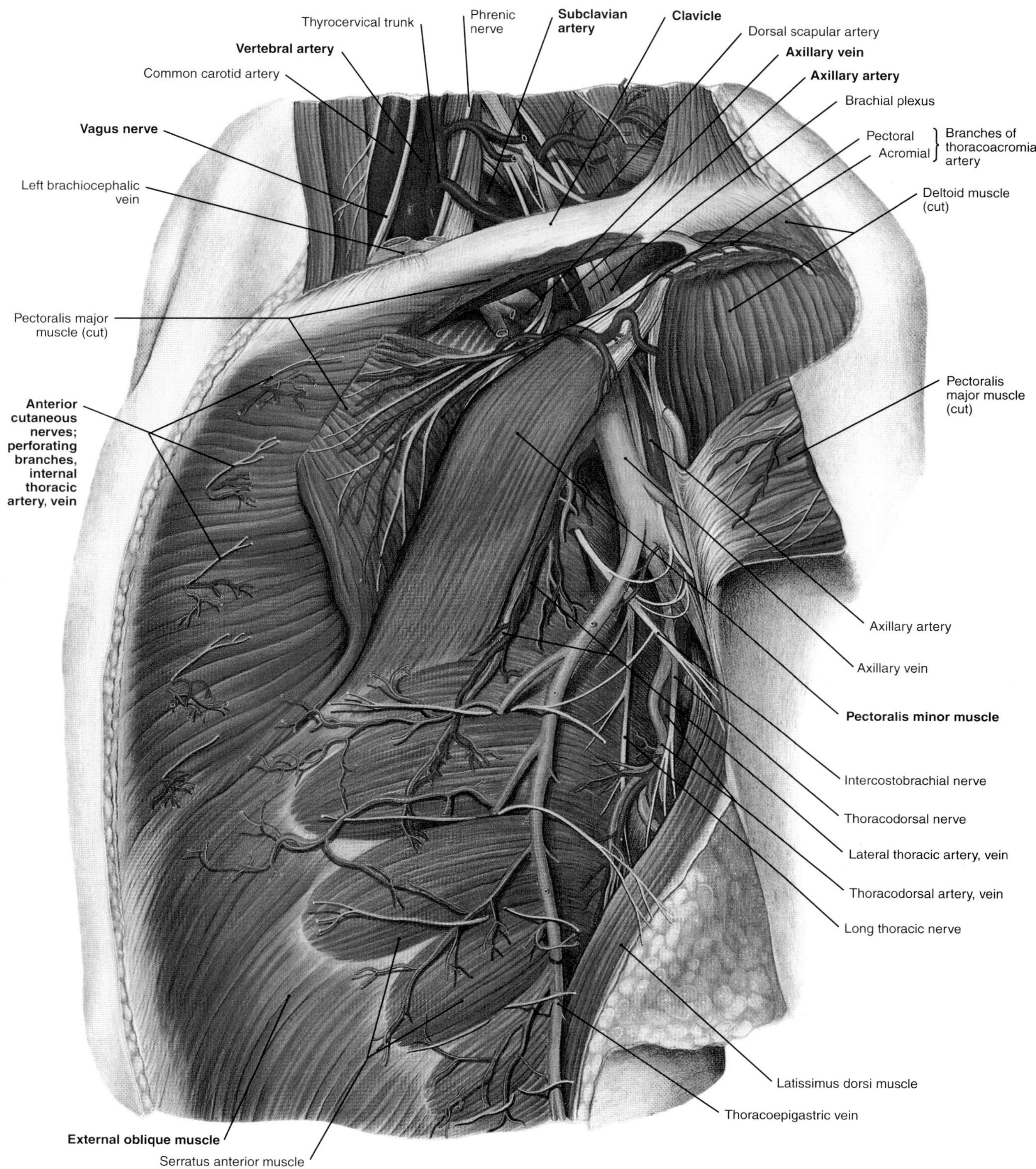
Thyrocervical trunk
Phrenic nerve
Subclavian artery
Clavicle
Dorsal scapular artery
Vertebral artery
Axillary vein
Common carotid artery
Axillary artery
Brachial plexus
Vagus nerve
Pectoral
Acromial
Branches of thoracoacromial artery
Left brachiocephalic vein
Deltoid muscle (cut)
Pectoralis major muscle (cut)
Pectoralis major muscle (cut)
Anterior cutaneous nerves; perforating branches, internal thoracic artery, vein
Axillary artery
Axillary vein
Pectoralis minor muscle
Intercostobrachial nerve
Thoracodorsal nerve
Lateral thoracic artery, vein
Thoracodorsal artery, vein
Long thoracic nerve
Latissimus dorsi muscle
Thoracoepigastric vein
External oblique muscle
Serratus anterior muscle

Figure 21 Axilla (Left): Deep Vessels and Nerves

NOTE: (1) The subclavian artery becomes the axillary artery distal to the clavicle.

(2) The pectoralis minor muscle is capable of elevating the ribs if the coracoid attachment is fixed or of protracting the scapula if the costal attachment is fixed.

(3) The axillary artery is surrounded by the three cords of the brachial plexus.

(4) The thoracoacromial artery divides into **pectoral, acromial, deltoid,** and small **clavicular** branches.

(5) The intercostobrachial nerve (T2) pierces the second intercostal space in its course toward the axilla and arm, and it communicates with the medial brachial cutaneous nerve.

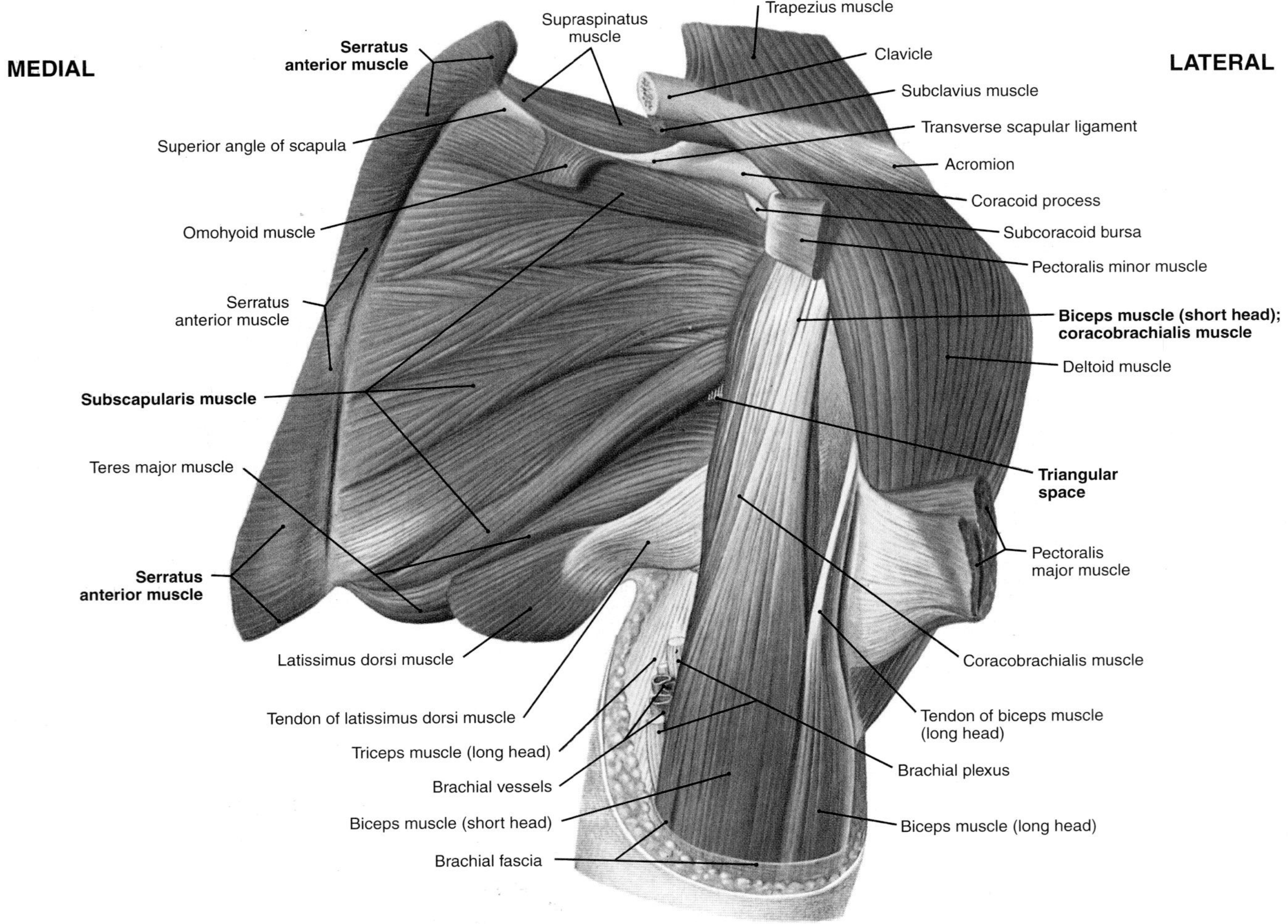
MEDIAL
LATERAL
Serratus anterior muscle
Supraspinatus muscle
Trapezius muscle
Clavicle
Subclavius muscle
Transverse scapular ligament
Acromion
Coracoid process
Subcoracoid bursa
Pectoralis minor muscle
Superior angle of scapula
Omohyoid muscle
Serratus anterior muscle
Biceps muscle (short head); coracobrachialis muscle
Deltoid muscle
Subscapularis muscle
Teres major muscle
Triangular space
Pectoralis major muscle
Serratus anterior muscle
Latissimus dorsi muscle
Coracobrachialis muscle
Tendon of latissimus dorsi muscle
Tendon of biceps muscle (long head)
Triceps muscle (long head)
Brachial plexus
Brachial vessels
Biceps muscle (short head)
Biceps muscle (long head)
Brachial fascia

Figure 22 Muscles of Anterior Aspect of the Shoulder (Left)

NOTE: (1) The large triangular mass of the subscapularis muscle occupying the concave subscapular fossa. From this broad origin, its fibers converge toward the humerus, where it inserts on the lesser tubercle.

(2) The subscapularis along with the other muscles that constitute the "rotator cuff" (supraspinatus, infraspinatus, and teres minor) help to stabilize the shoulder joint by keeping the head of the humerus in the glenoid fossa.

(3) Both the short head of the biceps and the coracobrachialis have a common origin from the coracoid process.

Muscle	Origin	Insertion	Innervation	Action
Subscapularis	Subscapular fossa of the scapula	Lesser tubercle of the humerus	Upper and lower subscapular nerves (C5, C6) from posterior cord of brachial plexus	Medial rotation of the humerus
Latissimus dorsi	Thoracolumbar fascia; spinous processes of lower six thoracic and lumbar vertebrae, and the sacrum	Bottom of the intertubercular sulcus of the humerus	Thoracodorsal nerve (C6, C7, C8) from posterior cord of brachial plexus	Extends, adducts, and medially rotates the humerus
Deltoid	Lateral third of clavicle; the acromion; spine of the scapula	Deltoid tubercle on lateral surface of humerus	Axillary nerve (C5, C6) from posterior cord of brachial plexus	Abduction of the humerus; anterior fibers assist in flexion and posterior fibers in extension of the humerus

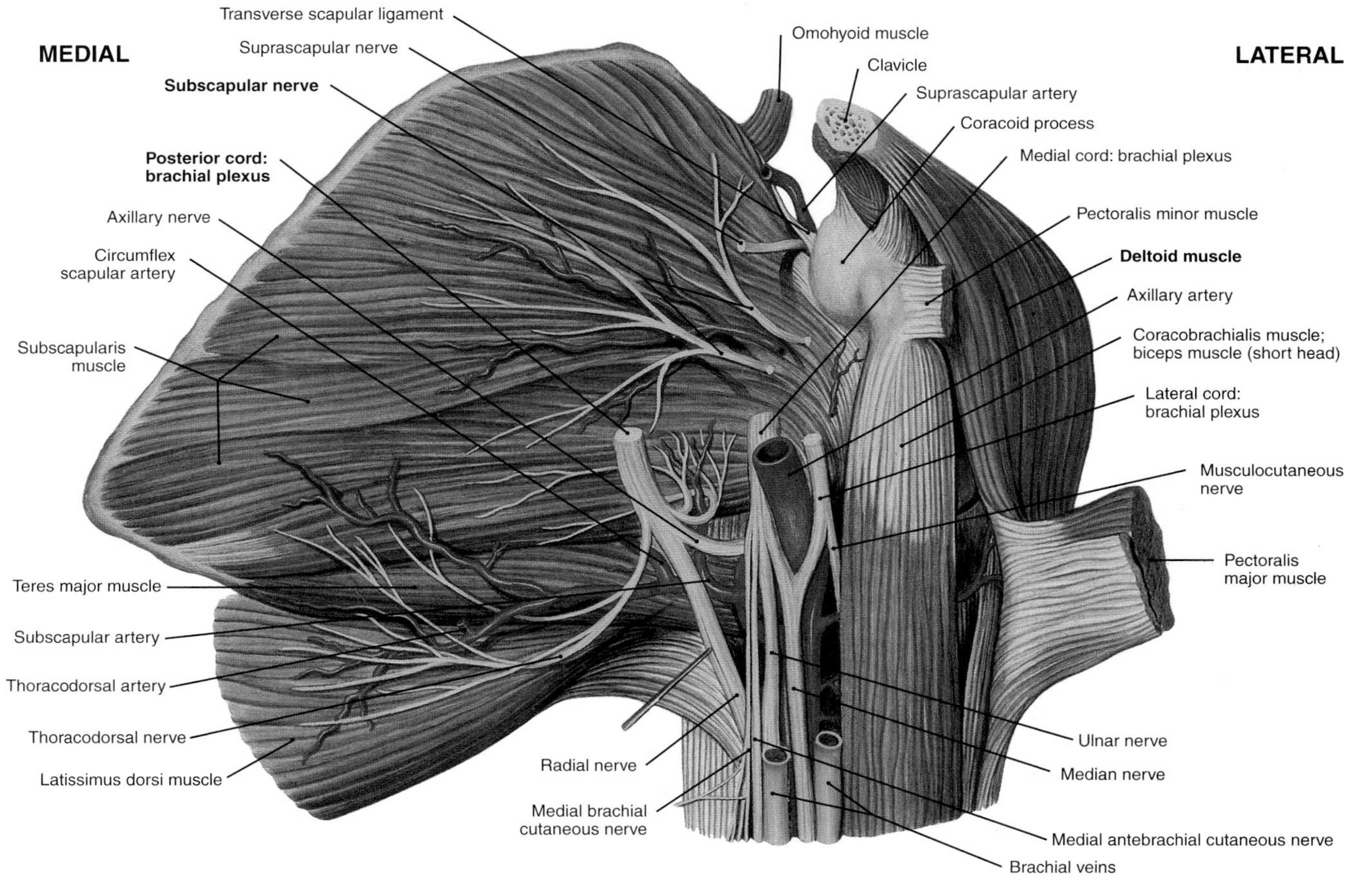
MEDIAL
LATERAL
Transverse scapular ligament
Suprascapular nerve
Subscapular nerve
Posterior cord: brachial plexus
Axillary nerve
Circumflex scapular artery
Subscapularis muscle
Teres major muscle
Subscapular artery
Thoracodorsal artery
Thoracodorsal nerve
Latissimus dorsi muscle
Radial nerve
Medial brachial cutaneous nerve
Omohyoid muscle
Clavicle
Suprascapular artery
Coracoid process
Medial cord: brachial plexus
Pectoralis minor muscle
Deltoid muscle
Axillary artery
Coracobrachialis muscle; biceps muscle (short head)
Lateral cord: brachial plexus
Musculocutaneous nerve
Pectoralis major muscle
Ulnar nerve
Median nerve
Medial antebrachial cutaneous nerve
Brachial veins

Figure 23.1 Nerves and Vessels of Anterior Aspect of the Shoulder (Left)

NOTE: (1) The relationships of the medial, lateral, and posterior cords of the brachial plexus to the axillary artery.

(2) The posterior cord and its axillary and radial terminal nerves have been pulled medially from behind the axillary artery in this dissection.

(3) The median nerve formed by contributions from the lateral and medial cords. Observe that the median nerve, its two roots of origin and the ulnar and musculocutaneous nerves outline an **M** formation on the anterior aspect of the axillary artery.

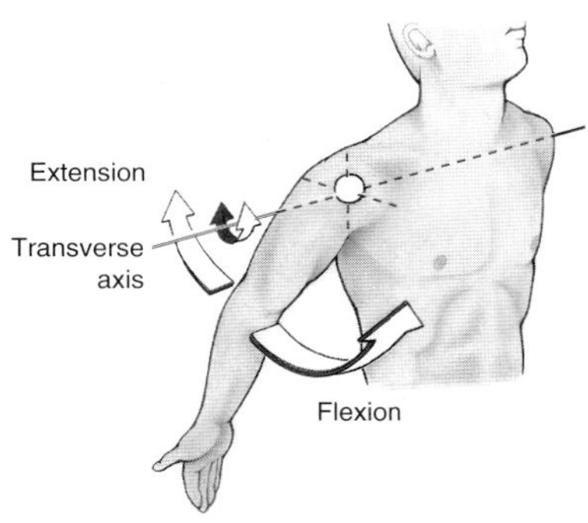
Extension
Transverse axis
Flexion

Figure 23.2 Shoulder Joint: Flexion and Extension

In **flexion** the upper limb is moved anteriorly (forward), while in **extension** the limb moves posteriorly (backward) in reference to the transverse axis.

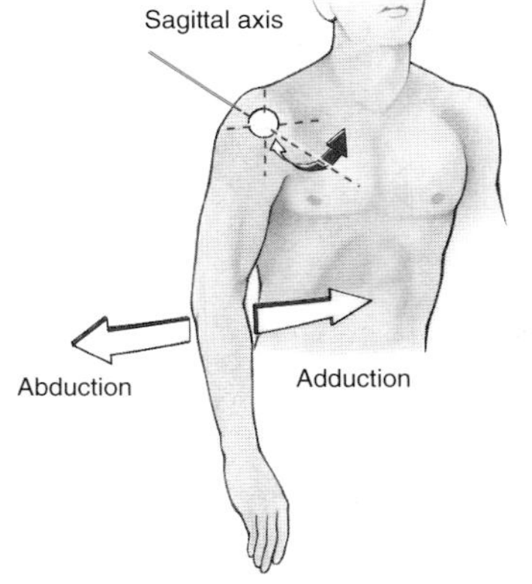
Sagittal axis
Abduction
Adduction

Figure 23.3 Shoulder Joint: Abduction and Adduction

In **abduction,** the upper limb is moved laterally, or away from the midline of the body, with reference to the sagittal axis. In **adduction,** the upper limb is moved medially, or toward the midline of the body.

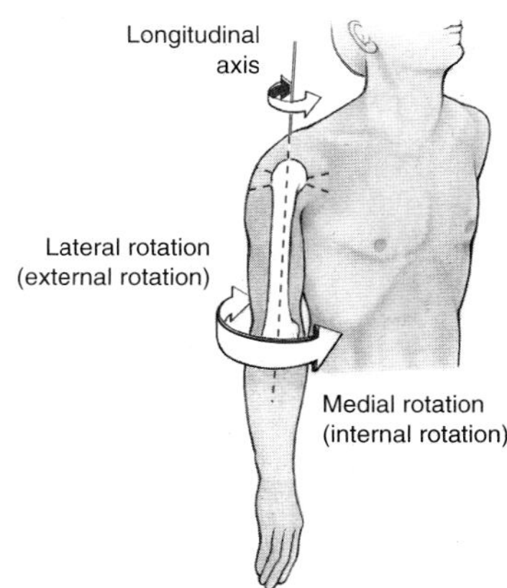
Longitudinal axis
Lateral rotation (external rotation)
Medial rotation (internal rotation)

Figure 23.4 Shoulder Joint: Medial and Lateral Rotation

Medial rotation at the shoulder joint occurs when the humerus is rotated internally (medially) with reference to the long or longitudinal axis of the bone. In contrast, **lateral rotation** of the upper limb moves the humerus (arm) externally or laterally.

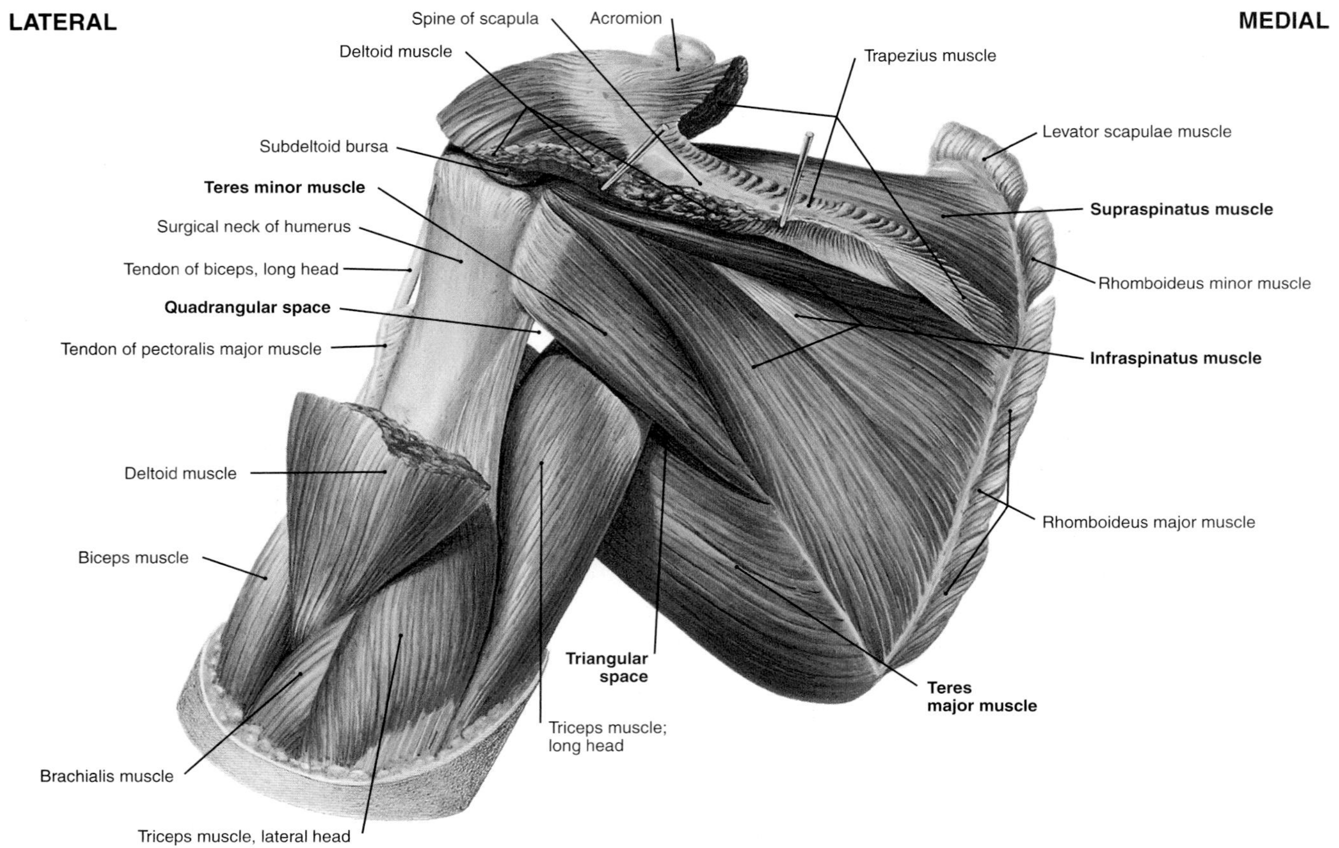
LATERAL
MEDIAL
Spine of scapula
Acromion
Deltoid muscle
Trapezius muscle
Subdeltoid bursa
Levator scapulae muscle
Teres minor muscle
Supraspinatus muscle
Surgical neck of humerus
Tendon of biceps, long head
Rhomboideus minor muscle
Quadrangular space
Tendon of pectoralis major muscle
Infraspinatus muscle
Deltoid muscle
Rhomboideus major muscle
Biceps muscle
Triangular space
Teres major muscle
Triceps muscle; long head
Brachialis muscle
Triceps muscle, lateral head

Figure 24 Posterior Scapular Muscles (Left)

NOTE: (1) The supraspinatus, infraspinatus, and teres minor muscles all course laterally from the dorsal scapula, and all are considered "rotator cuff" muscles.

(2) These three muscles insert in sequence from above downward on the greater tubercle of the humerus.

(3) The long head of the triceps intersects a space between the teres major and teres minor muscles, forming a **quadrangular space** laterally and a **triangular space** medially.

(4) The posterior humeral circumflex artery and the axillary nerve pass through the quadrangular space (see Fig. 43).

(5) The circumflex scapular branch of the subscapular artery passes through the triangular space (Fig. 25.1).

(6) Since the lateral border of the quadrangular space is the surgical neck of the humerus, the axillary nerve and posterior humeral circumflex artery are in danger if the bone is fractured at this site.

Muscle	Origin	Insertion	Innervation	Action
Supraspinatus	Supraspinatus fossa of the scapula	Highest facet of the greater tubercle of the humerus	Suprascapular nerve (C5)	Initiates abduction of the arm; rotates the humerus laterally
Infraspinatus	Infraspinatus fossa of the scapula	Middle part of greater tubercle of humerus	Suprascapular nerve (C5, C6)	Rotates the humerus laterally
Teres major	Lower lateral border and inferior angle of the scapula	Crest of lesser tubercle and medial lip of intertubercular sulcus of humerus	Lower subscapular nerve (C5, C6)	Adducts and medially rotates the humerus; assists in extension of the arm
Teres minor	Upper part of the lateral border of the scapula	Lower part of the greater tubercle of the humerus	Axillary nerve (C5)	Rotates humerus laterally; weakly adducts humerus

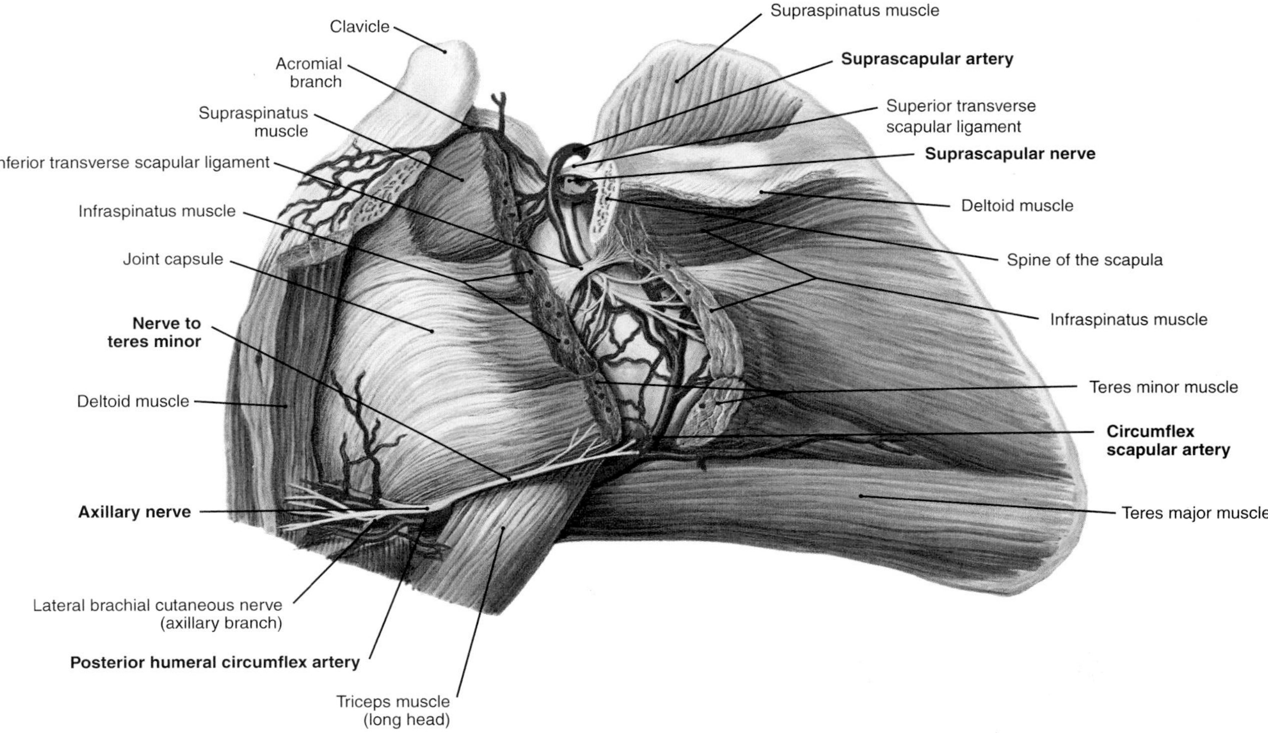
LATERAL
MEDIA
Clavicle
Acromial branch
Supraspinatus muscle
Inferior transverse scapular ligament
Infraspinatus muscle
Joint capsule
Nerve to teres minor
Deltoid muscle
Axillary nerve
Lateral brachial cutaneous nerve (axillary branch)
Posterior humeral circumflex artery
Triceps muscle (long head)
Supraspinatus muscle
Suprascapular artery
Superior transverse scapular ligament
Suprascapular nerve
Deltoid muscle
Spine of the scapula
Infraspinatus muscle
Teres minor muscle
Circumflex scapular artery
Teres major muscle

Figure 25.1 Nerves and Vessels of Posterior Scapular Region (Left)

NOTE: (1) The **superior** transverse scapular ligament bridges the scapular notch, and the suprascapular nerve passes beneath the ligament while the suprascapular artery usually passes above it to reach the supraspinatus fossa.

(2) Both the suprascapular nerve and artery pass beneath the **inferior** transverse scapular ligament to reach the infraspinatus fossa.

(3) The axillary nerve supplies four structures: (a) the teres minor muscle, (b) the deltoid muscle, (c) the capsule of the shoulder joint, and (d) the skin over the shoulder joint.

(4) The axillary nerve and posterior humeral circumflex artery from the dorsal view. These two structures have passed through the quadrangular space, whereas the circumflex scapular artery reaches the infraspinatus fossa through the triangular space.

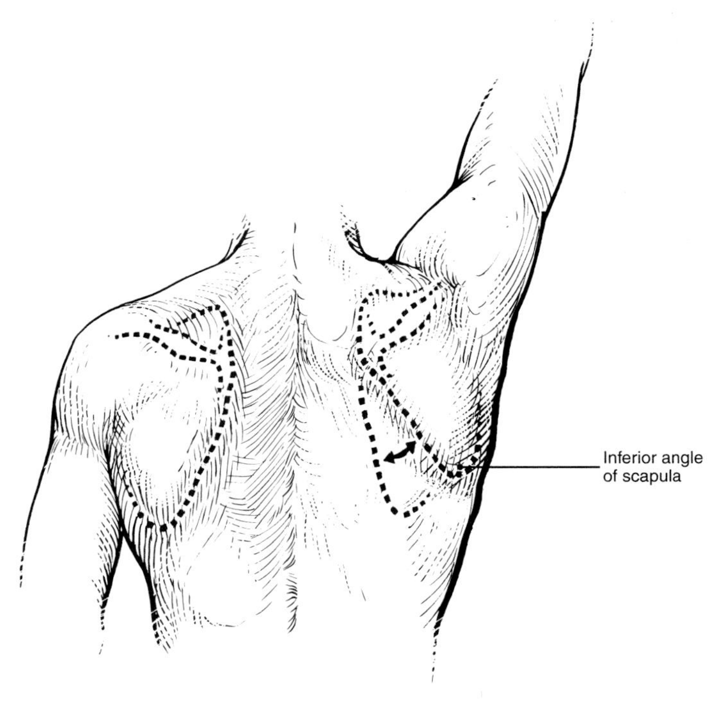
Inferior angle of scapula

Figure 25.2 Abduction of the Upper Limb

NOTE: (1) The first 20 degrees of abduction is performed by the supraspinatus muscle.

(2) From 20 to 90 degrees, abduction is almost exclusively the action of the deltoid muscle.

(3) Continuing beyond 90 degrees to 180 degrees (as shown in this figure), the vertebral border and inferior angle of the scapula must rotate laterally as the upper limb is elevated.

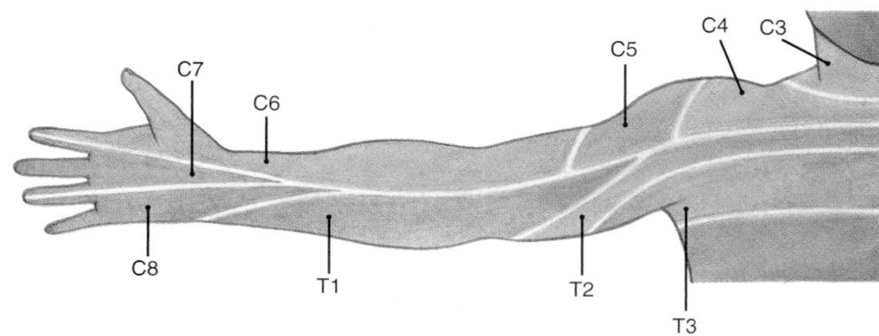
C4
C3
C5
C7
C6
C8
T1
T2
T3

Figure 26.1 Cutaneous Innervation and Dermatomes of the Upper Limb (Anterior Aspect)

NOTE: (1) An area of skin surface that receives innervation from any single spinal nerve is called a **dermatome**.

(2) The solid lines on this figure and on Figure 26.2 are the boundaries between dermatomes. The boundary between C5 and C6 laterally and T1 and T2 medially is called the **anterior axial line**.

(3) The dermatomes on the anterior aspect of the limb commence over the anterior lateral surface of the brachium with the C5 dermatome.

(4) Continuing down laterally in the forearm is the C6 dermatome, the palmar and radial hand is C7, the ulnar aspect of the hand is C8, and then sequentially up the medial surface of the forearm and hand are the T1 and T2 dermatomes.

(5) Although there is overlap between adjacent dermatomes (such as between C5 and C6), **there is no overlap across the axial** line (such as between C6 and T1). This has important clinical significance, because differences in sensation across the axial line might help localize a problem in the spinal cord.

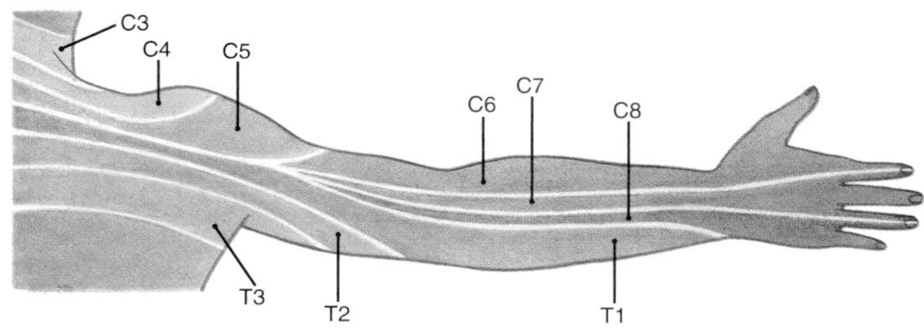
C3
C4
C5
C6
C7
C8
T3
T2
T1

Figure 26.2 Cutaneous Innervation and Dermatomes of the Upper Limb (Posterior Aspect)

NOTE: (1) Dermatomes on the posterior surface of the upper limb start at the proximal lateral region of the arm with the C5 dermatome.

(2) The C6 dermatome continues down the radial aspect of the forearm and hand; it includes the dorsal thumb and the radial part of the index finger.

(3) The C7 dermatome includes the posterior aspect of the middle finger and the adjacent halves of the index and ring fingers, as well as a strip of skin over the intermediate parts of the posterior hand and forearm.

(4) The C8 dermatome includes the little finger and the adjacent part of the ring finger and the ulnar part of the hand, along with a thin region of forearm skin.

(5) Continuing sequentially up the posterior aspect of the medial (ulnar) side of the forearm and arm are the T1 and T2 dermatomes.

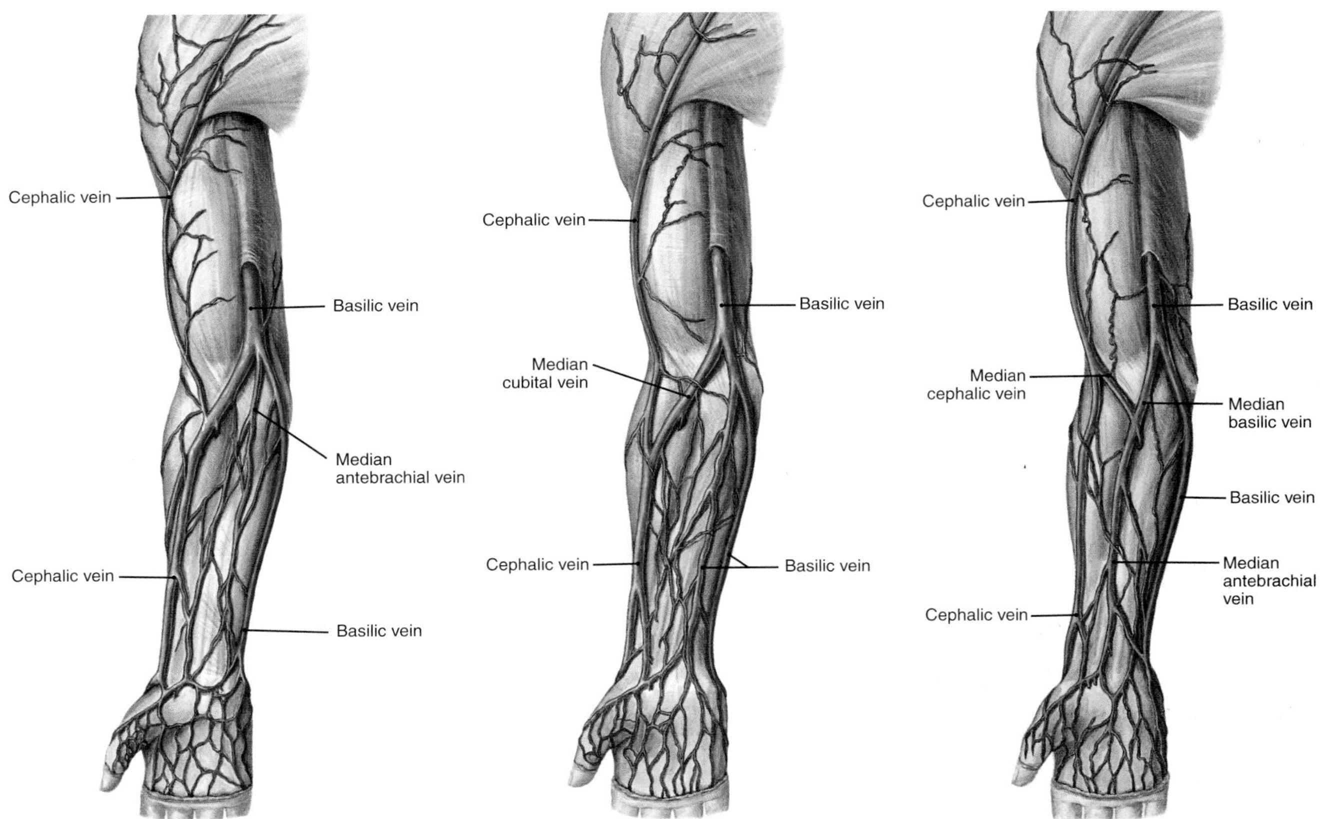

Cephalic vein
Basilic vein
Median antebrachial vein
Cephalic vein
Basilic vein
Cephalic vein
Basilic vein
Median cubital vein
Cephalic vein
Basilic vein
Cephalic vein
Basilic vein
Median cephalic vein
Median basilic vein
Basilic vein
Median antebrachial vein
Cephalic vein

Figure 27.1 Variations in the Venous Pattern of the Upper Extremity

NOTE: Superficial veins are variable and are of significance clinically. The median cubital vein is often used for the withdrawal of blood and the injection of fluids into the vascular system. Care must be taken not to injure the median nerve or puncture the brachial artery, which lie deep to the median cubital vein and the underlying bicipital aponeurosis.

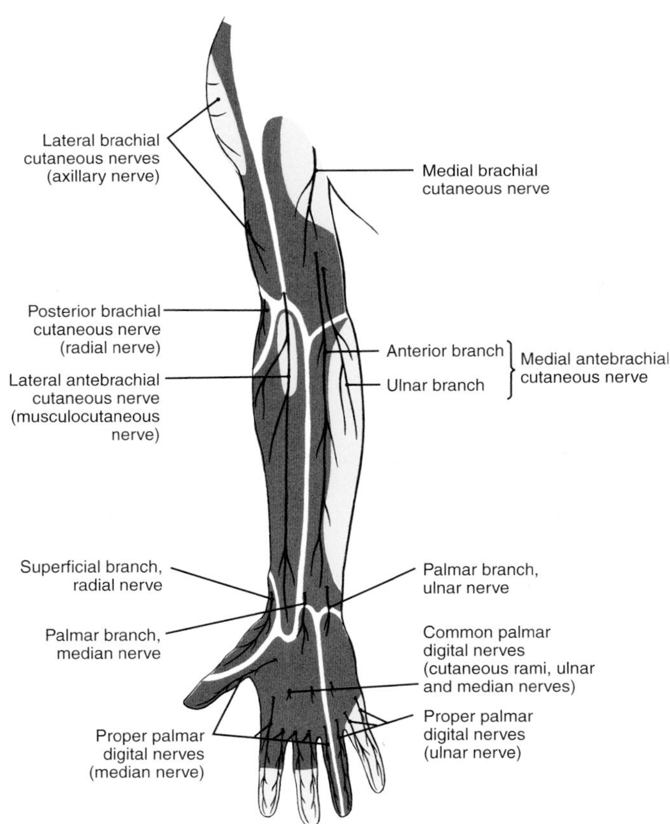

Lateral brachial cutaneous nerves (axillary nerve)
Medial brachial cutaneous nerve
Posterior brachial cutaneous nerve (radial nerve)
Anterior branch
Ulnar branch
Medial antebrachial cutaneous nerve
Lateral antebrachial cutaneous nerve (musculocutaneous nerve)
Superficial branch, radial nerve
Palmar branch, ulnar nerve
Palmar branch, median nerve
Common palmar digital nerves (cutaneous rami, ulnar and median nerves)
Proper palmar digital nerves (median nerve)
Proper palmar digital nerves (ulnar nerve)

Figure 27.2 Cutaneous Fields and the Courses of Cutaneous Nerves in the Superficial Fascia: Anterior Aspect of the Upper Limb

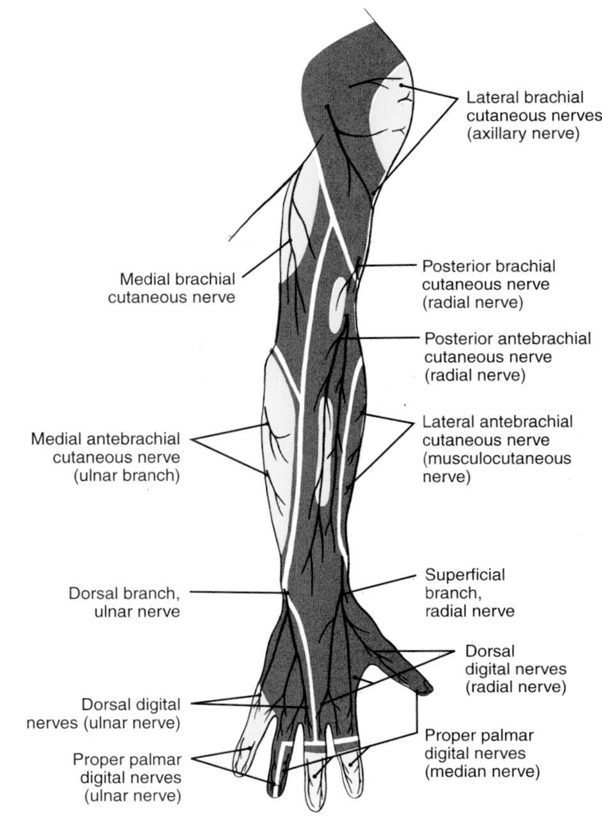

Lateral brachial cutaneous nerves (axillary nerve)
Medial brachial cutaneous nerve
Posterior brachial cutaneous nerve (radial nerve)
Posterior antebrachial cutaneous nerve (radial nerve)
Medial antebrachial cutaneous nerve (ulnar branch)
Lateral antebrachial cutaneous nerve (musculocutaneous nerve)
Dorsal branch, ulnar nerve
Superficial branch, radial nerve
Dorsal digital nerves (radial nerve)
Dorsal digital nerves (ulnar nerve)
Proper palmar digital nerves (ulnar nerve)
Proper palmar digital nerves (median nerve)

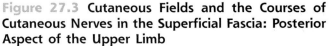

Figure 27.3 Cutaneous Fields and the Courses of Cutaneous Nerves in the Superficial Fascia: Posterior Aspect of the Upper Limb

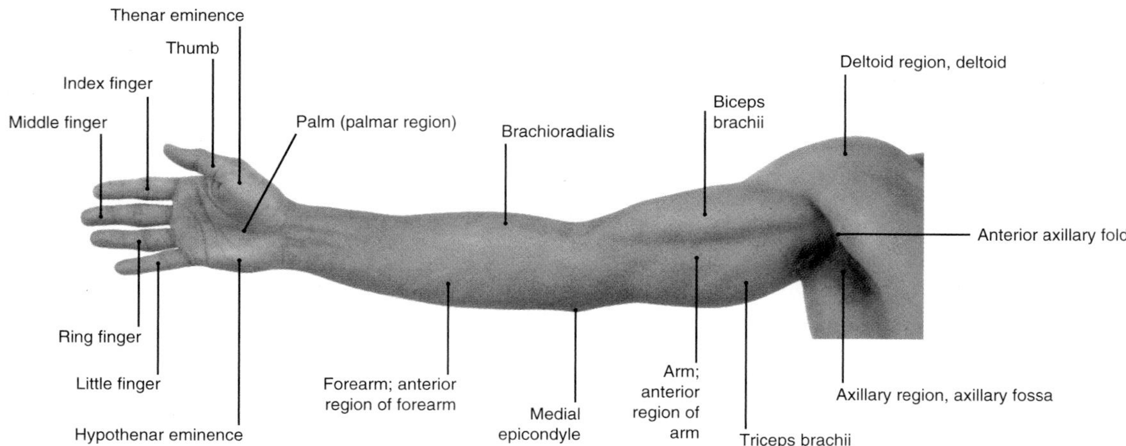
Thenar eminence
Thumb
Index finger
Middle finger
Palm (palmar region)
Brachioradialis
Biceps brachii
Deltoid region, deltoid
Anterior axillary fold
Ring finger
Little finger
Hypothenar eminence
Forearm; anterior region of forearm
Medial epicondyle
Arm; anterior region of arm
Triceps brachii
Axillary region, axillary fossa

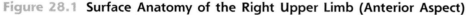

Figure 28.1 Surface Anatomy of the Right Upper Limb (Anterior Aspect)

NOTE: (1) The vertically oriented **medial bicipital furrow** along the arm. The **basilica vein** and the **medial antebrachial cutaneous nerve** course beneath the skin along this furrow. More deeply are found the brachial artery and vein and the **median** and **ulnar nerves**;

(2) The **cubital fossa** in front of the elbow joint, between the bellies of the flexor and extensor muscles in the upper forearm.

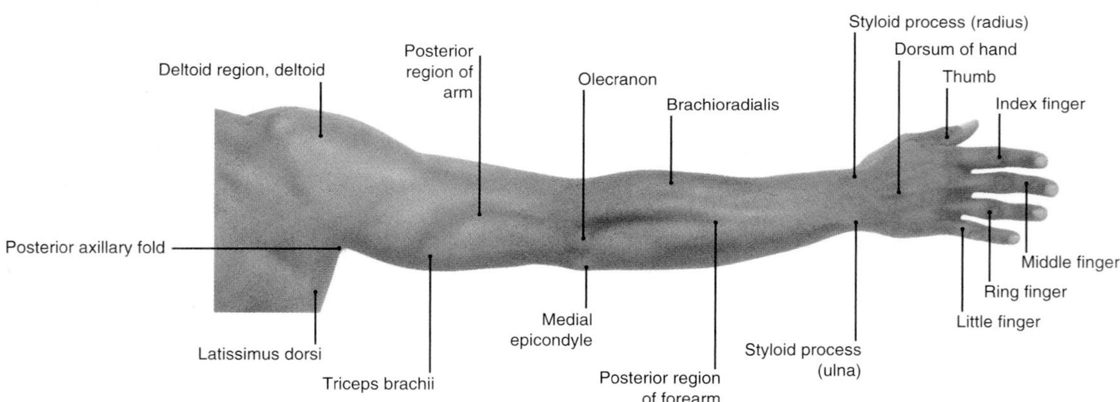
Deltoid region, deltoid
Posterior region of arm
Olecranon
Brachioradialis
Styloid process (radius)
Dorsum of hand
Thumb
Index finger
Posterior axillary fold
Middle finger
Ring finger
Little finger
Latissimus dorsi
Triceps brachii
Medial epicondyle
Posterior region of forearm
Styloid process (ulna)

Figure 28.2 Surface Anatomy of the Right Upper Limb (Posterior Aspect)

NOTE: (1) The surface contours of the **biceps brachii** and **brachioradialis** muscles and the surface projections of the olecranon and the medial epicondyle in the elbow region.

(2) The distal sharp ends of both the radius and ulna end in a **styloid process**. They are frequently fractured by severe trauma at the wrist.

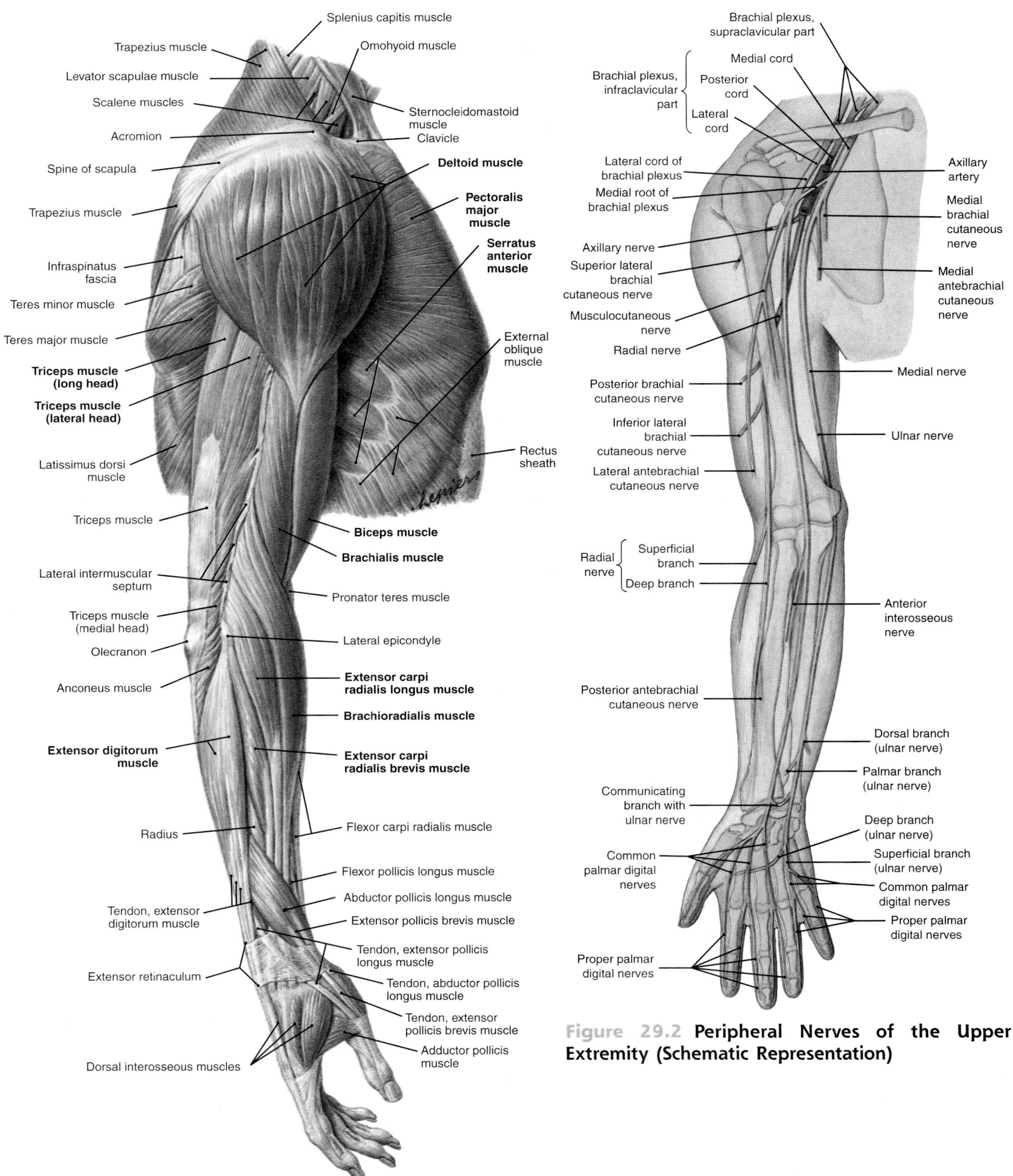

Splenius capitis muscle
Trapezius muscle
Omohyoid muscle
Levator scapulae muscle
Scalene muscles
Sternocleidomastoid muscle
Acromion
Clavicle
Spine of scapula
Deltoid muscle
Trapezius muscle
Pectoralis major muscle
Serratus anterior muscle
Infraspinatus fascia
Teres minor muscle
Teres major muscle
External oblique muscle
Triceps muscle (long head)
Triceps muscle (lateral head)
Rectus sheath
Latissimus dorsi muscle
Triceps muscle
Biceps muscle
Brachialis muscle
Lateral intermuscular septum
Pronator teres muscle
Triceps muscle (medial head)
Lateral epicondyle
Olecranon
Anconeus muscle
Extensor carpi radialis longus muscle
Brachioradialis muscle
Extensor digitorum muscle
Extensor carpi radialis brevis muscle
Radius
Flexor carpi radialis muscle
Flexor pollicis longus muscle
Abductor pollicis longus muscle
Tendon, extensor digitorum muscle
Extensor pollicis brevis muscle
Tendon, extensor pollicis longus muscle
Extensor retinaculum
Tendon, abductor pollicis longus muscle
Tendon, extensor pollicis brevis muscle
Adductor pollicis muscle
Dorsal interosseous muscles
Brachial plexus, supraclavicular part
Medial cord
Brachial plexus, infraclavicular part
Posterior cord
Lateral cord
Lateral cord of brachial plexus
Axillary artery
Medial root of brachial plexus
Medial brachial cutaneous nerve
Axillary nerve
Superior lateral brachial cutaneous nerve
Medial antebrachial cutaneous nerve
Musculocutaneous nerve
Radial nerve
Medial nerve
Posterior brachial cutaneous nerve
Inferior lateral brachial cutaneous nerve
Ulnar nerve
Lateral antebrachial cutaneous nerve
Radial nerve
Superficial branch
Deep branch
Anterior interosseous nerve
Posterior antebrachial cutaneous nerve
Dorsal branch (ulnar nerve)
Palmar branch (ulnar nerve)
Communicating branch with ulnar nerve
Deep branch (ulnar nerve)
Common palmar digital nerves
Superficial branch (ulnar nerve)
Common palmar digital nerves
Proper palmar digital nerves
Proper palmar digital nerves

Figure 29.1 Muscles of the Thorax and Right Upper Extremity (Lateral View)

Figure 29.2 Peripheral Nerves of the Upper Extremity (Schematic Representation)

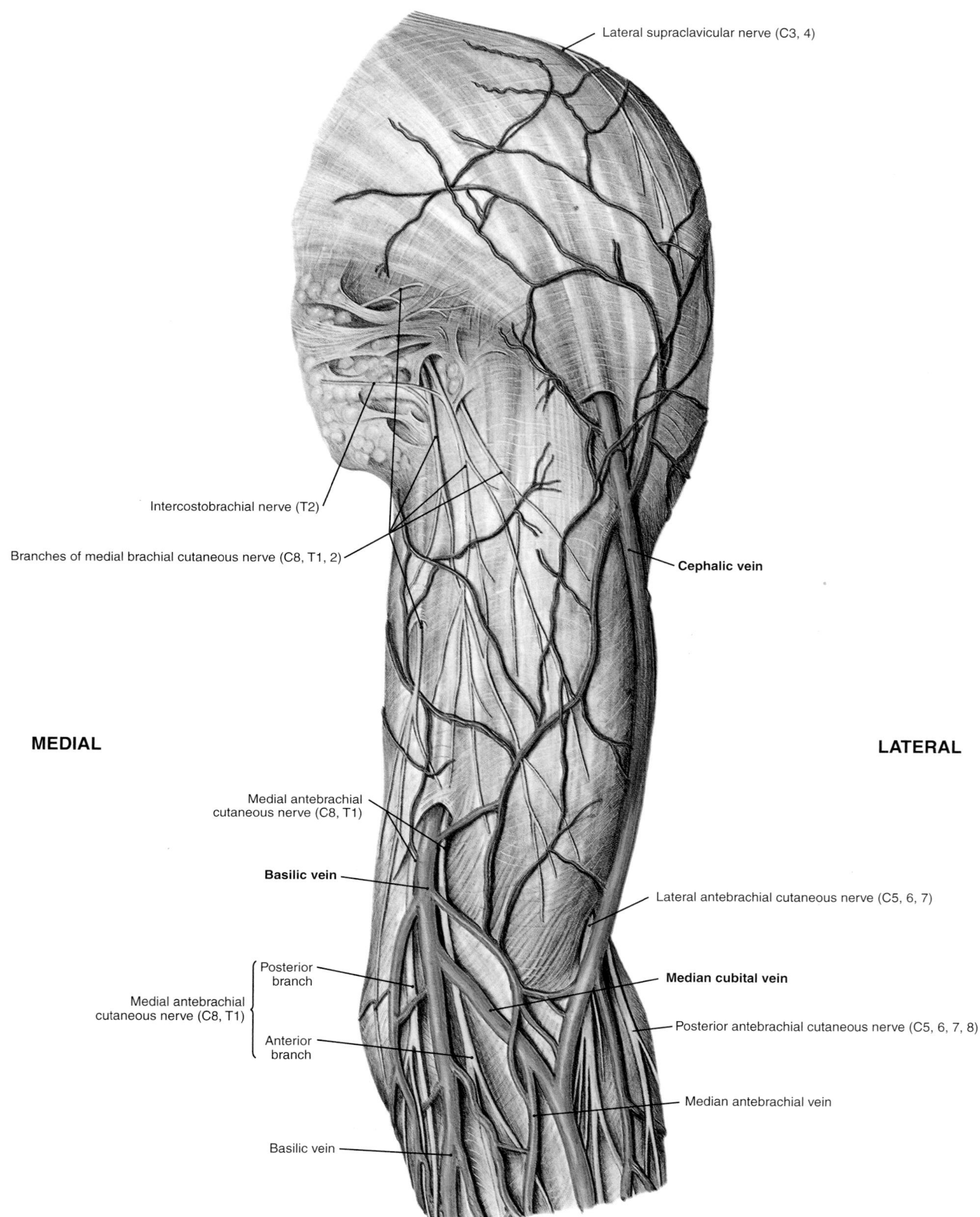
Lateral supraclavicular nerve (C3, 4)
Intercostobrachial nerve (T2)
Branches of medial brachial cutaneous nerve (C8, T1, 2)
Cephalic vein
MEDIAL
LATERAL
Medial antebrachial cutaneous nerve (C8, T1)
Basilic vein
Lateral antebrachial cutaneous nerve (C5, 6, 7)
Posterior branch
Medial antebrachial cutaneous nerve (C8, T1)
Anterior branch
Median cubital vein
Posterior antebrachial cutaneous nerve (C5, 6, 7, 8)
Median antebrachial vein
Basilic vein

Figure 30 Arm; Superficial Veins and Cutaneous Nerves of the Left Upper Limb (Anterior Surface)

NOTE: (1) The **basilic vein** ascends on the medial (ulnar) aspect of the arm, pierces the deep fascia, and at the lower border of the teres major, joins the brachial veins to form the axillary vein.

(2) In contrast, the **cephalic vein** ascends along the lateral aspect of the arm toward the axillary vein, which it joins deep to the deltopectoral triangle.

(3) The principal sensory nerves of the anterior arm region are the **medial brachial cutaneous** and **intercostobrachial nerves.**

Superficial Dissection of the Arm (Posterior View)

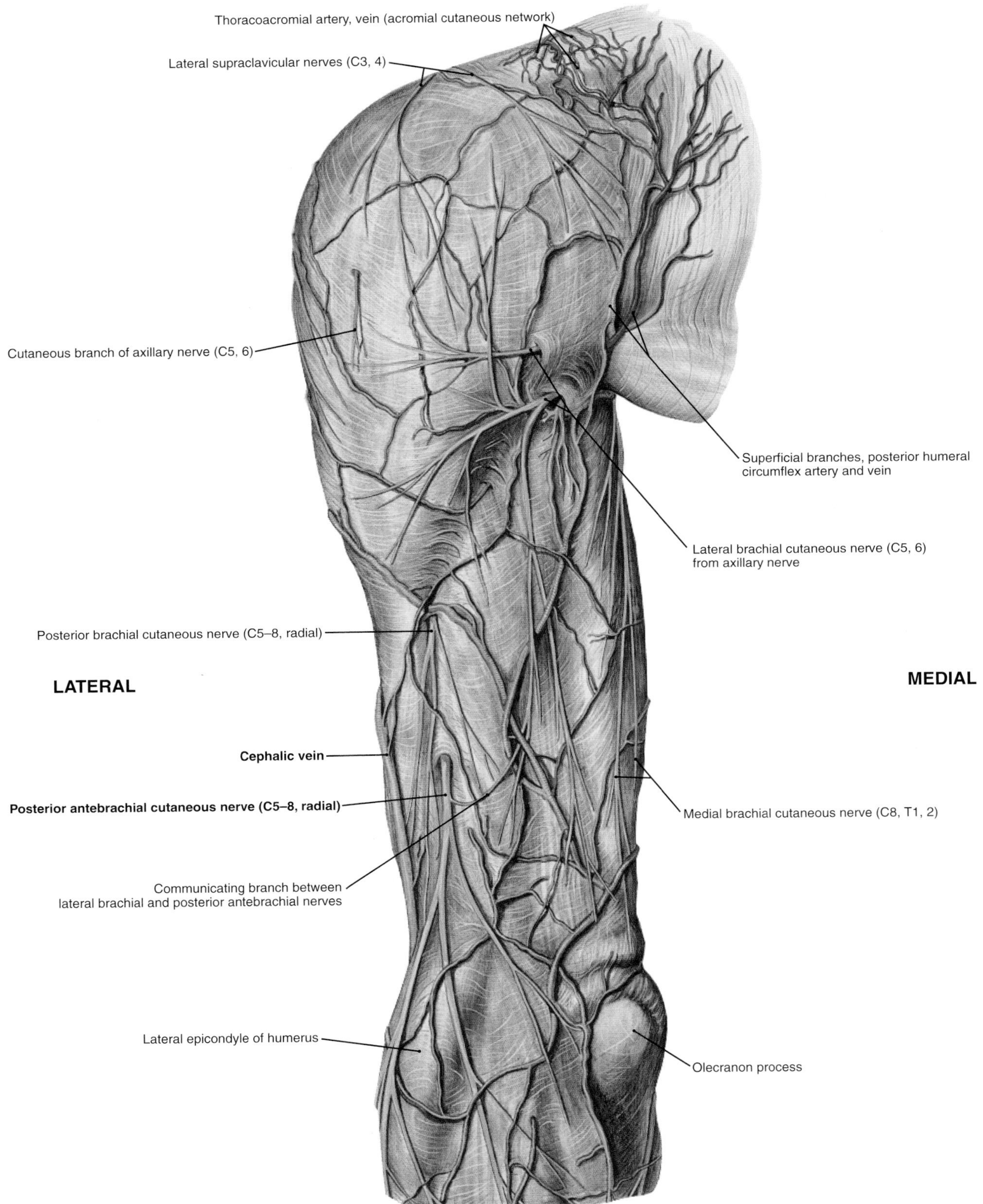
Thoracoacromial artery, vein (acromial cutaneous network)
Lateral supraclavicular nerves (C3, 4)
Cutaneous branch of axillary nerve (C5, 6)
Superficial branches, posterior humeral circumflex artery and vein
Lateral brachial cutaneous nerve (C5, 6) from axillary nerve
Posterior brachial cutaneous nerve (C5–8, radial)
LATERAL
MEDIAL
Cephalic vein
Posterior antebrachial cutaneous nerve (C5–8, radial)
Medial brachial cutaneous nerve (C8, T1, 2)
Communicating branch between lateral brachial and posterior antebrachial nerves
Lateral epicondyle of humerus
Olecranon process

Figure 31 Arm; Superficial Veins, and Cutaneous Nerves of Left Upper Limb (Posterior Surface)

NOTE: (1) The posterior arm region receives cutaneous innervation from the **radial** (posterior brachial cutaneous nerve) and **axillary** (lateral brachial cutaneous nerve) nerves. Both are derived from the posterior cord of the brachial plexus.

(2) The **posterior antebrachial cutaneous nerve** (from the radial nerve) perforates the lateral head of the triceps about 5 cm above the elbow. Upon piercing the superficial fascia, it sends cutaneous branches to the posterior surface of the forearm, as well as a communicating branch to the cutaneous rami of the axillary nerve.

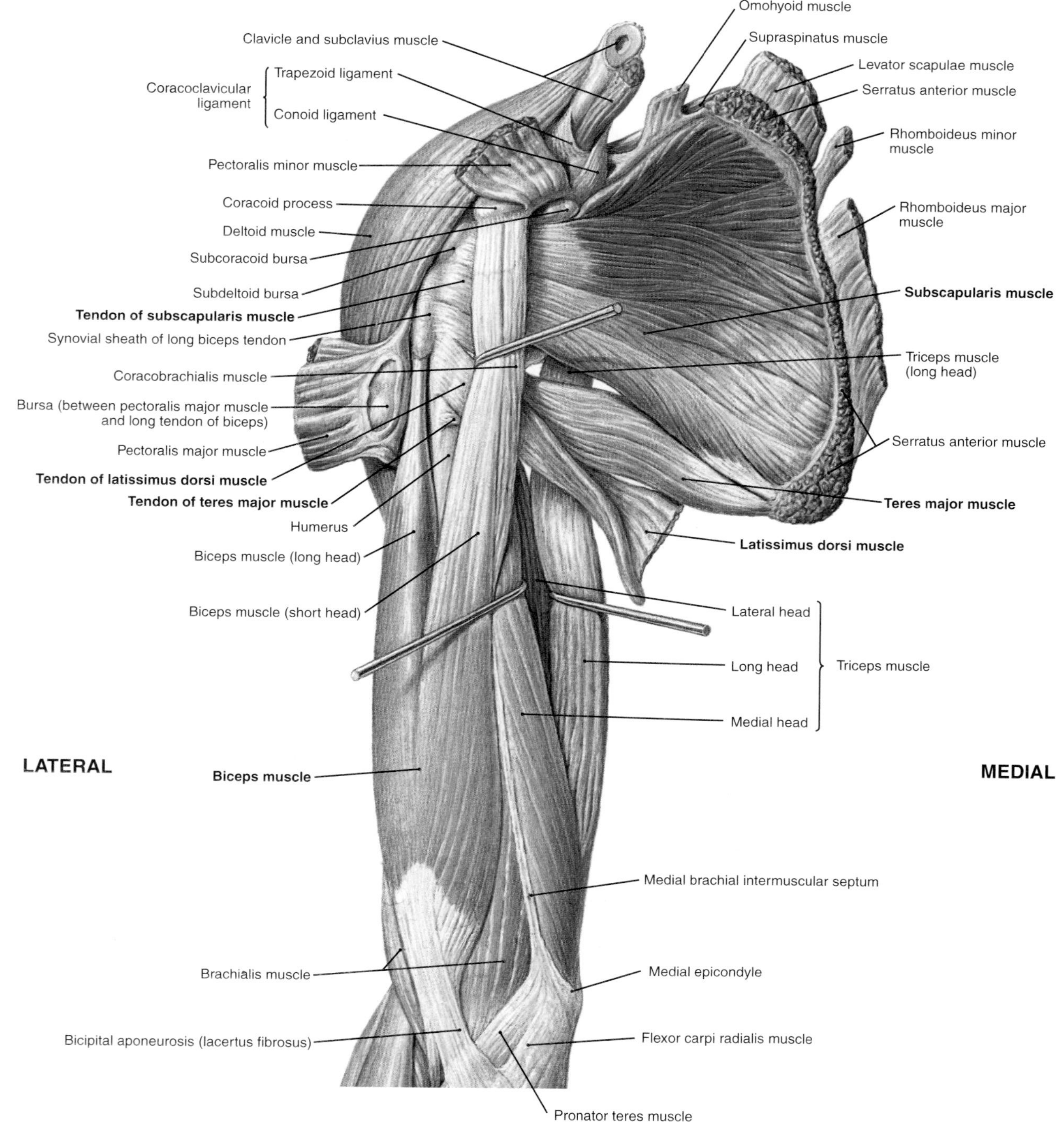
Omohyoid muscle
Supraspinatus muscle
Clavicle and subclavius muscle
Levator scapulae muscle
Serratus anterior muscle
Coracoclavicular ligament
Trapezoid ligament
Conoid ligament
Rhomboideus minor muscle
Pectoralis minor muscle
Coracoid process
Rhomboideus major muscle
Deltoid muscle
Subcoracoid bursa
Subdeltoid bursa
Subscapularis muscle
Tendon of subscapularis muscle
Synovial sheath of long biceps tendon
Triceps muscle (long head)
Coracobrachialis muscle
Bursa (between pectoralis major muscle and long tendon of biceps)
Pectoralis major muscle
Serratus anterior muscle
Tendon of latissimus dorsi muscle
Tendon of teres major muscle
Teres major muscle
Humerus
Latissimus dorsi muscle
Biceps muscle (long head)
Biceps muscle (short head)
Lateral head
Long head
Triceps muscle
Medial head
LATERAL
Biceps muscle
MEDIAL
Medial brachial intermuscular septum
Brachialis muscle
Medial epicondyle
Bicipital aponeurosis (lacertus fibrosus)
Flexor carpi radialis muscle
Pronator teres muscle

Figure 32 Muscles of the Right Shoulder and Arm (Anterior View)

NOTE: (1) The insertion of the subscapularis muscle on the lesser tubercle of the humerus. Distal to this, from medial to lateral, insert the teres major, latissimus dorsi, and pectoralis major muscles.

(2) The pectoralis minor, coracobrachialis, and short head of the biceps all attach to the coracoid process.

(3) The tendon of insertion of the pectoralis major muscle and the long tendon of the biceps muscle are usually separated by a bursa.

(4) From its origin on the coracoid process, the short head of the biceps courses inferiorly and laterally across the tendons of the subscapularis and latissimus dorsi to join the belly of the long head.

(5) The biceps is a very powerful supinator of the forearm and it is an efficient flexor of the forearm, especially when the forearm is supinated.

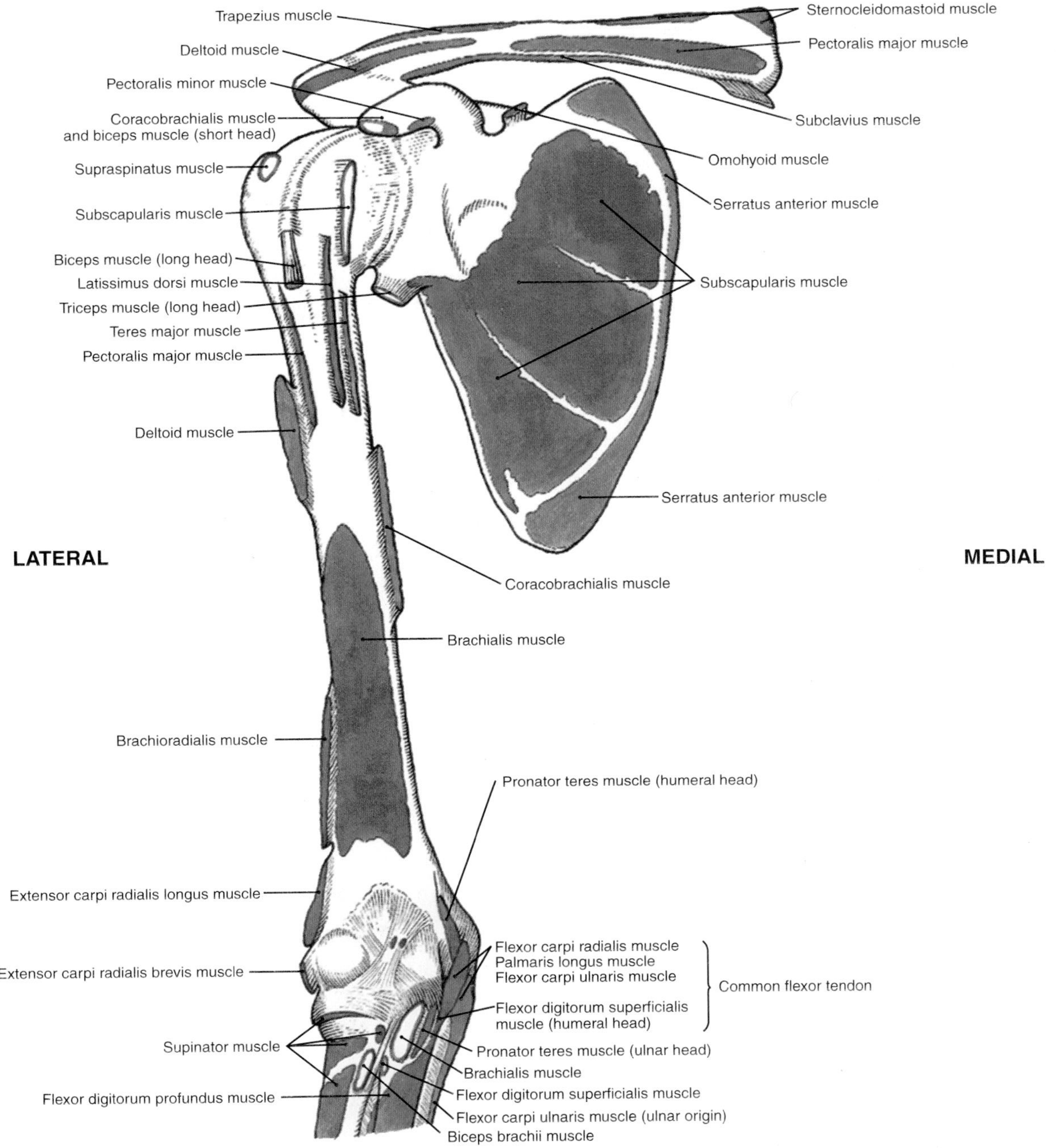
Trapezius muscle
Deltoid muscle
Pectoralis minor muscle
Coracobrachialis muscle and biceps muscle (short head)
Supraspinatus muscle
Subscapularis muscle
Biceps muscle (long head)
Latissimus dorsi muscle
Triceps muscle (long head)
Teres major muscle
Pectoralis major muscle
Deltoid muscle
Sternocleidomastoid muscle
Pectoralis major muscle
Subclavius muscle
Omohyoid muscle
Serratus anterior muscle
Subscapularis muscle
Serratus anterior muscle
LATERAL
MEDIAL
Coracobrachialis muscle
Brachialis muscle
Brachioradialis muscle
Pronator teres muscle (humeral head)
Extensor carpi radialis longus muscle
Extensor carpi radialis brevis muscle
Flexor carpi radialis muscle
Palmaris longus muscle
Flexor carpi ulnaris muscle
Flexor digitorum superficialis muscle (humeral head)
Common flexor tendon
Supinator muscle
Pronator teres muscle (ulnar head)
Brachialis muscle
Flexor digitorum profundus muscle
Flexor digitorum superficialis muscle
Flexor carpi ulnaris muscle (ulnar origin)
Biceps brachii muscle

Figure 33 **Anterior View of Bones of the Upper Limb (Including the Proximal End of the Radius and Ulna) Showing Attachments of Muscles**

NOTE: (1) The broad **origin** of the subscapularis muscle in the subscapular fossa of the scapula. Its **insertion** on the lesser tubercle of the humerus is proximal to the insertions of the latissimus dorsi and teres major muscles.

(2) The biceps muscle extends across both the shoulder and elbow joints, but the coracobrachialis muscle crosses only the shoulder joint.

(3) The tendon of the long head of the biceps commences within the capsule of the shoulder joint and immediately becomes enclosed within a sheath formed by the synovial membrane of the joint.

(4) Upon emerging from the joint capsule, the tendon of the long head of the biceps descends in the intertubercular sulcus (bicipital groove). Inflammation of the synovial sheath of this tendon within the sulcus can be exceedingly painful because the tendon is closely bound to bone in this region.

(5) The latissimus dorsi and teres major insert on the humerus medial to the tendon of the long head of the biceps, whereas the pectoralis major inserts lateral to it.

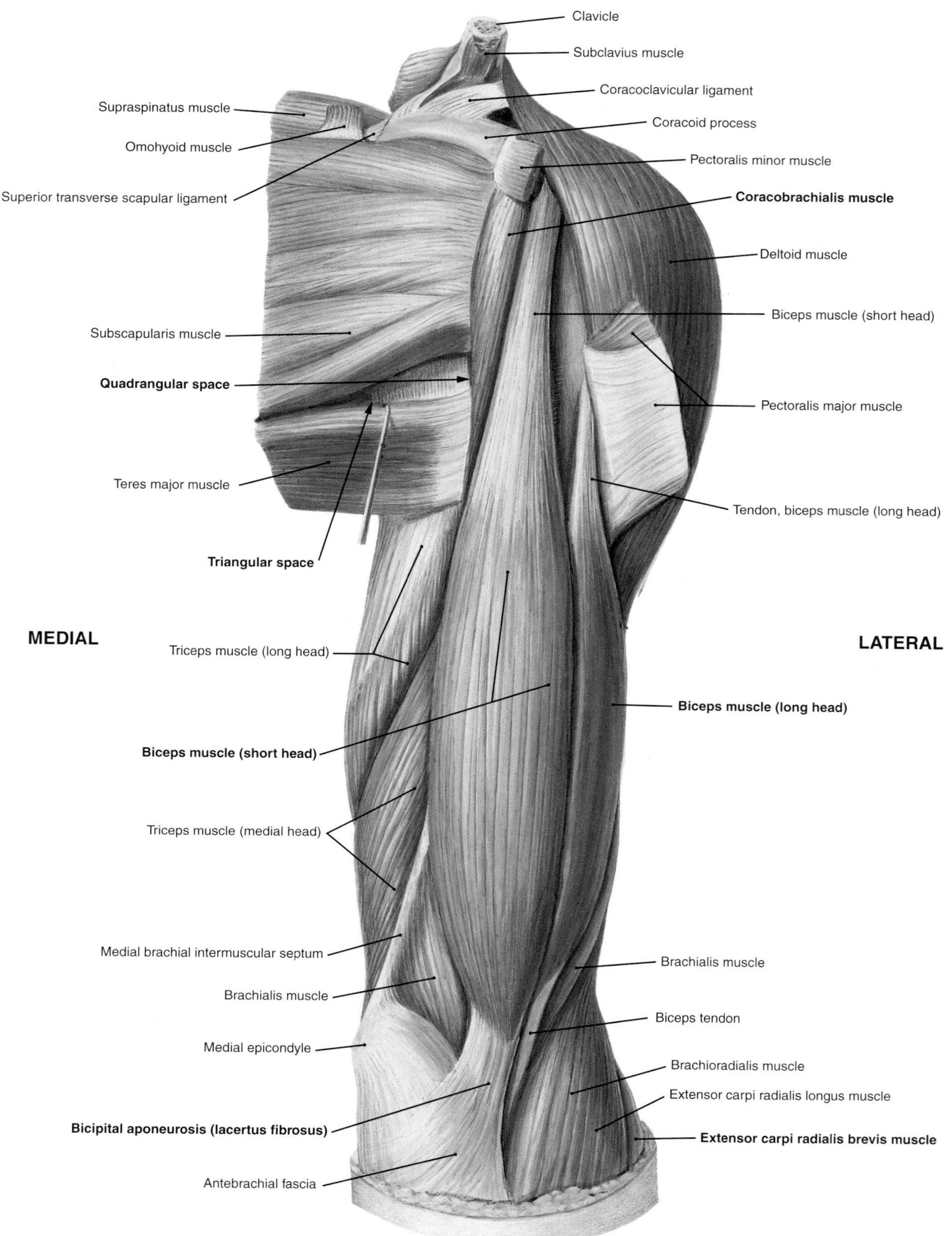
Clavicle
Subclavius muscle
Coracoclavicular ligament
Coracoid process
Pectoralis minor muscle
Coracobrachialis muscle
Deltoid muscle
Biceps muscle (short head)
Pectoralis major muscle
Tendon, biceps muscle (long head)
Supraspinatus muscle
Omohyoid muscle
Superior transverse scapular ligament
Subscapularis muscle
Quadrangular space
Teres major muscle
Triangular space
MEDIAL
LATERAL
Triceps muscle (long head)
Biceps muscle (long head)
Biceps muscle (short head)
Triceps muscle (medial head)
Medial brachial intermuscular septum
Brachialis muscle
Brachialis muscle
Biceps tendon
Medial epicondyle
Brachioradialis muscle
Extensor carpi radialis longus muscle
Bicipital aponeurosis (lacertus fibrosus)
Extensor carpi radialis brevis muscle
Antebrachial fascia

Figure 34 **Superficial View of Muscles on the Anterior Aspect of the Left Arm**

Muscle	Origin	Insertion	Innervation	Action
Biceps brachii	Long head: Supraglenoid tubercle of the scapula. Short head: Coracoid process of the scapula	Tuberosity of the radius and the bicipital aponeurosis	Musculocutaneous nerve (C5, C6)	Flexes and supinates the forearm; long head can also assist in flexing the humerus.

Muscles of the Anterior Arm (Deep Dissection)

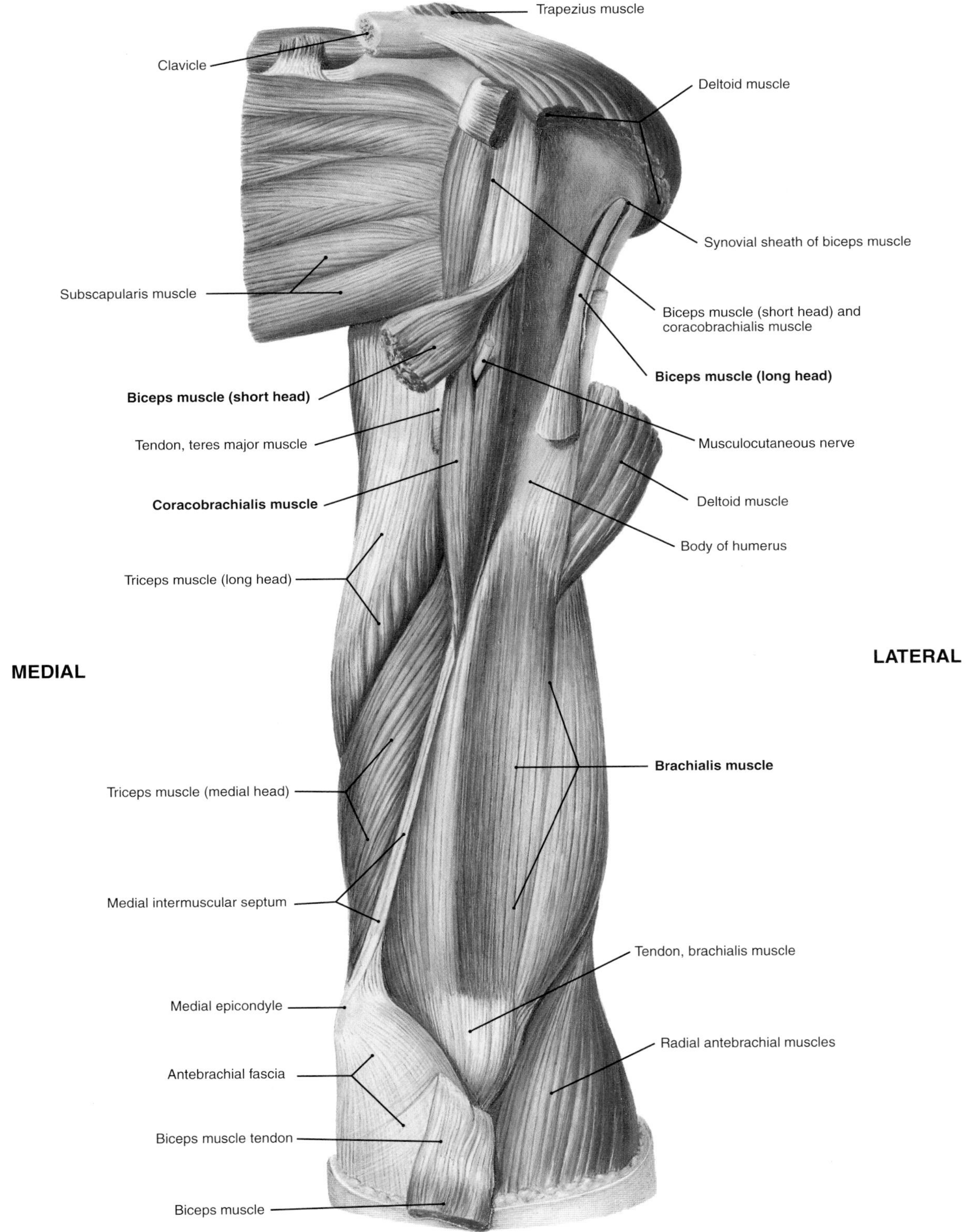
Trapezius muscle
Clavicle
Deltoid muscle
Synovial sheath of biceps muscle
Subscapularis muscle
Biceps muscle (short head) and coracobrachialis muscle
Biceps muscle (long head)
Biceps muscle (short head)
Tendon, teres major muscle
Musculocutaneous nerve
Deltoid muscle
Coracobrachialis muscle
Body of humerus
Triceps muscle (long head)
MEDIAL
LATERAL
Brachialis muscle
Triceps muscle (medial head)
Medial intermuscular septum
Tendon, brachialis muscle
Medial epicondyle
Radial antebrachial muscles
Antebrachial fascia
Biceps muscle tendon
Biceps muscle

Figure 35 Deep View of Muscles on the Anterior Aspect of the Left Arm

Muscle	Origin	Insertion	Innervation	Action
Brachialis	Distal half of anterior surface of the humerus	Tuberosity of the ulna and anterior surface of the coronoid process	Musculocutaneous nerve and often a small branch of the radial nerve (C5, C6)	Powerful flexor of the forearm
Coracobrachialis	Coracoid process of the scapula	Along the medial surface of the humerus near its middle	Musculocutaneous nerve (C6, C7)	Flexes and adducts the arm

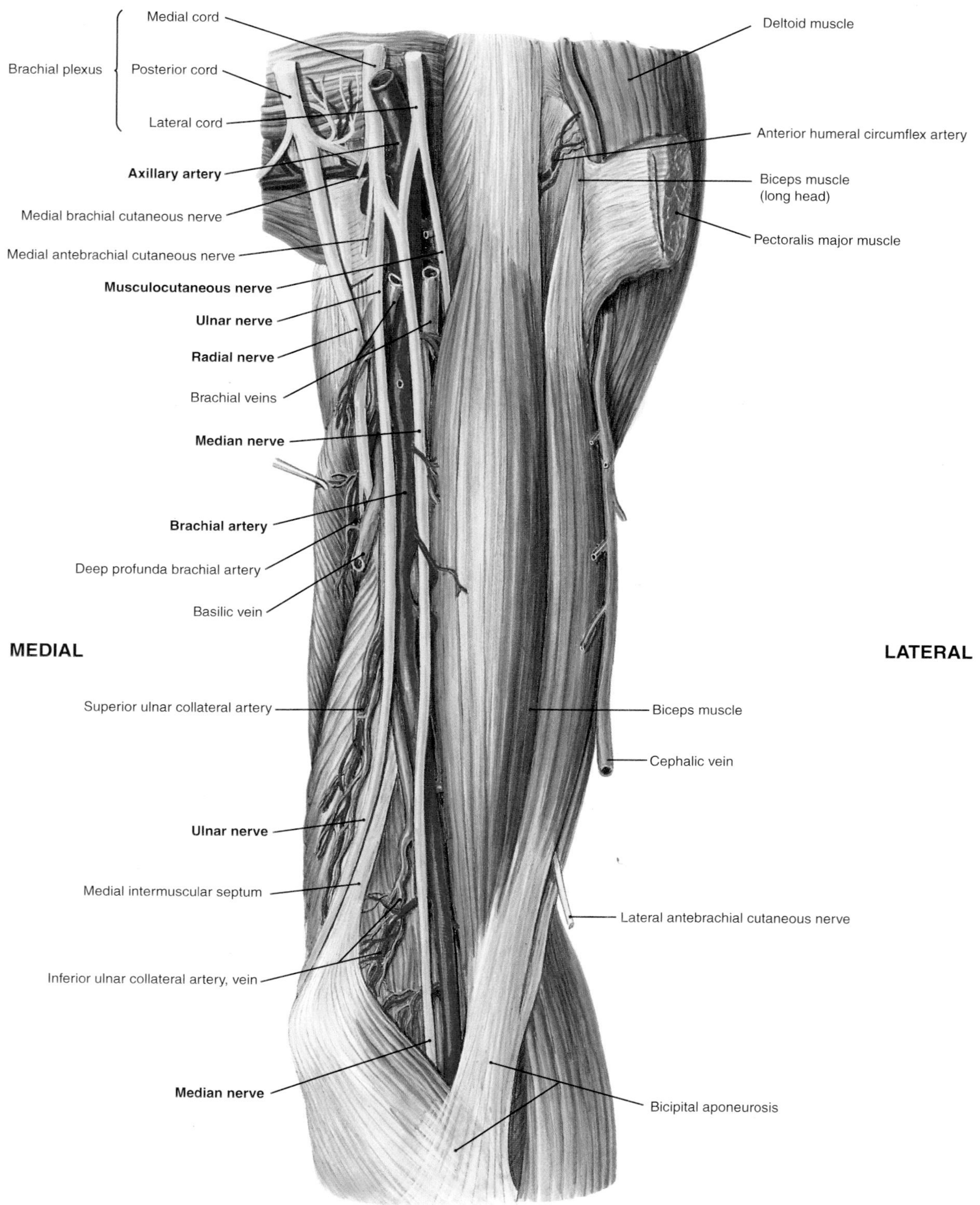
Brachial plexus
Medial cord
Posterior cord
Lateral cord
Axillary artery
Medial brachial cutaneous nerve
Medial antebrachial cutaneous nerve
Musculocutaneous nerve
Ulnar nerve
Radial nerve
Brachial veins
Median nerve
Brachial artery
Deep profunda brachial artery
Basilic vein
MEDIAL
Superior ulnar collateral artery
Ulnar nerve
Medial intermuscular septum
Inferior ulnar collateral artery, vein
Median nerve
Deltoid muscle
Anterior humeral circumflex artery
Biceps muscle
(long head)
Pectoralis major muscle
LATERAL
Biceps muscle
Cephalic vein
Lateral antebrachial cutaneous nerve
Bicipital aponeurosis

Figure 36 **Vessels and Nerves of the Anterior Arm (Left)**

NOTE: (1) The **median nerve** crosses the brachial artery anteriorly from lateral to medial just above the cubital fossa.

(2) The median nerve arises by two roots, one each from the medial and lateral cords of the brachial plexus. The lateral cord then continues downward as the **musculocutaneous nerve**, whereas the medial cord becomes the **ulnar nerve** distal to the axilla.

(3) At the origin of the median nerve, its two roots and the musculocutaneous and ulnar nerves combine to form an outline that resembles the letter M.

(4) Neither the ulnar nor the median nerve gives off branches in the arm region.

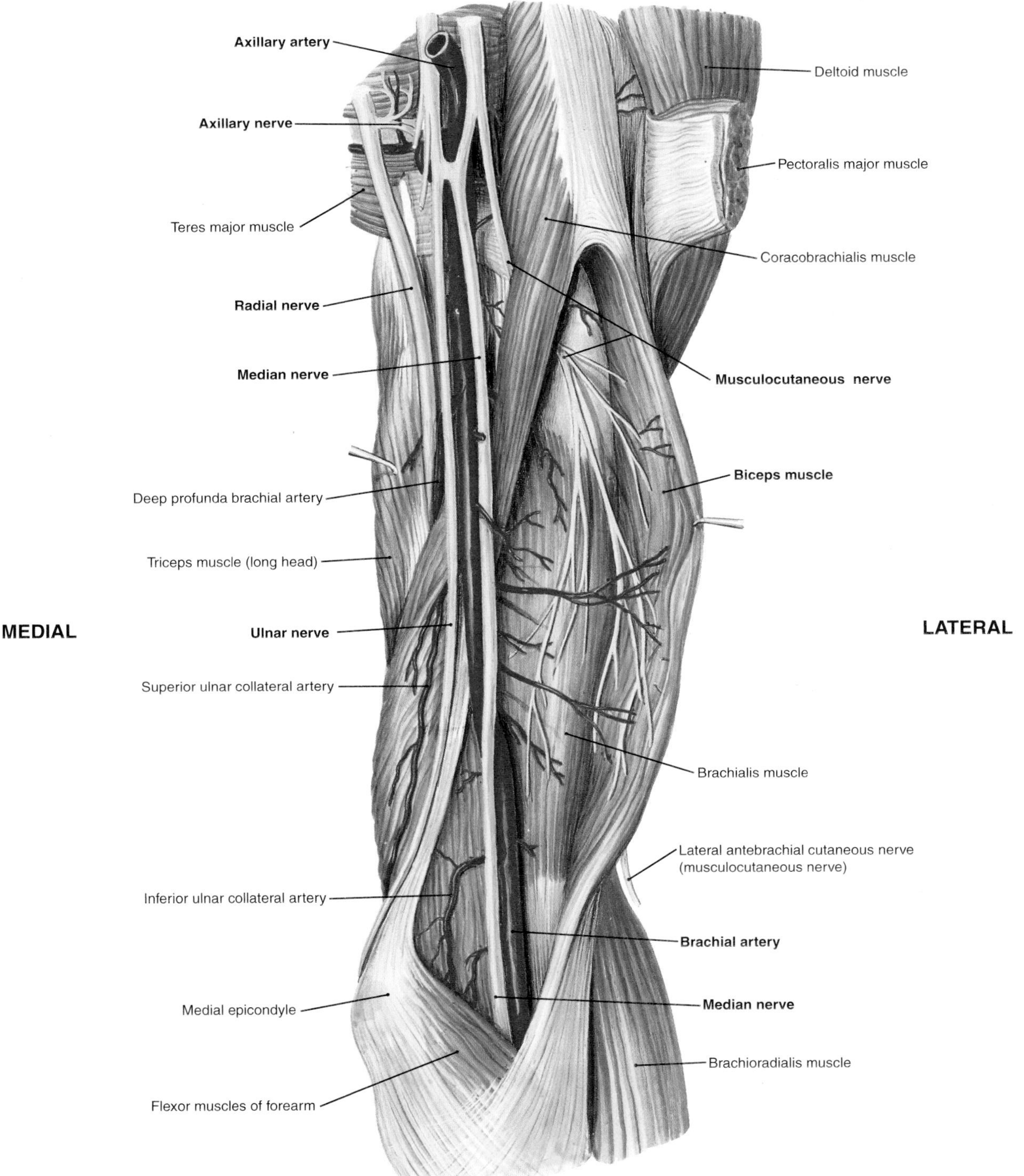
Axillary artery
Axillary nerve
Teres major muscle
Radial nerve
Median nerve
Deep profunda brachial artery
Triceps muscle (long head)
MEDIAL
Ulnar nerve
Superior ulnar collateral artery
Inferior ulnar collateral artery
Medial epicondyle
Flexor muscles of forearm
Deltoid muscle
Pectoralis major muscle
Coracobrachialis muscle
Musculocutaneous nerve
Biceps muscle
LATERAL
Brachialis muscle
Lateral antebrachial cutaneous nerve
(musculocutaneous nerve)
Brachial artery
Median nerve
Brachioradialis muscle

Figure 37 Nerves and Arteries of the Anterior Left Arm (Deep Dissection)

NOTE: (1) The musculocutaneous nerve descends from the lateral cord and perforates the coracobrachialis muscle, which it supplies.

(2) The short head of the biceps muscle has been pulled aside to reveal the musculocutaneous nerve more deeply between the biceps and brachialis muscles, both of which it supplies. This nerve continues into the forearm as the **lateral antebrachial cutaneous nerve**.

(3) The superficial course of the brachial artery in the arm. Its branches include the profunda (deep) brachial artery and the superior and inferior ulnar collateral arteries, in addition to its muscular branches.

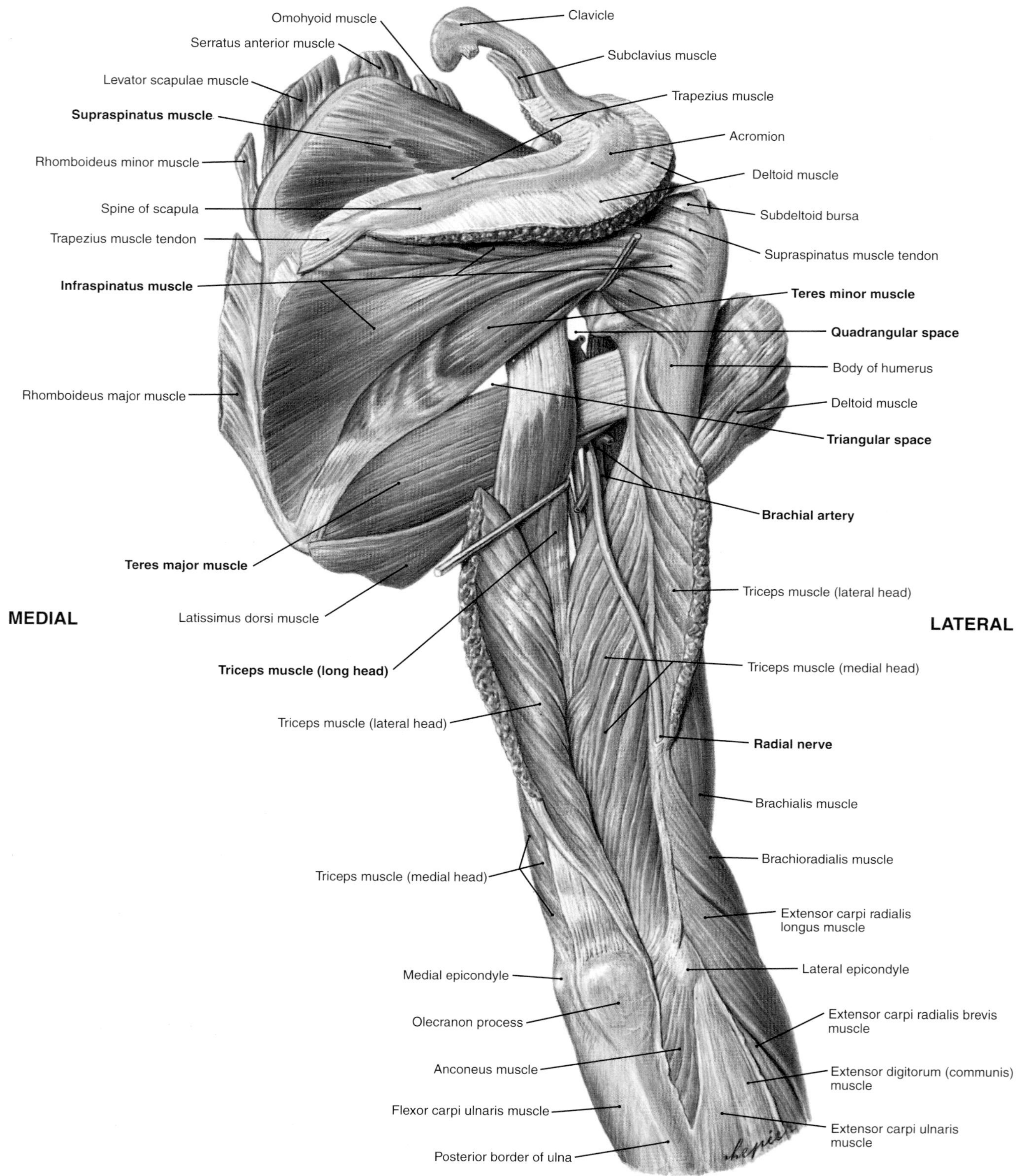
Omohyoid muscle
Serratus anterior muscle
Levator scapulae muscle
Supraspinatus muscle
Rhomboideus minor muscle
Spine of scapula
Trapezius muscle tendon
Infraspinatus muscle
Rhomboideus major muscle
Teres major muscle
MEDIAL
Latissimus dorsi muscle
Triceps muscle (long head)
Triceps muscle (lateral head)
Triceps muscle (medial head)
Medial epicondyle
Olecranon process
Anconeus muscle
Flexor carpi ulnaris muscle
Posterior border of ulna
Clavicle
Subclavius muscle
Trapezius muscle
Acromion
Deltoid muscle
Subdeltoid bursa
Supraspinatus muscle tendon
Teres minor muscle
Quadrangular space
Body of humerus
Deltoid muscle
Triangular space
Brachial artery
Triceps muscle (lateral head)
LATERAL
Triceps muscle (medial head)
Radial nerve
Brachialis muscle
Brachioradialis muscle
Extensor carpi radialis longus muscle
Lateral epicondyle
Extensor carpi radialis brevis muscle
Extensor digitorum (communis) muscle
Extensor carpi ulnaris muscle

Figure 38 Muscles of the Shoulder and Deep Arm (Posterior View)

NOTE: (1) The deltoid muscle and the lateral head of the triceps have been severed, thereby exposing the course of the radial nerve in the upper arm.

(2) The sequential insertions of the supraspinatus, infraspinatus, and teres minor on the greater tubercle of the humerus.

(3) The boundaries of the quadrangular space: **medial,** long head of triceps; **lateral**, the humerus; **superior,** teres minor, and **inferior**, teres major. The axillary nerve and posterior humeral circumflex vessels course through the space.

(4) The boundaries of the triangular space: **superior**, teres minor; **inferior**, teres major; and **lateral**, long head of triceps. The circumflex scapular vessels course through the space.

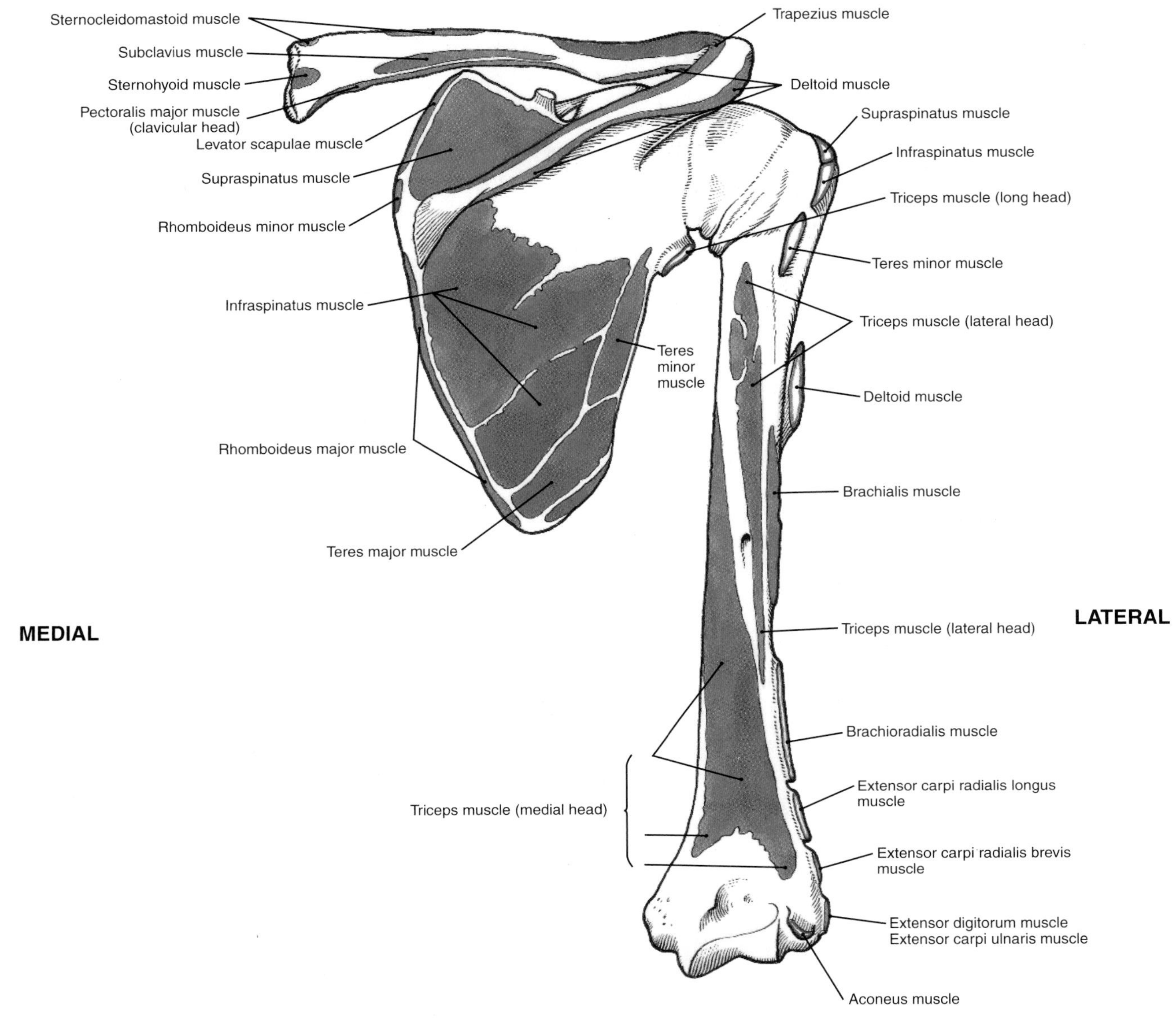
Sternocleidomastoid muscle
Subclavius muscle
Sternohyoid muscle
Pectoralis major muscle (clavicular head)
Levator scapulae muscle
Supraspinatus muscle
Rhomboideus minor muscle
Infraspinatus muscle
Rhomboideus major muscle
Teres major muscle
Teres minor muscle
Trapezius muscle
Deltoid muscle
Supraspinatus muscle
Infraspinatus muscle
Triceps muscle (long head)
Teres minor muscle
Triceps muscle (lateral head)
Deltoid muscle
Brachialis muscle
MEDIAL
LATERAL
Triceps muscle (lateral head)
Brachioradialis muscle
Extensor carpi radialis longus muscle
Triceps muscle (medial head)
Extensor carpi radialis brevis muscle
Extensor digitorum muscle
Extensor carpi ulnaris muscle
Aconeus muscle

Figure 39 **Posterior View of the Clavicle, Scapula, and Humerus Showing Muscle Attachments**

Muscle	Origin	Insertion	Innervation	Action
Triceps brachii	**Long head:** Infraglenoid tubercle of the scapula. **Lateral head:** Posterior surface and lateral border of the humerus and the lateral intermuscular septum. **Medial head:** Posterior surface and medial border of the humerus and the medial intermuscular septum.	Posterior part of the olecranon process of the ulna and the deep fascia of the dorsal forearm	Radial nerve (C7, C8)	All three heads extend the forearm at the elbow joint; the long head also extends the humerus at the shoulder joint

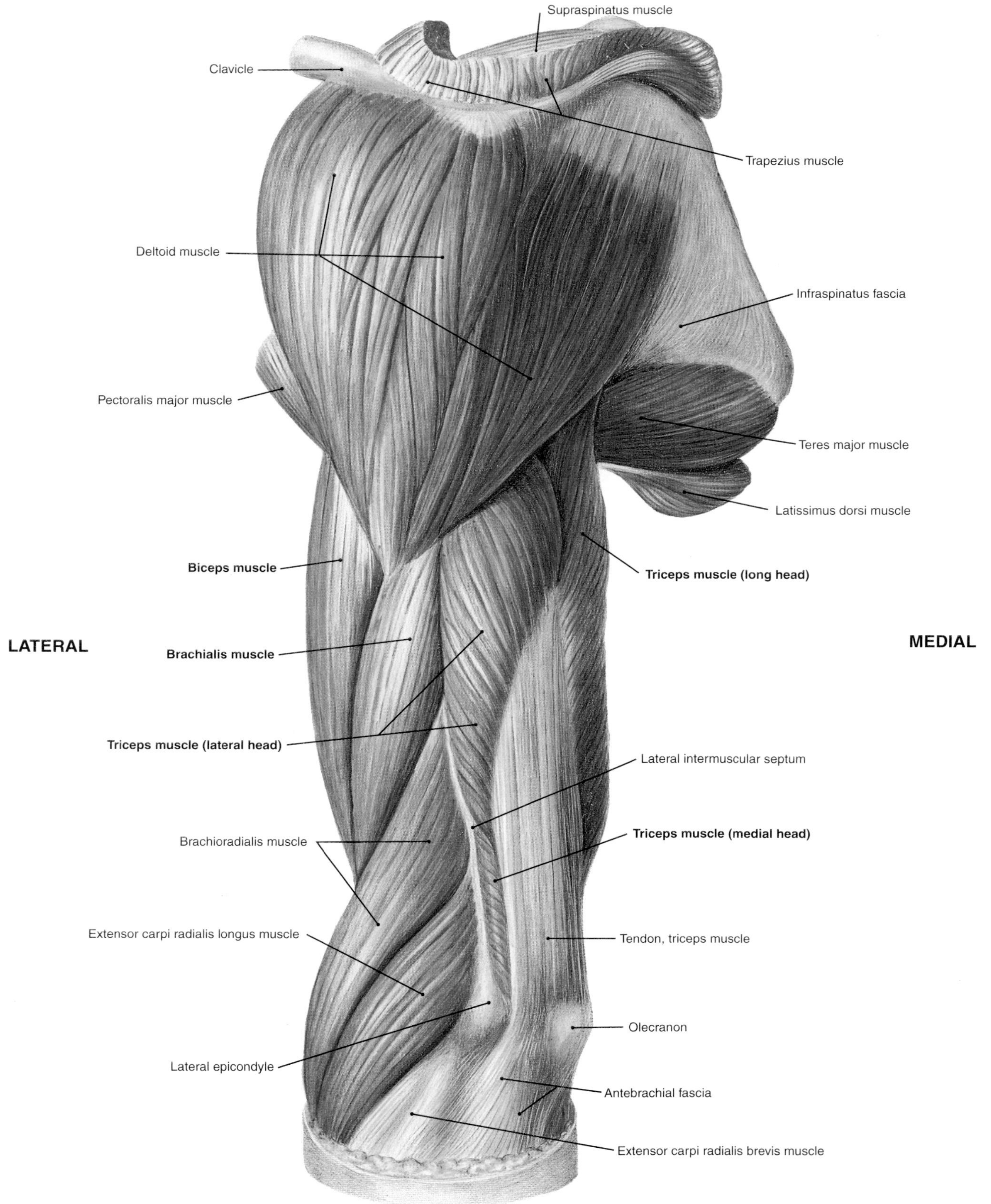
Supraspinatus muscle
Clavicle
Trapezius muscle
Deltoid muscle
Infraspinatus fascia
Pectoralis major muscle
Teres major muscle
Latissimus dorsi muscle
Biceps muscle
Triceps muscle (long head)
LATERAL
Brachialis muscle
MEDIAL
Triceps muscle (lateral head)
Lateral intermuscular septum
Brachioradialis muscle
Triceps muscle (medial head)
Extensor carpi radialis longus muscle
Tendon, triceps muscle
Olecranon
Lateral epicondyle
Antebrachial fascia
Extensor carpi radialis brevis muscle

Figure 40 **Muscles of the Arm (Lateral View)**

NOTE: (1) The deltoid muscle acting as a whole abducts the arm. The clavicular portion flexes and medially rotates the arm, whereas the scapular part extends and laterally rotates the arm.

(2) The lateral intermuscular septum separates the anterior muscular compartment from the posterior muscular compartment.

(3) The sequential origin of the brachioradialis and extensor carpi radialis longus from the humerus above the lateral epicondyle; the extensor carpi radialis brevis arises directly from the lateral epicondyle.

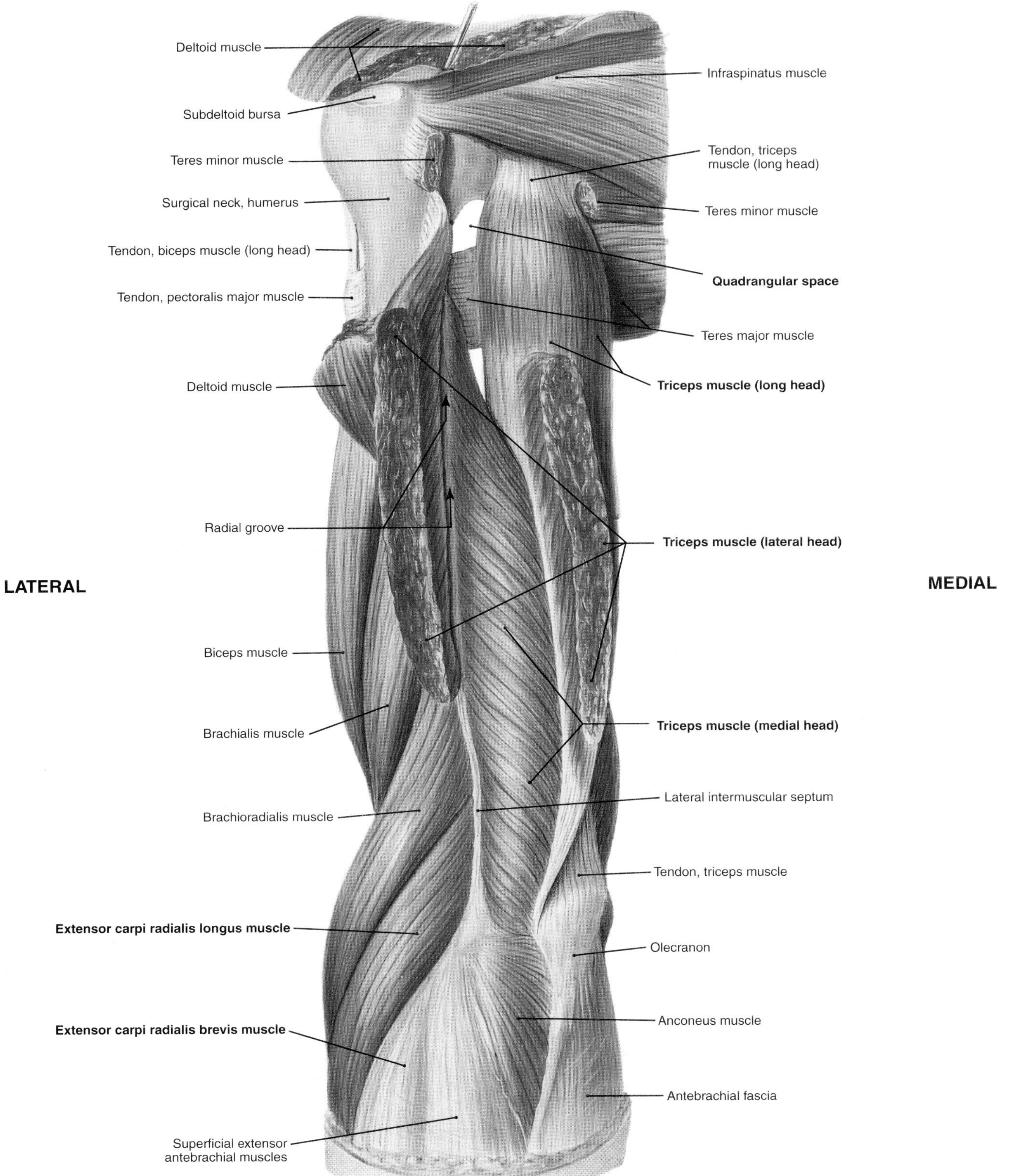
Deltoid muscle
Subdeltoid bursa
Teres minor muscle
Surgical neck, humerus
Tendon, biceps muscle (long head)
Tendon, pectoralis major muscle
Deltoid muscle
Radial groove
LATERAL
Biceps muscle
Brachialis muscle
Brachioradialis muscle
Extensor carpi radialis longus muscle
Extensor carpi radialis brevis muscle
Superficial extensor antebrachial muscles
Infraspinatus muscle
Tendon, triceps muscle (long head)
Teres minor muscle
Quadrangular space
Teres major muscle
Triceps muscle (long head)
Triceps muscle (lateral head)
MEDIAL
Triceps muscle (medial head)
Lateral intermuscular septum
Tendon, triceps muscle
Olecranon
Anconeus muscle
Antebrachial fascia

Figure 41 Deep Muscles of the Arm and Shoulder (Posterior View)

NOTE: (1) Much of the deltoid and teres minor muscles has been removed in this dissection, and the lateral head of the triceps muscle was transected and reflected. Observe the radial groove between the medial and lateral heads of the triceps.

(2) The broad origin of the medial and lateral heads of the triceps from the posterior surface of the humerus (see Fig. 39).

Posterior Arm: Vessels and Nerves (Superficial Dissection)

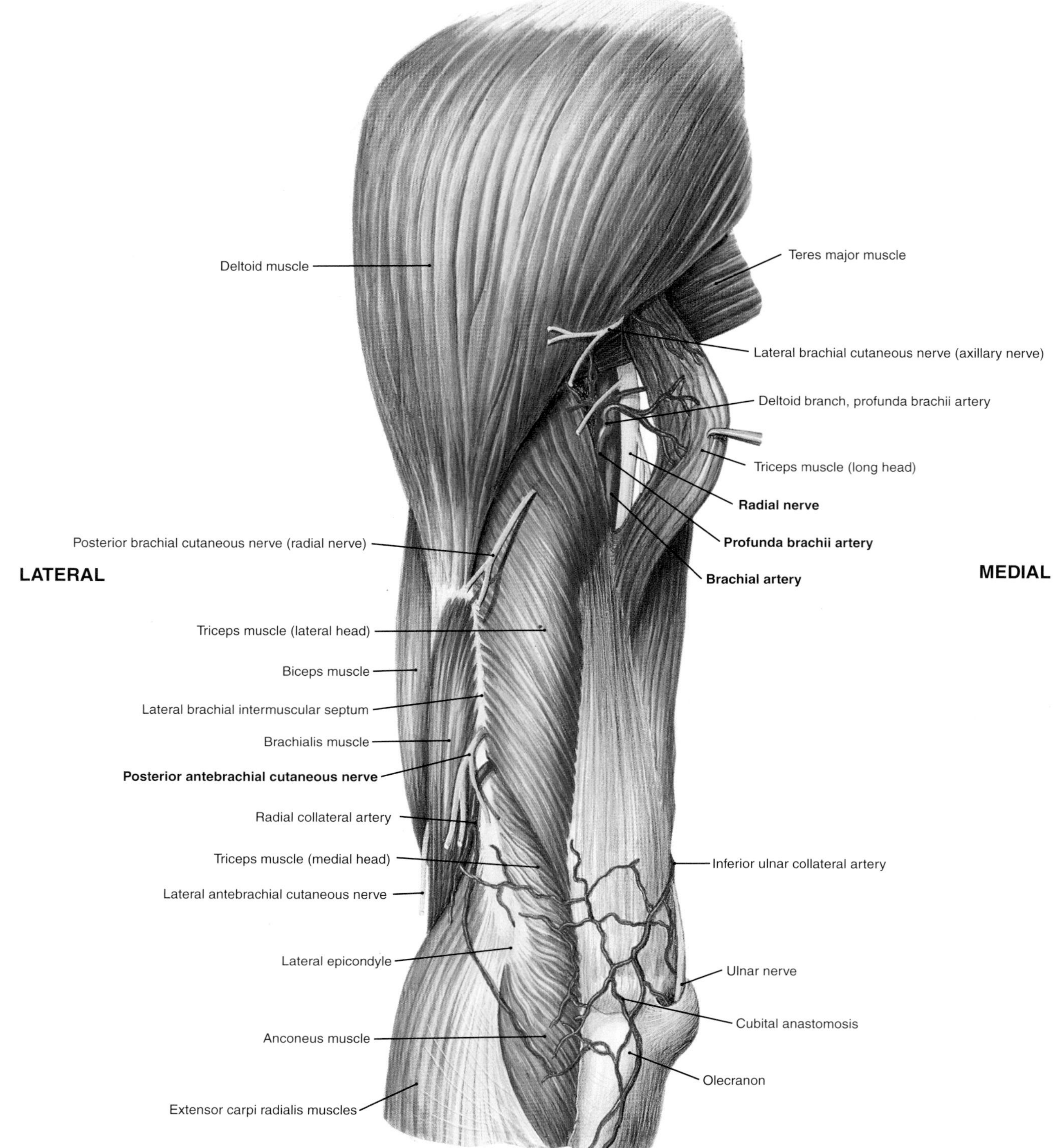
Deltoid muscle
Teres major muscle
Lateral brachial cutaneous nerve (axillary nerve)
Deltoid branch, profunda brachii artery
Triceps muscle (long head)
Radial nerve
Profunda brachii artery
Brachial artery
Posterior brachial cutaneous nerve (radial nerve)
LATERAL
MEDIAL
Triceps muscle (lateral head)
Biceps muscle
Lateral brachial intermuscular septum
Brachialis muscle
Posterior antebrachial cutaneous nerve
Radial collateral artery
Triceps muscle (medial head)
Lateral antebrachial cutaneous nerve
Inferior ulnar collateral artery
Lateral epicondyle
Ulnar nerve
Cubital anastomosis
Anconeus muscle
Olecranon
Extensor carpi radialis muscles

Figure 42 Nerves and Arteries of the Left Posterior Arm (Superficial Branches)

NOTE: (1) The origin of the profunda brachii artery from the brachial artery and its relationship to the radial nerve. The long head of the triceps has been pulled medially.

(2) The relationship of the ulnar nerve to the olecranon process and the vascular anastomosis around the elbow.

(3) Both the posterior brachial and posterior antebrachial nerves of the radial nerve perforate the lateral head of the triceps muscle to reach the superficial fascia and skin.

(4) The site of attachment of the deltoid muscle on the humerus, and the relationship of this attachment to the uppermost fibers of the brachialis muscle, the lateral intermuscular septum, and the lateral head of the triceps muscle (see Fig. 39)

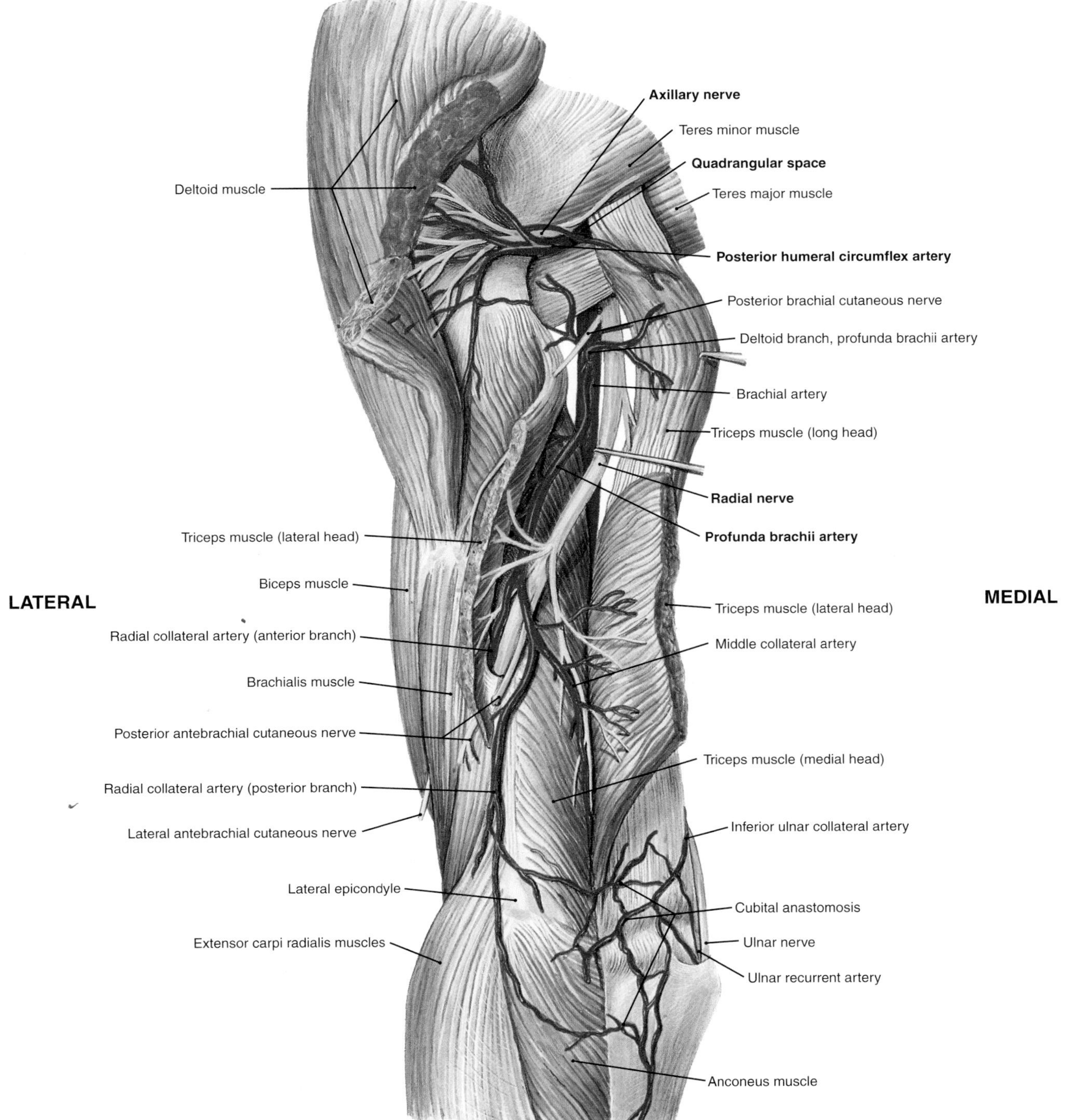
Axillary nerve
Teres minor muscle
Quadrangular space
Teres major muscle
Deltoid muscle
Posterior humeral circumflex artery
Posterior brachial cutaneous nerve
Deltoid branch, profunda brachii artery
Brachial artery
Triceps muscle (long head)
Radial nerve
Profunda brachii artery
Triceps muscle (lateral head)
Biceps muscle
LATERAL
MEDIAL
Triceps muscle (lateral head)
Radial collateral artery (anterior branch)
Middle collateral artery
Brachialis muscle
Posterior antebrachial cutaneous nerve
Triceps muscle (medial head)
Radial collateral artery (posterior branch)
Inferior ulnar collateral artery
Lateral antebrachial cutaneous nerve
Lateral epicondyle
Cubital anastomosis
Extensor carpi radialis muscles
Ulnar nerve
Ulnar recurrent artery
Anconeus muscle

Figure 43 **Deep Nerves and Arteries of the Posterior Arm**

NOTE: (1) The course of the axillary nerve and posterior humeral circumflex artery through the quadrangular space to reach the deltoid and dorsal shoulder region.

(2) The course of the radial nerve and profunda brachii artery along the radial (spiral) groove to the posterior brachial region. This groove lies along the body of the humerus between the origins of the lateral and medial heads of the triceps muscle.

(3) The common insertion of the three heads of the triceps muscle onto the olecranon process of the ulna.

(4) In addition to a **deltoid branch**, which anastomoses with the posterior humeral circumflex artery and helps supply the long head of the triceps along with the deltoid muscle, the profunda brachii artery gives off the **middle and radial collateral arteries.**

(5) The latter two vessels and the **superior and inferior ulnar collateral** branches of the brachial artery are the four descending vessels that participate in the anastomosis around the elbow joint (see Fig. 42).

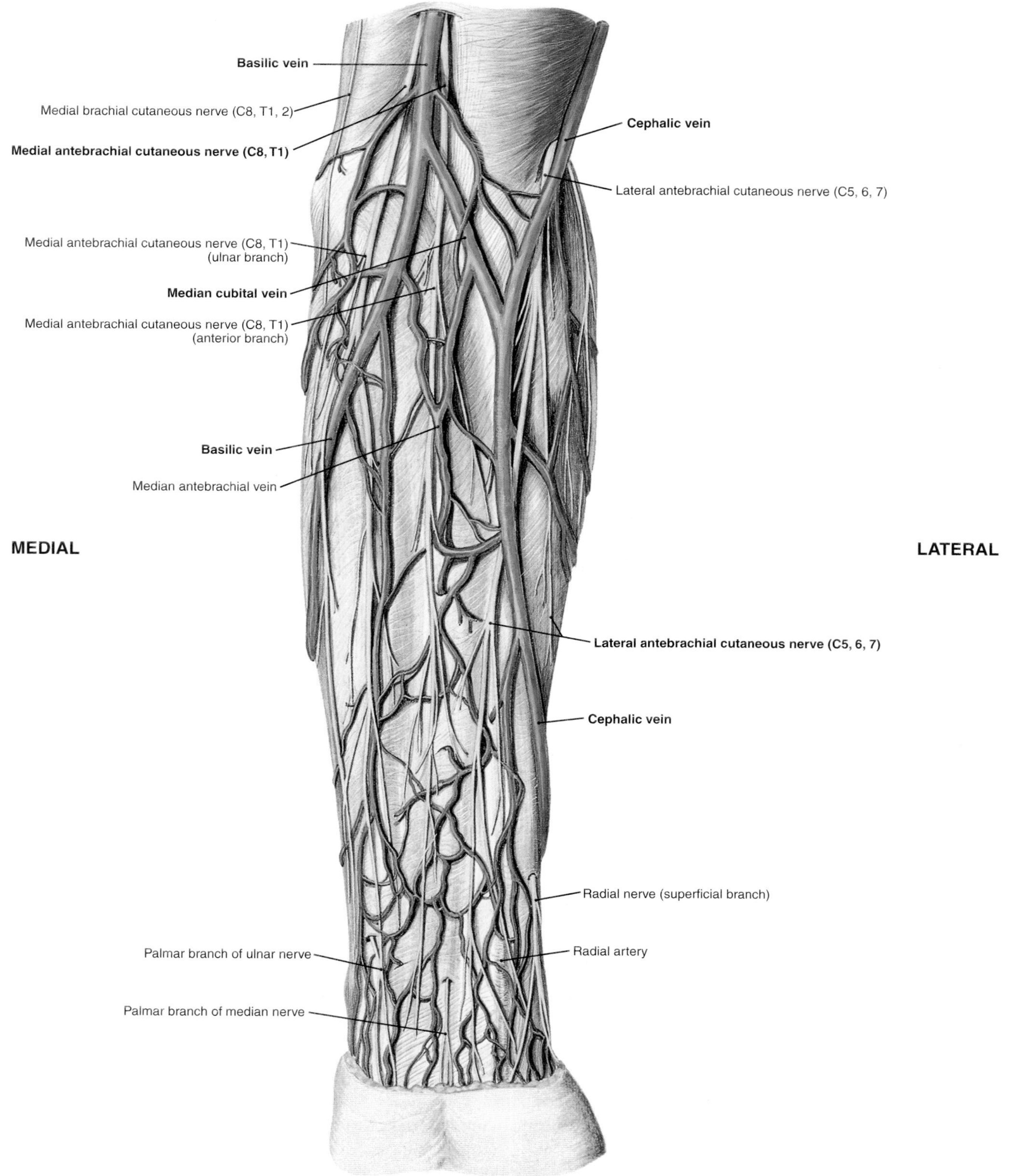
Basilic vein
Medial brachial cutaneous nerve (C8, T1, 2)
Medial antebrachial cutaneous nerve (C8, T1)
Cephalic vein
Lateral antebrachial cutaneous nerve (C5, 6, 7)
Medial antebrachial cutaneous nerve (C8, T1) (ulnar branch)
Median cubital vein
Medial antebrachial cutaneous nerve (C8, T1) (anterior branch)
Basilic vein
Median antebrachial vein
MEDIAL
LATERAL
Lateral antebrachial cutaneous nerve (C5, 6, 7)
Cephalic vein
Radial nerve (superficial branch)
Radial artery
Palmar branch of ulnar nerve
Palmar branch of median nerve

Figure 44 **Forearm; Superficial Veins, and Cutaneous Nerves of Left Upper Limb (Anterior Surface)**

NOTE: (1) The median cubital vein joins the cephalic and basilic veins in the cubital fossa.

(2) The main sensory nerves of the anterior forearm are the medial antebrachial cutaneous nerve (derived from the medial cord of the brachial plexus) and the lateral antebrachial cutaneous nerve, which is a continuation of the musculocutaneous nerve.

(3) The medial antebrachial cutaneous nerve courses with the basilic vein, while the lateral antebrachial cutaneous nerve lies next to the cephalic vein at the elbow.

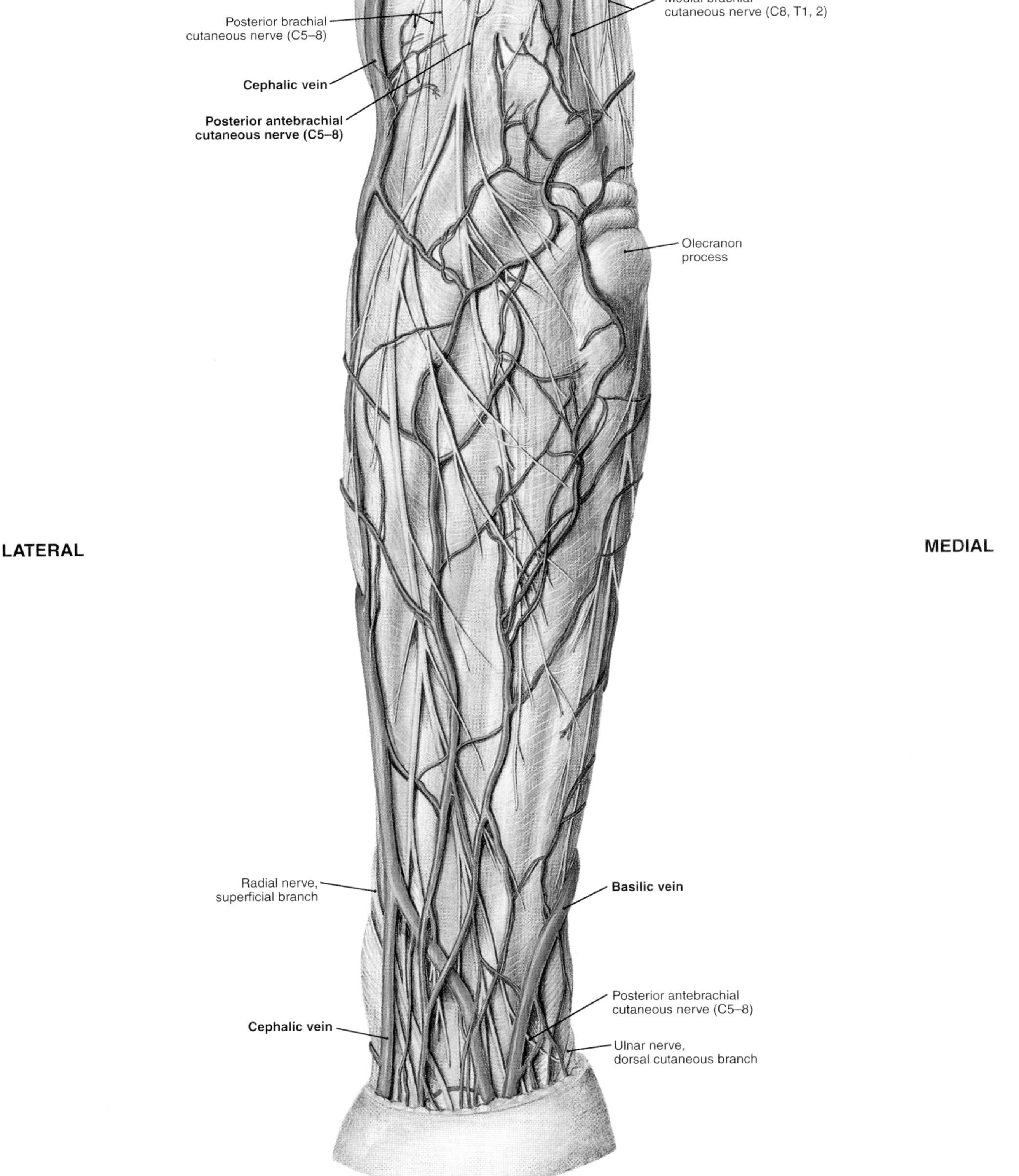
Posterior brachial cutaneous nerve (C5–8)
Cephalic vein
Posterior antebrachial cutaneous nerve (C5–8)
Medial brachial cutaneous nerve (C8, T1, 2)
Olecranon process
LATERAL
MEDIAL
Radial nerve, superficial branch
Basilic vein
Posterior antebrachial cutaneous nerve (C5–8)
Cephalic vein
Ulnar nerve, dorsal cutaneous branch

Figure 45 **Forearm: Superficial Veins and Cutaneous Nerves of the Left Upper Limb (Posterior Surface)**

NOTE: (1) Branches of the radial nerve (posterior antebrachial cutaneous and superficial radial) contribute the principal innervation to the skin on the posterior aspect of the forearm.

(2) At the wrist, the dorsal branch of the ulnar nerve passes backward onto the dorsal surfaces of the wrist and hand.

(3) The basilic vein arises on the ulnar (or medial) side of the dorsum of the hand and wrist, while the cephalic vein arises on the radial (lateral) side.

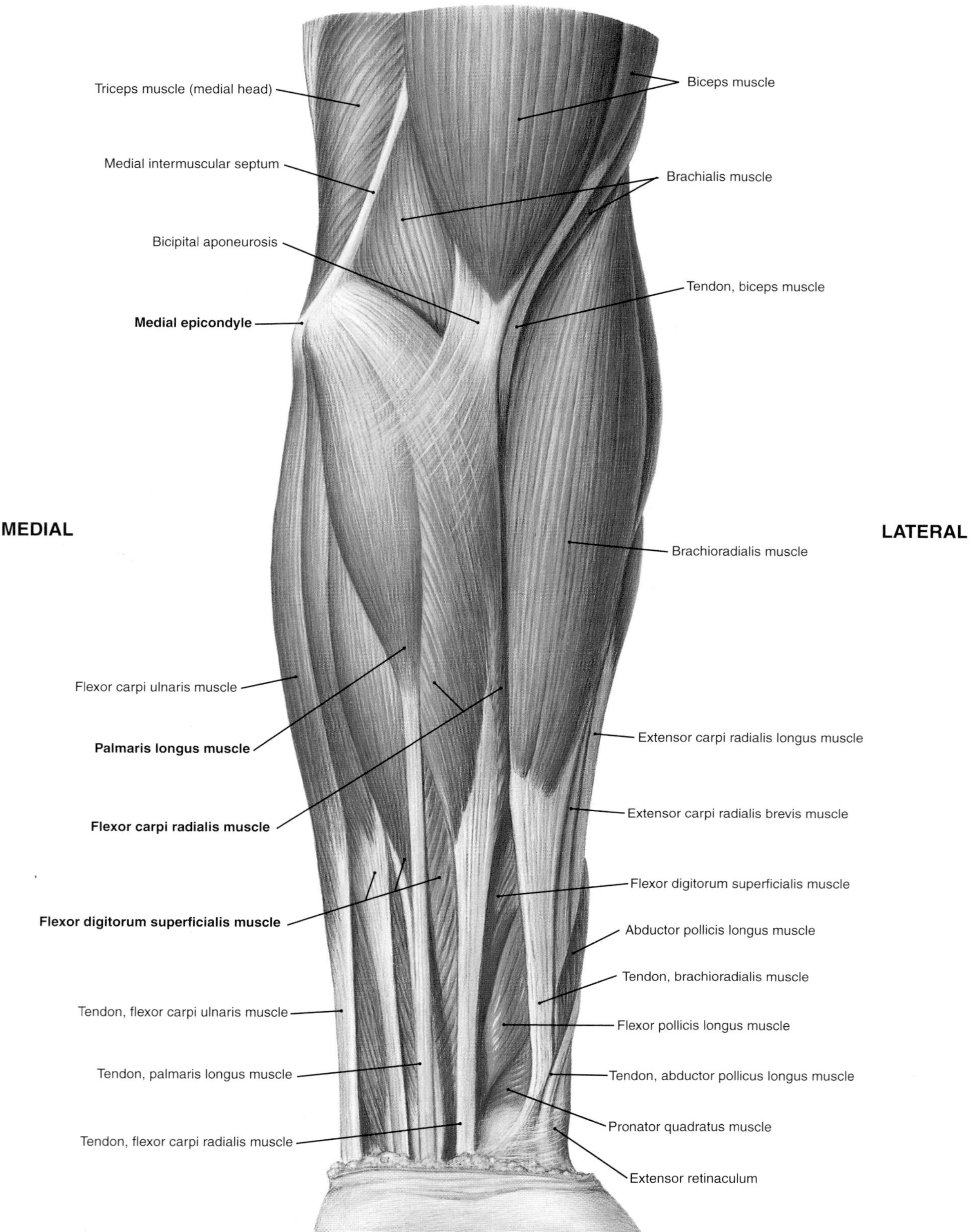
Triceps muscle (medial head)
Biceps muscle
Medial intermuscular septum
Brachialis muscle
Bicipital aponeurosis
Tendon, biceps muscle
Medial epicondyle
MEDIAL
LATERAL
Brachioradialis muscle
Flexor carpi ulnaris muscle
Palmaris longus muscle
Extensor carpi radialis longus muscle
Flexor carpi radialis muscle
Extensor carpi radialis brevis muscle
Flexor digitorum superficialis muscle
Flexor digitorum superficialis muscle
Abductor pollicis longus muscle
Tendon, brachioradialis muscle
Tendon, flexor carpi ulnaris muscle
Flexor pollicis longus muscle
Tendon, palmaris longus muscle
Tendon, abductor pollicus longus muscle
Pronator quadratus muscle
Tendon, flexor carpi radialis muscle
Extensor retinaculum

Figure 46 **Left Anterior Forearm Muscles, Superficial Group**

NOTE: (1) The brachioradialis muscle is studied with the posterior forearm muscles and is not included with the flexor muscles of the anterior forearm.

(2) The anterior forearm muscles arise from the medial epicondyle of the humerus and include the pronator teres (not labeled, see Fig. 47) **flexor carpi radialis, palmaris longus,** and **flexor carpi ulnaris.** Beneath these is the **flexor digitorum superficialis.**

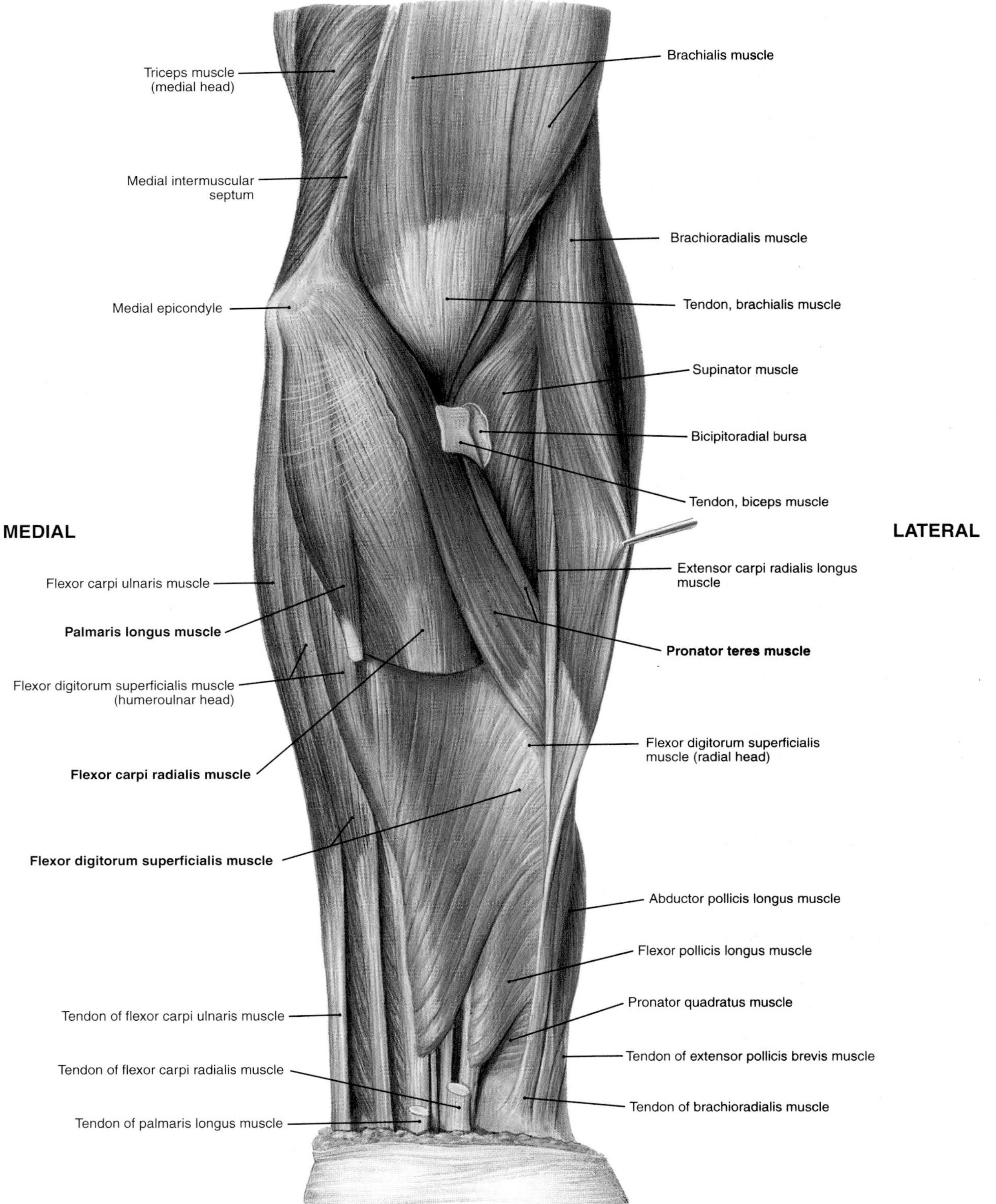
Triceps muscle (medial head)
Brachialis muscle
Medial intermuscular septum
Brachioradialis muscle
Medial epicondyle
Tendon, brachialis muscle
Supinator muscle
Bicipitoradial bursa
Tendon, biceps muscle
MEDIAL
LATERAL
Extensor carpi radialis longus muscle
Flexor carpi ulnaris muscle
Palmaris longus muscle
Pronator teres muscle
Flexor digitorum superficialis muscle (humeroulnar head)
Flexor digitorum superficialis muscle (radial head)
Flexor carpi radialis muscle
Flexor digitorum superficialis muscle
Abductor pollicis longus muscle
Flexor pollicis longus muscle
Pronator quadratus muscle
Tendon of flexor carpi ulnaris muscle
Tendon of extensor pollicis brevis muscle
Tendon of flexor carpi radialis muscle
Tendon of brachioradialis muscle
Tendon of palmaris longus muscle

Figure 47 Flexor Digitorum Superficialis Muscle and Related Muscles (Left)

NOTE: (1) The palmaris longus, flexor carpi radialis, and insertion of the biceps have been cut to reveal the flexor digitorum superficialis and pronator teres.

(2) The triangular cubital fossa is bounded medially by the superficial flexors and laterally by the extensors. Its floor is the brachialis muscle.

(3) The pronator teres arises by two heads: a larger **humeral head** from the medial epicondyle and a much smaller **ulnar head** from the coronoid process. It crosses the forearm obliquely to insert on the shaft of the radius.

(4) The flexor digitorum superficialis arises broadly from the humerus and ulna medially (humeral–ulnar head) and from the anterior border of the radius laterally (radial head).

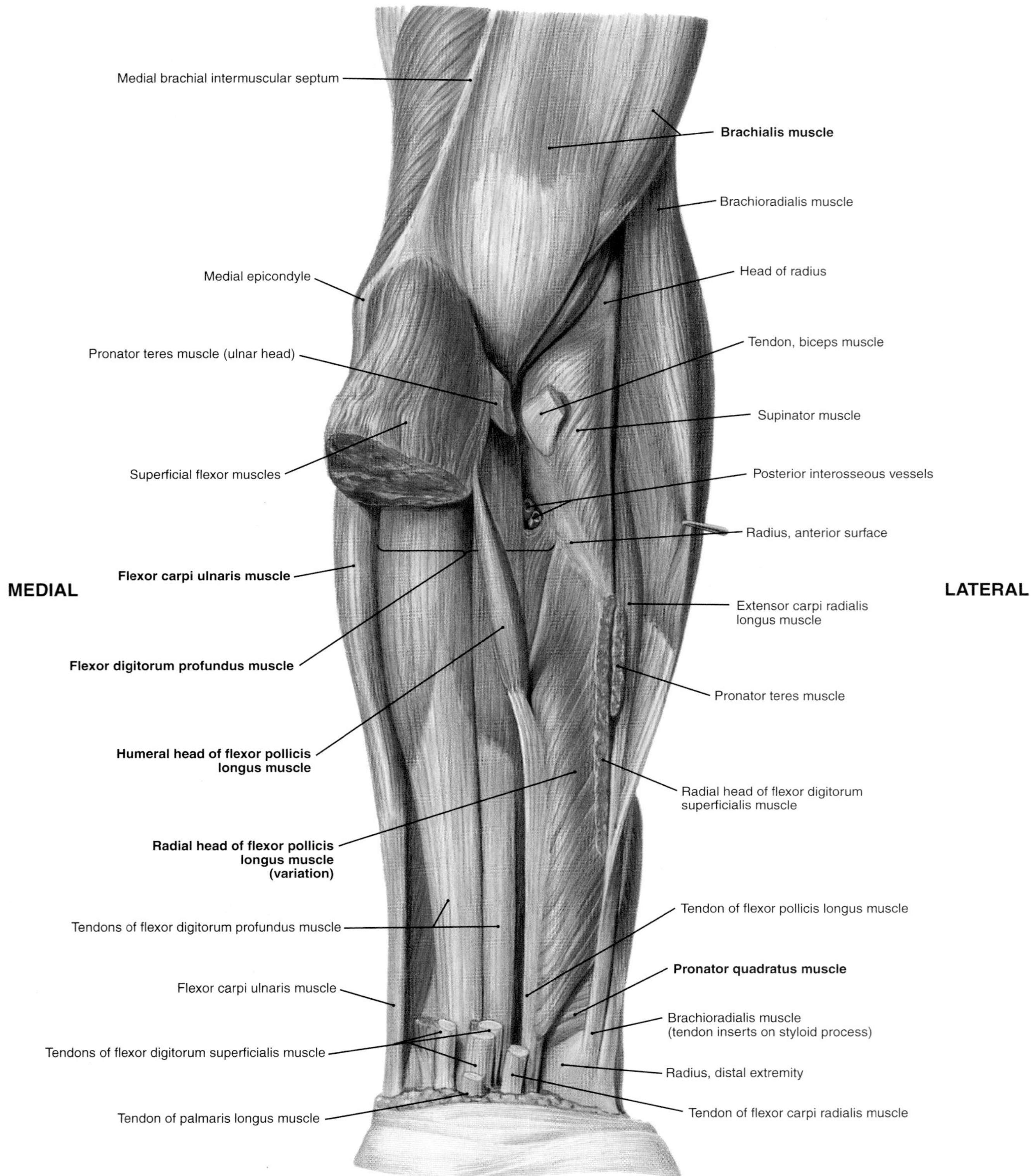
Medial brachial intermuscular septum
Brachialis muscle
Brachioradialis muscle
Medial epicondyle
Head of radius
Pronator teres muscle (ulnar head)
Tendon, biceps muscle
Supinator muscle
Superficial flexor muscles
Posterior interosseous vessels
Radius, anterior surface
MEDIAL
Flexor carpi ulnaris muscle
LATERAL
Extensor carpi radialis longus muscle
Flexor digitorum profundus muscle
Pronator teres muscle
Humeral head of flexor pollicis longus muscle
Radial head of flexor digitorum superficialis muscle
Radial head of flexor pollicis longus muscle (variation)
Tendon of flexor pollicis longus muscle
Tendons of flexor digitorum profundus muscle
Pronator quadratus muscle
Flexor carpi ulnaris muscle
Brachioradialis muscle (tendon inserts on styloid process)
Tendons of flexor digitorum superficialis muscle
Radius, distal extremity
Tendon of palmaris longus muscle
Tendon of flexor carpi radialis muscle

Figure 48 Left Anterior Forearm Muscles, Deep Group

NOTE: (1) The superficial anterior forearm muscles have been removed to reveal the three muscles of the deep group: the flexor digitorum profundus, the flexor pollicis longus, and the pronator quadratus.

(2) The pronator quadratus is a small quadrangular muscle situated at the distal end of the forearm beneath the tendons of the flexor digitorum profundus and flexor pollicis longus. It is partially shown in this dissection and can be seen better in Fig. 67.1.

(3) In this drawing, the tendons of the flexor digitorum profundus to the ring and little fingers and those to the middle and index fingers appear fused at the wrist, as if they were two structures rather than four.

Anterior Forearm Muscles: Complete Chart

FLEXOR MUSCLES OF FOREARM: SUPERFICIAL GROUP

Muscle	Origin	Insertion	Innervation	Action
Pronator teres	**Humeral head:** Medial epicondyle of humerus. **Ulnar head:** Coronoid process of ulna	Midway along the lateral surface of the radius	Median nerve (C6, C7) (enters the forearm by passing between the two heads)	Pronates and flexes the forearm
Flexor carpi radialis	Medial epicondyle of humerus	Base of the second metacarpal bone	Median nerve (C6, C7)	Flexes the hand at the wrist joint; abducts the hand (radially deviates the hand)
Palmaris longus	Medial epicondyle of humerus	Anterior flexor retinaculum and the palmar aponeurosis	Median nerve (C6, C7)	Flexes the hand at the wrist and tenses the palmar aponeurosis
Flexor digitorum superficialis	**Humeroulnar head:** Medial epicondyle of humerus and the coronoid process of ulna. **Radial head:** Anterior surface of the radius below the radial tuberosity.	By four long tendons onto the sides of the middle phalanx of the four medial fingers	Median nerve (C7, C8, T1)	Flexes the middle and proximal phalanges of the four medial fingers; also flexes the wrist
Flexor carpi ulnaris	**Humeral head:** Medial epicondyle of the humerus. **Ulnar head:** Medial margin of the olecranon, and upper posterior border of the ulna	Pisiform bone and by ligaments to the hamate and fifth metacarpal bone	Ulnar nerve (C7, C8)	Flexes the hand at the wrist joint; adducts the hand (ulnar deviates the hand)

FLEXOR MUSCLES OF THE FOREARM: DEEP GROUP

Muscle	Origin	Insertion	Innervation	Action
Flexor digitorum profundus	Upper three-fourths of the anterior and medial aspects of the ulna and the ulnar half of the interosseous membrane	Anterior surface of the base of the distal phalanx of the four medial fingers	Median nerve by its interosseous branch; and the ulnar nerve (C8, T1)	Flexes the distal phalanx of the four medial fingers; and also flexes the hand at the wrist
Flexor pollicis longus	**Radial head:** Anterior surface of radius and the adjacent part of the interosseous membrane. **Humeral head:** Medial epicondyle of humerus or the coronoid process of the ulna	Base of the distal phalanx of the thumb	Median nerve by its interosseous branch (C8, T1)	Flexes the distal phalanx and helps in flexing the proximal phalanx of the thumb
Pronator quadratus	Distal fourth of anterior surface of the ulna	Distal fourth of anterior surface of the radius	Median nerve by its interosseous branch (C8, T1)	Pronates the hand

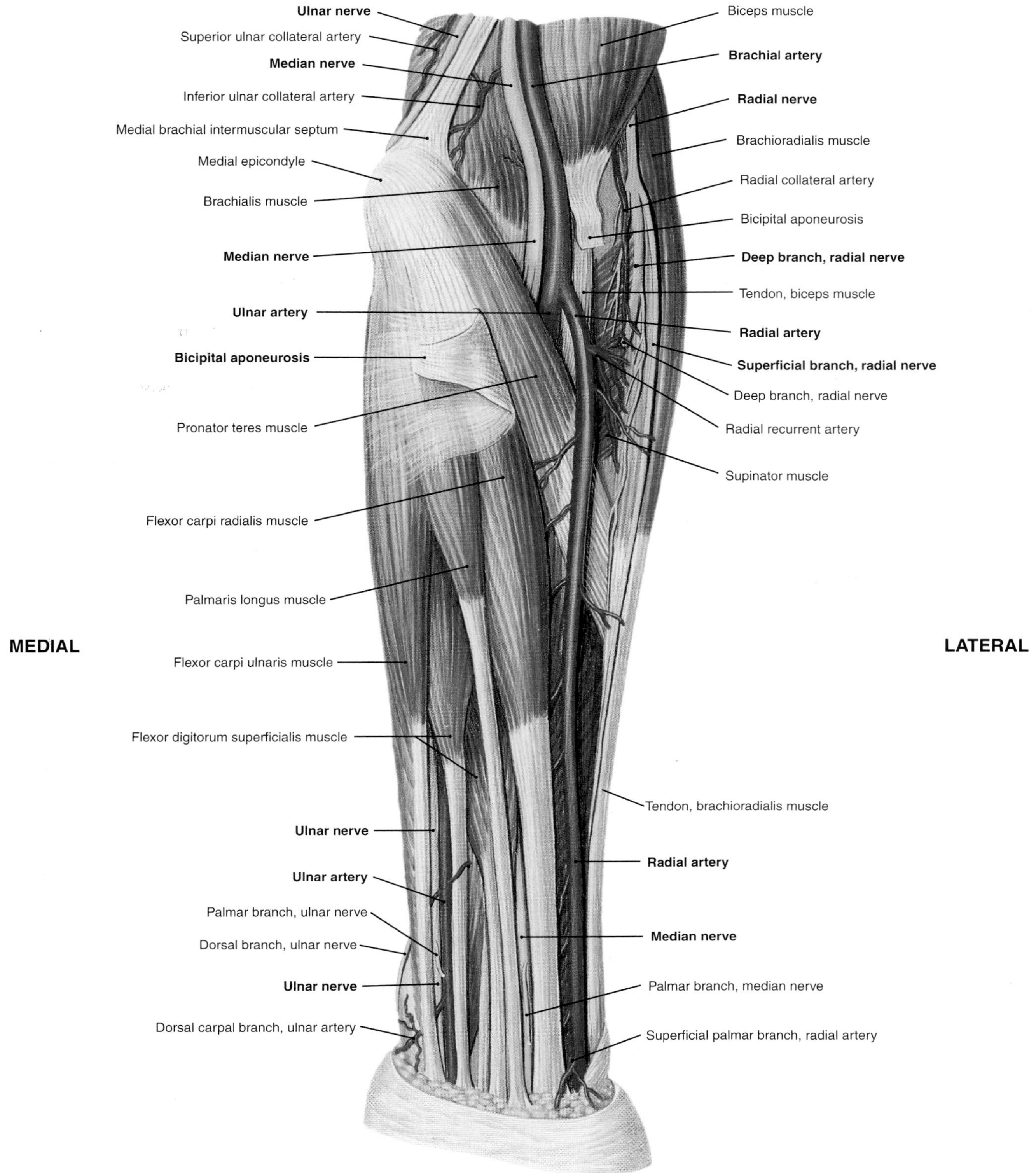
Ulnar nerve
Superior ulnar collateral artery
Median nerve
Inferior ulnar collateral artery
Medial brachial intermuscular septum
Medial epicondyle
Brachialis muscle
Median nerve
Ulnar artery
Bicipital aponeurosis
Pronator teres muscle
Flexor carpi radialis muscle
Palmaris longus muscle
MEDIAL
Flexor carpi ulnaris muscle
Flexor digitorum superficialis muscle
Ulnar nerve
Ulnar artery
Palmar branch, ulnar nerve
Dorsal branch, ulnar nerve
Ulnar nerve
Dorsal carpal branch, ulnar artery
Biceps muscle
Brachial artery
Radial nerve
Brachioradialis muscle
Radial collateral artery
Bicipital aponeurosis
Deep branch, radial nerve
Tendon, biceps muscle
Radial artery
Superficial branch, radial nerve
Deep branch, radial nerve
Radial recurrent artery
Supinator muscle
LATERAL
Tendon, brachioradialis muscle
Radial artery
Median nerve
Palmar branch, median nerve
Superficial palmar branch, radial artery

Figure 50 Anterior Dissection of the Left Forearm Vessels and Nerves, Stage 1

NOTE: (1) The bicipital aponeurosis has been reflected to reveal the underlying median nerve, brachial artery, and tendon of insertion of the biceps brachii muscle.

(2) The brachioradialis muscle has been pulled laterally (toward the radial side) to expose the course of the radial artery and the division of the radial nerve into its superficial and deep branches.

(3) The radial artery, as it descends in the forearm, courses anterior to the biceps brachii muscle, the supinator muscle, the tendon of insertion of the pronator teres, and the belly of the flexor pollicis longus (the latter is not labeled in this figure, but can be seen in Fig. 51).

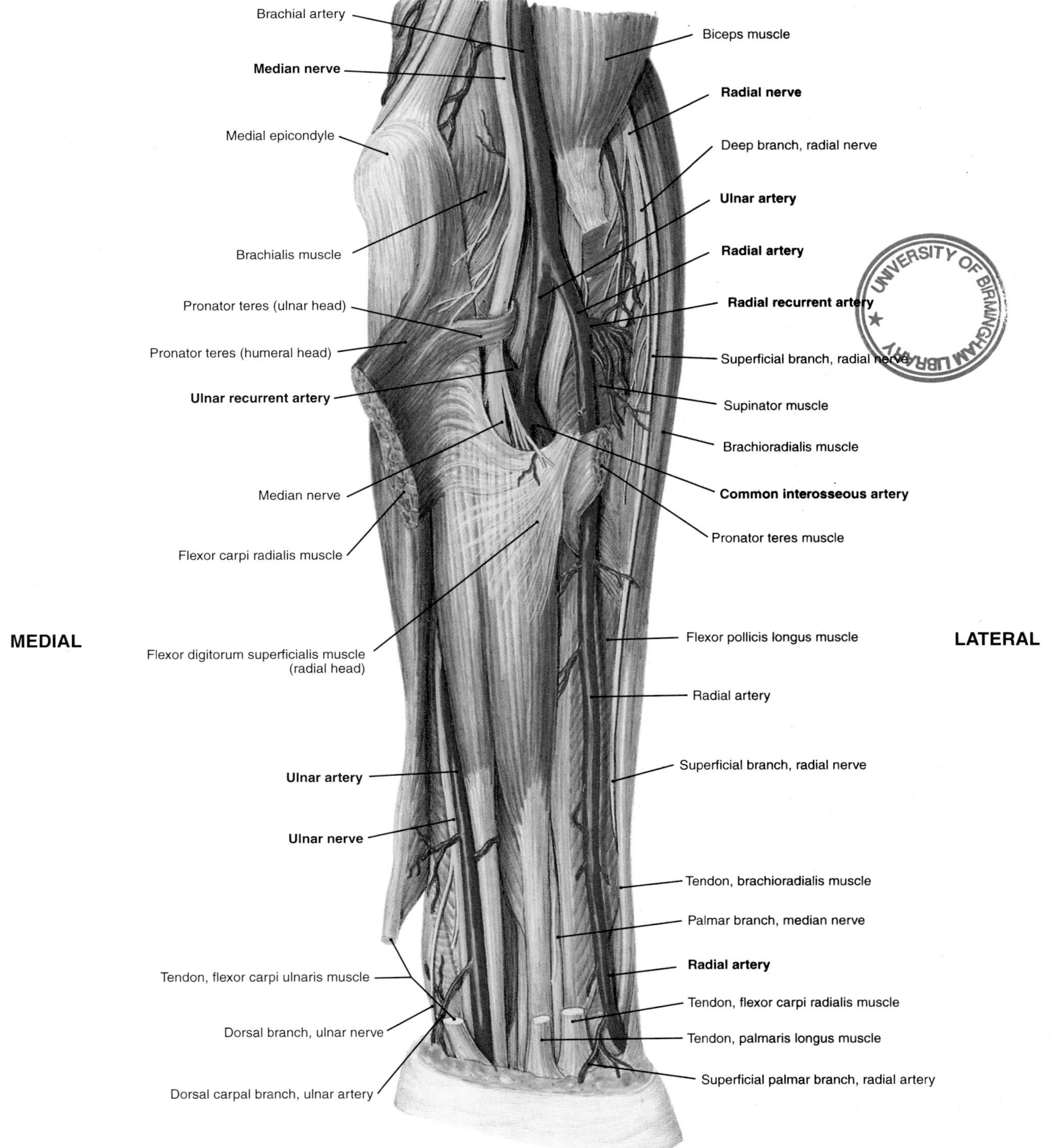
Brachial artery
Median nerve
Medial epicondyle
Brachialis muscle
Pronator teres (ulnar head)
Pronator teres (humeral head)
Ulnar recurrent artery
Median nerve
Flexor carpi radialis muscle
MEDIAL
Flexor digitorum superficialis muscle (radial head)
Ulnar artery
Ulnar nerve
Tendon, flexor carpi ulnaris muscle
Dorsal branch, ulnar nerve
Dorsal carpal branch, ulnar artery
Biceps muscle
Radial nerve
Deep branch, radial nerve
Ulnar artery
Radial artery
Radial recurrent artery
Superficial branch, radial nerve
Supinator muscle
Brachioradialis muscle
Common interosseous artery
Pronator teres muscle
Flexor pollicis longus muscle
LATERAL
Radial artery
Superficial branch, radial nerve
Tendon, brachioradialis muscle
Palmar branch, median nerve
Radial artery
Tendon, flexor carpi radialis muscle
Tendon, palmaris longus muscle
Superficial palmar branch, radial artery

Figure 51 Anterior Dissection of the Left Forearm Vessels and Nerves, Stage 2

NOTE: (1) The pronator teres and flexor carpi radialis muscles are reflected just below the cubital fossa to show the bifurcation of the brachial artery into the ulnar and radial arteries.

(2) At the wrist, the tendon of the flexor carpi ulnaris muscle is severed and pulled aside to expose the ulnar nerve and artery.

(3) The median nerve lies deep to the flexor digitorum superficialis muscle along much of its course in the forearm, but just above the wrist it usually becomes visible between the tendons. Observe that the tendons of the flexor pollicis longus and flexor carpi radialis are on its **radial side** and the tendons of the palmaris longus and flexor digitorum superficialis **are on its ulnar side.**

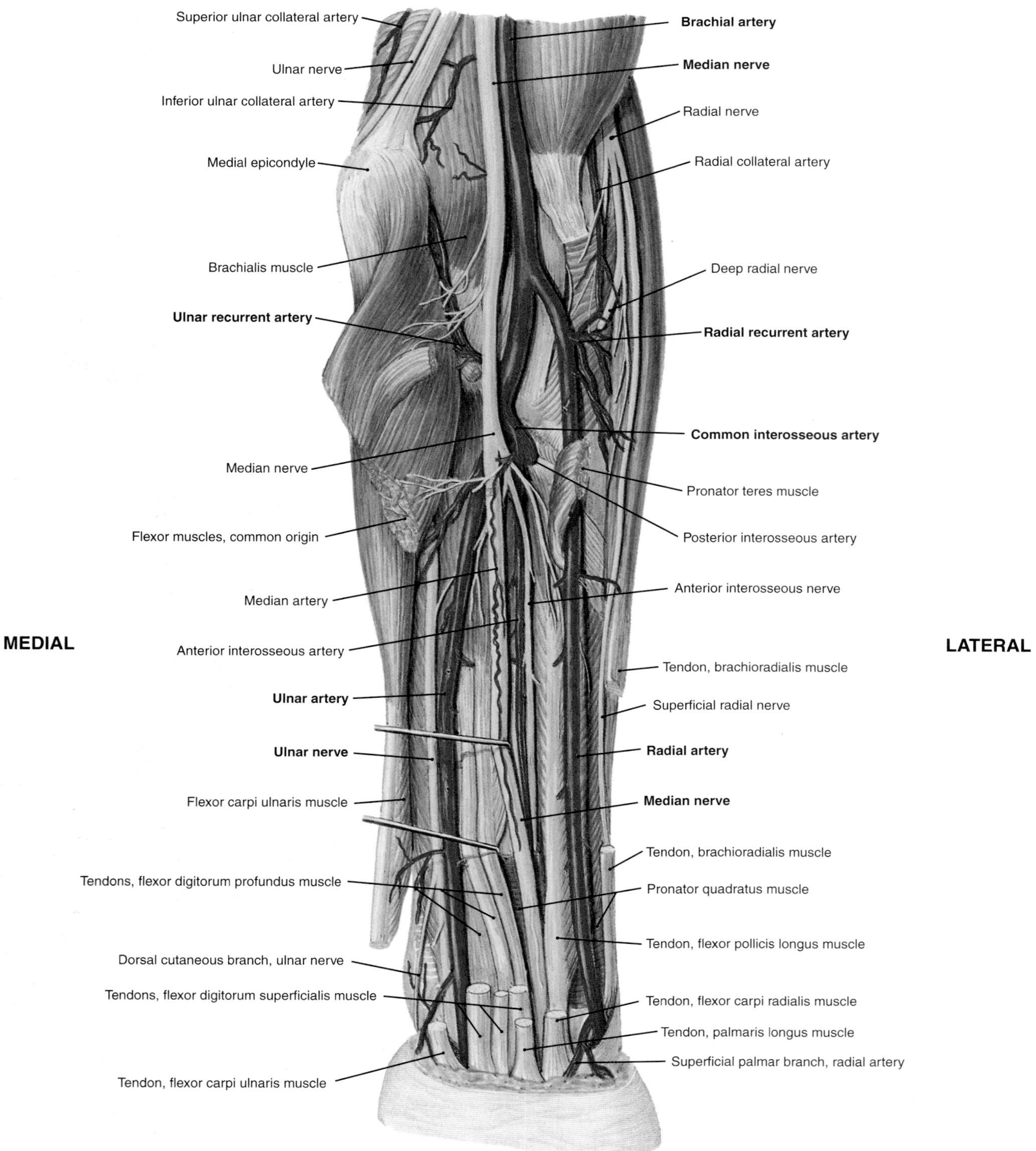
Superior ulnar collateral artery
Ulnar nerve
Inferior ulnar collateral artery
Medial epicondyle
Brachialis muscle
Ulnar recurrent artery
Median nerve
Flexor muscles, common origin
Median artery
MEDIAL
Anterior interosseous artery
Ulnar artery
Ulnar nerve
Flexor carpi ulnaris muscle
Tendons, flexor digitorum profundus muscle
Dorsal cutaneous branch, ulnar nerve
Tendons, flexor digitorum superficialis muscle
Tendon, flexor carpi ulnaris muscle
Brachial artery
Median nerve
Radial nerve
Radial collateral artery
Deep radial nerve
Radial recurrent artery
Common interosseous artery
Pronator teres muscle
Posterior interosseous artery
Anterior interosseous nerve
LATERAL
Tendon, brachioradialis muscle
Superficial radial nerve
Radial artery
Median nerve
Tendon, brachioradialis muscle
Pronator quadratus muscle
Tendon, flexor pollicis longus muscle
Tendon, flexor carpi radialis muscle
Tendon, palmaris longus muscle
Superficial palmar branch, radial artery

Figure 52 Anterior Dissection of the Left Forearm Vessels and Nerves, Stage 3

NOTE: (1) The division of the **brachial artery** into the **radial** and **ulnar arteries** at the lower end of the cubital fossa.

(2) The **common interosseous artery** branches from the **ulnar artery** and divides almost immediately into the **anterior and posterior interosseous arteries.**

(3) The courses of the ulnar and median nerves. In the lower half of the forearm, the **ulnar nerve** descends with the ulnar artery, whereas the median nerve descends in front of the anterior interosseous nerve and artery.

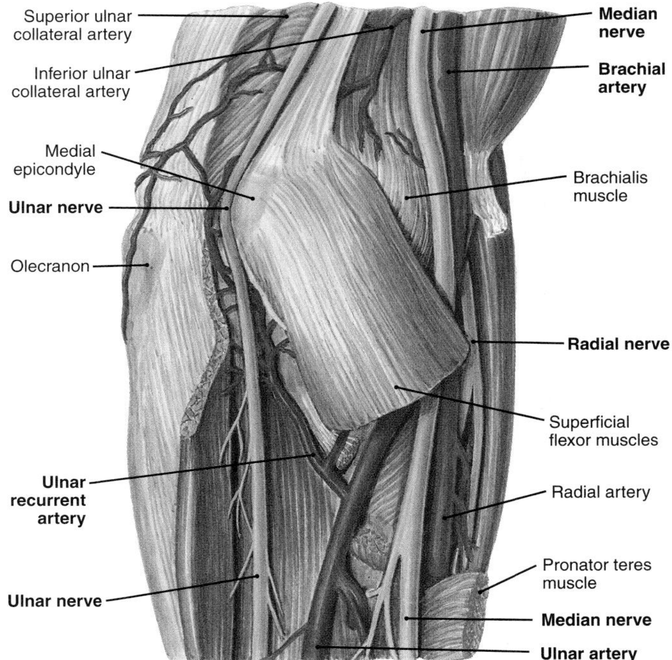
Superior ulnar collateral artery
Inferior ulnar collateral artery
Medial epicondyle
Ulnar nerve
Olecranon
Ulnar recurrent artery
Ulnar nerve
Median nerve
Brachial artery
Brachialis muscle
Radial nerve
Superficial flexor muscles
Radial artery
Pronator teres muscle
Median nerve
Ulnar artery

Figure 53.1 Nerves and Arteries at the Elbow (Medial View)

NOTE: The **ulnar nerve** enters the forearm directly behind the medial epicondyle, and at this site it is closely related to the **ulnar recurrent artery**.

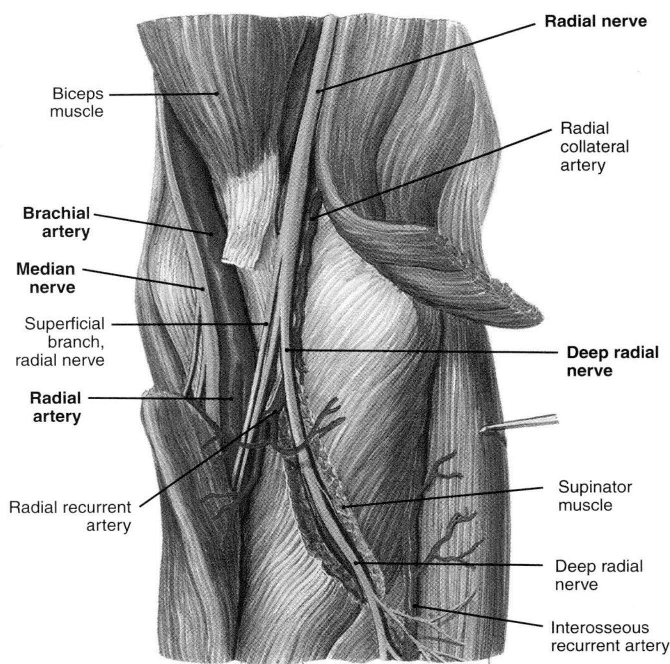
Biceps muscle
Brachial artery
Median nerve
Superficial branch, radial nerve
Radial artery
Radial recurrent artery
Radial nerve
Radial collateral artery
Deep radial nerve
Supinator muscle
Deep radial nerve
Interosseous recurrent artery

Figure 53.2 Nerves and Arteries at the Elbow (Lateral View)

NOTE: The **deep radial nerve** passes into the forearm in front of the lateral part of the elbow joint. It then courses dorsally through the supinator muscle to supply the posterior forearm muscles.

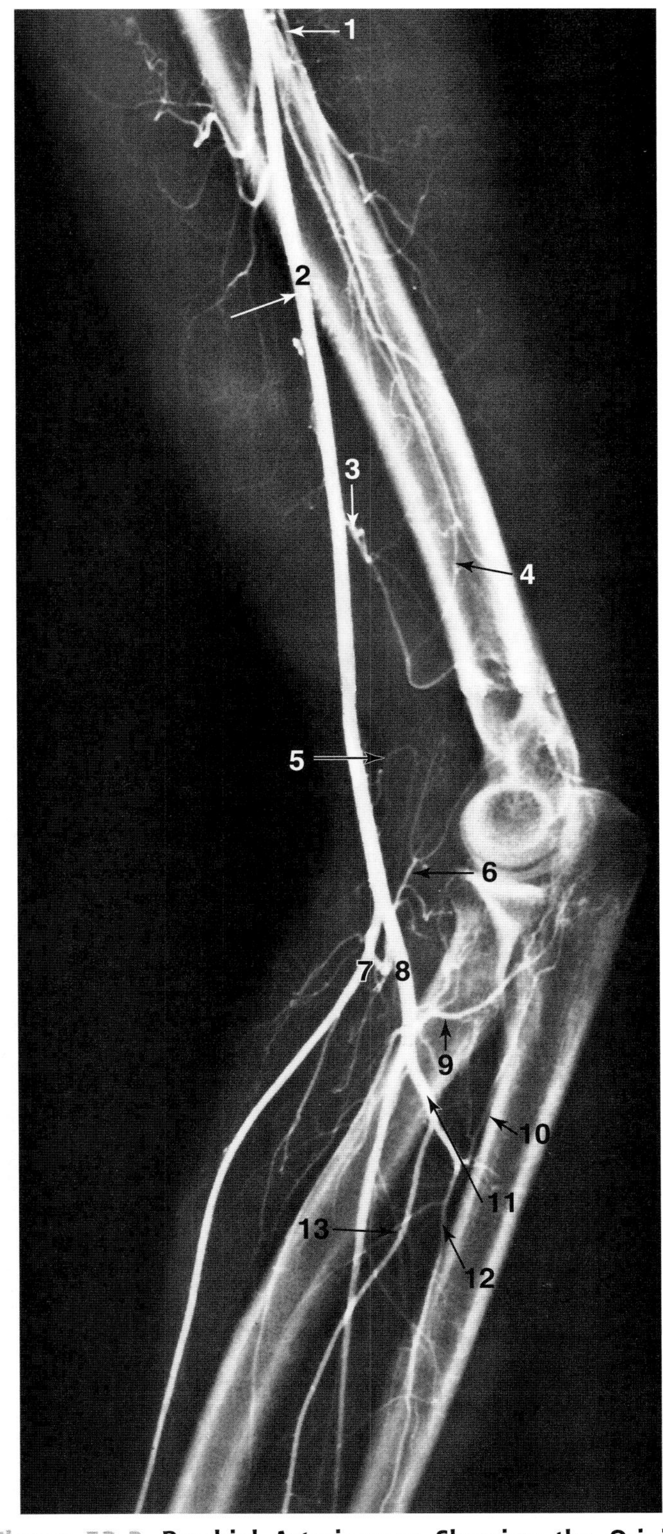
1
2
3
4
5
6
7
8
9
10
11
12
13

Figure 53.3 Brachial Arteriogram Showing the Origins of the Vessels That Supply the Elbow and Forearm

1. Profunda brachii artery
2. Brachial artery
3. Superior ulnar collateral artery
4. Radial collateral artery
5. Inferior ulnar collateral artery
6. Radial recurrent artery
7. Radial artery
8. Ulnar artery
9. Ulnar recurrent artery
10. Interosseous recurrent artery
11. Common interosseous artery
12. Posterior interosseous artery
13. Anterior interosseous artery

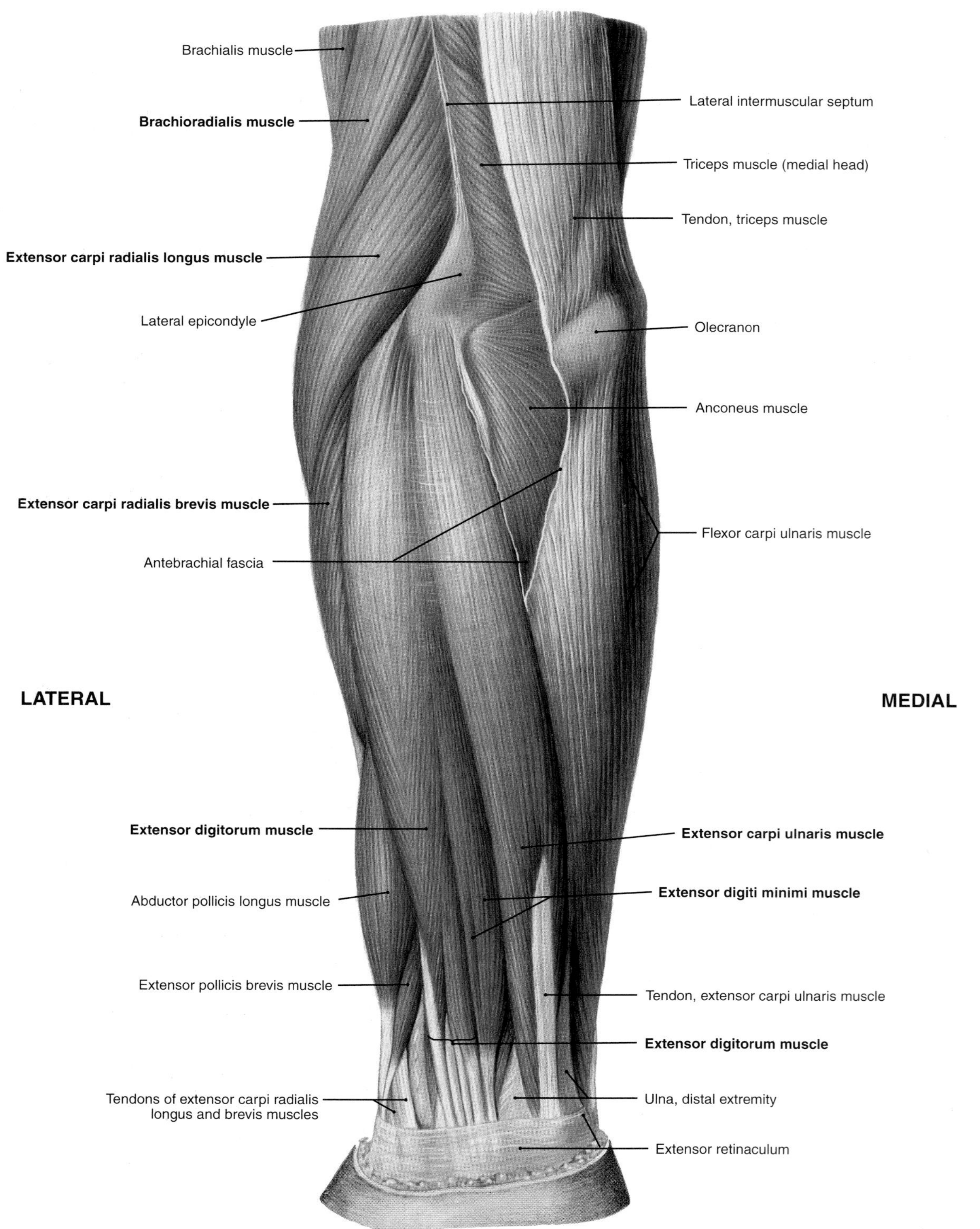
Brachialis muscle
Brachioradialis muscle
Extensor carpi radialis longus muscle
Lateral epicondyle
Extensor carpi radialis brevis muscle
Antebrachial fascia
LATERAL
Extensor digitorum muscle
Abductor pollicis longus muscle
Extensor pollicis brevis muscle
Tendons of extensor carpi radialis longus and brevis muscles
Lateral intermuscular septum
Triceps muscle (medial head)
Tendon, triceps muscle
Olecranon
Anconeus muscle
Flexor carpi ulnaris muscle
MEDIAL
Extensor carpi ulnaris muscle
Extensor digiti minimi muscle
Tendon, extensor carpi ulnaris muscle
Extensor digitorum muscle
Ulna, distal extremity
Extensor retinaculum

Figure 54 Posterior Muscles of the Left Forearm, Superficial Group (Posterior View)

NOTE: The superficial radial group of extensor muscles of the forearm include the **brachioradialis muscle** and the **extensors carpi radialis longus and brevis.**

Muscle	Origin	Insertion	Innervation	Action
Brachioradialis	Upper two-thirds of lateral supracondylar ridge of humerus	Lateral aspect of the base of the styloid process of the radius	Radial nerve (C5, C6)	Flexes the forearm when the forearm is semipronated

Superficial Extensor Muscles of the Forearm (Lateral View)

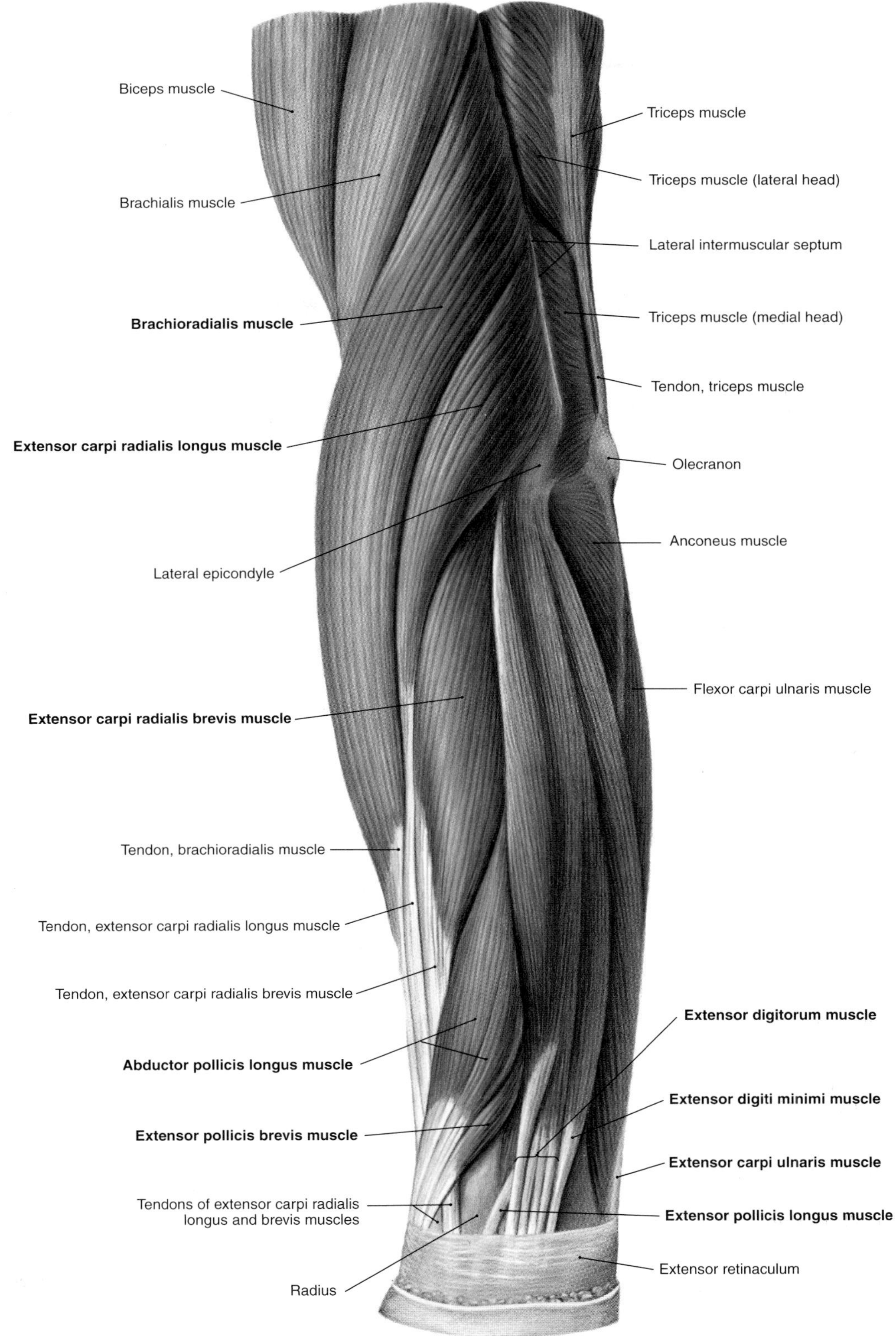
Biceps muscle
Brachialis muscle
Brachioradialis muscle
Extensor carpi radialis longus muscle
Lateral epicondyle
Extensor carpi radialis brevis muscle
Tendon, brachioradialis muscle
Tendon, extensor carpi radialis longus muscle
Tendon, extensor carpi radialis brevis muscle
Abductor pollicis longus muscle
Extensor pollicis brevis muscle
Tendons of extensor carpi radialis longus and brevis muscles
Radius
Triceps muscle
Triceps muscle (lateral head)
Lateral intermuscular septum
Triceps muscle (medial head)
Tendon, triceps muscle
Olecranon
Anconeus muscle
Flexor carpi ulnaris muscle
Extensor digitorum muscle
Extensor digiti minimi muscle
Extensor carpi ulnaris muscle
Extensor pollicis longus muscle
Extensor retinaculum

Figure 55 **Posterior Muscles of the Left Forearm, Superficial Group (Lateral View)**

Muscle	Origin	Insertion	Innervation	Action
Extensor carpi radialis longus	Lower third of lateral supracondylar ridge of humerus	Dorsal surface of the base of the second metacarpal bone	Radial nerve (C6, C7)	Extends the hand; abducts the hand at the wrist (radial deviation)
Extensor carpi radialis brevis	Lateral epicondyle of humerus	Dorsal surface of the base of the third metacarpal bone	Radial nerve (C6, C7)	Extends the hand; abducts the hand at the wrist (radial deviation)

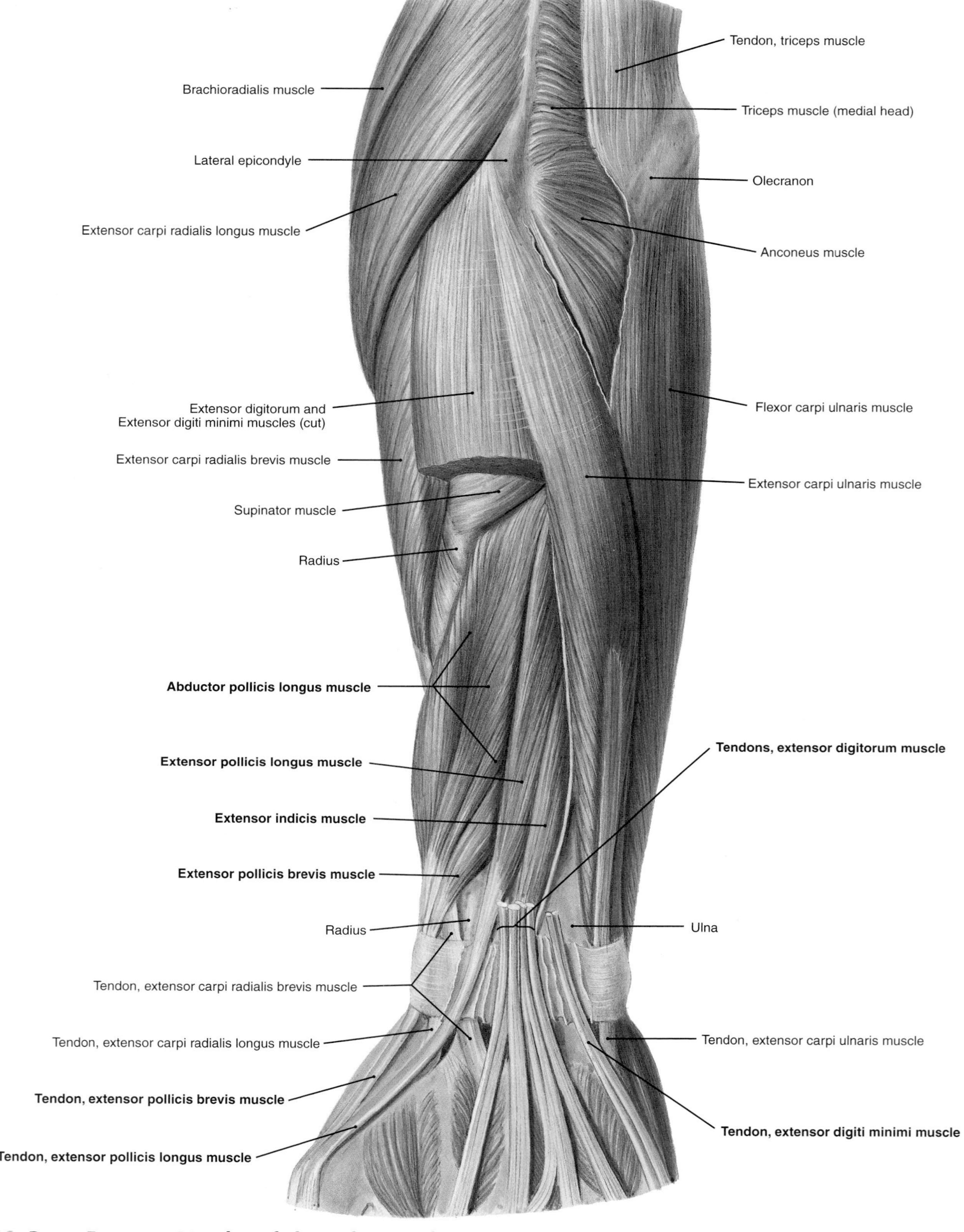
Tendon, triceps muscle
Brachioradialis muscle
Triceps muscle (medial head)
Lateral epicondyle
Olecranon
Extensor carpi radialis longus muscle
Anconeus muscle
Extensor digitorum and
Extensor digiti minimi muscles (cut)
Flexor carpi ulnaris muscle
Extensor carpi radialis brevis muscle
Extensor carpi ulnaris muscle
Supinator muscle
Radius
Abductor pollicis longus muscle
Tendons, extensor digitorum muscle
Extensor pollicis longus muscle
Extensor indicis muscle
Extensor pollicis brevis muscle
Radius
Ulna
Tendon, extensor carpi radialis brevis muscle
Tendon, extensor carpi radialis longus muscle
Tendon, extensor carpi ulnaris muscle
Tendon, extensor pollicis brevis muscle
Tendon, extensor digiti minimi muscle
Tendon, extensor pollicis longus muscle

Figure 56 Deep Extensor Muscles of the Left Posterior Forearm

NOTE: Four other muscles complete the **superficial** extensor muscles on the posterior aspect of the forearm. These are the **extensor digitorum, extensor digiti minimi, extensor carpi ulnaris,** and the **anconeus.** There are also five **deep** extensor muscles: the **abductor pollicis longus, extensor pollicis longus** and **brevis, extensor indicis,** and the **supinator** muscle.

Chart of Posterior Forearm Muscles

SUPERFICIAL EXTENSOR FOREARM MUSCLES

Muscle	Origin	Insertion	Innervation	Action
Extensor digitorum	Lateral epicondyle of humerus	Dorsum of middle and distal phalanges of the four fingers	Posterior interosseous branch of the radial nerve (C7, C8)	Extends the fingers and the hand
Extensor digiti minimi	Lateral epicondyle of humerus	Dorsal digital expansion of little finger	Posterior interosseous branch of the radial nerve (C7, C8)	Extends the little finger and the hand
Extensor carpi ulnaris	Lateral epicondyle of humerus	Medial side of the base of the fifth metacarpal bone	Posterior interosseous branch of the radial nerve (C7, C8)	Extends and adducts the hand (ulnar deviation)
Anconeus	Lateral epicondyle of humerus	Lateral side of olecranon and shaft of ulna	Radial nerve (C7, C8, T1)	Helps to extend the forearm at the elbow joint

DEEP EXTENSOR FOREARM MUSCLES

Muscle	Origin	Insertion	Innervation	Action
Extensor pollicis longus	Posterior shaft of ulna and interosseous membrane	Base of the distal phalanx of the thumb	Posterior interosseous branch of the radial nerve (C7, C8)	Extends the thumb, and to a minor extent, the hand
Extensor pollicis brevis	Posterior surface of radius and interosseous membrane	Base of the proximal phalanx of the thumb	Posterior interosseous branch of the radial nerve (C7, C8)	Extends the proximal phalanx and metacarpal bone of thumb
Abductor pollicis longus	Posterior surfaces of both radius and ulna and interosseous membrane	Radial side of base of the first metacarpal bone, and on the trapezoid bone	Posterior interosseous branch of the radial nerve (C7, C8)	Abducts and assists in extending the thumb
Extensor indicis	Posterior surface of the ulna and interosseous membrane	Into the extensor hood of the index finger	Posterior interosseous branch of the radial nerve (C7, C8)	Extends the index finger and helps extend the hand
Supinator	Lateral epicondyle of humerus; radial collateral ligament; supinator crest of ulna	Lateral surface of the proximal third of the radius	Posterior interosseous branch of the radial nerve (C6)	Rotates the radius to supinate the hand and forearm

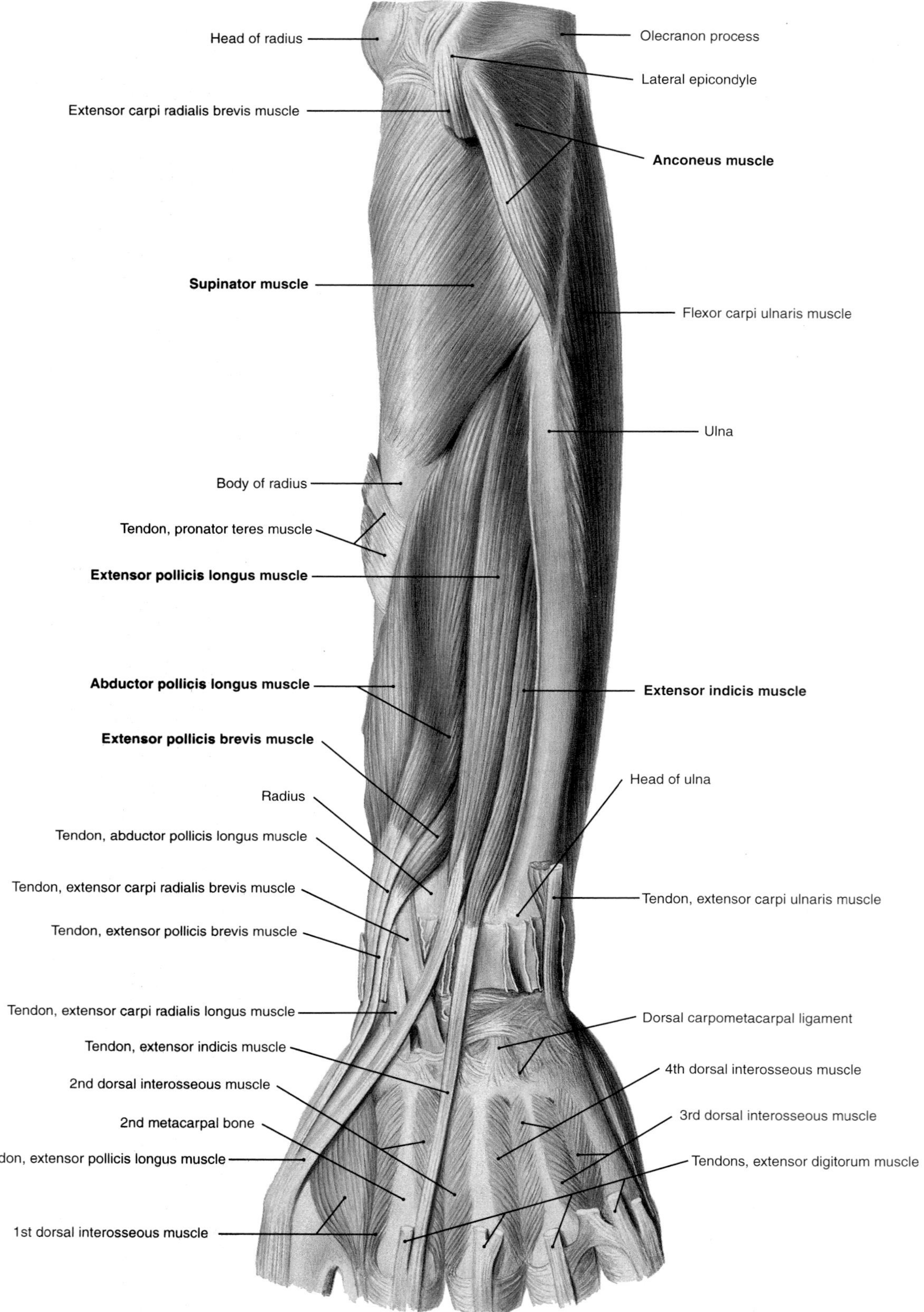
Head of radius
Extensor carpi radialis brevis muscle
Supinator muscle
Body of radius
Tendon, pronator teres muscle
Extensor pollicis longus muscle
Abductor pollicis longus muscle
Extensor pollicis brevis muscle
Radius
Tendon, abductor pollicis longus muscle
Tendon, extensor carpi radialis brevis muscle
Tendon, extensor pollicis brevis muscle
Tendon, extensor carpi radialis longus muscle
Tendon, extensor indicis muscle
2nd dorsal interosseous muscle
2nd metacarpal bone
Tendon, extensor pollicis longus muscle
1st dorsal interosseous muscle
Olecranon process
Lateral epicondyle
Anconeus muscle
Flexor carpi ulnaris muscle
Ulna
Extensor indicis muscle
Head of ulna
Tendon, extensor carpi ulnaris muscle
Dorsal carpometacarpal ligament
4th dorsal interosseous muscle
3rd dorsal interosseous muscle
Tendons, extensor digitorum muscle

Figure 58 **Left Posterior Forearm Muscles, Deep Group**

NOTE: (1) The three thumb muscles (abductor pollicis longus and extensors pollicis brevis and longus) are exposed when the extensor digitorum, extensor digiti minimi, and extensor carpi ulnaris are removed.

(2) The extensor indicis courses to the index finger, and the supinator is a broad muscle that stretches across the upper forearm from the humerus and ulna to the upper third of the radius.

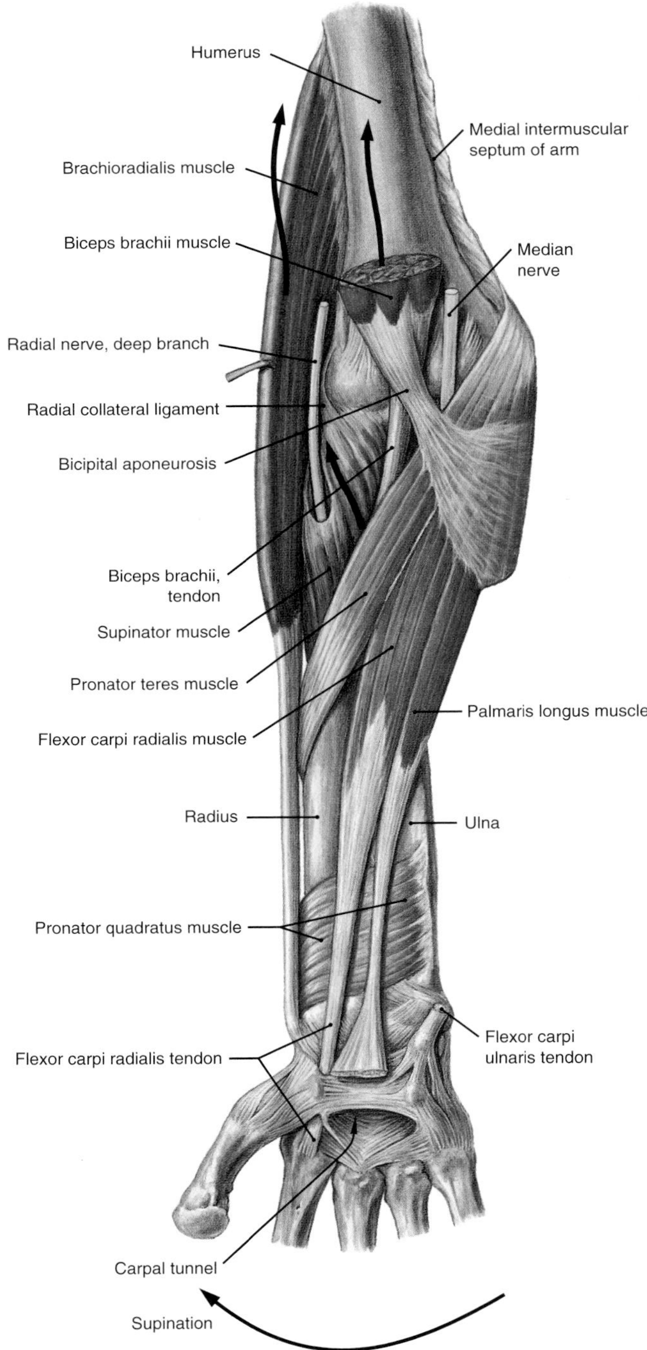
Humerus
Medial intermuscular septum of arm
Brachioradialis muscle
Biceps brachii muscle
Median nerve
Radial nerve, deep branch
Radial collateral ligament
Bicipital aponeurosis
Biceps brachii, tendon
Supinator muscle
Pronator teres muscle
Flexor carpi radialis muscle
Palmaris longus muscle
Radius
Ulna
Pronator quadratus muscle
Flexor carpi ulnaris tendon
Flexor carpi radialis tendon
Carpal tunnel
Supination

Figure 59.1 **Supinated Right Forearm (Anterior Aspect)**

NOTE: (1) Supination involves turning the pronated forearm and hand over, resulting in the palm being oriented anteriorly and the thumb directed laterally.

(2) In supination, the head of the radius rotates within the annular ligament at the proximal radioulnar joint. The radius then assumes a position lateral to and parallel with the ulna.

(3) The principal muscles that supinate the forearm are the supinator and biceps brachii muscle. In addition, it is thought that the brachioradialis muscle assists in this action, but this has been questioned.

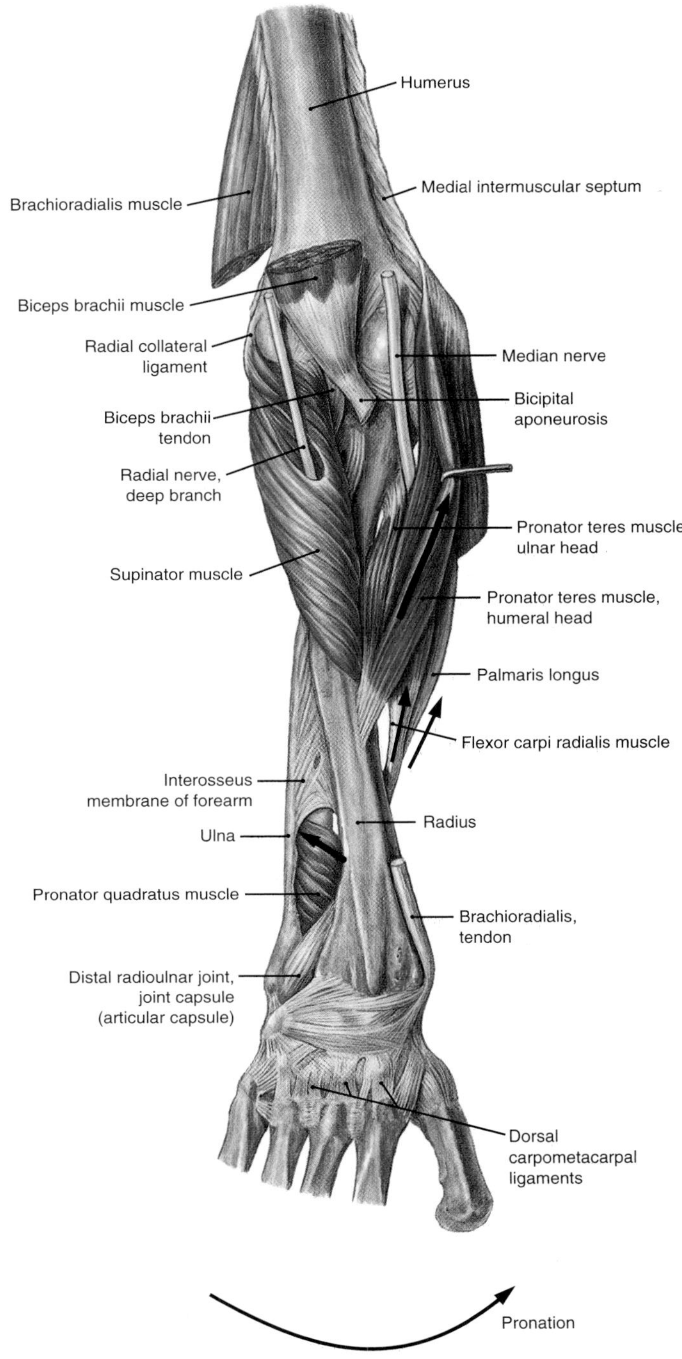
Humerus
Brachioradialis muscle
Medial intermuscular septum
Biceps brachii muscle
Radial collateral ligament
Median nerve
Biceps brachii tendon
Bicipital aponeurosis
Radial nerve, deep branch
Pronator teres muscle, ulnar head
Supinator muscle
Pronator teres muscle, humeral head
Palmaris longus
Flexor carpi radialis muscle
Interosseus membrane of forearm
Ulna
Radius
Pronator quadratus muscle
Brachioradialis, tendon
Distal radioulnar joint, joint capsule (articular capsule)
Dorsal carpometacarpal ligaments
Pronation

Figure 59.2 **Pronated Right Forearm (Anterior Aspect)**

NOTE: (1) Pronation is the act of turning the supinated forearm and hand over, after which the palm becomes oriented posteriorly and the thumb directed medially.

(2) In pronation of the forearm and hand, the radius turns obliquely across the anterior aspect of the ulna. The proximal end of the radius is still lateral to the ulna, but the distal end is medial to it.

(3) The muscles producing pronation are the **pronator teres** and the **pronator quadratus.** In addition, the **flexor carpi radialis** and the **palmaris longus** may assist.

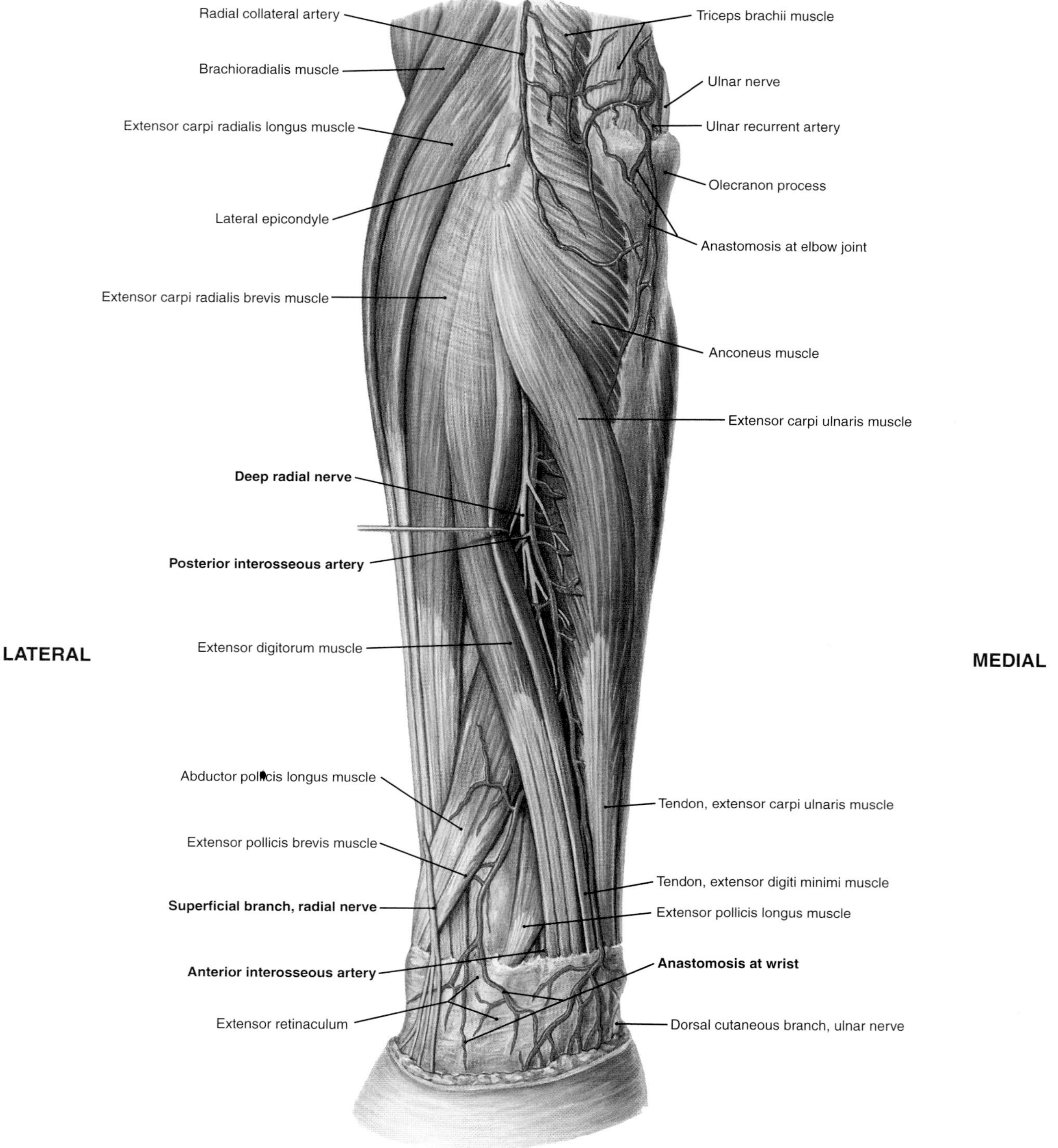
Radial collateral artery
Brachioradialis muscle
Extensor carpi radialis longus muscle
Lateral epicondyle
Extensor carpi radialis brevis muscle
Deep radial nerve
Posterior interosseous artery
LATERAL
Extensor digitorum muscle
Abductor pollicis longus muscle
Extensor pollicis brevis muscle
Superficial branch, radial nerve
Anterior interosseous artery
Extensor retinaculum
Triceps brachii muscle
Ulnar nerve
Ulnar recurrent artery
Olecranon process
Anastomosis at elbow joint
Anconeus muscle
Extensor carpi ulnaris muscle
MEDIAL
Tendon, extensor carpi ulnaris muscle
Tendon, extensor digiti minimi muscle
Extensor pollicis longus muscle
Anastomosis at wrist
Dorsal cutaneous branch, ulnar nerve

Figure 60 Nerves and Arteries of the Left Posterior Forearm

NOTE: (1) The extensor digiti minimi and extensor digitorum have been separated from the extensor carpi ulnaris to expose the **posterior interosseous artery** and the **deep radial nerve.**

(2) The posterior interosseous artery is derived in the anterior compartment of the forearm from the common interosseous artery, a branch of the ulnar artery, which divides into anterior and posterior interosseous branches (see Fig. 17.1).

(3) The posterior interosseous branch passes over the proximal border of the interosseous membrane to achieve the posterior compartment, and it descends with the deep radial nerve between the superficial and deep extensor forearm muscles.

(4) In the distal forearm, the posterior interosseous artery anastomoses with terminal branches of the anterior interosseous artery to help form the carpal anastomosis at the wrist.

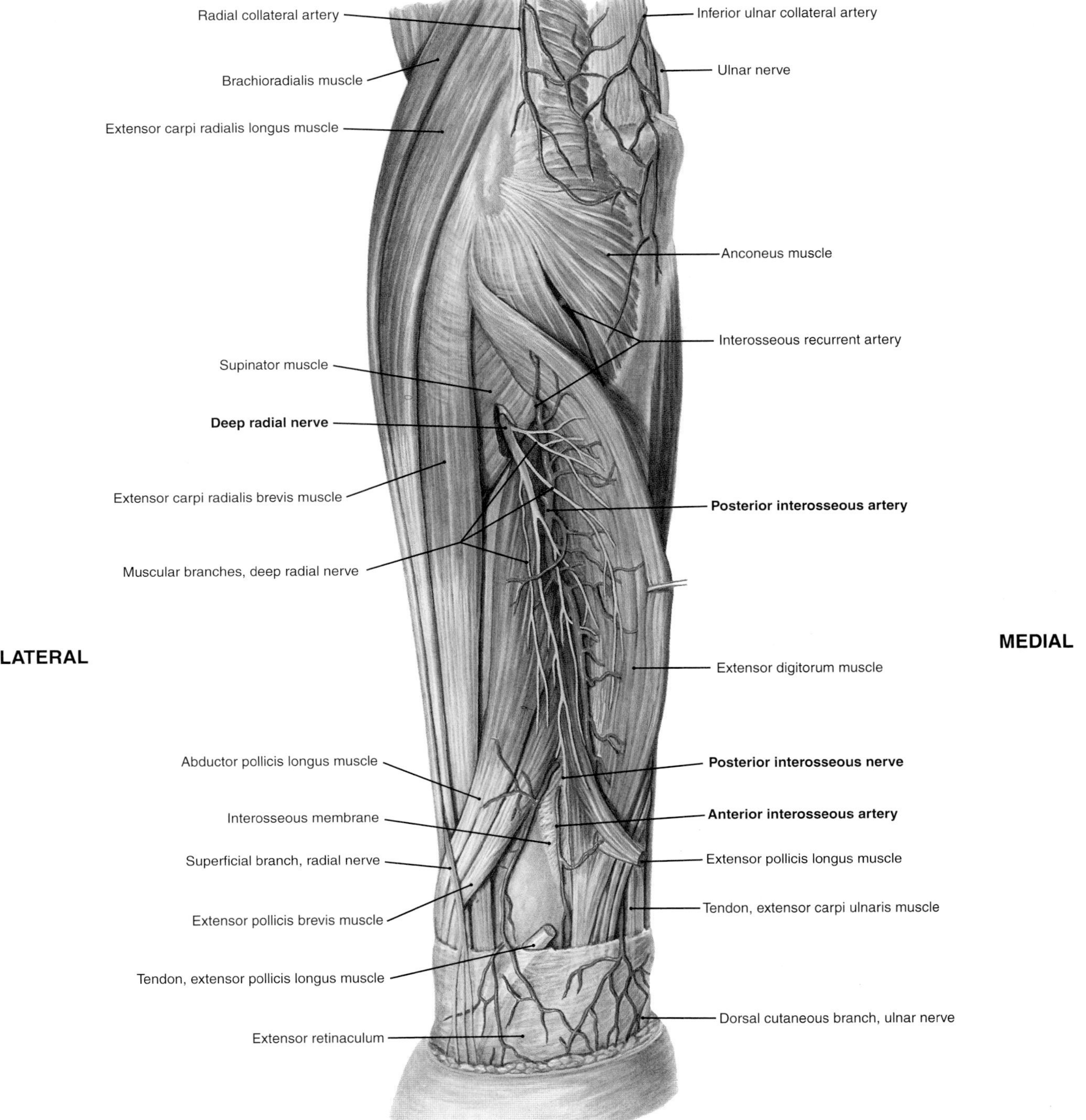
Radial collateral artery
Brachioradialis muscle
Extensor carpi radialis longus muscle
Supinator muscle
Deep radial nerve
Extensor carpi radialis brevis muscle
Muscular branches, deep radial nerve
LATERAL
Abductor pollicis longus muscle
Interosseous membrane
Superficial branch, radial nerve
Extensor pollicis brevis muscle
Tendon, extensor pollicis longus muscle
Extensor retinaculum
Inferior ulnar collateral artery
Ulnar nerve
Anconeus muscle
Interosseous recurrent artery
Posterior interosseous artery
MEDIAL
Extensor digitorum muscle
Posterior interosseous nerve
Anterior interosseous artery
Extensor pollicis longus muscle
Tendon, extensor carpi ulnaris muscle
Dorsal cutaneous branch, ulnar nerve

Figure 61 **Nerves and Arteries of the Left Posterior Forearm (Deep Dissection)**

NOTE: (1) The extensor digitorum muscle is separated from the extensor carpi radialis brevis and pulled medially to reveal the **posterior interosseous artery** and **deep radial nerve.**

(2) After the radial nerve leaves the radial groove of the humerus in the lower brachium, it divides into superficial and deep branches.

(3) The **superficial branch** descends along the lateral side of the forearm under cover of the brachioradialis muscle and becomes a sensory nerve to the dorsum of the hand.

(4) The **deep branch** enters the posterior forearm by piercing through the supinator muscle and, coursing along the dorsum of the interosseous membrane, is called the **posterior interosseous nerve.** It supplies all the deep posterior forearm muscles and descends deep to the extensor pollicis longus muscle, which has been cut in this dissection.

Dorsum of the Hand: Superficial Vessels and Nerves and Tendon Sheaths

Dorsal digital nerves
Cephalic vein
Intercapitular veins
Dorsal venous network
Dorsal branch, ulnar nerve
Basilic vein
Superficial branch, radial nerve
Cephalic vein
Posterior antebrachial cutaneous nerve (from radial)

Figure 62.1 Superficial Veins and Nerves of the Dorsum of the Left Hand

NOTE: (1) The **cephalic vein** originates on the radial side of the dorsum of the hand, whereas the **basilic vein** arises on the ulnar side.

(2) The **superficial radial** nerve supplies the dorsum of the radial $3^{1/2}$ digits, whereas the **dorsal branch of the ulnar nerve** supplies the dorsum of the ulnar $1^{1/2}$ digits.

(3) The dorsum of the distal phalanx (not dissected) of the radial $3^{1/2}$ digits is supplied by the **median nerve,** but the same region on the ulnar $1^{1/2}$ digits is supplied by the **ulnar nerve.**

(4) There is a profuse venous plexus on the dorsal surface of the hand, but very few and small superficial veins on the palmar surface. This is beneficial because the frequent mechanical pressures to which the palmar surface is subjected could injure surface vessels.

(5) Adjacent branches of the radial and ulnar nerve frequently communicate. Observe that the posterior antebrachial cutaneous branches usually terminate at the wrist.

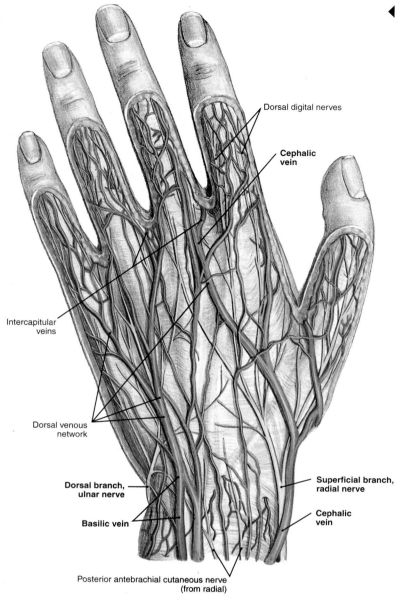

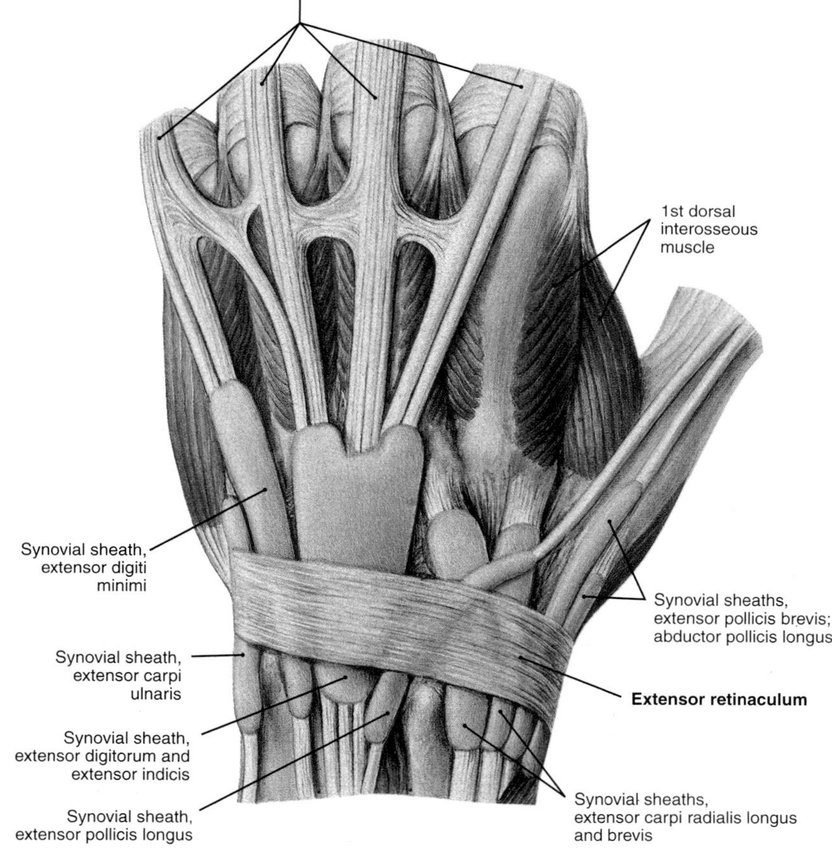

Tendons, extensor digitorum muscle
1st dorsal interosseous muscle
Synovial sheath, extensor digiti minimi
Synovial sheaths, extensor pollicis brevis; abductor pollicis longus
Synovial sheath, extensor carpi ulnaris
Extensor retinaculum
Synovial sheath, extensor digitorum and extensor indicis
Synovial sheath, extensor pollicis longus
Synovial sheaths, extensor carpi radialis longus and brevis

Figure 62.2 Extensor Tendons and Their Synovial Sheaths of the Left Dorsal Wrist

NOTE: (1) A synovial sheath is a double mesothelial-lined envelope that surrounds a tendon, allowing it to move more freely beneath the retinaculum.

(2) There are six synovial compartments on the dorsum of the wrist. From radial to ulnar these contain the tendons of:

(a) Extensor pollicis brevis and abductor pollicis longus
(b) Extensor carpi radialis longus and brevis
(c) Extensor pollicis longus
(d) Extensor digitorum and extensor indicis
(e) Extensor digiti minimi
(f) Extensor carpi ulnaris.

Figure 63.1 Arteries of the Left Dorsal Wrist and Hand (Deep View)

NOTE: (1) The transverse course of the dorsal carpal branch of the radial artery.

(2) The princeps pollicis branch of the radial artery coursing deep to the first dorsal interosseous muscle.

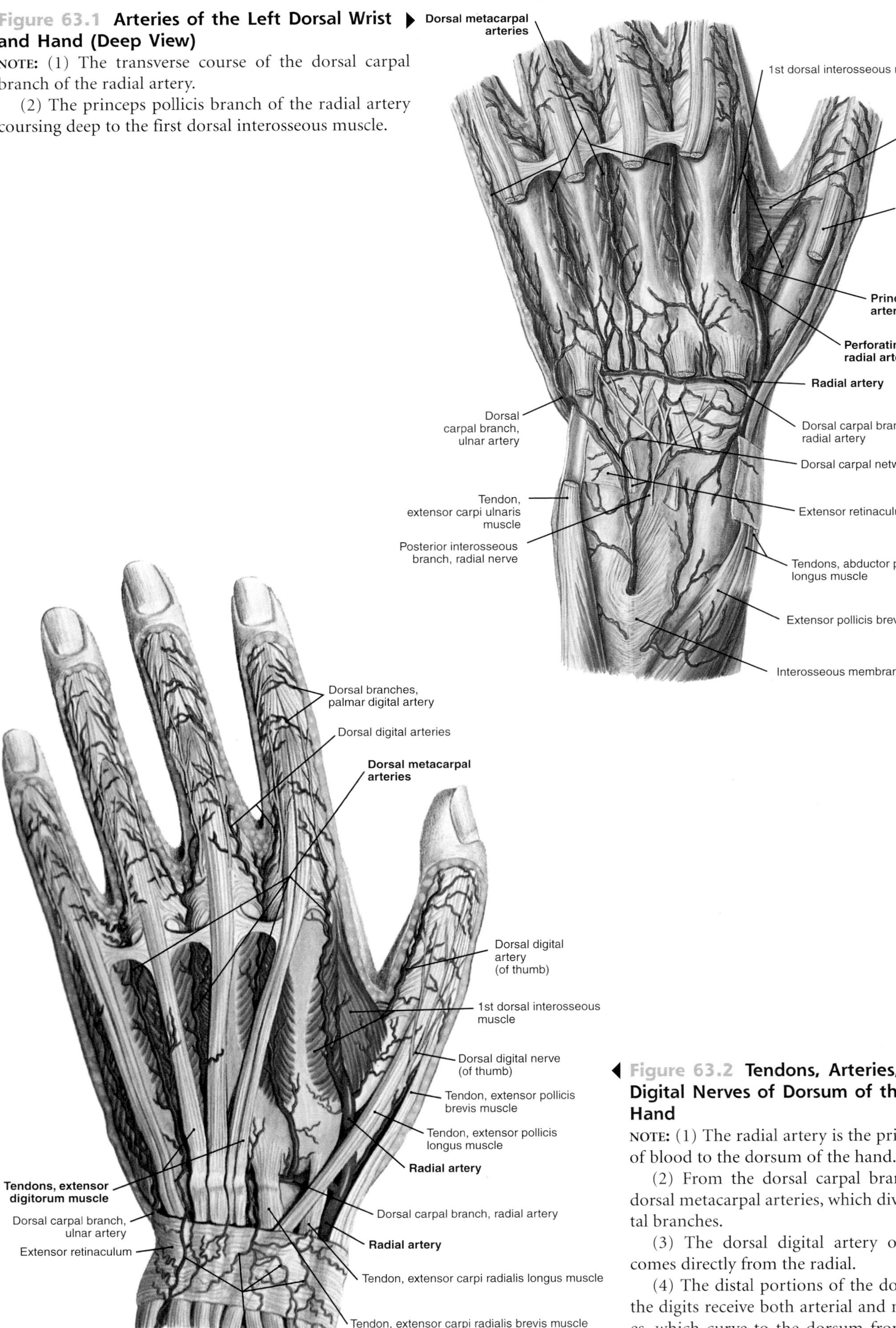

Dorsal metacarpal arteries
1st dorsal interosseous muscle
Adductor pollicis muscle
Tendon, extensor pollicis longus muscle
Princeps pollicis artery
Perforating branch, radial artery
Radial artery
Dorsal carpal branch, ulnar artery
Dorsal carpal branch, radial artery
Dorsal carpal network
Tendon, extensor carpi ulnaris muscle
Extensor retinaculum
Posterior interosseous branch, radial nerve
Tendons, abductor pollicis longus muscle
Extensor pollicis brevis muscle
Interosseous membrane
Dorsal branches, palmar digital artery
Dorsal digital arteries
Dorsal metacarpal arteries
Dorsal digital artery (of thumb)
1st dorsal interosseous muscle
Dorsal digital nerve (of thumb)
Tendon, extensor pollicis brevis muscle
Tendon, extensor pollicis longus muscle
Radial artery
Tendons, extensor digitorum muscle
Dorsal carpal branch, radial artery
Dorsal carpal branch, ulnar artery
Radial artery
Extensor retinaculum
Tendon, extensor carpi radialis longus muscle
Tendon, extensor carpi radialis brevis muscle
Dorsal carpal network

Figure 63.2 Tendons, Arteries, and Digital Nerves of Dorsum of the Left Hand

NOTE: (1) The radial artery is the principal source of blood to the dorsum of the hand.

(2) From the dorsal carpal branch stem the dorsal metacarpal arteries, which divide into digital branches.

(3) The dorsal digital artery of the thumb comes directly from the radial.

(4) The distal portions of the dorsal aspect of the digits receive both arterial and nerve branches, which curve to the dorsum from the palmar aspect of the fingers.

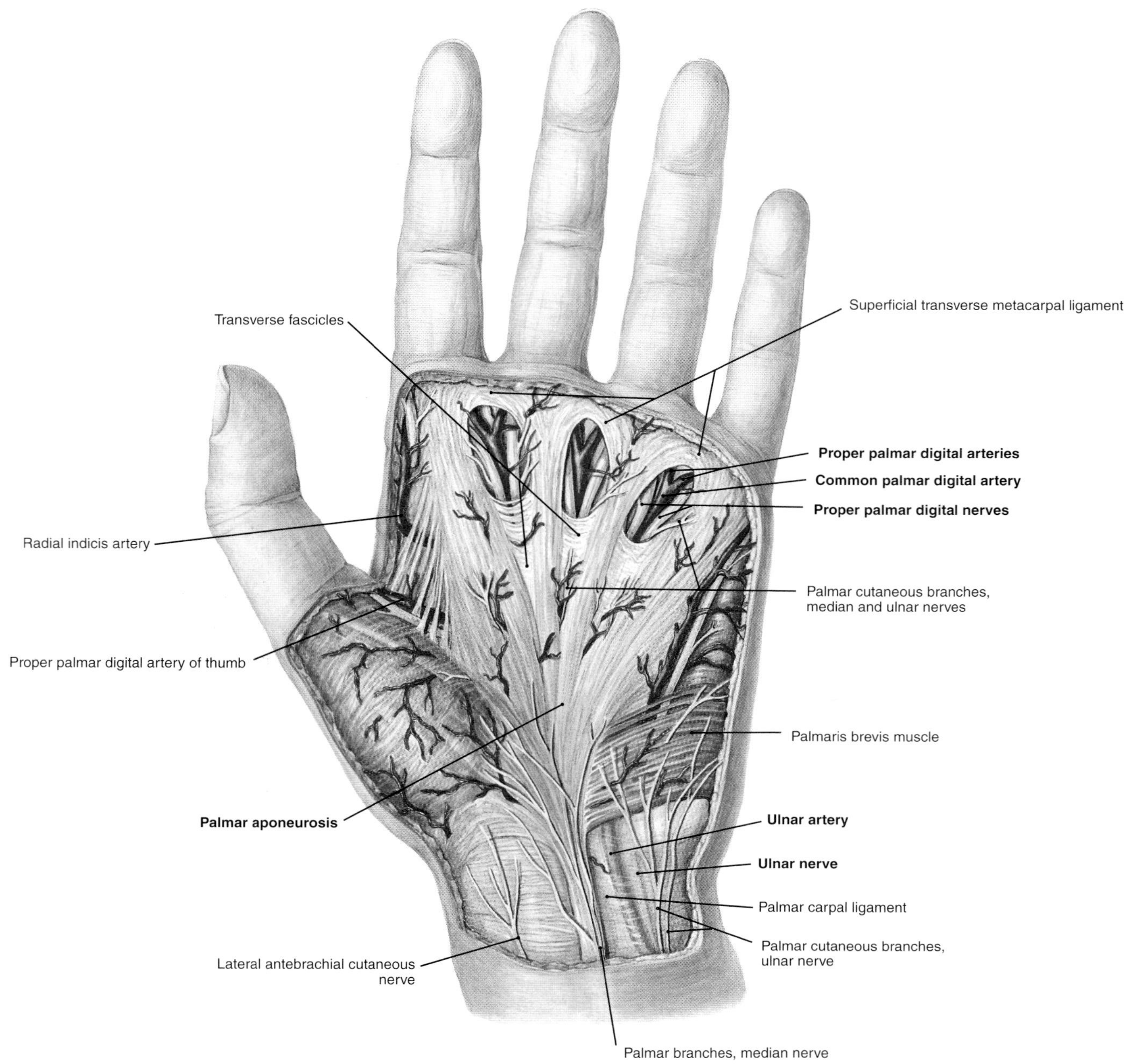
Transverse fascicles
Superficial transverse metacarpal ligament
Proper palmar digital arteries
Common palmar digital artery
Proper palmar digital nerves
Radial indicis artery
Palmar cutaneous branches, median and ulnar nerves
Proper palmar digital artery of thumb
Palmaris brevis muscle
Palmar aponeurosis
Ulnar artery
Ulnar nerve
Palmar carpal ligament
Palmar cutaneous branches, ulnar nerve
Lateral antebrachial cutaneous nerve
Palmar branches, median nerve

Figure 64 Superficial Nerves and Arteries of the Palm of the Left Hand

NOTE: (1) The thick fibrous palmar aponeurosis, which protects the palmar vessels and nerves and strengthens the midportion of the palm.

(2) The radial two-thirds of the palm is innervated by the median nerve, whereas the ulnar third is supplied by the ulnar nerve.

(3) The superficial exposure of vessels and nerves in the distal palm, where the palmar aponeurosis is deficient.

THENAR (THUMB) MUSCLES OF HAND

Muscle	Origin	Insertion	Innervation	Action
Abductor pollicis brevis	Flexor retinaculum and the tubercle of the trapezium	Base of proximal phalanx of thumb; dorsal digital expansion of thumb	Median nerve (C8, T1)	Abducts thumb
Opponens pollicis	Flexor retinaculum and the tubercles of the scaphoid and trapezium bones	Whole length of lateral border of metacarpal bone of the thumb	Median nerve (C8, T1) and often a small branch of deep ulnar nerve	Opposes the thumb to the other fingers

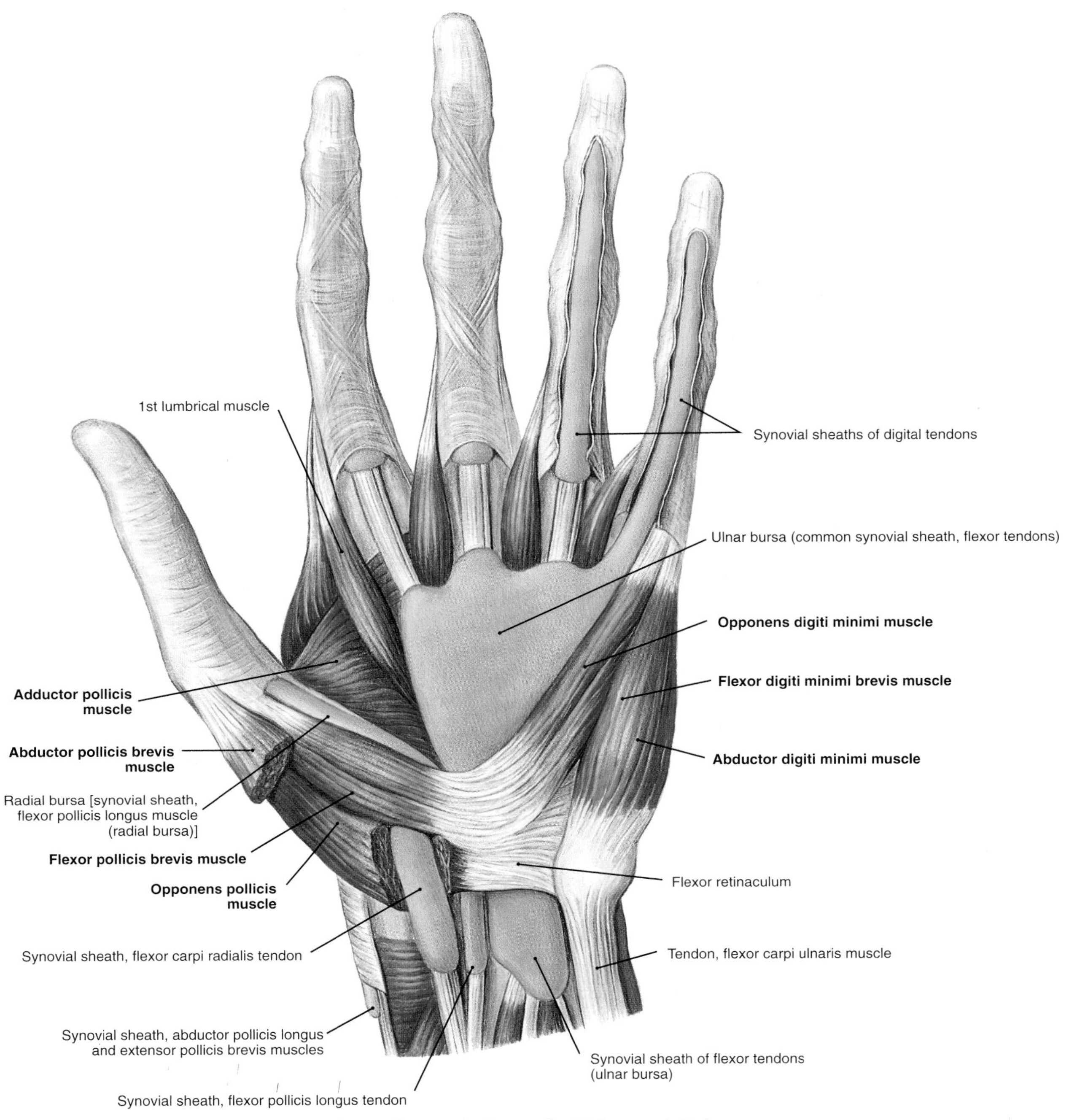
1st lumbrical muscle
Synovial sheaths of digital tendons
Ulnar bursa (common synovial sheath, flexor tendons)
Opponens digiti minimi muscle
Flexor digiti minimi brevis muscle
Abductor digiti minimi muscle
Adductor pollicis muscle
Abductor pollicis brevis muscle
Radial bursa [synovial sheath, flexor pollicis longus muscle (radial bursa)]
Flexor pollicis brevis muscle
Opponens pollicis muscle
Flexor retinaculum
Synovial sheath, flexor carpi radialis tendon
Tendon, flexor carpi ulnaris muscle
Synovial sheath, abductor pollicis longus and extensor pollicis brevis muscles
Synovial sheath of flexor tendons (ulnar bursa)
Synovial sheath, flexor pollicis longus tendon

Figure 65 Muscles, Synovial Sheaths, and Tendons of the Left Wrist and Palm

THENAR MUSCLES (CONT.)

Muscle	Origin	Insertion	Innervation	Action
Flexor pollicis brevis	**Superficial head:** Flexor retinaculum and tubercle of the trapezium. **Deep head:** Trapezoid and capitate bones.	Radial side of the base of the proximal phalanx of the thumb	**Superficial head:** Median nerve (C8, T1). **Deep head:** Deep branch of ulnar nerve (C8, T1).	Flexes proximal phalanx of thumb; flexes metacarpal bone and rotates it medially
Adductor pollicis	**Oblique head:** Capitate bone and bases of second and third metacarpal bones. **Transverse head:** Palmar surface of third metacarpal bone.	Ulnar side of base of proximal phalanx of thumb	Deep branch of ulnar nerve (C8, T1)	Adducts the thumb

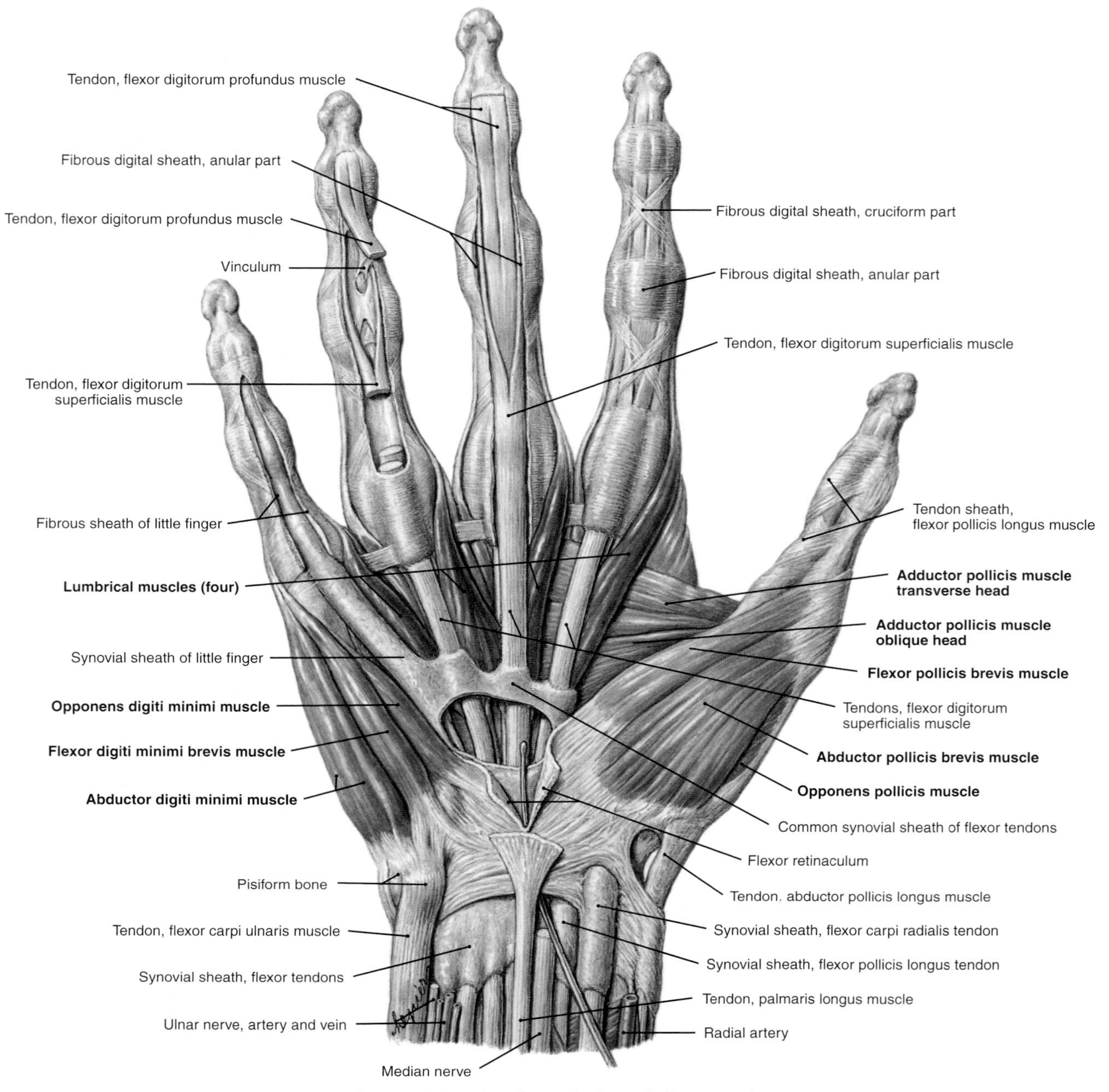
Tendon, flexor digitorum profundus muscle
Fibrous digital sheath, anular part
Tendon, flexor digitorum profundus muscle
Vinculum
Tendon, flexor digitorum superficialis muscle
Fibrous sheath of little finger
Lumbrical muscles (four)
Synovial sheath of little finger
Opponens digiti minimi muscle
Flexor digiti minimi brevis muscle
Abductor digiti minimi muscle
Pisiform bone
Tendon, flexor carpi ulnaris muscle
Synovial sheath, flexor tendons
Ulnar nerve, artery and vein
Median nerve
Fibrous digital sheath, cruciform part
Fibrous digital sheath, anular part
Tendon, flexor digitorum superficialis muscle
Tendon sheath, flexor pollicis longus muscle
Adductor pollicis muscle transverse head
Adductor pollicis muscle oblique head
Flexor pollicis brevis muscle
Tendons, flexor digitorum superficialis muscle
Abductor pollicis brevis muscle
Opponens pollicis muscle
Common synovial sheath of flexor tendons
Flexor retinaculum
Tendon. abductor pollicis longus muscle
Synovial sheath, flexor carpi radialis tendon
Synovial sheath, flexor pollicis longus tendon
Tendon, palmaris longus muscle
Radial artery

Figure 66 **Muscles of the Right Hand**

HYPOTHENAR (LITTLE FINGER) MUSCLES OF HAND

Muscle	Origin	Insertion	Innervation	Action
Palmaris brevis (see Fig. 64)	Palmar aponeurosis and the flexor retinaculum	Into the dermis on the ulnar side of the hand	Ulnar nerve, superficial branch (C8, T1)	Helps tense the skin over the hypothenar muscles
Abductor digiti minimi	Pisiform bone and tendon of flexor carpi ulnaris	Base of proximal phalanx and dorsal aponeurosis of little finger	Ulnar nerve, deep branch (C8, T1)	Abducts the little finger
Flexor digiti minimi	Hamulus of the hamate bone and flexor retinaculum	Base of proximal phalanx of the little finger	Ulnar nerve, deep branch (C8, T1)	Flexes the little finger at metacarpophalangeal joint
Opponens digiti minimi	Hamulus of the hamate bone and flexor retinaculum	Ulnar side of fifth metacarpal bone	Ulnar nerve, deep branch (C8, T1)	Brings the little finger into opposition with the thumb

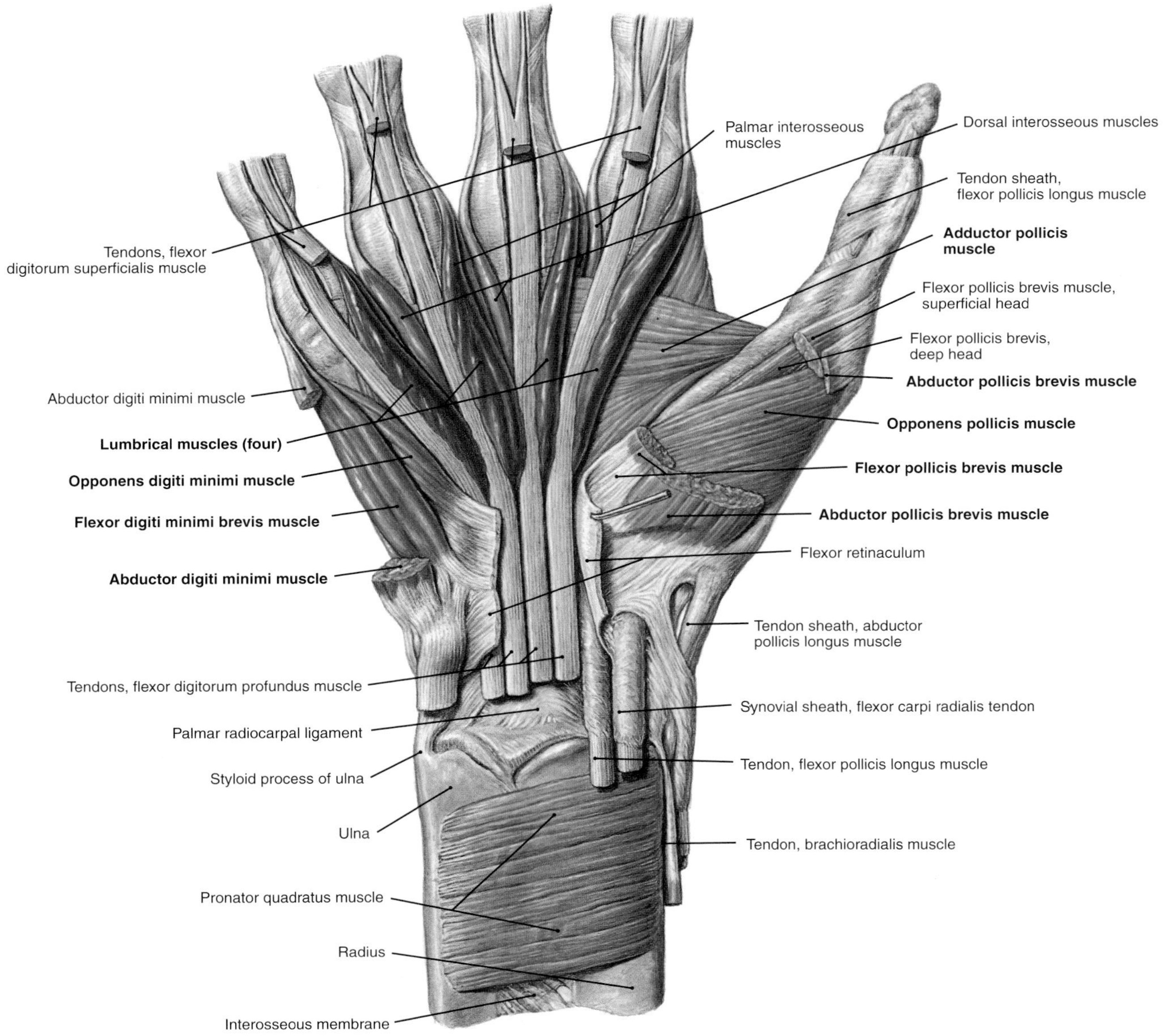

Tendons, flexor digitorum superficialis muscle
Palmar interosseous muscles
Dorsal interosseous muscles
Tendon sheath, flexor pollicis longus muscle
Adductor pollicis muscle
Flexor pollicis brevis muscle, superficial head
Flexor pollicis brevis, deep head
Abductor pollicis brevis muscle
Abductor digiti minimi muscle
Opponens pollicis muscle
Lumbrical muscles (four)
Flexor pollicis brevis muscle
Opponens digiti minimi muscle
Abductor pollicis brevis muscle
Flexor digiti minimi brevis muscle
Flexor retinaculum
Abductor digiti minimi muscle
Tendon sheath, abductor pollicis longus muscle
Tendons, flexor digitorum profundus muscle
Synovial sheath, flexor carpi radialis tendon
Palmar radiocarpal ligament
Styloid process of ulna
Tendon, flexor pollicis longus muscle
Ulna
Tendon, brachioradialis muscle
Pronator quadratus muscle
Radius
Interosseous membrane

Figure 67.1 **Deep Muscles of the Right Hand (Palmar View)**

NOTE: (1) The tendon of the flexor digitorum superficialis divides into two slips and allows the flexor digitorum profundus to pass and insert onto the distal phalanx.

(2) In the fingers the tendons are encased in a synovial sheath and then bound by both crossed and transverse (cruciform and annular) fibrous sheaths (see Fig. 66).

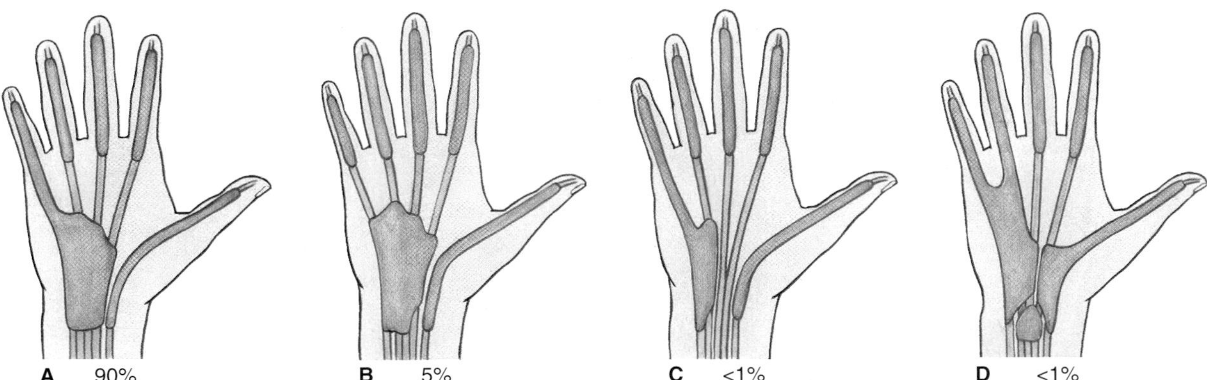
A 90%
B 5%
C <1%
D <1%

Figure 67.2a-d **Variations in the Synovial Tendon Sheathes within the Carpal Tunnel and Hand**

NOTE that because of these variations the hand surgeon must be careful when repairing carpal tunnel syndrome, since infections spread rapidly within the synovial sheathes of the hand.

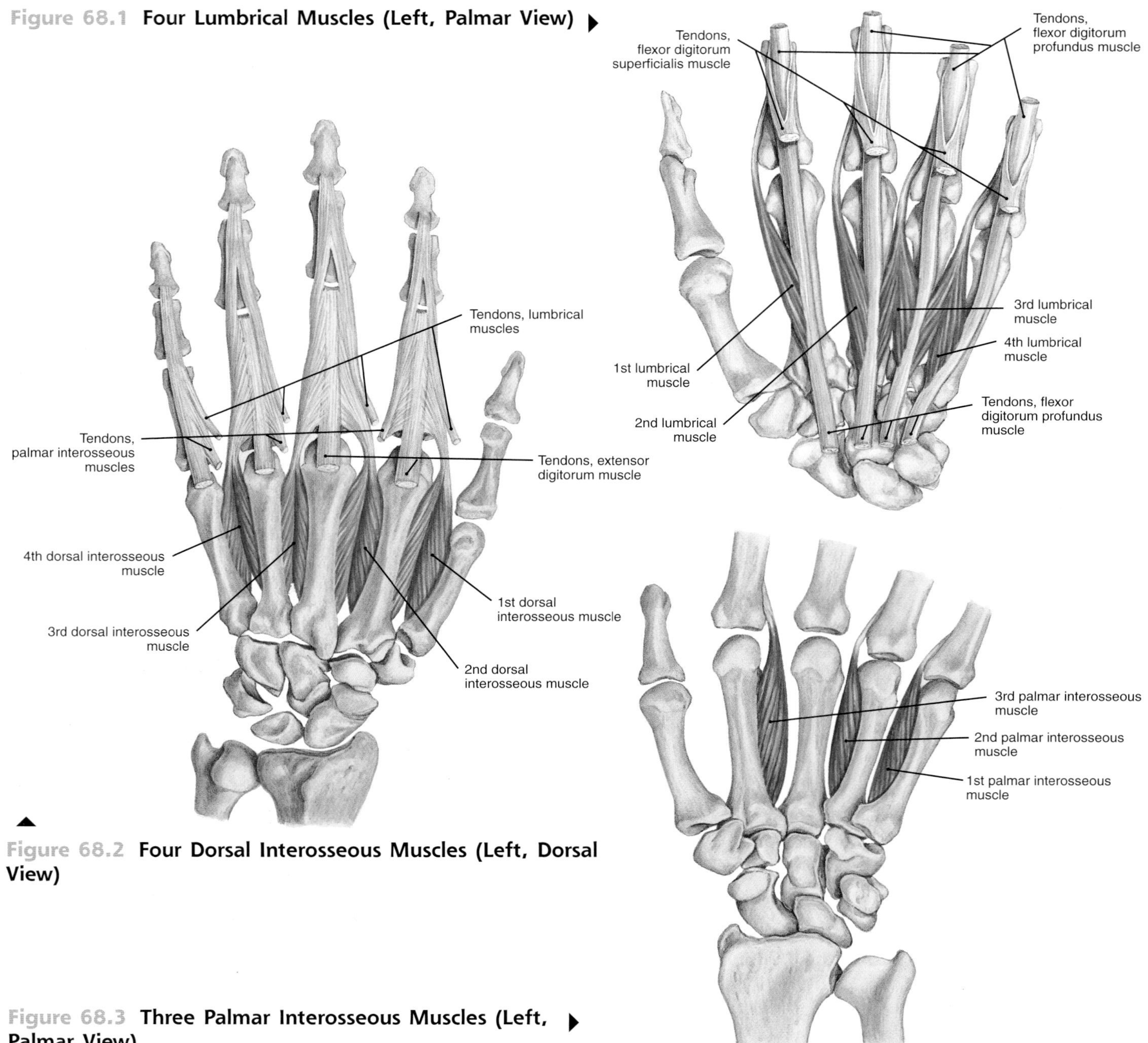
Tendons, flexor digitorum superficialis muscle
Tendons, flexor digitorum profundus muscle
3rd lumbrical muscle
4th lumbrical muscle
1st lumbrical muscle
2nd lumbrical muscle
Tendons, flexor digitorum profundus muscle
Tendons, lumbrical muscles
Tendons, palmar interosseous muscles
Tendons, extensor digitorum muscle
4th dorsal interosseous muscle
1st dorsal interosseous muscle
3rd dorsal interosseous muscle
2nd dorsal interosseous muscle
3rd palmar interosseous muscle
2nd palmar interosseous muscle
1st palmar interosseous muscle

Figure 68.1 **Four Lumbrical Muscles (Left, Palmar View)**

Figure 68.2 **Four Dorsal Interosseous Muscles (Left, Dorsal View)**

Figure 68.3 **Three Palmar Interosseous Muscles (Left, Palmar View)**

LUMBRICAL MUSCLES (FIGS. 66, 67.1, 68.1, 69.1)

Muscle	Origin	Insertion	Innervation	Action
Lumbrical muscles (four)	Four tendons of flexor digitorum profundus muscle	Radial side of dorsal digital expansion, second, third, fourth, and fifth digits	Radial two lumbricals (first and second): median nerve Ulnar two lumbricals (third and fourth): ulnar nerve	Flex metacarpophalangeal joints; extend interphalangeal joints

INTEROSSEOUS MUSCLES (FIGS. 68.2, 68.3)

Muscle	Origin	Insertion	Innervation	Action
Dorsal interossei (four)	Each arises by two heads from the adjacent sides of metacarpal bones	Bases of the proximal phalanges and the dorsal expansions of the second, third, and fourth fingers	Ulnar nerve, deep palmar branch (C8, T1)	Abduct fingers; flex at metacarpophalangeal joints and extend at interphalangeal joints
Palmar interossei (three)	Each arises by one head from the second, fourth, and fifth metacarpal bones	Dorsal digital expansions of the second, fourth, and fifth fingers	Ulnar nerve, deep palmar branch (C8, T1)	Adduct fingers; flex at metacarpophalangeal joints and extend at interphalangeal joints

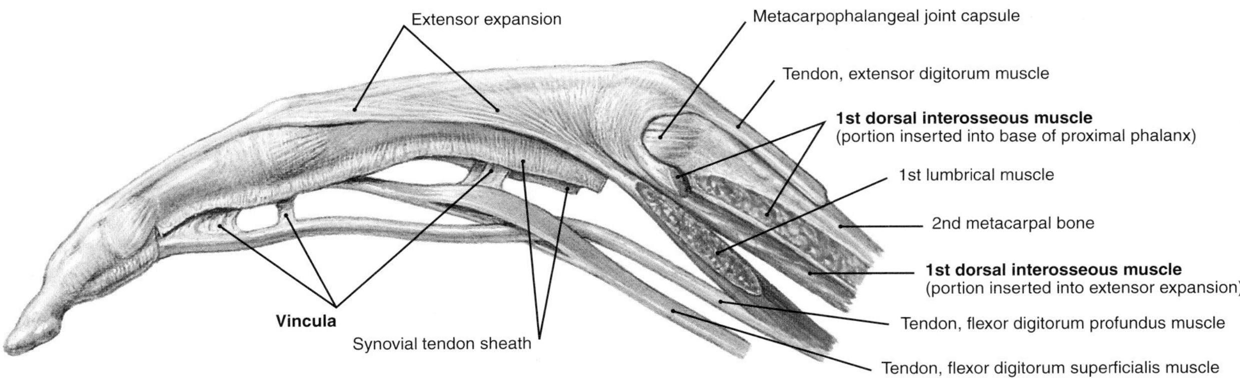
Extensor expansion
Metacarpophalangeal joint capsule
Tendon, extensor digitorum muscle
1st dorsal interosseous muscle
(portion inserted into base of proximal phalanx)
1st lumbrical muscle
2nd metacarpal bone
1st dorsal interosseous muscle
(portion inserted into extensor expansion)
Tendon, flexor digitorum profundus muscle
Tendon, flexor digitorum superficialis muscle
Vincula
Synovial tendon sheath

Figure 69.1 Tendon Insertions, Index Finger of Right Hand (Radial Side)

NOTE: (1) The dorsal interosseous and lumbrical muscles join fibers from the extensor tendon in the formation of the dorsal extensor expansion.

(2) The vincula are remnants of mesotendons and attach both superficial and deep tendons to the digital sheath.

(3) The tendon of the flexor digitorum superficialis splits to allow the tendon of the flexor digitorum profundus to reach the distal phalanx.

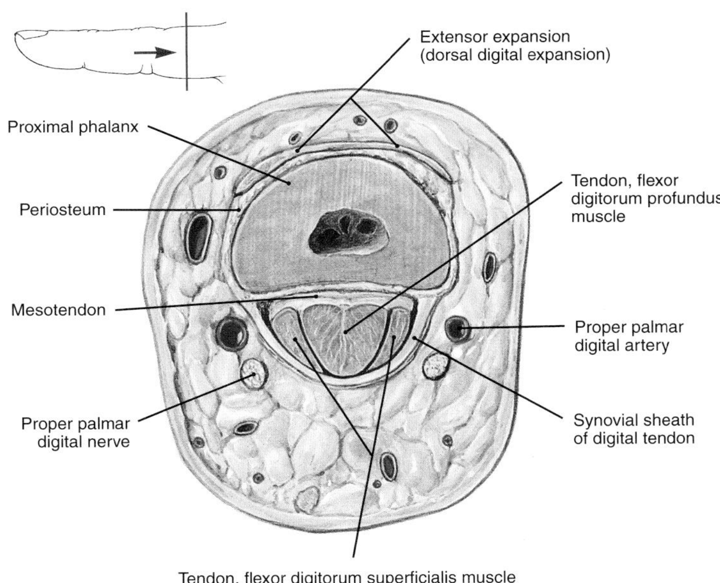
Extensor expansion
(dorsal digital expansion)
Proximal phalanx
Periosteum
Mesotendon
Proper palmar
digital nerve
Tendon, flexor
digitorum profundus
muscle
Proper palmar
digital artery
Synovial sheath
of digital tendon
Tendon, flexor digitorum superficialis muscle

Figure 69.2 Cross Section of the Middle Finger through the Proximal Phalanx

NOTE: (1) The extensor expansion (or extensor hood) over the dorsal aspect of the proximal phalanx and part of the middle phalanx.

(2) Into the extensor expansion blend the tendon of the extensor digitorum and the tendons of insertion of the adjacent interosseous and lumbrical muscles.

(3) The synovial sheath on the palmar side of the phalanx, which surrounds the superficial and deep flexor tendons of the digit.

Figure 69.3 Cross Section of the Middle Finger through the Middle Phalanx

NOTE: (1) The location of the proper digital arteries and nerves within the subcutaneous tissue on the sides of the deep flexor tendon.

(2) Knowing the location of these neurovascular structures is important both for the application of local anesthesia to the digit and for the cessation of severe bleeding.

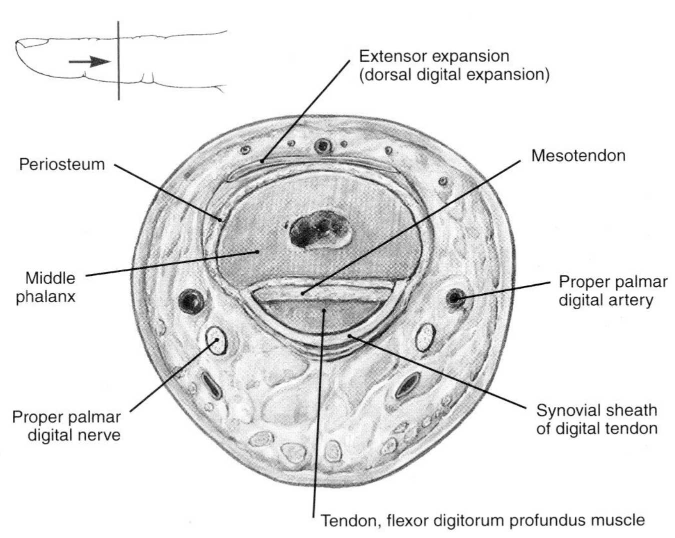
Extensor expansion
(dorsal digital expansion)
Periosteum
Mesotendon
Middle
phalanx
Proper palmar
digital artery
Proper palmar
digital nerve
Synovial sheath
of digital tendon
Tendon, flexor digitorum profundus muscle

Palm of the Hand: Nerves and Arteries (Superficial Dissection)

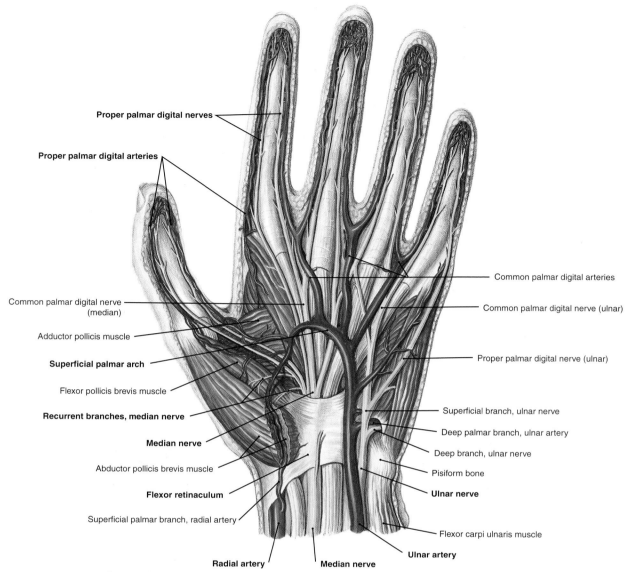

Proper palmar digital nerves
Proper palmar digital arteries
Common palmar digital arteries
Common palmar digital nerve (median)
Common palmar digital nerve (ulnar)
Adductor pollicis muscle
Superficial palmar arch
Proper palmar digital nerve (ulnar)
Flexor pollicis brevis muscle
Recurrent branches, median nerve
Superficial branch, ulnar nerve
Deep palmar branch, ulnar artery
Median nerve
Deep branch, ulnar nerve
Abductor pollicis brevis muscle
Pisiform bone
Flexor retinaculum
Ulnar nerve
Superficial palmar branch, radial artery
Flexor carpi ulnaris muscle
Ulnar artery
Radial artery
Median nerve

Figure 70.1 **Nerves and Arteries of the Left Palm, Superficial Palmar Arch**

NOTE: (1) The **median nerve** enters the palm beneath the flexor retinaculum and supplies the muscles of the thenar eminence: abductor pollicis brevis, opponens pollicis, and the superficial head of the flexor pollicis brevis.

(2) The **median nerve** also supplies the radial (lateral) two lumbrical muscles as well as the palmar surface of the lateral hand and lateral $3^1/_2$ fingers.

(3) The superficial location of the **recurrent branches of the median nerve,** which supply the thenar muscles. Just deep to the superficial fascia, these branches are easily injured.

(4) The **ulnar nerve** enters the palm superficial to the flexor retinaculum, and it supplies the ulnar $1^1/_2$ fingers and **all** the remaining muscles in the hand.

(5) The **superficial palmar arterial arch** is derived principally from the ulnar artery. The arch is completed by the **palmar branch of the radial artery.** From the arch three or four **common palmar digital arteries** course distally and divide into **proper palmar digital arteries.** These accompany the corresponding digital nerves along the fingers.

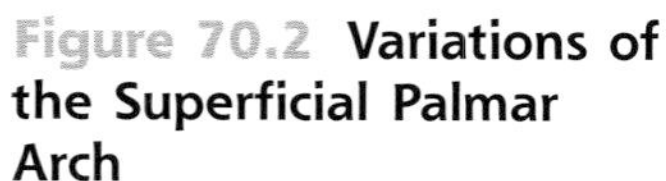

Figure 70.2 **Variations of the Superficial Palmar Arch**

A: Complete arch

B: Ulnar three fingers supplied by the ulnar artery

C: All fingers supplied by ulnar artery

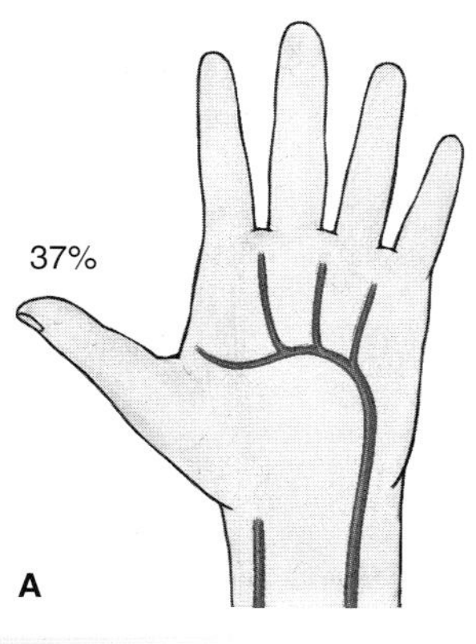
37%
A

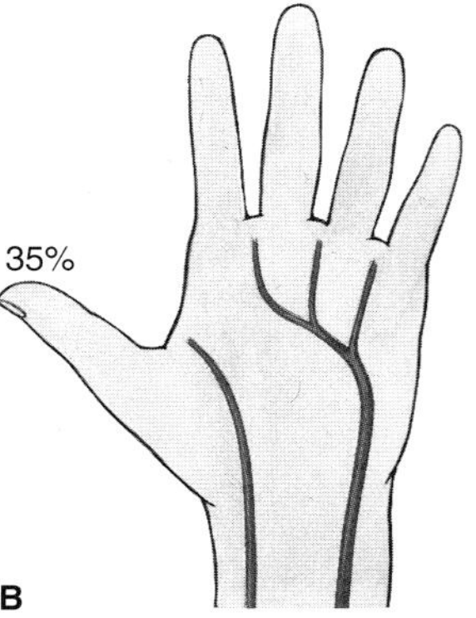
35%
B

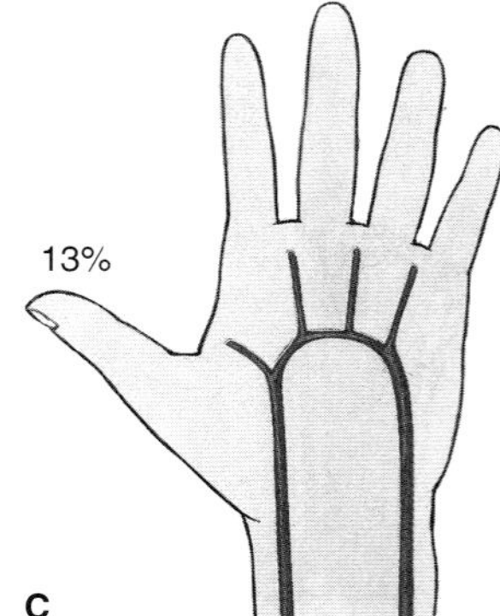
13%
C

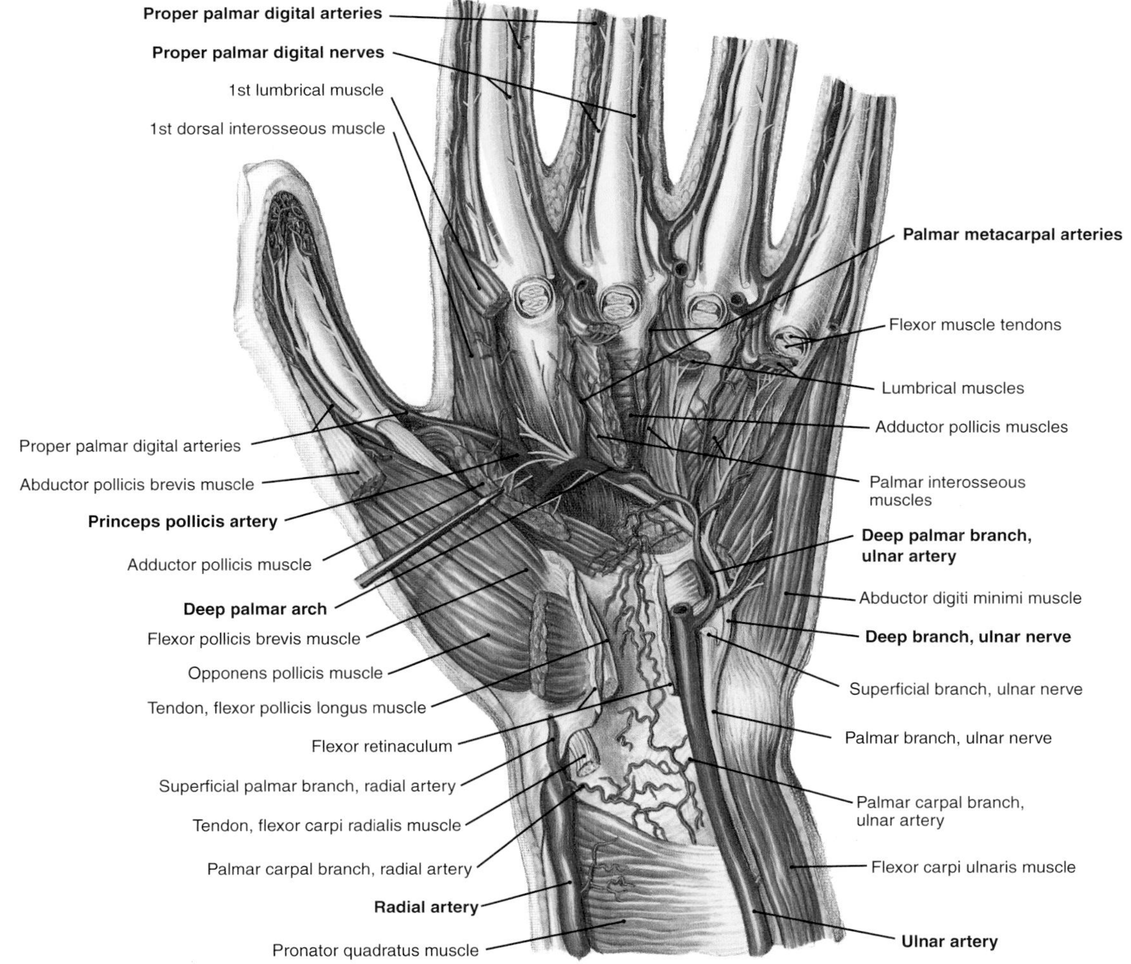
Proper palmar digital arteries
Proper palmar digital nerves
1st lumbrical muscle
1st dorsal interosseous muscle
Palmar metacarpal arteries
Flexor muscle tendons
Lumbrical muscles
Adductor pollicis muscles
Palmar interosseous muscles
Deep palmar branch, ulnar artery
Abductor digiti minimi muscle
Deep branch, ulnar nerve
Superficial branch, ulnar nerve
Palmar branch, ulnar nerve
Palmar carpal branch, ulnar artery
Flexor carpi ulnaris muscle
Ulnar artery
Proper palmar digital arteries
Abductor pollicis brevis muscle
Princeps pollicis artery
Adductor pollicis muscle
Deep palmar arch
Flexor pollicis brevis muscle
Opponens pollicis muscle
Tendon, flexor pollicis longus muscle
Flexor retinaculum
Superficial palmar branch, radial artery
Tendon, flexor carpi radialis muscle
Palmar carpal branch, radial artery
Radial artery
Pronator quadratus muscle

Figure 71.1 Nerves and Arteries of the Left Palm, Deep Palmar Arch

NOTE: (1) The **radial artery** at the wrist enters the hand dorsally through the "anatomical snuff box" (see Figs. 54 and 55) and then passes distally, perforates the two heads of first dorsal interosseous muscle, and reaches the palm of the hand.

(2) In the palm, the radial artery forms the **deep palmar arch,** uniting medially with the **deep palmar branch** of the ulnar artery.

(3) From the deep arch arise the **palmar metacarpal arteries** as well as the **princeps pollicis artery**.

(4) The **deep branch of the ulnar nerve** courses with the deep palmar arterial arch. It supplies all the muscles in the deep palm.

(5) There is a rich anastomosis between the superficial and deep arches and between the ulnar and radial arteries.

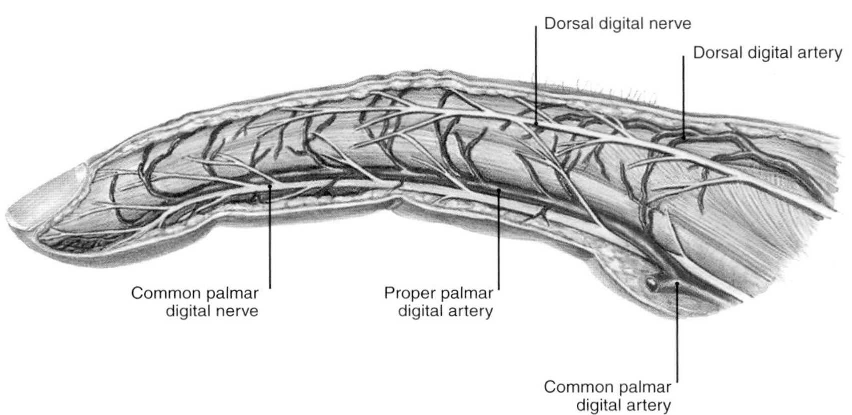
Dorsal digital nerve
Dorsal digital artery
Common palmar digital nerve
Proper palmar digital artery
Common palmar digital artery

Figure 71.2 Nerves and Arteries of the Index Finger

NOTE: The **dorsal digital nerve and artery** extend only two-thirds the length of the finger. The distal third is supplied by the **palmar digital nerve and artery,** which also supplies the entire palmar surface.

Arteries and Nerves of the Hand; Variations in the Deep Palmar Arch

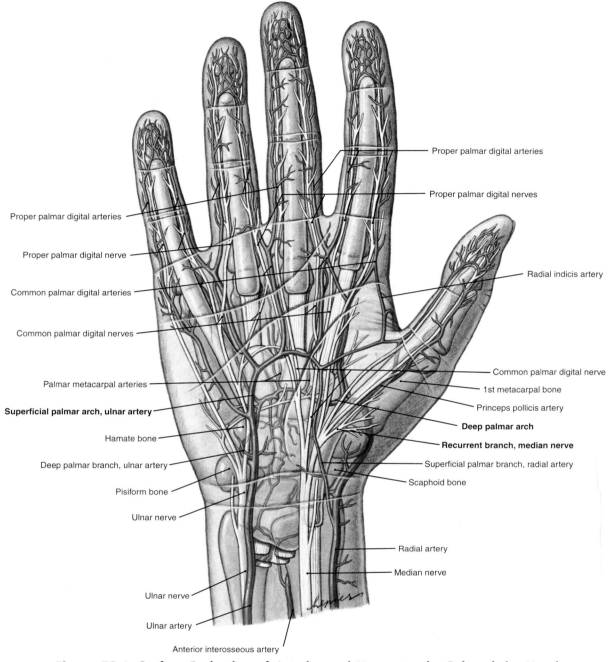

Proper palmar digital arteries
Proper palmar digital nerves
Proper palmar digital arteries
Proper palmar digital nerve
Common palmar digital arteries
Common palmar digital nerves
Radial indicis artery
Common palmar digital nerve
Palmar metacarpal arteries
1st metacarpal bone
Princeps pollicis artery
Superficial palmar arch, ulnar artery
Deep palmar arch
Hamate bone
Recurrent branch, median nerve
Deep palmar branch, ulnar artery
Superficial palmar branch, radial artery
Scaphoid bone
Pisiform bone
Ulnar nerve
Radial artery
Median nerve
Ulnar nerve
Ulnar artery
Anterior interosseous artery

Figure 72.1 **Surface Projection of Arteries and Nerves to the Palm of the Hand**

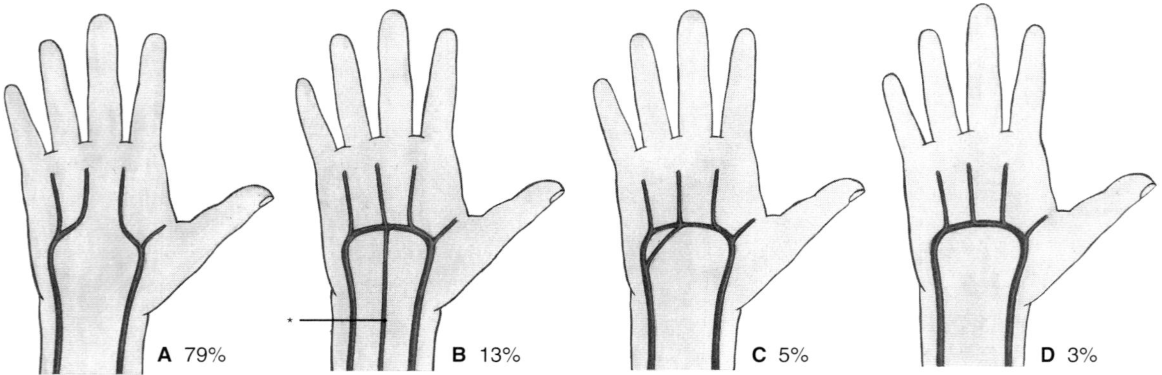
A 79%
B 13%
C 5%
D 3%

Figure 72.2 **Variations in the Formation of the Deep Palmar Arch**

A: Complete deep palmar arch
B: Double ulnar contribution
C: Anastomosis with anterior interosseous artery
D: Radial two digits supplied by the radial artery, ulnar three digits supplied by the ulnar artery.

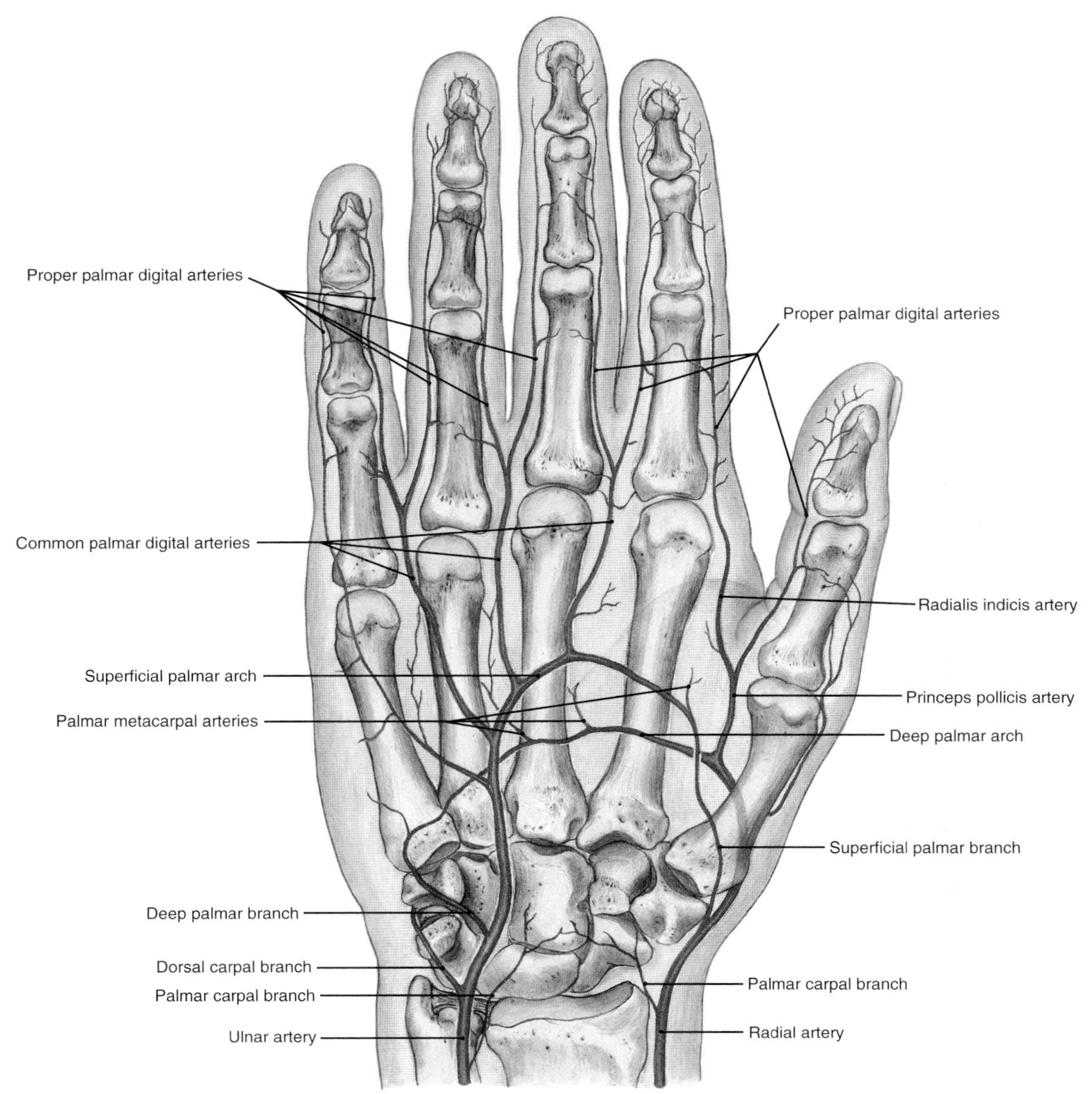
Proper palmar digital arteries
Proper palmar digital arteries
Common palmar digital arteries
Radialis indicis artery
Superficial palmar arch
Palmar metacarpal arteries
Princeps pollicis artery
Deep palmar arch
Superficial palmar branch
Deep palmar branch
Dorsal carpal branch
Palmar carpal branch
Palmar carpal branch
Ulnar artery
Radial artery

Figure 73.1 **Arteries of the Right Hand Showing the Palmar Arterial Arches**

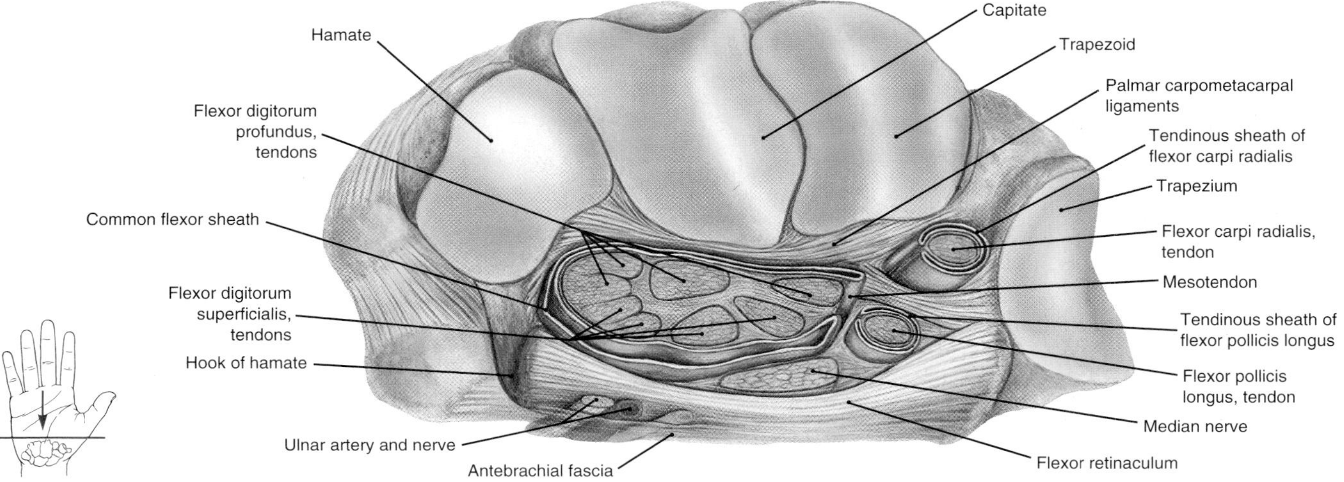
Hamate
Capitate
Trapezoid
Palmar carpometacarpal ligaments
Flexor digitorum profundus, tendons
Tendinous sheath of flexor carpi radialis
Trapezium
Common flexor sheath
Flexor carpi radialis, tendon
Mesotendon
Flexor digitorum superficialis, tendons
Tendinous sheath of flexor pollicis longus
Hook of hamate
Flexor pollicis longus, tendon
Median nerve
Ulnar artery and nerve
Antebrachial fascia
Flexor retinaculum

Figure 73.2 **Transverse Section through the Right Wrist Showing the Carpal Tunnel and Its Contents**

NOTE that the median nerve can be compressed and thereby be functionally compromised if there is edema or fibrosis due to trauma within the carpal tunnel (carpal tunnel syndrome). In this condition weakness is experienced in muscles innervated by the median nerve.

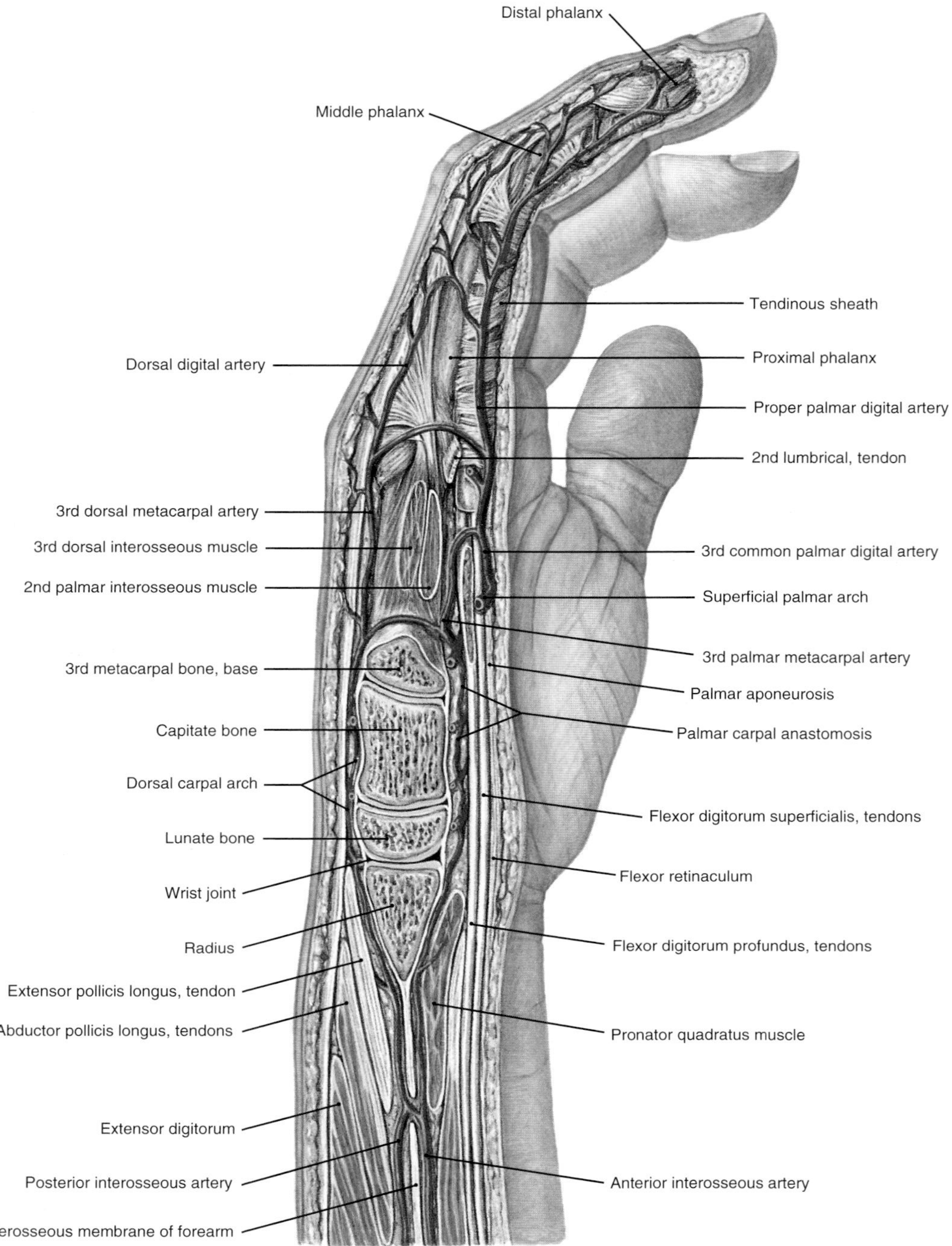
Distal phalanx
Middle phalanx
Tendinous sheath
Dorsal digital artery
Proximal phalanx
Proper palmar digital artery
2nd lumbrical, tendon
3rd dorsal metacarpal artery
3rd dorsal interosseous muscle
3rd common palmar digital artery
2nd palmar interosseous muscle
Superficial palmar arch
3rd palmar metacarpal artery
3rd metacarpal bone, base
Palmar aponeurosis
Capitate bone
Palmar carpal anastomosis
Dorsal carpal arch
Flexor digitorum superficialis, tendons
Lunate bone
Flexor retinaculum
Wrist joint
Radius
Flexor digitorum profundus, tendons
Extensor pollicis longus, tendon
Abductor pollicis longus, tendons
Pronator quadratus muscle
Extensor digitorum
Posterior interosseous artery
Anterior interosseous artery
Interosseous membrane of forearm

Figure 74 Sagittal Section through the Middle Finger: Right Hand (Ulnar View)

NOTE: (1) There is a rich blood supply and abundant anastomoses along the entire extent of the finger.

(2) The second palmar interosseous muscle of the ring finger and the third dorsal interosseous muscle of the middle finger.

(3) The skeletal continuum from proximal to distal: radius, lunate and capitate bones; the third metacarpal; and the proximal, middle, and distal phalanges.

(4) The anastomosis just proximal to the wrist joint between the anterior and posterior interosseous arteries.

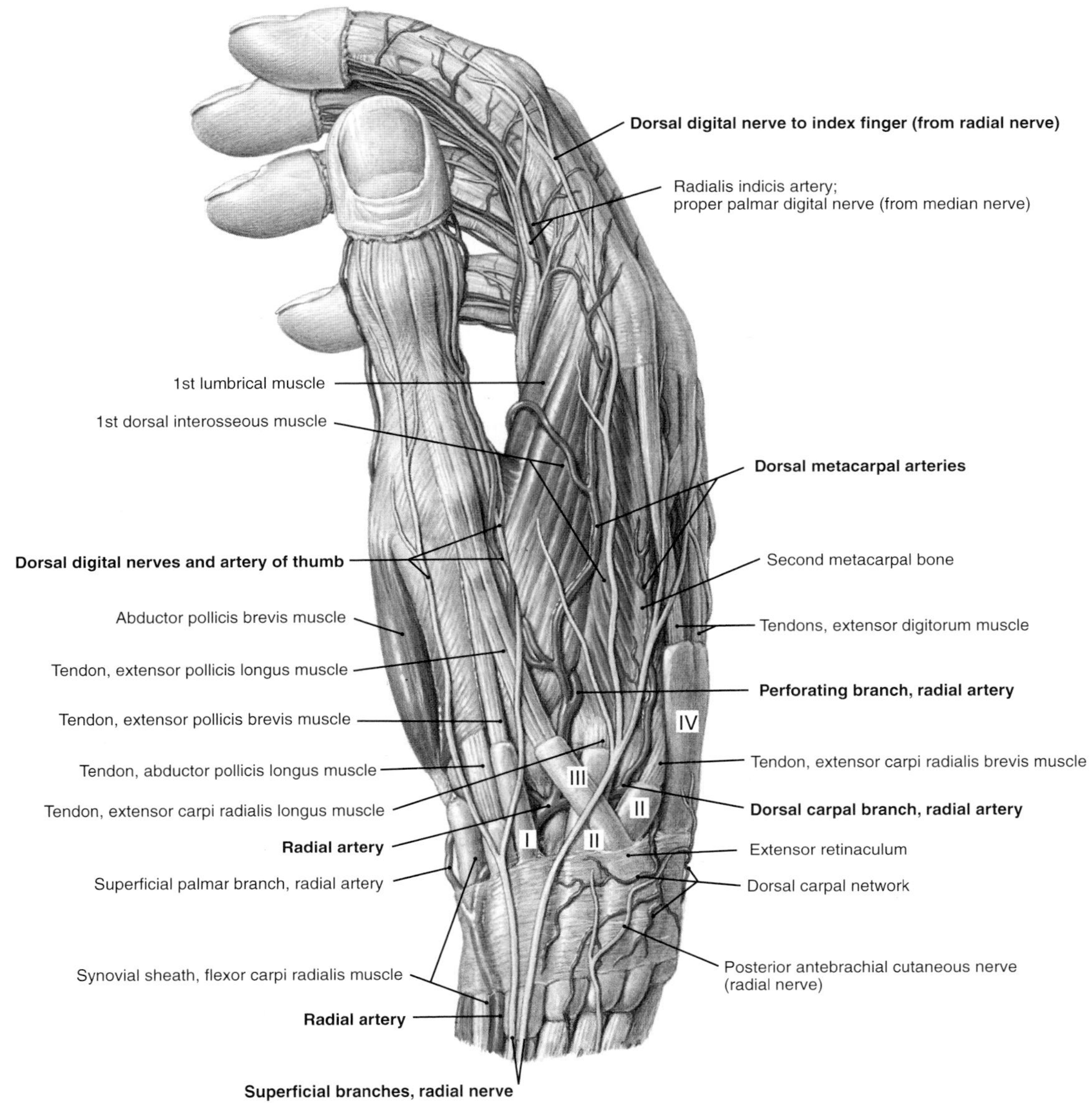
Dorsal digital nerve to index finger (from radial nerve)
Radialis indicis artery;
proper palmar digital nerve (from median nerve)
1st lumbrical muscle
1st dorsal interosseous muscle
Dorsal metacarpal arteries
Dorsal digital nerves and artery of thumb
Second metacarpal bone
Abductor pollicis brevis muscle
Tendons, extensor digitorum muscle
Tendon, extensor pollicis longus muscle
Perforating branch, radial artery
Tendon, extensor pollicis brevis muscle
IV
Tendon, extensor carpi radialis brevis muscle
Tendon, abductor pollicis longus muscle
III
Tendon, extensor carpi radialis longus muscle
Dorsal carpal branch, radial artery
II
I
Radial artery
Extensor retinaculum
Superficial palmar branch, radial artery
Dorsal carpal network
Posterior antebrachial cutaneous nerve
(radial nerve)
Synovial sheath, flexor carpi radialis muscle
Radial artery
Superficial branches, radial nerve
I—IV = Synovial tendon sheaths
I = Abductor pollicis longus and extensor pollicis
brevis tendon sheaths
II = Extensor carpi radialis longus and brevis tendon sheaths
IIII = Extensor pollicis longus tendon sheath
IV = Extensor digitorum and extensor indicis tendon sheath

Figure 75 Superficial Nerves, Arteries, and Tendons on the Radial Aspect of the Right Hand

NOTE: (1) Only the skin and superficial fascia have been removed in this dissection, and the cutaneous nerves and superficial arteries to the thumb, radial side of the index finger, and dorsum of the hand have been retained.

(2) The **superficial branches of the radial nerve** to the hand (see Figs. 44, 61, and 62.1). These supply the dorsum of the thumb, nearly to the tip, as well as the lateral (radial) half of the dorsum of the hand.

(3) The radial nerve also supplies the proximal part of the dorsum of the index, middle, and lateral half of the ring fingers, as far as the proximal interphalangeal joint because the median nerve sends branches around the digits to supply the more distal parts of the fingers.

(4) The distribution of the radial artery to the thumb and dorsum of the hand (see Figs. 63.1 and 63.2). Observe: (a) the **dorsal digital branch** to the thumb; (b) the **radial indicis branch** to the index finger; (c) the **perforating branch** that penetrates between the two heads of the first dorsal interosseous muscle; and (d) the **dorsal carpal branch,** from which the dorsal metacarpal arteries arise.

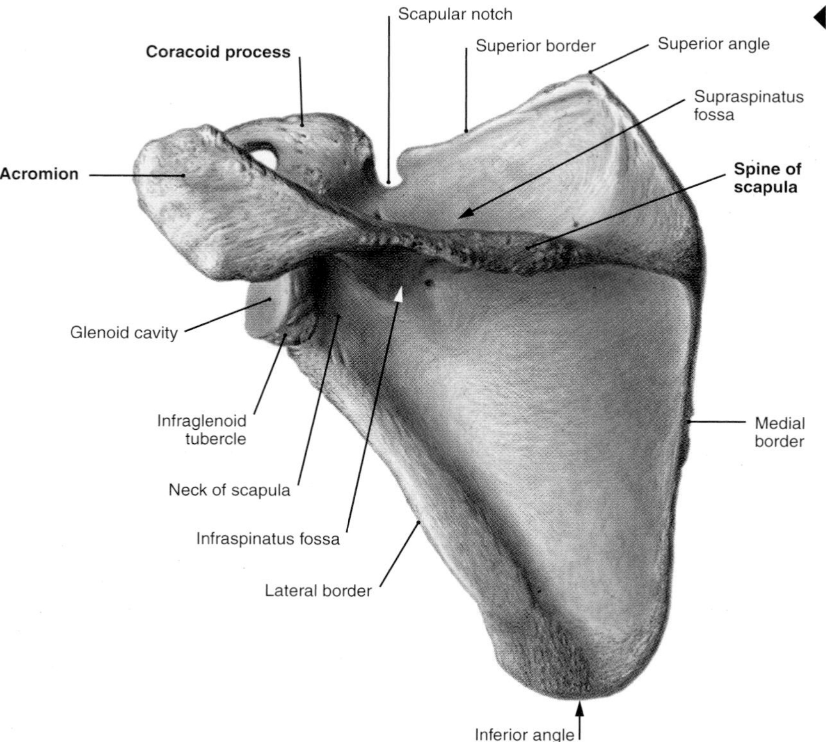
Scapular notch
Coracoid process
Superior border
Superior angle
Supraspinatus fossa
Acromion
Spine of scapula
Glenoid cavity
Infraglenoid tubercle
Medial border
Neck of scapula
Infraspinatus fossa
Lateral border
Inferior angle

Figure 76.1 Left Scapula (Dorsal Surface)

NOTE: (1) The socket for the head of the humerus is formed by the glenoid cavity.

(2) The acromion and coracoid process give additional protection to the socket superiorly, anteriorly, and posteriorly.

(3) The spine of the scapula separates the dorsal surface into supraspinatus and infraspinatus fossae.

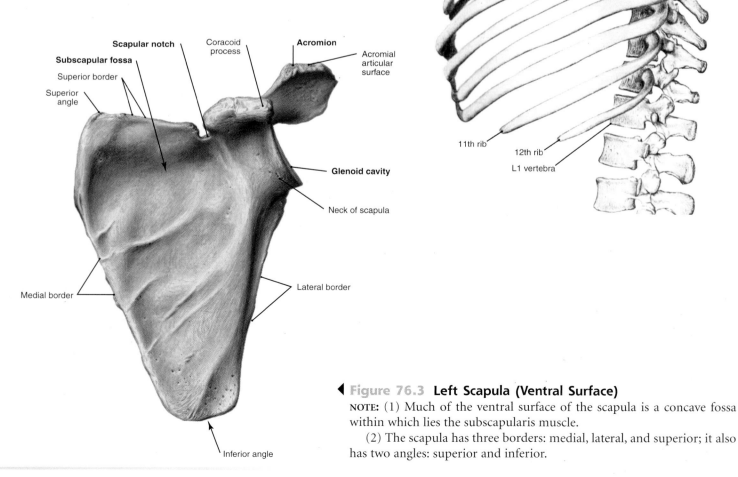

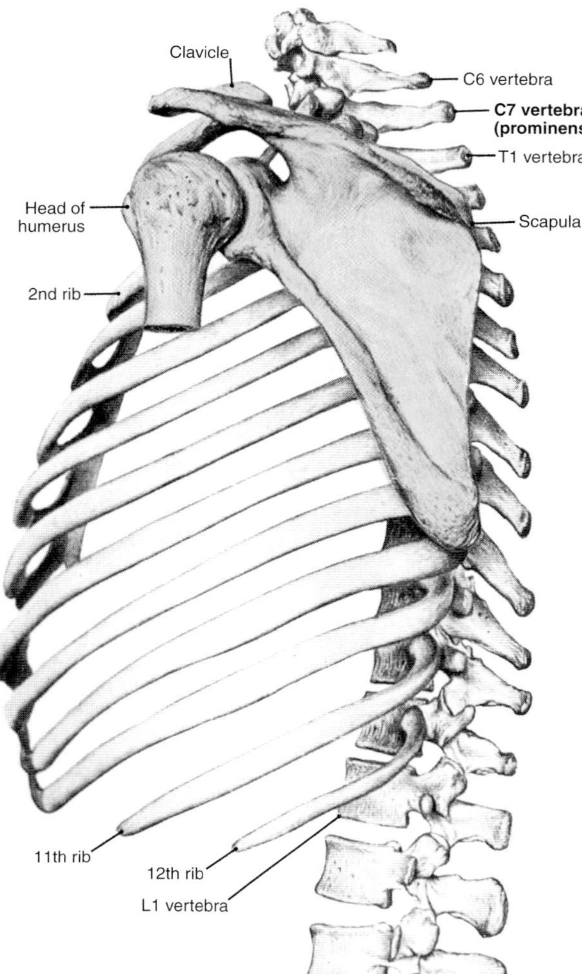
Clavicle
C6 vertebra
C7 vertebra (prominens)
T1 vertebra
Head of humerus
Scapula
2nd rib
11th rib
12th rib
L1 vertebra

Figure 76.2 Skeleton of Trunk with Scapula and Humerus

NOTE: (1) The triangular-shaped scapula articulates with the head of the humerus and the clavicle.

(2) The medial border of the scapula is attached to the vertebral column by muscles and not by an osseous joint.

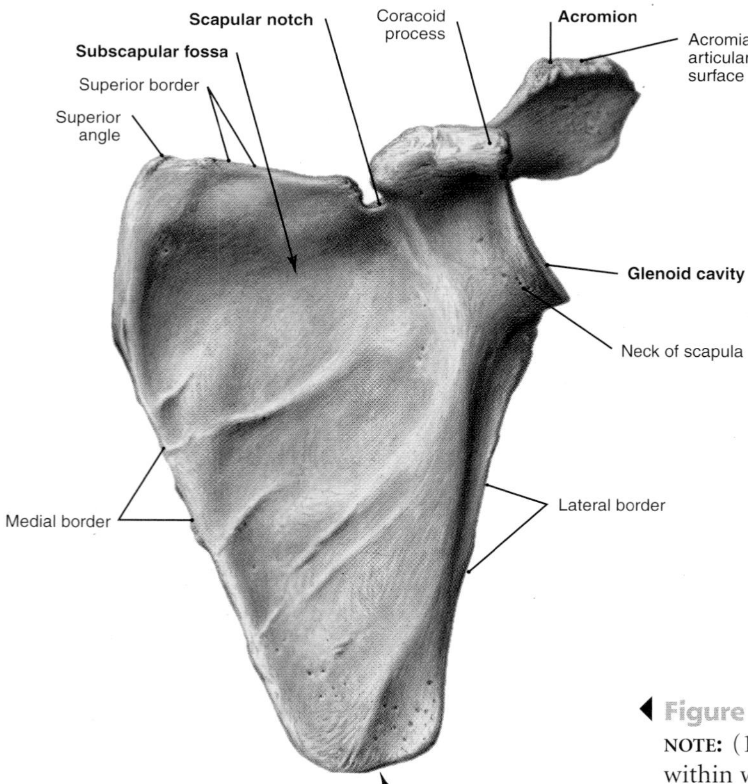
Scapular notch
Subscapular fossa
Superior border
Superior angle
Coracoid process
Acromion
Acromial articular surface
Glenoid cavity
Neck of scapula
Medial border
Lateral border
Inferior angle

Figure 76.3 Left Scapula (Ventral Surface)

NOTE: (1) Much of the ventral surface of the scapula is a concave fossa within which lies the subscapularis muscle.

(2) The scapula has three borders: medial, lateral, and superior; it also has two angles: superior and inferior.

Figures 77.1 and 77.2 Left Humerus

NOTE: (1) The hemispheric head of the humerus articulates with the glenoid cavity of the scapula.

(2) The surgical neck of the humerus is frequently a site of fractures.

(3) On the greater tubercle insert the supraspinatus, infraspinatus, and teres minor, in that order. On the lesser tubercle inserts the subscapularis. These four muscles form the **rotator cuff.**

(4) Within the intertubercular sulcus passes the tendon of the long head of the biceps.

(5) Adjacent to the **radial groove** courses the radial **nerve,** which is endangered by fractures of the humerus.

(6) Injury to the radial nerve in the arm results in a condition called **wrist drop,** because innervation to the extensors of the wrist and fingers is lost.

(7) The distal extremity of the humerus articulates with the radius and ulna, the **capitulum** with the head of the radius, and the **trochlea** with the trochlear notch of the ulna.

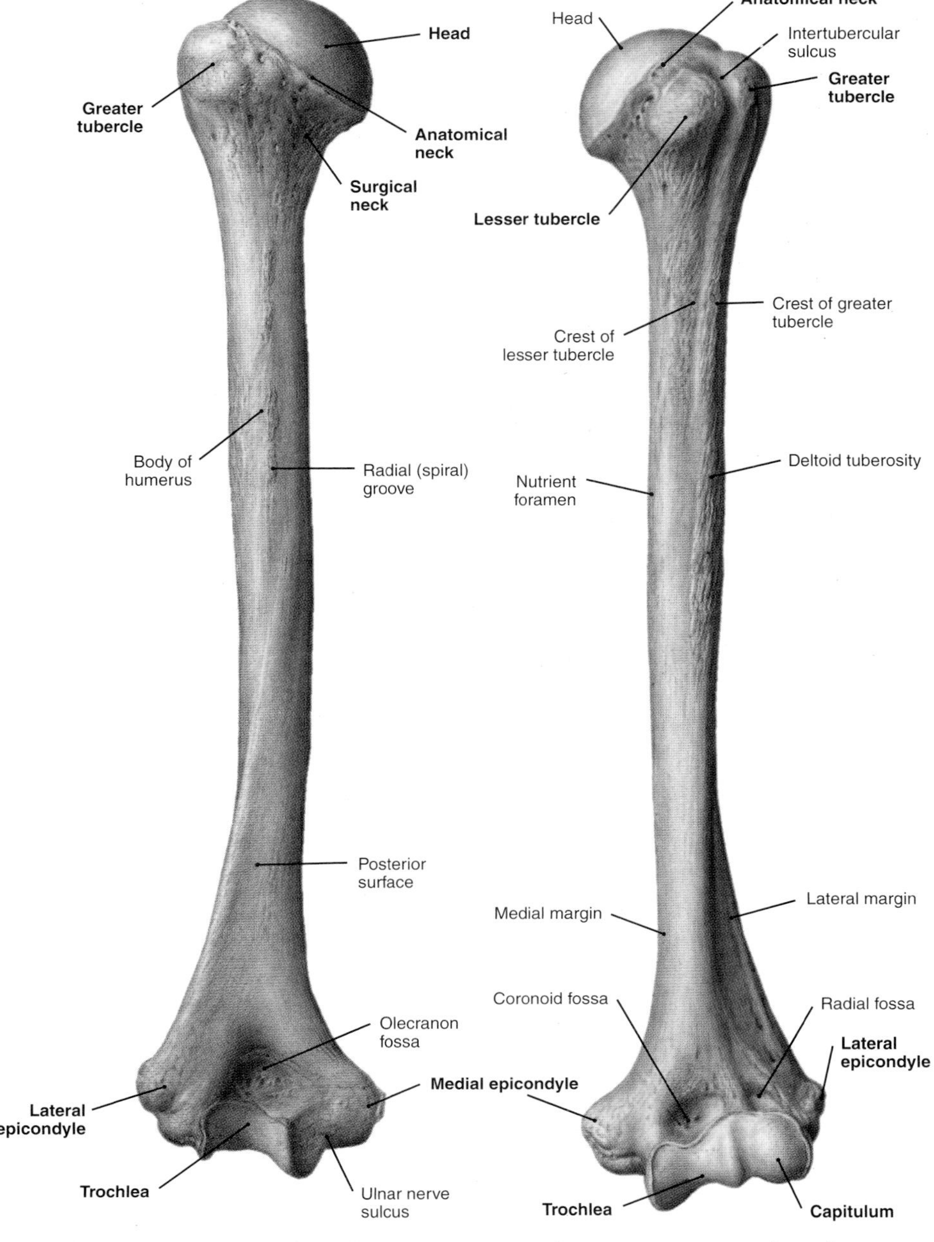
Head
Greater tubercle
Anatomical neck
Surgical neck
Body of humerus
Radial (spiral) groove
Posterior surface
Olecranon fossa
Lateral epicondyle
Medial epicondyle
Trochlea
Ulnar nerve sulcus
Head
Anatomical neck
Intertubercular sulcus
Greater tubercle
Lesser tubercle
Crest of greater tubercle
Crest of lesser tubercle
Deltoid tuberosity
Nutrient foramen
Medial margin
Lateral margin
Coronoid fossa
Radial fossa
Lateral epicondyle
Trochlea
Capitulum

Figure 77.1 Posterior View

Figure 77.2 Anterior View

Lesser tubercle
Intertubercular sulcus
Anatomical neck
For supraspinatus muscle
Greater tubercle
Head of humerus
For infraspinatus muscle
For teres minor muscle

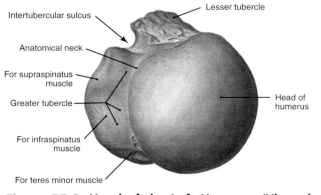

Figure 77.3 Head of the Left Humerus (Viewed from Above)

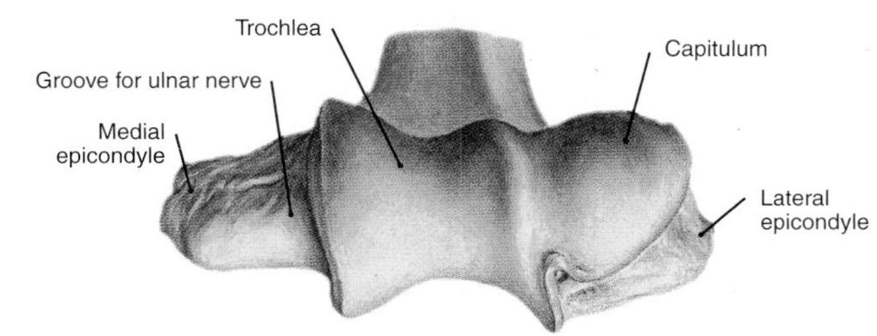
Trochlea
Capitulum
Groove for ulnar nerve
Medial epicondyle
Lateral epicondyle

Figure 77.4 Distal Extremity of the Left Humerus (Viewed from Below)

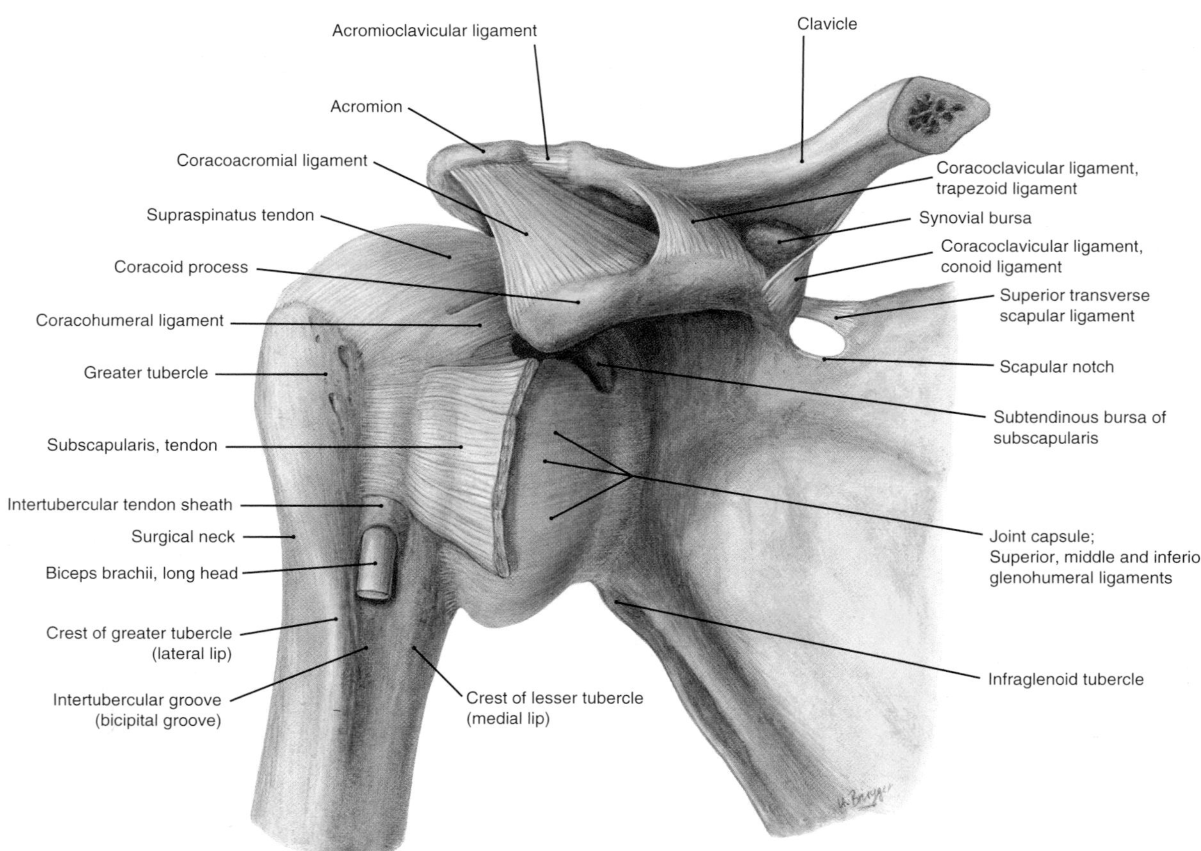
Acromioclavicular ligament
Clavicle
Acromion
Coracoacromial ligament
Supraspinatus tendon
Coracoid process
Coracohumeral ligament
Greater tubercle
Subscapularis, tendon
Intertubercular tendon sheath
Surgical neck
Biceps brachii, long head
Crest of greater tubercle (lateral lip)
Intertubercular groove (bicipital groove)
Crest of lesser tubercle (medial lip)
Coracoclavicular ligament, trapezoid ligament
Synovial bursa
Coracoclavicular ligament, conoid ligament
Superior transverse scapular ligament
Scapular notch
Subtendinous bursa of subscapularis
Joint capsule; Superior, middle and inferior glenohumeral ligaments
Infraglenoid tubercle

Figure 78.1 Ligaments of the Right Shoulder (Glenohumeral) Joint (Anterior View)

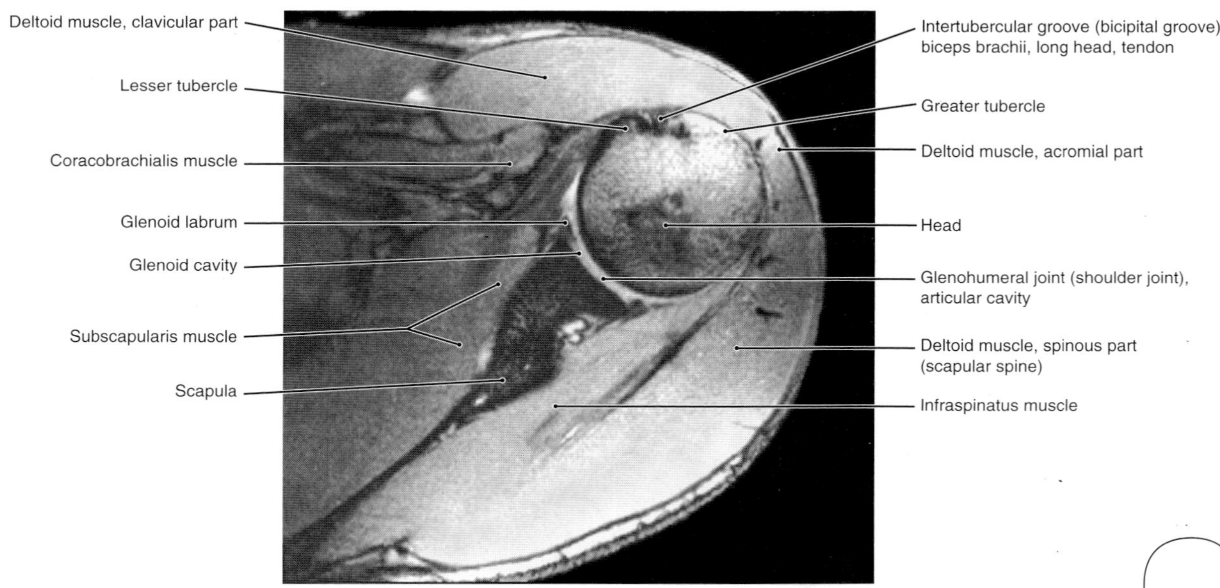
Deltoid muscle, clavicular part
Lesser tubercle
Coracobrachialis muscle
Glenoid labrum
Glenoid cavity
Subscapularis muscle
Scapula
Intertubercular groove (bicipital groove); biceps brachii, long head, tendon
Greater tubercle
Deltoid muscle, acromial part
Head
Glenohumeral joint (shoulder joint), articular cavity
Deltoid muscle, spinous part (scapular spine)
Infraspinatus muscle

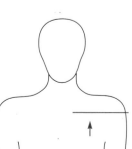

Figure 78.2 MRI Scan of the Left Shoulder Joint (Inferior View)

NOTE: (1) The upper limb is in a neutral position along the side of the chest, and the articular cavity is filled with air.

(2) The humeral head and the lesser and greater tubercles bounding the intertubercular groove within which courses the tendon of the long head of the biceps brachii muscle.

(3) The subscapularis and infraspinatus muscles, two of four muscles of the rotator cuff. The other two muscles (supraspinatus and teres minor) cannot be seen from this view.

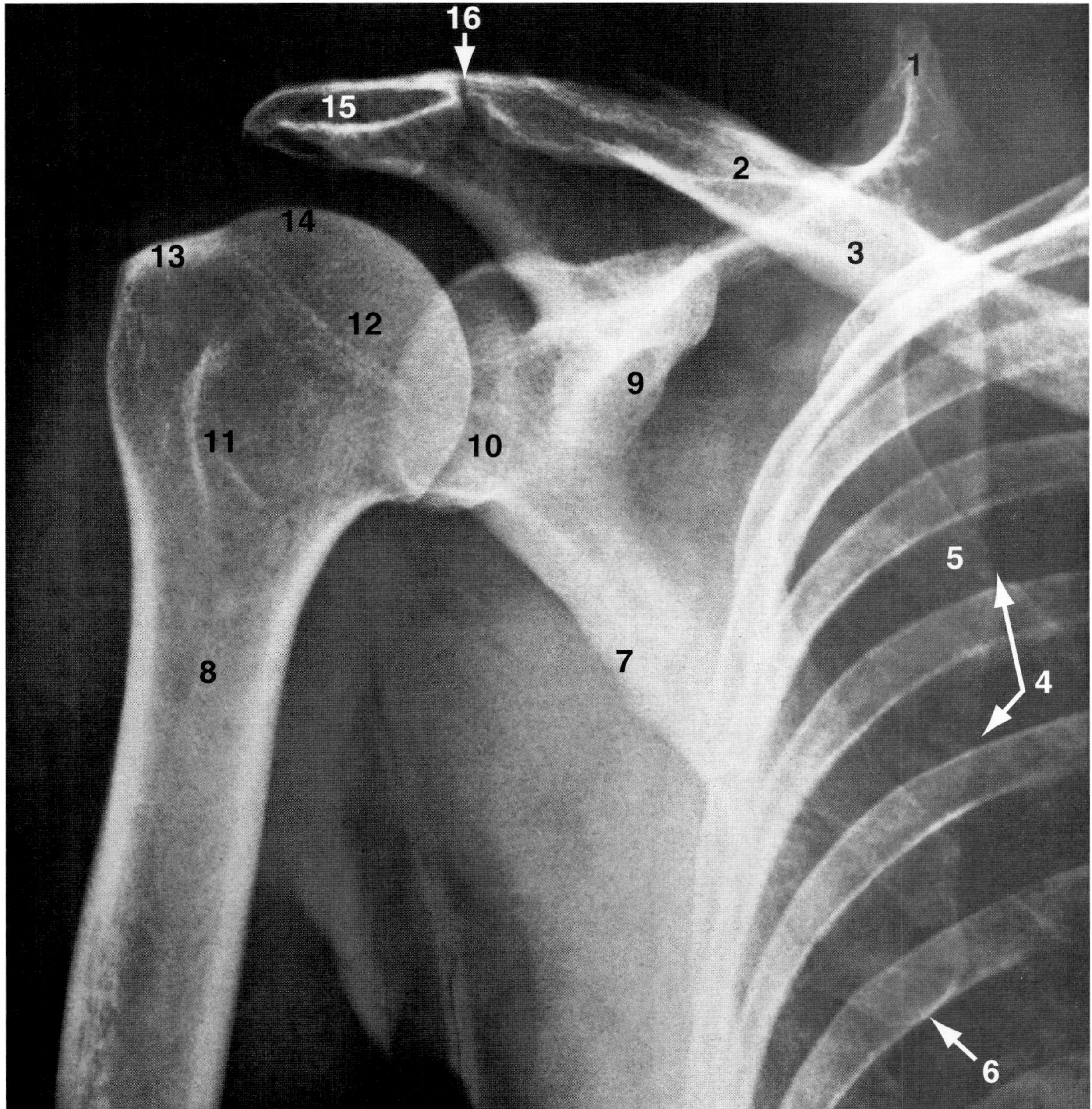
16
1
15
2
14
13
3
12
9
11
10
5
4
8
7
6

Figure 79 **Radiograph of the Right Shoulder Region**

1. Superior angle of scapula
2. Spine of scapula
3. Clavicle
4. Medial margin of scapula
5. Second rib
6. Inferior angle of scapula
7. Lateral margin of scapula
8. Surgical neck of humerus
9. Coracoid process
10. Glenoid cavity
11. Lesser tubercle
12. Anatomical neck of humerus
13. Greater tubercle
14. Head of humerus
15. Acromion
16. Acromioclavicular joint

NOTE: (1) The clavicle, scapula, and humerus are involved in radiography of the shoulder region. The acromioclavicular joint is a **planar** type formed by the lateral end of the clavicle and the medial border of the acromion.

(2) The glenohumeral, or shoulder, joint is remarkably loose and provides a free range of movement. Observe the wide separation between the humeral head and the glenoid cavity.

(3) Inferior **dislocations** of the head of the humerus are common because of minimal protection below. **A shoulder separation** results from a dislocation of the acromion under the lateral edge of the clavicle due to a strong blow to the lateral side of the joint.

(4) The hemispheric smooth surface of the humeral head. Covered with hyalin cartilage, the head of the humerus is slightly constricted at the anatomical neck, where a line separates the articular part superomedially from the greater and lesser tubercles below.

(5) Below these tubercles, the humerus shows another constriction, called the surgical neck, where fractures frequently occur.

(From Wicke, 6th ed.)

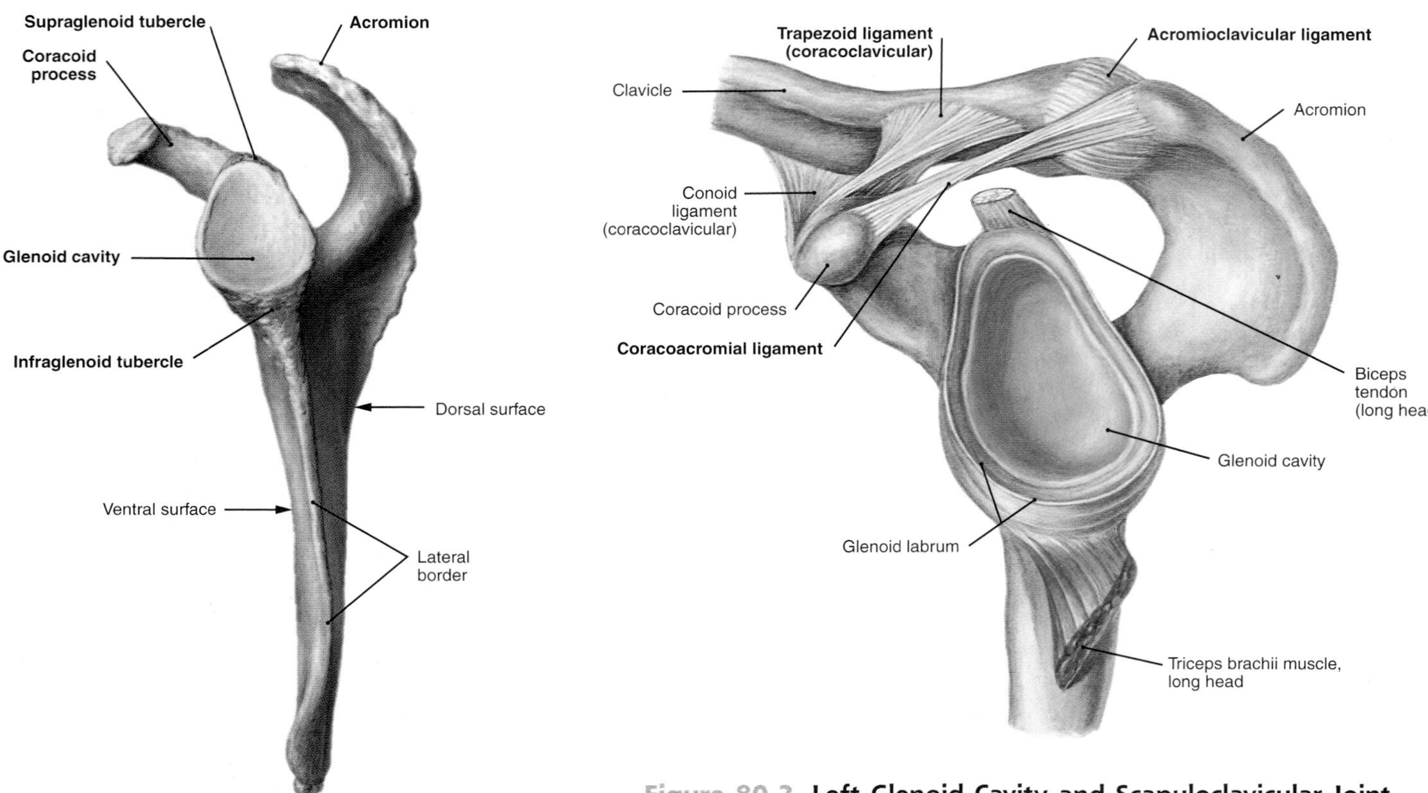
Supraglenoid tubercle
Acromion
Coracoid process
Glenoid cavity
Infraglenoid tubercle
Dorsal surface
Ventral surface
Lateral border
Trapezoid ligament (coracoclavicular)
Acromioclavicular ligament
Clavicle
Acromion
Conoid ligament (coracoclavicular)
Coracoid process
Coracoacromial ligament
Biceps tendon (long heac
Glenoid cavity
Glenoid labrum
Triceps brachii muscle, long head

Figure 80.1 Left Scapula (Lateral View)

NOTE: (1) The supraglenoid and infraglenoid tubercles from which arise the long heads of the biceps and triceps muscles (see Fig. 80.2)

(2) The anteriorly projecting coracoid process to which are attached the pectoralis minor, short head of biceps, and coracobrachialis muscles.

Figure 80.2 Left Glenoid Cavity and Scapuloclavicular Joint (Lateral View)

NOTE: (1) The glenoid cavity was exposed by removing the articular capsule at the glenoid labrum.

(2) The attachments at the supraglenoid (long head of biceps) and infraglenoid (long head of triceps) tubercles have been left intact.

(3) The shallowness of the glenoid cavity is somewhat deepened (3 to 6 mm) by the glenoid labrum.

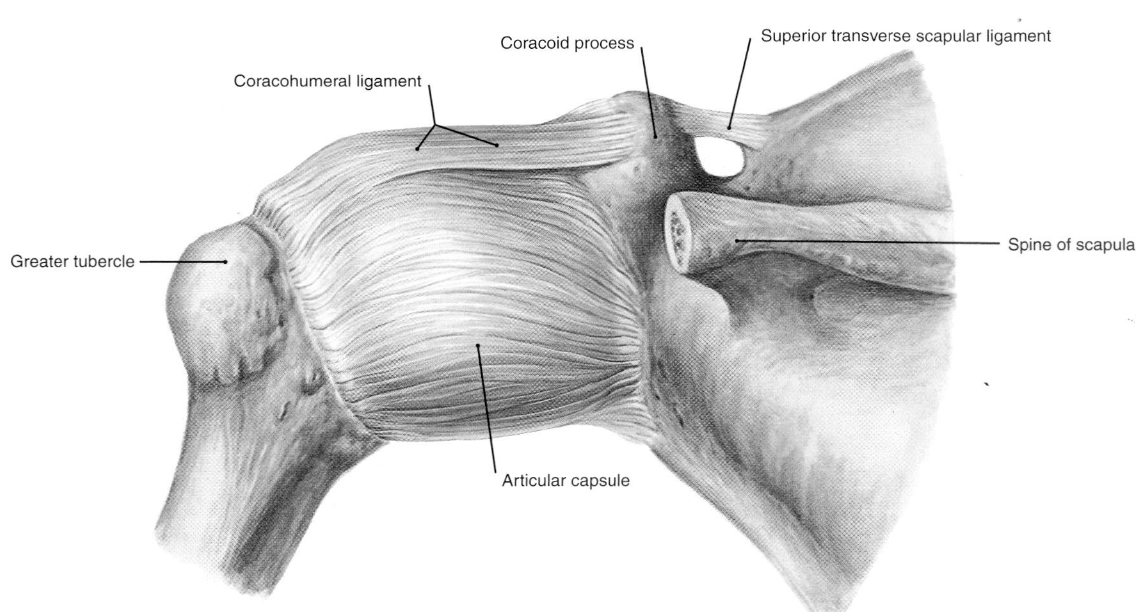
Coracoid process
Superior transverse scapular ligament
Coracohumeral ligament
Greater tubercle
Spine of scapula
Articular capsule

Figure 80.3 Capsule of Left Shoulder Joint (Posterior View)

NOTE: (1) The articular capsule completely surrounds the joint. It is attached beyond the glenoid cavity on the scapula above and to the anatomical neck of the humerus below.

(2) The superior part of the capsule is further strengthened by the coracohumeral ligament.

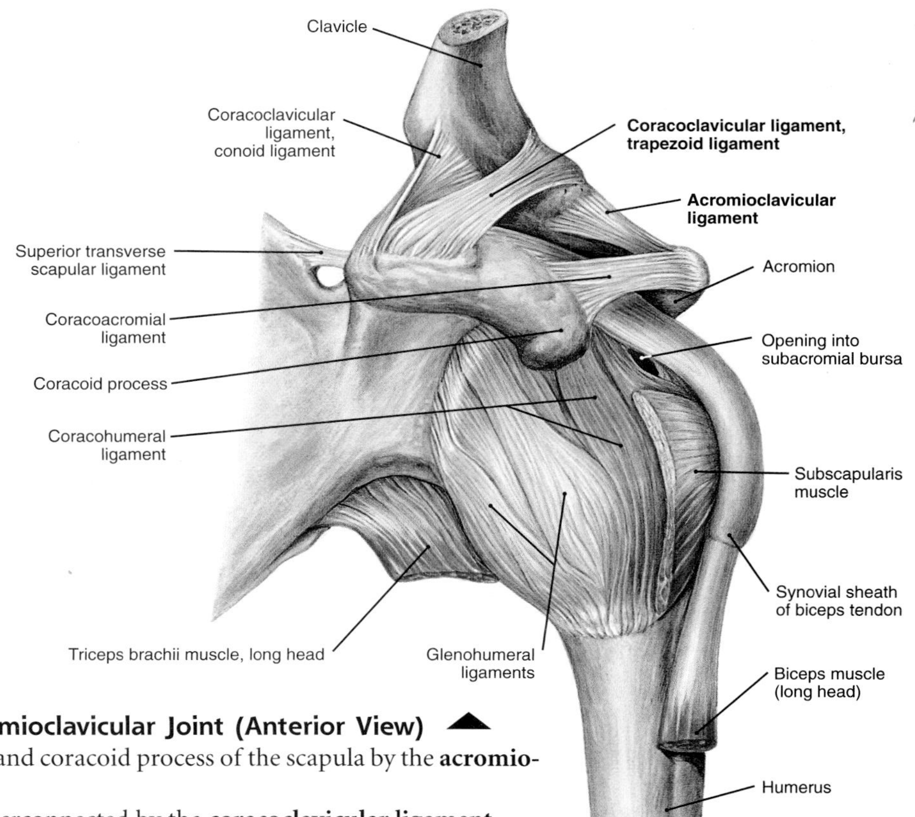
Clavicle
Coracoclavicular ligament, conoid ligament
Coracoclavicular ligament, trapezoid ligament
Acromioclavicular ligament
Superior transverse scapular ligament
Acromion
Coracoacromial ligament
Opening into subacromial bursa
Coracoid process
Coracohumeral ligament
Subscapularis muscle
Synovial sheath of biceps tendon
Triceps brachii muscle, long head
Glenohumeral ligaments
Biceps muscle (long head)
Humerus

Figure 81.1 Left Shoulder Joint and Acromioclavicular Joint (Anterior View)

NOTE: (1) The clavicle is attached to the acromion and coracoid process of the scapula by the **acromioclavicular** and **coracoclavicular ligaments.**

(2) The acromion and coracoid process are interconnected by the **coracoclavicular ligament.**

(3) Neither the acromion nor the clavicle attach to the humerus, but the glenoid labrum and the coracoid process do.

(4) The acromion, coracoid process, and clavicle protect the shoulder from above. The joint is weakest inferiorly and anteriorly, the directions in which most dislocations occur.

(5) The **glenohumeral ligaments** are thickened bands that tend to strengthen the joint capsule anteriorly.

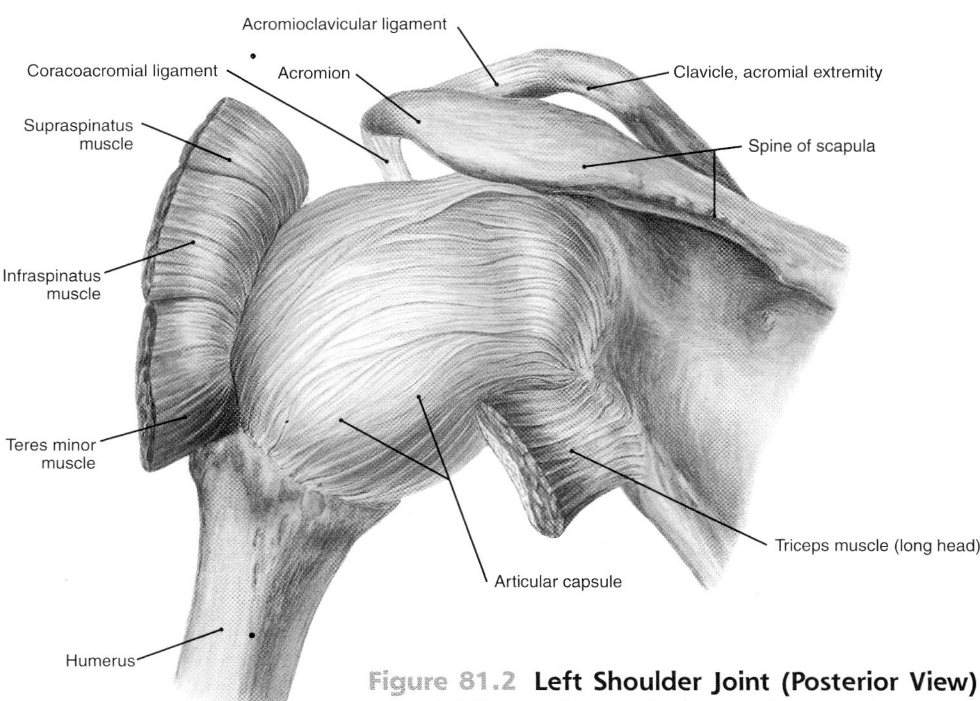
Acromioclavicular ligament
Coracoacromial ligament
Acromion
Clavicle, acromial extremity
Supraspinatus muscle
Spine of scapula
Infraspinatus muscle
Teres minor muscle
Triceps muscle (long head)
Articular capsule
Humerus

Figure 81.2 Left Shoulder Joint (Posterior View)

NOTE: (1) The tendons of the supraspinatus, infraspinatus, and teres minor blend with the joint capsule and form a muscular encasement to help maintain the humeral head in the socket.

(2) The long head of the triceps is attached close to the joint capsule. It is drawn even closer in abduction of the arm and helps prevent dislocation.

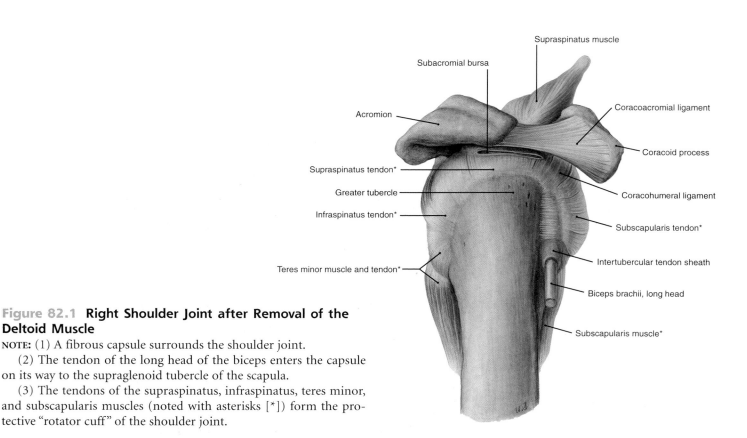

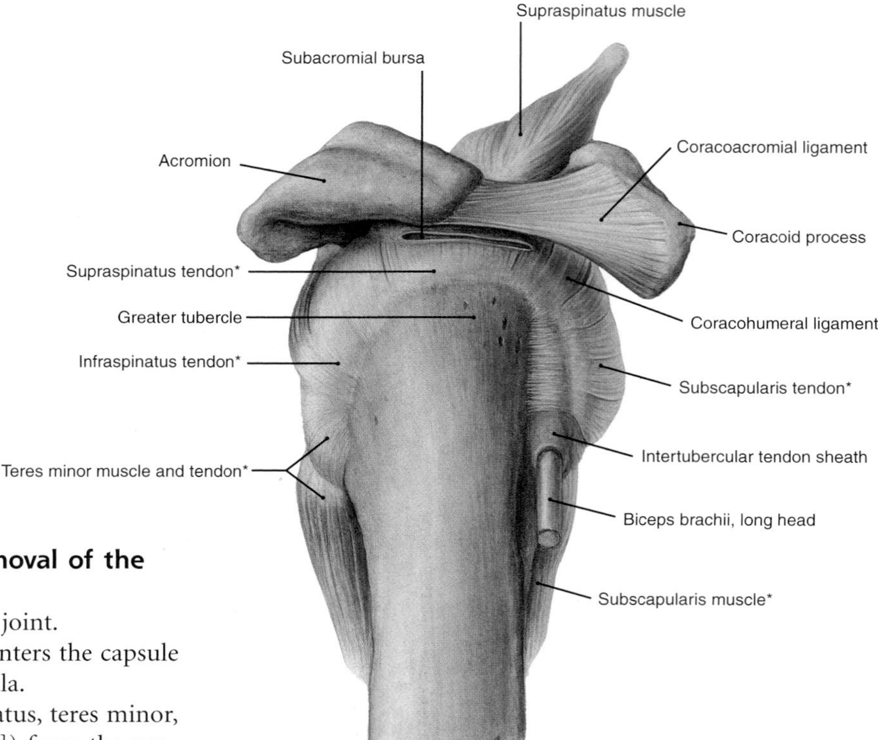
Supraspinatus muscle
Subacromial bursa
Acromion
Coracoacromial ligament
Coracoid process
Supraspinatus tendon*
Greater tubercle
Coracohumeral ligament
Infraspinatus tendon*
Subscapularis tendon*
Intertubercular tendon sheath
Teres minor muscle and tendon*
Biceps brachii, long head
Subscapularis muscle*

Figure 82.1 Right Shoulder Joint after Removal of the Deltoid Muscle

NOTE: (1) A fibrous capsule surrounds the shoulder joint.

(2) The tendon of the long head of the biceps enters the capsule on its way to the supraglenoid tubercle of the scapula.

(3) The tendons of the supraspinatus, infraspinatus, teres minor, and subscapularis muscles (noted with asterisks [*]) form the protective "rotator cuff" of the shoulder joint.

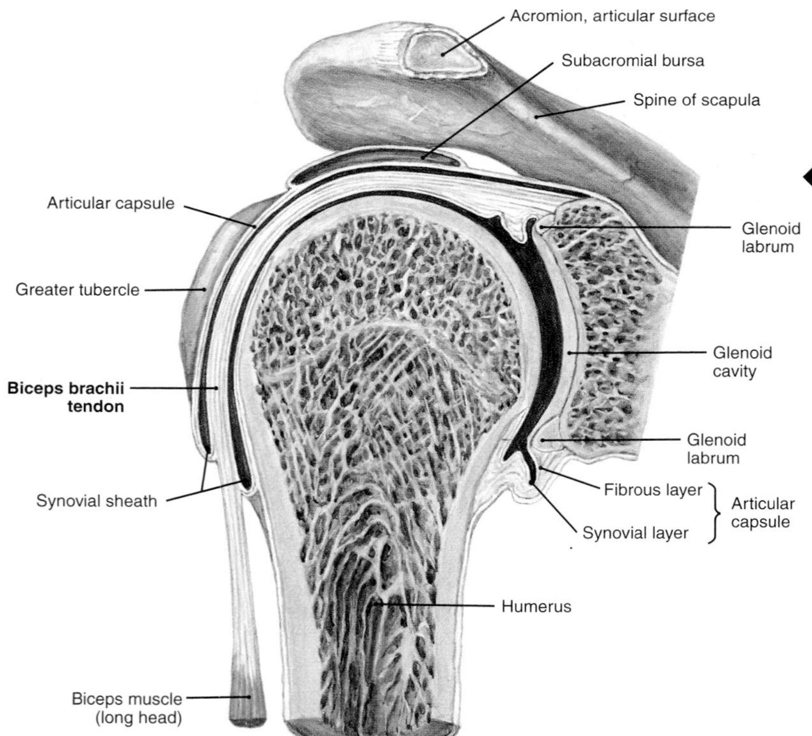
Acromion, articular surface
Subacromial bursa
Spine of scapula
Articular capsule
Glenoid labrum
Greater tubercle
Glenoid cavity
Biceps brachii tendon
Glenoid labrum
Fibrous layer
Synovial layer
Articular capsule
Synovial sheath
Humerus
Biceps muscle (long head)

Figure 82.2 Frontal Section through the Right Shoulder Joint

NOTE: (1) The tendon of the long head of the biceps is enclosed by a synovial sheath. Although the tendon passes through the joint, it is not within the synovial cavity.

(2) The capsule of the joint is composed of a dense outer fibrous layer and a thin synovial inner layer.

(3) A bursa is a sac lined by a synovial-like membrane. They are found at sites subjected to friction and usually do not communicate with the joint cavity.

(4) In the shoulder, bursae are found between the capsule and muscle tendons such as the subscapularis, infraspinatus, and deltoid. The **subacromial bursa** lies deep to the coracoid and acromial processes.

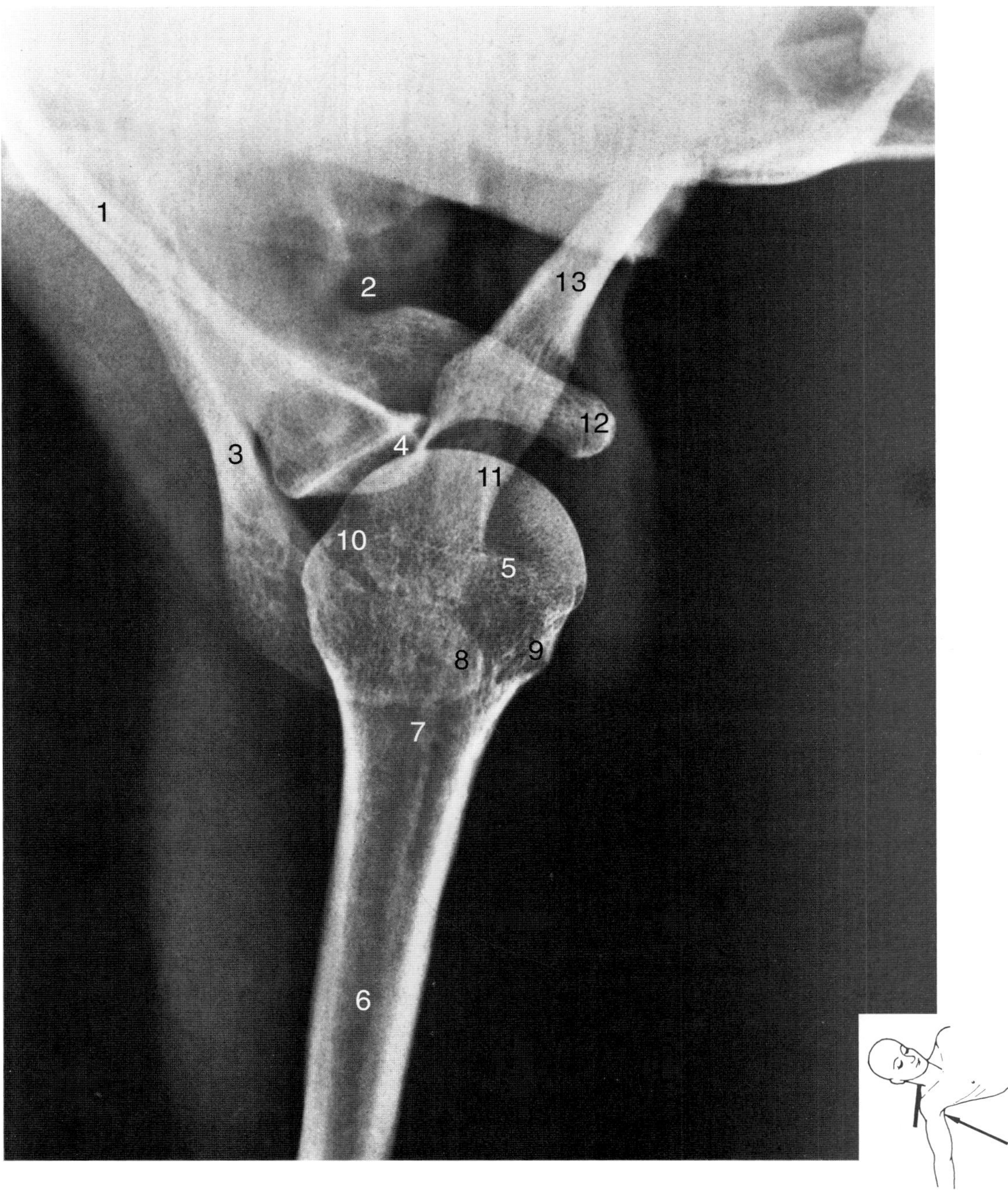
1
2
13
12
3
4
11
10
5
9
8
7
6

Figure 83 Radiograph of the Right Shoulder Joint

NOTE: This is an axial (longitudinal) view of the shoulder joint with the scapula and clavicle superior and the shaft of the humerus projecting inferiorly.

1. Scapula
2. Scapular notch
3. Spine of the scapula
4. Glenoid fossa
5. Greater tubercle
6. Shaft of the humerus
7. Surgical neck of the humerus
8. Acromion
9. Lesser tubercle
10. Anatomical neck of the humerus
11. Head of the humerus
12. Coracoid process
13. Clavicle

(From Wicke, 6th ed.)

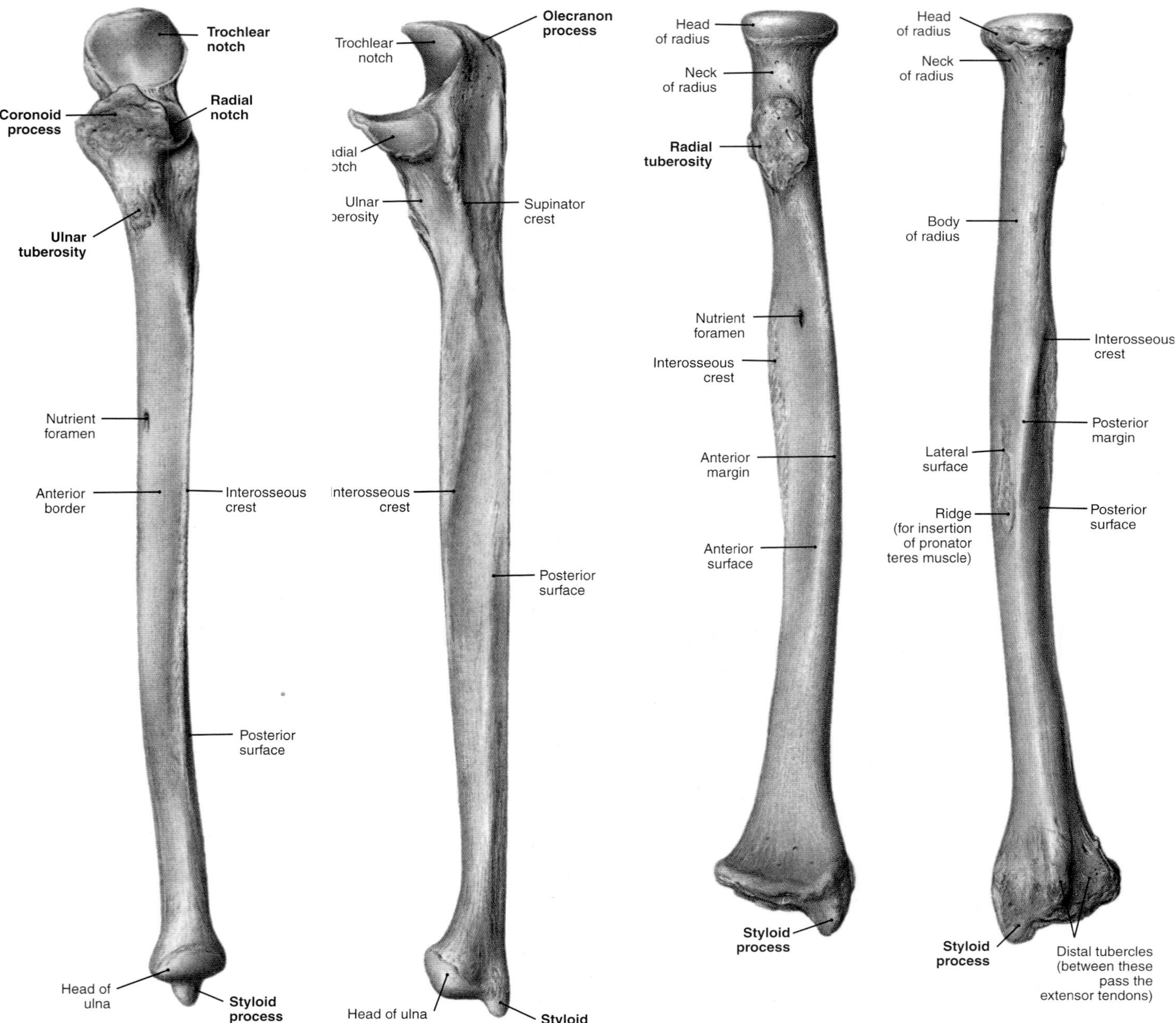

Trochlear notch
Radial notch
Coronoid process
Ulnar tuberosity
Nutrient foramen
Anterior border
Interosseous crest
Posterior surface
Head of ulna
Styloid process
Olecranon process
Trochlear notch
Supinator crest
Posterior surface
Head of ulna
Styloid process
Head of radius
Neck of radius
Radial tuberosity
Nutrient foramen
Interosseous crest
Anterior margin
Anterior surface
Styloid process
Head of radius
Neck of radius
Body of radius
Interosseous crest
Posterior margin
Lateral surface
Ridge (for insertion of pronator teres muscle)
Posterior surface
Styloid process
Distal tubercles (between these pass the extensor tendons)

Figure 84.1 **Anterior Ulna**

Figure 84.2 **Lateral Ulna**

Figure 84.3 **Anterior Radius**

Figure 84.4 **Posterior Radius**

Left Ulna (Figs. 84.1 and 84.2)

NOTE: (1) The ulna is the medial bone of forearm. It has a superior extremity, a body or shaft, and an inferior extremity.

(2) The **superior extremity** contains the **olecranon** and **coronoid processes** and two cavities: the **radial notch** for articulation with the radius and the **trochlear notch** for the trochlea of the humerus.

(3) The brachialis muscle inserts on the tuberosity of the ulna.

(4) Along the **body** of the ulna attaches the interosseous membrane.

(5) The **distal extremity** is marked by the **ulnar head** laterally and the **styloid process** posteromedially.

Left Radius (Figs. 84.3 and 84.4)

NOTE: (1) The radius is situated lateral to the ulna, and it has a body and two extremities. Proximally, it attaches to both the humerus and ulna. Distally, it articulates with the carpal bones (scaphoid, lunate, and triquetrum) and with the ulna.

(2) The **proximal extremity** contains a cylindrical head that articulates with both the **capitulum** of the humerus and the **radial notch** of the ulna.

(3) Onto the **radial tuberosity** inserts the tendon of the biceps brachii.

(4) Onto the **styloid process** attaches the brachioradialis muscle and the radial collateral ligament of the radiocarpal joint.

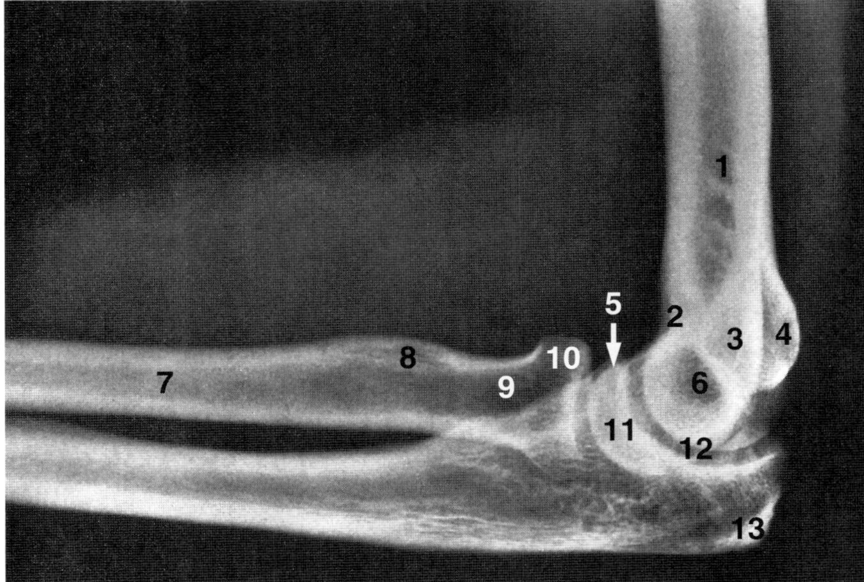
1
2
3
4
5
6
7
8
9
10
11
12
13

Figure 85.1 Radiograph of the Left Elbow Joint in an Adult (Lateral View)
(From Wicke, 6th ed.)

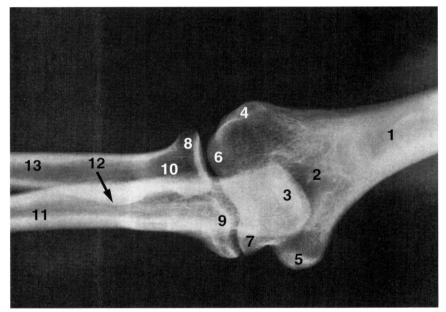

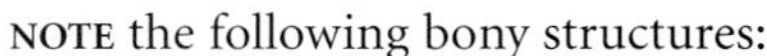

NOTE the following bony structures:
1. Body of humerus
2. Radial fossa
3. Olecranon fossa
4. Medial epicondyle
5. Coronoid process of ulna
6. Trochlea of humerus
7. Body of radius
8. Radial tuberosity
9. Neck of radius
10. Head of radius
11. Capitulum of humerus
12. Trochlear notch
13. Olecranon

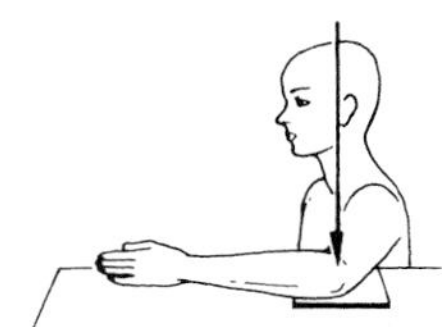

Figure 85.2 Radiograph of the Right Elbow Joint in an Adult (Anteroposterior View)
(From Wicke, 6th ed.)

NOTE the following bony structures:
1. Body of humerus
2. Olecranon fossa
3. Olecranon
4. Lateral epicondyle
5. Medial epicondyle
6. Capitulum of humerus
7. Trochlea of humerus
8. Head of radius
9. Coronoid process of ulna
10. Neck of radius
11. Ulna
12. Radial tuberosity
13. Body of radius

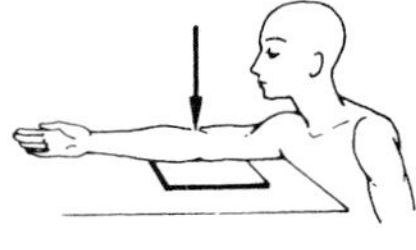

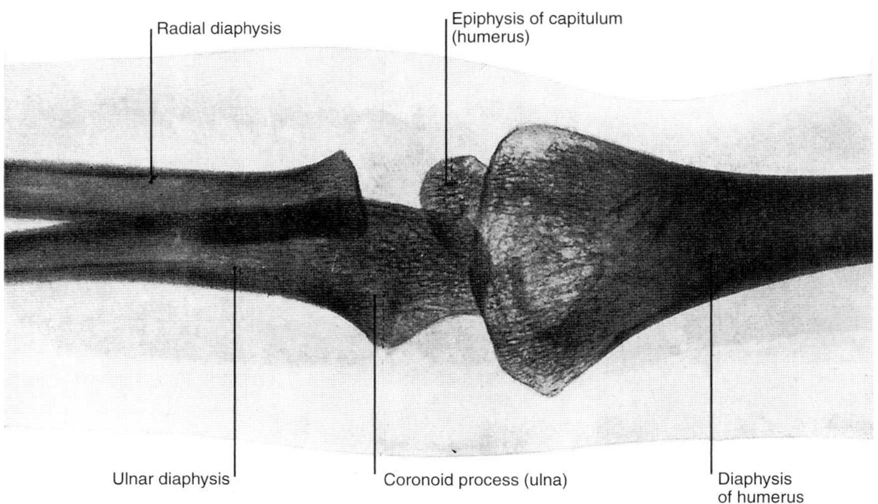
Radial diaphysis
Epiphysis of capitulum (humerus)
Ulnar diaphysis
Coronoid process (ulna)
Diaphysis of humerus

Figure 85.3 **Radiograph of the Elbow Joint in a $5\frac{1}{2}$-Year-Old Boy**

NOTE: (1) The shaft of a long bone is called the **diaphysis,** whereas a center of ossification, distinct from the shaft and usually at the end of a long bone, is called an **epiphysis.**

(2) The epiphysis of the head of the radius is as yet not formed in the $5\frac{1}{2}$-year-old child, whereas ossification has started in the humeral capitulum.

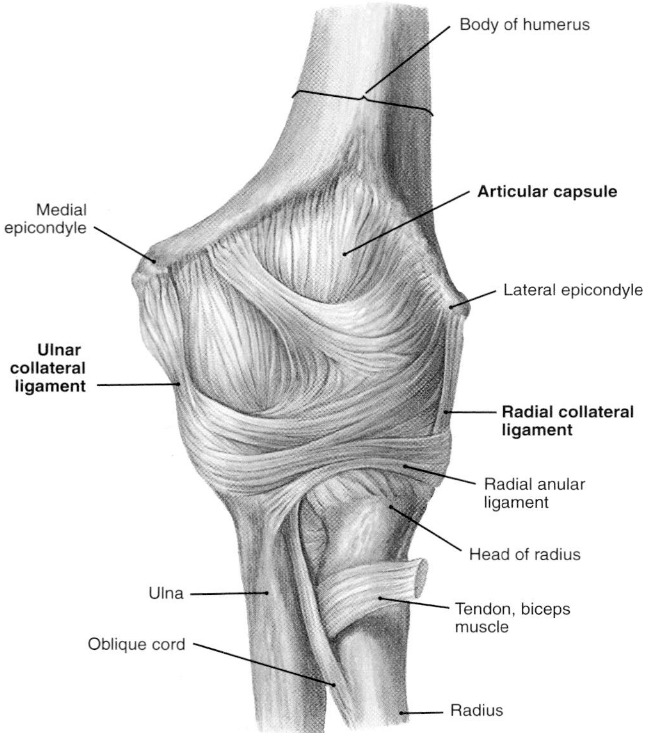
Body of humerus
Articular capsule
Medial epicondyle
Lateral epicondyle
Ulnar collateral ligament
Radial collateral ligament
Radial anular ligament
Head of radius
Ulna
Tendon, biceps muscle
Oblique cord
Radius

Figure 86.1 Left Elbow Joint (Anterior View)

NOTE: (1) The elbow joint is a hinge, or ginglymus, joint.

(2) The **trochlea** of the humerus is received in the trochlear notch of the ulna.

(3) The capitulum of the humerus articulates with the head of the radius.

(4) The articular capsule is loose but is thickened medially and laterally by the ulnar and **radial collateral** ligaments

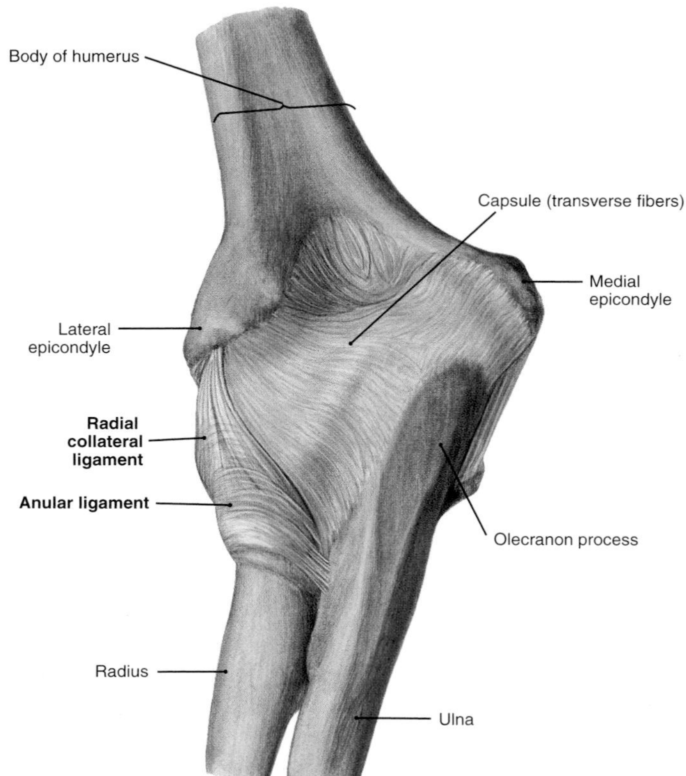
Body of humerus
Capsule (transverse fibers)
Medial epicondyle
Lateral epicondyle
Radial collateral ligament
Anular ligament
Olecranon process
Radius
Ulna

Figure 86.2 Left Elbow Joint (Posterolateral View)

NOTE: (1) The fan-shaped **radial collateral ligament** attaches above to the lateral epicondyle and blends with the capsule.

(2) The upper border of the **radial anular ligament** also blends with the joint capsule.

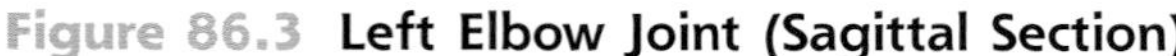

Figure 86.3 Left Elbow Joint (Sagittal Section)

NOTE: (1) The adaptation of the trochlea of the humerus with the trochlear notch of the ulna allows only flexion and extension, not lateral displacement.

(2) The posterior surface of the olecranon is separated from the skin by a subcutaneous bursa and the insertion of the triceps.

(3) **Fractures** of the distal end of the humerus occur most often from falls on the outstretched hand, because the force is transmitted through the bones of the forearm to the humerus.

(4) **Fractures** of the olecranon result from direct trauma to the bone by a fall on the point of the elbow.

(5) **Posterior dislocation** of the ulna and attached radius is the most common dislocation at the elbow joint, again from falls on the outstretched and abducted hand.

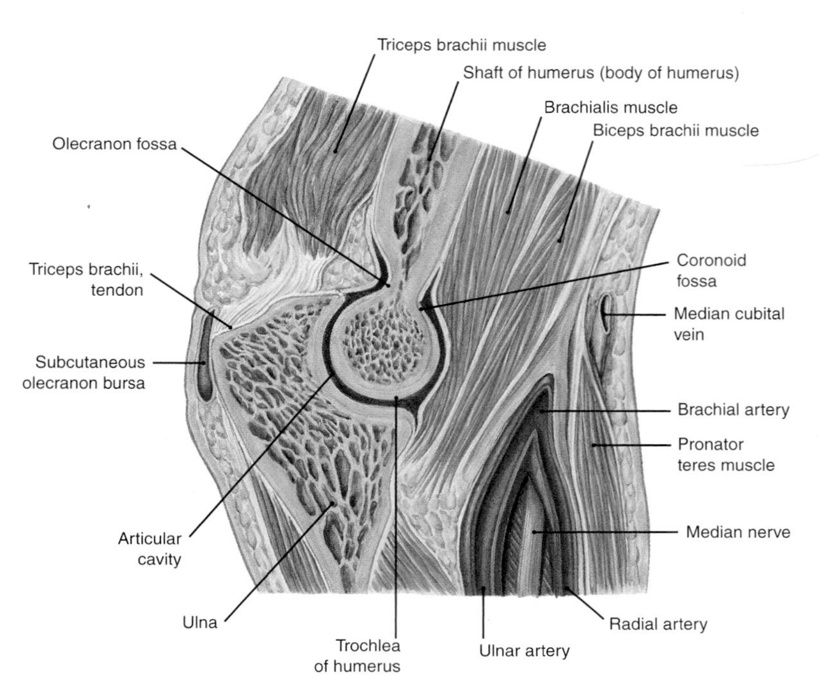
Triceps brachii muscle
Shaft of humerus (body of humerus)
Brachialis muscle
Biceps brachii muscle
Olecranon fossa
Triceps brachii, tendon
Coronoid fossa
Median cubital vein
Subcutaneous olecranon bursa
Brachial artery
Pronator teres muscle
Median nerve
Articular cavity
Ulna
Trochlea of humerus
Ulnar artery
Radial artery

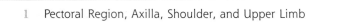

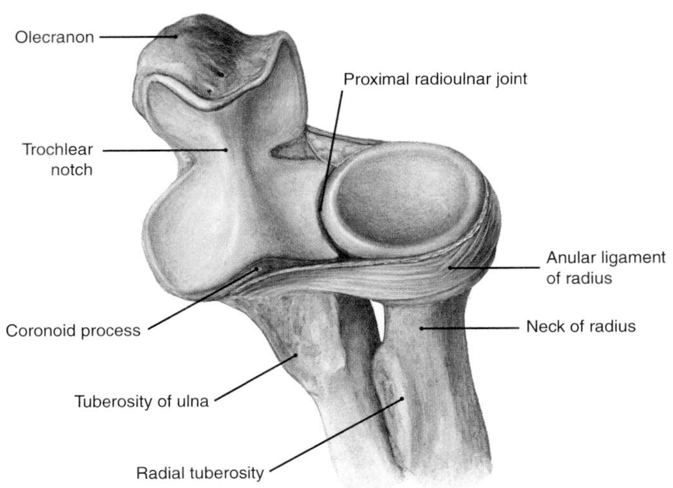
Olecranon
Proximal radioulnar joint
Trochlear notch
Anular ligament of radius
Coronoid process
Neck of radius
Tuberosity of ulna
Radial tuberosity

Figure 87.1 Left Proximal Radioulnar Joint

NOTE: (1) This anterior view of the proximal radioulnar joint (oriented similar to Fig. 86.1) shows the anular ligament surrounding the head of the radius. The ligament attaches to the ulna both anteriorly and posteriorly.

(2) The radial tuberosity onto which inserts the biceps brachii and the olecranon where the triceps brachii inserts

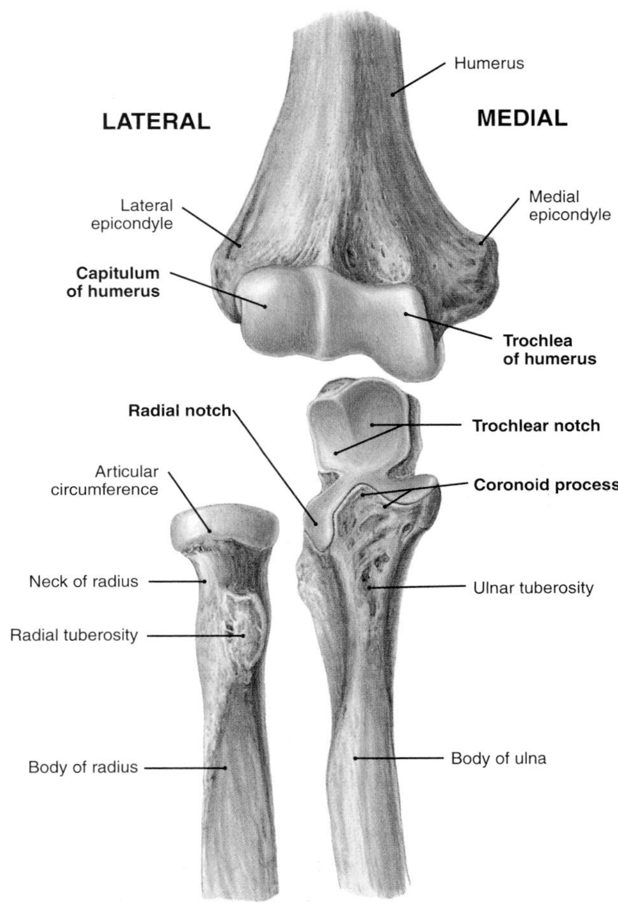
Humerus
LATERAL
MEDIAL
Lateral epicondyle
Medial epicondyle
Capitulum of humerus
Trochlea of humerus
Radial notch
Trochlear notch
Articular circumference
Coronoid process
Neck of radius
Ulnar tuberosity
Radial tuberosity
Body of radius
Body of ulna

Figure 87.2 Bones of the Right Elbow and Radioulnar Joints (Anterior View)

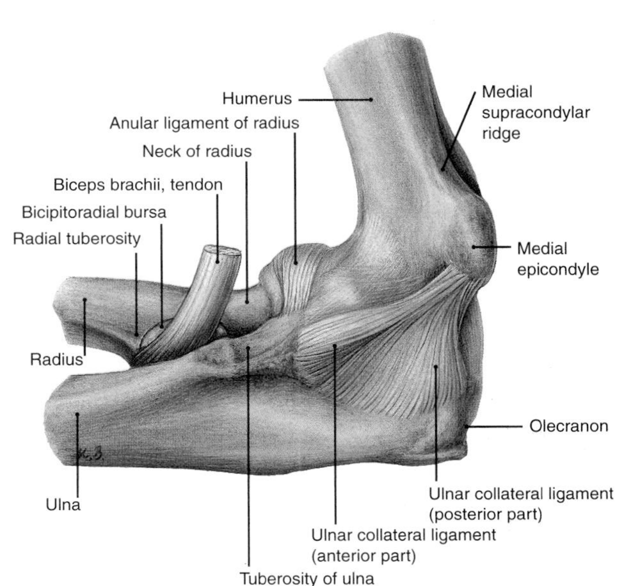
Humerus
Anular ligament of radius
Neck of radius
Biceps brachii, tendon
Bicipitoradial bursa
Radial tuberosity
Medial supracondylar ridge
Medial epicondyle
Radius
Olecranon
Ulna
Ulnar collateral ligament (posterior part)
Ulnar collateral ligament (anterior part)
Tuberosity of ulna

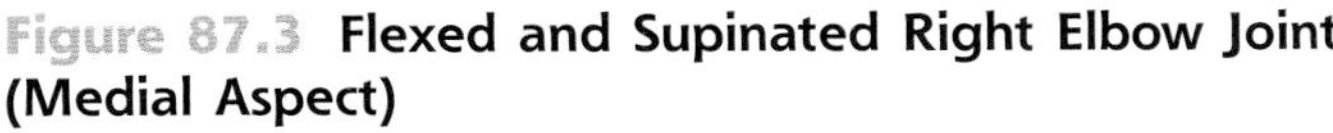

Figure 87.3 Flexed and Supinated Right Elbow Joint (Medial Aspect)

NOTE: (1) The anterior and posterior parts of the ulnar (medial) collateral ligament.

(2) The anular ligament encasing the head of the radius.

(3) The insertion of the biceps brachii tendon onto the tuberosity of the radius.

(4) The olecranon of the ulna onto which the triceps brachii (not shown) inserts.

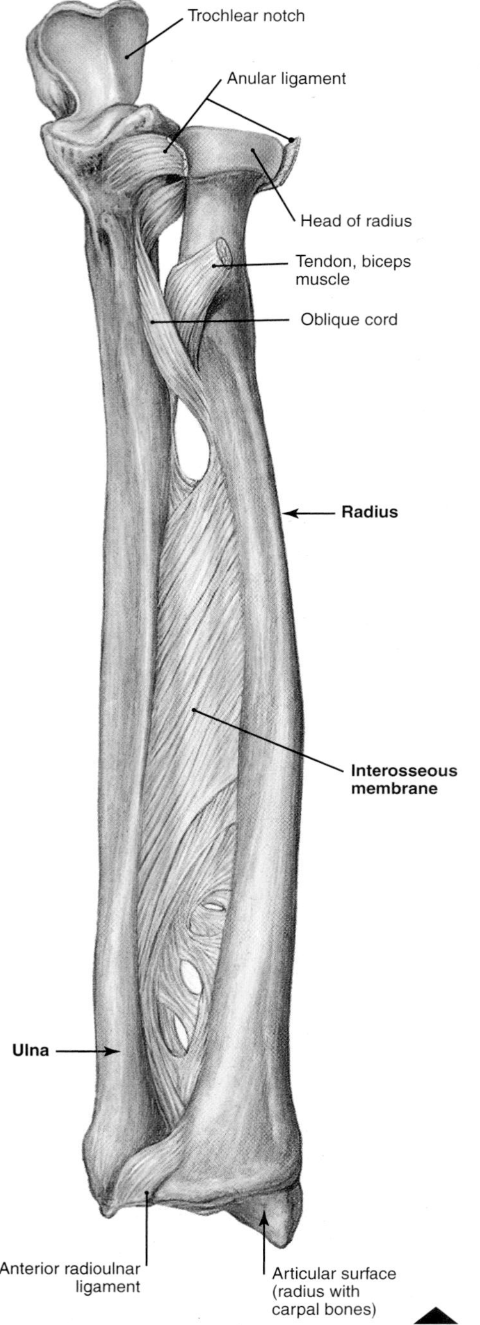

Trochlear notch
Anular ligament
Head of radius
Tendon, biceps muscle
Oblique cord
Radius
Interosseous membrane
Ulna
Anterior radioulnar ligament
Articular surface (radius with carpal bones)

Figure 88.1 Radioulnar Joints (Anterior View, Left)

NOTE: (1) The radius and ulna articulate proximally, along the shafts of the two bones, and distally.

(2) Proximally the head of the radius rotates within the radial notch of the ulna (pivot or trochoid joint).

(3) The **annular ligament,** attached at both ends to the ulna, encircles the head of the radius, protecting the joint.

(4) The interosseous membrane extends obliquely between the shafts of the two bones, whereas distally the head of the ulna attaches to the ulnar notch of the radius.

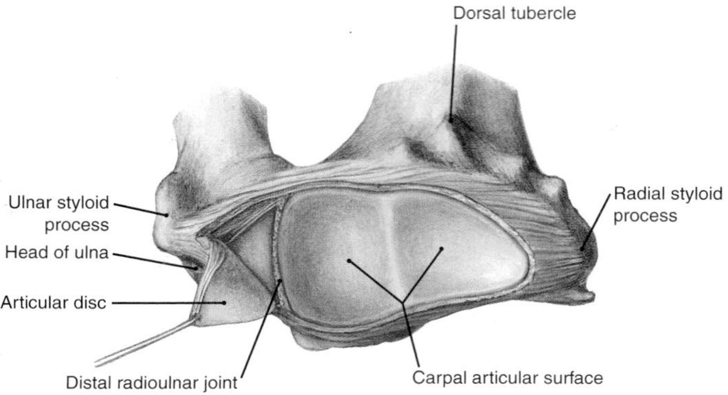

Dorsal tubercle
Ulnar styloid process
Head of ulna
Articular disc
Distal radioulnar joint
Carpal articular surface
Radial styloid process

Figure 88.2 Right Radioulnar Joint

NOTE: (1) The lateral surface of the distal radius and the medial surface of the distal ulna form the distal radioulnar joint.

(2) The synovial cavity at this joint is L-shaped and is interposed between the distal end of the ulna and an articular disk. This cavity extends superiorly between the lateral surface of the distal radius and the medial surface of the distal ulna.

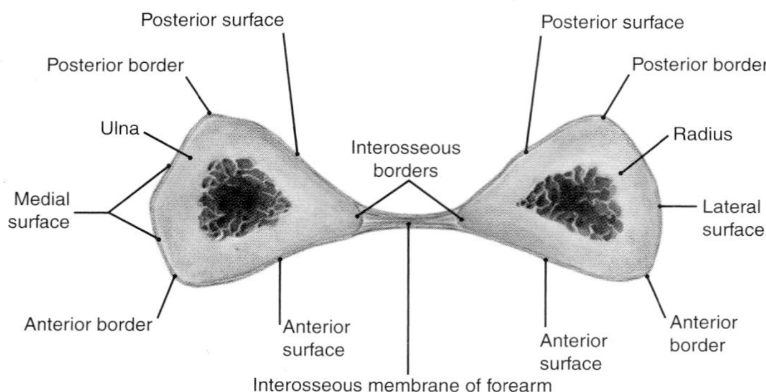

Posterior surface
Posterior border
Ulna
Medial surface
Anterior border
Anterior surface
Interosseous borders
Interosseous membrane of forearm
Posterior surface
Posterior border
Radius
Lateral surface
Anterior surface
Anterior border

Figure 88.3 Bones of the Forearm (Transverse Section)

NOTE: (1) The interosseous membrane between the shafts of the radius and ulna. This membrane greatly strengthens the bony structures of the forearm.

(2) If a significant force ascends in the forearm (such as from a fall onto the outstretched hand) the interosseous membrane helps to dissipate the impact of the fall. It does this by transmitting a part of the force to the other bone, thereby helping to prevent fractures of the forearm bones.

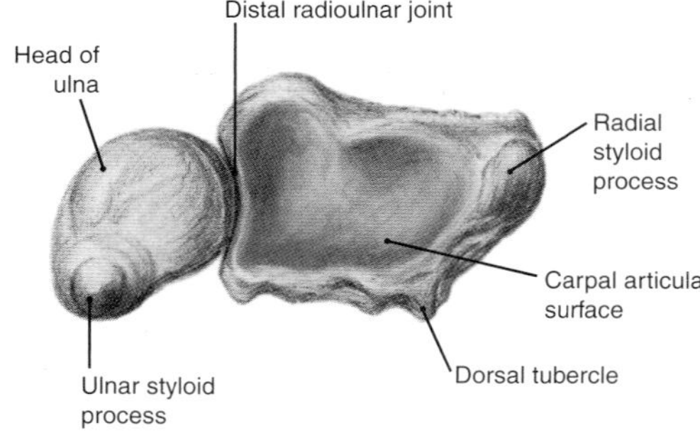

Distal radioulnar joint
Head of ulna
Radial styloid process
Carpal articular surface
Dorsal tubercle
Ulnar styloid process

Figure 88.4 Distal Aspect of the Left Radius and Ulna

NOTE that the distal extremity of both bones is marked by a styloid process. Between the lateral side of the distal end of the ulna and the medial side of the wide lower end of the radius is located the distal radioulnar joint.

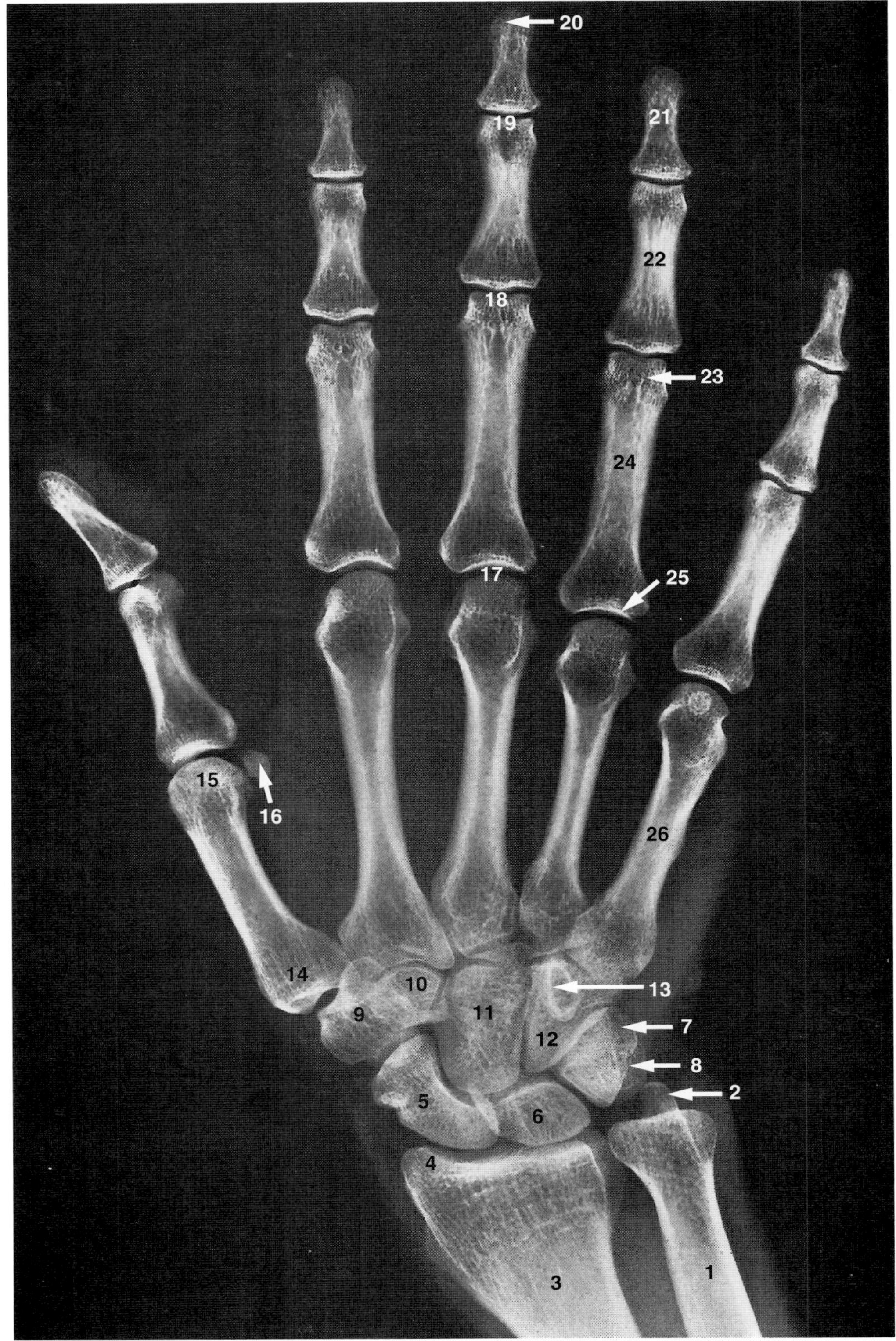
20
19
21
22
18
23
24
17
25
15
16
26
14
10
13
11
9
12
7
8
2
5
6
4
3
1

Figure 89 Radiograph of the Right Wrist and Hand (Dorsopalmar View)

1. Ulna
2. Styloid process of ulna
3. Radius
4. Styloid process of radius
5. Scaphoid
6. Lunate
7. Triquetral
8. Pisiform
9. Trapezium
10. Trapezoid
11. Capitate
12. Hamate
13. Hamulus of hamate
14. Base of first metacarpal bone
15. Head of first metacarpal bone
16. Sesamoid bone
17. Metacarpophalangeal joint
18. Proximal interphalangeal joint
19. Distal interphalangeal joint
20. Tuberosity of distal phalanx
21. Distal phalanx
22. Middle phalanx
23. Head of phalanx
24. Proximal phalanx
25. Base of phalanx
26. Fifth metacarpal bone

(From Wicke, 6th ed.)

Figure 90.1 Skeleton of the Right Wrist and Hand (Palmar View)

NOTE: (1) **Carpal bones**: 8; **metacarpal bones**: 5; **phalanges**: 14 (thumb has 2, each of the other 4 fingers has 3)

(2) **Carpal bones**, lateral to medial:

Proximal Row	**Distal Row**
Scaphoid	Trapezium
Lunate	Trapezoid
Triquetrum	Capitate
Pisiform	Hamate

3) **Metacarpal bones:**

(a) First is shortest

(b) Second is longest

(c) Each has a **base** (carpal end), a **body**, and a **head** (distal end)

(4) **Phalanges:**

(a) Those of four medial fingers are set in transverse rows—**proximal, middle** and **distal.**

(b) The thumb has only a proximal and a distal phalanx.

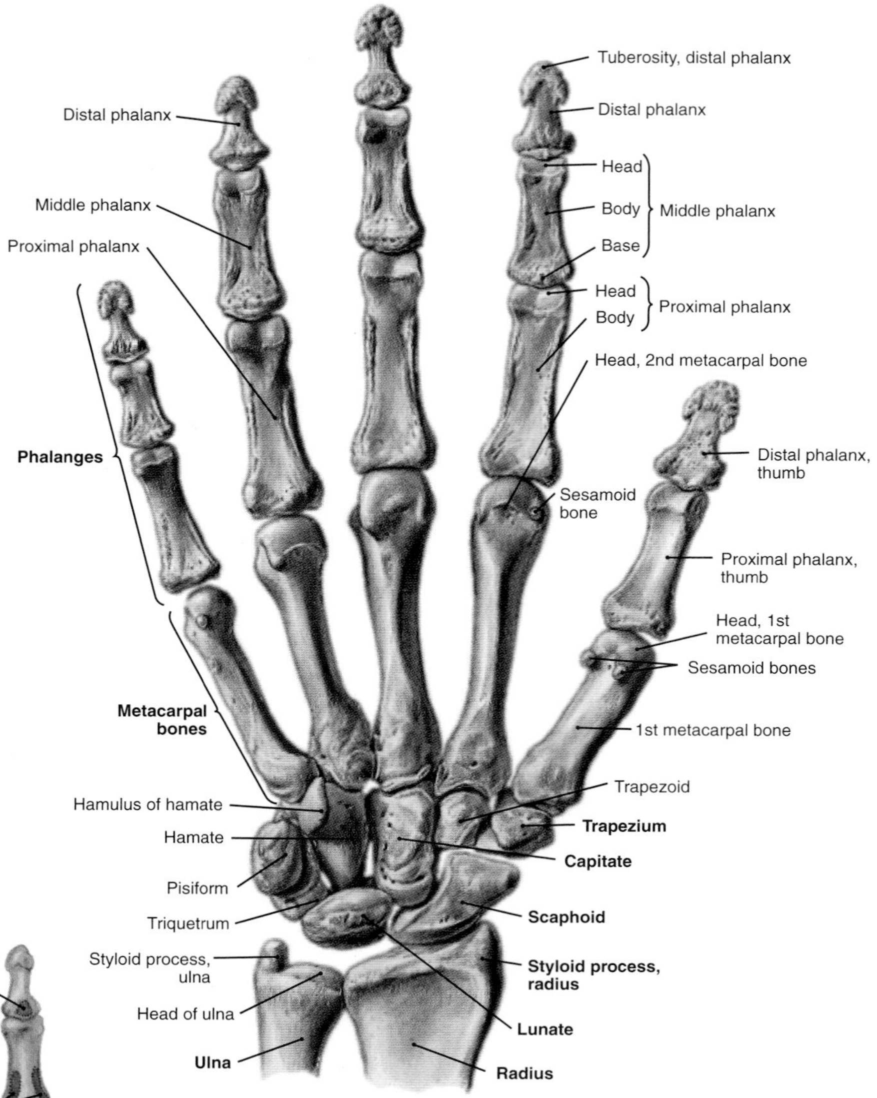

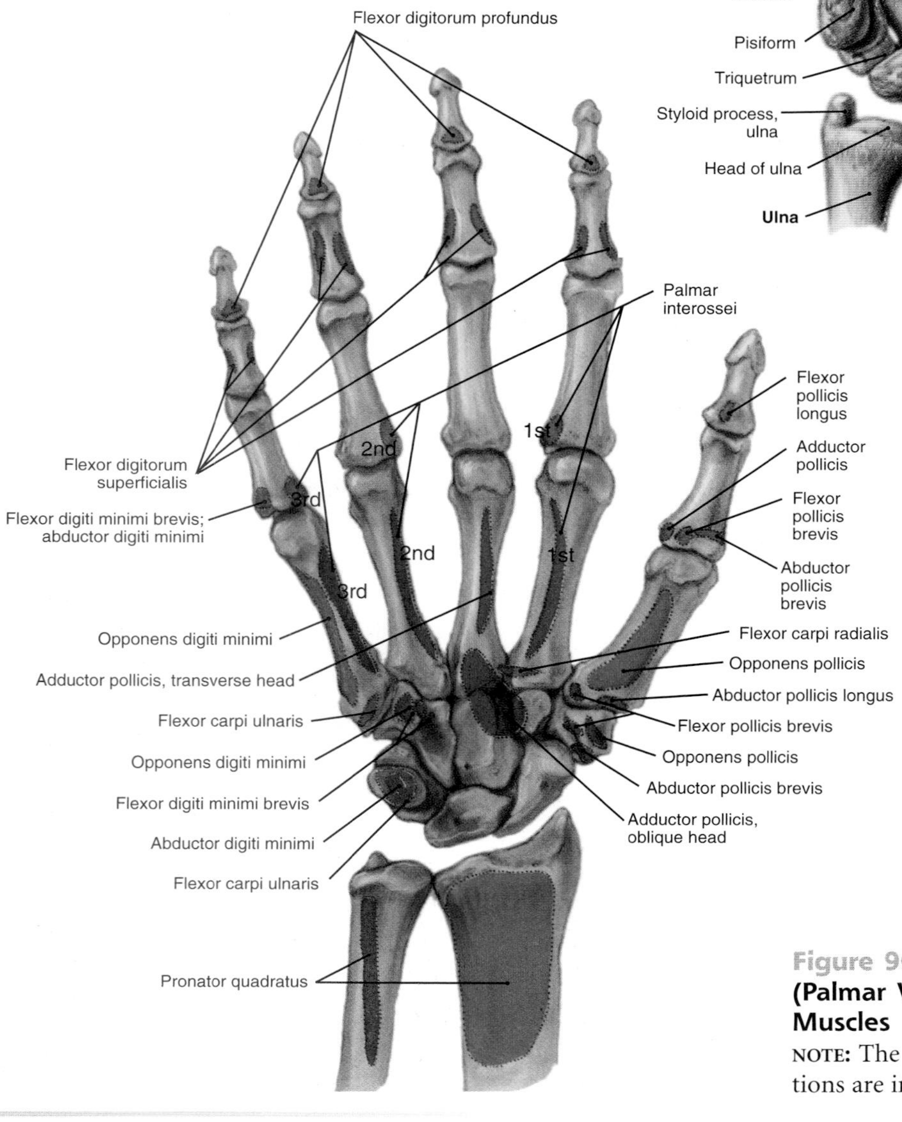

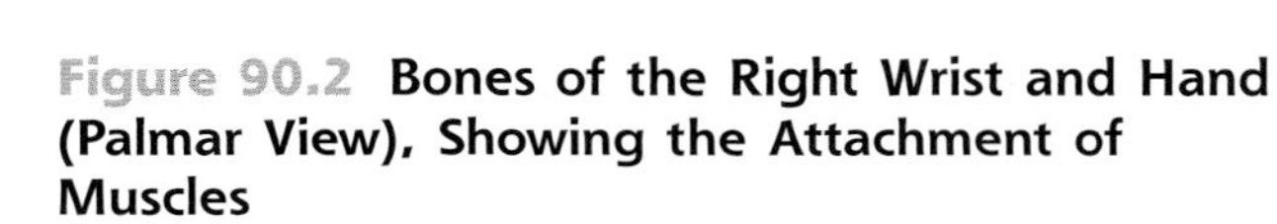

Tuberosity, distal phalanx
Distal phalanx
Head
Body
Base
Middle phalanx
Head
Body
Proximal phalanx
Head, 2nd metacarpal bone
Distal phalanx
Middle phalanx
Proximal phalanx
Phalanges
Distal phalanx, thumb
Sesamoid bone
Proximal phalanx, thumb
Head, 1st metacarpal bone
Sesamoid bones
1st metacarpal bone
Metacarpal bones
Trapezoid
Hamulus of hamate
Trapezium
Hamate
Capitate
Pisiform
Triquetrum
Scaphoid
Styloid process, ulna
Styloid process, radius
Head of ulna
Lunate
Ulna
Radius
Flexor digitorum profundus
Palmar interossei
Flexor pollicis longus
Adductor pollicis
Flexor pollicis brevis
Abductor pollicis brevis
Flexor digitorum superficialis
Flexor digiti minimi brevis; abductor digiti minimi
1st
2nd
3rd
2nd
1st
3rd
Opponens digiti minimi
Adductor pollicis, transverse head
Flexor carpi ulnaris
Opponens digiti minimi
Flexor digiti minimi brevis
Abductor digiti minimi
Flexor carpi ulnaris
Pronator quadratus
Flexor carpi radialis
Opponens pollicis
Abductor pollicis longus
Flexor pollicis brevis
Opponens pollicis
Abductor pollicis brevis
Adductor pollicis, oblique head

Figure 90.2 Bones of the Right Wrist and Hand (Palmar View), Showing the Attachment of Muscles

NOTE: The origins of muscles are in RED, whereas the insertions are in BLUE.

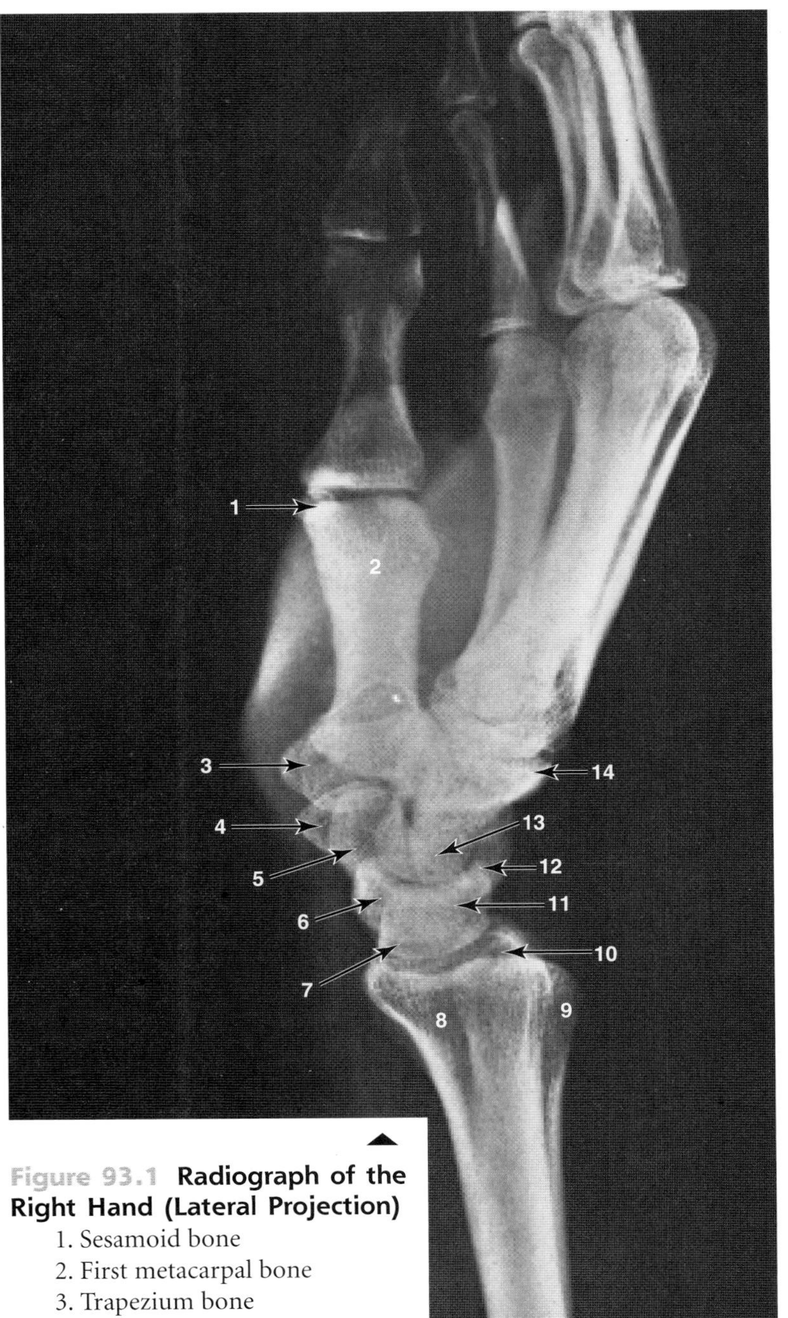
1
2
3
4
5
6
7
8
9
10
11
12
13
14

Figure 93.1 Radiograph of the Right Hand (Lateral Projection)

1. Sesamoid bone
2. First metacarpal bone
3. Trapezium bone
4. Tuberosity of scaphoid bone
5. Pisiform bone
6. Styloid process of radius
7. Scaphoid bone
8. Radius
9. Ulna
10. Styloid process of ulna
11. Lunate bone
12. Triquetral bone
13. Head of capitate bone
14. Hamate bone

(From Wicke, 6th ed.)

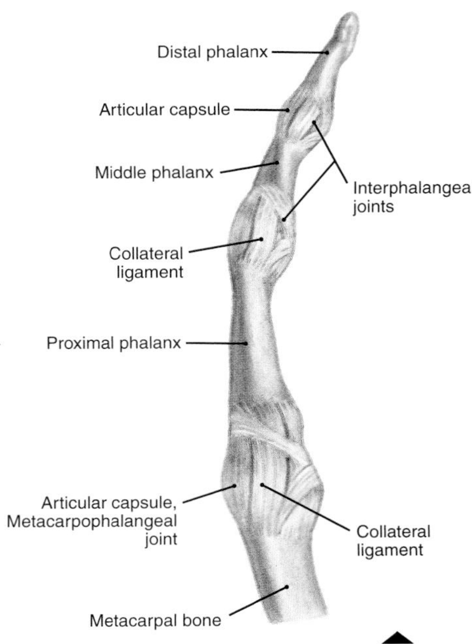
Distal phalanx
Articular capsule
Middle phalanx
Interphalangeal joints
Collateral ligament
Proximal phalanx
Articular capsule, Metacarpophalangeal joint
Collateral ligament
Metacarpal bone

Figure 93.2 Joints and Ligaments of the Middle Finger

NOTE: The articular capsules of the joints in the fingers are strengthened by longitudinally oriented collateral ligaments.

Figure 93.3 Coronal (Frontal) Section through the Left Wrist Joints

NOTE: (1) The articular disk at the distal end of the ulna.

(2) The radiocarpal joint consists of the radius and articular disk proximally and the scaphoid, lunate, and triquetrum distally.

(3) The midcarpal joint that extends between the proximal and distal rows of carpal bones.

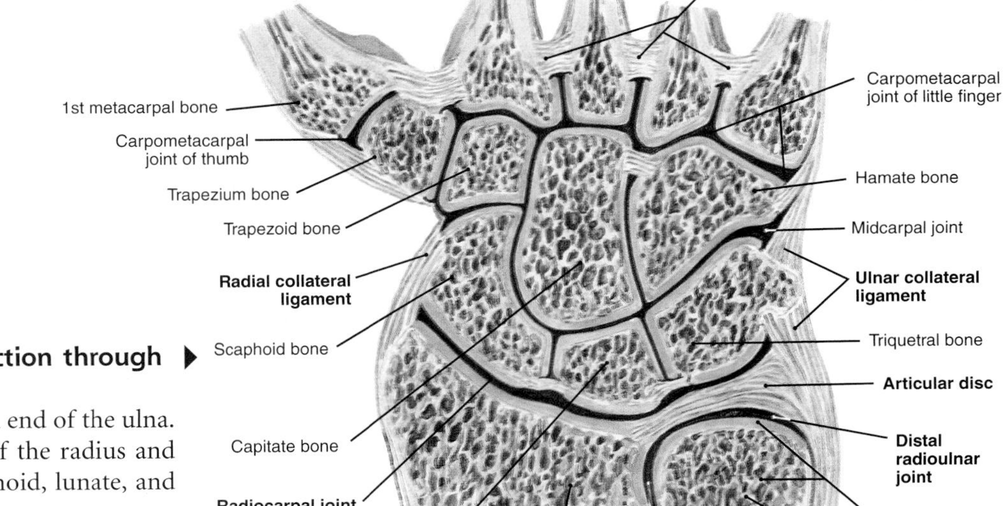
Interosseous metacarpal ligaments
1st metacarpal bone
Carpometacarpal joint of thumb
Trapezium bone
Trapezoid bone
Radial collateral ligament
Scaphoid bone
Capitate bone
Radiocarpal joint
Lunate bone
Radius
Distal radioulnar joint
Carpometacarpal joint of little finger
Hamate bone
Midcarpal joint
Ulnar collateral ligament
Triquetral bone
Articular disc
Distal radioulnar joint
Head of ulna
Ulna

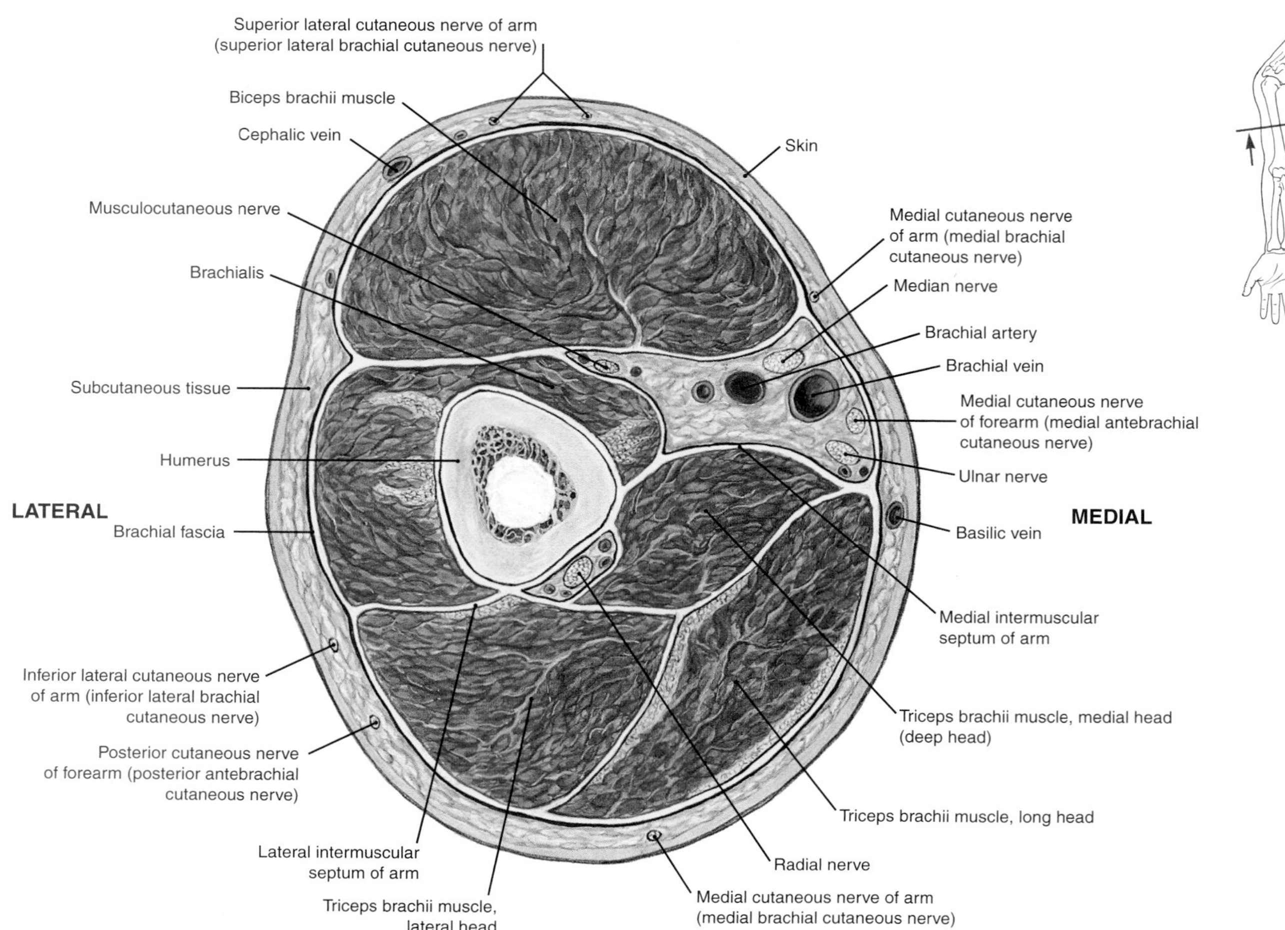
Superior lateral cutaneous nerve of arm
(superior lateral brachial cutaneous nerve)
Biceps brachii muscle
Cephalic vein
Skin
Musculocutaneous nerve
Medial cutaneous nerve of arm (medial brachial cutaneous nerve)
Brachialis
Median nerve
Brachial artery
Subcutaneous tissue
Brachial vein
Medial cutaneous nerve of forearm (medial antebrachial cutaneous nerve)
Humerus
Ulnar nerve
LATERAL
MEDIAL
Brachial fascia
Basilic vein
Medial intermuscular septum of arm
Inferior lateral cutaneous nerve of arm (inferior lateral brachial cutaneous nerve)
Triceps brachii muscle, medial head (deep head)
Posterior cutaneous nerve of forearm (posterior antebrachial cutaneous nerve)
Triceps brachii muscle, long head
Lateral intermuscular septum of arm
Radial nerve
Triceps brachii muscle, lateral head
Medial cutaneous nerve of arm (medial brachial cutaneous nerve)

Figure 94.1 Cross Section of the Right Upper Extremity through the Middle of the Humerus

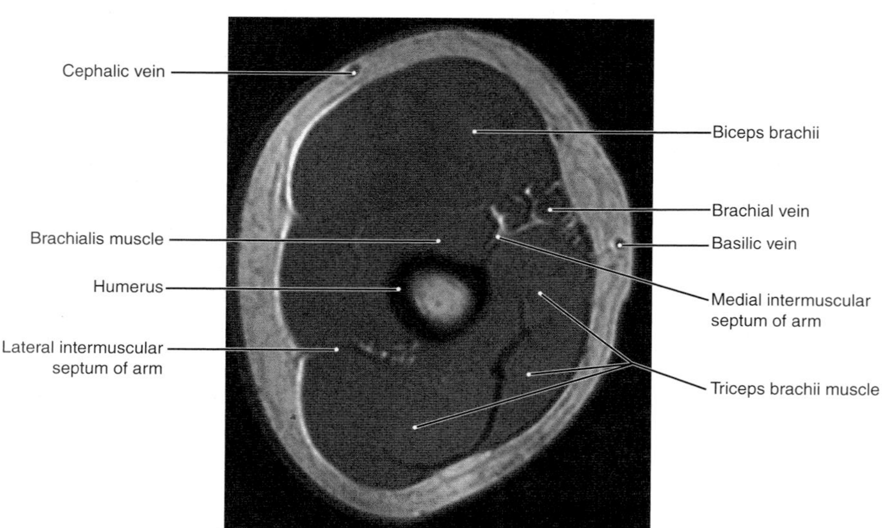
Cephalic vein
Biceps brachii
Brachial vein
Brachialis muscle
Basilic vein
Humerus
Medial intermuscular septum of arm
Lateral intermuscular septum of arm
Triceps brachii muscle

Figure 94.2 Magnetic Resonance Image (MRI) of the Right Upper Limb through the Middle of the Humerus

NOTE that this MRI may be compared with the cross section in Figure 94.1.

Cross Sections of the Upper Limb: Elbow and Upper Forearm

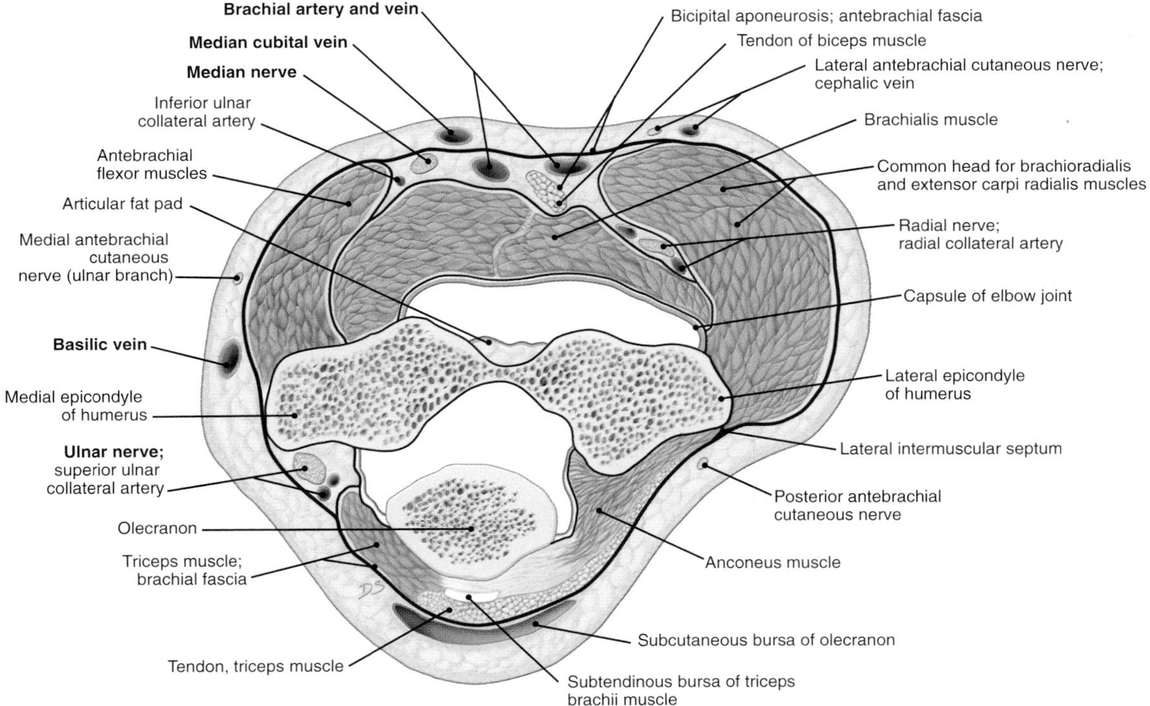
Brachial artery and vein
Median cubital vein
Median nerve
Inferior ulnar collateral artery
Antebrachial flexor muscles
Articular fat pad
Medial antebrachial cutaneous nerve (ulnar branch)
Basilic vein
Medial epicondyle of humerus
Ulnar nerve; superior ulnar collateral artery
Olecranon
Triceps muscle; brachial fascia
Tendon, triceps muscle
Bicipital aponeurosis; antebrachial fascia
Tendon of biceps muscle
Lateral antebrachial cutaneous nerve; cephalic vein
Brachialis muscle
Common head for brachioradialis and extensor carpi radialis muscles
Radial nerve; radial collateral artery
Capsule of elbow joint
Lateral epicondyle of humerus
Lateral intermuscular septum
Posterior antebrachial cutaneous nerve
Anconeus muscle
Subcutaneous bursa of olecranon
Subtendinous bursa of triceps brachii muscle

Figure 95.1 Cross Section through the Right Upper Extremity at the Level of the Elbow Joint

NOTE: (1) The ulnar nerve and superior ulnar collateral artery lie behind the medial epicondyle of the humerus, medial to the olecranon of the ulna.

(2) The median nerve lies to the ulnar (medial) side of the brachial vein and artery in the cubital fossa, and all three structures lie deep to the cubital fascia and median cubital vein.

(3) At this level, the radial nerve and radial collateral artery lie between the common origins of the extensor muscles and the deeply located brachialis muscle.

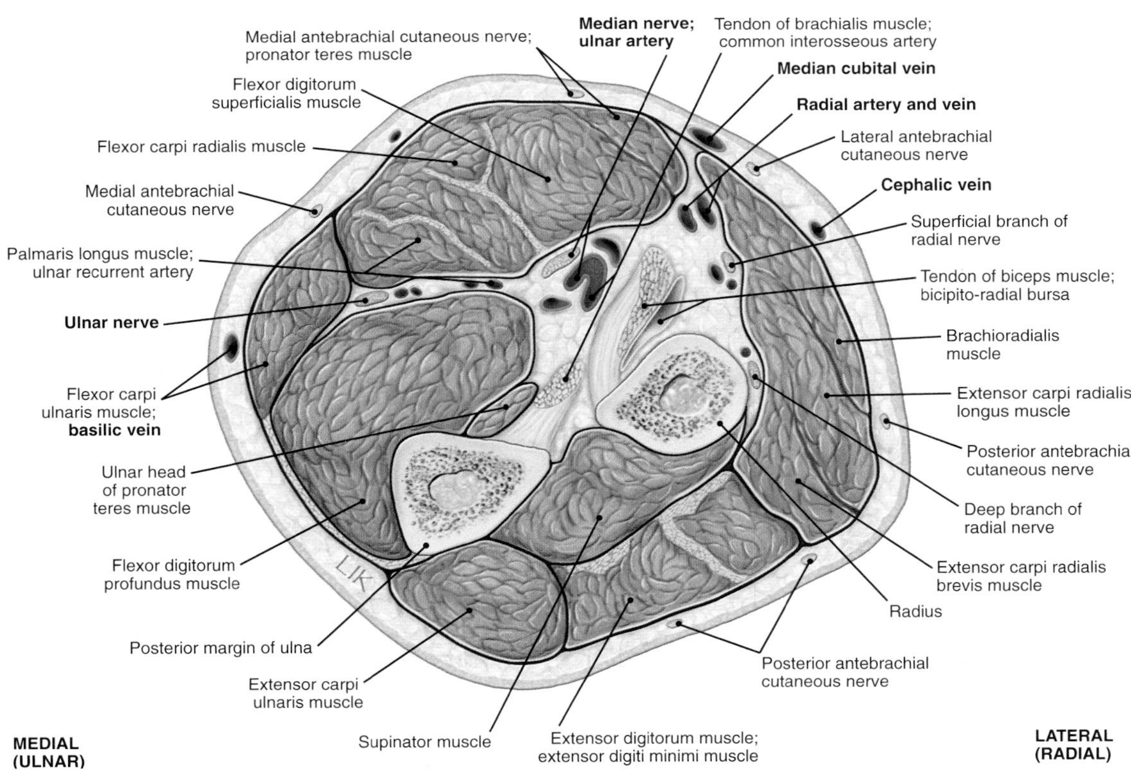
Medial antebrachial cutaneous nerve; pronator teres muscle
Median nerve; ulnar artery
Tendon of brachialis muscle; common interosseous artery
Median cubital vein
Radial artery and vein
Flexor digitorum superficialis muscle
Flexor carpi radialis muscle
Lateral antebrachial cutaneous nerve
Medial antebrachial cutaneous nerve
Cephalic vein
Superficial branch of radial nerve
Palmaris longus muscle; ulnar recurrent artery
Tendon of biceps muscle; bicipito-radial bursa
Ulnar nerve
Brachioradialis muscle
Flexor carpi ulnaris muscle; basilic vein
Extensor carpi radialis longus muscle
Posterior antebrachial cutaneous nerve
Ulnar head of pronator teres muscle
Deep branch of radial nerve
Flexor digitorum profundus muscle
Extensor carpi radialis brevis muscle
Radius
Posterior margin of ulna
Posterior antebrachial cutaneous nerve
Extensor carpi ulnaris muscle
Supinator muscle
Extensor digitorum muscle; extensor digiti minimi muscle
MEDIAL (ULNAR)
LATERAL (RADIAL)

Figure 95.2 Cross Section through the Proximal Third of the Right Forearm

NOTE: (1) The common interosseous artery branching from the ulnar artery and the insertions of the biceps brachii and brachialis muscles to the radius and ulna, respectively.

(2) The radial nerve has already divided into its superficial and deep branches.

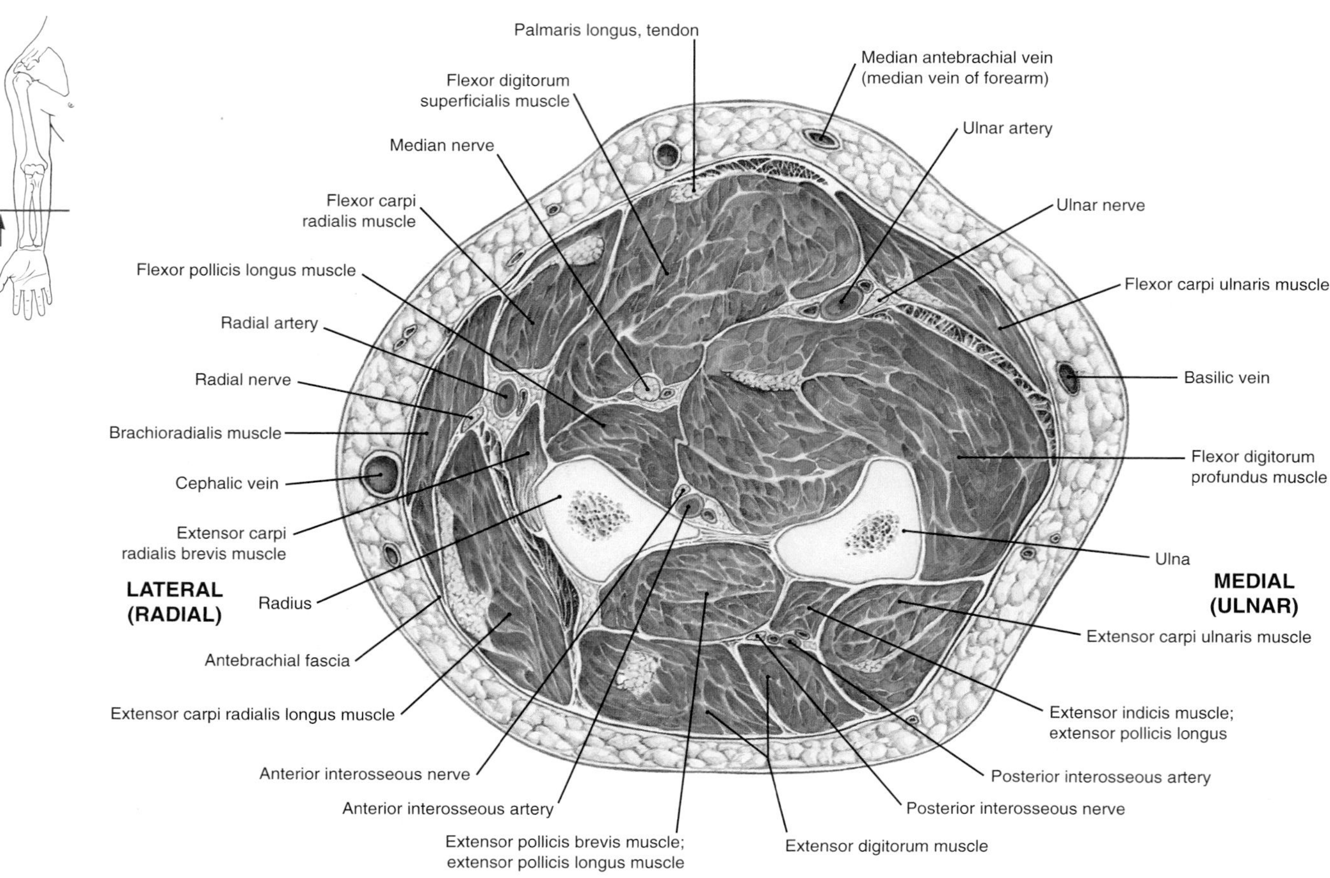
Palmaris longus, tendon
Median antebrachial vein (median vein of forearm)
Flexor digitorum superficialis muscle
Ulnar artery
Median nerve
Ulnar nerve
Flexor carpi radialis muscle
Flexor pollicis longus muscle
Flexor carpi ulnaris muscle
Radial artery
Basilic vein
Radial nerve
Brachioradialis muscle
Flexor digitorum profundus muscle
Cephalic vein
Extensor carpi radialis brevis muscle
Ulna
LATERAL (RADIAL)
Radius
MEDIAL (ULNAR)
Extensor carpi ulnaris muscle
Antebrachial fascia
Extensor carpi radialis longus muscle
Extensor indicis muscle; extensor pollicis longus
Anterior interosseous nerve
Posterior interosseous artery
Anterior interosseous artery
Posterior interosseous nerve
Extensor pollicis brevis muscle; extensor pollicis longus muscle
Extensor digitorum muscle

Figure 96.1 Cross Section through the Middle Third of the Right Forearm

NOTE: (1) At this level, the ulna, radius, interosseous membrane, and intermuscular septum clearly delineate the **posterior compartment,** extending dorsally and laterally, from the **anterior compartment** located anteriorly and medially.

(2) The **median nerve** coursing down the forearm deep to the flexor digitorum superficialis and anterior to the flexor digitorum profundus and flexor pollicis longus.

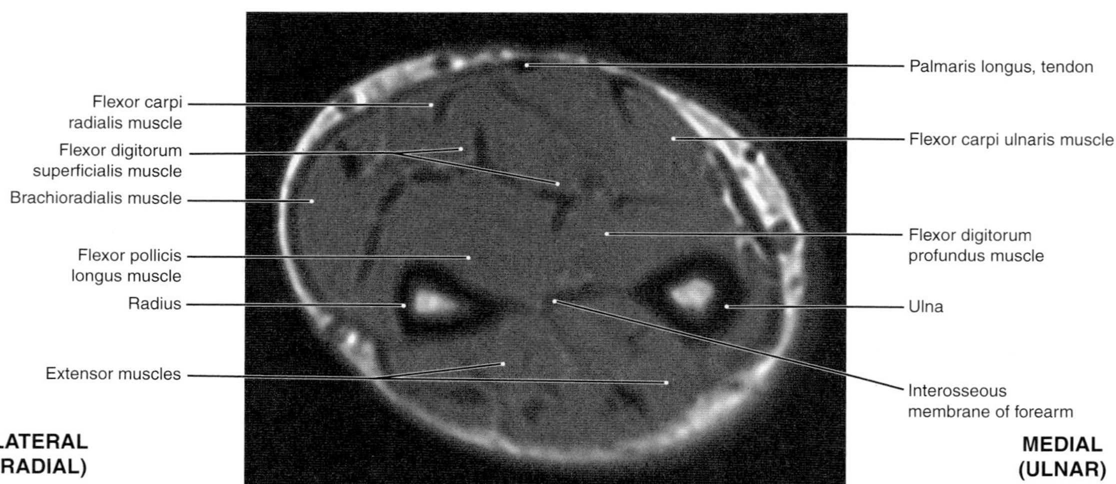
Palmaris longus, tendon
Flexor carpi radialis muscle
Flexor carpi ulnaris muscle
Flexor digitorum superficialis muscle
Brachioradialis muscle
Flexor digitorum profundus muscle
Flexor pollicis longus muscle
Radius
Ulna
Extensor muscles
Interosseous membrane of forearm
LATERAL (RADIAL)
MEDIAL (ULNAR)

Figure 96.2 Transverse MRI Section through the Middle of the Forearm

NOTE that this figure should be compared with Fig. 96.1. Observe the locations of the anterior and posterior forearm muscle groups and judge where the important vessels and nerves would be found in the MRI.

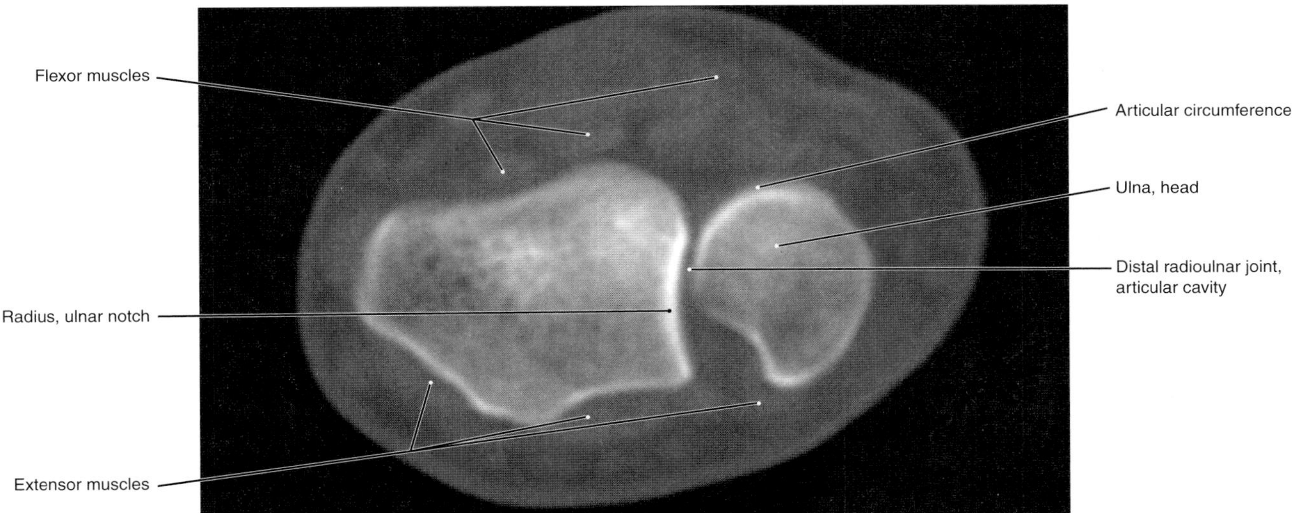
Flexor muscles
Articular circumference
Ulna, head
Distal radioulnar joint, articular cavity
Radius, ulnar notch
Extensor muscles

Figure 97.1 CT of the Right Distal Radioulnar Joint

NOTE: (1) The **head of the ulna** fits into the **ulnar notch** of the radius and the articular cavity of the distal radioulnar joint between.

(2) The distal end of the radius is large, while its proximal end is relatively small. In contrast, the distal end of the ulna is small in comparison to the proximal end at the elbow joint. Compare with the bones in Figs. 98.1 and 98.2.

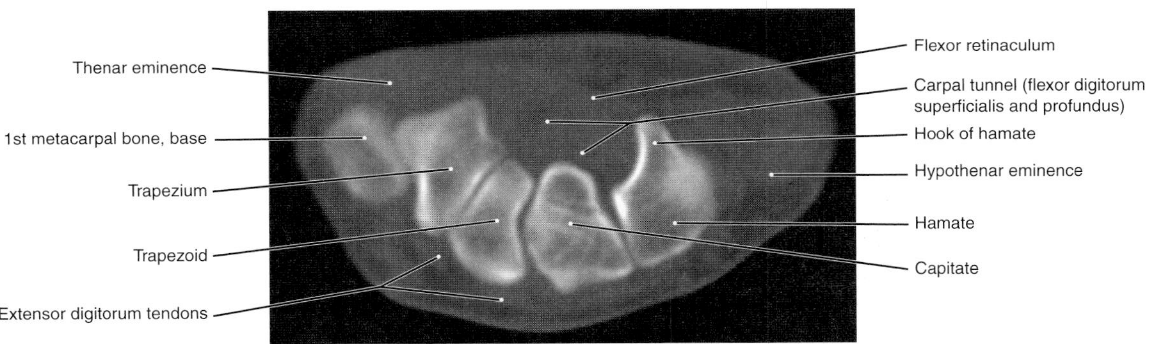
Thenar eminence
1st metacarpal bone, base
Trapezium
Trapezoid
Extensor digitorum tendons
Flexor retinaculum
Carpal tunnel (flexor digitorum superficialis and profundus)
Hook of hamate
Hypothenar eminence
Hamate
Capitate

Figure 97.2 CT of the Right Wrist

NOTE: (1) This image is taken at the level of the distal row of carpal bones (from lateral to medial: trapezium, trapezoid, capitate, and hamate).

(2) The base of the first metacarpal bone as it articulates proximally with the trapezium to form the carpometacarpal joint of the thumb. Compare this figure with the radiograph in Figure 89.

(3) The hook (hamulus) of the hamate bone projects from the palmar surface of the bone. It can be felt through the skin over the proximal part of the hypothenar eminence.

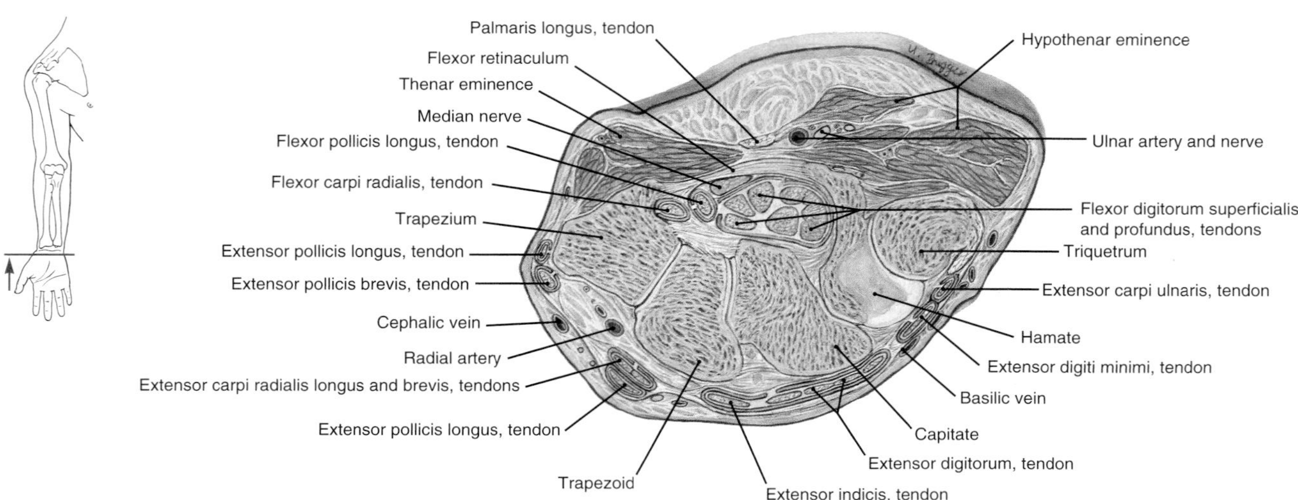
Palmaris longus, tendon
Flexor retinaculum
Thenar eminence
Median nerve
Flexor pollicis longus, tendon
Flexor carpi radialis, tendon
Trapezium
Extensor pollicis longus, tendon
Extensor pollicis brevis, tendon
Cephalic vein
Radial artery
Extensor carpi radialis longus and brevis, tendons
Extensor pollicis longus, tendon
Trapezoid
Extensor indicis, tendon
Extensor digitorum, tendon
Capitate
Basilic vein
Extensor digiti minimi, tendon
Hamate
Extensor carpi ulnaris, tendon
Triquetrum
Flexor digitorum superficialis and profundus, tendons
Ulnar artery and nerve
Hypothenar eminence

Figure 98.1 Transverse Section through the Wrist Joint

NOTE: (1) This cross section is at the level of the distal row of carpal bones. Compare the carpal bones in this section with the figures in Plate 91.

(2) The locations of the **median nerve** in the **carpal tunnel** and the ulnar nerve and artery superficial to the carpal tunnel adjacent to the hypothenar muscles;

(3) The strong **flexor retinaculum** bounds the carpal tunnel anteriorly, while the carpal bones bound the tunnel posteriorly. In addition to the median nerve, the flexor tendons enter the hand within the tunnel;

(4) Significant trauma to this region of the hand can result in excessive pressure on the median nerve; this condition is called **carpal tunnel syndrome,** and it severely limits the functions of the thenar muscles supplied by the median nerve.

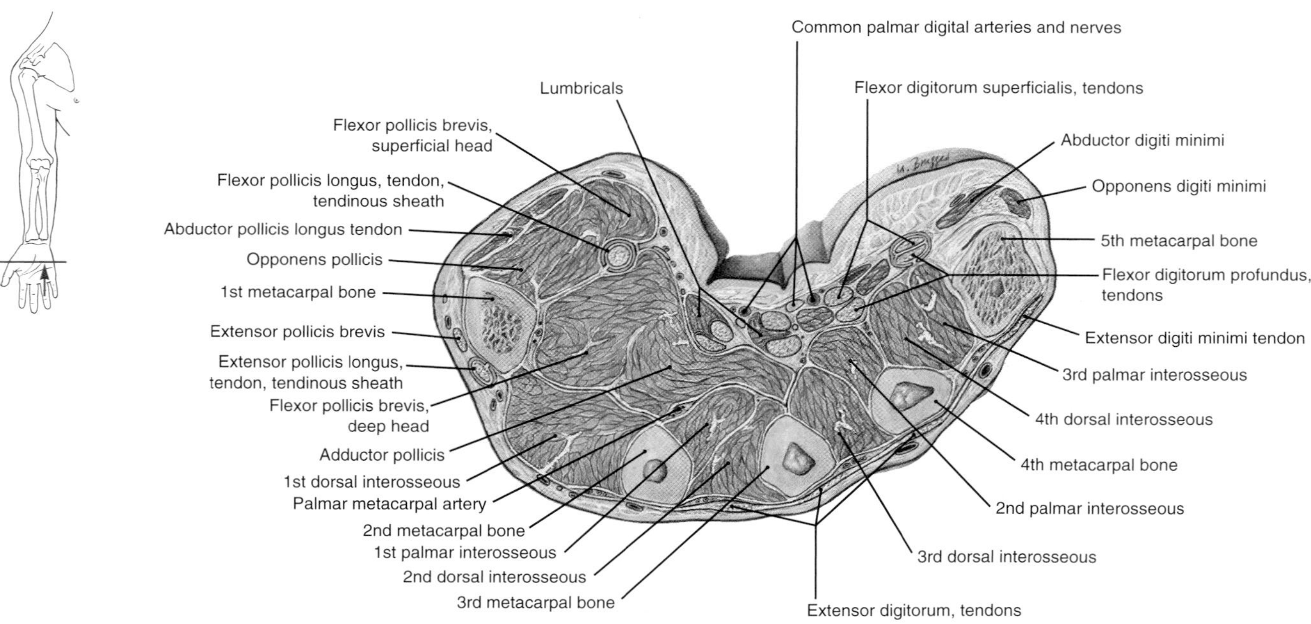
Common palmar digital arteries and nerves
Lumbricals
Flexor digitorum superficialis, tendons
Flexor pollicis brevis, superficial head
Flexor pollicis longus, tendon, tendinous sheath
Abductor pollicis longus tendon
Opponens pollicis
1st metacarpal bone
Extensor pollicis brevis
Extensor pollicis longus, tendon, tendinous sheath
Flexor pollicis brevis, deep head
Adductor pollicis
1st dorsal interosseous
Palmar metacarpal artery
2nd metacarpal bone
1st palmar interosseous
2nd dorsal interosseous
3rd metacarpal bone
Extensor digitorum, tendons
3rd dorsal interosseous
2nd palmar interosseous
4th metacarpal bone
4th dorsal interosseous
3rd palmar interosseous
Extensor digiti minimi tendon
Flexor digitorum profundus, tendons
5th metacarpal bone
Opponens digiti minimi
Abductor digiti minimi

Figure 98.2 Cross Section of the Right Hand through the Metacarpal Bones

NOTE: (1) The four **dorsal interosseous muscles** that act as abductors of the fingers and fill the intervals between the metacarpal bones.

(2) The three **palmar interosseous muscles** that serve as adductors of the fingers.

(3) The **thenar muscles** on the radial side of the hand and the **hypothenar muscles** on the ulnar side.

(4) There are seven **interosseous muscles,** three palmar, and four dorsal. In addition to flexing the metacarpophalangeal joints, these muscles abduct and adduct the fingers. The thumb has its own abductors and adductor and the little finger has its own abductor. This accounts for adduction and abduction actions for the five fingers.

Figure 99.1 Cross Section of the Middle Finger through the Proximal Phalanx

NOTE: (1) The extensor expansion (or extensor hood) over the dorsal aspect of the proximal phalanx and part of the middle phalanx.

(2) Into the extensor expansion blend the tendon of the extensor digitorum and the tendons of insertion of the adjacent interosseous and lumbrical muscles.

(3) The synovial sheath on the palmar side of the phalanx, which surrounds the superficial and deep flexor tendons of the digit.

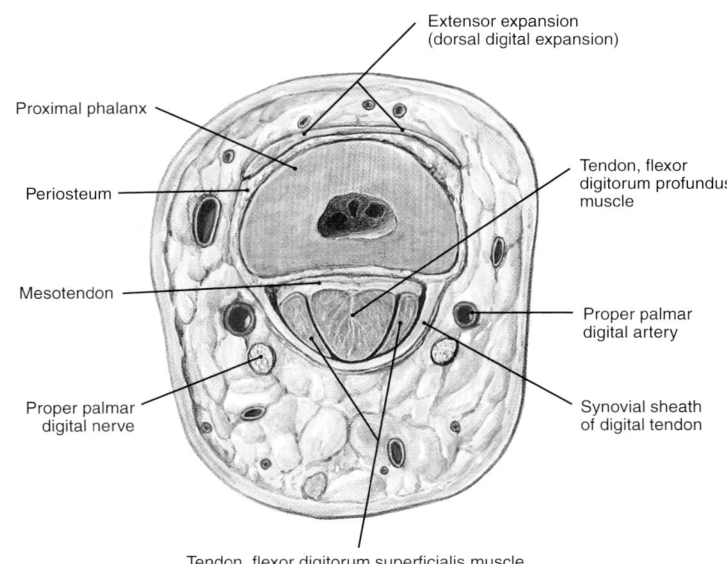
Extensor expansion
(dorsal digital expansion)
Proximal phalanx
Tendon, flexor
digitorum profundus
muscle
Periosteum
Mesotendon
Proper palmar
digital artery
Proper palmar
digital nerve
Synovial sheath
of digital tendon
Tendon, flexor digitorum superficialis muscle

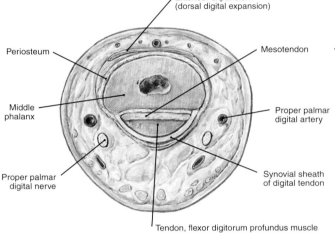

Extensor expansion
(dorsal digital expansion)
Periosteum
Mesotendon
Middle
phalanx
Proper palmar
digital artery
Proper palmar
digital nerve
Synovial sheath
of digital tendon
Tendon, flexor digitorum profundus muscle

Figure 99.2 Cross Section of the Middle Finger through the Middle Phalanx

NOTE: (1) The locations of the proper digital arteries and nerves within the subcutaneous tissue on the sides of the deep flexor tendon.

(2) Knowing the location of these neurovascular structures is important both for the application of local anesthesia to the digit and for the cessation of severe bleeding.

Figure 99.3 Longitudinal Section through a Flexed Finger

NOTE: The location of the flexion creases in relation to the corresponding joints.

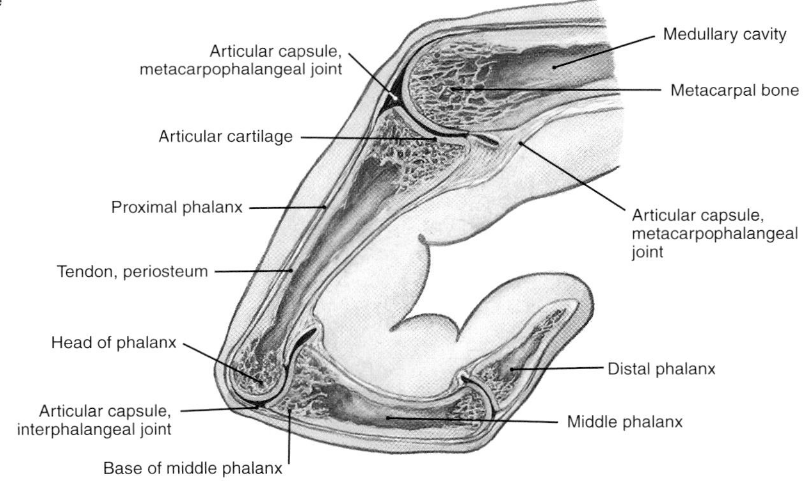
Articular capsule,
metacarpophalangeal joint
Medullary cavity
Metacarpal bone
Articular cartilage
Proximal phalanx
Articular capsule,
metacarpophalangeal
joint
Tendon, periosteum
Head of phalanx
Distal phalanx
Articular capsule,
interphalangeal joint
Middle phalanx
Base of middle phalanx

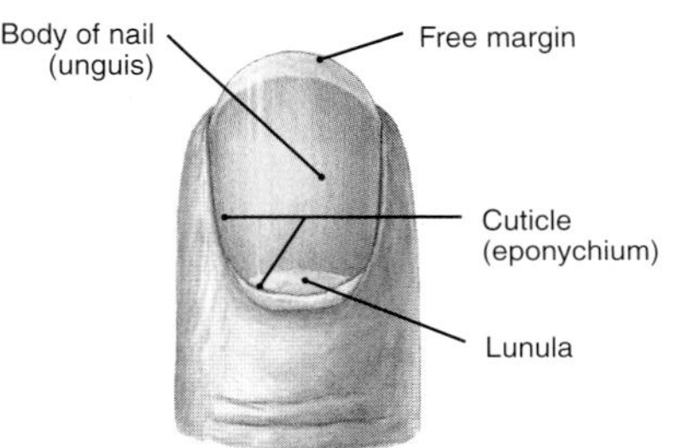
Body of nail
(unguis)
Free margin
Cuticle
(eponychium)
Lunula

Figure 99.4 Fingernail, Normal Position (Dorsal View)

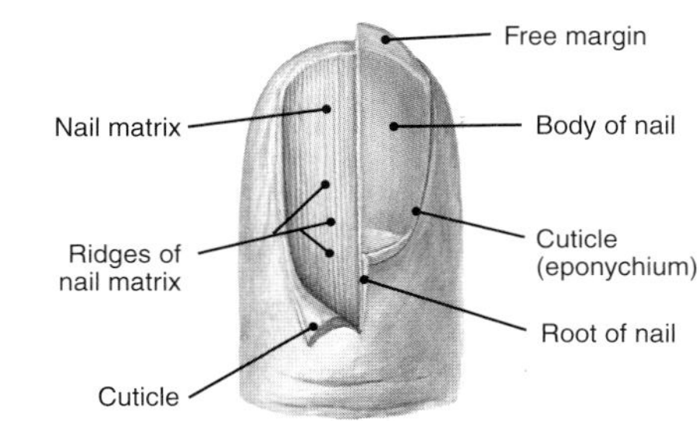
Free margin
Nail matrix
Body of nail
Ridges of
nail matrix
Cuticle
(eponychium)
Root of nail
Cuticle

Figure 99.5 Left Half of Finger Nailbed Exposed

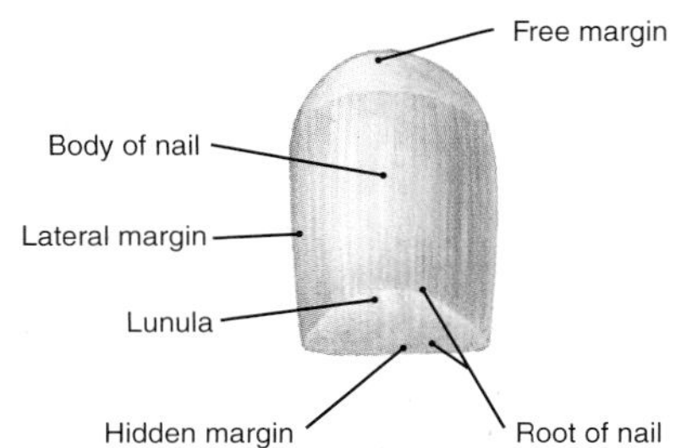
Free margin
Body of nail
Lateral margin
Lunula
Hidden margin
Root of nail

Figure 99.6 Body of Fingernail Removed from the Nailbed

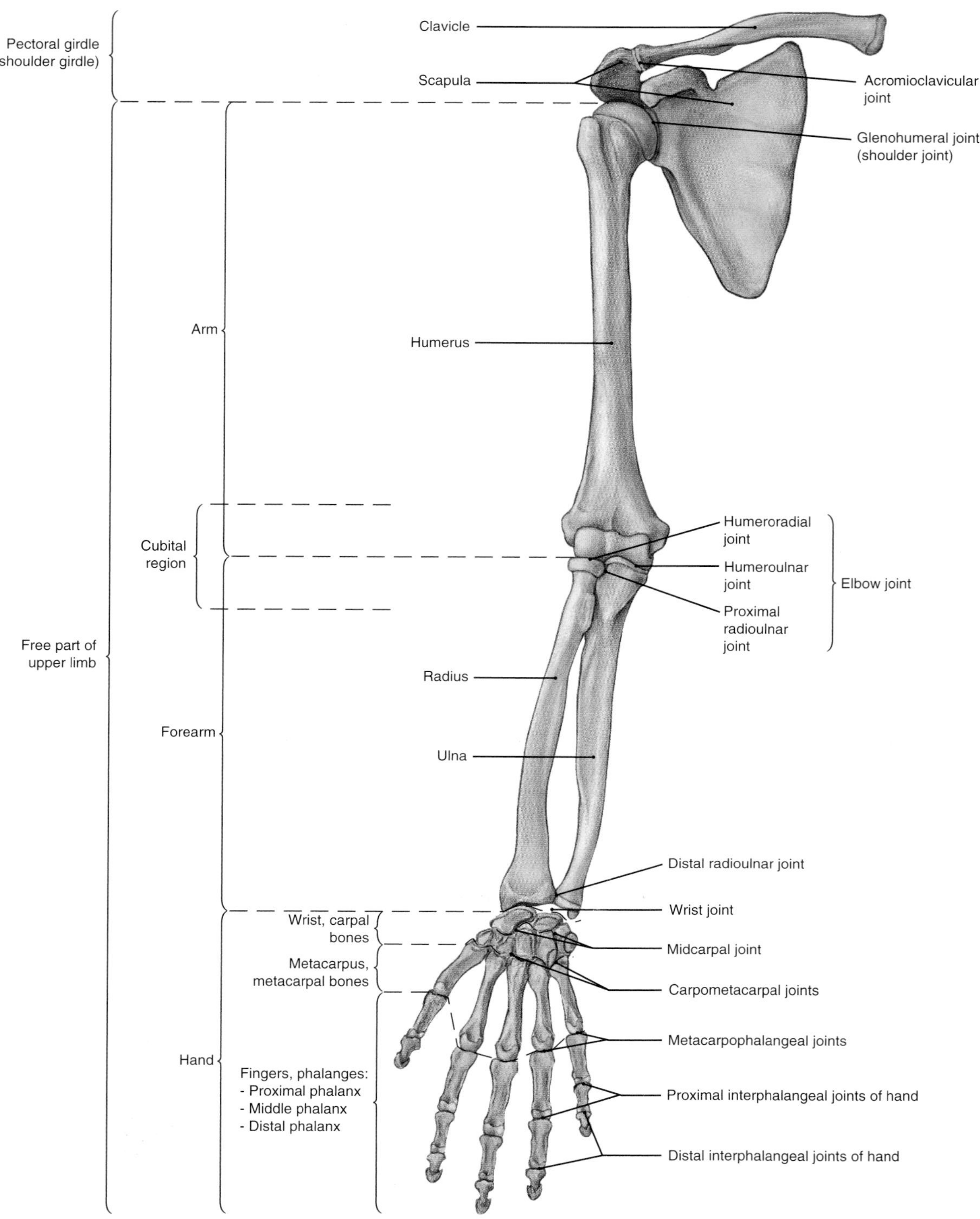

Pectoral girdle (shoulder girdle)
Clavicle
Scapula
Acromioclavicular joint
Glenohumeral joint (shoulder joint)
Arm
Humerus
Cubital region
Humeroradial joint
Humeroulnar joint
Proximal radioulnar joint
Elbow joint
Free part of upper limb
Radius
Forearm
Ulna
Distal radioulnar joint
Wrist joint
Wrist, carpal bones
Midcarpal joint
Metacarpus, metacarpal bones
Carpometacarpal joints
Metacarpophalangeal joints
Hand
Fingers, phalanges:
- Proximal phalanx
- Middle phalanx
- Distal phalanx
Proximal interphalangeal joints of hand
Distal interphalangeal joints of hand

Figure 100 Bones and Joints of the Upper Limb, Including the Pectoral Girdle

NOTE that this skeletal view shows the anterior aspect of the right upper limb and pectoral girdle. The bones are labeled on the left and the joints are labeled to the right.

THE THORAX

2

PLATES

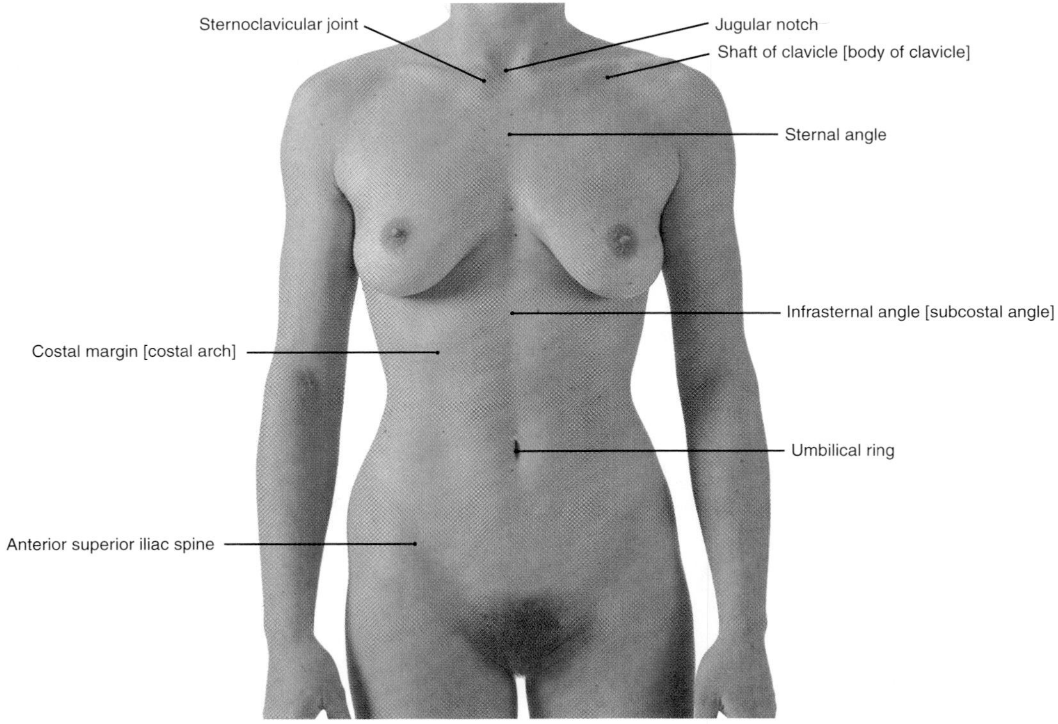
Sternoclavicular joint
Jugular notch
Shaft of clavicle [body of clavicle]
Sternal angle
Infrasternal angle [subcostal angle]
Costal margin [costal arch]
Umbilical ring
Anterior superior iliac spine

Figure 101.1 Surface Anatomy of the Thoracic and Abdominal Walls in a Young Female
NOTE that prominent bony structures are labeled along with the jugular notch and umbilicus.

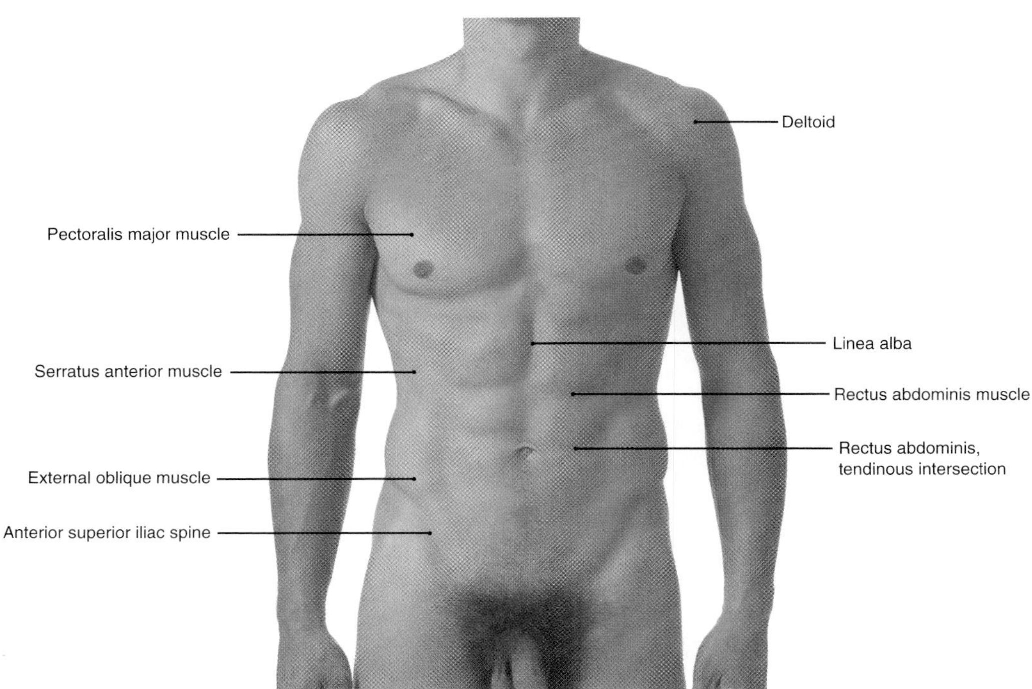
Deltoid
Pectoralis major muscle
Linea alba
Serratus anterior muscle
Rectus abdominis muscle
Rectus abdominis,
tendinous intersection
External oblique muscle
Anterior superior iliac spine

Figure 101.2 Surface Anatomy of the Thoracic and Abdominal Walls in a Young Male
NOTE that the surface contours of prominent muscles are labeled.

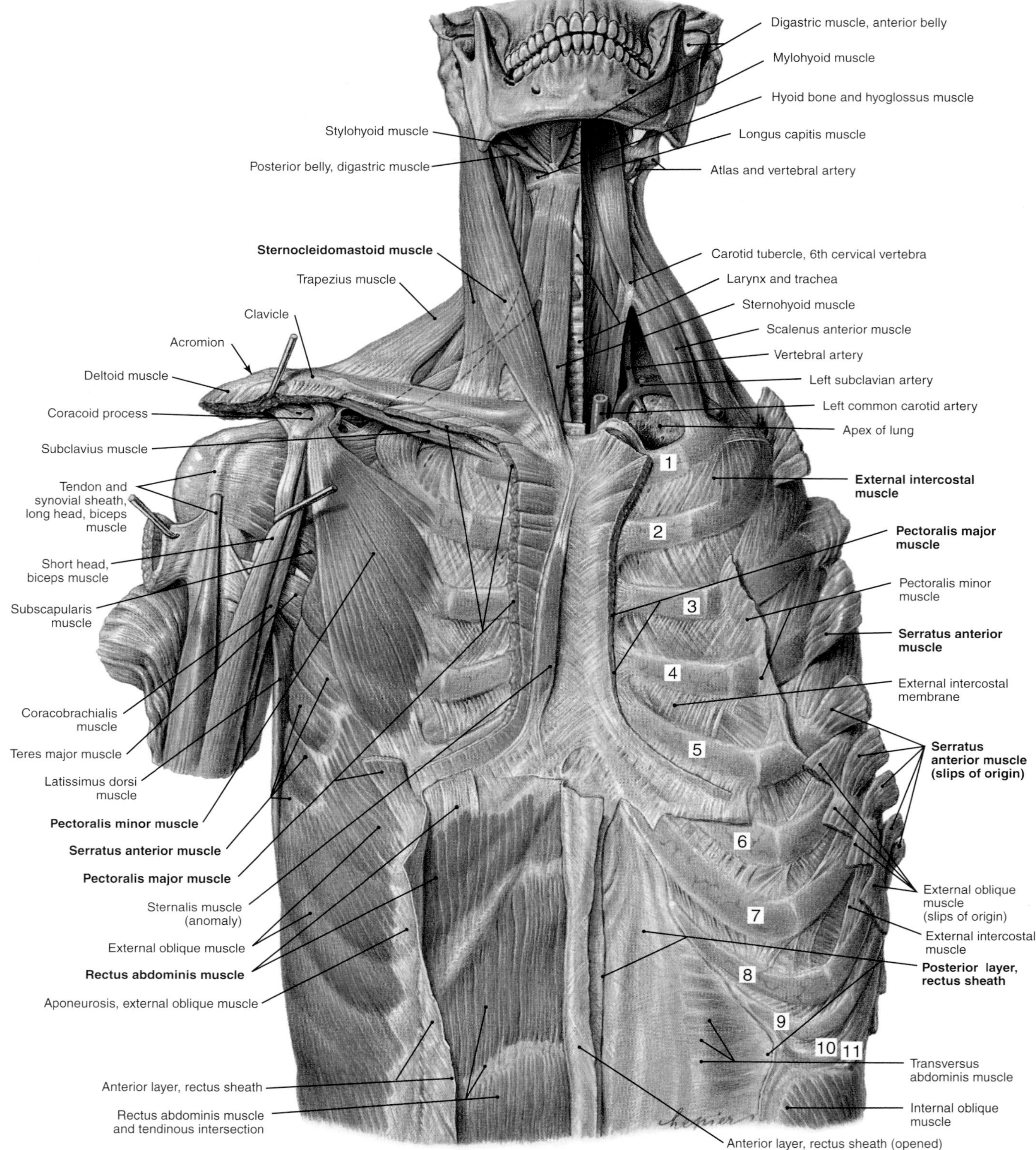

Digastric muscle, anterior belly
Mylohyoid muscle
Hyoid bone and hyoglossus muscle
Longus capitis muscle
Atlas and vertebral artery
Stylohyoid muscle
Posterior belly, digastric muscle
Sternocleidomastoid muscle
Trapezius muscle
Clavicle
Acromion
Deltoid muscle
Coracoid process
Subclavius muscle
Tendon and synovial sheath, long head, biceps muscle
Short head, biceps muscle
Subscapularis muscle
Coracobrachialis muscle
Teres major muscle
Latissimus dorsi muscle
Pectoralis minor muscle
Serratus anterior muscle
Pectoralis major muscle
Sternalis muscle (anomaly)
External oblique muscle
Rectus abdominis muscle
Aponeurosis, external oblique muscle
Anterior layer, rectus sheath
Rectus abdominis muscle and tendinous intersection
Carotid tubercle, 6th cervical vertebra
Larynx and trachea
Sternohyoid muscle
Scalenus anterior muscle
Vertebral artery
Left subclavian artery
Left common carotid artery
Apex of lung
External intercostal muscle
Pectoralis major muscle
Pectoralis minor muscle
Serratus anterior muscle
External intercostal membrane
Serratus anterior muscle (slips of origin)
External oblique muscle (slips of origin)
External intercostal muscle
Posterior layer, rectus sheath
Transversus abdominis muscle
Internal oblique muscle
Anterior layer, rectus sheath (opened)
1
2
3
4
5
6
7
8
9
10
11

Figure 102 Musculature of the Anterior Thoracic Wall Deep to the Pectoralis Major and the Adjacent Cervical and Abdominal Muscles

NOTE: (1) On the right side (reader's left), the anterior thoracic wall and upper arm are shown after removal of the pectoralis major muscle.

(2) On the left (reader's right), the upper limb and the superficial trunk and cervical muscles have been removed, exposing the ribs and intercostal tissues.

Muscle	Origin	Insertion	Innervation	Action
Subclavius	First rib and its cartilage at their junction	Groove on the lower surface of middle third of the clavicle	Nerve to subclavius from upper trunk of brachial plexus (C5, C6)	Depresses and pulls clavicle forward

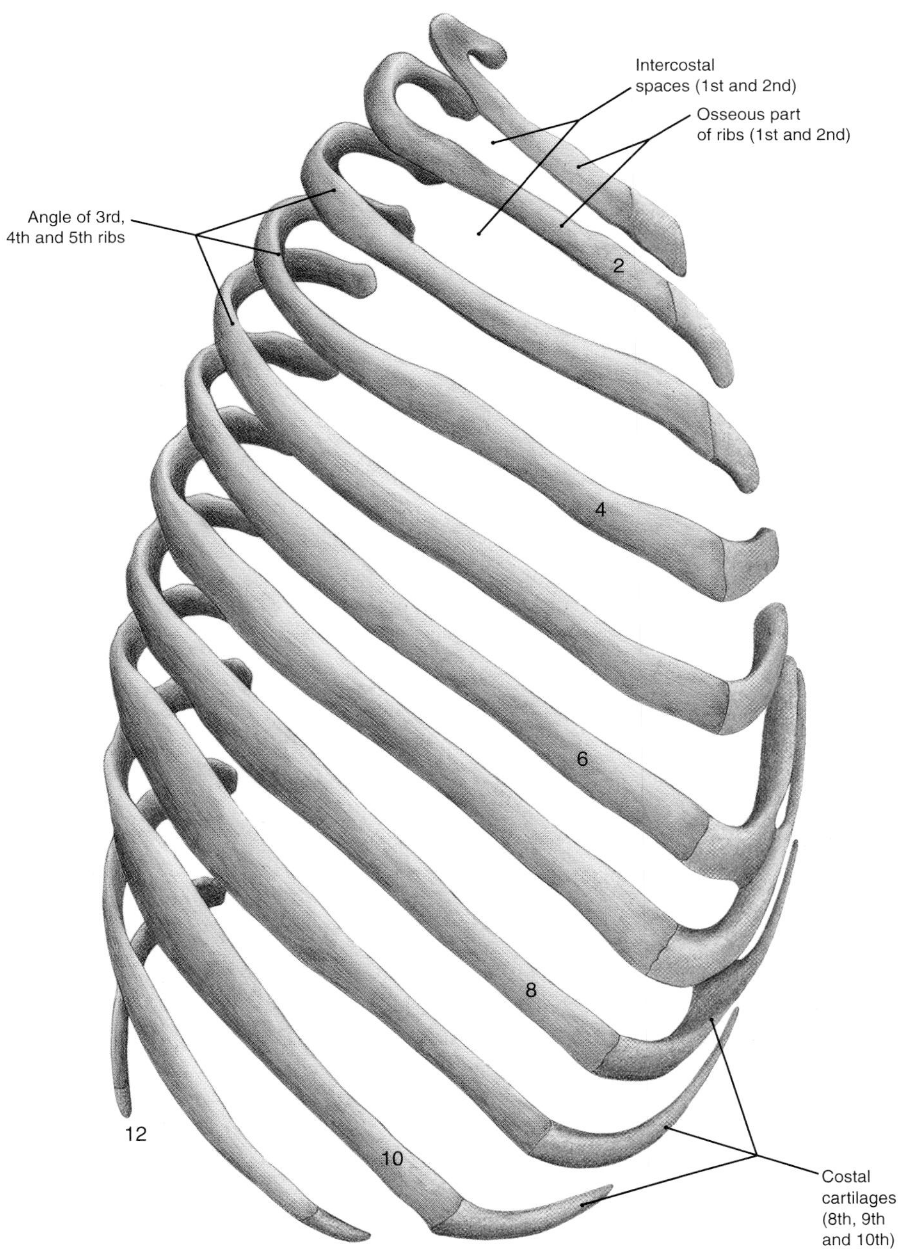
Intercostal spaces (1st and 2nd)
Osseous part of ribs (1st and 2nd)
Angle of 3rd, 4th and 5th ribs
2
4
6
8
10
12
Costal cartilages (8th, 9th and 10th)

Figure 103 Twelve Right Ribs Showing the Natural Contour of the Thoracic Cage (Lateral View)

NOTE: (1) The posterior end of each rib is located more superiorly than the costal end that attaches to the costal cartilage; thus, as each rib leaves its vertebral articulation, it courses around the chest in a rounded, descending manner.

(2) Ribs 5 to 10 are longer than ribs 1 to 4 and 11 and 12. The latter two ribs are considered "floating ribs" because they do not attach to the sternum or the costal margin.

Muscle	Origin	Insertion	Innervation	Action
External intercostal (11 muscles)	Lower border of a rib	Upper border of the rib below	Intercostal nerves	Elevate the ribs; active during normal inspiration
	Within intercostal space, each extends from the tubercle of the rib dorsally to the cartilage of the rib ventrally			
Internal intercostal (11 muscles)	Ridge on the inner surface near lower border of rib	Upper border of the rib below	Intercostal nerves	Elevate the ribs; active during inspiration and expiration
	Within intercostal space, each extends from the sternum ventrally to the angle of the rib dorsally			

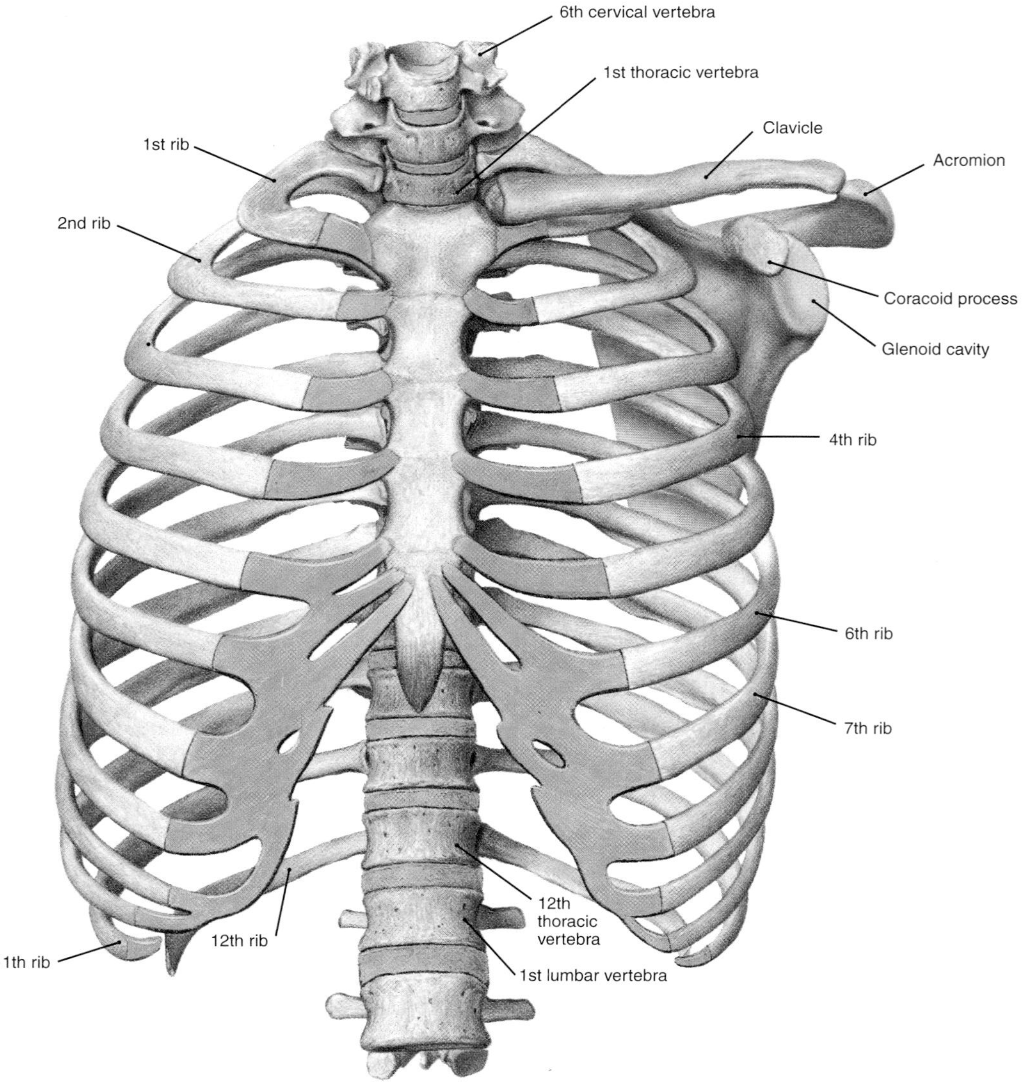
6th cervical vertebra
1st thoracic vertebra
Clavicle
Acromion
1st rib
2nd rib
Coracoid process
Glenoid cavity
4th rib
6th rib
7th rib
12th thoracic vertebra
12th rib
11th rib
1st lumbar vertebra

Figure 104.1 Thoracic Skeleton (Anterior View)

Left clavicle and scapula are shown in yellow; costal cartilages and intervertebral disks are in blue.

NOTE: (1) The skeleton of the thorax protects the thoracic organs. It is formed by 12 pairs of ribs that articulate posteriorly with the 12 thoracic vertebrae. Anteriorly, the bony parts of the ribs are continued as cartilages, the upper 7 pairs of which are attached directly to the sternum.

(2) The bony parts of the ribs fall progressively more lateral to the sternum from above downward, resulting in longer costal cartilages in lower ribs than in higher ones.

(3) The thoracic cage is narrow superiorly at its inlet, but is more broad inferiorly, where it is closer to abdominal structures.

Figure 104.2 Sternoclavicular and the First Two Sternocostal Joints

NOTE: (1) The sternoclavicular joint is formed by the junction of the clavicle with (a) the upper lateral aspect of the manubrium and (b) the cartilage of the first rib.

(2) An articular disk is interposed between the clavicle and the sternum, and an articular capsule and fibrous ligamentous bands protect the joint.

(3) The cartilages of the second to the seventh ribs (see Fig. 104.1) articulate with the sternum by movable (diarthrodial) joints. The cartilage of the first rib, however, directly joins the sternum and, without a joint cavity, forms an immovable joint (synarthrosis).

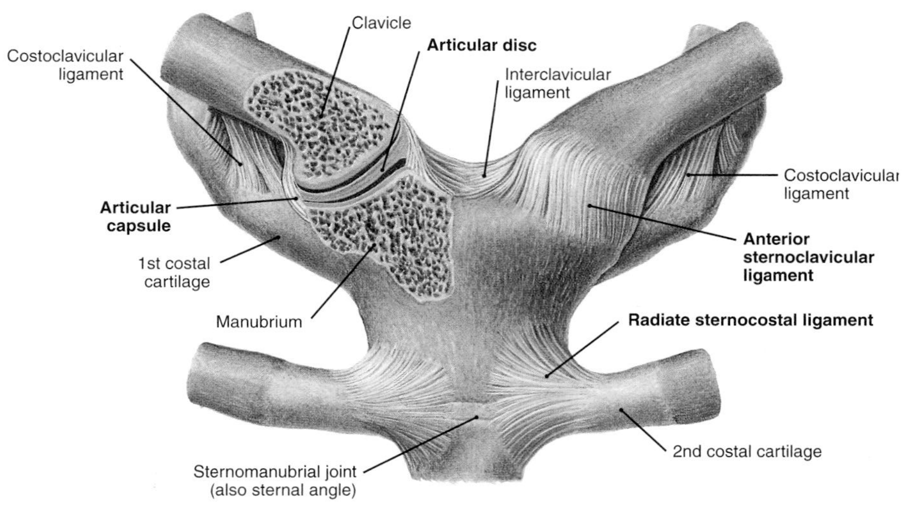
Clavicle
Articular disc
Costoclavicular ligament
Interclavicular ligament
Costoclavicular ligament
Articular capsule
Anterior sternoclavicular ligament
1st costal cartilage
Manubrium
Radiate sternocostal ligament
2nd costal cartilage
Sternomanubrial joint (also sternal angle)

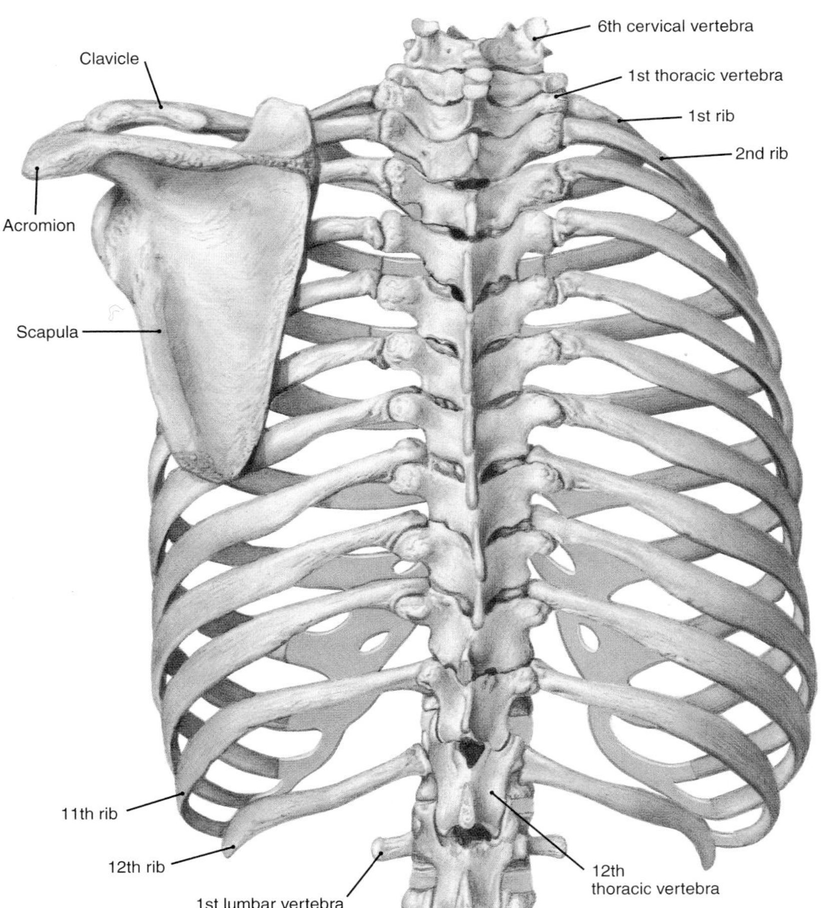
6th cervical vertebra
Clavicle
1st thoracic vertebra
1st rib
2nd rib
Acromion
Scapula
11th rib
12th rib
1st lumbar vertebra
12th thoracic vertebra

Figure 105.1 Thoracic Skeleton (Posterior View)

Left clavicle and scapula are shown in yellow.

NOTE: (1) The posterior skeleton of the thoracic cage consists of 12 thoracic vertebrae and the posterior parts of 12 pairs of ribs.

(2) The extremity on the head of typical ribs possesses two articular facets separated by a crest (see Fig. 106: eighth rib).

(3) These two facets articulate with the bodies of two adjacent vertebrae, whereas the crest is attached to the intervertebral disk. The lower facet articulates with the vertebra that corresponds with the rib, whereas the upper facet articulates with the adjacent vertebra above.

(4) The crest between the facets articulates with the intervertebral disk.

(5) The scapula affords some bony protection posteriorly to the upper lateral aspect of the thoracic cage.

Figure 105.2 Sternum (Anterior View)

NOTE: (1) The sternum consists of the manubrium, the body, and the xiphoid process and forms the middle portion of the anterior thoracic wall.

(2) The manubrium articulates with the body at the **sternal angle.** The xiphoid process is thin and often cartilaginous.

(3) The concave jugular notch, two clavicular notches, and first costal notches on the manubrium.

Figure 105.3 Sternum (Lateral View)

NOTE: (1) The clavicle and the first rib articulate with the manubrium. The second rib articulates at the sternal angle. The third to the sixth ribs articulate with the body of the sternum, whereas the seventh rib joins the sternum at the junction of the xiphoid process.

(2) A line projected backward through the sternal angle crosses at the fourth thoracic level, whereas the xiphisternal junction lies at T9.

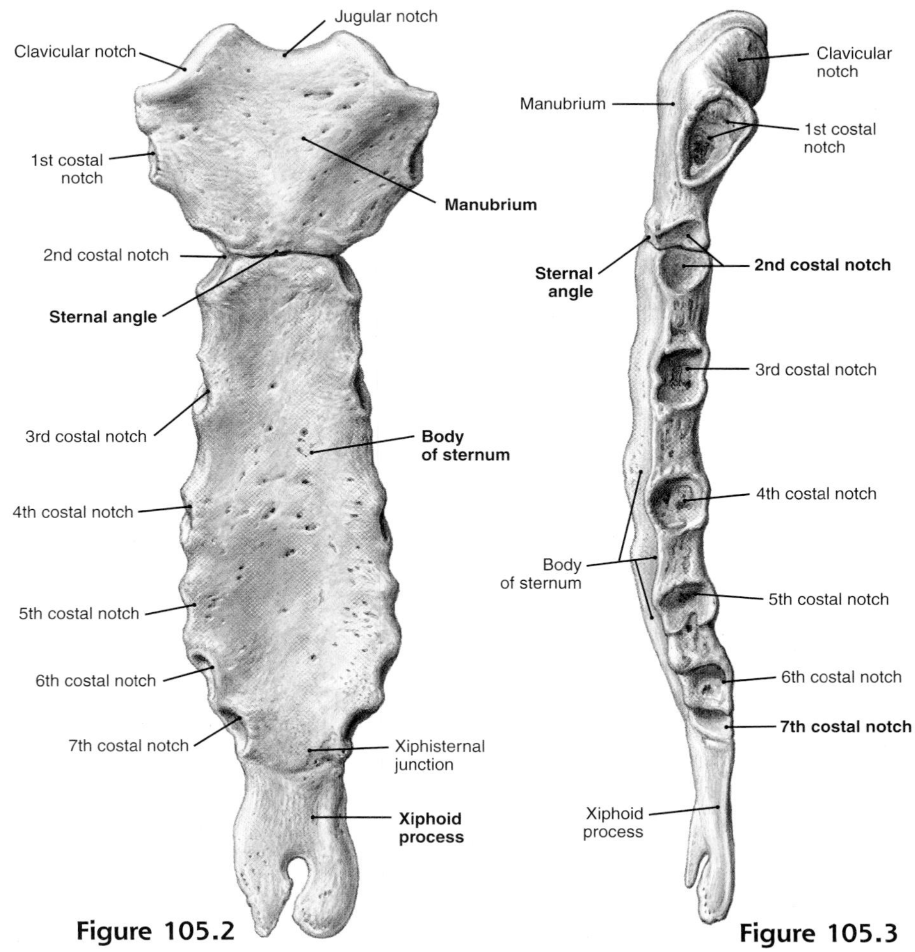
Jugular notch
Clavicular notch
1st costal notch
Manubrium
2nd costal notch
Sternal angle
3rd costal notch
Body of sternum
4th costal notch
5th costal notch
6th costal notch
7th costal notch
Xiphisternal junction
Xiphoid process
Clavicular notch
Manubrium
1st costal notch
Sternal angle
2nd costal notch
3rd costal notch
4th costal notch
Body of sternum
5th costal notch
6th costal notch
7th costal notch
Xiphoid process

Figure 105.2

Figure 105.3

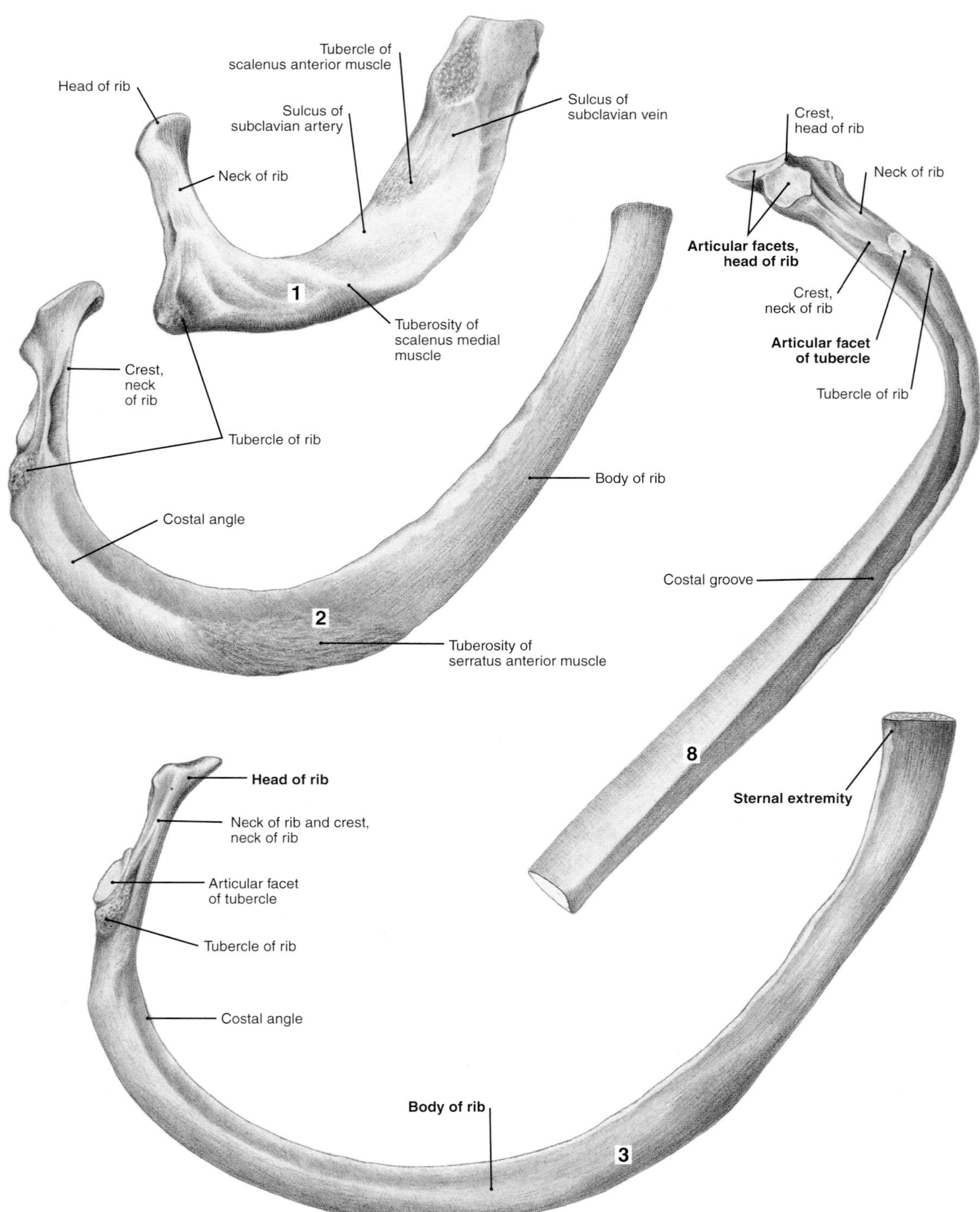
Tubercle of
scalenus anterior muscle
Head of rib
Sulcus of
subclavian artery
Sulcus of
subclavian vein
Neck of rib
1
Tuberosity of
scalenus medial
muscle
Crest,
neck
of rib
Tubercle of rib
Costal angle
2
Tuberosity of
serratus anterior muscle
Body of rib
Crest,
head of rib
Neck of rib
Articular facets,
head of rib
Crest,
neck of rib
Articular facet
of tubercle
Tubercle of rib
Costal groove
8
Head of rib
Neck of rib and crest,
neck of rib
Articular facet
of tubercle
Tubercle of rib
Costal angle
Body of rib
3
Sternal extremity

Figure 106 First, Second, Third, and Eighth Right Ribs

NOTE: (1) The superior surfaces of the first, second, and third ribs are illustrated, whereas the inferior surface of the eighth rib is shown.

(2) Each rib has a vertebral extremity directed posteriorly and a sternal extremity directed anteriorly. The body of the rib is the shaft that stretches between the extremities.

(3) The vertebral end is marked by a **head,** a **neck,** and a **tubercle.** The head contains two facets for articulation with the bodies of the thoracic vertebrae, whereas the tubercle has a nonarticular roughened elevation and an articular facet, which attaches to the transverse process of thoracic vertebrae.

(4) The 1st, 2nd, 10th, 11th, and 12th ribs present certain structural differences from the 3rd through the 9th ribs. The 1st rib is the most curved, and the 2nd is shaped similar to the 1st, but it is longer. The 10th, 11th, and 12th ribs also have only a single facet on the rib head.

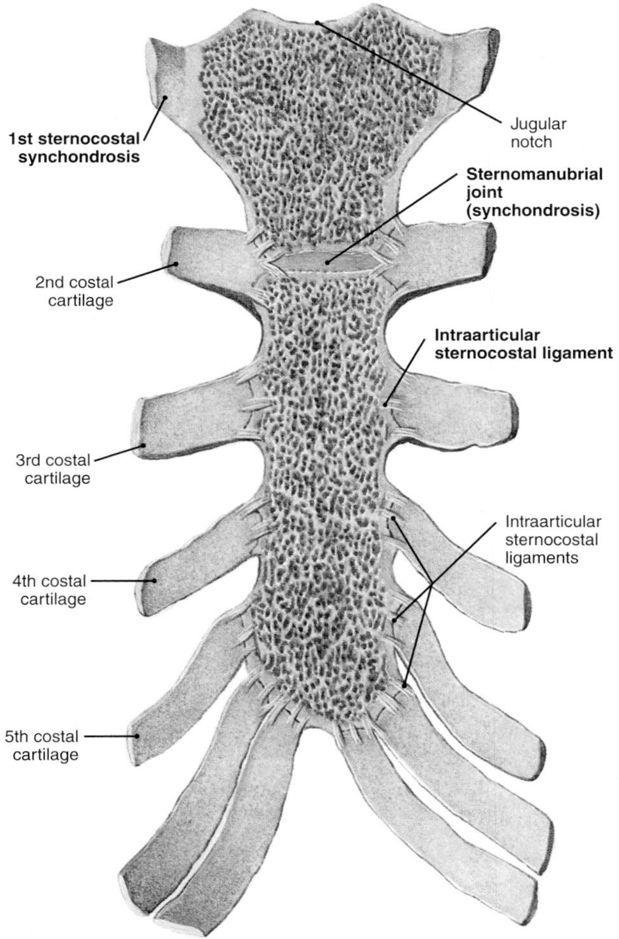
1st sternocostal synchondrosis
Jugular notch
Sternomanubrial joint (synchondrosis)
2nd costal cartilage
Intraarticular sternocostal ligament
3rd costal cartilage
Intraarticular sternocostal ligaments
4th costal cartilage
5th costal cartilage

Figure 107.1 Sternocostal Articulations, Frontal Section (Posterior View)

NOTE: (1) The articulations of the first pair of ribs do not have joint cavities, but are directly cartilaginous unions (synchondroses), similar to the joint between the manubrium and body of the sternum.

(2) Each of the other sternocostal joints contains a true joint cavity surrounded by a capsule. Intraarticular sternocostal ligaments also attach the rib cartilage to the sternum. These are most frequently found at the junctions of the second and third cartilages with the sternum, but may also be seen in lower sternocostal joints.

Figure 107.2 Left Clavicle (Inferior View) ▼

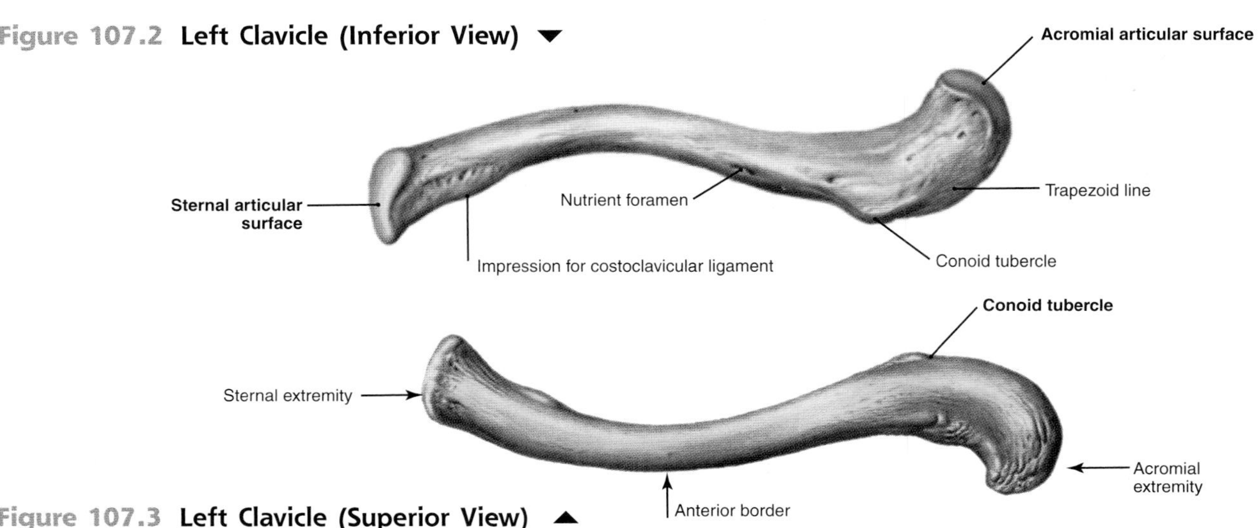
Acromial articular surface
Sternal articular surface
Nutrient foramen
Trapezoid line
Impression for costoclavicular ligament
Conoid tubercle
Conoid tubercle
Sternal extremity
Acromial extremity
Anterior border

Figure 107.3 Left Clavicle (Superior View) ▲

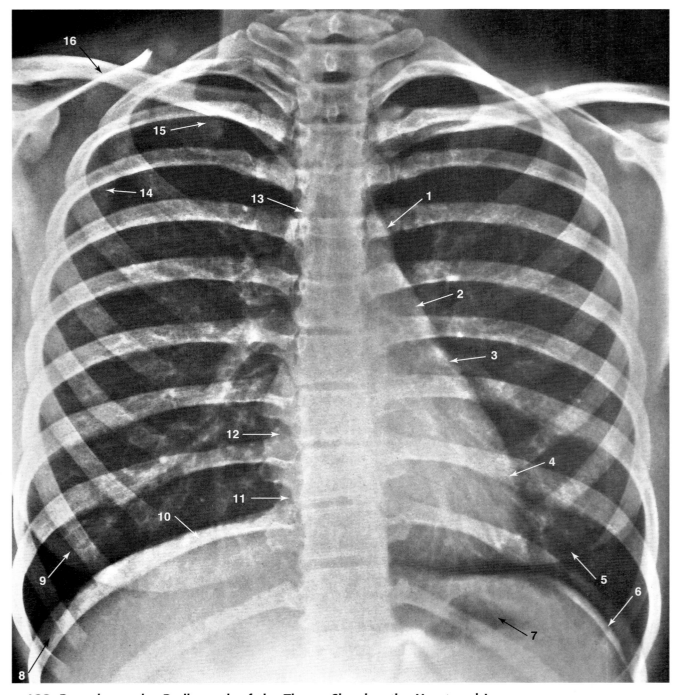

Figure 108 Posterioanterior Radiograph of the Thorax Showing the Heart and Lungs
NOTE: (1) The contour of the heart and great vessels: arch of aorta (1), pulmonary trunk (2), inferior vena cava (11), and superior vena cava (13), and the relationship of these structures to the vertebral column.

(2) The left margin of the heart is formed by the left auricle (3) and left ventricle (4), and it slopes toward the apex, which usually lies about 9 cm to the left of the midsternal line, deep to the fifth intercostal space.

(3) The right margin of the heart (12) projects as a curved line slightly to the right of the vertebral column (and sternum). Observe that the heart rests on the diaphragm (6), and note the contours of the left (5) and right (9) breasts.

(From Wicke, 6th ed.)

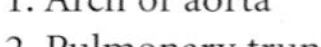

1. Arch of aorta
2. Pulmonary trunk
3. Left auricle
4. Left ventricle
5. Contour of left breast
6. Diaphragm
7. Air in fundus of stomach
8. Costodiaphragmatic recess
9. Contour of right breast
10. Diaphragm
11. Inferior vena cava
12. Right atrium
13. Superior vena cava
14. Medial border of scapula
15. First rib
16. Right clavicle

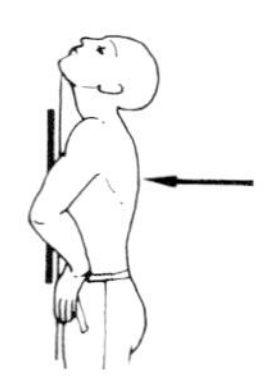

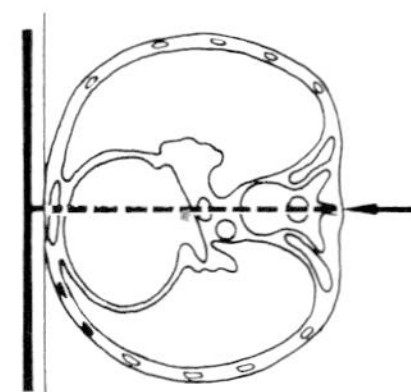

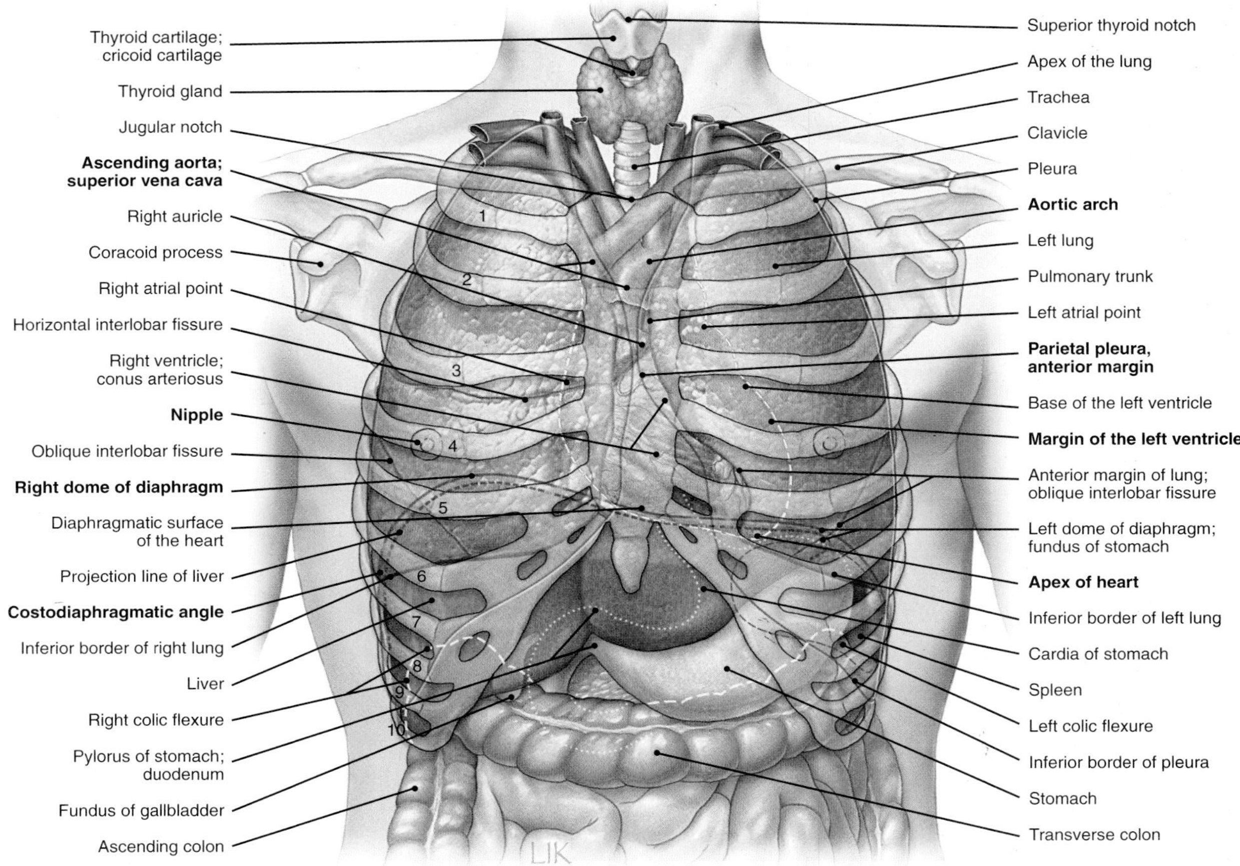
Thyroid cartilage; cricoid cartilage
Thyroid gland
Jugular notch
Ascending aorta; superior vena cava
Right auricle
Coracoid process
Right atrial point
Horizontal interlobar fissure
Right ventricle; conus arteriosus
Nipple
Oblique interlobar fissure
Right dome of diaphragm
Diaphragmatic surface of the heart
Projection line of liver
Costodiaphragmatic angle
Inferior border of right lung
Liver
Right colic flexure
Pylorus of stomach; duodenum
Fundus of gallbladder
Ascending colon
Superior thyroid notch
Apex of the lung
Trachea
Clavicle
Pleura
Aortic arch
Left lung
Pulmonary trunk
Left atrial point
Parietal pleura, anterior margin
Base of the left ventricle
Margin of the left ventricle
Anterior margin of lung; oblique interlobar fissure
Left dome of diaphragm; fundus of stomach
Apex of heart
Inferior border of left lung
Cardia of stomach
Spleen
Left colic flexure
Inferior border of pleura
Stomach
Transverse colon
1
2
3
4
5
6
7
8
9
10

Figure 109.1 Thoracic and Upper Abdominal Viscera Projected onto the Anterior Surface of the Body

NOTE: (1) The outline of the heart and great vessels (white broken line) deep to the anterior border of the lungs.

(2) The liver, lying below the diaphragm, extends upward as high as the fourth interspace on the right, and to the fifth interspace on the left (red broken line).

(3) The superficial location of the superior vena cava and ascending aorta just deep to the manubrium of the sternum.

(4) A triangular region containing the great vessels above and a lower triangular region over the heart (area of superficial cardiac dullness) are not covered by pleura.

(5) The reflections of the pleura over the lungs. Observe that the anterior margins of the lung and pleura on the left side are indented to form the cardiac notch.

(6) The position of the nipple over the fourth rib (or fourth intercostal space) in the male and in the young female. Observe also the apex of the heart deep to the fifth interspace.

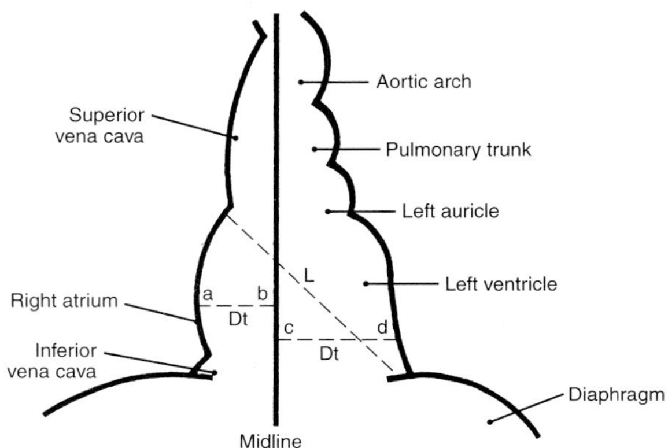
Aortic arch
Superior vena cava
Pulmonary trunk
Left auricle
Left ventricle
Right atrium
Inferior vena cava
Diaphragm
Midline
a
b
c
d
Dt
Dt
L

Figure 109.2 Shadow Outline of Heart and Great Vessels in Radiograph of the Thorax

Dt: Transverse diameter (normal)
a to b: about 4 cm
c to d: about 9 cm

L: Longitudinal axis of heart: 15 to 16 cm
(measured from the upper end of the right atrial shadow to the apex of the heart)

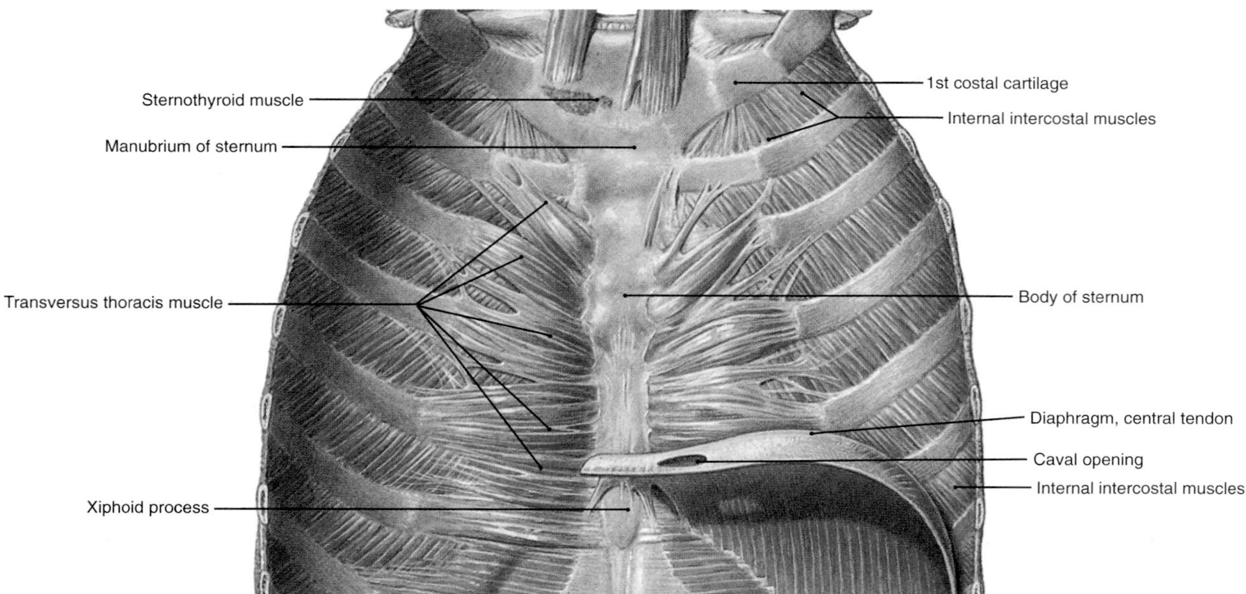
Sternothyroid muscle
Manubrium of sternum
Transversus thoracis muscle
Xiphoid process
1st costal cartilage
Internal intercostal muscles
Body of sternum
Diaphragm, central tendon
Caval opening
Internal intercostal muscles

Figure 110.1 Internal Surface of the Thoracic Cage (Anterior Part)

NOTE: (1) The transversus thoracis muscle. It arises from the inferior half of the body of the sternum and the xiphoid process. Its fibers course laterally and superiorly to insert on the inner surfaces of the second to the sixth ribs and their costal cartilages.

(2) The intercostal nerves supply the transversus thoracis muscle and its fascicles depress the costal cartilages to which the fibers attach.

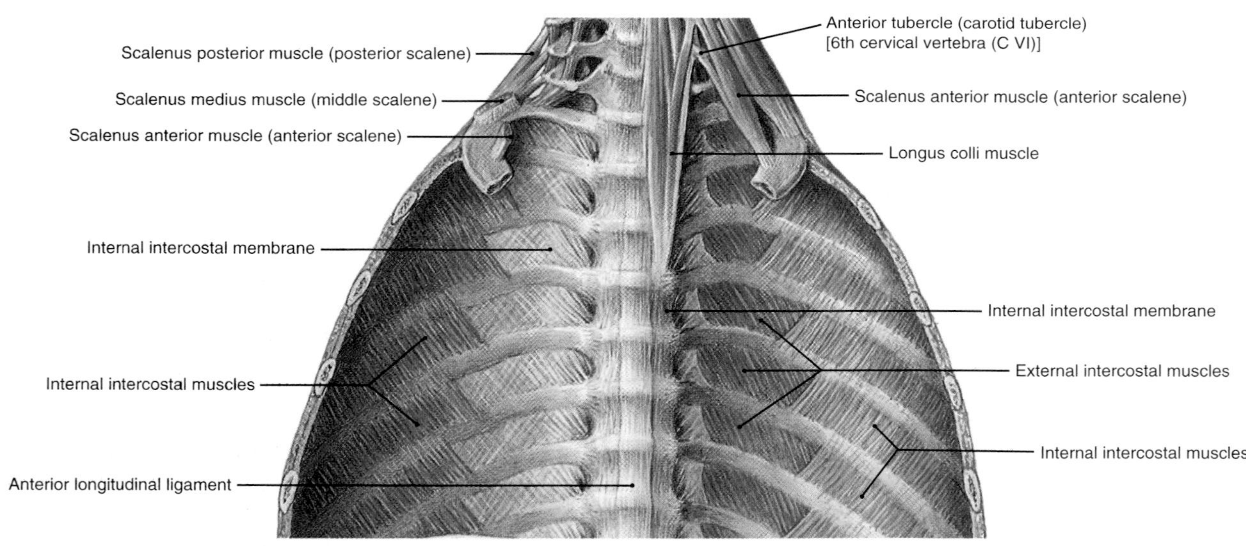
Scalenus posterior muscle (posterior scalene)
Scalenus medius muscle (middle scalene)
Scalenus anterior muscle (anterior scalene)
Internal intercostal membrane
Internal intercostal muscles
Anterior longitudinal ligament
Anterior tubercle (carotid tubercle)
[6th cervical vertebra (C VI)]
Scalenus anterior muscle (anterior scalene)
Longus colli muscle
Internal intercostal membrane
External intercostal muscles
Internal intercostal muscles

Figure 110.2 Internal Surface of the Thoracic Cage (Posterior Part)

NOTE: (1) The internal intercostal muscle fibers can be seen to extend between the ribs as far posteriorly as the bodies of the thoracic vertebrae.

(2) In contrast to the external intercostal muscle fibers, the internal intercostal 1 muscle fibers are replaced by the internal intercostal membrane medial to the posterior costal angles of the ribs and as far as the bodies of the thoracic vertebrae.

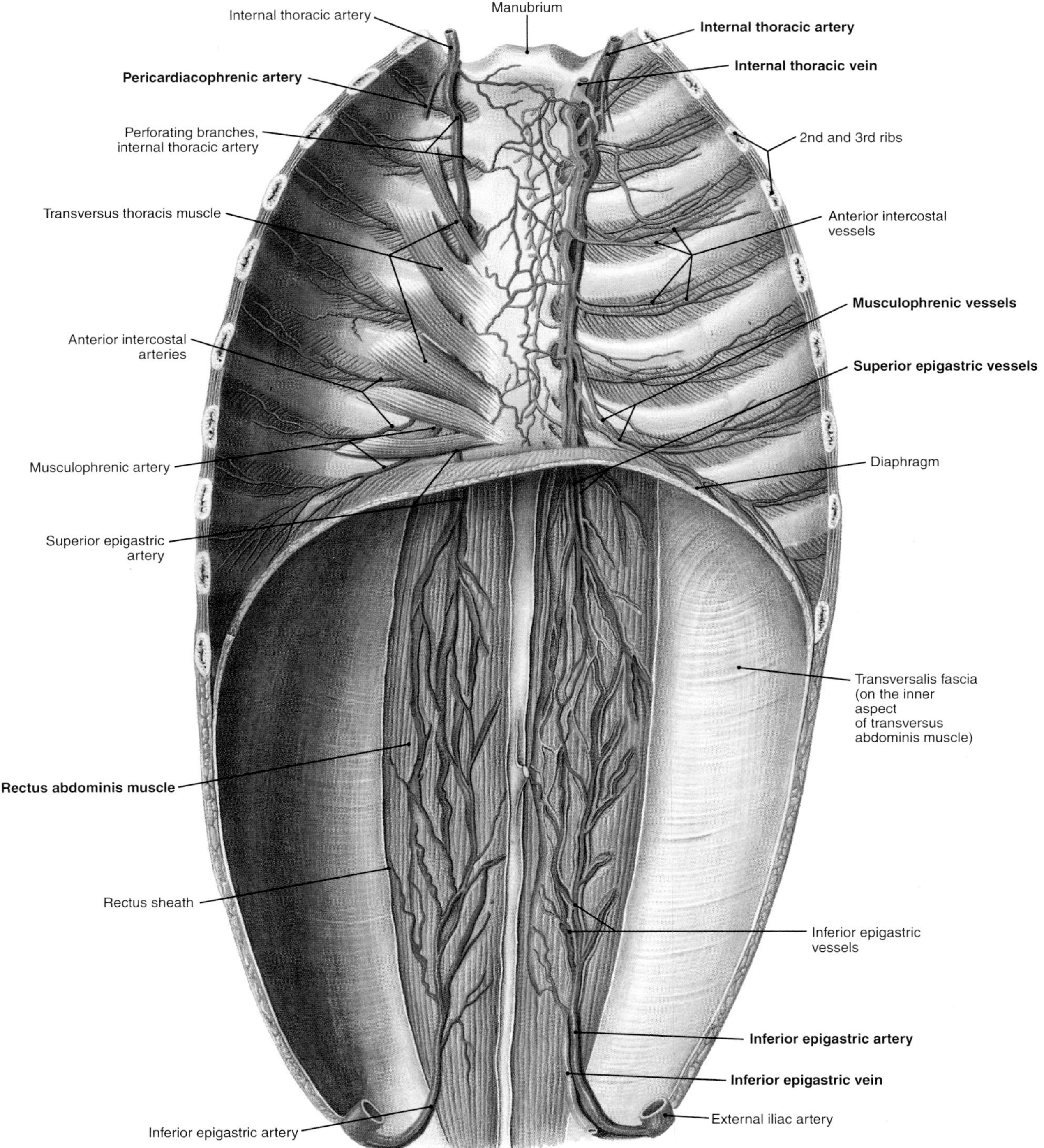

Internal thoracic artery
Manubrium
Internal thoracic artery
Pericardiacophrenic artery
Internal thoracic vein
Perforating branches, internal thoracic artery
2nd and 3rd ribs
Transversus thoracis muscle
Anterior intercostal vessels
Musculophrenic vessels
Anterior intercostal arteries
Superior epigastric vessels
Musculophrenic artery
Diaphragm
Superior epigastric artery
Transversalis fascia (on the inner aspect of transversus abdominis muscle)
Rectus abdominis muscle
Rectus sheath
Inferior epigastric vessels
Inferior epigastric artery
Inferior epigastric vein
External iliac artery
Inferior epigastric artery

Figure 111 Muscles and Blood Vessels of the Thoracic and Abdominal Wall, Viewed from the Inside

NOTE: (1) The principal vessels dissected include the **internal thoracic** and **inferior epigastric** arteries and veins and their terminal branches.

(2) The internal thoracic artery is a branch of the subclavian artery, and it descends behind the costal cartilages along the inner surface of the anterior thoracic wall in front of the transversus thoracis muscle and parallel to the margin of the sternum.

(3) The internal thoracic artery gives rise to (a) the pericardiacophrenic artery, (b) small vessels to the thymus and to bronchial structures, (c) perforating branches to the chest wall, (d) anterior intercostal branches, and finally it terminates as (e) the **musculophrenic** and **superior epigastric arteries.**

(4) The superior epigastric artery anastomoses with the **inferior epigastric artery**, a branch of the external iliac artery. The anastomosis occurs within the rectus abdominis muscle.

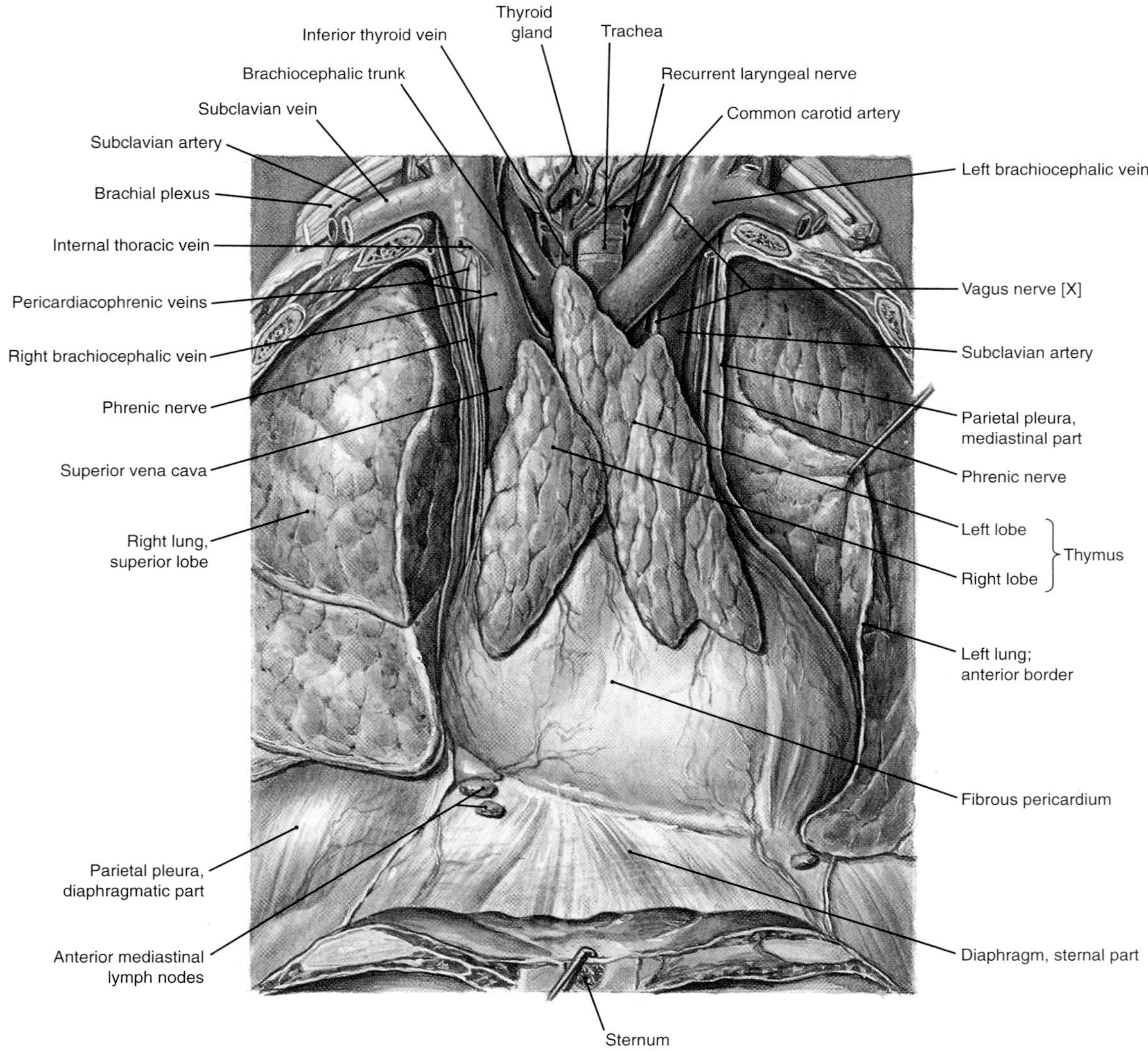

Thyroid gland
Inferior thyroid vein
Trachea
Brachiocephalic trunk
Recurrent laryngeal nerve
Subclavian vein
Common carotid artery
Subclavian artery
Left brachiocephalic vein
Brachial plexus
Internal thoracic vein
Pericardiacophrenic veins
Vagus nerve [X]
Right brachiocephalic vein
Subclavian artery
Phrenic nerve
Parietal pleura, mediastinal part
Superior vena cava
Phrenic nerve
Right lung, superior lobe
Left lobe
Thymus
Right lobe
Left lung; anterior border
Fibrous pericardium
Parietal pleura, diaphragmatic part
Anterior mediastinal lymph nodes
Diaphragm, sternal part
Sternum

Figure 112.1 Thymus in an Adolescent
NOTE that the chest wall is removed and the parietal pleura has been opened.

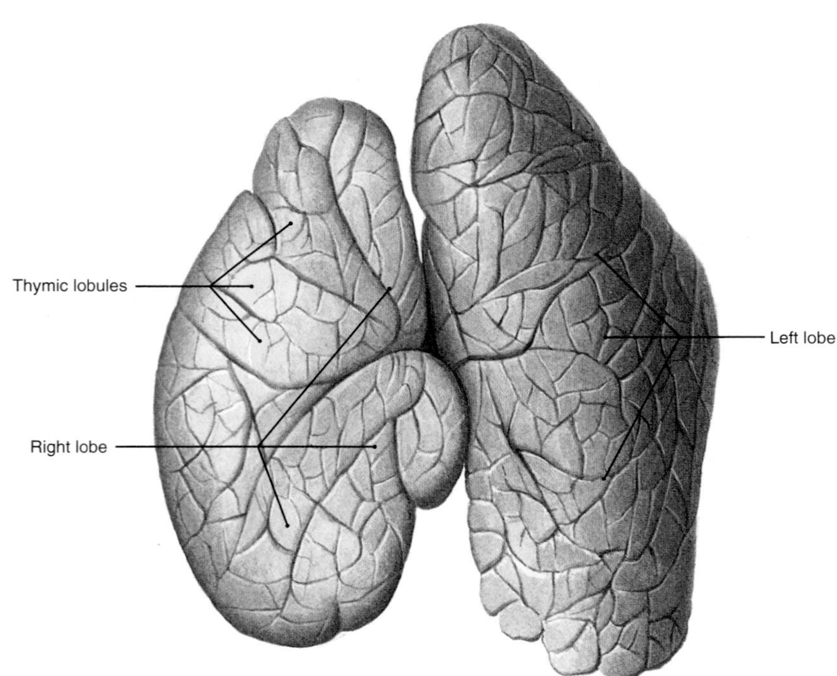

Thymic lobules
Left lobe
Right lobe

Figure 112.2 Thymus of a 2-Year-Old Child
NOTE: (1) The thymus is the central organ of the immune-lymphoid system.

(2) At birth it weighs under 15 g and at puberty it has grown to about 35 g. In the adult it diminishes in size, becoming atrophic and being replaced by fat.

(3) The thymus lies in the anterior and superior mediastina, and it receives branches from the internal thoracic and inferior thyroid arteries. Its veins drain into the brachiocephalic, internal thoracic, and inferior thyroid veins.

(4) The thymus differentiates lymphocytes into thymocytes (T cells), which are released into peripheral blood and become capable of cell-mediated immunologic responses to antigenic foreign substances. Also, these cells act with B lymphocytes for humoral responses.

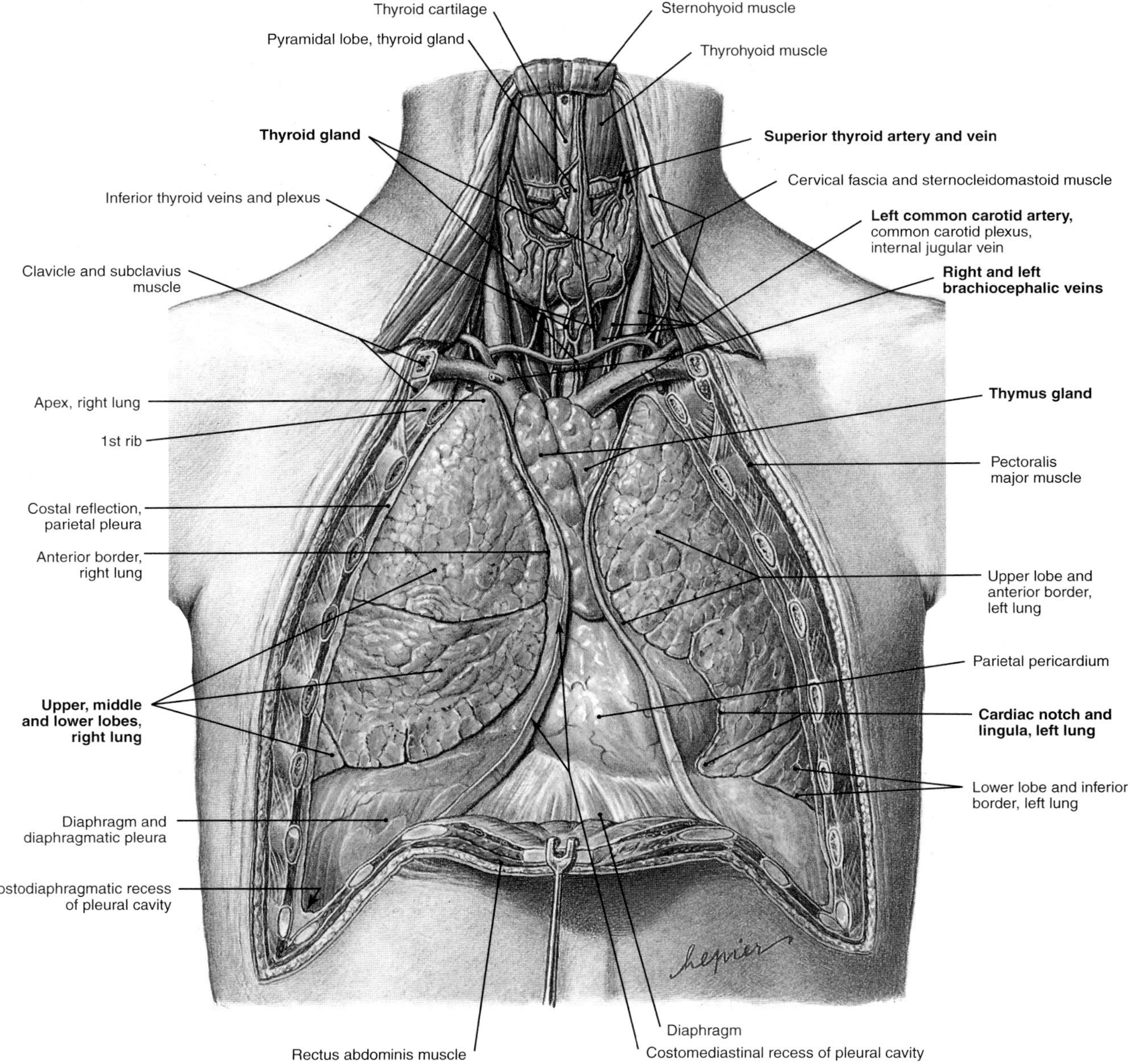
Thyroid cartilage
Sternohyoid muscle
Pyramidal lobe, thyroid gland
Thyrohyoid muscle
Thyroid gland
Superior thyroid artery and vein
Cervical fascia and sternocleidomastoid muscle
Inferior thyroid veins and plexus
Left common carotid artery, common carotid plexus, internal jugular vein
Clavicle and subclavius muscle
Right and left brachiocephalic veins
Apex, right lung
Thymus gland
1st rib
Pectoralis major muscle
Costal reflection, parietal pleura
Anterior border, right lung
Upper lobe and anterior border, left lung
Parietal pericardium
Upper, middle and lower lobes, right lung
Cardiac notch and lingula, left lung
Lower lobe and inferior border, left lung
Diaphragm and diaphragmatic pleura
Costodiaphragmatic recess of pleural cavity
Diaphragm
Rectus abdominis muscle
Costomediastinal recess of pleural cavity

Figure 113 Thoracic Viscera and the Root of the Neck (Anterior Exposure)

NOTE: (1) The anterior thoracic wall has been removed along with the medial parts of both clavicles to reveal the normal position of the heart, lungs, thymus, and thyroid gland. The great vessels in the superior aperture of the thorax are also exposed.

(2) The parietal pleura has been removed anteriorly. The thymus is situated between the two lungs superiorly, whereas inferiorly is found the bare area of the heart. Observe the **cardiac notch** along the anterior border of the left lung adjacent to the heart.

(3) The basal surface of both lungs and the inferior aspect of the heart rest on the diaphragm, whereas the apex of each lung extends superiorly above the level of the first rib.

(4) The rather transverse course in the superior mediastinum of the left brachiocephalic vein in contrast to the nearly vertical course of the right brachiocephalic vein. The two brachiocephalic veins join, deep to the thymus, to form the superior vena cava.

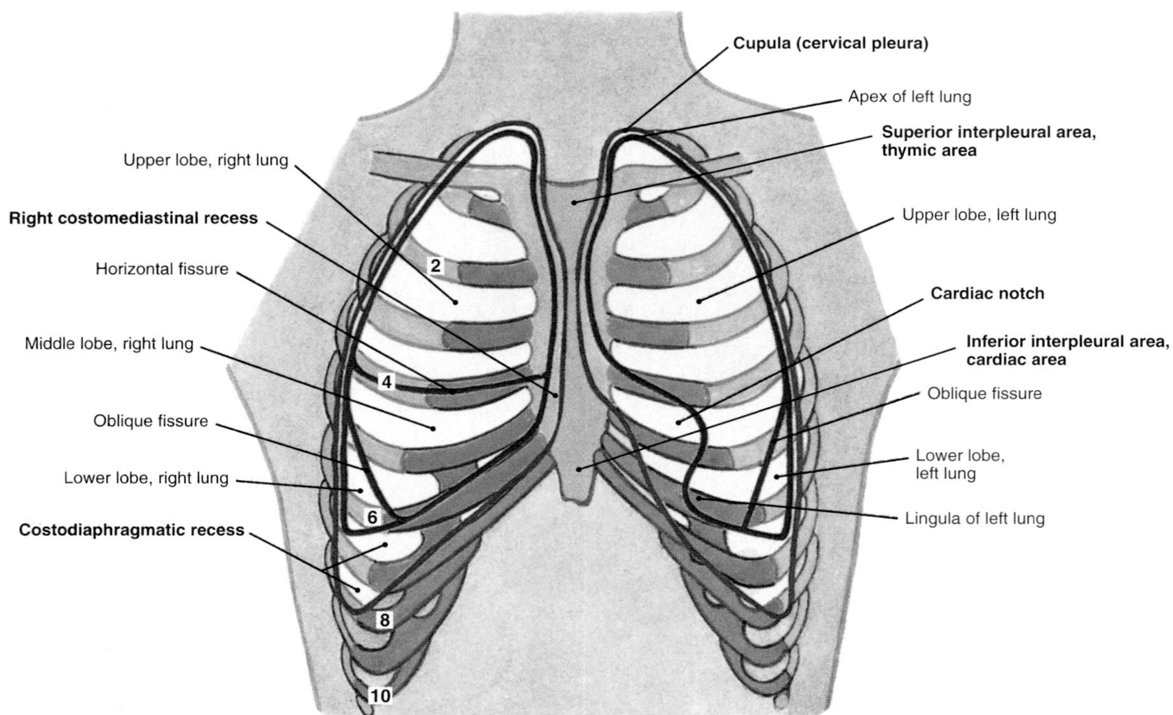
Cupula (cervical pleura)
Apex of left lung
Superior interpleural area, thymic area
Upper lobe, left lung
Cardiac notch
Inferior interpleural area, cardiac area
Oblique fissure
Lower lobe, left lung
Lingula of left lung
Upper lobe, right lung
Right costomediastinal recess
Horizontal fissure
Middle lobe, right lung
Oblique fissure
Lower lobe, right lung
Costodiaphragmatic recess
2
4
6
8
10

Figure 114.1 Parietal (Green) and Visceral (Red) Pleural Reflections Projected onto the Anterior Thoracic Wall

NOTE: (1) Each lung is invested by two layers of pleura that are continuous at the hilum of the lung, and thereby form an invaginated sac.

(2) The **parietal layer of pleura** (shown in green) is the outermost of the two layers, and it lines the inner surface of the thoracic wall and the superior surface of the diaphragm. The **visceral layer** of **pleura** closely invests and adheres to the surfaces of the lungs (in red).

(3) The potential space between the two pleural layers is called the **pleural cavity** and contains only a small amount of serous fluid in the healthy person, but it may contain considerable fluid and blood in pathologic conditions.

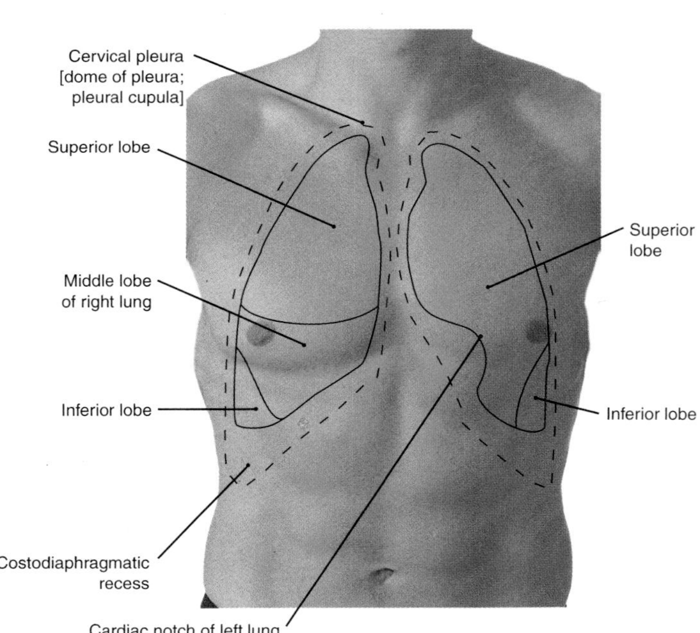
Cervical pleura [dome of pleura; pleural cupula]
Superior lobe
Middle lobe of right lung
Inferior lobe
Costodiaphragmatic recess
Cardiac notch of left lung
Superior lobe
Inferior lobe

Figure 114.2 Outline Directly onto the Anterior Thoracic Wall of Pleural Reflections

NOTE: The boundaries of the lungs are shown by solid lines, while those of the parietal pleura are shown by broken lines.

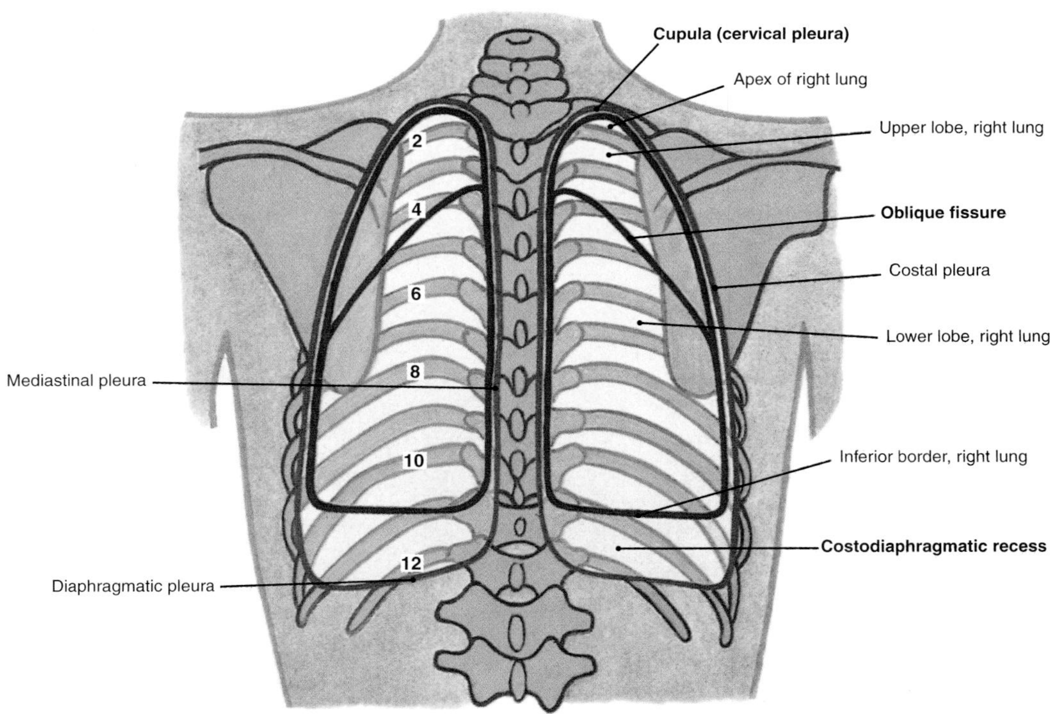
Cupula (cervical pleura)
Apex of right lung
Upper lobe, right lung
Oblique fissure
Costal pleura
Lower lobe, right lung
Mediastinal pleura
Inferior border, right lung
Costodiaphragmatic recess
Diaphragmatic pleura
2
4
6
8
10
12

Figure 115.1 Parietal (Green) and Visceral (Red) Pleural Reflections onto the Posterior Thoracic Wall

NOTE: (1) The parietal pleura is a continuous sheet, but parts of it are named in relation to their adjacent surfaces. Lining the inner surface of the ribs is the **costal pleura**, while the **diaphragmatic** and **mediastinal pleurae** are found on the surfaces of the diaphragm and mediastinum. Overlying the apex of each lung is the **cupula** or **cervical pleura**.

(2) Due to the curvature of the diaphragm, a narrow recess is formed around its periphery into which the lung (visceral pleura) does not extend. An important potential space lies between the costal and diaphragmatic pleurae called the **costodiaphragmatic recess**, which may be punctured and drained of fluid without damage to the lung tissue.

Figure 115.2 Outline of Pleural Reflections Directly onto the Posterior Thoracic Wall

NOTE: (1) The boundaries of the lungs are the solid lines, while the boundaries of the pleura are the broken (dash) lines.

(2) The "rib-level" relationships of the lungs (visceral pleura) and the parietal pleura are as follows:

	Visceral pleura	Parietal pleura
(a) Anterior (midclavicular line)	6th rib	8th rib
(b) Lateral (midaxillary line)	8th rib	10th rib
(c) Posterior (medial border of the scapula)	10th rib	12th rib
(Summary of Rib Levels)	Visceral Pleura	Ribs 6, 8, 10
	Parietal Pleura	Ribs 8, 10, 12

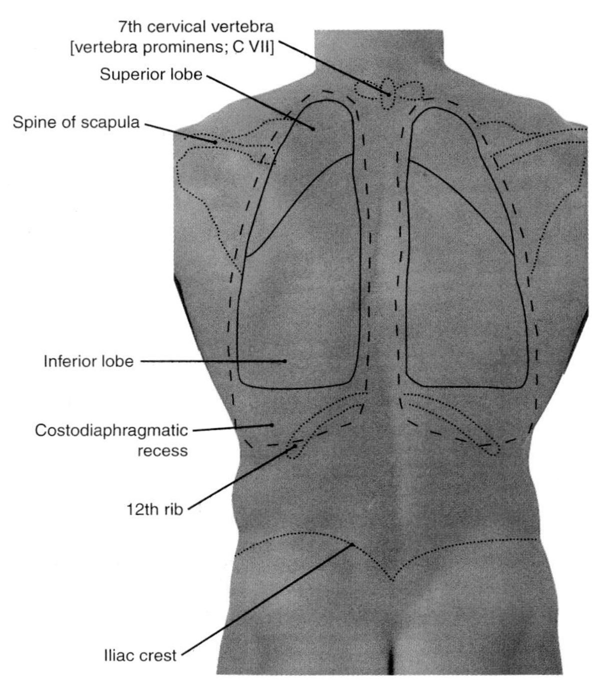
7th cervical vertebra
[vertebra prominens; C VII]
Superior lobe
Spine of scapula
Inferior lobe
Costodiaphragmatic
recess
12th rib
Iliac crest

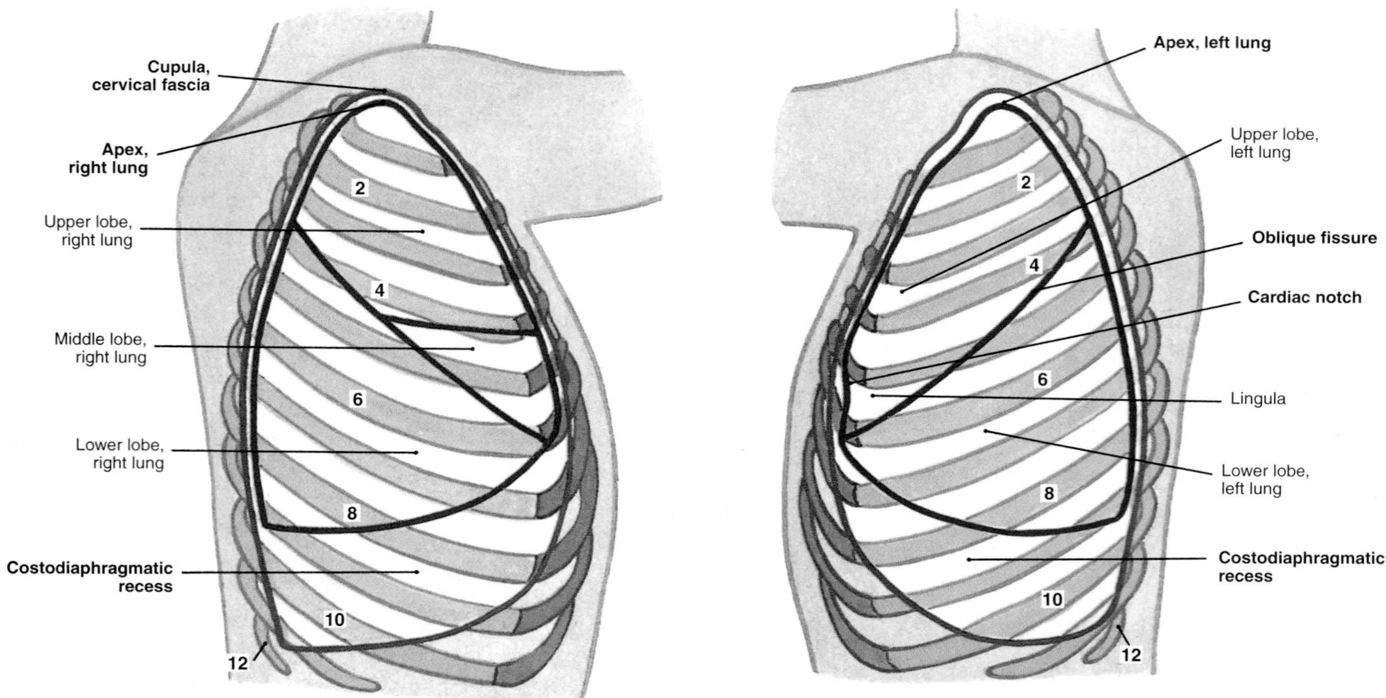
Cupula, cervical fascia
Apex, right lung
Upper lobe, right lung
Middle lobe, right lung
Lower lobe, right lung
Costodiaphragmatic recess
2
4
6
8
10
12
Apex, left lung
Upper lobe, left lung
Oblique fissure
Cardiac notch
Lingula
Lower lobe, left lung
Costodiaphragmatic recess

Figure 116.1 Right Lateral View **Figure 116.2 Left Lateral View**

Pleural Reflections (Green) and Lungs (Red) Projected onto Thoracic Wall

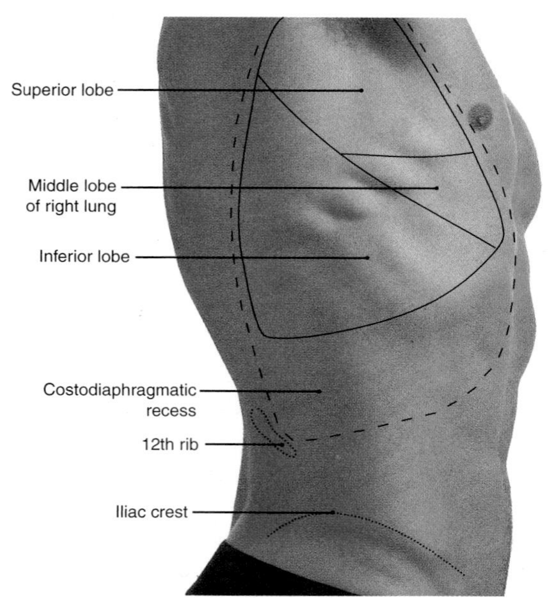
Superior lobe
Middle lobe of right lung
Inferior lobe
Costodiaphragmatic recess
12th rib
Iliac crest

Figure 116.3 Projection of Pleural and Pulmonary Borders (Right Lateral Aspect)

NOTE that the borders of the lung are shown by solid lines, while borders of the pleura are shown by broken (dashed) lines.

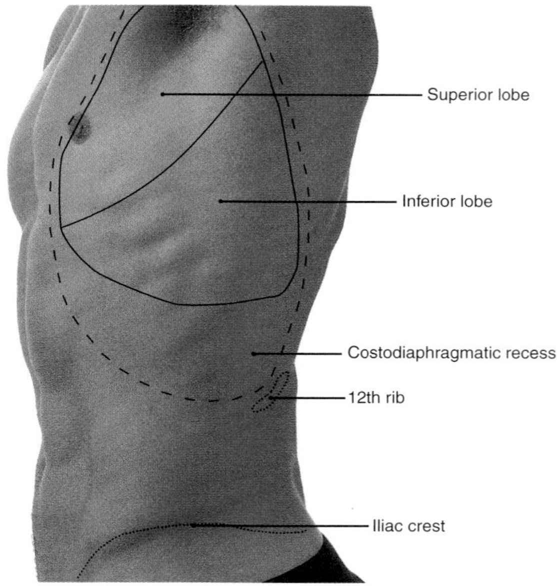
Superior lobe
Inferior lobe
Costodiaphragmatic recess
12th rib
Iliac crest

Figure 116.4 Projection of Pleural and Pulmonary Borders (Left Lateral Aspect)

NOTE that the borders of the lung are shown by solid lines, while borders of the pleura are shown by broken (dashed) lines.

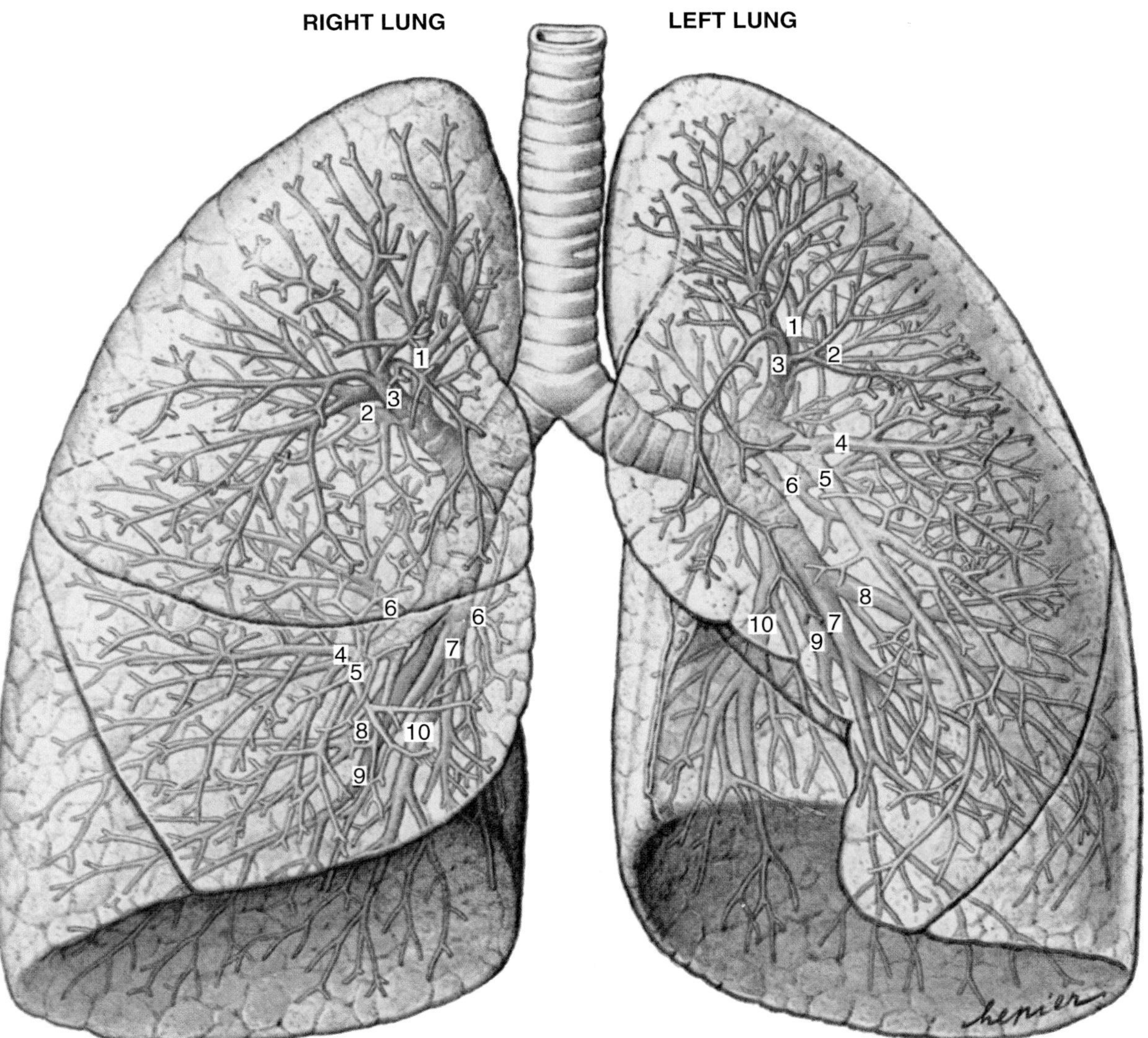
RIGHT LUNG
LEFT LUNG
1
2
3
4
5
6
6
7
8
9
10
1
2
3
4
5
6
7
8
9
10

Figure 117 Bronchial Tree and Its Lobar and Bronchopulmonary Divisions (Anterior View)

NOTE: (1) As the trachea divides, the **left primary bronchus** diverges at a greater angle than the **right primary bronchus** to reach the left lung. The left bronchus, therefore, is directed more transversely and the right bronchus more inferiorly.

(2) **On the right side** the upper lobar bronchus branches from the primary bronchus almost immediately, even above the pulmonary artery (eparterial), while the bronchus is directed toward the middle and lower lobes branches below the main stem of the pulmonary artery (hyparterial).

(3) **On the left side** the initial lobar bronchus, branching from the primary bronchus, is directed upward and lateral to the upper lobe segments and its lingular segments. The remaining lobar bronchus is directed inferiorly and soon divides into the segmental bronchi of the lower lobe.

(4) The segmental bronchi numbered in the figure above are as follows:

Right lung

1. Apical
2. Posterior
3. Anterior
4. Lateral
5. Medial
6. Superior
7. Medial basal
8. Anterior basal
9. Lateral basal
10. Posterior basal

Left lung

1. Apical
2. Posterior
3. Anterior
4. Superior lingular
5. Inferior lingular
6. Superior
7. Medial basal
8. Anterior basal
9. Lateral basal
10. Posterior basal

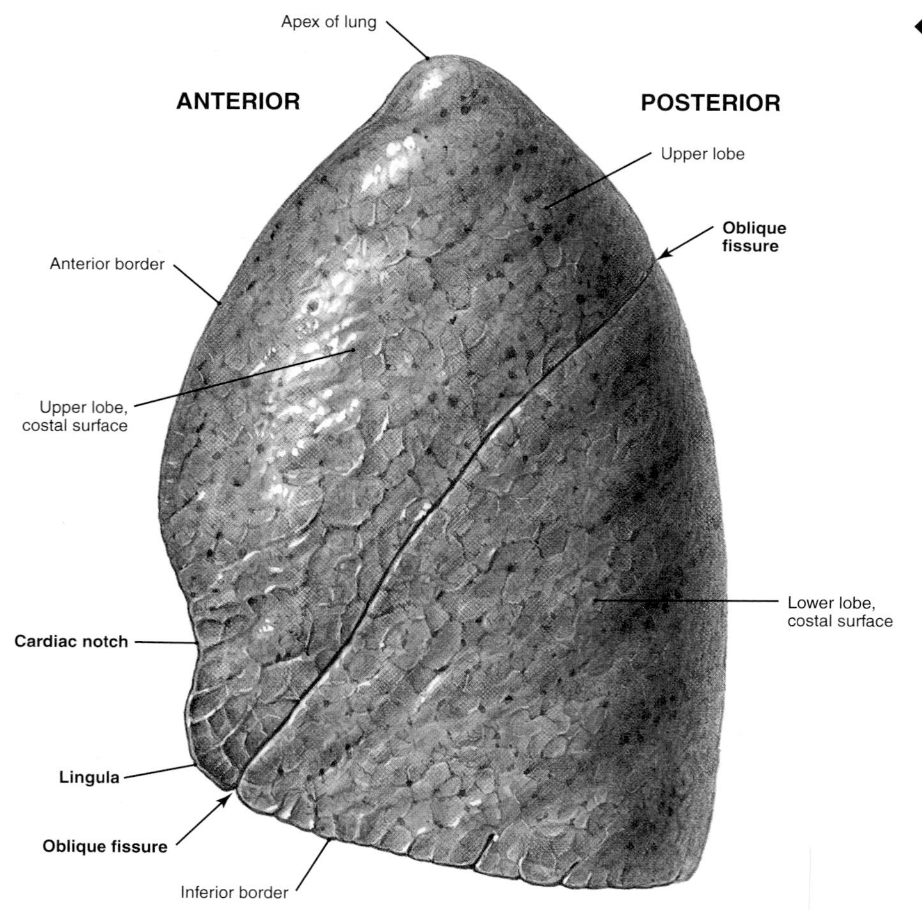
Apex of lung
ANTERIOR
POSTERIOR
Upper lobe
Oblique fissure
Anterior border
Upper lobe, costal surface
Lower lobe, costal surface
Cardiac notch
Lingula
Oblique fissure
Inferior border

Figure 118.1 Left Lung (Lateral View)

NOTE: (1) The lateral view of the left lung shows a rounded convex costal surface directed toward the thoracic wall and divided into upper and lower lobes by the **oblique fissure**.

(2) The **upper lobe** has a rounded apex, which is pointed above. The upper lobe forms virtually all of the **anterior border** of the left lung and, inferiorly, it is indented by the **cardiac notch**. A small tongue-like anterior projection below the cardiac notch is called the **lingula**.

(3) The **lower lobe** is somewhat larger than the upper, and its base is the **diaphragmatic surface** of the left lung. This is adapted to the dome shape of the diaphragm.

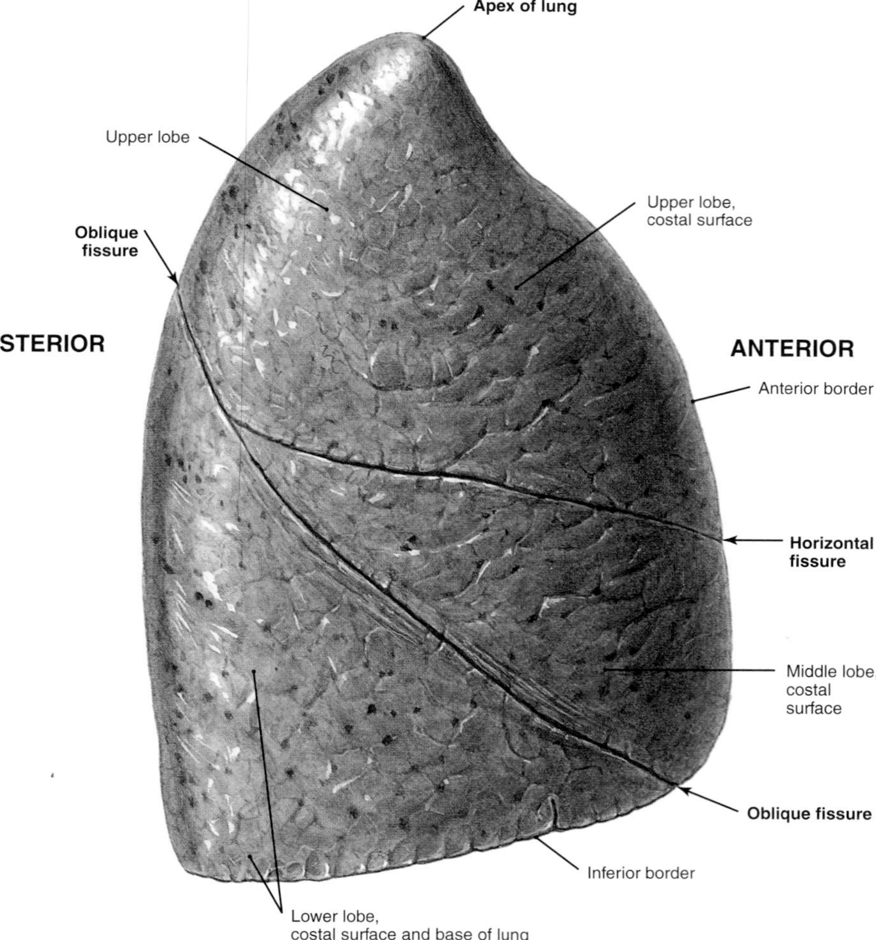
Apex of lung
Upper lobe
Upper lobe, costal surface
Oblique fissure
POSTERIOR
ANTERIOR
Anterior border
Horizontal fissure
Middle lobe, costal surface
Oblique fissure
Inferior border
Lower lobe, costal surface and base of lung

Figure 118.2 Right Lung (Lateral View)

NOTE: (1) The lateral or costal surface of the right lung is smooth and rounded and presents three lobes separated by two fissures. The **oblique fissure** separates the lower lobe from the middle and upper lobes and corresponds to the oblique fissure of the left lung. The **horizontal fissure** separates the upper and middle lobes.

(2) The upper lobe is capped by the apex of the lung. This lobe forms the upper two-thirds of the **anterior border.** The middle lobe forms the lower third of the anterior border, while the lower lobe (as in the left lung) constitutes the entire **inferior border** and diaphragmatic surface.

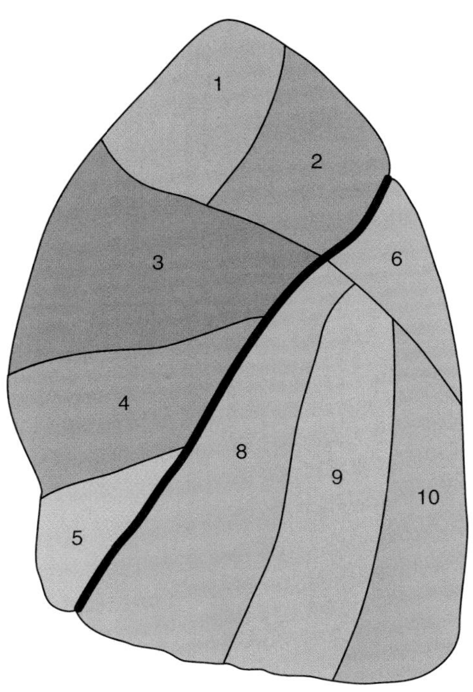
1
2
3
6
4
8
9
10
5

Figure 119.1 Left Lung, Bronchopulmonary Segments (Lateral View)

NOTE: (1) Bronchopulmonary segments are anatomical subdivisions of the lung, each supplied by its own segmental (tertiary) bronchus and artery and drained by intersegmental veins.

(2) The trachea divides into two primary bronchi, each of which serves an entire lung. The primary bronchi divide into secondary, or lobar, bronchi. There are two lobar bronchi on the left and three on the right, each supplying a separate lobe.

(3) Secondary bronchi divide into segmental or tertiary bronchi, distributed to the bronchopulmonary segments. Usual descriptions of the bronchopulmonary segments define 8 to 10 segments in the left lung.

(4) In the left lung, the segments are numbered and named as follows:

Upper lobe

1. Apical ⎤
2. Posterior ⎥ Frequently considered as a single segment
3. Anterior ⎦
4. Superior ⎤ Lingular
5. Inferior ⎦

Lower lobe

6. Superior
7. Medial basal ⎤ Usually considered as a single segment;
8. Anterior basal ⎦ medial basal cannot be seen from lateral view.
9. Lateral basal
10. Posterior basal

(5) In the left lower lobe the medial basal bronchus arises separately from the anterior basal bronchus in only about 13% of humans studied.

Figure 119.2 Right Lung, Bronchopulmonary Segments (Lateral View) ▶

NOTE: (1) Subdivision of the lungs into functional bronchopulmonary segments allows the surgeon to determine whether segments of lung might be resected in operations in preference to entire lobes.

(2) Although minor variations exist in the division of the bronchial tree, a consistency has become accepted in the naming of bronchopulmonary segmentation. The nomenclature used here was published by Jackson and Huber (Dis Chest 1943;9:319–326) and is now used because it is the simplest and most straightforward of those that have been suggested.

(3) The bronchopulmonary segments of the right lung are numbered and named as follows:

Upper lobe
1. Apical
2. Posterior
3. Anterior

Middle lobe
4. Lateral
5. Medial

Lower lobe
6. Superior
7. Medial basal (cannot be seen from lateral view)
8. Anterior basal
9. Lateral basal
10. Posterior basal

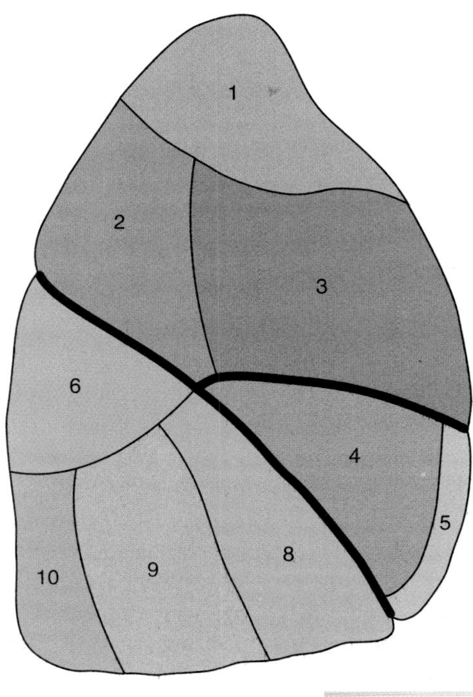
1
2
3
6
4
5
8
10
9

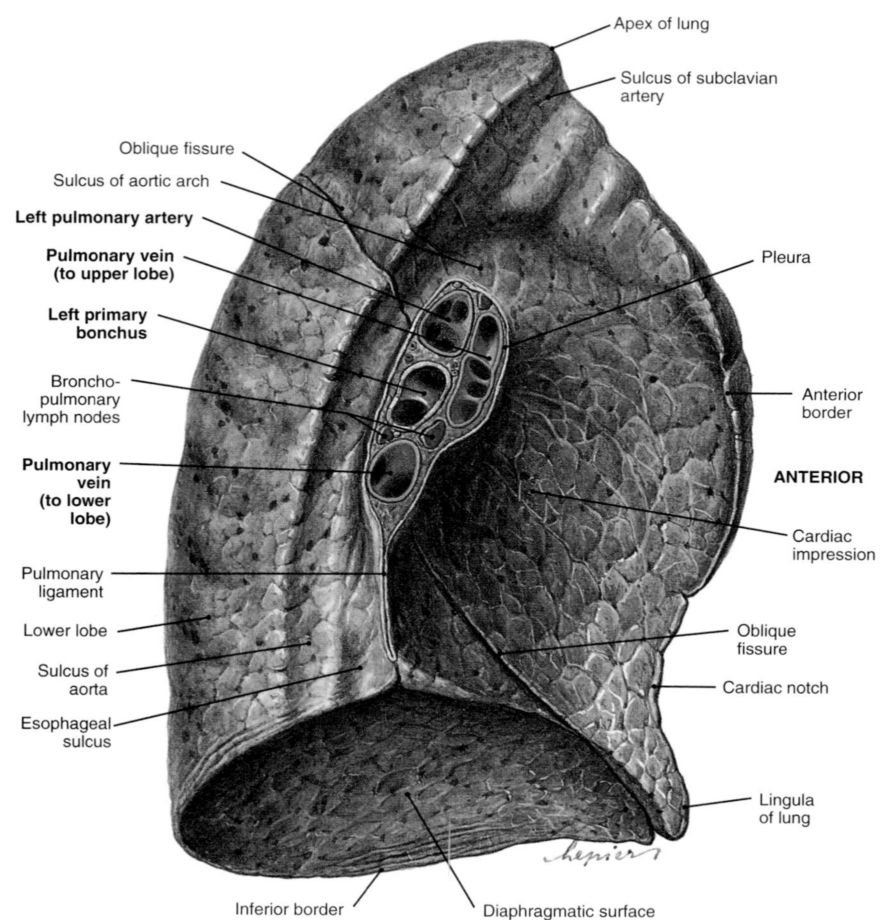
Apex of lung
Sulcus of subclavian artery
Oblique fissure
Sulcus of aortic arch
Left pulmonary artery
Pulmonary vein (to upper lobe)
Left primary bonchus
Broncho-pulmonary lymph nodes
Pulmonary vein (to lower lobe)
Pulmonary ligament
Lower lobe
Sulcus of aorta
Esophageal sulcus
Pleura
Anterior border
ANTERIOR
Cardiac impression
Oblique fissure
Cardiac notch
Lingula of lung
Inferior border
Diaphragmatic surface

Figure 120.1 Left Lung, Mediastinal and Diaphragmatic Surfaces

NOTE: (1) The concave diaphragmatic surface on the left lung covers most of the convex dome of the diaphragm, which is completely covered by parietal diaphragmatic pleura.

(2) The mediastinal (or medial) surface of the left lung is also concave and presents the contours of the organs of the mediastinum. The large anterior concavity is the cardiac impression. Observe the grooves for the aortic arch, the aorta, and the subclavian artery as well as the esophagus inferiorly.

(3) The structures at the hilum of the left lung include the **left pulmonary artery**, found superiorly, and below this the **left primary bronchus.** The **left pulmonary veins** lie anterior and inferior to the artery and bronchus. The **oblique fissure** completely divides the lung into two lobes.

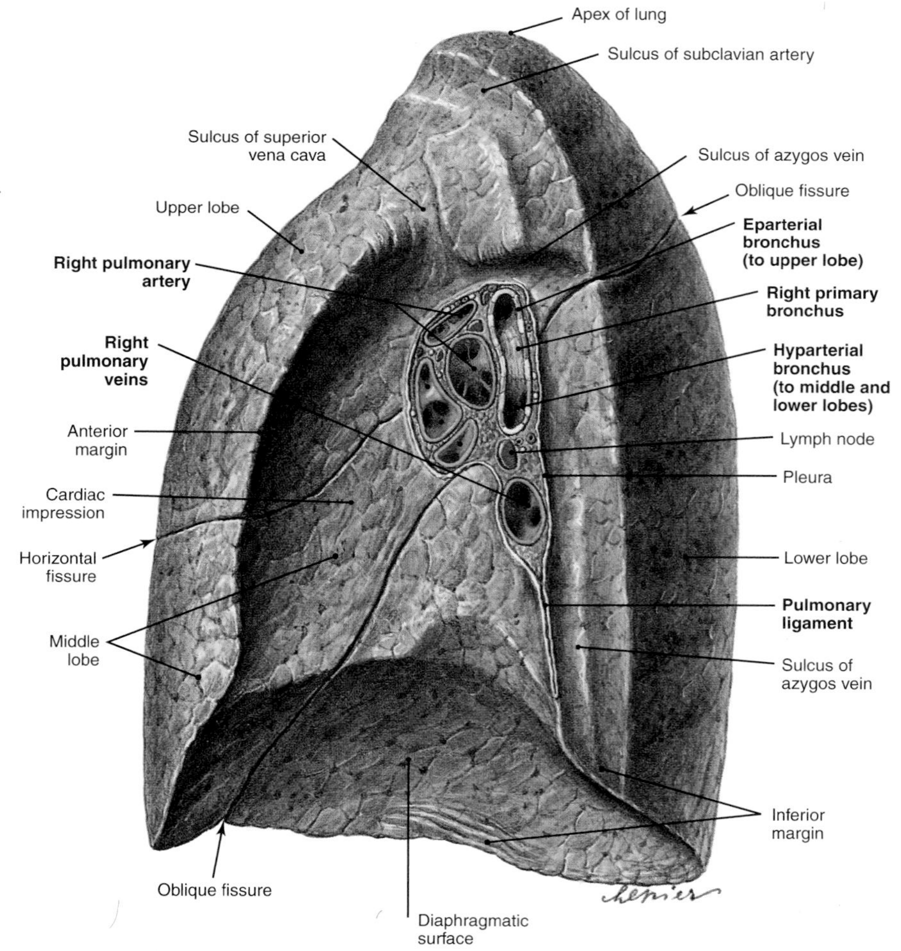
Apex of lung
Sulcus of subclavian artery
Sulcus of superior vena cava
Upper lobe
Right pulmonary artery
Right pulmonary veins
Anterior margin
Cardiac impression
Horizontal fissure
Middle lobe
Oblique fissure
Diaphragmatic surface
Sulcus of azygos vein
Oblique fissure
Eparterial bronchus (to upper lobe)
Right primary bronchus
Hyparterial bronchus (to middle and lower lobes)
Lymph node
Pleura
Lower lobe
Pulmonary ligament
Sulcus of azygos vein
Inferior margin

Figure 120.2 Right Lung, Mediastinal and Diaphragmatic Surfaces

NOTE: (1) The **diaphragmatic surface** of the right lung, similar to the left, is shaped to the contour of the diaphragm, while the **mediastinal surface** shows grooves for the superior vena cava and subclavian artery.

(2) Above the **hilum** of the right lung is the arched sulcus for the azygos vein, which continues inferiorly behind the hilum of the lung. The cardiac impression on the right lung is more shallow than on the left.

(3) The right bronchus frequently branches before the right pulmonary artery. Thus, often the most superior structure at the hilum of the right lung is the bronchus to the upper lobe (eparterial bronchus). The pulmonary artery lies anterior to the bronchus, while the pulmonary veins are located anterior and inferior to these structures.

(4) The root of the lung is ensheathed by parietal pleura, the layers of which come into contact below to form the **pulmonary ligament.** This extends from the inferior border of the hilum to a point just above the diaphragm.

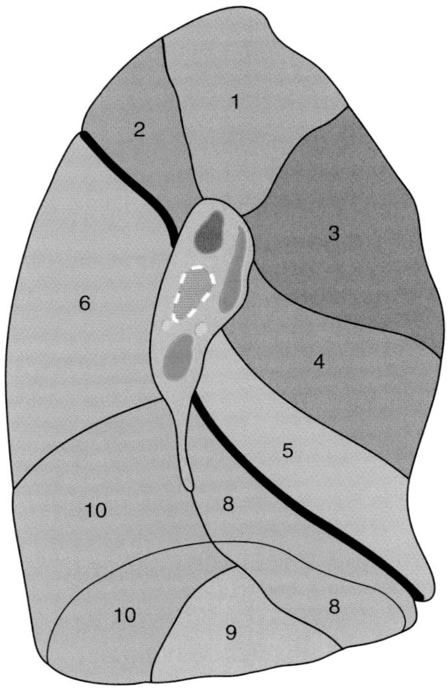
1
2
3
6
4
5
10
8
10
8
9

Figure 121.1 Left Lung: Bronchopulmonary Segments (Medial View)
NOTE: The bronchopulmonary segments of the left lung are identified as follows:

Upper lobe
1. Apical ⎤ Frequently considered
2. Posterior ⎦ as a single segment
3. Anterior
4. Superior ⎤ Lingular
5. Inferior ⎦

Lower lobe
6. Superior
7. Medial basal*
8. Anterior basal*
9. Lateral basal
10. Posterior basal

*The medial basal and anterior basal segments were at one time frequently considered as a single bronchopulmonary segment. Today, however, they have been recognized as separate segments in a majority of left lungs. Therefore, on this figure, the portion of segment 8 just inferior to the oblique fissure should be marked 7 and identified as medial basal.

Figures 121.1 and 121.2 Bronchopulmonary Segments: General Statements
NOTE: (1) Bronchopulmonary segments are separated by connective-tissue septa that are continuous with the visceral pleura. These septa maintain the air content of each segment and prevent leakage of air into adjacent segments.

(2) Each segment is pyramidal in shape. The apex of each pyramid is oriented toward the hilum of the lung, while the base faces the surface of the pulmonary lobe.

(3) It is important to know the bronchopulmonary segmental patterns in order, accurately, to read and interpret radiographs of the lungs.

(4) Knowledge of segmental anatomy is also important for the localization of pathologic conditions such as tumors, abscesses, or bronchiectasis or small foreign objects that have been aspirated into a lung.

Figure 121.2 Right Lung: Bronchopulmonary Segments (Medial View) ▶
NOTE: The bronchopulmonary segments of the right lung are identified as follows:

Upper lobe
1. Apical
2. Posterior
3. Anterior

Middle lobe
4. Lateral (not seen from this view)
5. Medial

Lower lobe
6. Superior
7. Medial basal
8. Anterior basal
9. Lateral basal
10. Posterior basal

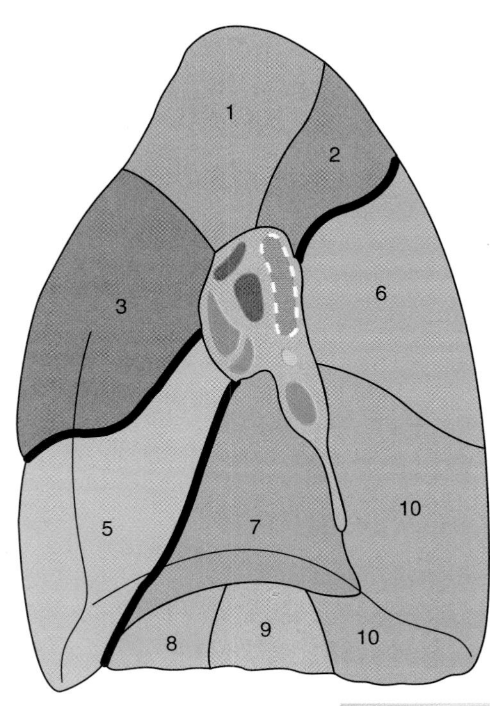
1
2
3
6
5
7
10
8
9
10

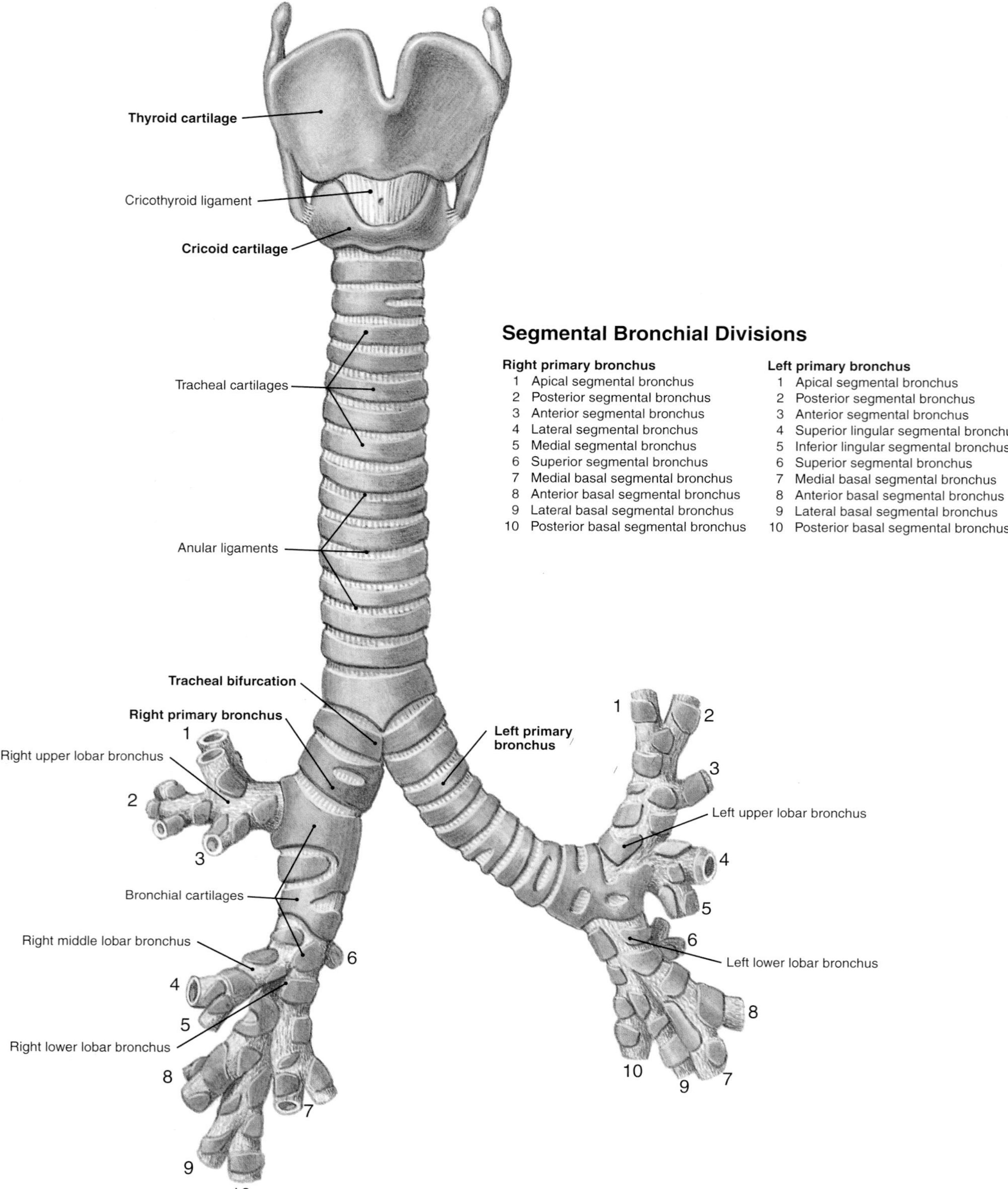
Thyroid cartilage
Cricothyroid ligament
Cricoid cartilage
Tracheal cartilages
Anular ligaments
Tracheal bifurcation
Right primary bronchus
Right upper lobar bronchus
Bronchial cartilages
Right middle lobar bronchus
Right lower lobar bronchus
Left primary bronchus
Left upper lobar bronchus
Left lower lobar bronchus
1
2
3
4
5
6
7
8
9
10
Segmental Bronchial Divisions
Right primary bronchus
1 Apical segmental bronchus
2 Posterior segmental bronchus
3 Anterior segmental bronchus
4 Lateral segmental bronchus
5 Medial segmental bronchus
6 Superior segmental bronchus
7 Medial basal segmental bronchus
8 Anterior basal segmental bronchus
9 Lateral basal segmental bronchus
10 Posterior basal segmental bronchus
Left primary bronchus
1 Apical segmental bronchus
2 Posterior segmental bronchus
3 Anterior segmental bronchus
4 Superior lingular segmental bronchus
5 Inferior lingular segmental bronchus
6 Superior segmental bronchus
7 Medial basal segmental bronchus
8 Anterior basal segmental bronchus
9 Lateral basal segmental bronchus
10 Posterior basal segmental bronchus

Figure 122 Anterior Aspect of Larynx, Trachea, and Bronchi

NOTE: (1) The **trachea** bifurcates into two **principal** (primary) **bronchi**. These then divide into **lobar** (secondary) **bronchi,** which give rise to **segmental** (tertiary) **bronchi.**

(2) The larynx is located in the anterior aspect of the neck, and its thyroid and cricoid cartilages can be felt through the skin.

(3) The **thyroid cartilage,** projected posteriorly, lies at the level of the fourth and fifth cervical vertebrae, while the **cricoid cartilage** is at the sixth cervical level.

(4) The trachea commences at the lower end of the cricoid cartilage and extends slightly more than 4 in. before bifurcating into the two primary bronchi at the level of T4–T5 intervertebral disc. Two inches of the trachea lie above the suprasternal notch in the neck, and about 2 in. of trachea are within the thorax above the tracheal bifurcation.

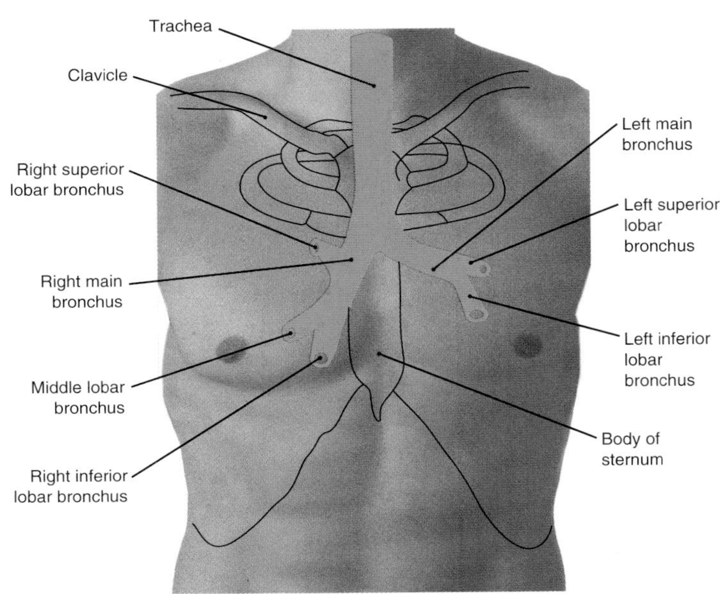
Trachea
Clavicle
Right superior lobar bronchus
Right main bronchus
Middle lobar bronchus
Right inferior lobar bronchus
Left main bronchus
Left superior lobar bronchus
Left inferior lobar bronchus
Body of sternum

Figure 123.1 Surface Projection of the Trachea and Bronchi in a Living Person

NOTE that the bifurcation occurs at approximately the level of the sternal angle located anteriorly on the sternum.

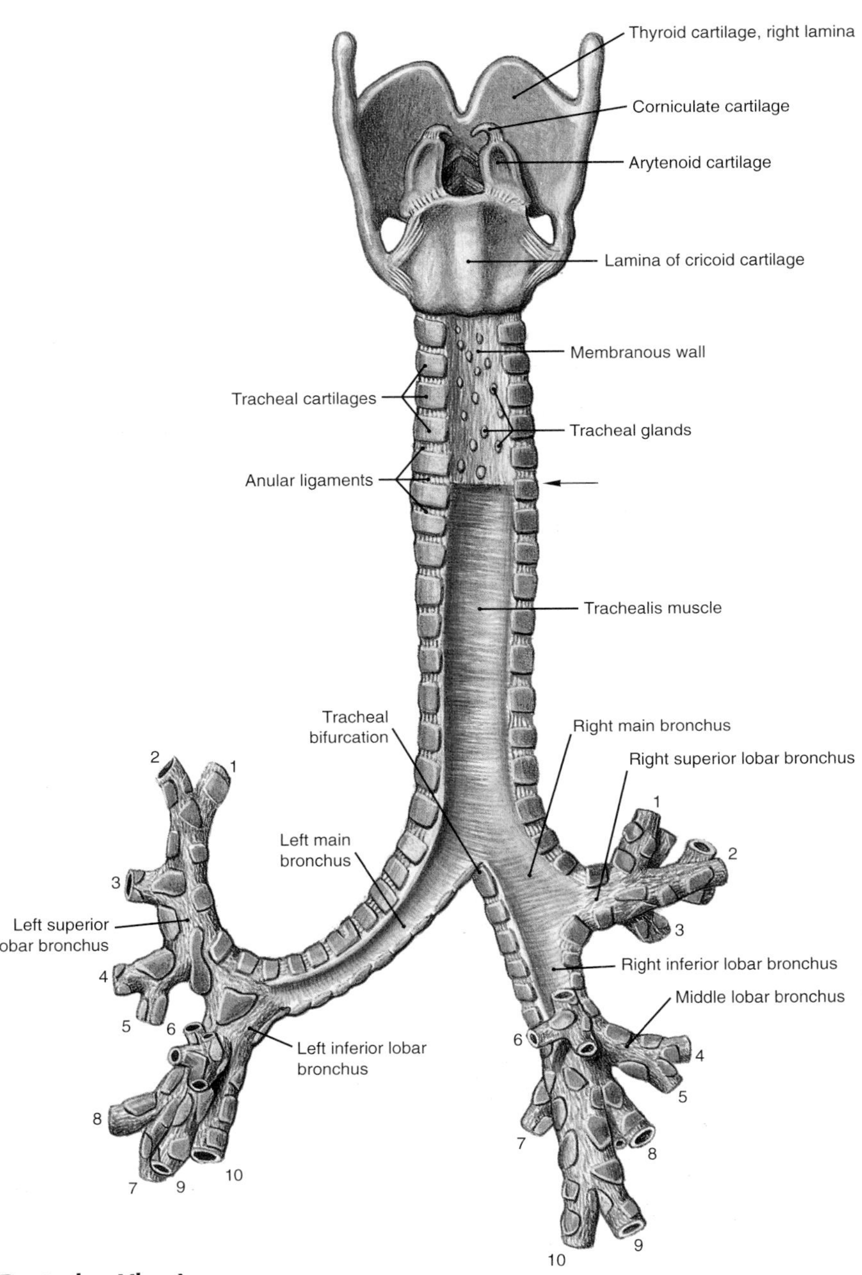
Thyroid cartilage, right lamina
Corniculate cartilage
Arytenoid cartilage
Lamina of cricoid cartilage
Membranous wall
Tracheal cartilages
Tracheal glands
Anular ligaments
Trachealis muscle
Tracheal bifurcation
Right main bronchus
Right superior lobar bronchus
Left main bronchus
Left superior lobar bronchus
Right inferior lobar bronchus
Middle lobar bronchus
Left inferior lobar bronchus
1
2
3
4
5
6
7
8
9
10

Figure 123.2 Opened Trachea and Bronchi (Posterior View)

NOTE: (1) The numbers refer to the bronchopulmonary segments listed in Plate 122.

(2) Below the arrow, observe the trachealis muscle along the posterior surface of the trachea. It is composed of nonstriated muscle fibers, and it extends along the posterior surface of the bronchi.

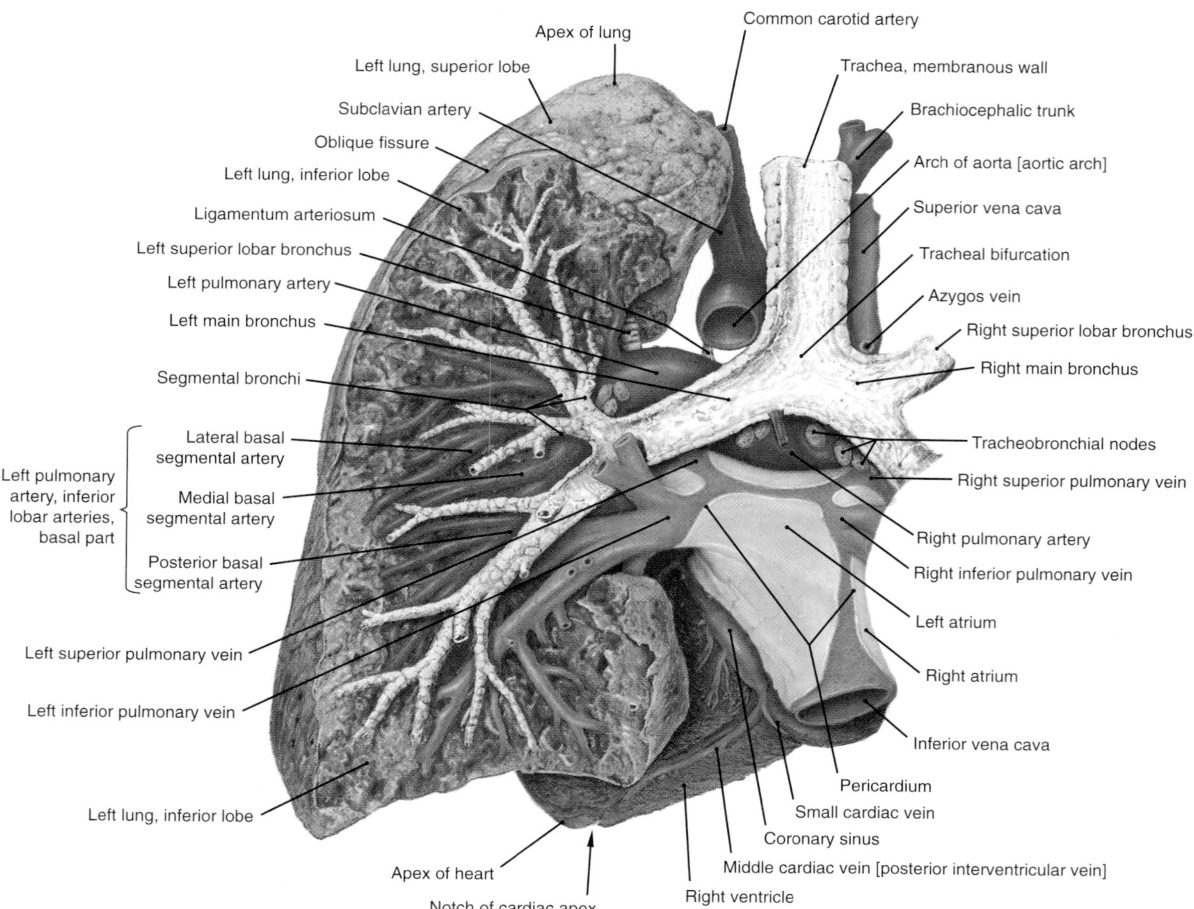

Apex of lung
Common carotid artery
Left lung, superior lobe
Trachea, membranous wall
Subclavian artery
Brachiocephalic trunk
Oblique fissure
Arch of aorta [aortic arch]
Left lung, inferior lobe
Superior vena cava
Ligamentum arteriosum
Tracheal bifurcation
Left superior lobar bronchus
Azygos vein
Left pulmonary artery
Right superior lobar bronchus
Left main bronchus
Right main bronchus
Segmental bronchi
Tracheobronchial nodes
Left pulmonary artery, inferior lobar arteries, basal part
Lateral basal segmental artery
Right superior pulmonary vein
Medial basal segmental artery
Posterior basal segmental artery
Right pulmonary artery
Right inferior pulmonary vein
Left atrium
Left superior pulmonary vein
Right atrium
Left inferior pulmonary vein
Inferior vena cava
Pericardium
Small cardiac vein
Left lung, inferior lobe
Coronary sinus
Middle cardiac vein [posterior interventricular vein]
Apex of heart
Right ventricle
Notch of cardiac apex

Figure 124.1 Dissected Hilum of the Left Lung (Posterior View)
NOTE that the bronchus is more posterior to the pulmonary vessels.

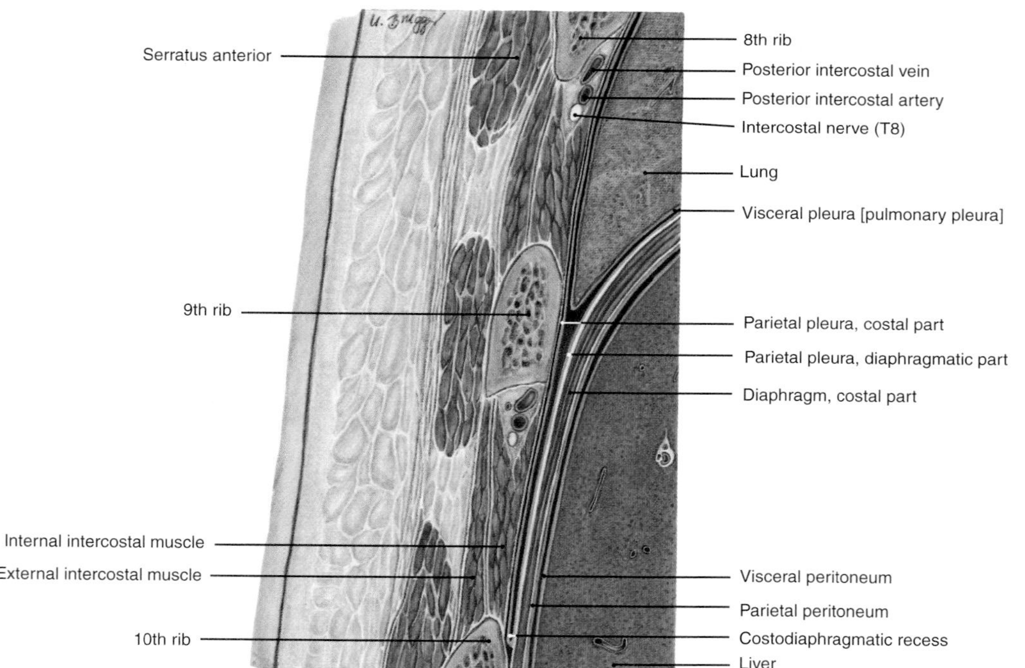

Serratus anterior
8th rib
Posterior intercostal vein
Posterior intercostal artery
Intercostal nerve (T8)
Lung
Visceral pleura [pulmonary pleura]
9th rib
Parietal pleura, costal part
Parietal pleura, diaphragmatic part
Diaphragm, costal part
Internal intercostal muscle
External intercostal muscle
Visceral peritoneum
Parietal peritoneum
10th rib
Costodiaphragmatic recess
Liver

Figure 124.2 Costodiaphragmatic Recess (Frontal Section of Region)
NOTE: (1) The costodiaphragmatic recesses are located in the lowest lateral regions of the two pleural cavities.
(2) When aspiration of fluid is necessary, care must be taken not to puncture the liver or right lung on the right side, or the spleen or left lung on the left side.

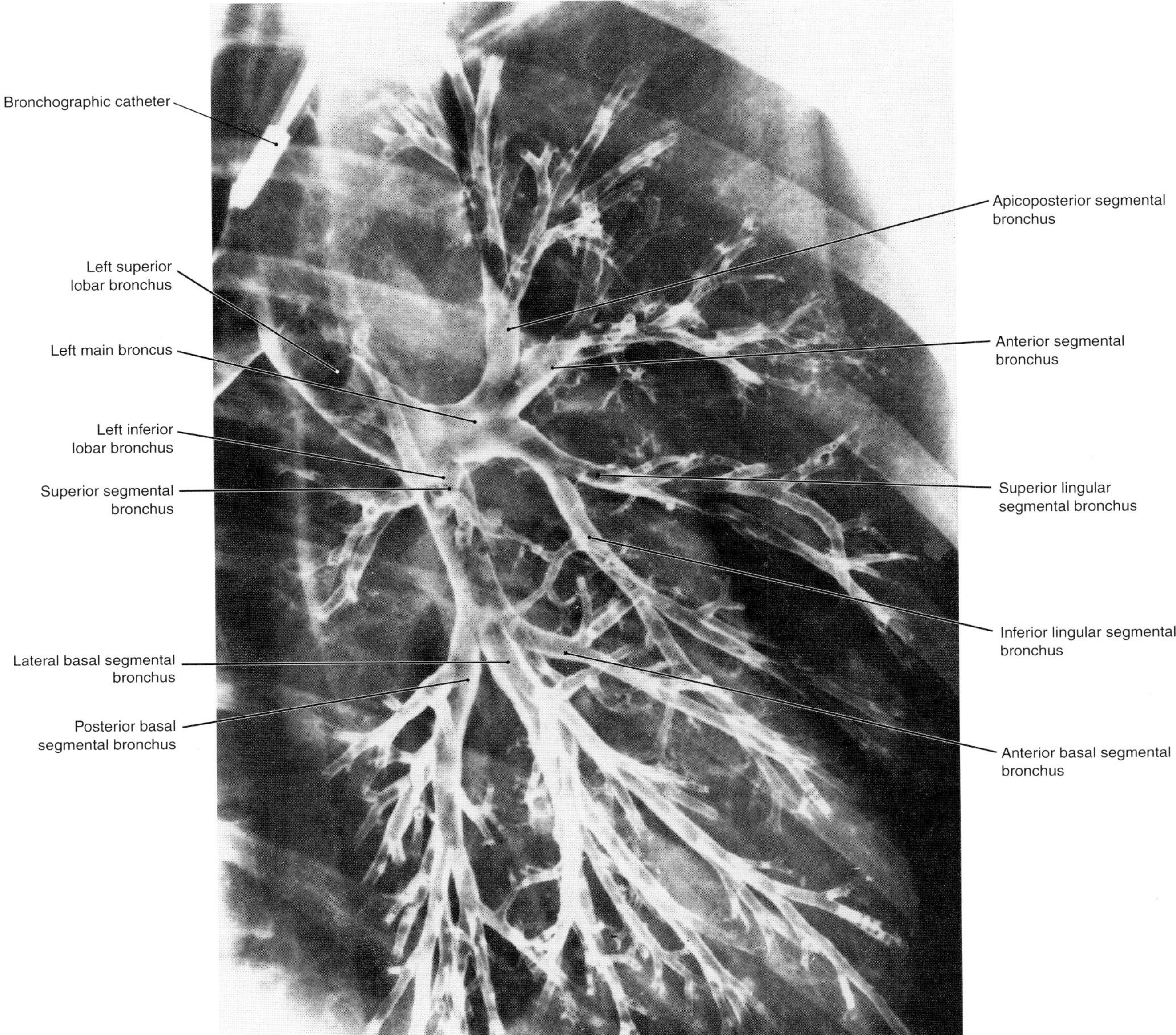
Bronchographic catheter
Left superior lobar bronchus
Left main broncus
Left inferior lobar bronchus
Superior segmental bronchus
Lateral basal segmental bronchus
Posterior basal segmental bronchus
Apicoposterior segmental bronchus
Anterior segmental bronchus
Superior lingular segmental bronchus
Inferior lingular segmental bronchus
Anterior basal segmental bronchus

Figure 125 Left Bronchogram Showing the Bronchial Tree

NOTE: (1) A bronchographic catheter was inserted into the trachea, through which a contrast medium powder was administered, allowing the bronchial tree to be visualized.

(2) The apical and posterior bronchopulmonary segmental bronchi (identified here as the apicoposterior segment) and the anterior segmental bronchus of the **superior lobe.**

(3) The superior and inferior segmental bronchi of the **lingular part** of the **superior lobe.**

(4) The superior, lateral basal, posterior basal, and lateral basal bronchopulmonary segmental bronchi of the **inferior lobe.** Note that the medial basal segmental bronchus of the inferior lobe is mostly missing in this bronchogram.

(5) Compare this bronchogram with Plate 117.

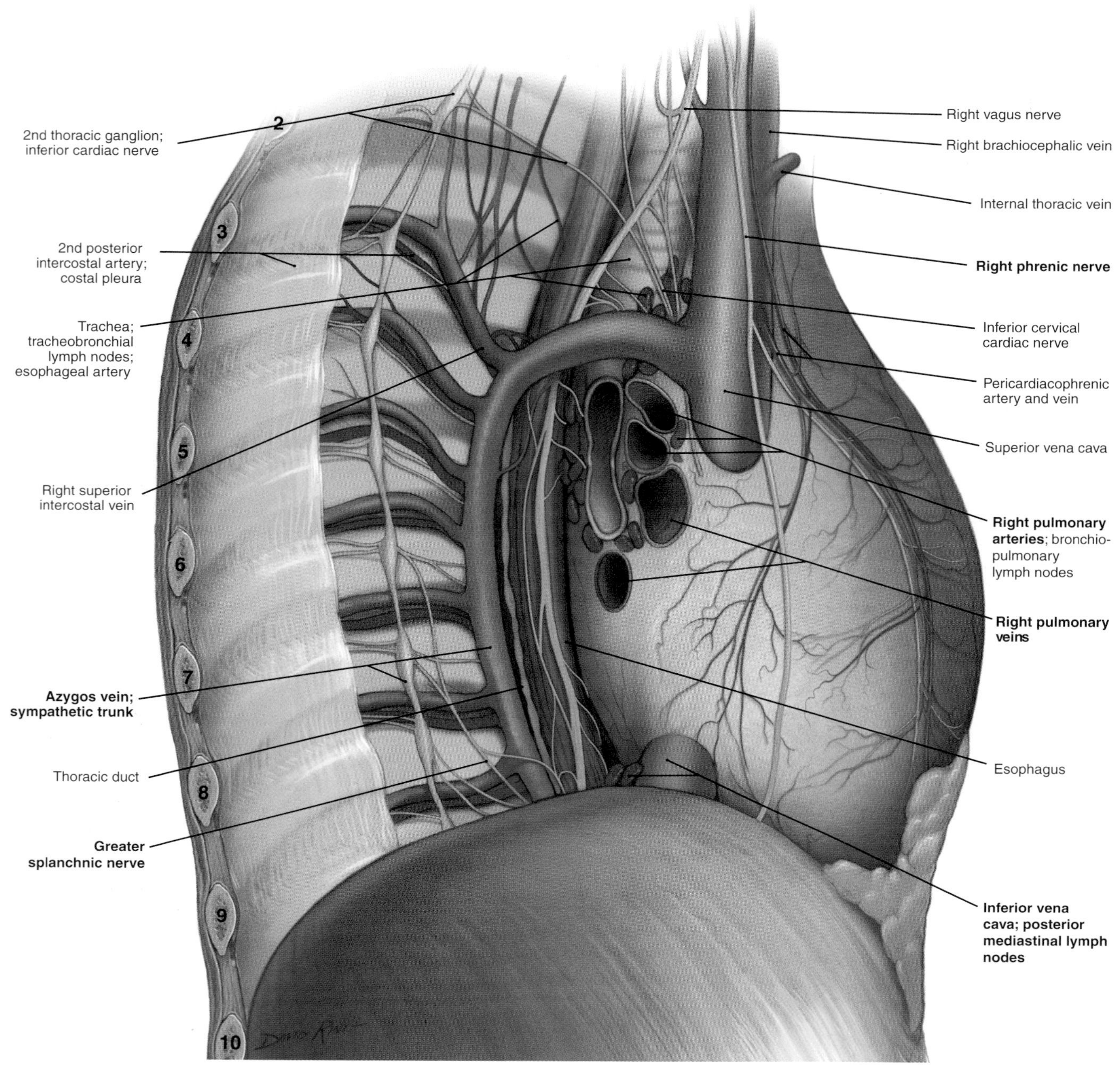
2nd thoracic ganglion; inferior cardiac nerve
2nd posterior intercostal artery; costal pleura
Trachea; tracheobronchial lymph nodes; esophageal artery
Right superior intercostal vein
Azygos vein; sympathetic trunk
Thoracic duct
Greater splanchnic nerve
Right vagus nerve
Right brachiocephalic vein
Internal thoracic vein
Right phrenic nerve
Inferior cervical cardiac nerve
Pericardiacophrenic artery and vein
Superior vena cava
Right pulmonary arteries; bronchio-pulmonary lymph nodes
Right pulmonary veins
Esophagus
Inferior vena cava; posterior mediastinal lymph nodes
2
3
4
5
6
7
8
9
10

Figure 126 Right Side of the Mediastinum with the Mediastinal Pleura and Some Costal Pleura Removed

NOTE: (1) The lung has been removed, the structures at the hilum transected, and the mediastinal pleura stripped away. This exposes the organs of the mediastinum, and their right lateral surface is presented.

(2) The right side of the heart is covered by pericardium and the course of the **phrenic nerve** and **pericardiacophrenic vessels** are visible.

(3) The ascending course of the **azygos vein,** its arch, and its junction with the superior vena cava.

(4) The **right vagus nerve** descends in the thorax behind the root of the right lung to form the **posterior pulmonary plexus.** It then helps form the **esophageal plexus** and leaves the thorax on the posterior aspect of the esophagus.

(5) The **dome of the diaphragm** on the right side as it takes the rounded form of the underlying liver. The inferior (diaphragmatic) surface of the heart rests on the diaphragm.

(6) The position of the thoracic **sympathetic chain** of ganglia coursing longitudinally along the inner surface of the thoracic wall. Observe the **greater thoracic splanchnic nerve.**

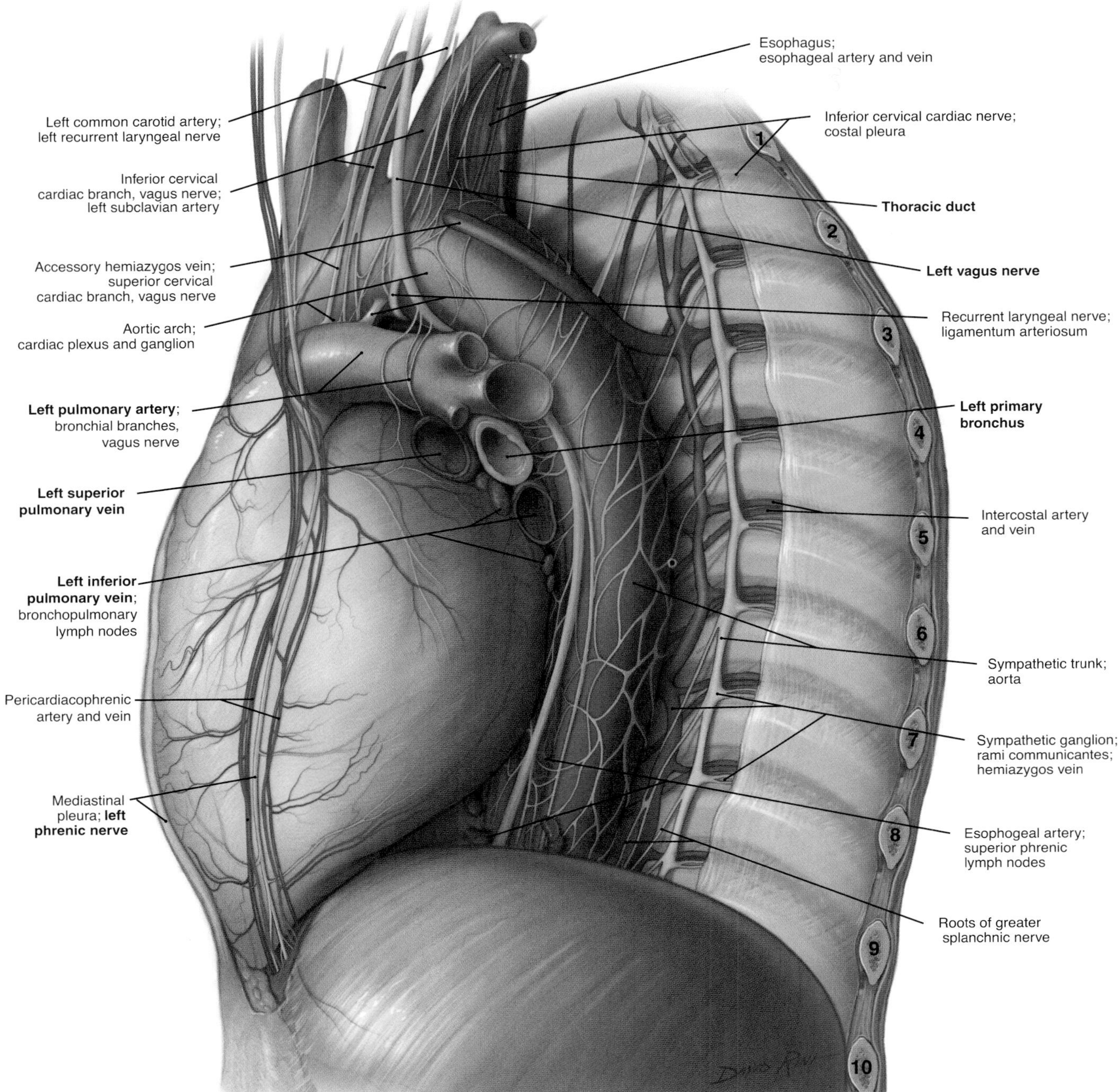
Left common carotid artery;
left recurrent laryngeal nerve
Inferior cervical
cardiac branch, vagus nerve;
left subclavian artery
Accessory hemiazygos vein;
superior cervical
cardiac branch, vagus nerve
Aortic arch;
cardiac plexus and ganglion
Left pulmonary artery;
bronchial branches,
vagus nerve
Left superior
pulmonary vein
Left inferior
pulmonary vein;
bronchopulmonary
lymph nodes
Pericardiacophrenic
artery and vein
Mediastinal
pleura; left
phrenic nerve
Esophagus;
esophageal artery and vein
Inferior cervical cardiac nerve;
costal pleura
Thoracic duct
Left vagus nerve
Recurrent laryngeal nerve;
ligamentum arteriosum
Left primary
bronchus
Intercostal artery
and vein
Sympathetic trunk;
aorta
Sympathetic ganglion;
rami communicantes;
hemiazygos vein
Esophageal artery;
superior phrenic
lymph nodes
Roots of greater
splanchnic nerve
1
2
3
4
5
6
7
8
9
10

Figure 127 Left Side of the Mediastinum with the Mediastinal Pleura and Some Costal Pleura Removed

NOTE: (1) With the left lung removed along with most of the mediastinal pleura, the structures of the mediastinal pleura and the structures of the mediastinum are observed from their left side.

(2) The **left phrenic nerve** and **pericardiacophrenic vessels** course to the diaphragm along the pericardial covering over the left side of the heart.

(3) The **aorta** ascends about 2 in. before it arches posteriorly and to the left of the vertebral column.

(4) The descending **thoracic aorta** commences at about the level of the fourth thoracic vertebra. As it descends, it comes to lie anterior to the vertebral column.

(5) The **intercostal arteries** branch directly from the thoracic aorta. The typical intercostal artery and vein course along the inferior border of their respective rib. Because the superior border of the ribs is free of vessels and nerves, it is a safer site for injection or drainage of the thorax.

(6) The **left vagus nerve** lies lateral to the aortic arch and gives off the **recurrent laryngeal branch,** which passes inferior to the **ligamentum arteriosum.** The main trunk then continues to descend, contributes to the esophageal plexus, and enters the abdomen on the anterior aspect of the esophagus.

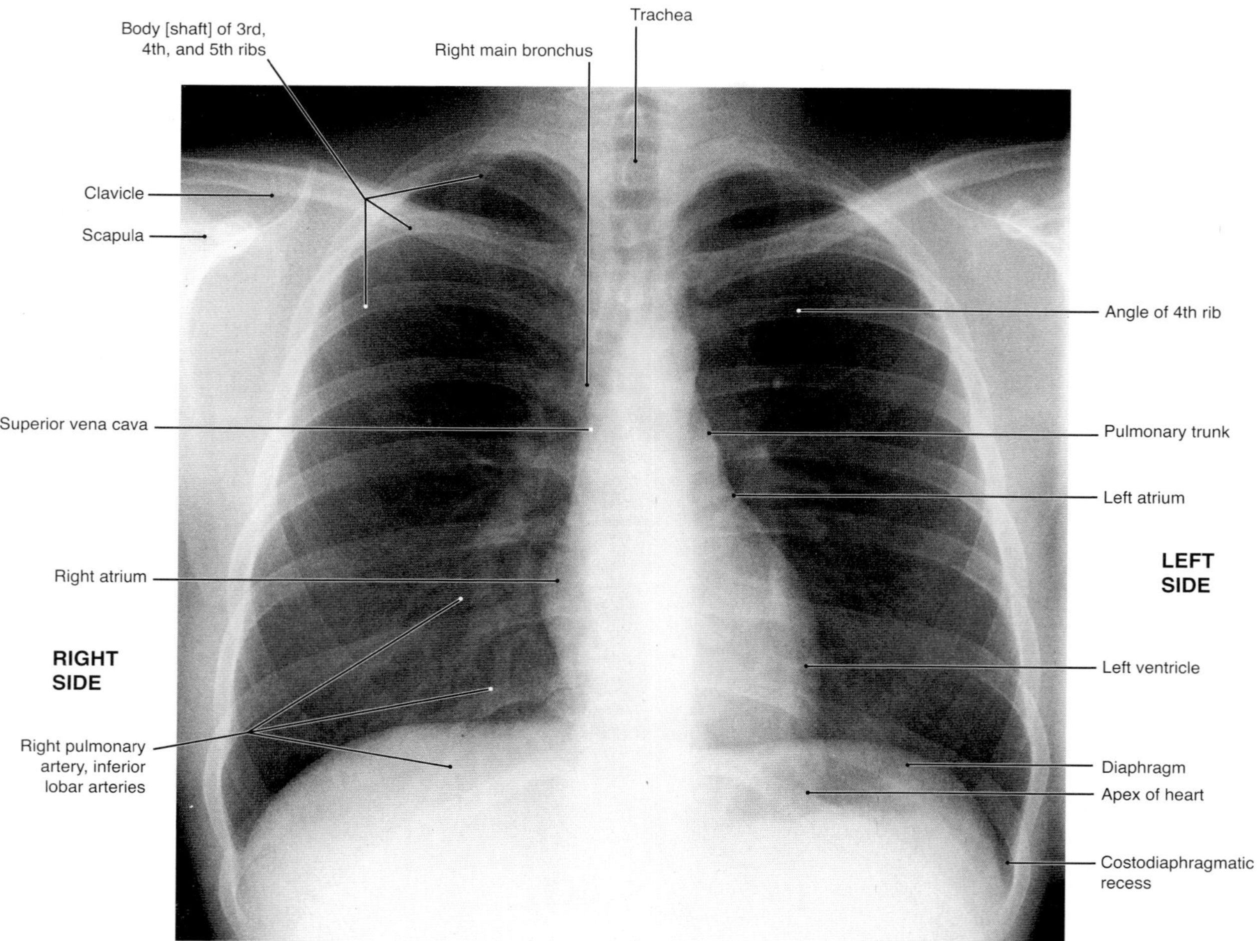
Body [shaft] of 3rd, 4th, and 5th ribs
Trachea
Right main bronchus
Clavicle
Scapula
Angle of 4th rib
Superior vena cava
Pulmonary trunk
Left atrium
LEFT SIDE
Right atrium
RIGHT SIDE
Left ventricle
Right pulmonary artery, inferior lobar arteries
Diaphragm
Apex of heart
Costodiaphragmatic recess

Figure 128.1 Posteroanterior Radiograph of the Thorax in a 27-Year-Old Male

NOTE: (1) A normal-appearing heart within the chest. Realize that it lies substernally with about two-thirds of the normal heart to the left of the midline and one-third to the right.

(2) Compare the labeled structures on the x-ray with those on the diagram seen in Figure 128.2.

(3) The right dome of the diaphragm is somewhat more superior than the dome on the left. This is because of the liver in the right upper abdomen.

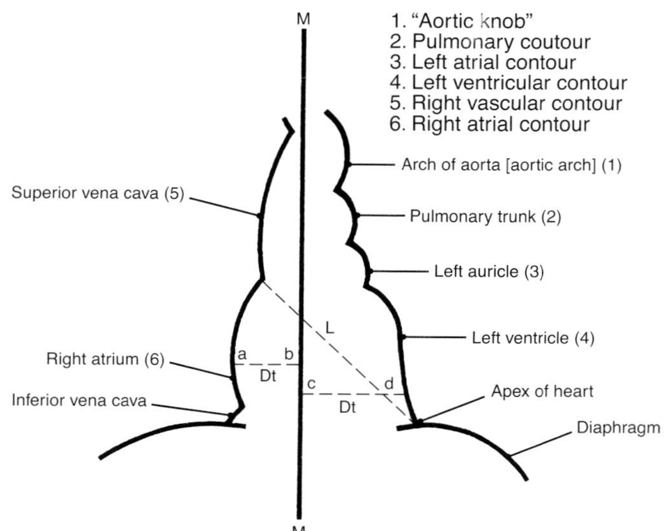
M
1. "Aortic knob"
2. Pulmonary coutour
3. Left atrial contour
4. Left ventricular contour
5. Right vascular contour
6. Right atrial contour
Arch of aorta [aortic arch] (1)
Superior vena cava (5)
Pulmonary trunk (2)
Left auricle (3)
L
Left ventricle (4)
Right atrium (6)
a
b
Dt
c
d
Dt
Inferior vena cava
Apex of heart
Diaphragm
M

Figure 128.2 Schematic Diagram of the Heart Seen in the Radiograph of Figure 128.1

NOTE: (1) The midline of the body (**M**) and the longitudinal (**Ld**) and transverse (**ab** + **cd**) dimensions (**Dt**) of the heart.

(2) Transverse diameter: ab + cd = 13 to 14 cm. Longitudinal axis (Ld): From the superior contour of the right atrium to the apex: 15 to 16 cm.

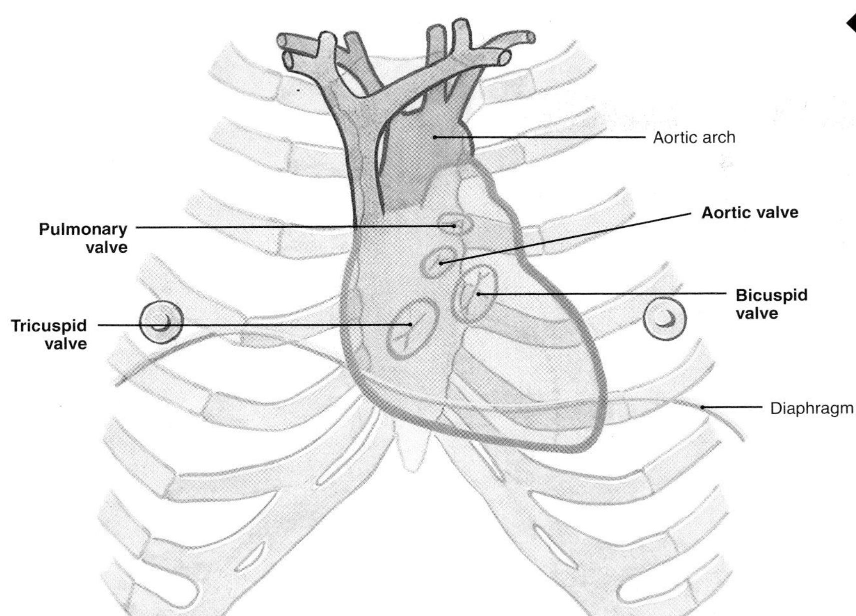
Aortic arch
Aortic valve
Pulmonary valve
Bicuspid valve
Tricuspid valve
Diaphragm

Figure 129.1 Projection of the Heart and Its Valves onto the Anterior Thoracic Wall

NOTE: (1) The **pulmonary valve** lies behind the sternal end of the third left costal cartilage. The **aortic valve** is behind the sternum at the level of the third intercostal space. The **mitral valve** (bicuspid) lies behind the fourth left sternocostal joint, and the **tricuspid valve** lies posterior to the middle of the sternum at the level of the fourth intercostal space.

(2) The unbroken blue line indicates the **area of deep cardiac dullness,** which produces a dull resonance by percussion. Lung tissue covers this area, but does not cover the area limited by the blue dotted line from which a less-resonant **superficial cardiac** dullness is obtained.

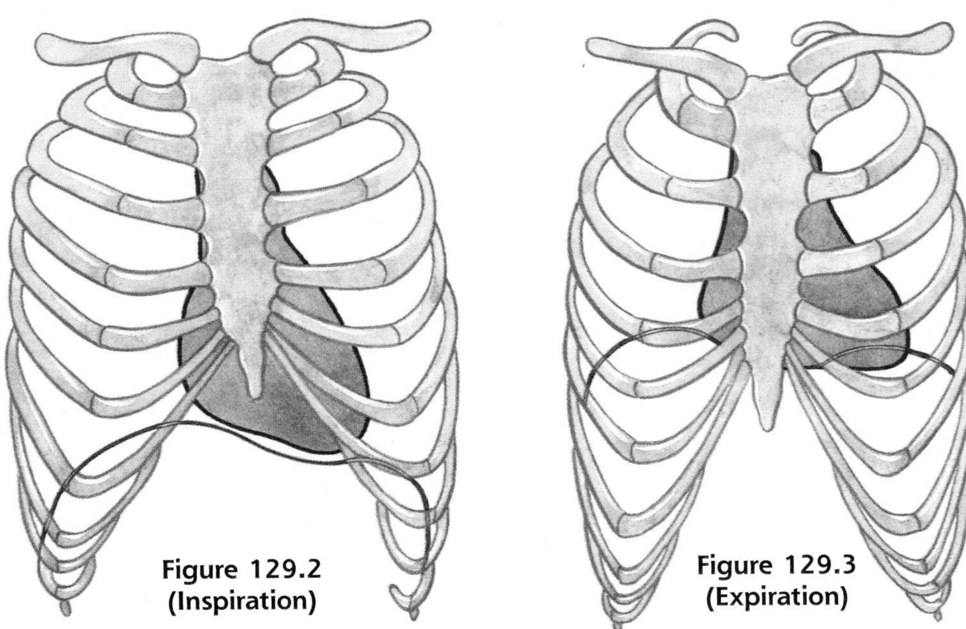
Figure 129.2 (Inspiration)
Figure 129.3 (Expiration)

Figures 129.2 and 129.3 Positions of the Heart during Full Inspiration (Fig. 129.2) and during Full Expiration (Fig. 129.3)

NOTE: (1) During **full inspiration** (Fig. 129.2).

(a) The thorax is enlarged by a lowering of the diaphragm due to contraction of its muscle fibers and by elevation and expansion of the thorax (ribs and sternum).

(b) The chest expands anteroposteriorly, transversely, and vertically, resulting in the heart becoming more oblong (i.e., its transverse diameter is decreased), and its apex and diaphragmatic surface are lowered.

(c) Inspiration is accompanied by relaxation of the anterior abdominal wall muscles, protrusion of the abdomen, and a lowering of abdominal viscera.

2) During **full expiration** (Fig. 129.3).

(a) The diaphragm is elevated because its muscle fibers relax and because the ribs and sternum contract the size of the thorax.

(b) With the capacity of the thoracic cage diminished, there is an elevation of the diaphragmatic surface of the heart and the apex of the heart. This results in an increase in the transverse diameter of the heart.

(c) Expiration is accompanied by contraction of the anterior abdominal wall muscles and an elevation of the abdominal viscera, which also pushes the relaxed diaphragm upward.

Brachiocephalic artery
Trachea
Thyroid gland
Left brachiocephalic vein
Left recurrent laryngeal nerve
Left common carotid artery
Right recurrent laryngeal nerve
Left phrenic nerve
Right vagus nerve
Left vagus nerve
Cardiac branches, left vagus nerve
Right brachiocephalic vein
Clavicle
Pectoralis minor muscle
Internal thoracic artery
Pectoralis major muscle
Pericardiacophrenic artery
Upper lobe, right lung
Aortic arch
Upper lobe, left lung
Superior vena cava
Cardiac plexus
Left phrenic nerve; pericardiacophrenic vessels
Right pericardiaco-phrenic vessels
4th and 5th ribs
Pericardial branch, right phrenic nerve
Middle lobe, right lung
Lower lobe, left lung
Lower lobe, right lung
Left phrenic nerve
Right phrenic nerve
Inferior border, left lung
Diaphragmatic pleura
Diaphragm
Pericardium
Left phrenic nerve branches
Costodiaphragmatic recess

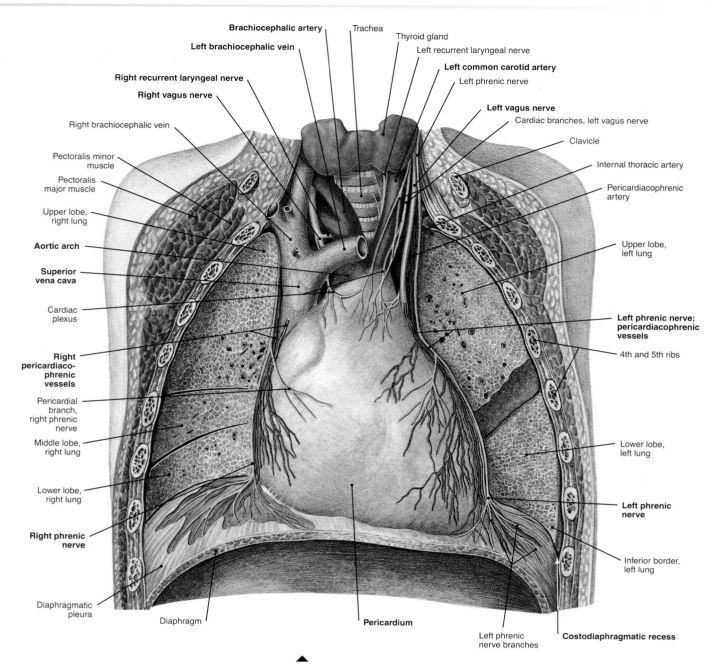

Figure 130.1 Adult Heart, Pericardium, and Superior Mediastinum (Anterior View)

NOTE: (1) In this frontal section, the anterior thoracic wall and the anterior part of the lungs and diaphragm have been removed, leaving the **pericardium** and its vessels and nerves intact. The **vagus nerves** and some of their branches are also shown.

(2) The **phrenic nerves** form in the neck (C3, C4, and C5) and descend with the pericardiacophrenic vessels to innervate the diaphragm, but they also send some sensory fibers to the pericardium.

(3) The pericardium is formed by an outer **fibrous layer,** which is lined by an inner serous sac. As the heart develops, it invaginates into the serous sac and becomes covered by a **visceral layer of serous pericardium** (epicardium) and a **parietal layer of serous pericardium.**

(4) The visceral layer clings closely to the heart, while the parietal layer lines the inner surface of the fibrous pericardium. The potential space between the visceral and parietal layers contains a little serous fluid and is called the **pericardial cavity.**

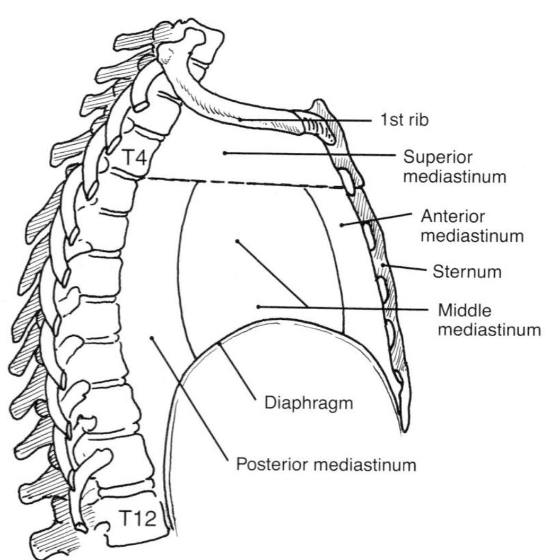
1st rib
T4
Superior mediastinum
Anterior mediastinum
Sternum
Middle mediastinum
Diaphragm
Posterior mediastinum
T12

Figure 130.2 Subdivisions of the Mediastinum

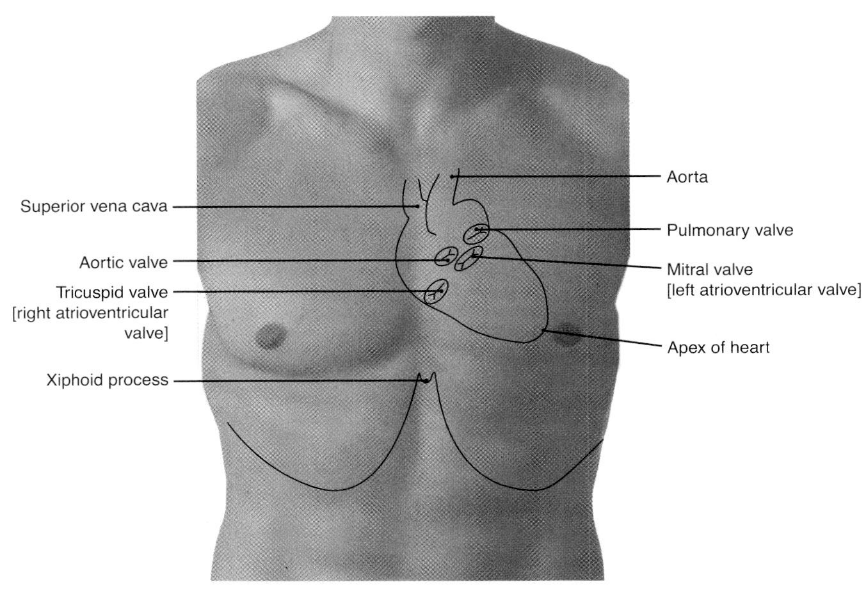
Superior vena cava
Aortic valve
Tricuspid valve
[right atrioventricular valve]
Xiphoid process
Aorta
Pulmonary valve
Mitral valve
[left atrioventricular valve]
Apex of heart

Figure 131.1 Projection of the Heart and Cardiac Valves onto the Thoracic Wall

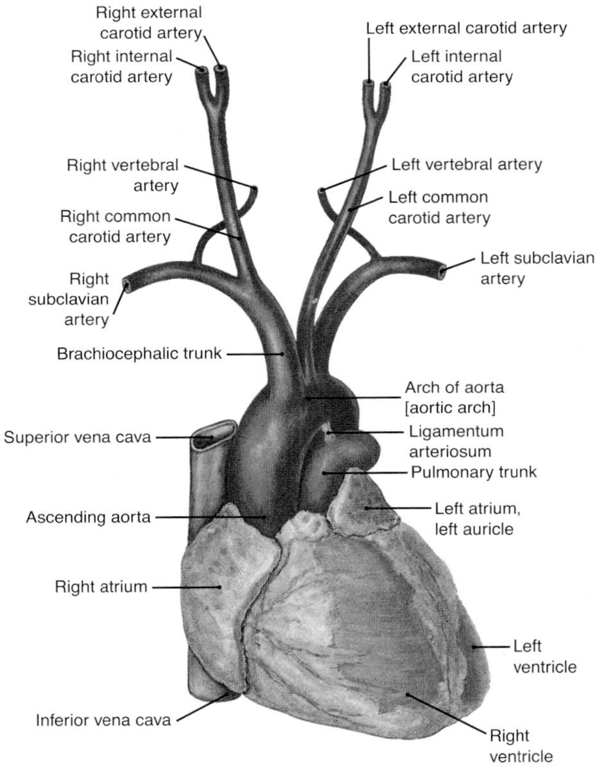
Right external carotid artery
Right internal carotid artery
Right vertebral artery
Right common carotid artery
Right subclavian artery
Brachiocephalic trunk
Superior vena cava
Ascending aorta
Right atrium
Inferior vena cava
Left external carotid artery
Left internal carotid artery
Left vertebral artery
Left common carotid artery
Left subclavian artery
Arch of aorta
[aortic arch]
Ligamentum arteriosum
Pulmonary trunk
Left atrium, left auricle
Left ventricle
Right ventricle

Figure 131.2 Heart, Aortic Arch, and the Great Arteries from the Arch

NOTE also the pulmonary trunk and the superior and inferior vena cavae.

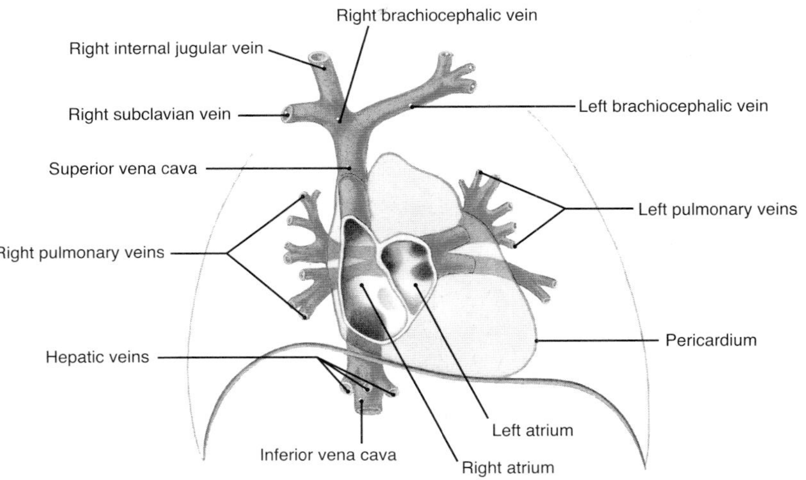
Right brachiocephalic vein
Right internal jugular vein
Right subclavian vein
Left brachiocephalic vein
Superior vena cava
Left pulmonary veins
Right pulmonary veins
Pericardium
Hepatic veins
Left atrium
Inferior vena cava
Right atrium

Figure 131.3 Great Veins That Drain into the Heart (Anterior View)

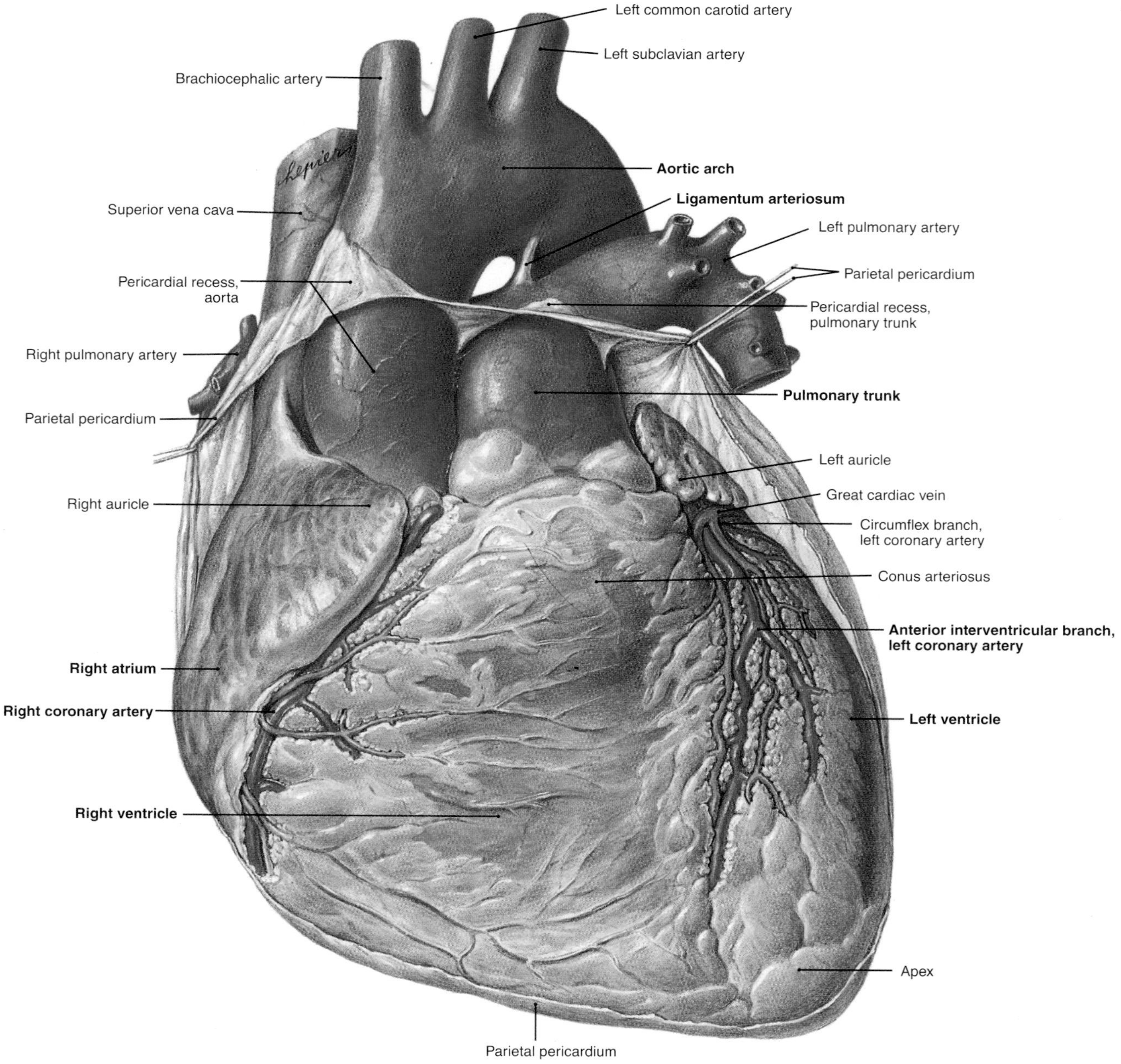
Left common carotid artery
Left subclavian artery
Brachiocephalic artery
Aortic arch
Ligamentum arteriosum
Superior vena cava
Left pulmonary artery
Parietal pericardium
Pericardial recess, aorta
Pericardial recess, pulmonary trunk
Right pulmonary artery
Pulmonary trunk
Parietal pericardium
Left auricle
Right auricle
Great cardiac vein
Circumflex branch, left coronary artery
Conus arteriosus
Anterior interventricular branch, left coronary artery
Right atrium
Right coronary artery
Left ventricle
Right ventricle
Apex
Parietal pericardium

Figure 132 Ventral View of the Heart and Great Vessels

NOTE: (1) The heart is a muscular organ in the middle mediastinum, and its **apex** points inferiorly, to the left, and slightly anteriorly. The **base** of the heart is opposite to the apex and is directed superiorly and to the right.

(2) The great vessels attach to the heart at its base, and the pericardium is reflected over these vessels at their origin.

(3) The anterior surface of the heart is its **sternocostal surface.** The auricular portion of the **right atrium** and much of the **right ventricle** is seen from this anterior view; also a small part of the **left ventricle** is visible along the left border.

(4) The **pulmonary trunk** originates from the right ventricle. To its right can be seen the **aorta,** which arises from the left ventricle. The **superior vena cava** can be seen opening into the upper aspect of the right atrium.

(5) The **ligamentum arteriosum.** This fibrous structure between the left pulmonary artery and the aorta is the remnant of the fetal **ductus arteriosus,** which, before birth, served to shunt blood directed to the lungs back into the aorta for systemic distribution.

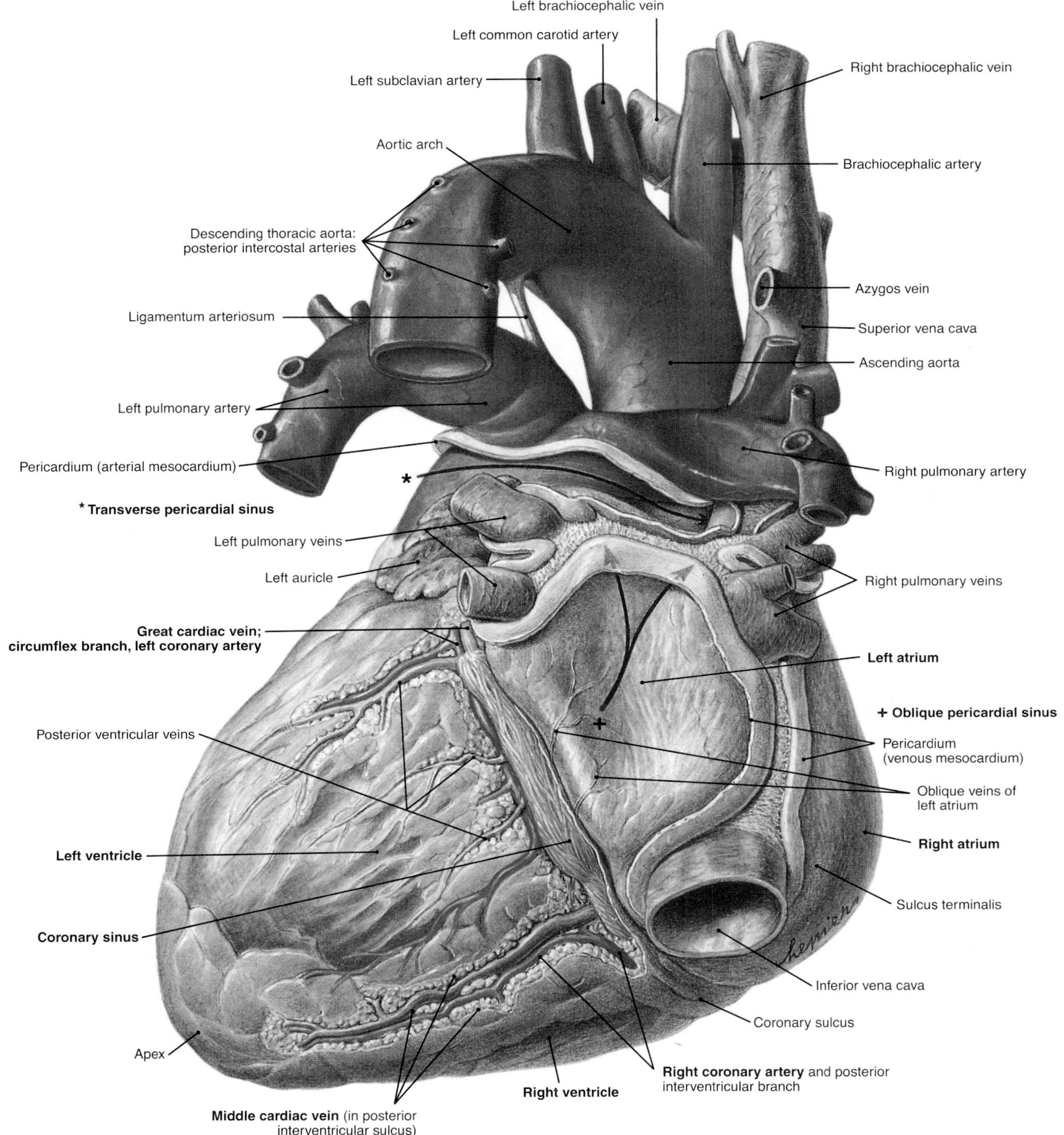

Left brachiocephalic vein
Left common carotid artery
Left subclavian artery
Right brachiocephalic vein
Aortic arch
Brachiocephalic artery
Descending thoracic aorta: posterior intercostal arteries
Azygos vein
Ligamentum arteriosum
Superior vena cava
Ascending aorta
Left pulmonary artery
Pericardium (arterial mesocardium)
Right pulmonary artery
*
* Transverse pericardial sinus
Left pulmonary veins
Left auricle
Right pulmonary veins
Great cardiac vein; circumflex branch, left coronary artery
Left atrium
+ Oblique pericardial sinus
+
Posterior ventricular veins
Pericardium (venous mesocardium)
Oblique veins of left atrium
Right atrium
Left ventricle
Sulcus terminalis
Coronary sinus
Inferior vena cava
Coronary sulcus
Apex
Right coronary artery and posterior interventricular branch
Right ventricle
Middle cardiac vein (in posterior interventricular sulcus)

Figure 133 The Heart and Great Vessels (Posterior View)

NOTE: (1) The two pericardial sinuses. The black horizontal arrow indicates the **transverse pericardial sinus,** which lies between the arterial mesocardium and the venous mesocardium. The vertical diverging double arrows lie in the **oblique pericardial sinus,** the boundary of which is limited by the pericardial reflections around the pulmonary veins.

(2) The transverse sinus can be identified by placing your index finger behind the pulmonary artery and aorta with the heart in place. The oblique sinus is open inferiorly and can be felt by cupping your fingers behind the heart and pushing upward; superiorly this sinus forms a closed cul-de-sac.

(3) The **coronary sinus** is a large vein, and it separates the posterior atrial and ventricular surfaces. The posterior atrial surface consists principally of the left atrium, into which flow the pulmonary veins, but also note the right atrium and its superior vena cava below and to the right.

(4) The posterior ventricular surface is formed principally by the left ventricle, and this surface lies over the diaphragm.

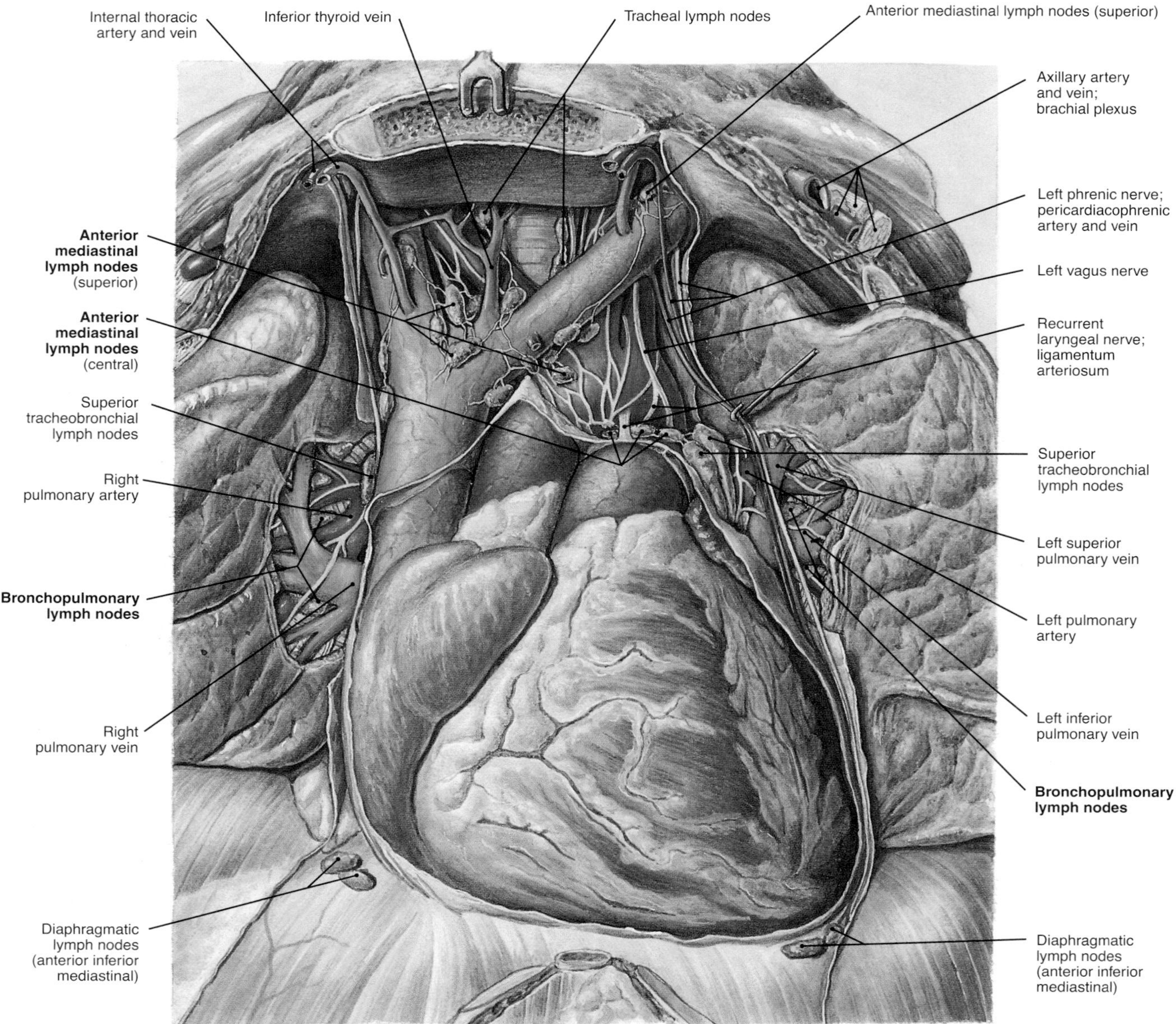
Internal thoracic artery and vein
Inferior thyroid vein
Tracheal lymph nodes
Anterior mediastinal lymph nodes (superior)
Axillary artery and vein; brachial plexus
Left phrenic nerve; pericardiacophrenic artery and vein
Left vagus nerve
Recurrent laryngeal nerve; ligamentum arteriosum
Superior tracheobronchial lymph nodes
Left superior pulmonary vein
Left pulmonary artery
Left inferior pulmonary vein
Bronchopulmonary lymph nodes
Diaphragmatic lymph nodes (anterior inferior mediastinal)
Anterior mediastinal lymph nodes (superior)
Anterior mediastinal lymph nodes (central)
Superior tracheobronchial lymph nodes
Right pulmonary artery
Bronchopulmonary lymph nodes
Right pulmonary vein
Diaphragmatic lymph nodes (anterior inferior mediastinal)

Figure 134 Lymphatics of the Thorax (Anterior Aspect)

NOTE: (1) The anterior thoracic wall was removed, along with the ventral portion of the fibrous pericardium. The anterior borders of the lungs have been pulled laterally to reveal the lymph nodes at the roots of the lungs.

(2) Removal of the thymus and its related fat and reflection of the manubrium superiorly, exposes the organs at the thoracic inlet and their associated lymphatics.

(3) Lymph nodes in the anterior part of the thorax may be divided into those associated with the thoracic cage (parietal) and those associated with the organs (visceral). Probably all the nodes indicated in this figure are visceral nodes.

(4) Situated ventrally are the **anterior mediastinal nodes,** which include a superior group, which lies ventral to the brachiocephalic veins and a more centrally located group that lies ventral to the arch of the aorta. Inferiorly, anterior diaphragmatic nodes are sometimes also classified as part of the anterior mediastinal nodes.

(5) Large numbers of lymph nodes are associated with the trachea, the bronchi, and the other structures at the root of the lung. These nodes have been aptly named **tracheal, tracheobronchial, bronchopulmonary,** and **pulmonary**.

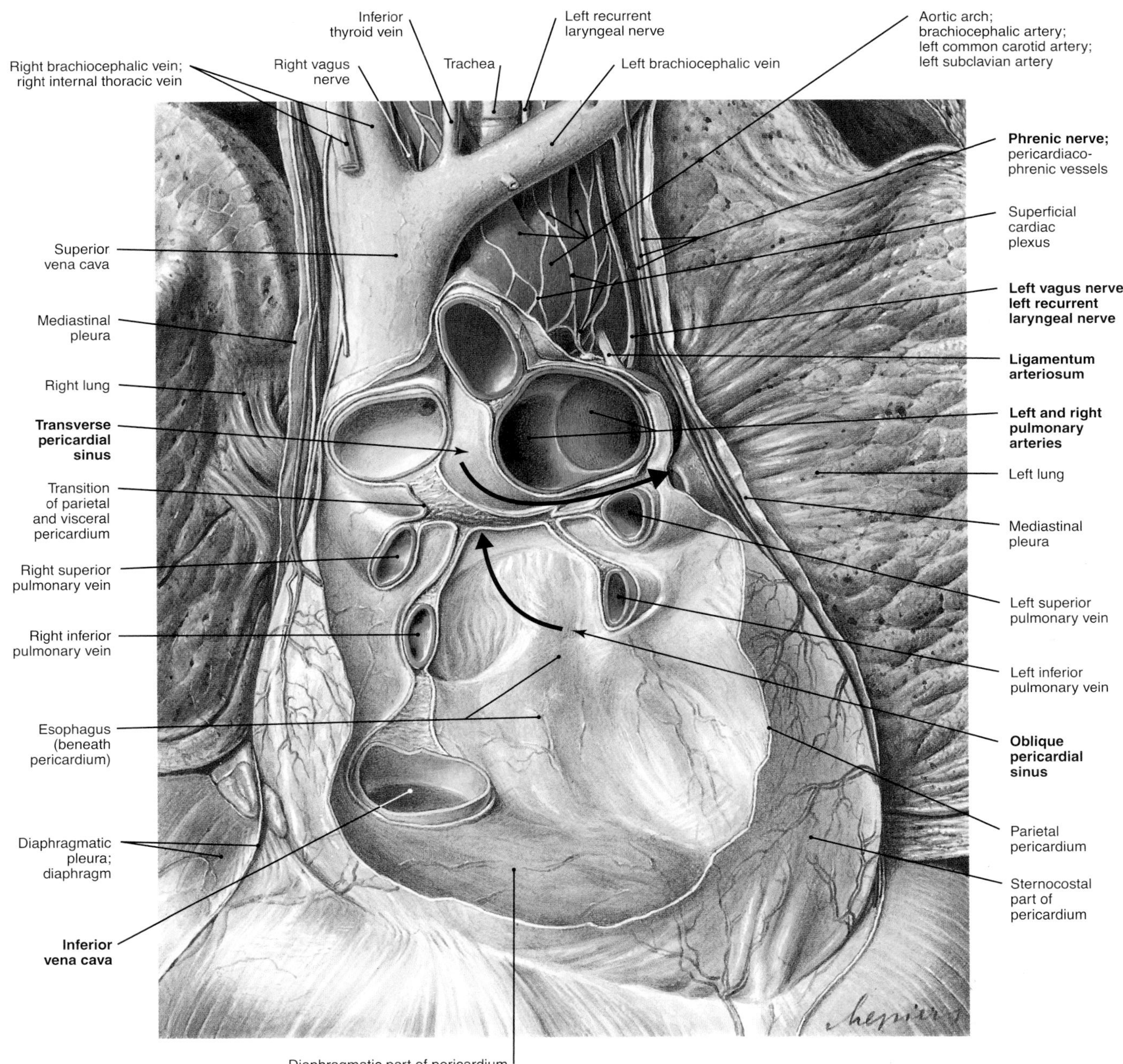
Inferior thyroid vein
Left recurrent laryngeal nerve
Aortic arch; brachiocephalic artery; left common carotid artery; left subclavian artery
Right brachiocephalic vein; right internal thoracic vein
Right vagus nerve
Trachea
Left brachiocephalic vein
Phrenic nerve; pericardiaco-phrenic vessels
Superficial cardiac plexus
Superior vena cava
Mediastinal pleura
Left vagus nerve; left recurrent laryngeal nerve
Ligamentum arteriosum
Right lung
Transverse pericardial sinus
Left and right pulmonary arteries
Left lung
Transition of parietal and visceral pericardium
Mediastinal pleura
Right superior pulmonary vein
Left superior pulmonary vein
Right inferior pulmonary vein
Left inferior pulmonary vein
Esophagus (beneath pericardium)
Oblique pericardial sinus
Parietal pericardium
Diaphragmatic pleura; diaphragm
Sternocostal part of pericardium
Inferior vena cava
Diaphragmatic part of pericardium

Figure 135 Interior of the Pericardium (Anterior View)

NOTE: (1) The pericardium has been opened anteriorly, and the heart has been severed from its attachment to the great vessels and removed. Eight vessels have been cut: the superior and inferior venae cavae, the four pulmonary veins, the pulmonary artery, and the aorta.

(2) The **oblique pericardial sinus** is located in the central portion of the posterior wall of the pericardium and is bounded by the pericardial reflections over the pulmonary veins and the venae cavae (venous mesocardium).

(3) With the heart in place and the pericardium opened anteriorly, the oblique pericardial sinus may be palpated by inserting several fingers behind the heart and probing superiorly until the blind pouch (cul-de-sac) of the sinus is felt.

(4) The **transverse pericardial sinus** lies behind the pericardial reflection surrounding the aorta and pulmonary artery (arterial mesocardium). It may be located by probing with the index finger from right to left immediately behind the pulmonary trunk.

(5) The site of bifurcation of the pulmonary trunk beneath the arch of the aorta and the course of the **left recurrent laryngeal nerve** beneath the **ligamentum arteriosum.**

Figure 136.1 Coronary Vessels (Anterior View)

NOTE: (1) Both the left and right coronary arteries arise from the ascending aorta. The **left coronary** is directed toward the left and soon divides into an **anterior interventricular branch,** which descends toward the apex, and a **circumflex branch,** which passes posteriorly to the back of the heart.

(2) The **right coronary** is directed toward the right and passes to the posterior heart within the coronary sulcus. In its course, branches from the right coronary supply the anterior surface of the right side (anterior cardiac artery). Its largest branch is the **posterior interventricular artery,** which courses toward the apex on the posterior or diaphragmatic surface of the heart.

(3) The principal veins of the heart drain into the **coronary sinus,** which flows into the right atrium. The distribution and course of the veins is similar to the arteries (see Figs. 137.1 and 137.2)

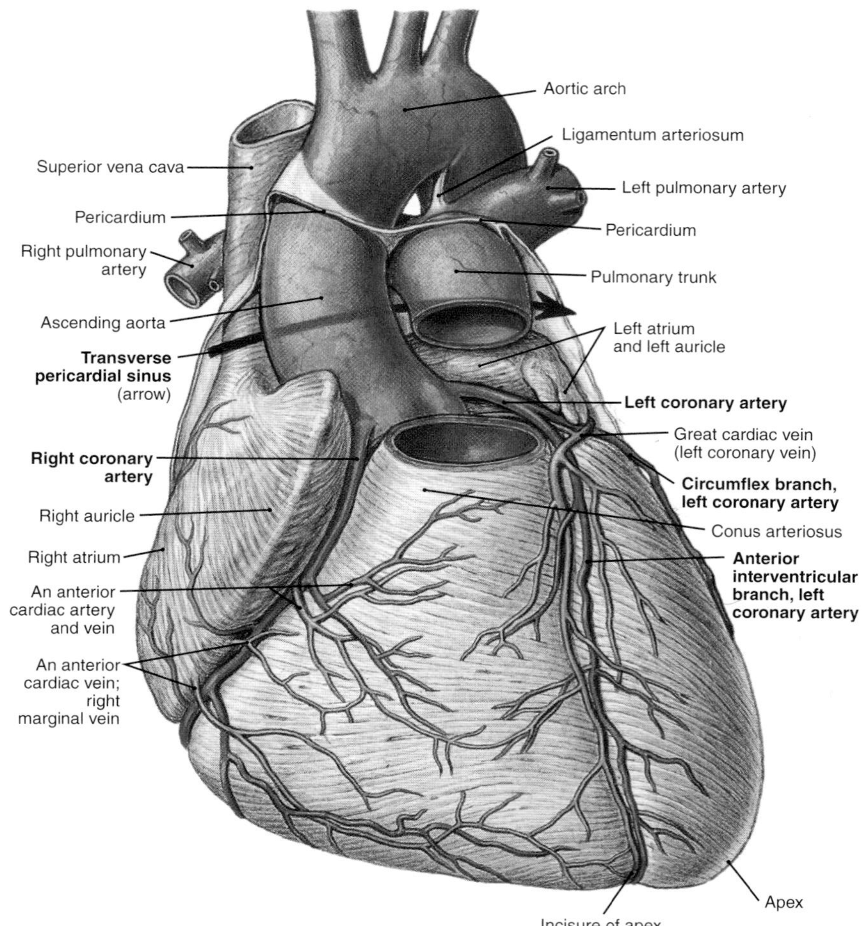
Aortic arch
Ligamentum arteriosum
Superior vena cava
Left pulmonary artery
Pericardium
Pericardium
Right pulmonary artery
Pulmonary trunk
Ascending aorta
Left atrium and left auricle
Transverse pericardial sinus (arrow)
Left coronary artery
Great cardiac vein (left coronary vein)
Right coronary artery
Circumflex branch, left coronary artery
Right auricle
Conus arteriosus
Right atrium
Anterior interventricular branch, left coronary artery
An anterior cardiac artery and vein
An anterior cardiac vein; right marginal vein
Apex
Incisure of apex

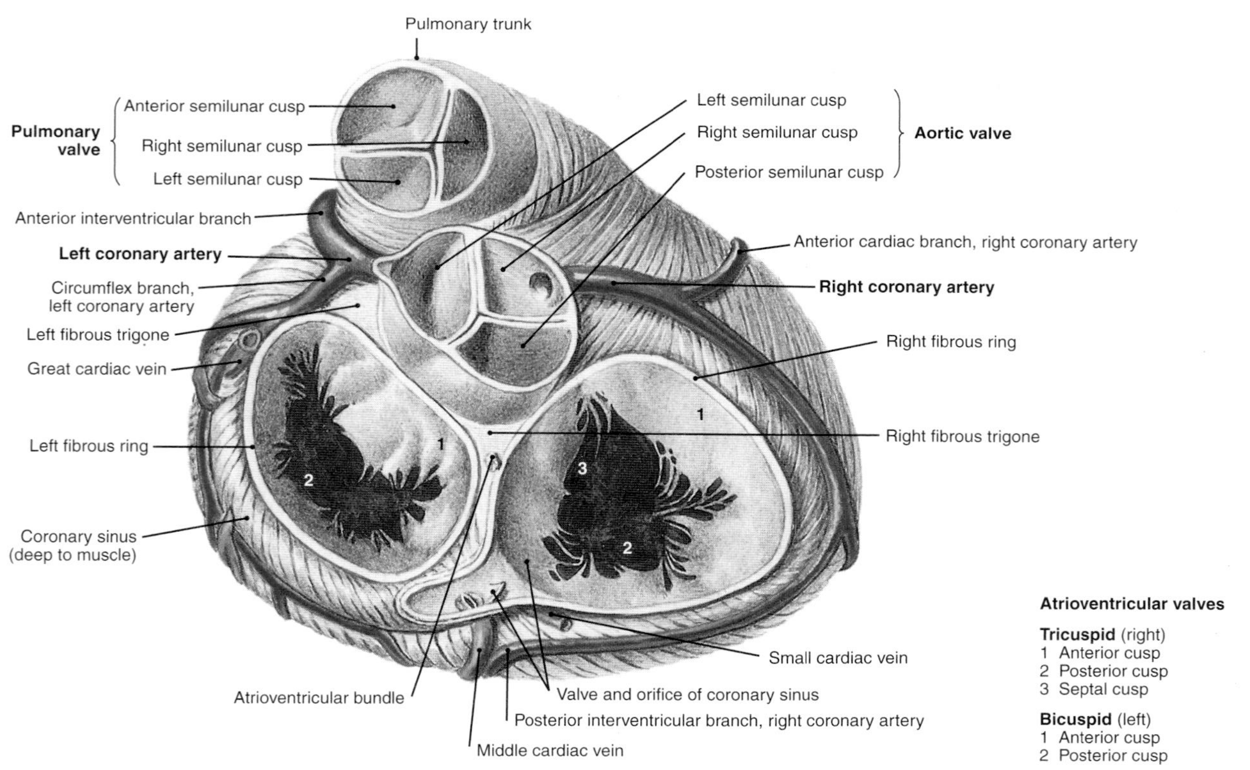
Pulmonary trunk
Pulmonary valve
Anterior semilunar cusp
Right semilunar cusp
Left semilunar cusp
Left semilunar cusp
Right semilunar cusp
Posterior semilunar cusp
Aortic valve
Anterior interventricular branch
Left coronary artery
Anterior cardiac branch, right coronary artery
Circumflex branch, left coronary artery
Right coronary artery
Left fibrous trigone
Right fibrous ring
Great cardiac vein
Left fibrous ring
Right fibrous trigone
Coronary sinus (deep to muscle)
1
2
1
3
2
Small cardiac vein
Atrioventricular bundle
Valve and orifice of coronary sinus
Posterior interventricular branch, right coronary artery
Middle cardiac vein
Atrioventricular valves
Tricuspid (right)
1 Anterior cusp
2 Posterior cusp
3 Septal cusp
Bicuspid (left)
1 Anterior cusp
2 Posterior cusp

Figure 136.2 Valves of the Heart and the Origin of the Coronary Vessels (Superior View)

NOTE that the left coronary artery arises from the aortic wall in the left aortic sinus behind the left semilunar cusp, and the right coronary stems from the aorta behind the right aortic sinus and right semilunar cusp.

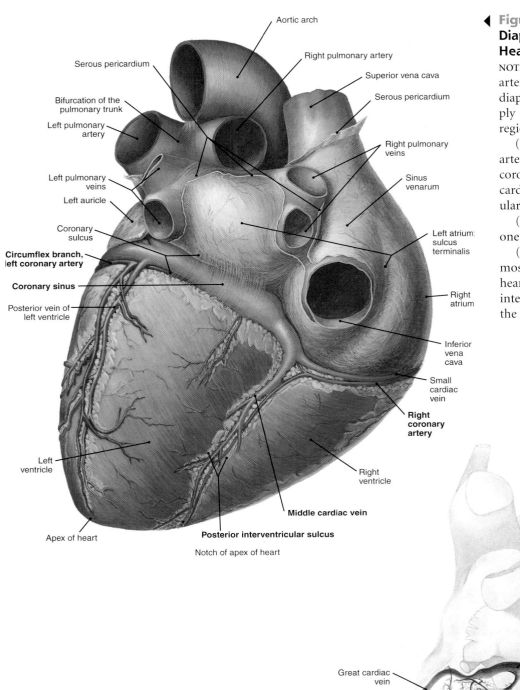

Aortic arch
Serous pericardium
Right pulmonary artery
Superior vena cava
Bifurcation of the pulmonary trunk
Serous pericardium
Left pulmonary artery
Right pulmonary veins
Left pulmonary veins
Sinus venarum
Left auricle
Coronary sulcus
Left atrium; sulcus terminalis
Circumflex branch, left coronary artery
Coronary sinus
Right atrium
Posterior vein of left ventricle
Inferior vena cava
Small cardiac vein
Right coronary artery
Left ventricle
Right ventricle
Middle cardiac vein
Apex of heart
Posterior interventricular sulcus
Notch of apex of heart

Figure 137.1 Coronary Vessels, Diaphragmatic Surface of the Heart

NOTE: (1) Both the left and right coronary arteries course around to the posterior or diaphragmatic surface of the heart to supply the left and right ventricles in that region.

(2) The posterior interventricular artery is usually a branch of the right coronary, and it courses with the middle cardiac vein in the posterior interventricular sulcus.

(3) The left coronary artery contributes one or more posterior ventricular arteries.

(4) The two coronary arteries anastomose on this posterior surface of the heart, and their anterior and posterior interventricular branches anastomose at the apex.

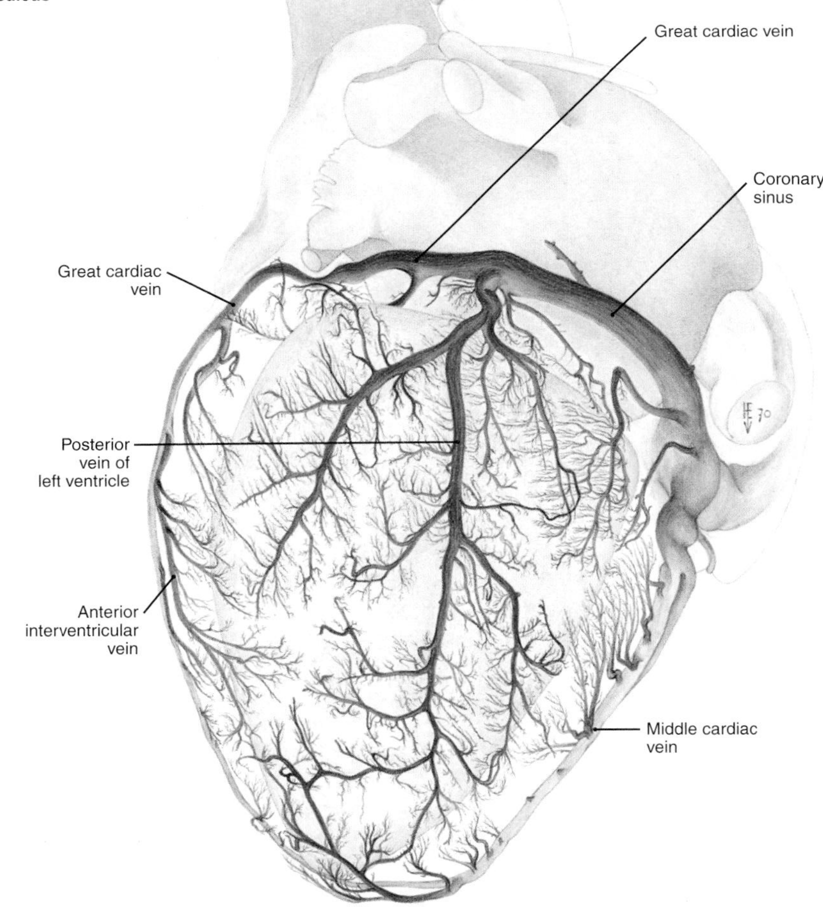
Great cardiac vein
Coronary sinus
Great cardiac vein
Posterior vein of left ventricle
Anterior interventricular vein
Middle cardiac vein

Figure 137.2 Venous Drainage of the Ventricles: Coronary Sinus

NOTE: (1) The left side and left margin of the heart are oriented forward such that the anterior interventricular vein is seen on the left and the middle cardiac vein is seen on the right.

(2) The anterior **interventricular vein** becomes the **great cardiac vein.** As the great cardiac vein courses in the coronary sulcus, it gradually enlarges to form the **coronary sinus** and receives the **posterior vein of the left ventricle.** The **middle cardiac vein,** which runs in the posterior interventricular sulcus, also drains directly into the coronary sinus.

(3) The coronary sinus opens into the right atrium.

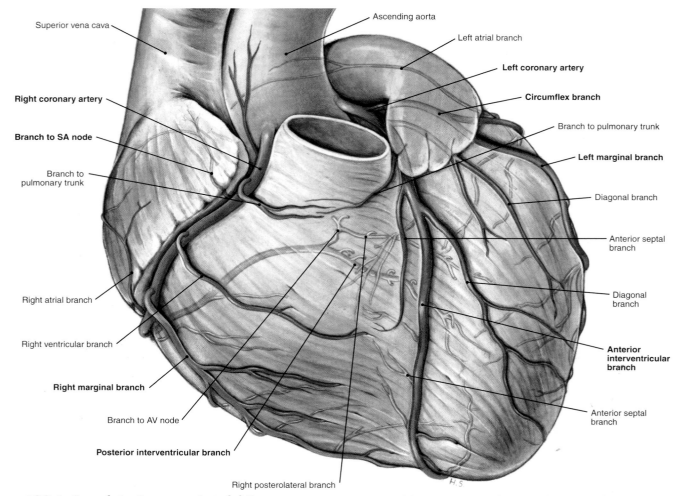

Superior vena cava
Ascending aorta
Left atrial branch
Left coronary artery
Circumflex branch
Right coronary artery
Branch to SA node
Branch to pulmonary trunk
Branch to pulmonary trunk
Left marginal branch
Diagonal branch
Anterior septal branch
Right atrial branch
Diagonal branch
Right ventricular branch
Anterior interventricular branch
Right marginal branch
Anterior septal branch
Branch to AV node
Posterior interventricular branch
Right posterolateral branch

Figure 138.1 Complete Coronary Arterial System ▲

NOTE: (1) Anastomoses between branches from the left and right coronary arteries (LCA and RCA) are visible in the substance of the posterior wall of the heart. These occur between the posterior interventricular branch of the RCA and the anterior interventricular branch of the LCA, which continues around the apex of the heart to the posterior wall.

(2) Vessels from the circumflex and left marginal branches of the LCA also anastomose with branches from the RCA in the posterior wall.

(3) Branches supplying the sinoatrial (SA) node and the atrioventricular (AV) node arise from the RCA. In about 35% of cases, however, the artery to the SA node comes from the circumflex branch of the LCA. Similarly, in about 20% of specimens, the vessel to the AV node is derived from the circumflex branch of the LCA. (From a drawing by Professor Helmut Ferner at the University of Vienna.)

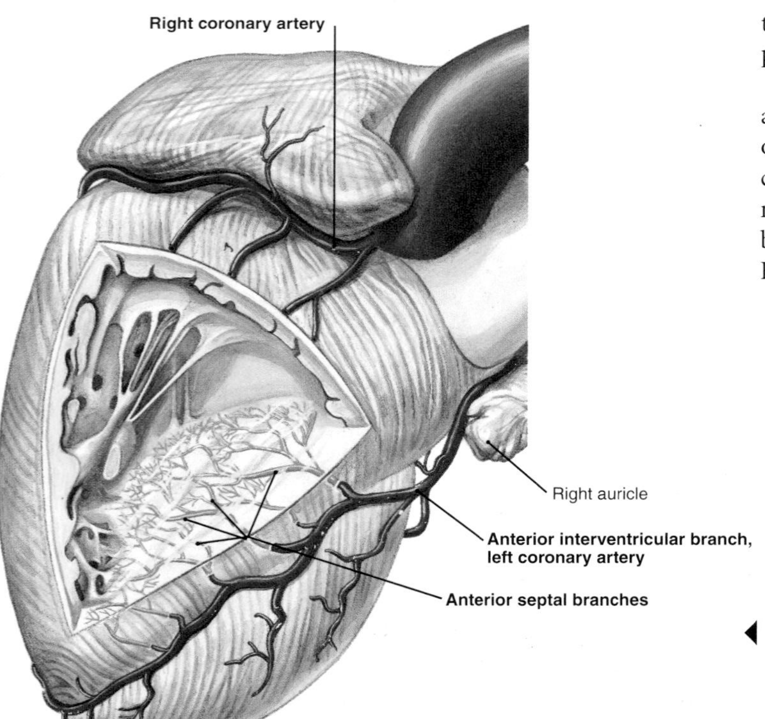
Right coronary artery
Right auricle
Anterior interventricular branch, left coronary artery
Anterior septal branches

◀ **Figure 138.2 Blood Supply to the Interventricular Septum**

NOTE that the **anterior septal branches** of the anterior interventricular artery course backward and downward to supply the interventricular septum.

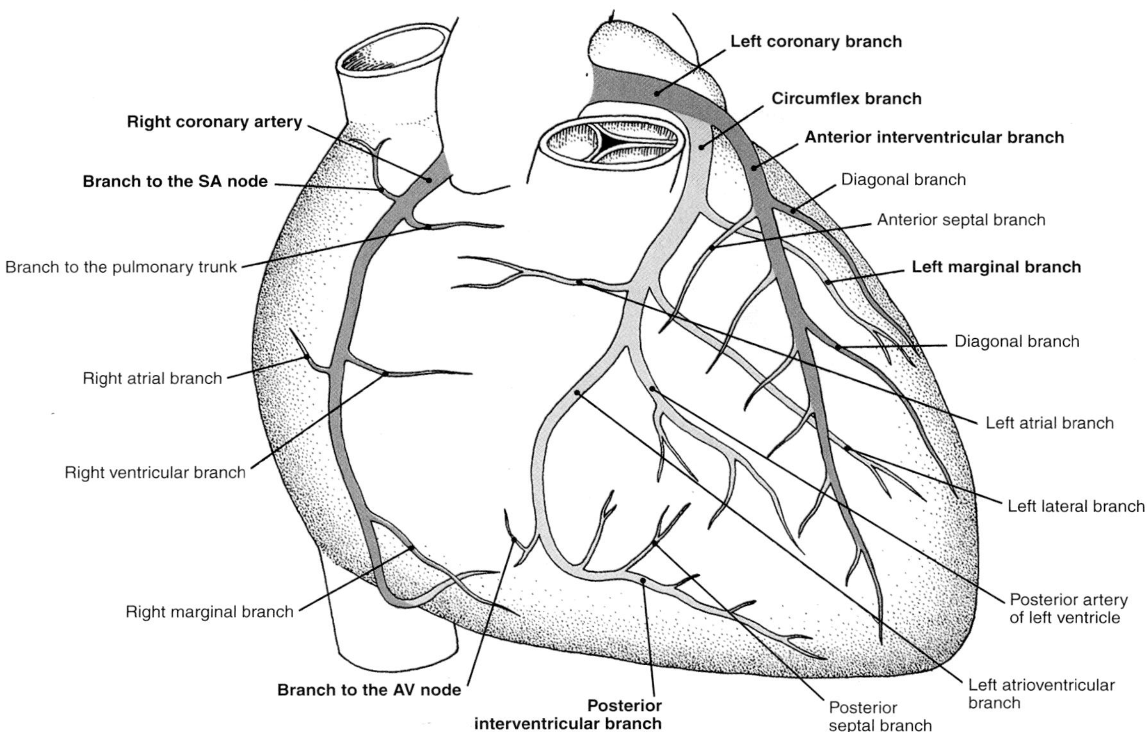

Left coronary branch
Circumflex branch
Anterior interventricular branch
Diagonal branch
Anterior septal branch
Left marginal branch
Diagonal branch
Left atrial branch
Left lateral branch
Posterior artery of left ventricle
Left atrioventricular branch
Posterior septal branch
Posterior interventricular branch
Branch to the AV node
Right marginal branch
Right ventricular branch
Right atrial branch
Branch to the pulmonary trunk
Branch to the SA node
Right coronary artery

Figure 139.1 Dominant Distribution to the Heart Wall from the Left Coronary Artery

NOTE that in hearts containing a dominant left coronary artery (10%), there is very little contribution from the right coronary artery to the posterior wall of the left ventricle. In these cases, the posterior interventricular artery arises from the left coronary artery as a continuation of the enlarged circumflex branch.

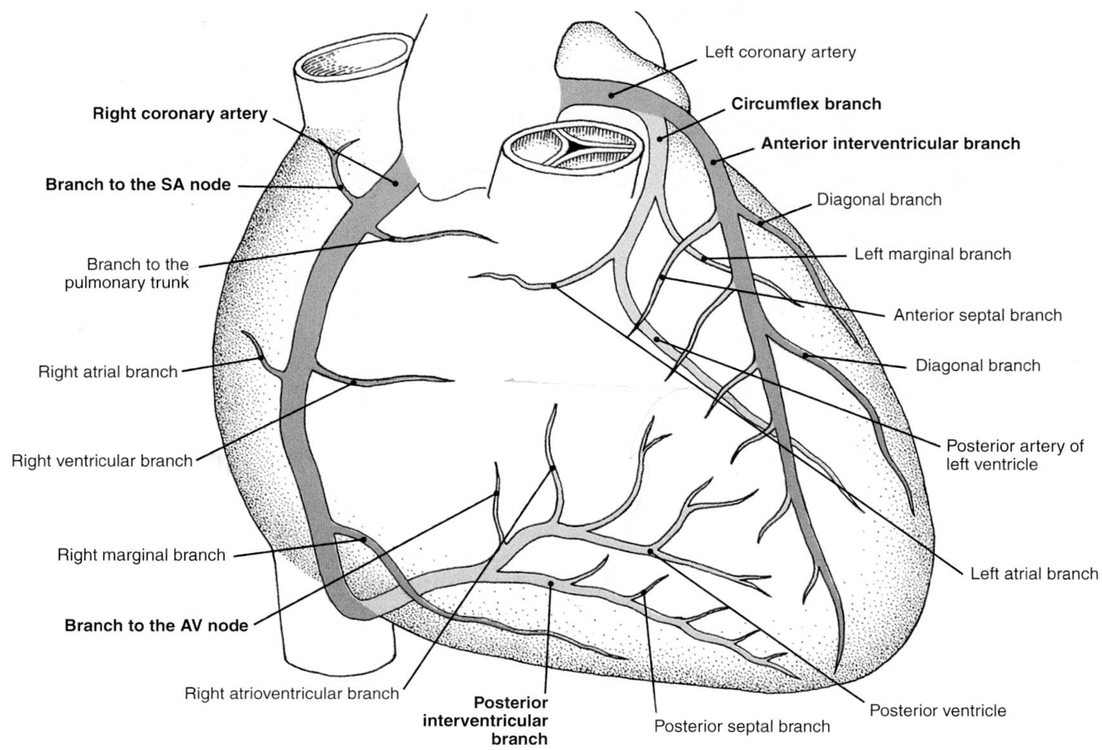

Left coronary artery
Circumflex branch
Anterior interventricular branch
Diagonal branch
Left marginal branch
Anterior septal branch
Diagonal branch
Posterior artery of left ventricle
Left atrial branch
Posterior ventricle
Posterior septal branch
Posterior interventricular branch
Right atrioventricular branch
Branch to the AV node
Right marginal branch
Right ventricular branch
Right atrial branch
Branch to the pulmonary trunk
Branch to the SA node
Right coronary artery

Figure 139.2 Dominant Distribution to the Heart Wall from the Right Coronary Artery

NOTE that in hearts containing a dominant right coronary artery, the posterior wall of the left ventricle receives a larger share of its blood from the right coronary artery when compared with a left dominant coronary heart. In these instances, the posterior interventricular artery arises from the right coronary artery and the circumflex and marginal branches of the left coronary are relatively smaller.

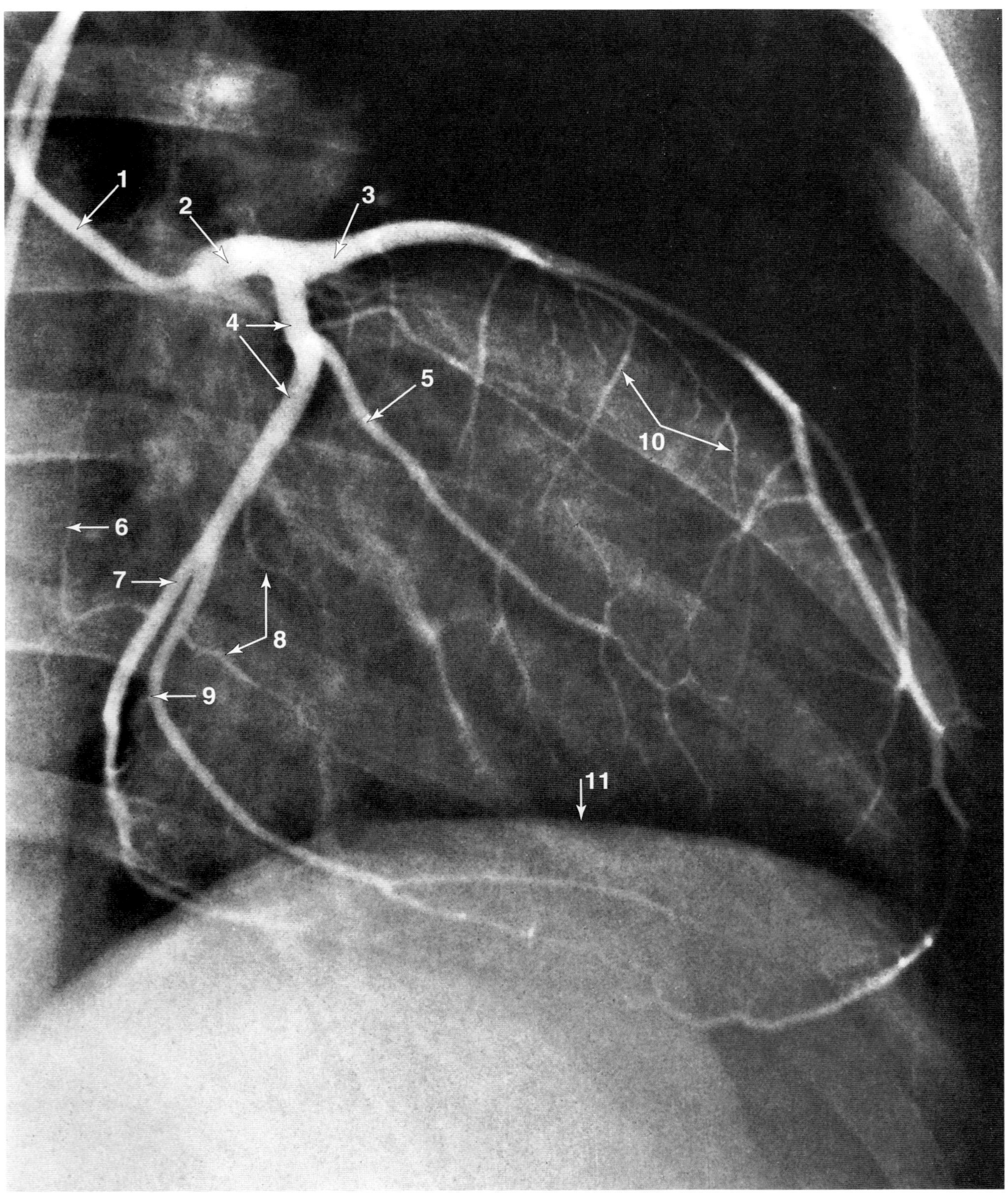
1
2
3
4
5
10
6
7
8
9
11

Figure 140 Left Coronary Arteriogram

NOTE that this arteriogram of the left coronary artery is viewed from a right anterior oblique direction.

1. Catheter
2. Left coronary artery
3. Anterior interventricular branch
4. Circumflex branch
5. Left marginal branch of circumflex
6. Posterior atrial branch
7. Left posterolateral branch of circumflex
8. Posterior ventricular branches
9. Posterior interventricular branch
10. Septal branches
11. Diaphragm

(From Wicke, 6th ed.)

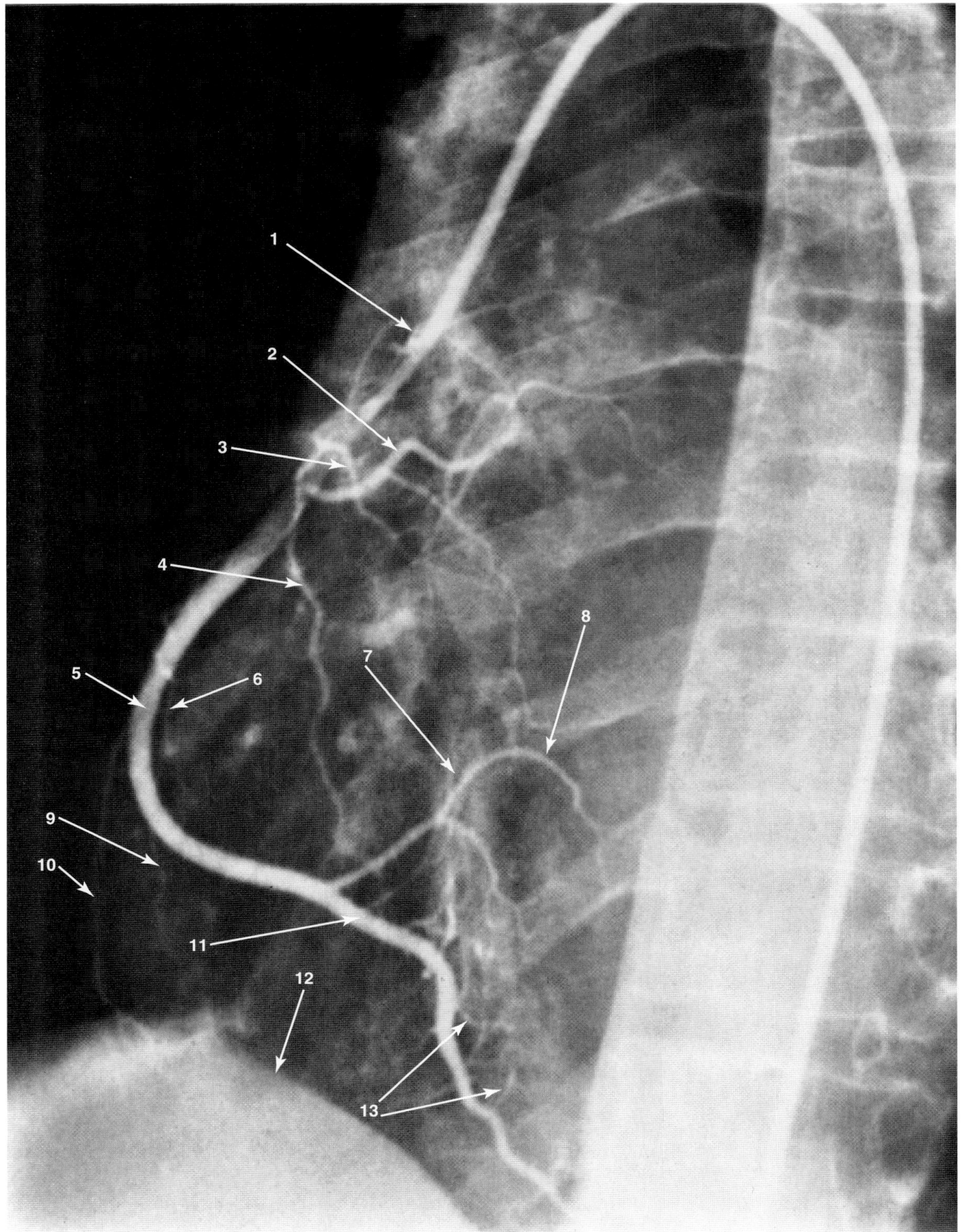
1
2
3
4
5
6
7
8
9
10
11
12
13

Figure 141 Right Coronary Arteriogram

NOTE that this arteriogram of the right coronary artery is viewed from the left anterior oblique direction.

1. Catheter
2. Sinoatrial node branch
3. Conus arteriosus branch
4. Anterior ventricular branch
5. Right coronary artery
6. Anterior ventricular branch
7. Atrioventricular node branch
8. Posterior ventricular branch
9. Posterior ventricular branch
10. Right marginal branch
11. Posterior interventricular branch
12. Diaphragm
13. Posterior septal branches

(From Wicke, 6th ed.)

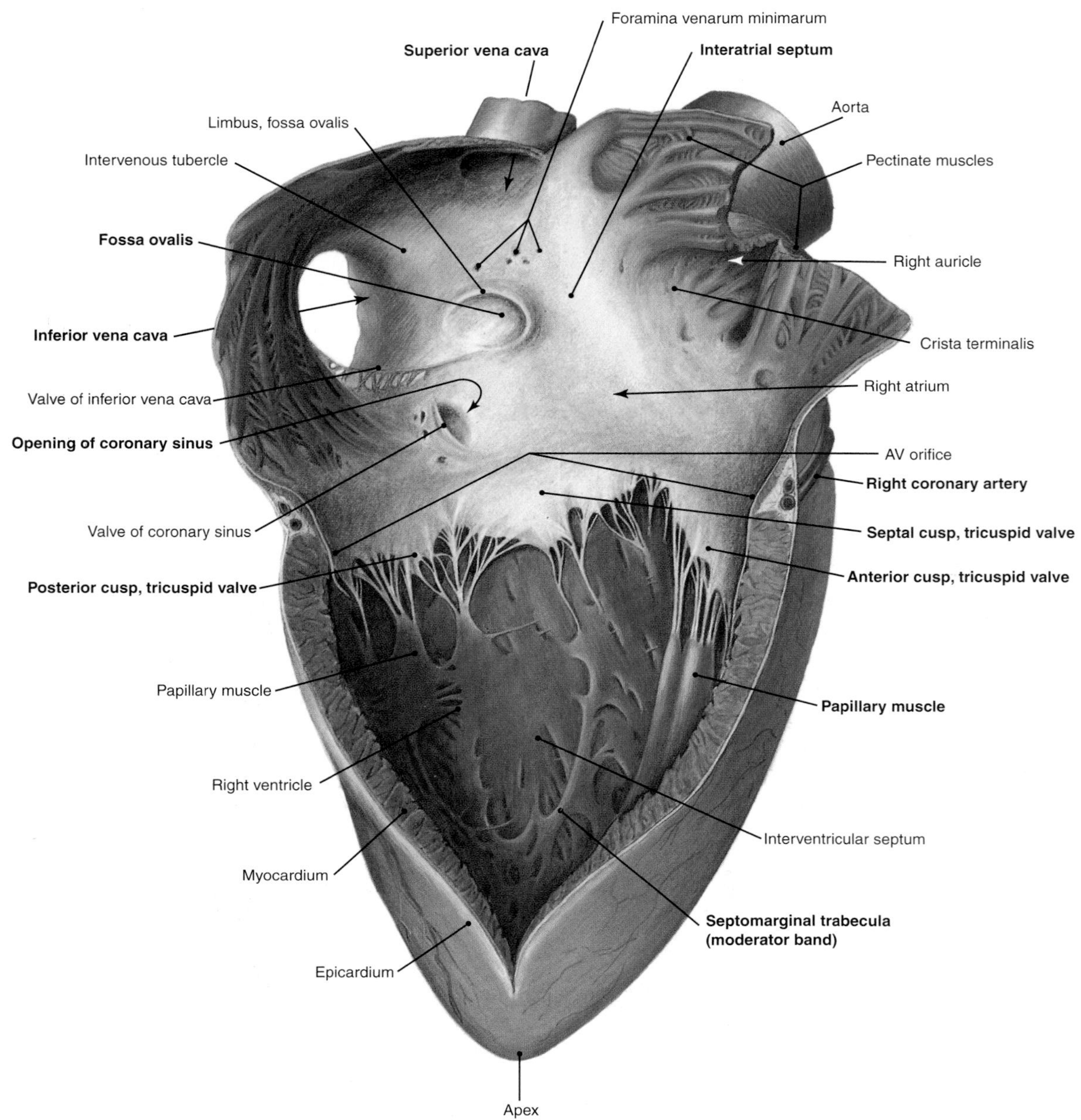
Foramina venarum minimarum
Superior vena cava
Interatrial septum
Aorta
Limbus, fossa ovalis
Intervenous tubercle
Pectinate muscles
Fossa ovalis
Right auricle
Inferior vena cava
Crista terminalis
Right atrium
Valve of inferior vena cava
Opening of coronary sinus
AV orifice
Right coronary artery
Septal cusp, tricuspid valve
Valve of coronary sinus
Anterior cusp, tricuspid valve
Posterior cusp, tricuspid valve
Papillary muscle
Papillary muscle
Right ventricle
Interventricular septum
Myocardium
Septomarginal trabecula
(moderator band)
Epicardium
Apex

Figure 142 Right Atrium and Right Ventricle

NOTE: (1) The right atrium consists of (a) a smooth area (at times called the **sinus venarum**) located between the openings of the superior vena cava and the inferior vena cava and (b) the **right auricle**, which is marked by parallel muscle ridges called the **pectinate muscles.**

(2) Opening into the right atrium are the **superior vena cava,** the **inferior vena cava,** the **coronary sinus,** and the small **venarum minimarum** (Thebesian veins).

(3) Crescent-shaped valves are found at the right atrial openings of both the inferior vena cava and the coronary sinus.

(4) The right atrioventricular (AV) opening is surrounded by the three cusps of the **tricuspid valve.** These are called the **anterior, posterior,** and **septal** cusps, and they are attached to the heart wall by way of the **chordae tendineae** and **papillary muscles.**

(5) The thickness of the right ventricular wall (4 to 5 mm) is about one-third that of the left ventricle (see Fig. 144). Normal right ventricular systolic blood pressure ranges between 25 and 30 mm Hg, and it is also much less than normal left ventricular systolic pressure, which ranges between 120 and 140 mm Hg.

(6) The **septomarginal trabecula** (moderator band) within which courses the right crus, or branch, of the **atrioventricular bundle** (of His).

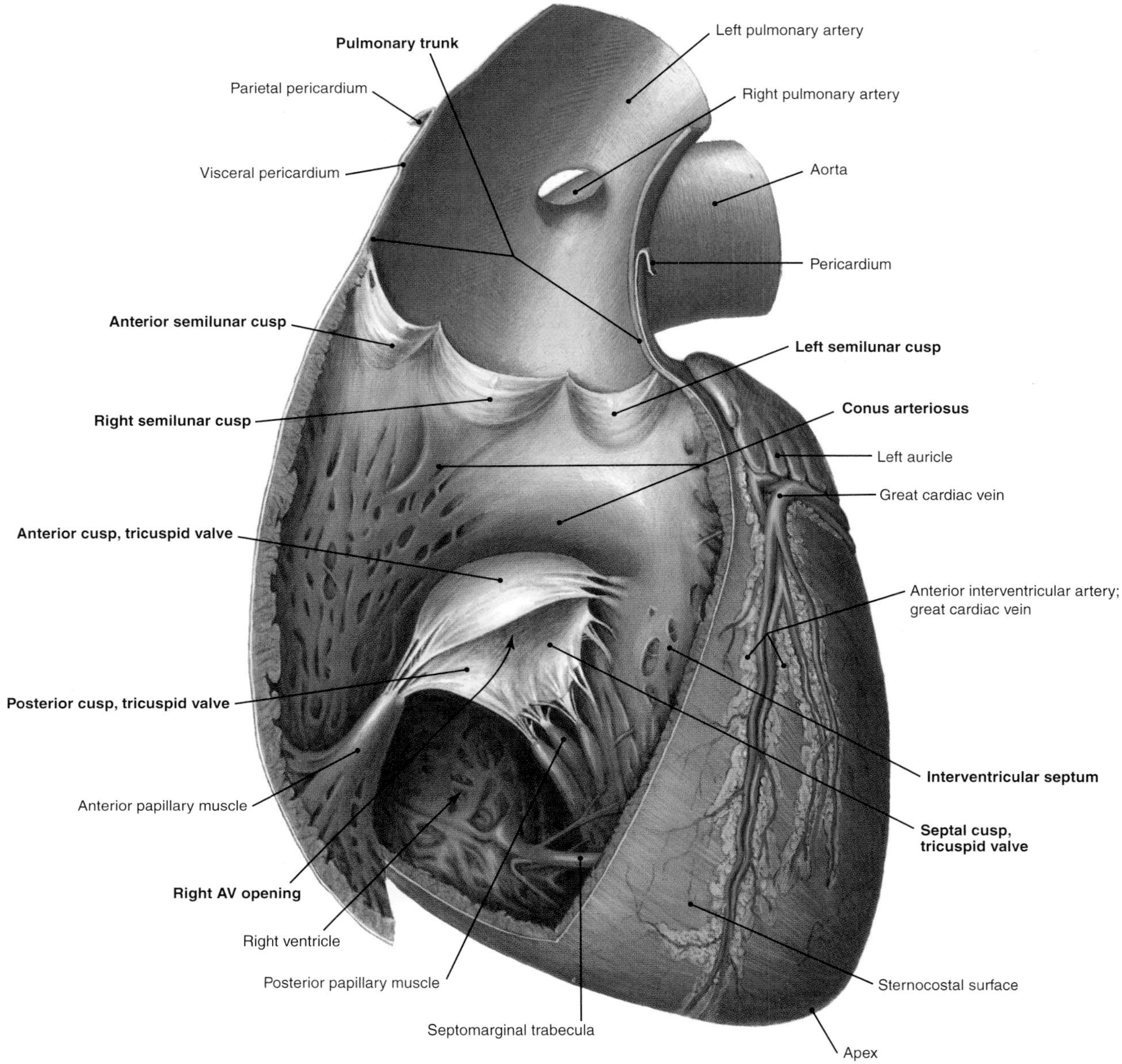
Pulmonary trunk
Parietal pericardium
Visceral pericardium
Left pulmonary artery
Right pulmonary artery
Aorta
Pericardium
Anterior semilunar cusp
Right semilunar cusp
Left semilunar cusp
Conus arteriosus
Left auricle
Great cardiac vein
Anterior cusp, tricuspid valve
Anterior interventricular artery; great cardiac vein
Posterior cusp, tricuspid valve
Interventricular septum
Anterior papillary muscle
Septal cusp, tricuspid valve
Right AV opening
Right ventricle
Posterior papillary muscle
Sternocostal surface
Septomarginal trabecula
Apex

Figure 143 Right Ventricle and Pulmonary Trunk

NOTE: (1) The musculature of the right ventricle has been cut along a V-shaped incision, thereby forming a flap in the anterior wall of the ventricle. As the flap is reflected to the right, the origin of the **pulmonary trunk** and the cusps of its valve are exposed.

(2) The three semilunar pulmonary cusps—the **right, left,** and **anterior** semilunar pulmonary cusps—are interposed between the right ventricle and the pulmonary artery. Together they comprise the **pulmonary valve.**

(3) The **septal, anterior,** and **posterior cusps** form the **right atrioventricular** (AV) or **tricuspid valve.** Note their attachments to the papillary muscles.

(4) The smooth surface of the right ventricular wall at the site of origin of the pulmonary trunk. This is called the **conus arteriosus** of the right ventricle.

(5) The attachment and shape of the tricuspid valve allow the cusps to open into the right ventricle when blood pressure in the atrium exceeds that in the ventricle. At some point during the cardiac cycle, ventricular pressure exceeds atrial pressure, and the cusps close. Blood is prevented from regurgitating into the atrium because the perimeter of the cusps is secured to the heart wall and the free edges of the cusps are attached to the papillary muscles in the ventricle below.

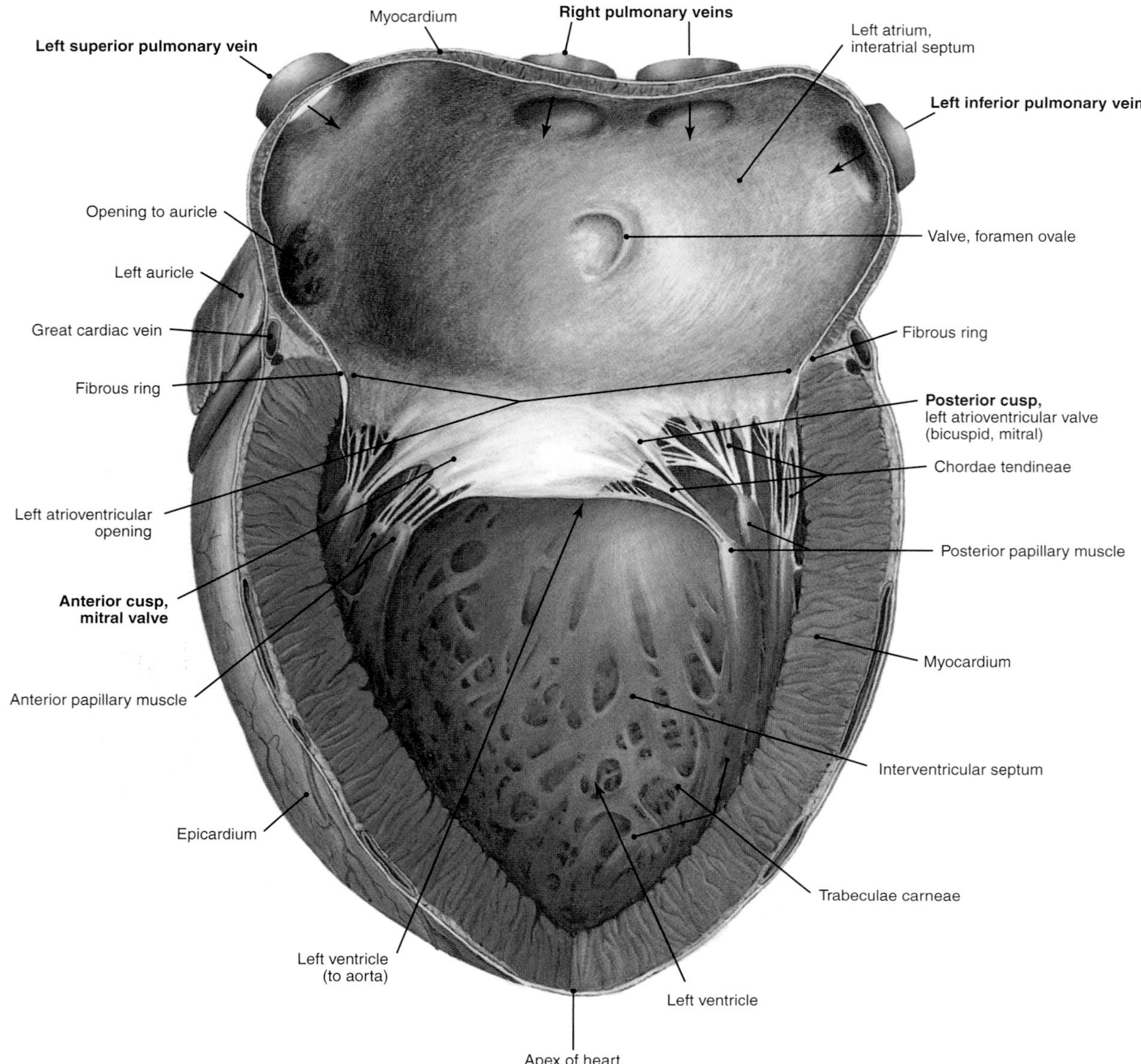
Myocardium
Right pulmonary veins
Left superior pulmonary vein
Left atrium, interatrial septum
Left inferior pulmonary vein
Opening to auricle
Valve, foramen ovale
Left auricle
Great cardiac vein
Fibrous ring
Fibrous ring
Posterior cusp, left atrioventricular valve (bicuspid, mitral)
Chordae tendineae
Left atrioventricular opening
Posterior papillary muscle
Anterior cusp, mitral valve
Myocardium
Anterior papillary muscle
Interventricular septum
Epicardium
Trabeculae carneae
Left ventricle (to aorta)
Left ventricle
Apex of heart

Figure 144 Left Atrium and Left Ventricle (Internal Surface)

NOTE: (1) In this specimen, the heart has been opened to expose the inner surface of the left atrium and left ventricle. Likewise, the left atrioventricular opening has been cut behind the **posterior cusp of the mitral valve,** thereby making that cusp visible.

(2) The left atrium receives the four **pulmonary veins** (two from each lung), while the left ventricle leads into the aorta (arrow).

(3) The **interatrial septum** on the left side is marked by the valve of the foramen ovale (falx septi), which represents the remnant of the **septum primum** during the development of the interatrial septum. The crescent-shaped structure around the border of the valve is the limbus of the fossa ovalis and is the remnant of the **septum secundum.**

(4) The mitral valve consists of **anterior** and **posterior cusps** (only the posterior is seen in this figure). The cusps are attached to the left ventricular wall by means of chordae tendineae and papillary muscles in a manner similar to that seen in the right ventricle.

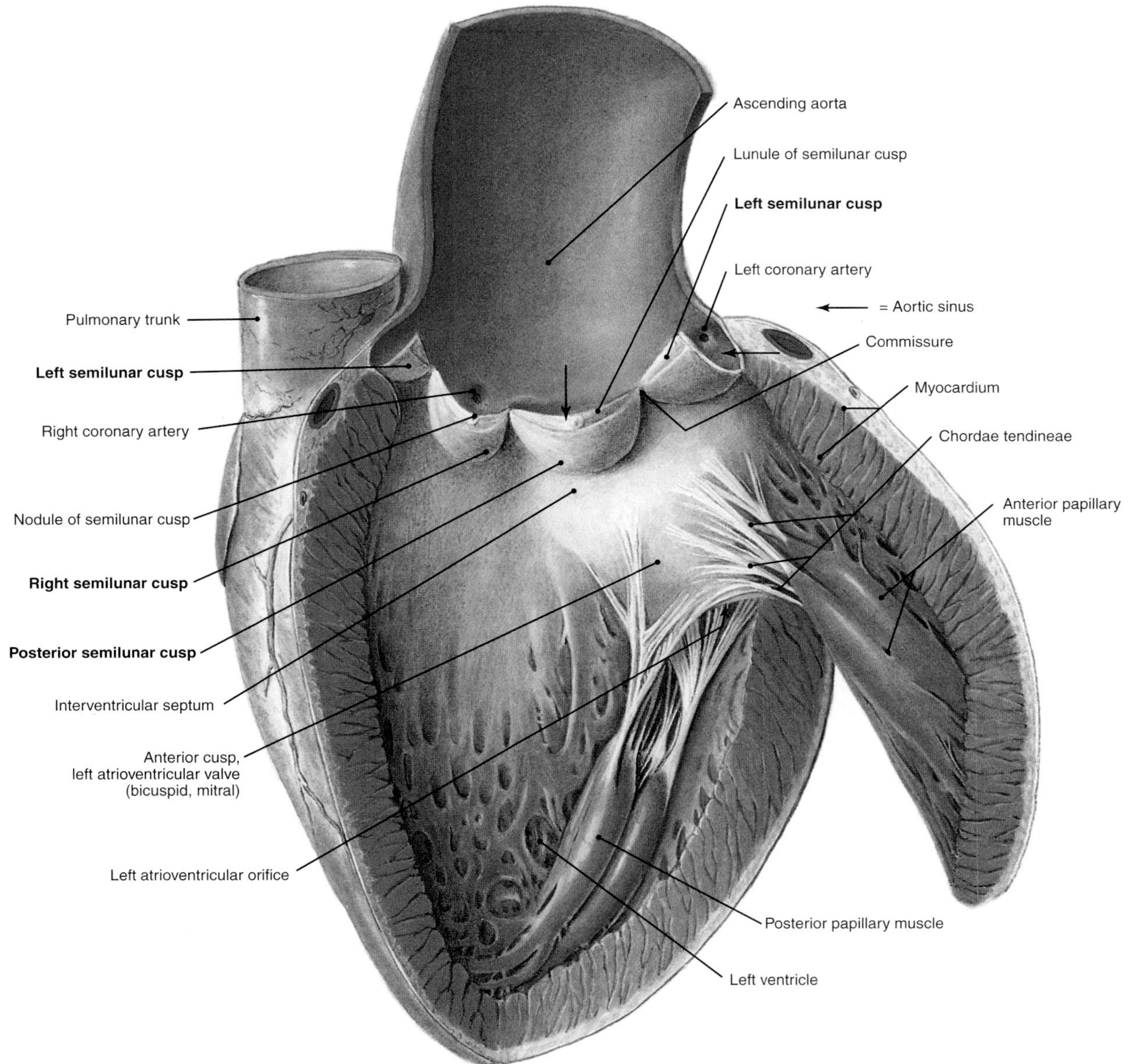
Ascending aorta
Lunule of semilunar cusp
Left semilunar cusp
Left coronary artery
= Aortic sinus
Commissure
Myocardium
Chordae tendineae
Anterior papillary muscle
Pulmonary trunk
Left semilunar cusp
Right coronary artery
Nodule of semilunar cusp
Right semilunar cusp
Posterior semilunar cusp
Interventricular septum
Anterior cusp, left atrioventricular valve (bicuspid, mitral)
Left atrioventricular orifice
Posterior papillary muscle
Left ventricle

Figure 145 Opened Left Ventricle and Aorta

NOTE: (1) In this dissection, the left ventricle was opened first to show the anterior and posterior papillary muscles that are related to the cusps of the left AV valve. A second cut was then made in the wall of the left ventricle (near the interventricular septum) that extends through the aortic opening to show the cusps of the **aortic valve.**

(2) The opening of the left coronary artery in the aortic wall behind the (cut) left **semilunar cusp**. Also see the opening of the right coronary artery behind the **right semilunar cusp.** The **posterior cusp** of the aortic valve is the noncoronary cusp.

(3) Between the cusps and the wall of the aorta are pockets called the **aortic sinuses.** These trap blood during the cardiac cycle, thereby closing the valve.

(4) Each cusp is marked by a thickened fibrocartilaginous **nodule** at the center of its free margin. Extending out from the nodule on each side of the cusp are clear crescentic areas of thinning of the free edges called **lunulae**, while the points at which two adjacent cusps come together are called **commissures**.

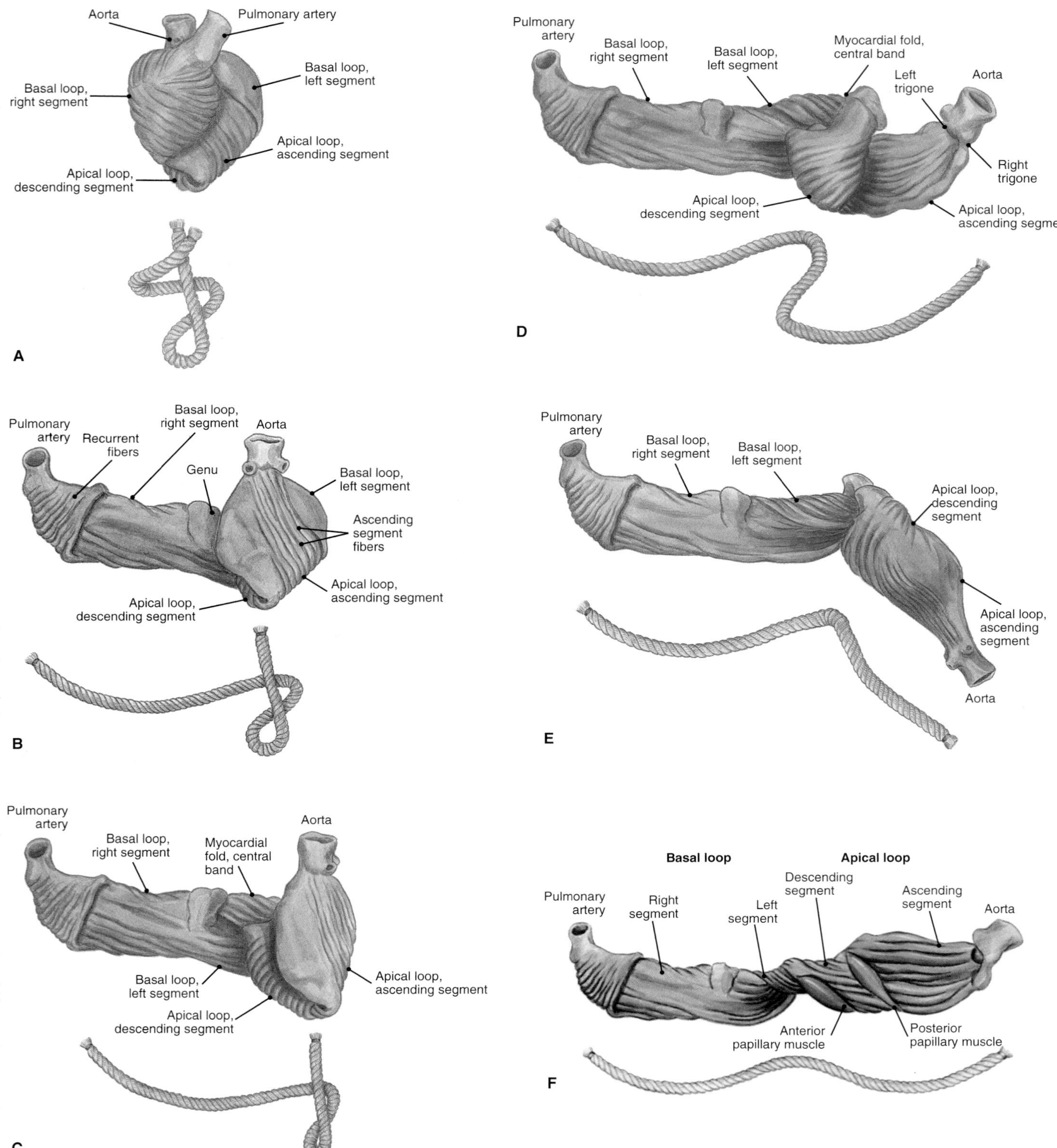

Aorta
Pulmonary artery
Basal loop, left segment
Basal loop, right segment
Apical loop, ascending segment
Apical loop, descending segment
A
Pulmonary artery
Basal loop, right segment
Basal loop, left segment
Myocardial fold, central band
Left trigone
Aorta
Right trigone
Apical loop, descending segment
Apical loop, ascending segment
D
Basal loop, right segment
Pulmonary artery
Recurrent fibers
Aorta
Genu
Basal loop, left segment
Ascending segment fibers
Apical loop, ascending segment
Apical loop, descending segment
B
Pulmonary artery
Basal loop, right segment
Basal loop, left segment
Apical loop, descending segment
Apical loop, ascending segment
Aorta
E
Pulmonary artery
Aorta
Basal loop, right segment
Myocardial fold, central band
Basal loop, left segment
Apical loop, ascending segment
Apical loop, descending segment
C
Basal loop
Apical loop
Descending segment
Pulmonary artery
Right segment
Left segment
Ascending segment
Aorta
Anterior papillary muscle
Posterior papillary muscle
F

Figure 146 A–F Progressive Unscrolling of the Cardiac Muscle That Forms the Heart (from F. Torrent-Guasp)

NOTE: (1) Upon unscrolling the muscle that forms the heart, the unfolded myocardium has a rope-like configuration (shown by the rope model) comprised of a **transverse basal loop,** with fibers running almost horizontally, and a **longitudinal apical loop,** with fibers that course almost vertically from apex to base. **Fig. 146A** shows the intact heart. **Fig. 146B** shows that detachment of the right ventricular free wall exposes the transverse orientation of the basal loop fibers. The pulmonary outflow tract is limited by **recurrent fibers** coming from the right free wall. These bend all along the anterior interventricular groove to ascend toward the ventricular base. A **genu** at the basal extreme of the posterior interventricular sulcus separates the right and left ventricles or segments of the basal loop.

(2) **Fig. 146C:** Further unfolding of the basal loop displays the **left basal segment,** beyond the genu (left), and exposes the central band **myocardial fold** by which fibers of the left segment, subendocardially, become nearly vertical fibers of the descending segment. These course deeper, subendocardially, toward the region of the apex, where they reflect and ascend to become the ascending segment fibers that connect to the aorta. In **Fig. 146D,** both **trigones of the aorta** are detached and the ascending segment is unfolded and moved laterally, thereby demonstrating the deeper descending segment of the apical loop. (**Continued next page.**)

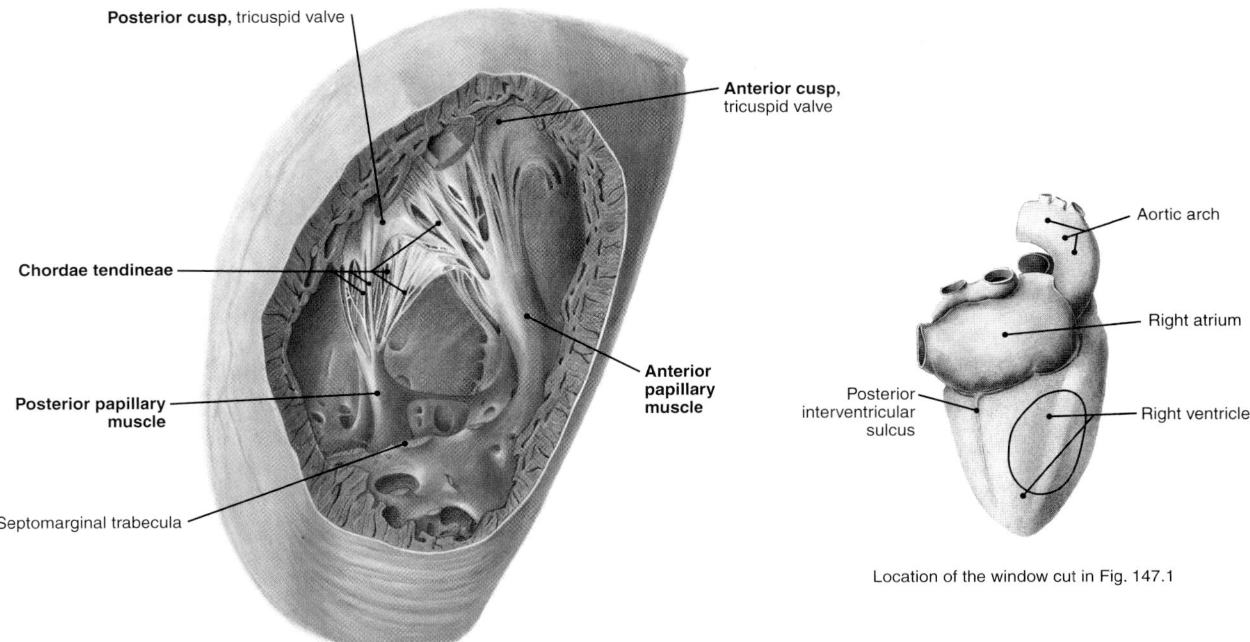
Posterior cusp, tricuspid valve
Anterior cusp, tricuspid valve
Chordae tendineae
Anterior papillary muscle
Posterior papillary muscle
Septomarginal trabecula
Aortic arch
Right atrium
Posterior interventricular sulcus
Right ventricle
Location of the window cut in Fig. 147.1

Figure 147.1 Right Ventricle: View of the Tricuspid Valve

NOTE: (1) The anterior and posterior cusps (two of the three) of the tricuspid valve and their attached papillary muscles are exposed.

(2) The **anterior papillary muscle** arises from the anterior and septal walls and attaches to both the anterior and posterior cusps, while the **posterior papillary muscle** arises from the anterior and septal walls and attaches to both the anterior and posterior cusps. Observe the septomarginal trabeculae, or moderator bands, that contain the atrioventricular bundle.

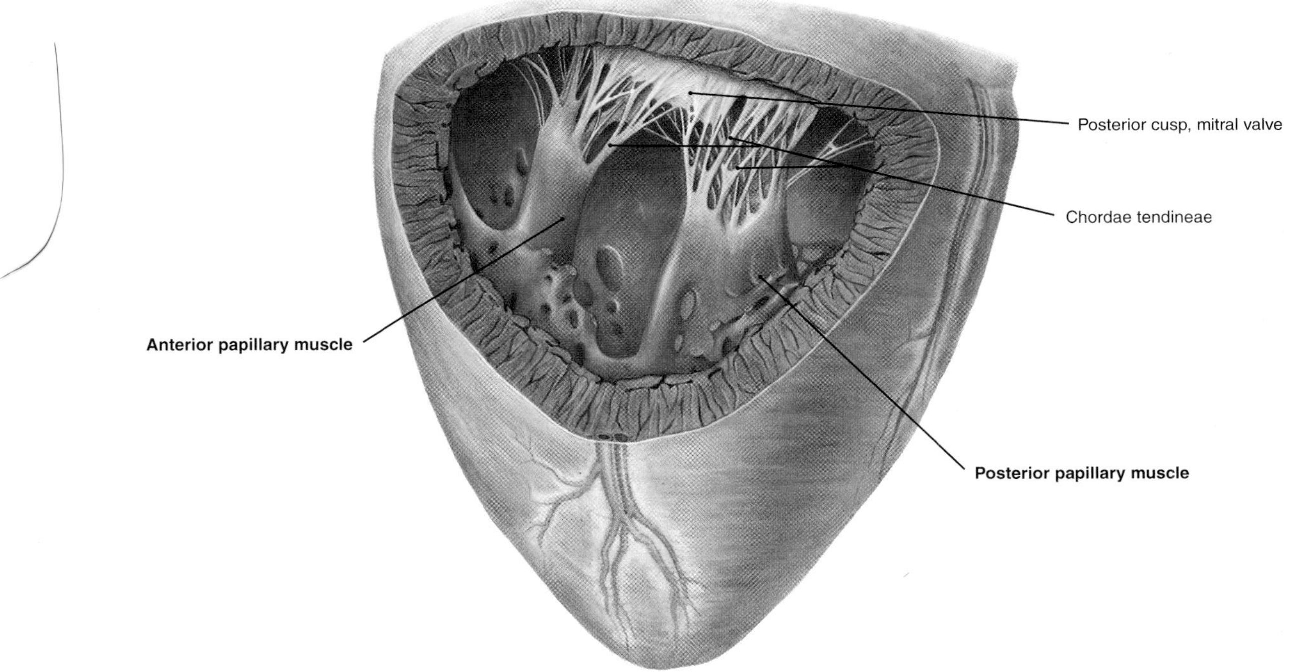
Posterior cusp, mitral valve
Chordae tendineae
Anterior papillary muscle
Posterior papillary muscle

Figure 147.2 Left Ventricle: View of the Mitral Valve

NOTE that the **posterior and anterior papillary muscles** attach to the cusps of the mitral valve.

(Continued from the previous page.)

(3) **Fig. 146E** shows the further unwrapping of the helix to clarify the apical loop that now is seen to be composed of the outer surfaces of descending and ascending segments. **Fig. 146F:** The complete transverse myocardial band is seen with the central muscle twist that separates the basal and apical loops. In this figure can be seen the anterior and posterior papillary muscles in the apical loop. The left component is the transverse basal loop, and the right component is the apical loop. Observe that before this folding, both segments have a transverse orientation. The oblique orientation of the serolied descending and ascending segments derives from the spiral architectural folding of the myocardial band between the basal and apical loops. (From Buckberg GD, Clemente CD, Cox JL, Coghlan HC, Castella M, Torrent-Guasp F, Gharib M. The structure and function of the helical heart and its buttress wrapping. IV. Concepts of dynamic function from the normal macroscopic helical structure. Semin Thorac Cardiovasc Surg 2001;14:342–357.)

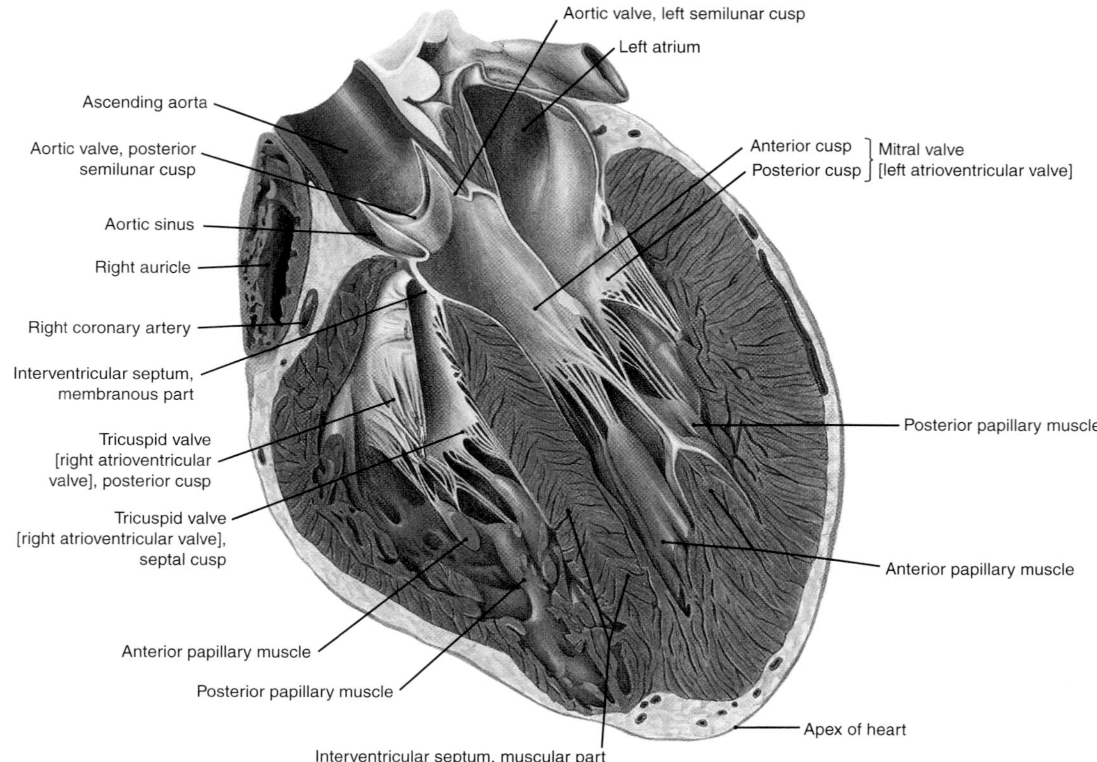
Aortic valve, left semilunar cusp
Left atrium
Ascending aorta
Aortic valve, posterior semilunar cusp
Anterior cusp
Posterior cusp
Mitral valve [left atrioventricular valve]
Aortic sinus
Right auricle
Right coronary artery
Interventricular septum, membranous part
Posterior papillary muscle
Tricuspid valve [right atrioventricular valve], posterior cusp
Tricuspid valve [right atrioventricular valve], septal cusp
Anterior papillary muscle
Anterior papillary muscle
Posterior papillary muscle
Apex of heart
Interventricular septum, muscular part

Figure 148.1 Frontal Section through the Heart

NOTE: (1) This frontal section exposes both atria and both ventricles.

(2) The right and left atrioventricular valves (tricuspid and mitral valves) and their cusps. Observe the papillary muscles attached to these cusps by way of the chordae tendineae (the latter are not labeled).

(3) The muscular and membranous parts of the interventricular septum. Observe the difference in thickness of the muscular walls of the two ventricles.

(4) The aorta emerging from the left ventricle and the cusps of the aortic valve.

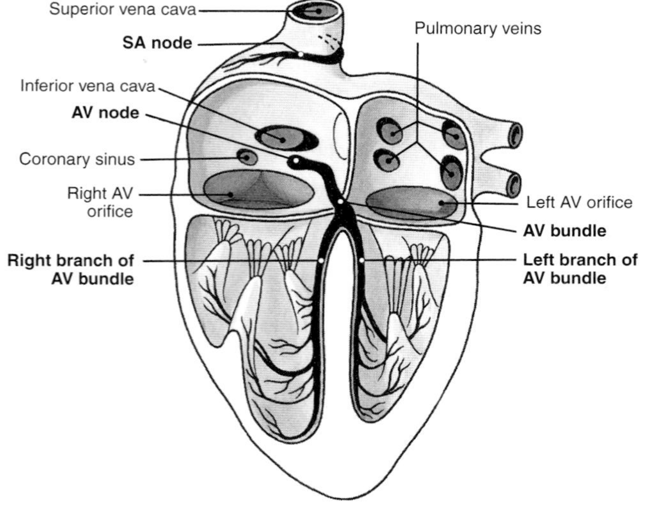
Superior vena cava
SA node
Pulmonary veins
Inferior vena cava
AV node
Coronary sinus
Right AV orifice
Left AV orifice
AV bundle
Right branch of AV bundle
Left branch of AV bundle

Figure 148.2 Diagram of the Conduction System of the Heart

NOTE: (1) The cardiac cycle begins at the SA (sinoatrial) node located in the sulcus terminalis between the superior vena cava and the right atrium.

(2) From this pacemaker, a wave of negativity (excitation) spreads over both atria and initiates atrial contraction, thereby increasing atrial blood pressure.

(3) When atrial pressure exceeds ventricular pressure, both atrioventricular (AV) valves open and blood rushes into both ventricles. Soon the impulse reaches the AV node and is passed along the AV bundle to the two ventricles, causing them to contract.

(4) When ventricular pressure exceeds atrial pressure, the AV valves close, and this can be heard with a stethoscope as the first of the two heart sounds of the heartbeat.

(5) Continued ventricular contraction forces the pulmonary and aortic valves to open, and blood rushes simultaneously into the pulmonary artery and the aorta.

(6) When the pressure in these vessels exceeds ventricular pressure, blood tends to rush back into the ventricles, but it gets trapped in the sinuses behind the semilunar cusps. This closes both the pulmonary and aortic valves, resulting in the second of the two heart sounds heard with the stethoscope.

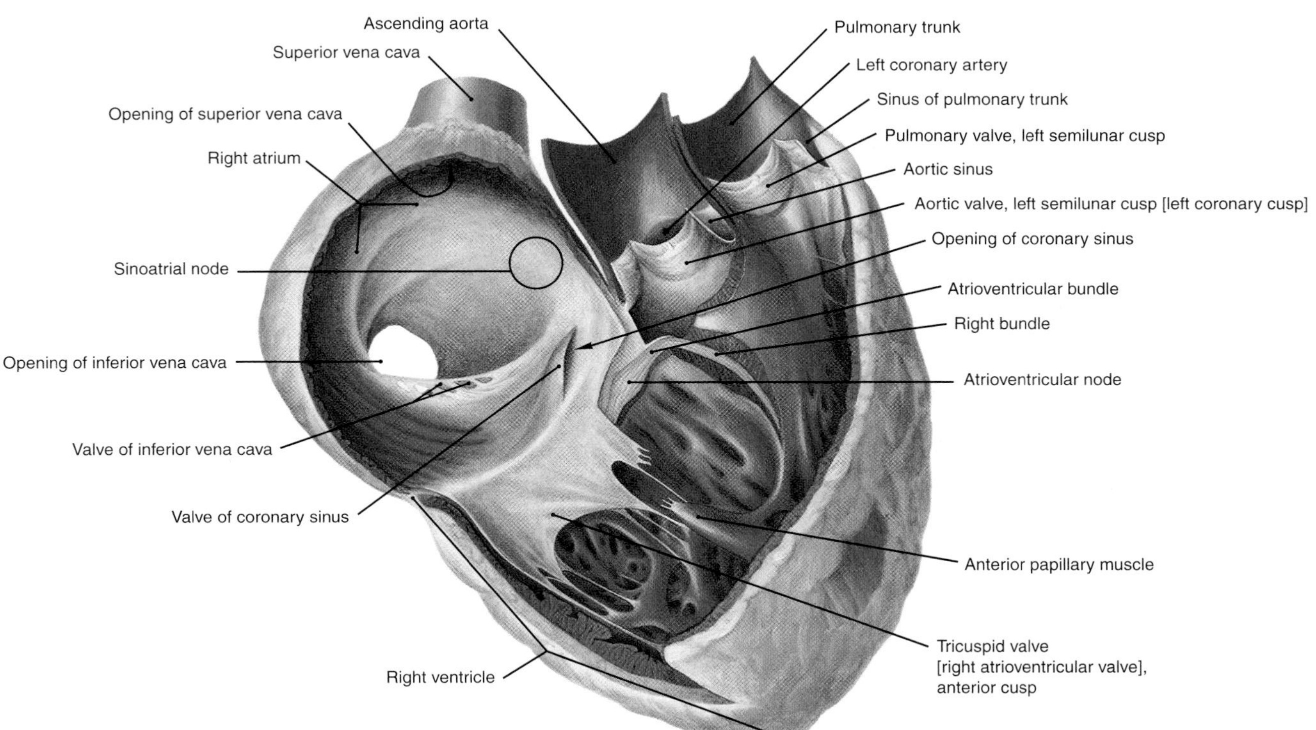
Ascending aorta
Superior vena cava
Opening of superior vena cava
Right atrium
Sinoatrial node
Opening of inferior vena cava
Valve of inferior vena cava
Valve of coronary sinus
Right ventricle
Pulmonary trunk
Left coronary artery
Sinus of pulmonary trunk
Pulmonary valve, left semilunar cusp
Aortic sinus
Aortic valve, left semilunar cusp [left coronary cusp]
Opening of coronary sinus
Atrioventricular bundle
Right bundle
Atrioventricular node
Anterior papillary muscle
Tricuspid valve
[right atrioventricular valve],
anterior cusp

Figure 149.1 Atrioventricular Bundle Dissected in the Right Ventricle

NOTE: (1) The atrioventricular (AV) bundle forms a part of the conduction system of the heart. It is formed by modified cardiac muscle fibers called Purkinje fibers. It commences at the AV node in the interatrial septum near the opening of the coronary sinus in the right atrium.

(2) The bundle is then directed toward the interventricular septum, where it divides into right and left branches. The **right** branch, dissected in this figure, courses in the wall of the right ventricle and is distributed toward the apex.

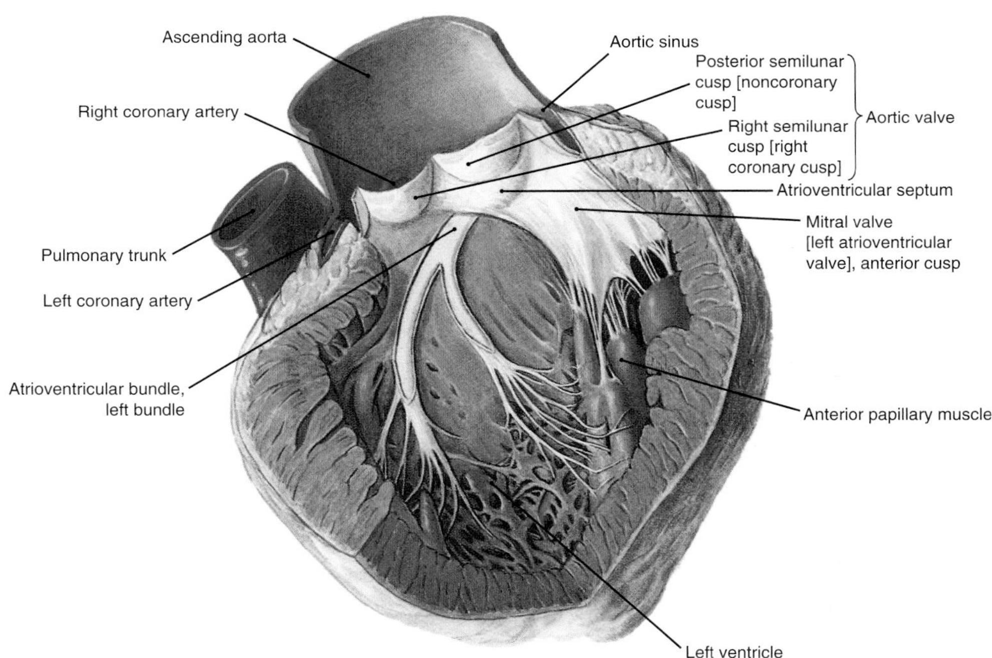
Ascending aorta
Right coronary artery
Pulmonary trunk
Left coronary artery
Atrioventricular bundle,
left bundle
Aortic sinus
Posterior semilunar
cusp [noncoronary
cusp]
Right semilunar
cusp [right
coronary cusp]
Aortic valve
Atrioventricular septum
Mitral valve
[left atrioventricular
valve], anterior cusp
Anterior papillary muscle
Left ventricle

Figure 149.2 Atrioventricular Bundle Dissected in the Left Ventricle

NOTE: (1) The left branch of the atrioventricular bundle is dissected on the left side of the interventricular wall. It commences as a rather wide band of tissue and soon divides into several strands. These fan out to become distributed among the papillary muscles and trabeculae carneae of the left ventricle.

(2) The conduction system of the heart transmits to the cardiac muscle the rhythmic impulses that characterize the rate of the heartbeat. This rhythm is superimposed on the natural contractile property of cardiac musculature, and the rate responds to regulation by cardiac nerves that innervate the heart.

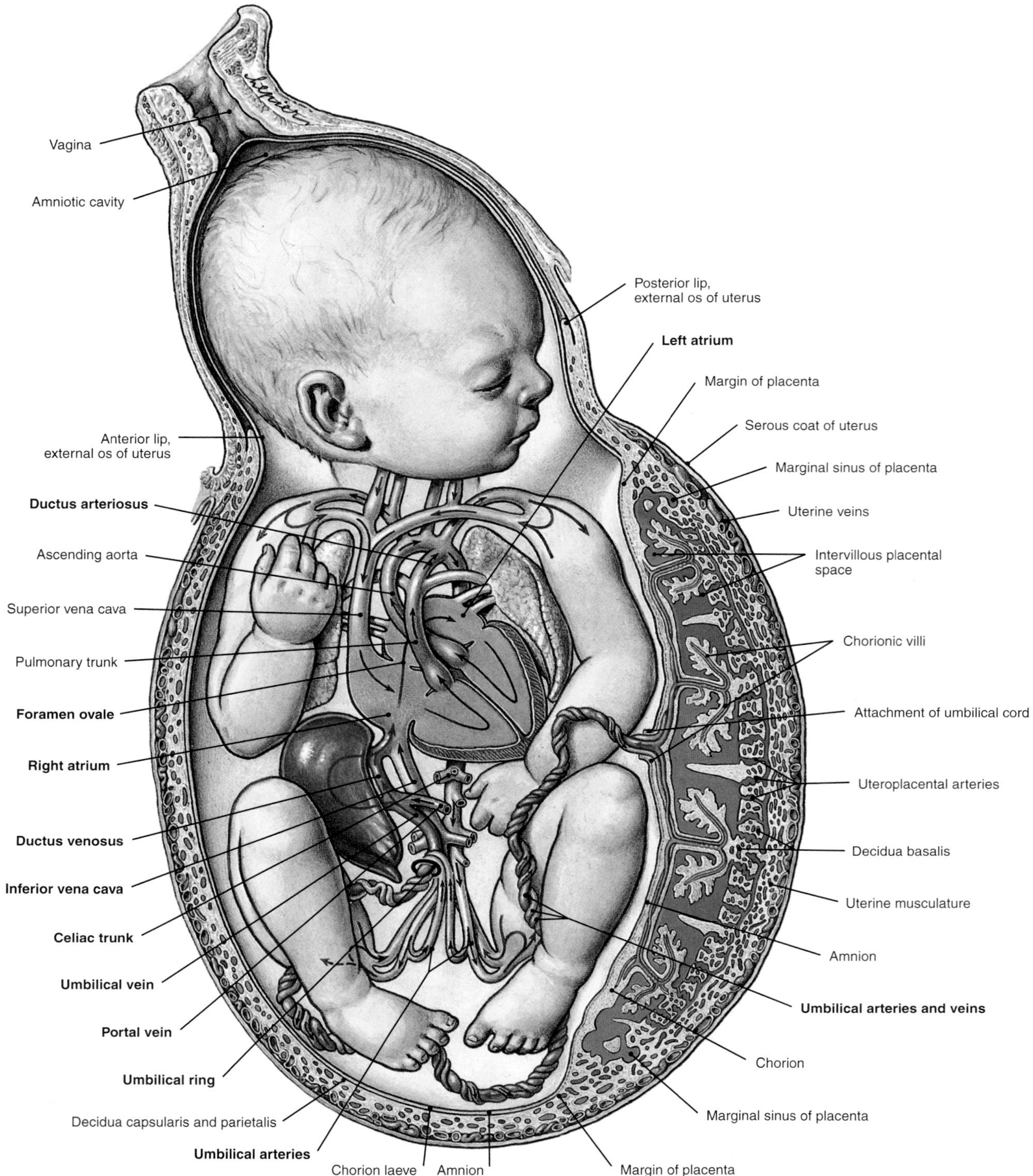
Vagina
Amniotic cavity
Posterior lip, external os of uterus
Left atrium
Margin of placenta
Serous coat of uterus
Marginal sinus of placenta
Uterine veins
Intervillous placental space
Chorionic villi
Attachment of umbilical cord
Uteroplacental arteries
Decidua basalis
Uterine musculature
Amnion
Umbilical arteries and veins
Chorion
Marginal sinus of placenta
Margin of placenta
Anterior lip, external os of uterus
Ductus arteriosus
Ascending aorta
Superior vena cava
Pulmonary trunk
Foramen ovale
Right atrium
Ductus venosus
Inferior vena cava
Celiac trunk
Umbilical vein
Portal vein
Umbilical ring
Decidua capsularis and parietalis
Umbilical arteries
Chorion laeve
Amnion

Figure 150 Circulation in the Fetus, as Seen in Utero

NOTE: In the fetus:

(1) Deoxygenated blood courses to the placenta by way of the **umbilical arteries.** It is then both nourished and oxygenated and leaves the placenta by way of the **umbilical vein.**

(2) Much of the oxygenated blood bypasses the liver, coursing from the umbilical vein, through the **ductus venosus,** to reach the inferior vena cava.

(3) From the inferior vena cava, blood enters the right atrium, as does blood from the superior vena cava. Right atrial blood bypasses the lungs by two routes:

(a) across to the left atrium through the **foramen ovale**, then to the left ventricle and out the aorta to the rest of the fetal body, and

(b) to the right ventricle, out the pulmonary artery and through the **ductus arteriosus** to reach the aorta, and then to the rest of the fetal body (also see, Fig. 151).

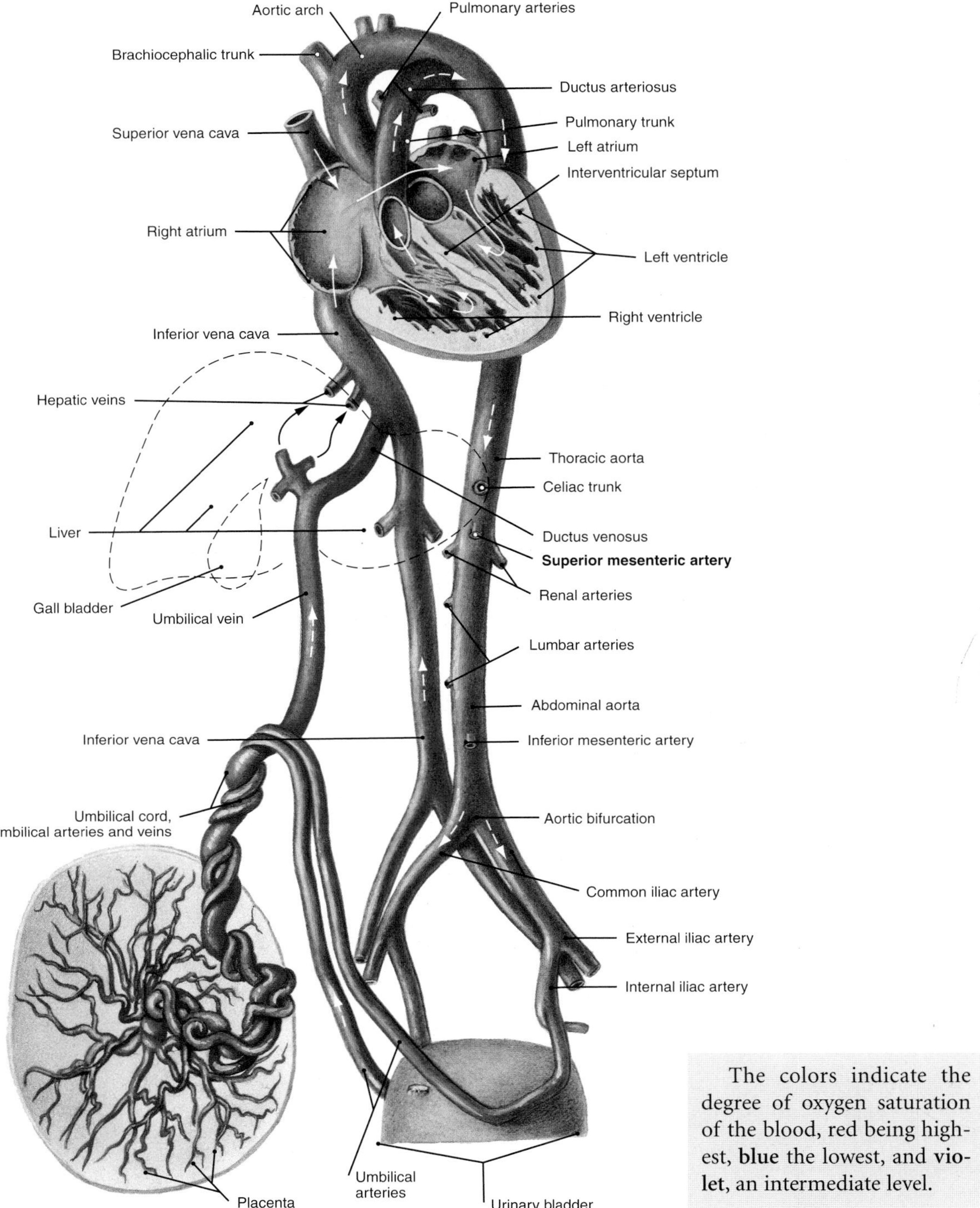
Aortic arch
Pulmonary arteries
Brachiocephalic trunk
Ductus arteriosus
Superior vena cava
Pulmonary trunk
Left atrium
Interventricular septum
Right atrium
Left ventricle
Right ventricle
Inferior vena cava
Hepatic veins
Thoracic aorta
Celiac trunk
Liver
Ductus venosus
Superior mesenteric artery
Gall bladder
Renal arteries
Umbilical vein
Lumbar arteries
Abdominal aorta
Inferior vena cava
Inferior mesenteric artery
Umbilical cord, umbilical arteries and veins
Aortic bifurcation
Common iliac artery
External iliac artery
Internal iliac artery
Placenta
Umbilical arteries
Urinary bladder

The colors indicate the degree of oxygen saturation of the blood, red being highest, **blue** the lowest, and **violet**, an intermediate level.

Figure 151 Diagrammatic Representation of the Circulation in the Fetus

NOTE: Changes in the vascular system after birth; because the newborn infant becomes dependent on the lungs for oxygen:

(1) Breathing commences and the lungs begin to function, thereby oxygenating the blood and removing carbon dioxide.

(2) The **foramen ovale** decreases in size, and blood ceases to cross from the right atrium to the left atrium.

(3) The **ductus arteriosus** that interconnected the pulmonary artery and aorta constricts and gradually closes to become a fibrous cord called the **ligamentum arteriosum.**

(4) The **umbilical arteries** cease to carry blood to the placenta, and they become fibrosed, to form the **medial umbilical ligaments.**

(5) The **umbilical vein** becomes fibrosed and forms the **ligamentum teres** (of the liver), while the **ductus venosus** is no longer functional and forms the **ligamentum venosum**.

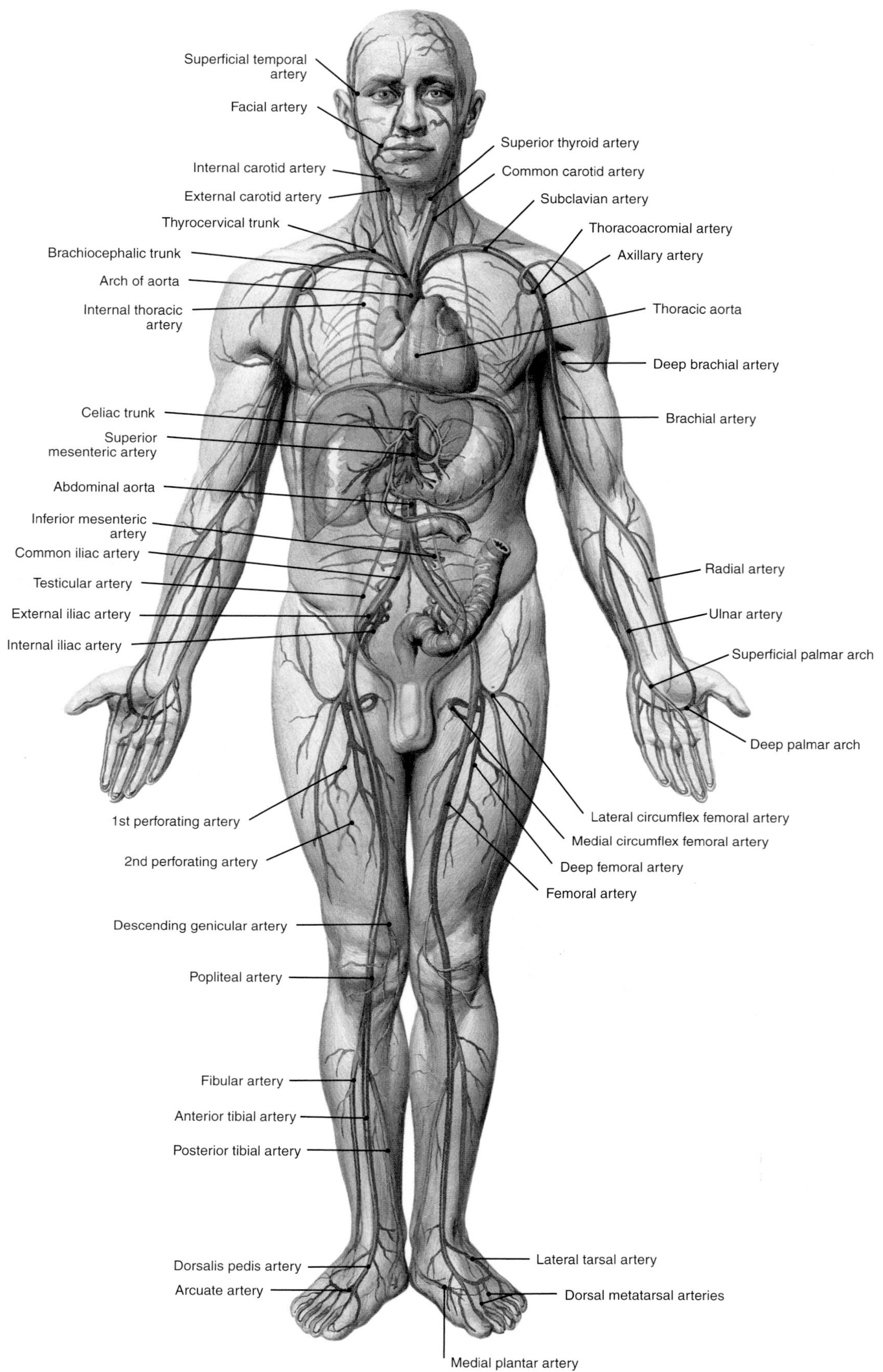
Superficial temporal artery
Facial artery
Internal carotid artery
External carotid artery
Thyrocervical trunk
Brachiocephalic trunk
Arch of aorta
Internal thoracic artery
Celiac trunk
Superior mesenteric artery
Abdominal aorta
Inferior mesenteric artery
Common iliac artery
Testicular artery
External iliac artery
Internal iliac artery
1st perforating artery
2nd perforating artery
Descending genicular artery
Popliteal artery
Fibular artery
Anterior tibial artery
Posterior tibial artery
Dorsalis pedis artery
Arcuate artery
Superior thyroid artery
Common carotid artery
Subclavian artery
Thoracoacromial artery
Axillary artery
Thoracic aorta
Deep brachial artery
Brachial artery
Radial artery
Ulnar artery
Superficial palmar arch
Deep palmar arch
Lateral circumflex femoral artery
Medial circumflex femoral artery
Deep femoral artery
Femoral artery
Lateral tarsal artery
Dorsal metatarsal arteries
Medial plantar artery

Figure 152 Adult Systemic Arterial System (Male)

NOTE: Most, but not all, of the named arteries in the systemic circulation are shown in this figure. In addition, the pulmonary arteries coursing to the lungs from the right ventricle are not included.

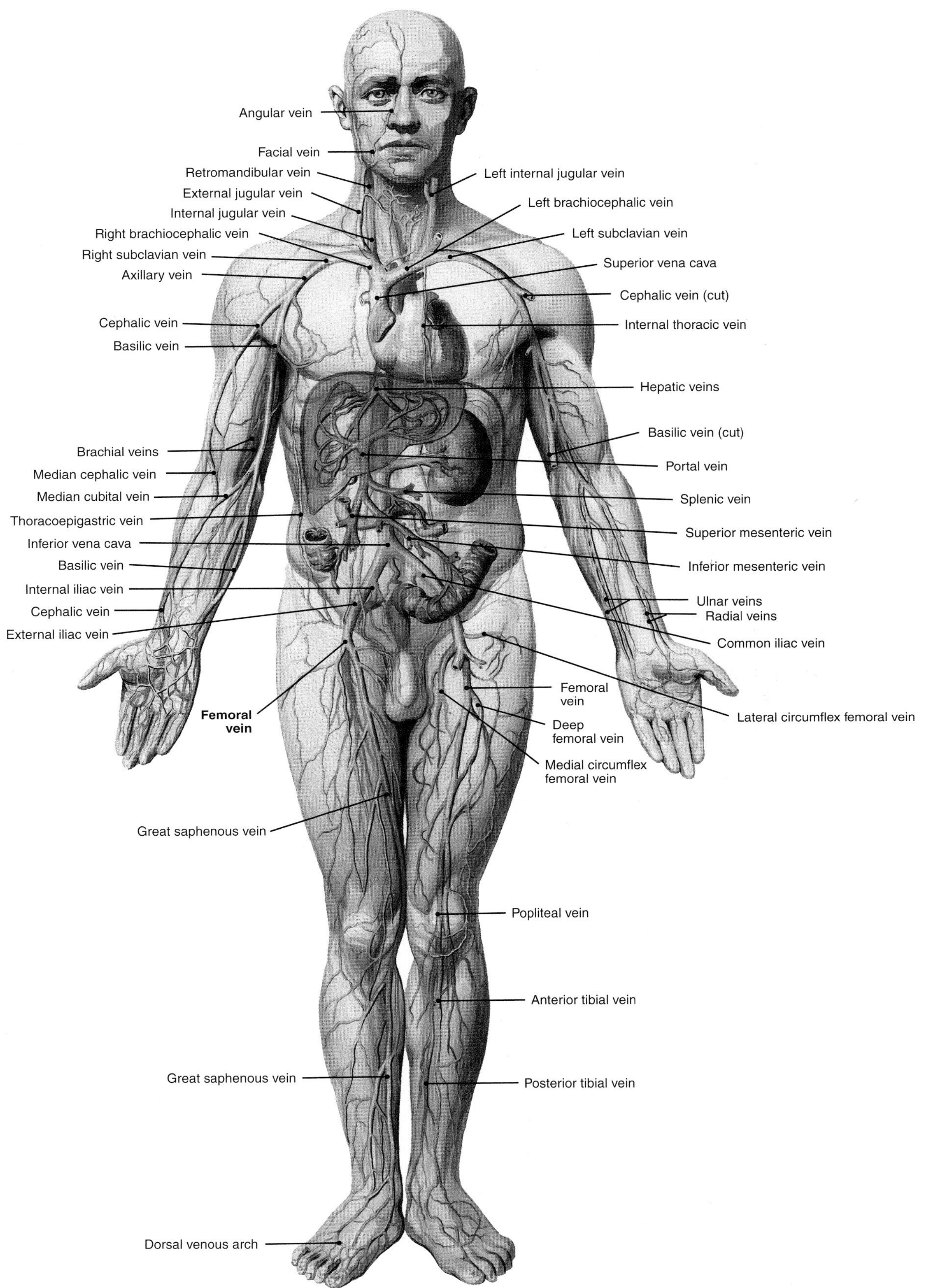
Angular vein
Facial vein
Retromandibular vein
External jugular vein
Internal jugular vein
Right brachiocephalic vein
Right subclavian vein
Axillary vein
Cephalic vein
Basilic vein
Brachial veins
Median cephalic vein
Median cubital vein
Thoracoepigastric vein
Inferior vena cava
Basilic vein
Internal iliac vein
Cephalic vein
External iliac vein
Femoral vein
Great saphenous vein
Great saphenous vein
Dorsal venous arch
Left internal jugular vein
Left brachiocephalic vein
Left subclavian vein
Superior vena cava
Cephalic vein (cut)
Internal thoracic vein
Hepatic veins
Basilic vein (cut)
Portal vein
Splenic vein
Superior mesenteric vein
Inferior mesenteric vein
Ulnar veins
Radial veins
Common iliac vein
Femoral vein
Lateral circumflex femoral vein
Deep femoral vein
Medial circumflex femoral vein
Popliteal vein
Anterior tibial vein
Posterior tibial vein

Figure 153 Adult Systemic and Portal Venous Systems (Male)
NOTE: Many, but not all, of the named veins are shown in this figure. The pulmonary veins that return blood to the left atrium from the lungs are not included. The portal system is shown in purple, while the other veins are shown in blue.

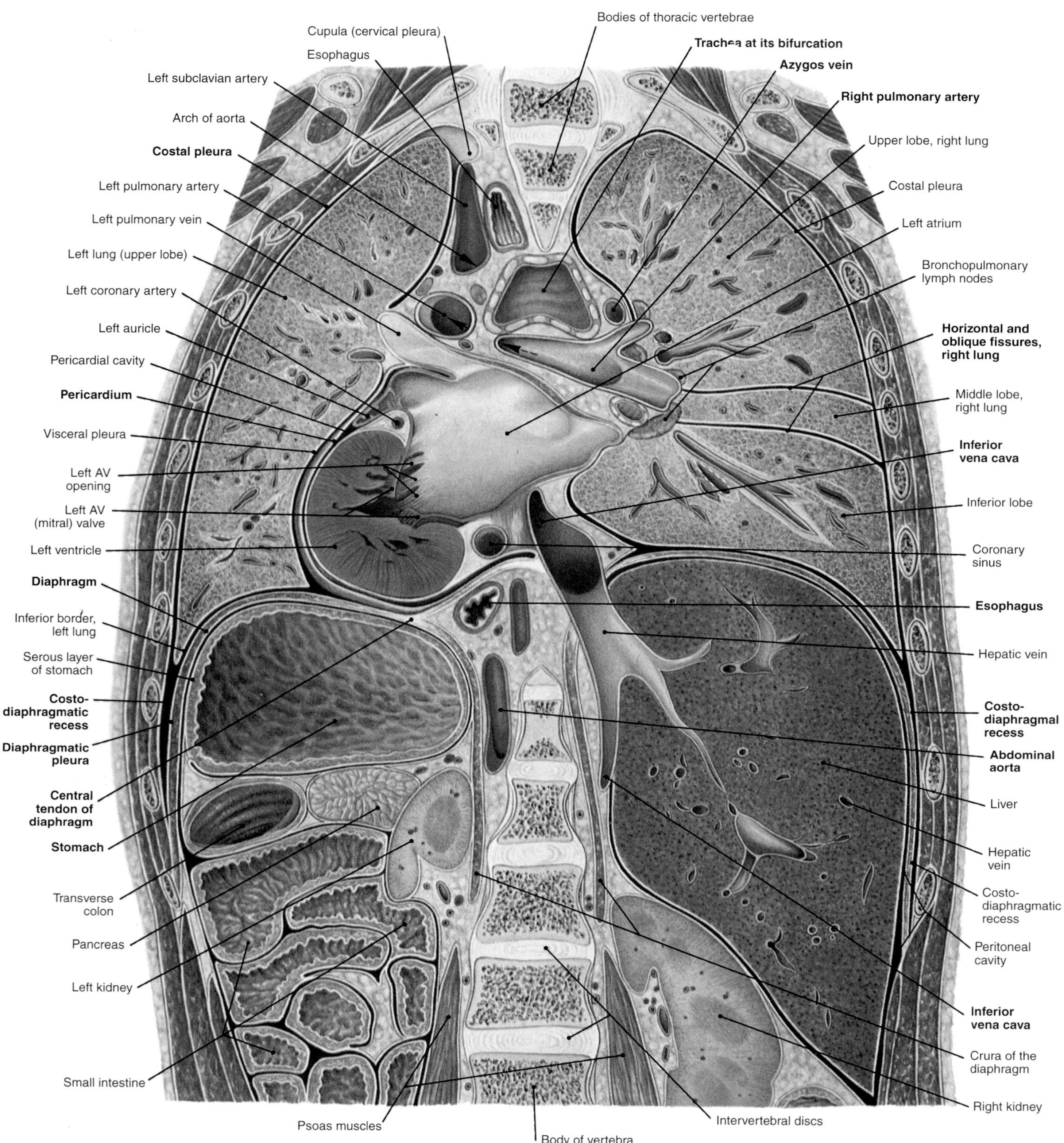
Cupula (cervical pleura)
Esophagus
Bodies of thoracic vertebrae
Trachea at its bifurcation
Azygos vein
Right pulmonary artery
Upper lobe, right lung
Costal pleura
Left atrium
Bronchopulmonary lymph nodes
Horizontal and oblique fissures, right lung
Middle lobe, right lung
Inferior vena cava
Inferior lobe
Coronary sinus
Esophagus
Hepatic vein
Costo-diaphragmal recess
Abdominal aorta
Liver
Hepatic vein
Costo-diaphragmatic recess
Peritoneal cavity
Inferior vena cava
Crura of the diaphragm
Right kidney
Left subclavian artery
Arch of aorta
Costal pleura
Left pulmonary artery
Left pulmonary vein
Left lung (upper lobe)
Left coronary artery
Left auricle
Pericardial cavity
Pericardium
Visceral pleura
Left AV opening
Left AV (mitral) valve
Left ventricle
Diaphragm
Inferior border, left lung
Serous layer of stomach
Costo-diaphragmatic recess
Diaphragmatic pleura
Central tendon of diaphragm
Stomach
Transverse colon
Pancreas
Left kidney
Small intestine
Psoas muscles
Body of vertebra
Intervertebral discs

Figure 154 Frontal Section of the Thorax and Abdomen from Behind (Dorsal View)

NOTE: (1) From this dorsal view, the right side of the specimen is on the reader's right. The pulmonary arteries and their branches are shown in blue, as are veins (such as the hepatic veins) that also carry blood with low levels of oxygen saturation.

(2) The anteroposterior plane of this frontal section in the thorax lies through the inferior vena cava and in front of the descending aorta. The esophagus is seen only in the superior mediastinum and at its entrance into the abdomen just below the diaphragm, while the trachea has been cut at its point of bifurcation.

Figure 155.1 Relationship of the Esophagus to the Aorta and Trachea, Viewed from Right Side

NOTE: (1) The **esophagus** commences above as an inferior extension of the pharynx, and it is initially in relationship with the larynx and thyroid gland.

(2) Its **middle third** courses in relation to the trachea, bronchi and the arch of the aorta, while its lower third descends with the thoracic aorta.

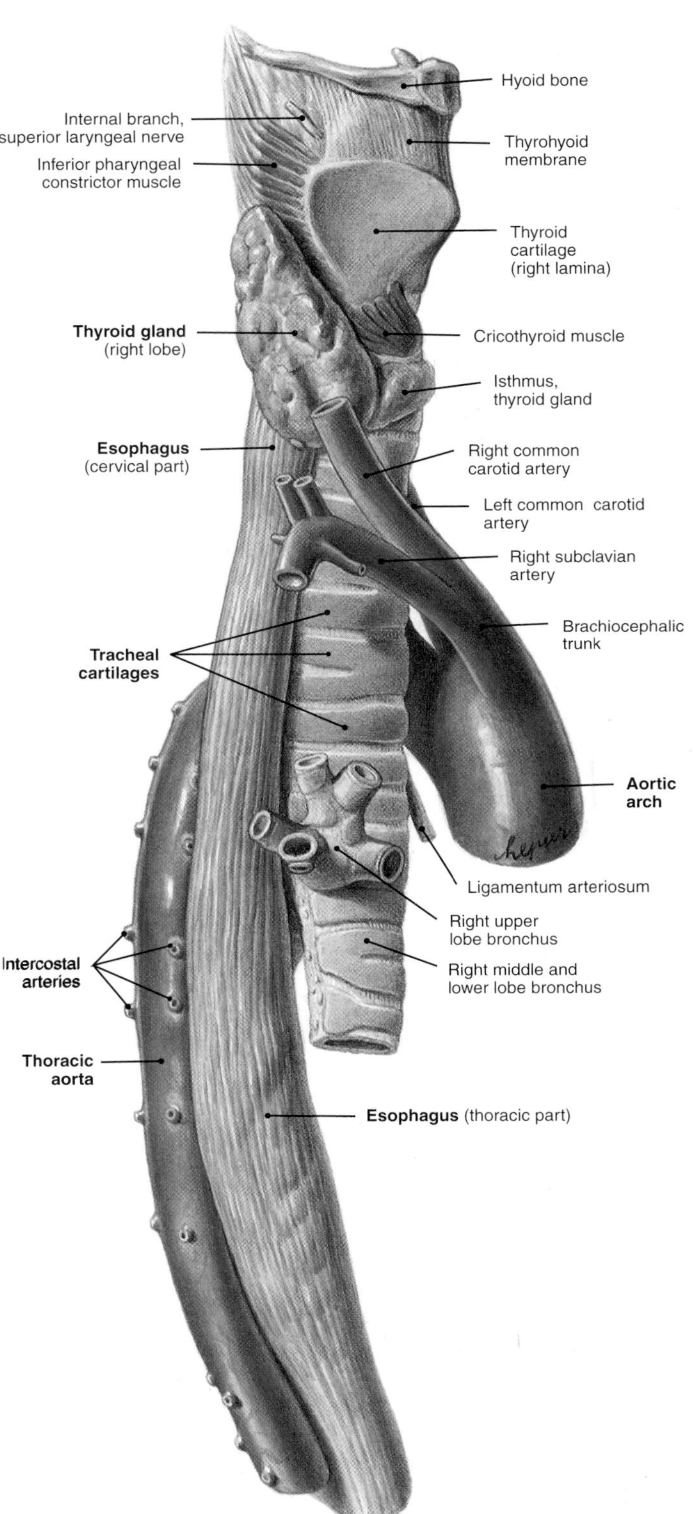

Hyoid bone
Internal branch, superior laryngeal nerve
Thyrohyoid membrane
Inferior pharyngeal constrictor muscle
Thyroid cartilage (right lamina)
Thyroid gland (right lobe)
Cricothyroid muscle
Isthmus, thyroid gland
Esophagus (cervical part)
Right common carotid artery
Left common carotid artery
Right subclavian artery
Brachiocephalic trunk
Tracheal cartilages
Aortic arch
Ligamentum arteriosum
Right upper lobe bronchus
Intercostal arteries
Right middle and lower lobe bronchus
Thoracic aorta
Esophagus (thoracic part)

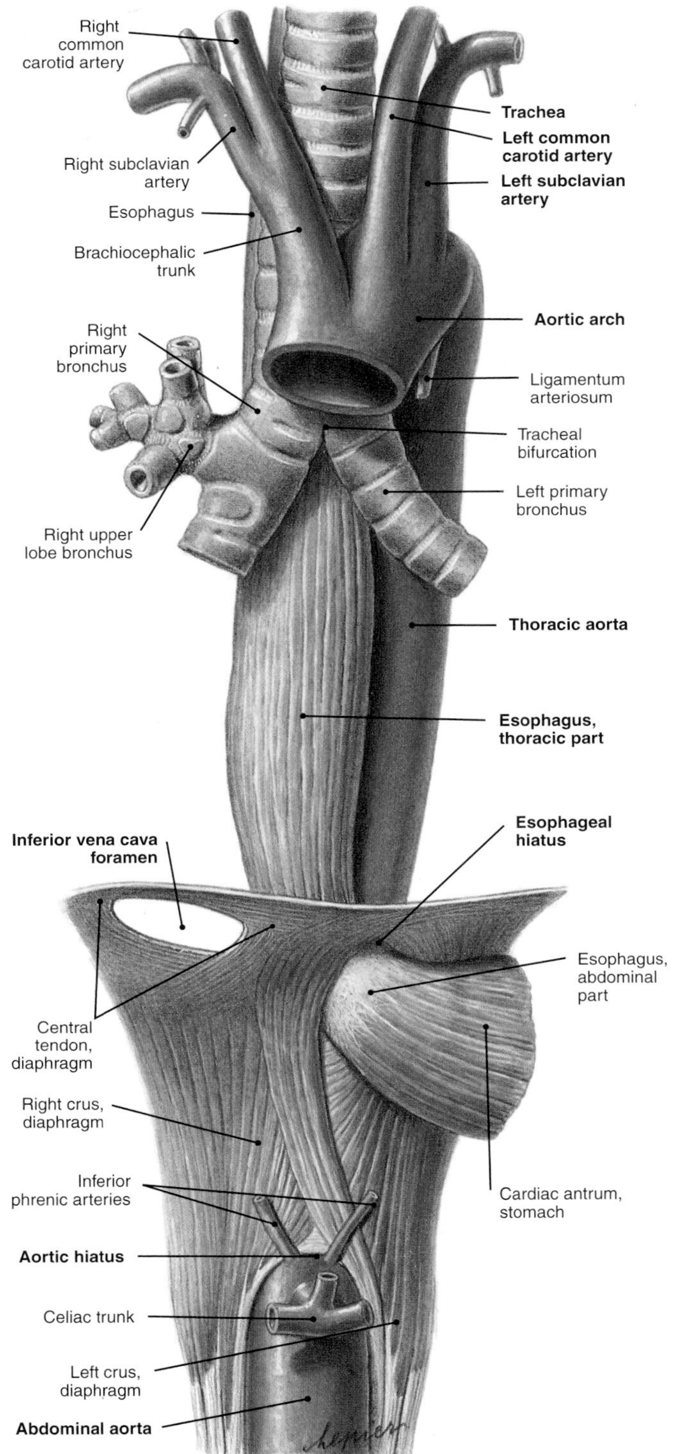

Right common carotid artery
Trachea
Left common carotid artery
Right subclavian artery
Left subclavian artery
Esophagus
Brachiocephalic trunk
Aortic arch
Right primary bronchus
Ligamentum arteriosum
Tracheal bifurcation
Left primary bronchus
Right upper lobe bronchus
Thoracic aorta
Esophagus, thoracic part
Inferior vena cava foramen
Esophageal hiatus
Esophagus, abdominal part
Central tendon, diaphragm
Right crus, diaphragm
Inferior phrenic arteries
Cardiac antrum, stomach
Aortic hiatus
Celiac trunk
Left crus, diaphragm
Abdominal aorta

Figure 155.2 Aorta and Lower Esophagus at the Tracheal Bifurcation and Diaphragm

NOTE: (1) At the level of the bifurcation of the trachea (T5), the esophagus lies between the trachea and the thoracic aorta. It then descends into the thorax with the aorta somewhat to its left. In the lower thorax, the esophagus bends to the left and crosses the aorta anteriorly from right to left.

(2) The esophagus enters the abdomen through the **esophageal hiatus** of the diaphragm, while the aorta passes through the **aortic hiatus.**

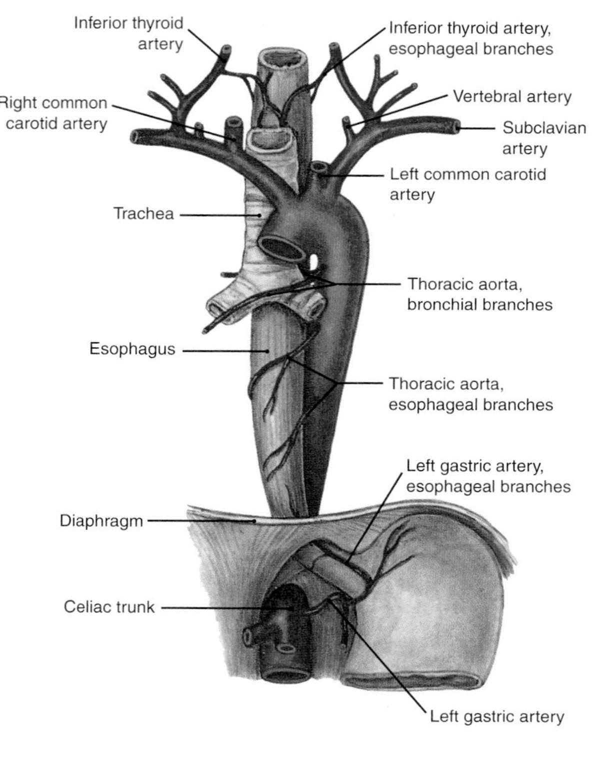
Inferior thyroid artery
Inferior thyroid artery, esophageal branches
Right common carotid artery
Vertebral artery
Subclavian artery
Left common carotid artery
Trachea
Thoracic aorta, bronchial branches
Esophagus
Thoracic aorta, esophageal branches
Left gastric artery, esophageal branches
Diaphragm
Celiac trunk
Left gastric artery

Figure 156.1 Arterial Blood Supply of the Esophagus

NOTE: (1) Because the esophagus is an elongated organ extending from the neck to the abdomen, it receives arterial blood from at least three sources:

(a) **In the neck**: most frequently from the **inferior thyroid** of the **thyrocervical trunk**, but it may come from the subclavian, or vertebral arteries or from the costocervical trunk.

(b) **In the thorax:** multiple **esophageal branches** coming directly from the **aorta.**

(c) **In the abdomen**: from the **inferior phrenic artery** or the **left gastric artery.**

(2) These vessels anastomose with each other in the substance of the esophagus.

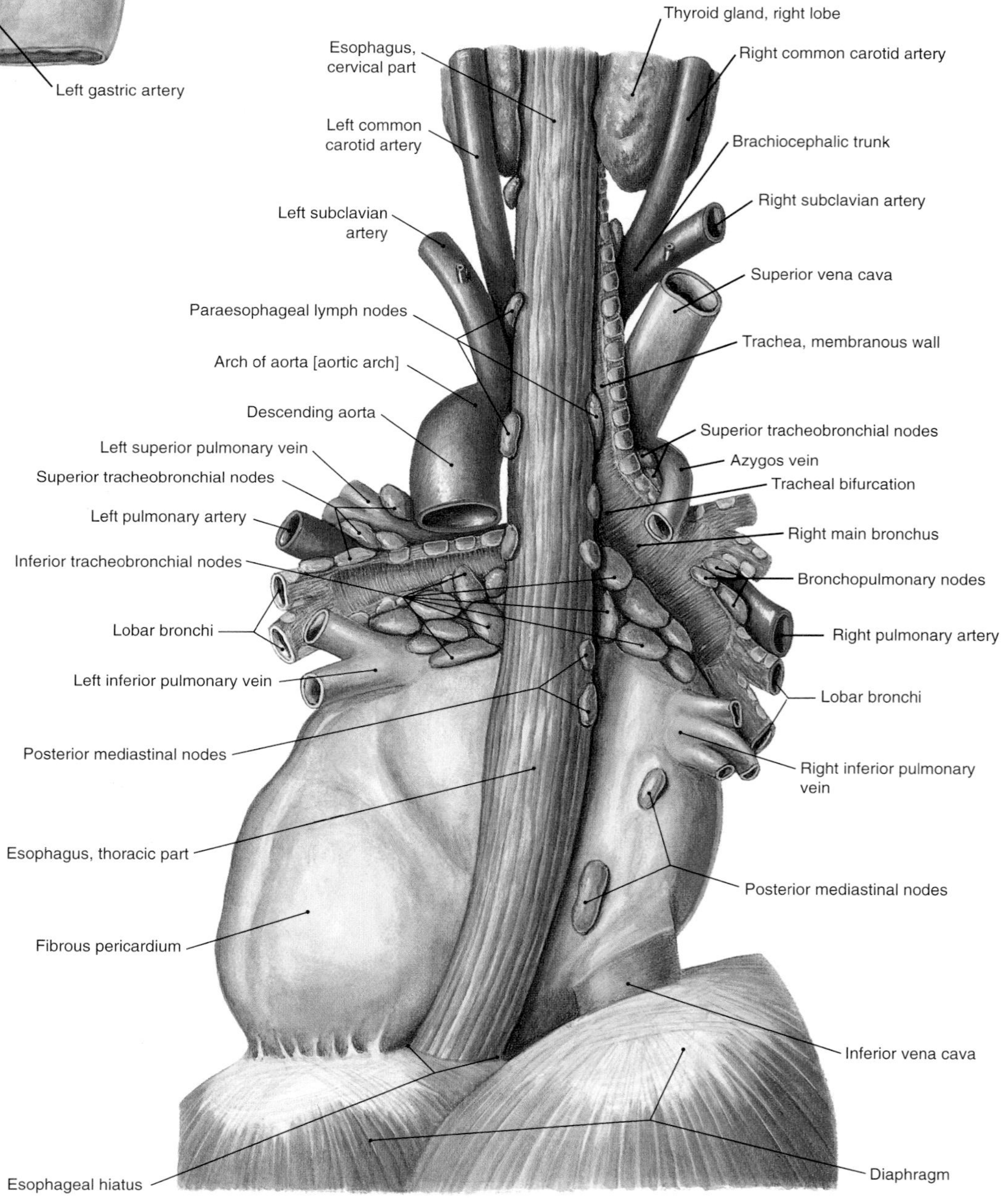

Thyroid gland, right lobe
Esophagus, cervical part
Right common carotid artery
Left common carotid artery
Brachiocephalic trunk
Left subclavian artery
Right subclavian artery
Superior vena cava
Paraesophageal lymph nodes
Trachea, membranous wall
Arch of aorta [aortic arch]
Descending aorta
Superior tracheobronchial nodes
Left superior pulmonary vein
Azygos vein
Superior tracheobronchial nodes
Tracheal bifurcation
Left pulmonary artery
Right main bronchus
Inferior tracheobronchial nodes
Bronchopulmonary nodes
Lobar bronchi
Right pulmonary artery
Left inferior pulmonary vein
Lobar bronchi
Posterior mediastinal nodes
Right inferior pulmonary vein
Esophagus, thoracic part
Posterior mediastinal nodes
Fibrous pericardium
Inferior vena cava
Esophageal hiatus
Diaphragm

Figure 156.2 Posterior View of the Esophagus and the Paraesophageal and Tracheobronchial Lymph Nodes

NOTE the large number of nodes near the bifurcation of the trachea (into the two primary bronchi). These many nodes may be located at this site for the receipt of macrophages coursing from the lungs, which may have ingested foreign elements from the air we breathe.

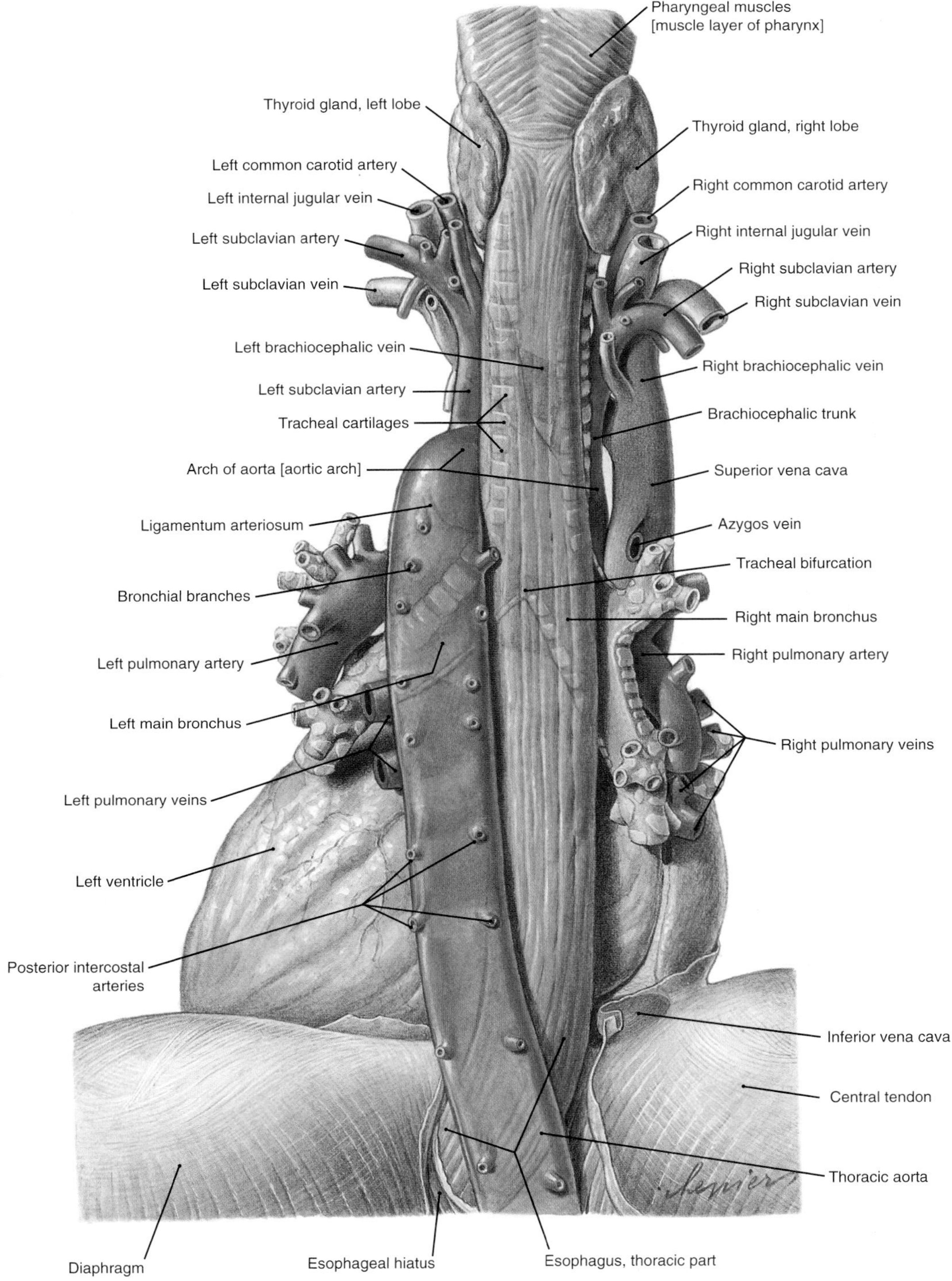
Pharyngeal muscles
[muscle layer of pharynx]
Thyroid gland, left lobe
Thyroid gland, right lobe
Left common carotid artery
Left internal jugular vein
Right common carotid artery
Right internal jugular vein
Left subclavian artery
Right subclavian artery
Left subclavian vein
Right subclavian vein
Left brachiocephalic vein
Right brachiocephalic vein
Left subclavian artery
Tracheal cartilages
Brachiocephalic trunk
Arch of aorta [aortic arch]
Superior vena cava
Ligamentum arteriosum
Azygos vein
Tracheal bifurcation
Bronchial branches
Right main bronchus
Left pulmonary artery
Right pulmonary artery
Left main bronchus
Right pulmonary veins
Left pulmonary veins
Left ventricle
Posterior intercostal
arteries
Inferior vena cava
Central tendon
Thoracic aorta
Diaphragm
Esophageal hiatus
Esophagus, thoracic part

Figure 157 Posterior View of the Esophagus, Aorta, and Pericardium

NOTE: (1) The origins of the intercostal arteries from the posterior aspect of the thoracic aorta.

(2) The relationship of the esophagus and the thoracic aorta is well shown in this dorsal view. Observe how the aorta courses posterior to the esophagus from left to right. It then descends in the midline ventral to the vertebral column to the level of L1, where it enters the posterior abdomen.

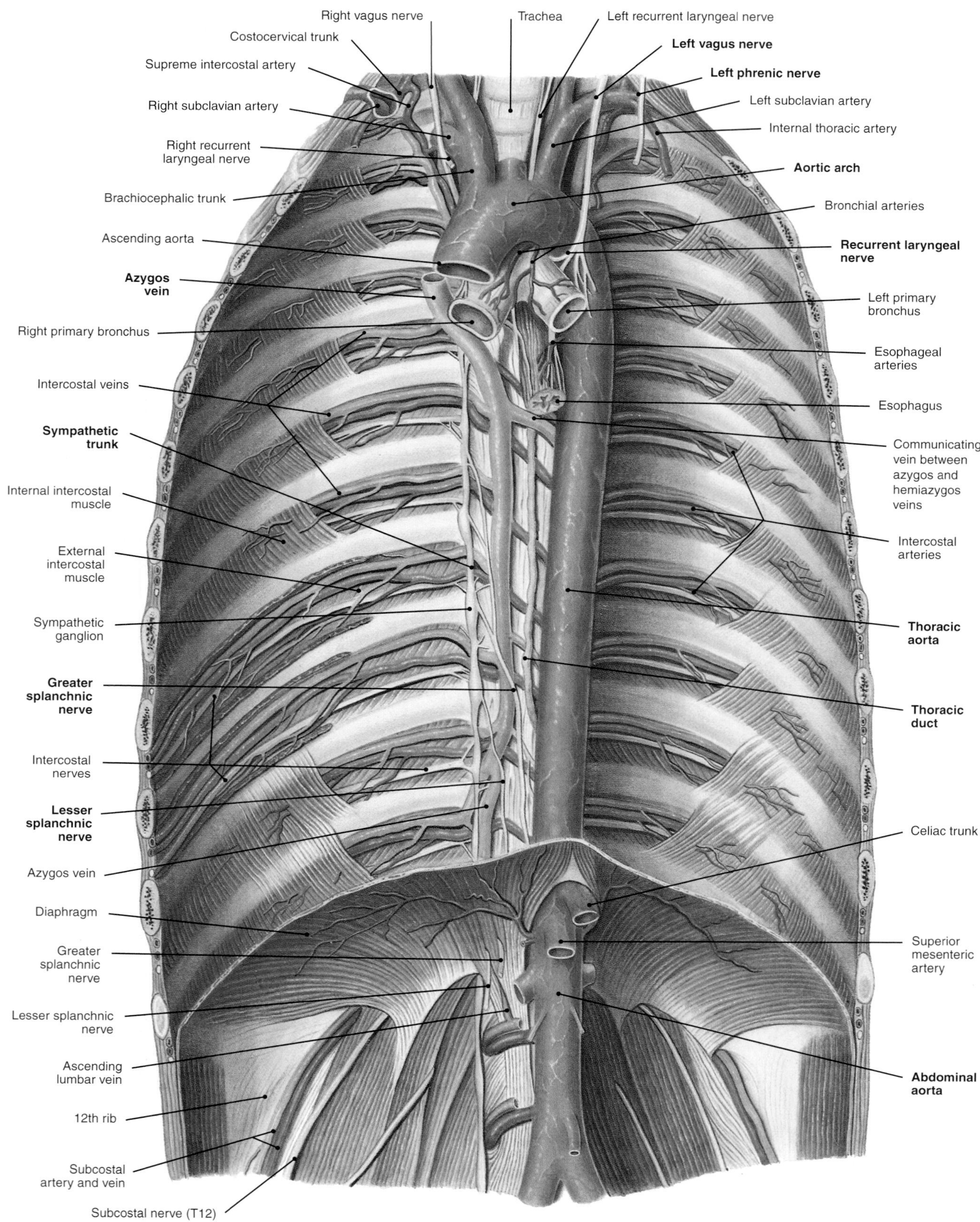
Right vagus nerve
Trachea
Left recurrent laryngeal nerve
Costocervical trunk
Left vagus nerve
Supreme intercostal artery
Left phrenic nerve
Right subclavian artery
Left subclavian artery
Internal thoracic artery
Right recurrent laryngeal nerve
Aortic arch
Brachiocephalic trunk
Bronchial arteries
Ascending aorta
Recurrent laryngeal nerve
Azygos vein
Left primary bronchus
Right primary bronchus
Esophageal arteries
Intercostal veins
Esophagus
Sympathetic trunk
Communicating vein between azygos and hemiazygos veins
Internal intercostal muscle
Intercostal arteries
External intercostal muscle
Sympathetic ganglion
Thoracic aorta
Greater splanchnic nerve
Thoracic duct
Intercostal nerves
Lesser splanchnic nerve
Celiac trunk
Azygos vein
Diaphragm
Superior mesenteric artery
Greater splanchnic nerve
Lesser splanchnic nerve
Ascending lumbar vein
Abdominal aorta
12th rib
Subcostal artery and vein
Subcostal nerve (T12)

Figure 158 Vessels and Nerves of the Dorsal Thoracic Wall

NOTE: (1) The aorta ascends from the left ventricle, arches behind the left pulmonary hilum, and descends through most of the thorax just to the left side of the vertebral column.

(2) In its course through the posterior mediastinum, the aorta gradually shifts toward the midline, which it has achieved when it traverses the diaphragm at the aortic hiatus to enter the abdomen.

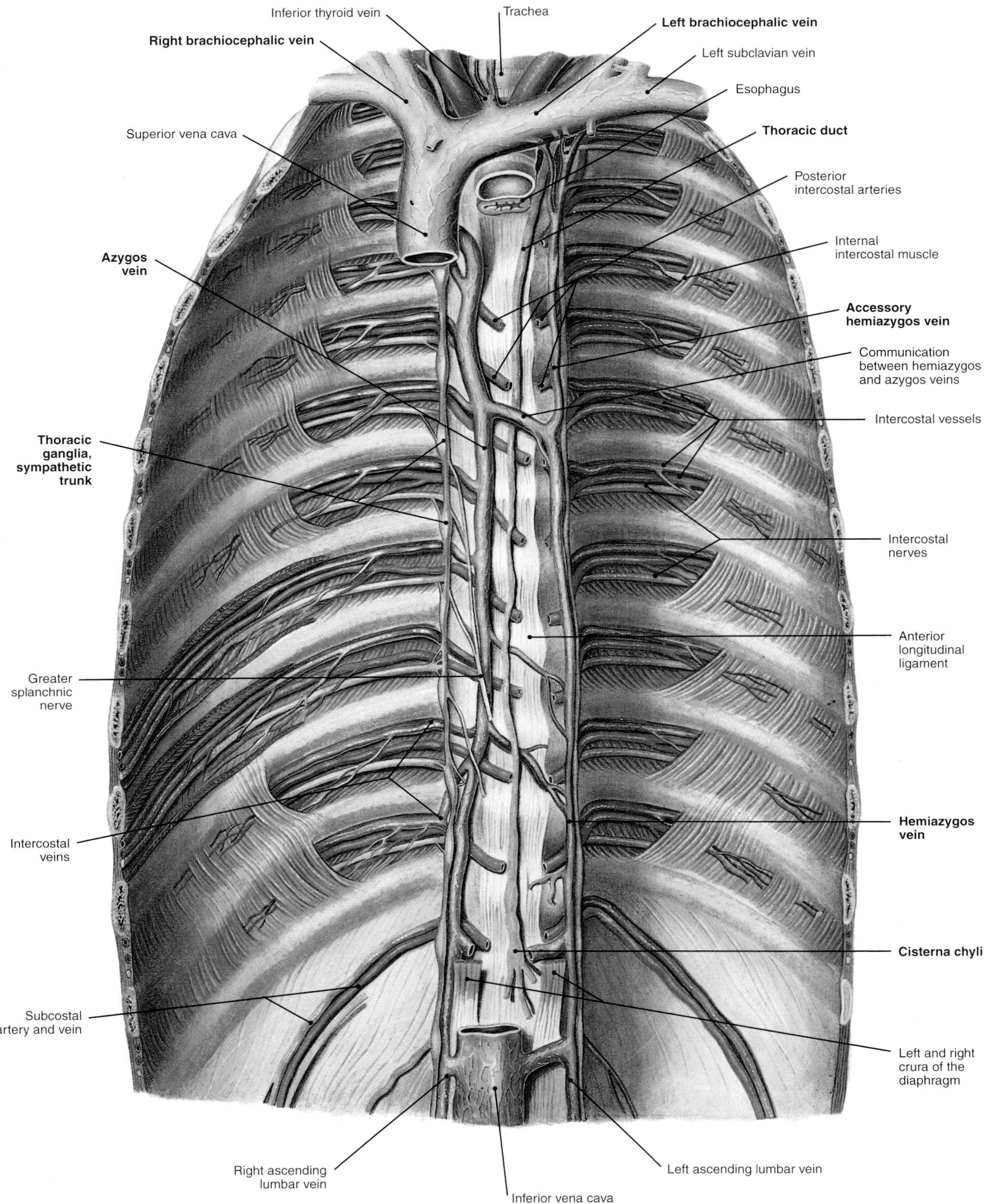
Inferior thyroid vein
Trachea
Left brachiocephalic vein
Right brachiocephalic vein
Left subclavian vein
Esophagus
Superior vena cava
Thoracic duct
Posterior intercostal arteries
Internal intercostal muscle
Azygos vein
Accessory hemiazygos vein
Communication between hemiazygos and azygos veins
Intercostal vessels
Thoracic ganglia, sympathetic trunk
Intercostal nerves
Anterior longitudinal ligament
Greater splanchnic nerve
Hemiazygos vein
Intercostal veins
Cisterna chyli
Subcostal artery and vein
Left and right crura of the diaphragm
Right ascending lumbar vein
Left ascending lumbar vein
Inferior vena cava

Figure 159 Azygos System of Veins, the Thoracic Duct, and Other Posterior Thoracic Wall Structures

NOTE: (1) With most of the organs of the thorax and mediastinum removed or cut, the **hemiazygos and accessory hemiazygos veins** to the left of the vertebral column are seen communicating across the midline with the larger **azygos vein.**

(2) The azygos vein is seen ascending in the right thorax to open into the superior vena cava.

(3) The **thoracic duct** arises from the cisterna chyli at the first lumbar level and ascends in the thorax anterior to the vertebral column.

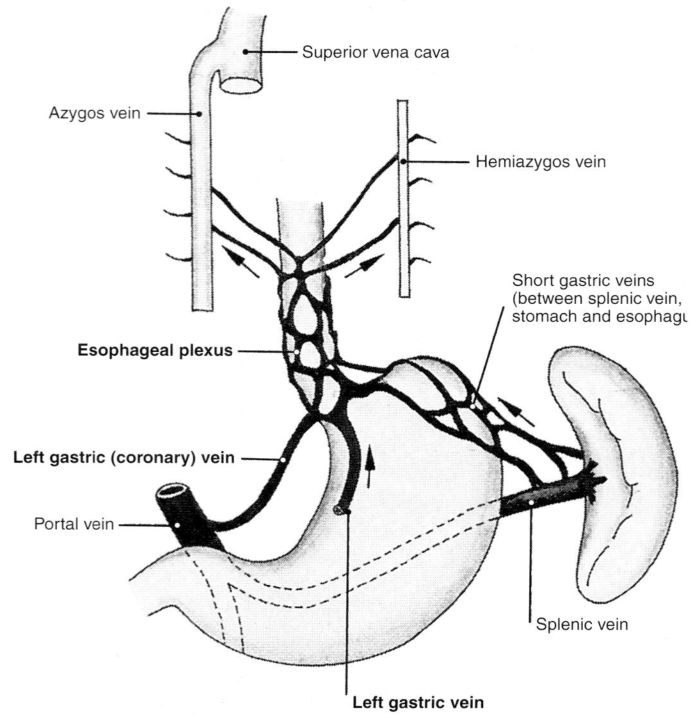
Superior vena cava
Azygos vein
Hemiazygos vein
Short gastric veins (between splenic vein, stomach and esophagu
Esophageal plexus
Left gastric (coronary) vein
Portal vein
Splenic vein
Left gastric vein

Figure 160.1 Anastomosis between the Portal Vein and the Superior Vena Cava through the Esophageal Venous Plexus

NOTE: (1) Veins from the **cervical part** of the esophagus drain into the inferior thyroid vein, while those from the **thoracic part** drain into the azygos, hemiazygos, and accessory hemiazygos veins.

(2) Veins from the **abdominal part** drain partially into the left gastric vein and partially into the azygos vein.

(3) This figure shows the anastomosis sometimes used to return blood from the portal vein to the inferior vena cava. Persons who have hypertension in the portal system may have blood diverted from the **portal vein** to the **coronary** and **left gastric veins**, then to the **hemiazygos** and **azygos veins**, and finally into the **superior vena cava.**

(4) This shunt of venous blood from the liver results in enlargement or varicosities of the esophageal veins, a condition that could lead to serious esophageal hemorrhage.

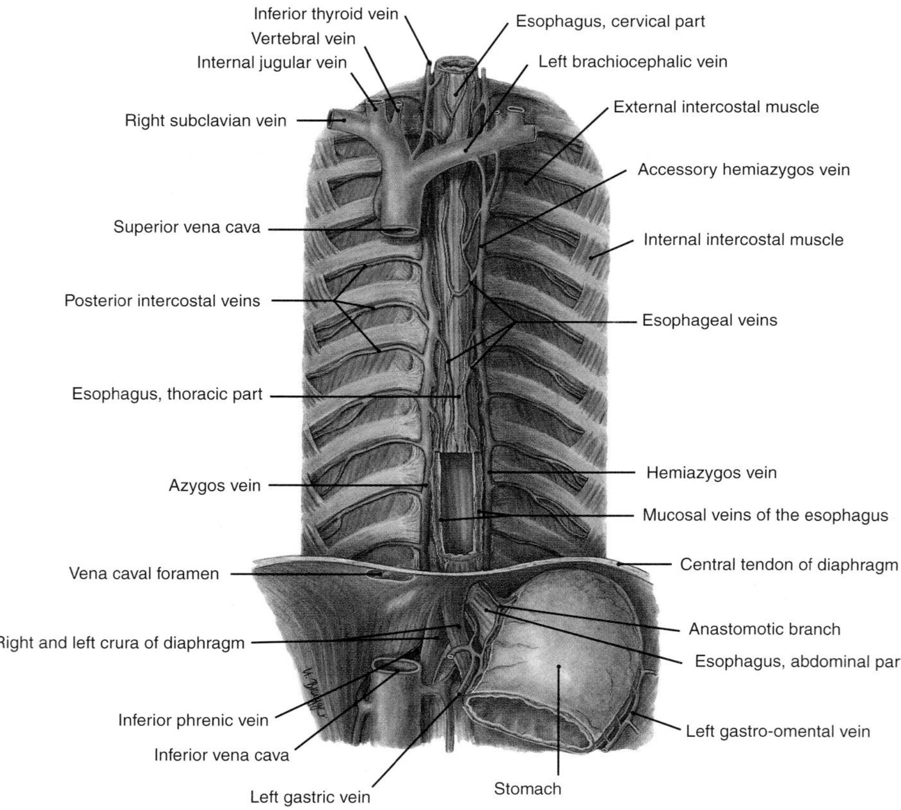
Inferior thyroid vein
Vertebral vein
Internal jugular vein
Right subclavian vein
Esophagus, cervical part
Left brachiocephalic vein
External intercostal muscle
Accessory hemiazygos vein
Superior vena cava
Internal intercostal muscle
Posterior intercostal veins
Esophageal veins
Esophagus, thoracic part
Azygos vein
Hemiazygos vein
Mucosal veins of the esophagus
Vena caval foramen
Central tendon of diaphragm
Right and left crura of diaphragm
Anastomotic branch
Esophagus, abdominal part
Inferior phrenic vein
Inferior vena cava
Left gastro-omental vein
Left gastric vein
Stomach

Figure 160.2 Veins That Drain the Esophagus
(Read NOTES that accompany Fig. 160.1.)

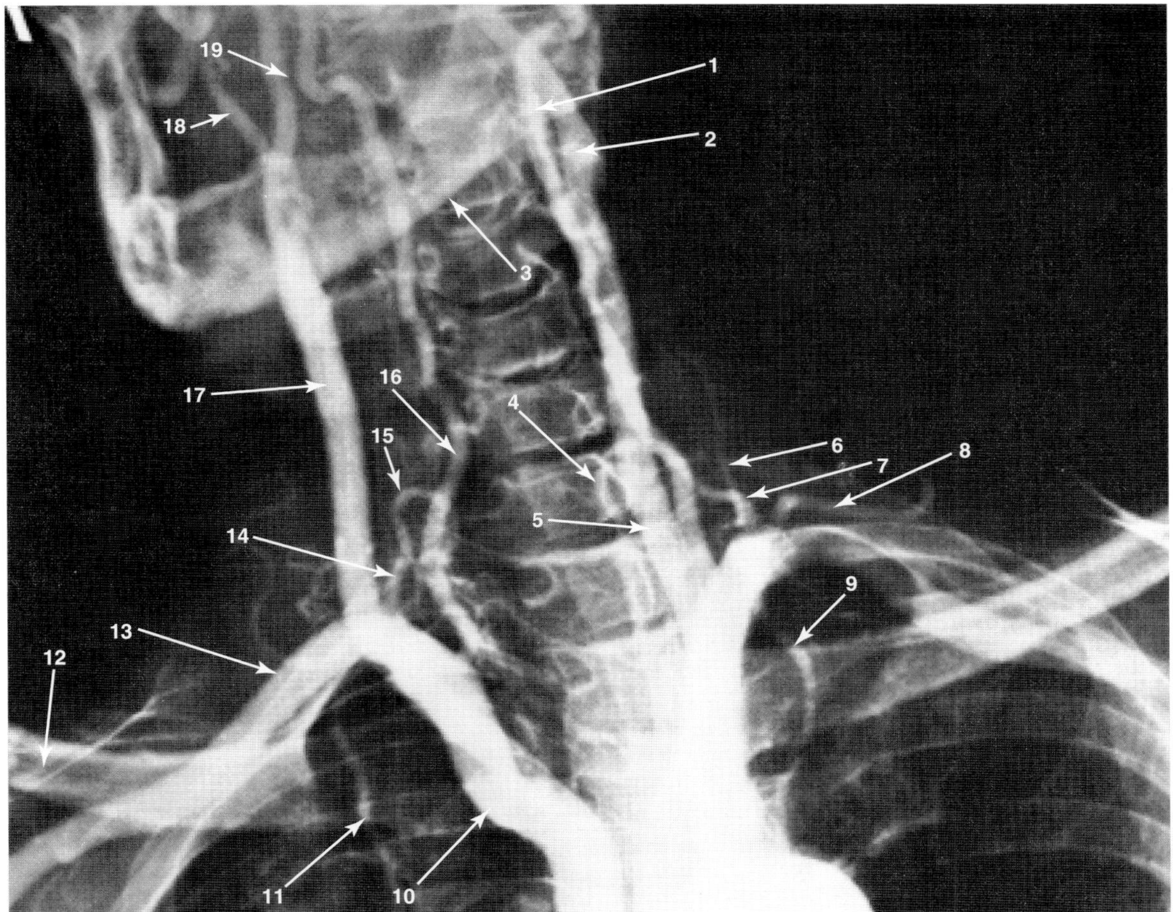
1
2
3
4
5
6
7
8
9
10
11
12
13
14
15
16
17
18
19

Figure 161.1 Angiogram of the Aortic Arch and Its Branches

1. Left vertebral artery
2. Left internal carotid artery
3. Body of the mandible
4. Left inferior thyroid artery
5. Left common carotid artery
6. Left ascending cervical artery
7. Left thyrocervical trunk
8. Left transverse cervical artery
9. Left internal thoracic artery
10. Brachiocephalic trunk
11. Right internal thoracic artery
12. Clavicle
13. Right subclavian artery
14. Right thyrocervical trunk
15. Right inferior thyroid artery
16. Right vertebral artery
17. Right common carotid artery
18. Right external carotid artery
19. Right internal carotid artery

(From Wicke, 6th ed.)

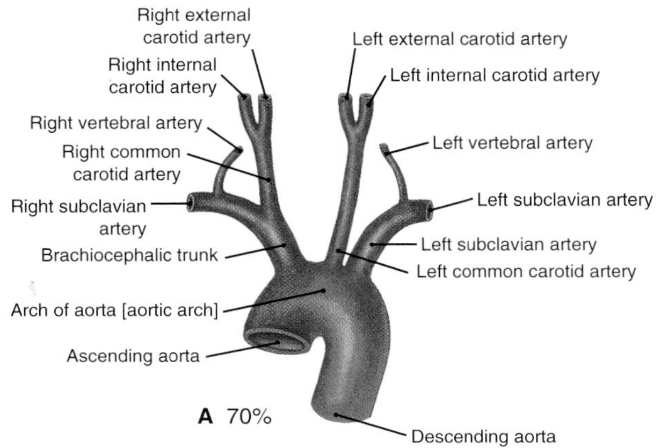
Right external carotid artery
Left external carotid artery
Right internal carotid artery
Left internal carotid artery
Right vertebral artery
Right common carotid artery
Left vertebral artery
Right subclavian artery
Left subclavian artery
Brachiocephalic trunk
Left subclavian artery
Left common carotid artery
Arch of aorta [aortic arch]
Ascending aorta
A 70%
Descending aorta

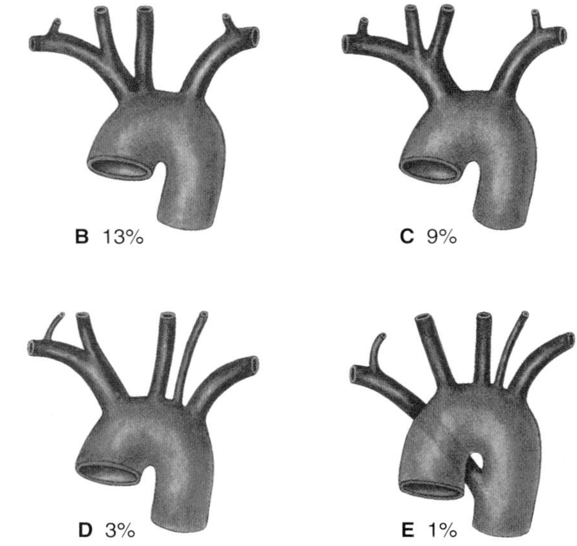
B 13%
C 9%
D 3%
E 1%

Figure 161.2 Variations in Branches from the Arch of the Aorta

A: Normal

B: Common origin of the brachiocephalic trunk and common carotid artery

C: Common stem for right vessel

D: Left vertebral from the aorta

E: Right subclavian arises below the aortic arch.

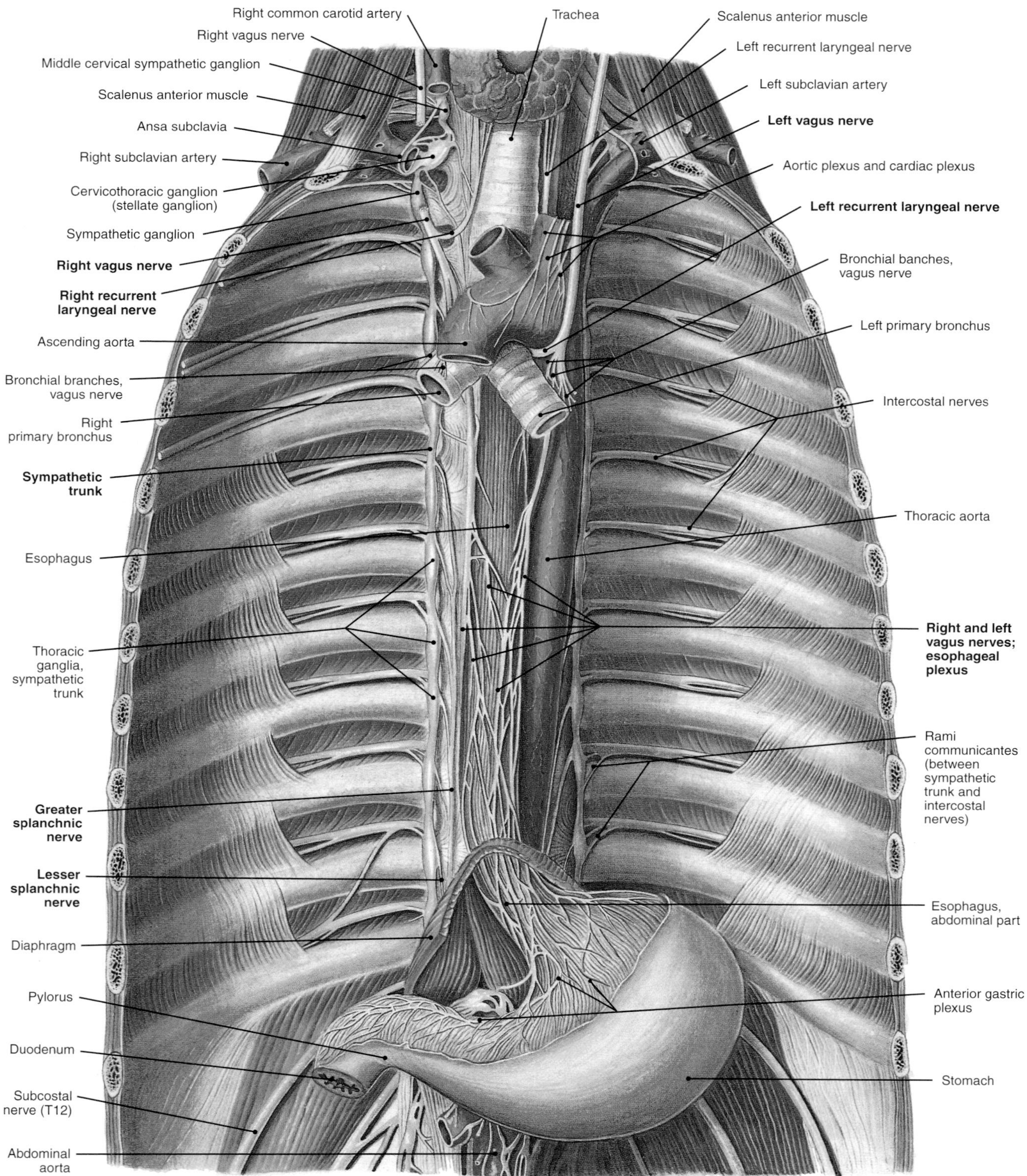
Right common carotid artery
Right vagus nerve
Middle cervical sympathetic ganglion
Scalenus anterior muscle
Ansa subclavia
Right subclavian artery
Cervicothoracic ganglion (stellate ganglion)
Sympathetic ganglion
Right vagus nerve
Right recurrent laryngeal nerve
Ascending aorta
Bronchial branches, vagus nerve
Right primary bronchus
Sympathetic trunk
Esophagus
Thoracic ganglia, sympathetic trunk
Greater splanchnic nerve
Lesser splanchnic nerve
Diaphragm
Pylorus
Duodenum
Subcostal nerve (T12)
Abdominal aorta
Trachea
Scalenus anterior muscle
Left recurrent laryngeal nerve
Left subclavian artery
Left vagus nerve
Aortic plexus and cardiac plexus
Left recurrent laryngeal nerve
Bronchial banches, vagus nerve
Left primary bronchus
Intercostal nerves
Thoracic aorta
Right and left vagus nerves; esophageal plexus
Rami communicantes (between sympathetic trunk and intercostal nerves)
Esophagus, abdominal part
Anterior gastric plexus
Stomach

Figure 162 Sympathetic Trunks and Vagus Nerves in the Thorax and Upper Abdomen

NOTE: (1) The ganglionated sympathetic trunks lie lateral to the bodies of the thoracic vertebrae on each side and are continued into the neck superiorly and the abdomen inferiorly.

(2) Each ganglion is connected to an intercostal nerve by means of **rami communicantes. White rami** consist principally of preganglionic sympathetic fibers coursing to the ganglia, while the **gray rami** carry postganglionic fibers back to the spinal nerves.

(3) The course of the vagus nerves in the thorax. Below the aortic arch they send branches to the bronchi and then descend to form much of the esophageal plexus.

(4) Below the diaphragm, most of the fibers of the **left vagus** form the **anterior gastric nerve,** while most of the fibers of the **right vagus** form the **posterior gastric nerve.**

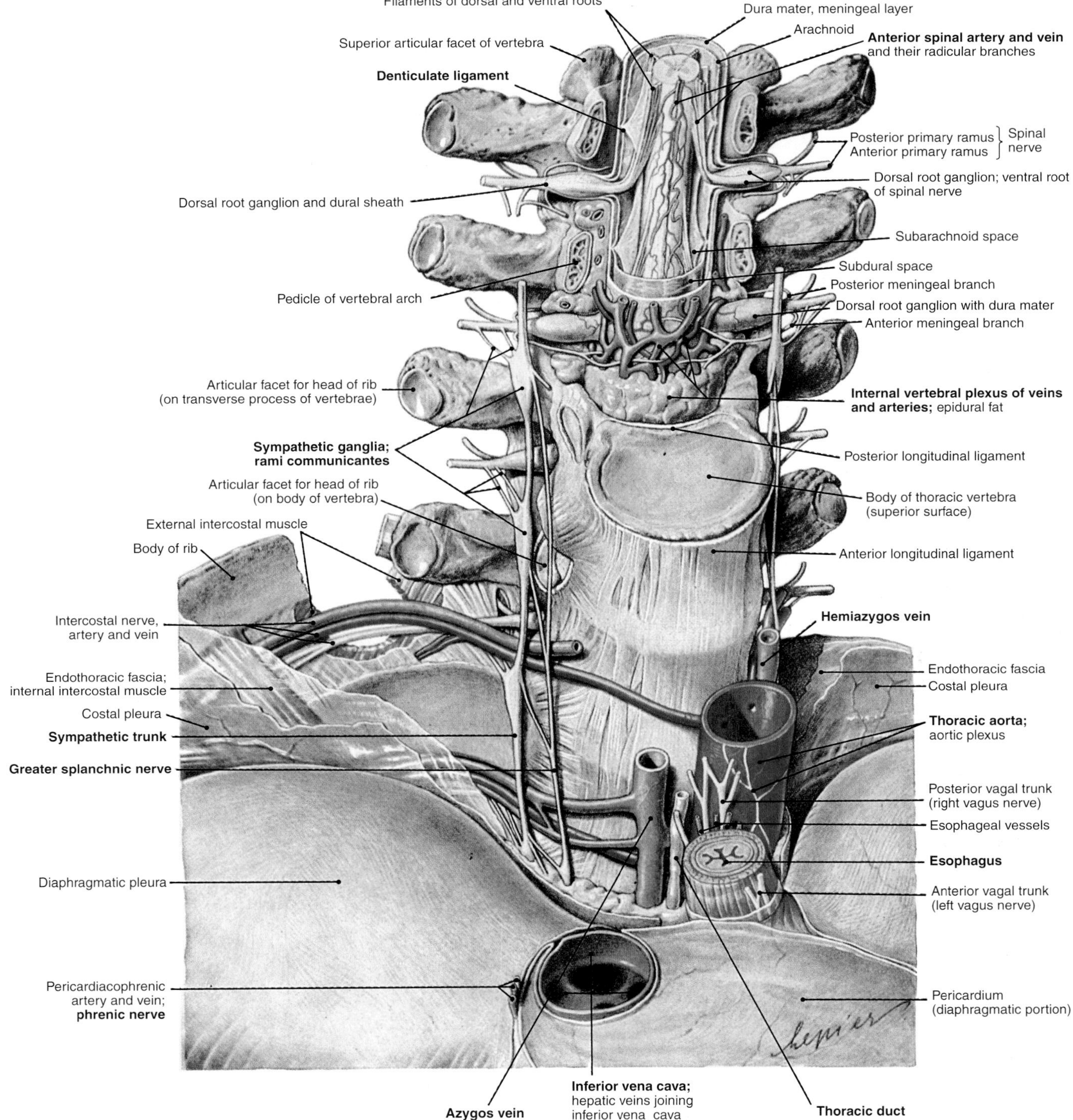
Filaments of dorsal and ventral roots
Dura mater, meningeal layer
Arachnoid
Superior articular facet of vertebra
Anterior spinal artery and vein and their radicular branches
Denticulate ligament
Posterior primary ramus
Anterior primary ramus
Spinal nerve
Dorsal root ganglion; ventral root of spinal nerve
Dorsal root ganglion and dural sheath
Subarachnoid space
Subdural space
Posterior meningeal branch
Pedicle of vertebral arch
Dorsal root ganglion with dura mater
Anterior meningeal branch
Articular facet for head of rib (on transverse process of vertebrae)
Internal vertebral plexus of veins and arteries; epidural fat
Sympathetic ganglia; rami communicantes
Posterior longitudinal ligament
Articular facet for head of rib (on body of vertebra)
Body of thoracic vertebra (superior surface)
External intercostal muscle
Body of rib
Anterior longitudinal ligament
Intercostal nerve, artery and vein
Hemiazygos vein
Endothoracic fascia; internal intercostal muscle
Endothoracic fascia
Costal pleura
Costal pleura
Thoracic aorta; aortic plexus
Sympathetic trunk
Greater splanchnic nerve
Posterior vagal trunk (right vagus nerve)
Esophageal vessels
Esophagus
Diaphragmatic pleura
Anterior vagal trunk (left vagus nerve)
Pericardiacophrenic artery and vein; phrenic nerve
Pericardium (diaphragmatic portion)
Azygos vein
Inferior vena cava; hepatic veins joining inferior vena cava
Thoracic duct

Figure 163 Anterior Dissection of Vertebral Column, Spinal Cord, and Prevertebral Structures at a Lower Thoracic Level

NOTE: (1) The internal vertebral plexus of veins and arteries that lie in the epidural space, where the epidural fat is also found. These should not be confused with the spinal vessels, which are situated in the pia mater and which are seen to be intimately applied to the spinal cord tissue.

(2) The ganglionated sympathetic chain observable here in the thoracic region receiving and giving communicating rami with the spinal nerves. Note also the formation of the greater splanchnic nerve and its descent prevertebrally into the abdomen.

(3) The aorta, inferior vena cava, azygos and hemiazygos veins, esophagus, and thoracic duct all lying anterior or somewhat to the left of the vertebral column and passing through the diaphragm.

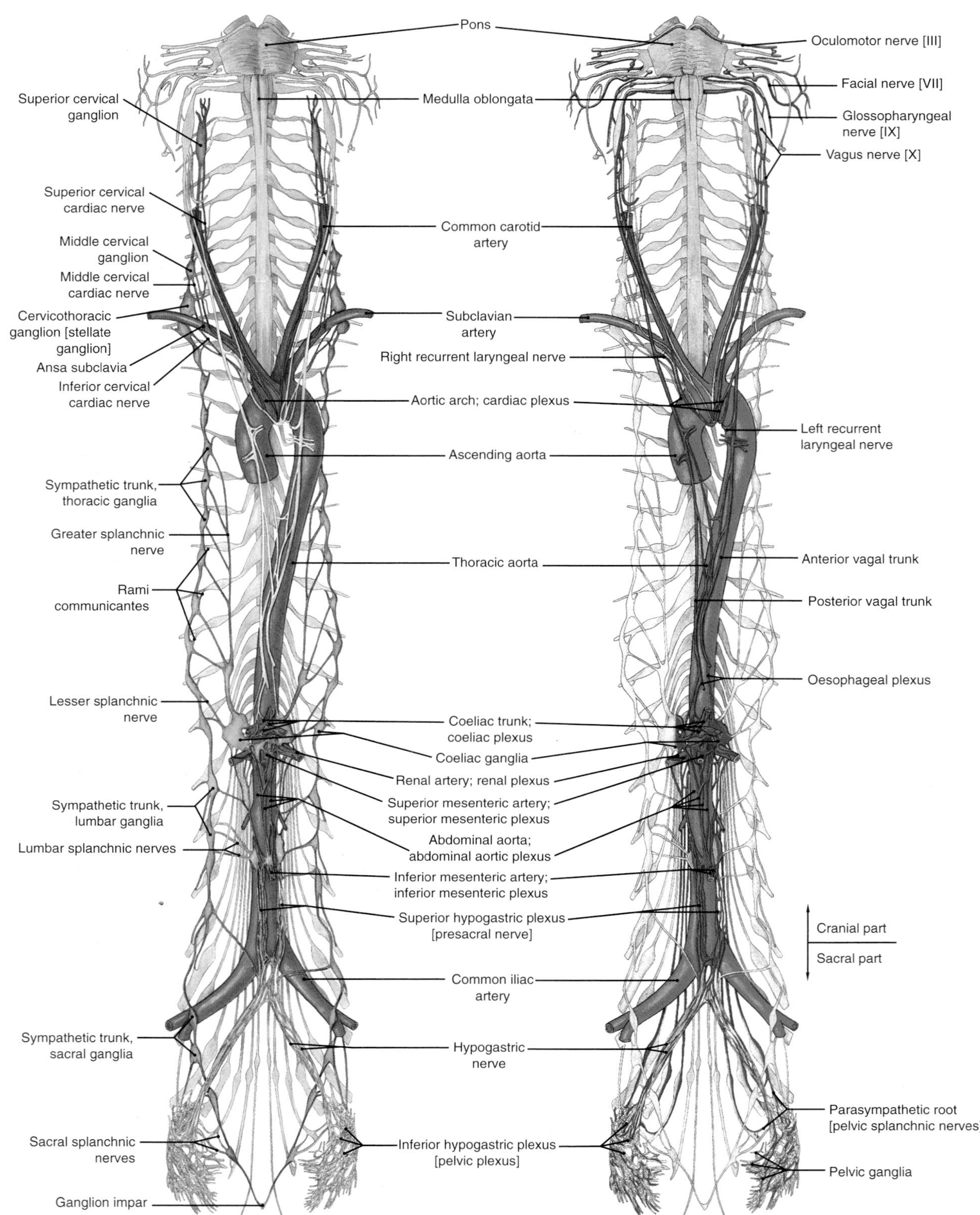
Pons
Superior cervical ganglion
Medulla oblongata
Oculomotor nerve [III]
Facial nerve [VII]
Glossopharyngeal nerve [IX]
Vagus nerve [X]
Superior cervical cardiac nerve
Middle cervical ganglion
Middle cervical cardiac nerve
Common carotid artery
Cervicothoracic ganglion [stellate ganglion]
Ansa subclavia
Inferior cervical cardiac nerve
Subclavian artery
Right recurrent laryngeal nerve
Aortic arch; cardiac plexus
Left recurrent laryngeal nerve
Ascending aorta
Sympathetic trunk, thoracic ganglia
Greater splanchnic nerve
Rami communicantes
Thoracic aorta
Anterior vagal trunk
Posterior vagal trunk
Oesophageal plexus
Lesser splanchnic nerve
Coeliac trunk; coeliac plexus
Coeliac ganglia
Renal artery; renal plexus
Superior mesenteric artery; superior mesenteric plexus
Sympathetic trunk, lumbar ganglia
Lumbar splanchnic nerves
Abdominal aorta; abdominal aortic plexus
Inferior mesenteric artery; inferior mesenteric plexus
Superior hypogastric plexus [presacral nerve]
Cranial part
Sacral part
Common iliac artery
Sympathetic trunk, sacral ganglia
Hypogastric nerve
Parasympathetic root [pelvic splanchnic nerves]
Sacral splanchnic nerves
Inferior hypogastric plexus [pelvic plexus]
Pelvic ganglia
Ganglion impar

Figure 164.1 Sympathetic Division of the Autonomic Nervous System

NOTE that the sympathetic chain and its ganglia and branches are shown in green. Preganglionic sympathetic fibers emerge from the spinal cord between the T1 and L3 spinal levels. Also called the **thoracolumbar outflow.**

Figure 164.2 Parasympathetic Division of the Autonomic Nervous System

NOTE that the parasympathetic fibers are shown in purple. Preganglionic fibers emerge from the central nervous system in cranial nerves III, VII, IX, and X and the sacral levels S2, S3, and S4. Also called **craniosacral outflow.**

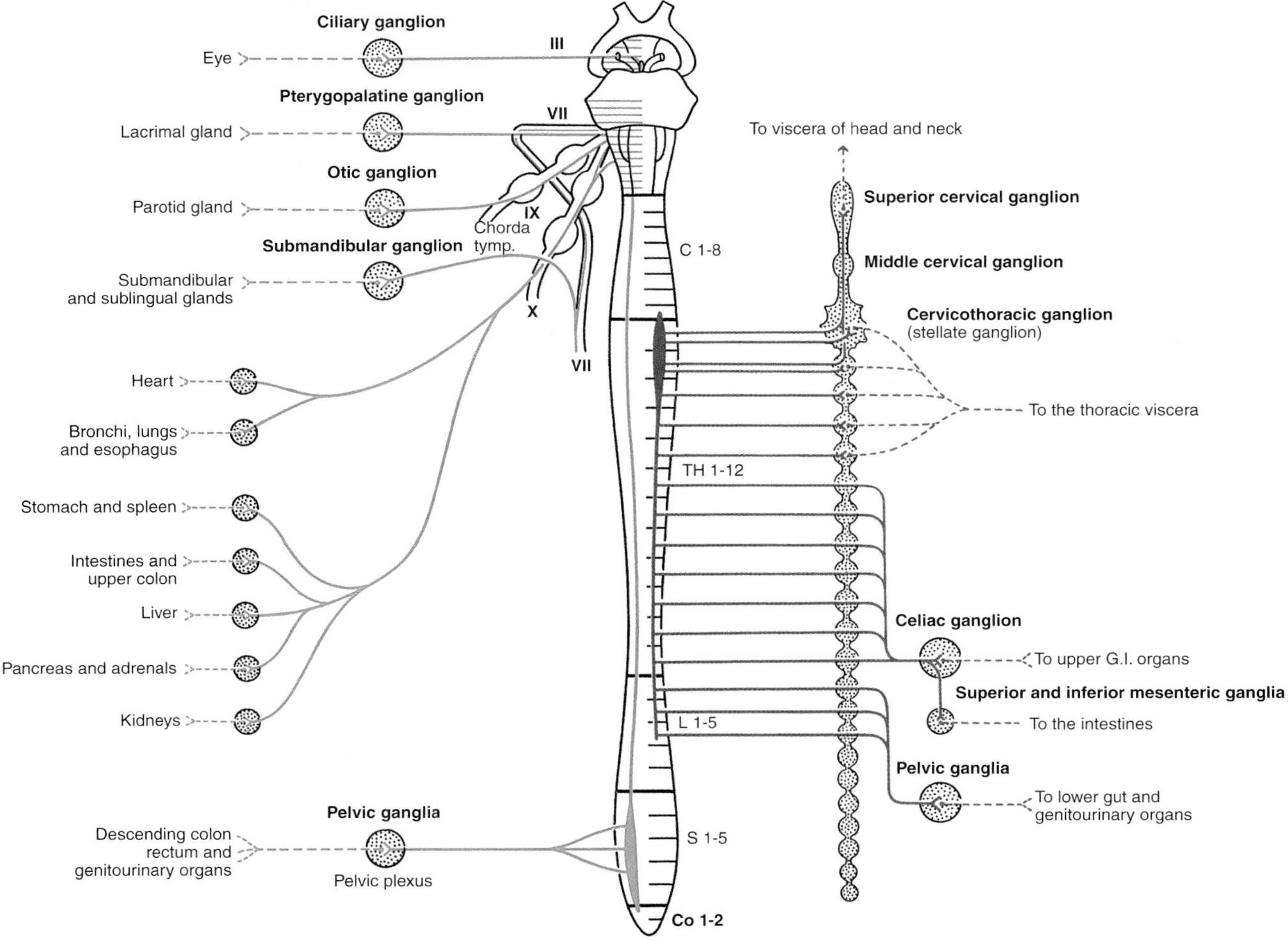

Ciliary ganglion
Eye
III
Pterygopalatine ganglion
VII
Lacrimal gland
To viscera of head and neck
Otic ganglion
Parotid gland
IX
Superior cervical ganglion
Chorda tymp.
Submandibular ganglion
C 1-8
Middle cervical ganglion
Submandibular and sublingual glands
X
Cervicothoracic ganglion (stellate ganglion)
VII
Heart
Bronchi, lungs and esophagus
To the thoracic viscera
TH 1-12
Stomach and spleen
Intestines and upper colon
Liver
Celiac ganglion
Pancreas and adrenals
To upper G.I. organs
Superior and inferior mesenteric ganglia
Kidneys
L 1-5
To the intestines
Pelvic ganglia
Pelvic ganglia
To lower gut and genitourinary organs
Descending colon rectum and genitourinary organs
S 1-5
Pelvic plexus
Co 1-2

Figure 165 Diagram of the Autonomic Nervous System

Blue = parasympathetic; red = sympathetic; solid lines = presynaptic neurons; broken lines = postsynaptic neurons.

NOTE: (1) The autonomic nervous system, by definition, is a two-motor neuron system with the neuron cell bodies of the *presynaptic neurons* (solid lines) somewhere within the central nervous system, and the cell bodies of the *postsynaptic neurons* (broken lines) located in ganglia distributed peripherally in the body.

(2) The autonomic nervous system is comprised of the nerve fibers, which supply all the glands and blood vessels of the body, including the heart. In so doing, all the smooth and cardiac muscle tissues (sometimes called involuntary muscles) are thereby innervated.

(3) The autonomic nervous system is composed of two major divisions, called the parasympathetic (in blue) and sympathetic (in red) divisions. The autonomic regulation of visceral function is, therefore, a dualistic control—i.e., most organs receive postganglionic fibers of both parasympathetic and sympathetic sources.

(4) The *parasympathetic division* is sometimes called a craniosacral outflow because the preganglionic cell bodies of this division lie in the brainstem and in the sacral segments of the spinal cord. Parasympathetic preganglionic fibers are found in four cranial nerves, III (oculomotor), VII (facial), IX (glossopharyngeal), and X (vagus) and in the second, third, and fourth sacral nerves.

(5) These *pre*ganglionic parasympathetic fibers then synapse with *post*ganglionic parasympathetic cell bodies in peripheral ganglia. From these ganglia the *post*ganglionic nerve fibers innervate the various organs.

(6) The *sympathetic division* is sometimes called the thoracolumbar outflow because the *pre*ganglionic sympathetic neuron cell bodies are located in the lateral horn of the spinal cord between the first thoracic spinal segment and the second or third lumbar spinal segment, (i.e., from T1 to L3).

(7) These *pre*ganglionic fibers emerge from the cord with their corresponding spinal roots and communicate with the sympathetic trunk and its ganglia, where some *pre*synaptic sympathetic fibers synapse with *post*ganglionic sympathetic neurons. Other presynaptic fibers (especially those of the upper thoracic segments) ascend in the sympathetic chain and synapse with *post*ganglionic neurons in the cervicothoracic and middle and superior cervical ganglia. *Post*ganglionic fibers from these latter ganglia are then distributed to the viscera of the head and neck. Still other *pre*synaptic sympathetic fibers do not synapse in the sympathetic chain of ganglia at all, but collect to form the splanchnic nerves. These nerves course to the collateral sympathetic ganglia (celiac, superior and inferior mesenteric, and aorticorenal ganglia), where they synapse with the *post*ganglionic neurons. The *post*ganglionic neurons of the sympathetic division then course to the viscera to supply sympathetic innervation.

(8) The functions of the parasympathetic and sympathetic divisions of the autonomic nervous system are antagonistic to each other. The parasympathetic division constricts the pupil, decelerates the heart, lowers blood pressure, relaxes the sphincters of the gut and contracts the longitudinal musculature of the hollow organs. It is the division that is active during periods of calm and tranquility, and it aids in digestion and absorption. In contrast, the *sympathetic division* dilates the pupil, accelerates the heart, increases blood pressure, contracts the sphincters of the gut and relaxes the longitudinal musculature of hollow organs. It is active when the organism is challenged. It prepares for fight and flight and generally comes to the individual's defense during periods of stress and adversity.

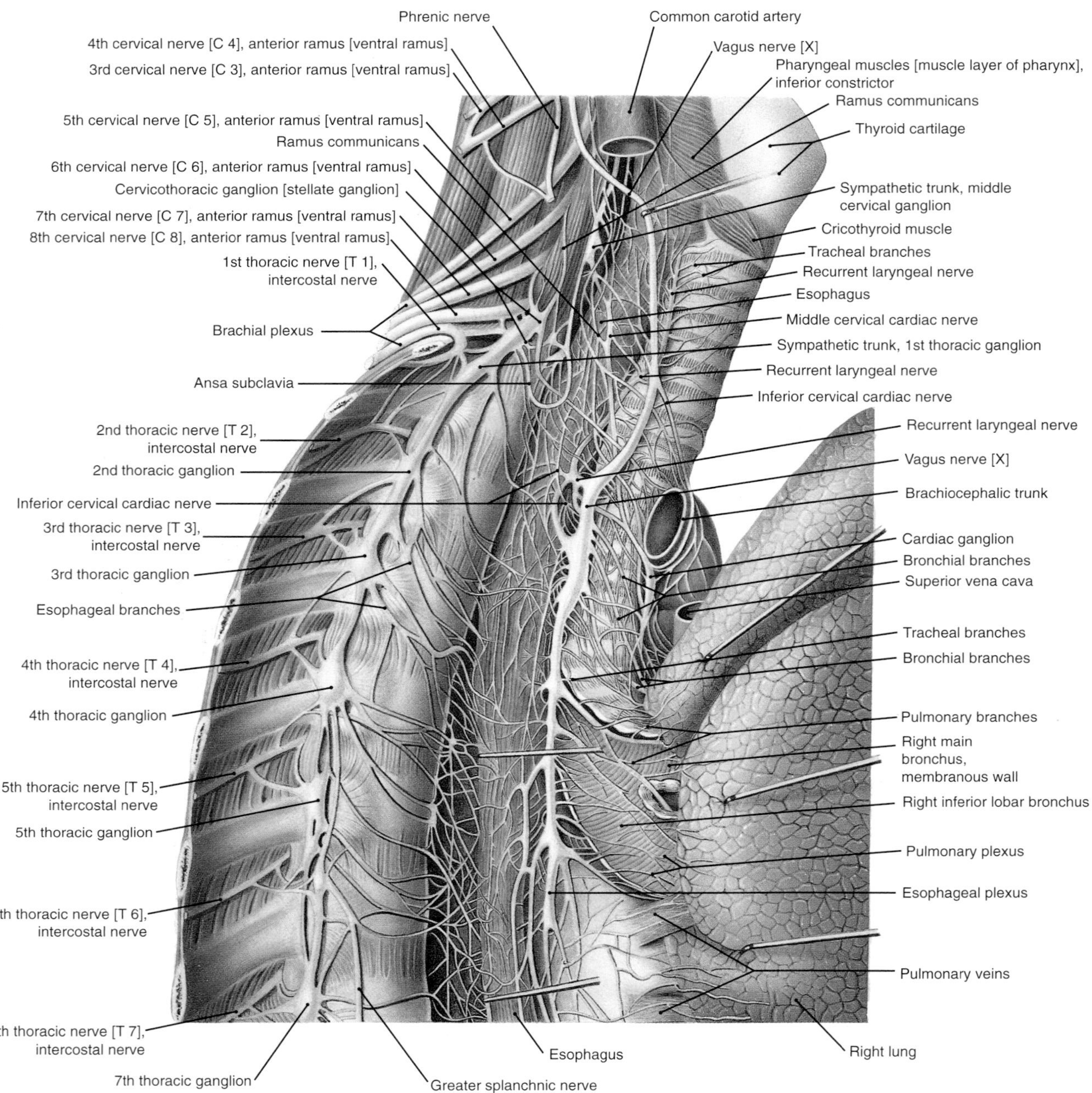

Phrenic nerve
Common carotid artery
4th cervical nerve [C 4], anterior ramus [ventral ramus]
3rd cervical nerve [C 3], anterior ramus [ventral ramus]
Vagus nerve [X]
Pharyngeal muscles [muscle layer of pharynx], inferior constrictor
Ramus communicans
5th cervical nerve [C 5], anterior ramus [ventral ramus]
Ramus communicans
Thyroid cartilage
6th cervical nerve [C 6], anterior ramus [ventral ramus]
Cervicothoracic ganglion [stellate ganglion]
Sympathetic trunk, middle cervical ganglion
7th cervical nerve [C 7], anterior ramus [ventral ramus]
8th cervical nerve [C 8], anterior ramus [ventral ramus]
Cricothyroid muscle
1st thoracic nerve [T 1], intercostal nerve
Tracheal branches
Recurrent laryngeal nerve
Esophagus
Brachial plexus
Middle cervical cardiac nerve
Sympathetic trunk, 1st thoracic ganglion
Recurrent laryngeal nerve
Ansa subclavia
Inferior cervical cardiac nerve
2nd thoracic nerve [T 2], intercostal nerve
Recurrent laryngeal nerve
2nd thoracic ganglion
Vagus nerve [X]
Inferior cervical cardiac nerve
Brachiocephalic trunk
3rd thoracic nerve [T 3], intercostal nerve
Cardiac ganglion
Bronchial branches
3rd thoracic ganglion
Superior vena cava
Esophageal branches
Tracheal branches
Bronchial branches
4th thoracic nerve [T 4], intercostal nerve
4th thoracic ganglion
Pulmonary branches
Right main bronchus, membranous wall
5th thoracic nerve [T 5], intercostal nerve
Right inferior lobar bronchus
5th thoracic ganglion
Pulmonary plexus
Esophageal plexus
6th thoracic nerve [T 6], intercostal nerve
Pulmonary veins
7th thoracic nerve [T 7], intercostal nerve
Esophagus
Right lung
7th thoracic ganglion
Greater splanchnic nerve

Figure 166 Autonomic Nervous System: Cervical and Upper Thoracic Regions

NOTE: (1) The organs of the posterior mediastinum are viewed from the right side by pulling the lungs forward and removing certain of the organs.

(2) Observe the two major nerve trunks and their associated complexes: the right vagus nerve situated more anteriorly and the sympathetic trunk descending more posteriorly in the thorax adjacent to the costovertebral joints.

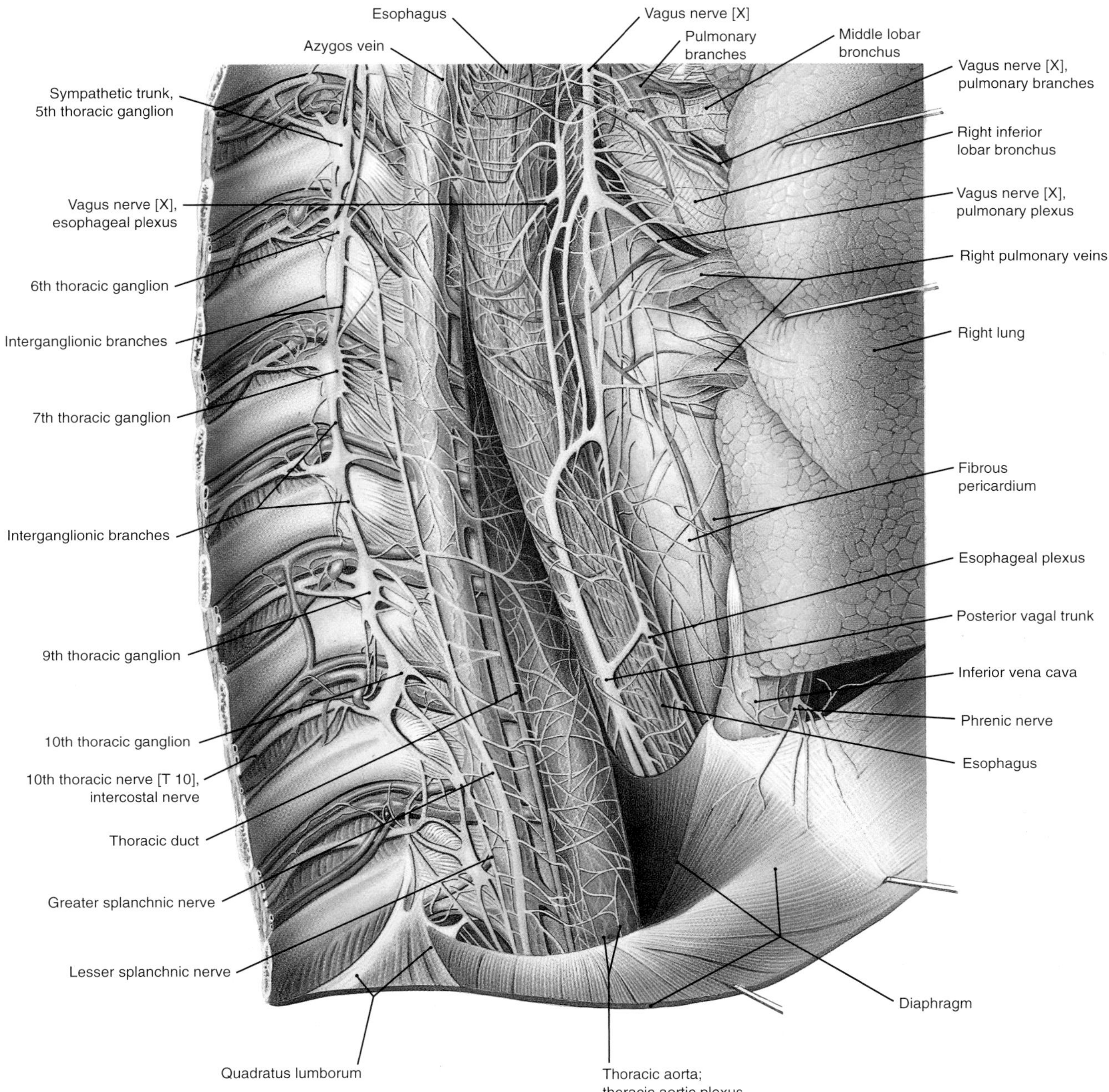
Esophagus
Azygos vein
Vagus nerve [X]
Pulmonary branches
Middle lobar bronchus
Sympathetic trunk, 5th thoracic ganglion
Vagus nerve [X], pulmonary branches
Right inferior lobar bronchus
Vagus nerve [X], esophageal plexus
Vagus nerve [X], pulmonary plexus
Right pulmonary veins
6th thoracic ganglion
Interganglionic branches
Right lung
7th thoracic ganglion
Fibrous pericardium
Interganglionic branches
Esophageal plexus
Posterior vagal trunk
9th thoracic ganglion
Inferior vena cava
Phrenic nerve
10th thoracic ganglion
Esophagus
10th thoracic nerve [T 10], intercostal nerve
Thoracic duct
Greater splanchnic nerve
Lesser splanchnic nerve
Diaphragm
Quadratus lumborum
Thoracic aorta; thoracic aortic plexus

Figure 167 Autonomic Nervous System: Lower Thoracic Region

NOTE: (1) The formation of the greater and lesser splanchnic nerves. The greater splanchnic nerve is derived from preganglionic sympathetic fibers that emerge from sympathetic ganglia T5 to T9 or T10, whereas the lesser splanchnic nerve is derived from ganglia T10 and T11.

(2) The right vagus nerve after contributing parasympathetic fibers to the esophageal plexus becomes the posterior vagal trunk dorsal to the esophagus as that organ passes through the diaphragm.

Thoracic Duct and Lymphatic Drainage

Left brachiocephalic vein
Left jugular lymphatic trunk
Right jugular lymphatic trunk
Thoracic duct, arch
Internal jugular vein
Left subclavian lymphatic trunk
Right lymphatic duct
Subclavian vein
Right subclavian lymphatic trunk
Subclavian vein
Right brachiocephalic vein
Thoracic duct
Superior vena cava
Thoracic duct
Diaphragm, left crus
Cisterna chyli
Right lumbar lymphatic trunk
Left lumbar lymphatic trunk
Intestinal lymphatic trunk

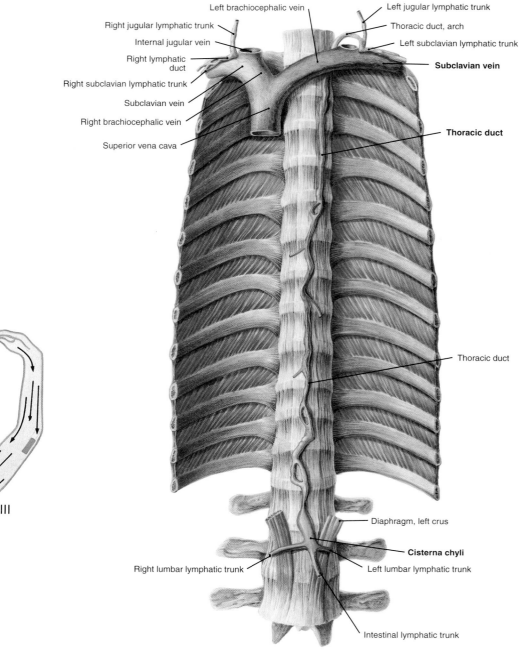

Figure 168.2 Thoracic Duct: Its Origin and Course

NOTE: (1) The **thoracic duct** collects lymph from most of the body regions and conveys it back into the bloodstream. The duct originates in the abdomen anterior to the second lumbar vertebra at the **cisterna chyli.**

(2) The thoracic duct enters the thorax through the **aortic hiatus** of the diaphragm, slightly to the right of the midline. Within the posterior mediastinum of the thorax, still coursing just ventral to the vertebral column, it gradually crosses the midline from right to left.

(3) The duct then ascends into the root of the neck on the left side and opens into the **left subclavian vein** near the junction of the **left internal jugular vein.**

(4) The **right lymphatic duct** receives lymph from the right side of the head, neck, and trunk and from the right upper extremity. It empties into the **right subclavian vein.**

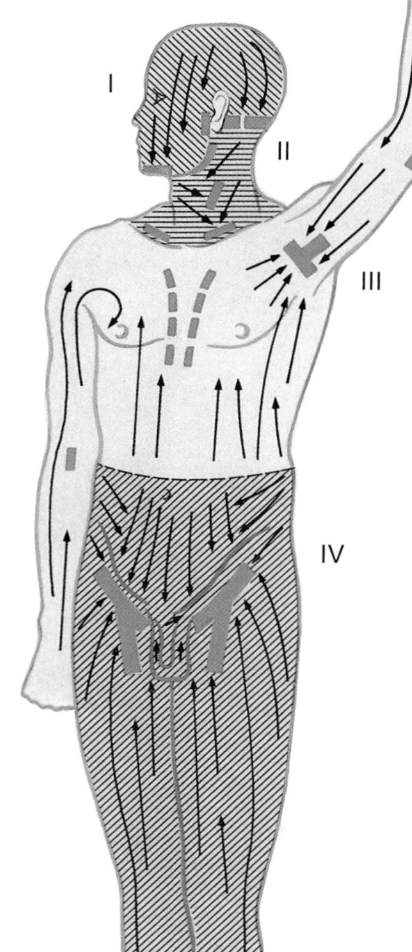
I
II
III
IV

→ = Direction of flow of lymph in the following large areas of the body:
I = Head
II = Neck
III = Upper extremity and thorax
IV = Lower trunk and lower extremity
■ = Siote sof lymphatic channel convergence

Figure 168.1 Diagram of Lymphatic Channel Flow

Figure 169.1 Certain Lymphatics of the Head, Abdomen, Pelvis, and Limbs

NOTE: (1) In addition to its physiologic importance in returning tissue fluids and cells to the blood vascular system, the lymphatic system may serve as pathways for the spread of disease.

(2) Lymph channels may be used as preformed tubes for the spread of infectious diseases as well as metastatic cells from established tumors.

(3) Enlarged or painful lymph nodes are often clinical signs of disease processes elsewhere in the body or of the lymphoid organs themselves.

(4) This figure shows the lymphatic channels that drain the upper limb into axillary nodes and those of the lower limb into the inguinal nodes. Also seen are the iliac and lumbar nodes, as well as the mesenteric nodes. Not shown are the deep nodes of the head, neck, and thorax or many of the visceral nodes of the thorax, abdomen, and pelvis.

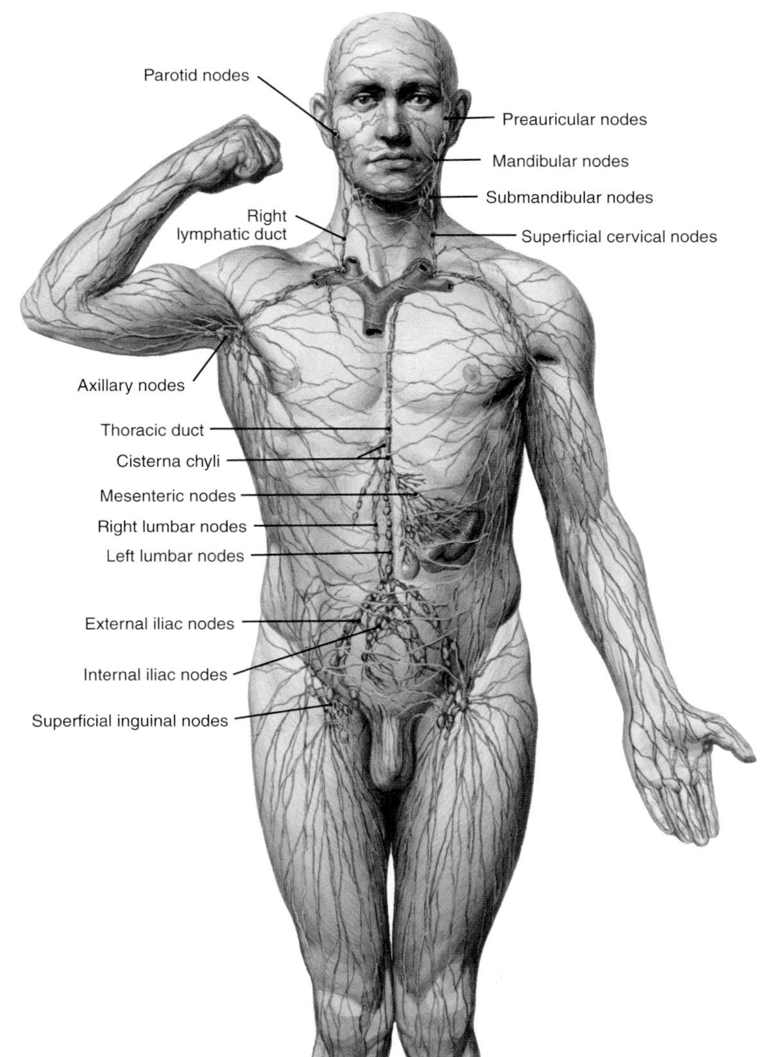

Parotid nodes
Preauricular nodes
Mandibular nodes
Submandibular nodes
Right lymphatic duct
Superficial cervical nodes
Axillary nodes
Thoracic duct
Cisterna chyli
Mesenteric nodes
Right lumbar nodes
Left lumbar nodes
External iliac nodes
Internal iliac nodes
Superficial inguinal nodes

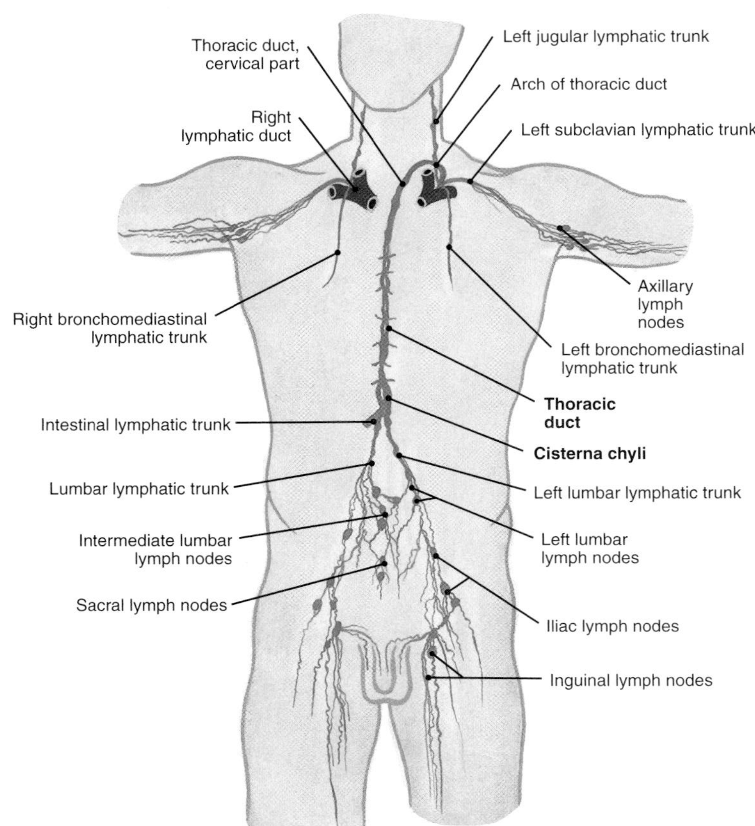

Thoracic duct, cervical part
Right lymphatic duct
Left jugular lymphatic trunk
Arch of thoracic duct
Left subclavian lymphatic trunk
Axillary lymph nodes
Right bronchomediastinal lymphatic trunk
Left bronchomediastinal lymphatic trunk
Thoracic duct
Intestinal lymphatic trunk
Cisterna chyli
Lumbar lymphatic trunk
Left lumbar lymphatic trunk
Intermediate lumbar lymph nodes
Left lumbar lymph nodes
Sacral lymph nodes
Iliac lymph nodes
Inguinal lymph nodes

Figure 169.2 Large Lymphatic Vessels

NOTE: (1) The **inguinal lymph nodes** drain the lower limb. The inguinal nodes drain into the **iliac nodes,** which also receive lymph from the pelvic organs.

(2) The iliac nodes drain into the **right** and **left lumbar nodes.** The lumbar lymphatic trunks join the **intestinal trunk(s)** to form the **cisterna chyli,** which opens into the **thoracic duct.**

(3) The thoracic duct receives the **left jugular** and **left subclavian trunks** as well as the **left bronchomediastinal trunk** before it opens into the **left subclavian vein.**

(4) The **right lymphatic duct** drains the **right jugular trunk** and the **right subclavian trunk** (shown but not labeled), as well as the **right bronchomediastinal** trunk before opening into the **right subclavian vein.**

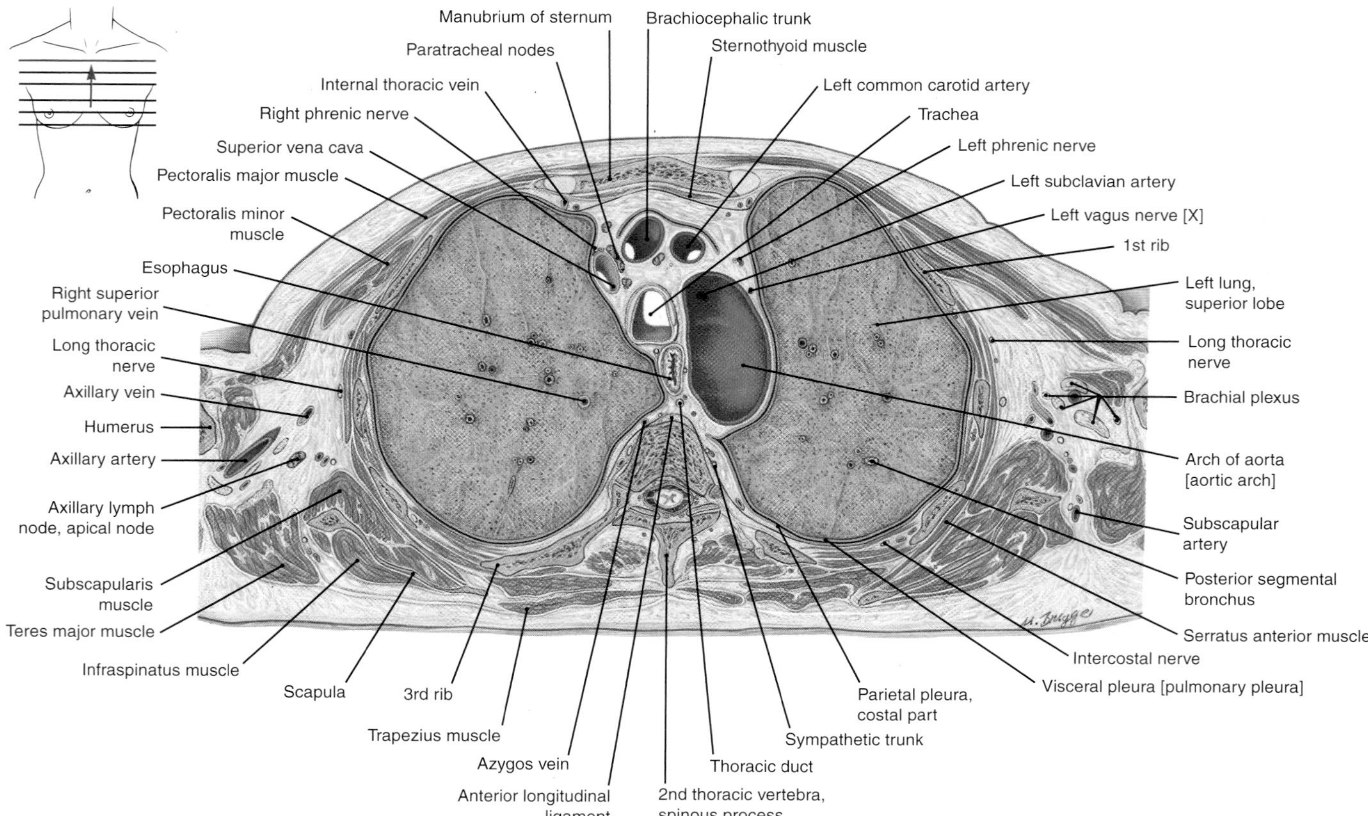

Manubrium of sternum
Brachiocephalic trunk
Paratracheal nodes
Sternothyoid muscle
Internal thoracic vein
Left common carotid artery
Right phrenic nerve
Trachea
Superior vena cava
Left phrenic nerve
Pectoralis major muscle
Left subclavian artery
Pectoralis minor muscle
Left vagus nerve [X]
1st rib
Esophagus
Left lung, superior lobe
Right superior pulmonary vein
Long thoracic nerve
Long thoracic nerve
Brachial plexus
Axillary vein
Humerus
Axillary artery
Arch of aorta [aortic arch]
Axillary lymph node, apical node
Subscapular artery
Subscapularis muscle
Posterior segmental bronchus
Teres major muscle
Serratus anterior muscle
Intercostal nerve
Infraspinatus muscle
Visceral pleura [pulmonary pleura]
Scapula
3rd rib
Parietal pleura, costal part
Trapezius muscle
Sympathetic trunk
Azygos vein
Thoracic duct
Anterior longitudinal ligament
2nd thoracic vertebra, spinous process

Figure 170.1 Horizontal Section through the Thorax at the Level of the Arch of the Aorta (Caudal View)

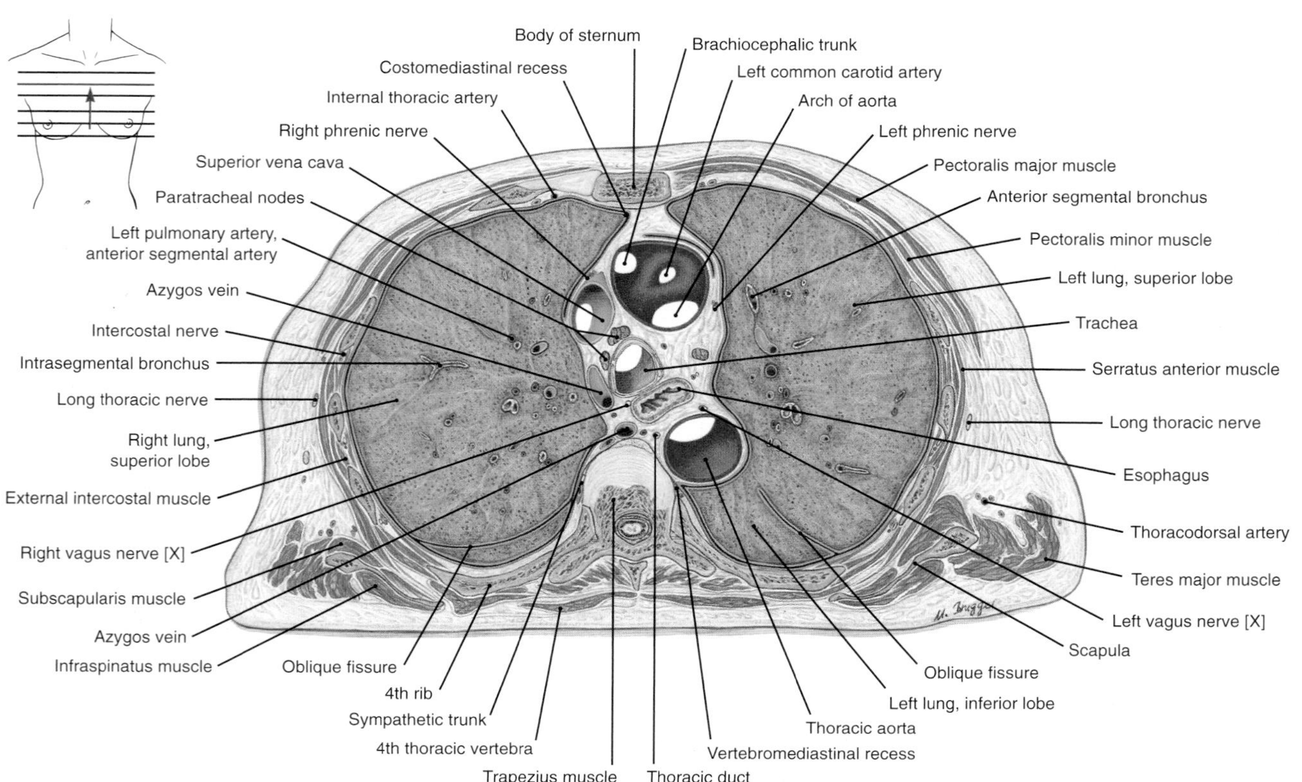

Body of sternum
Brachiocephalic trunk
Costomediastinal recess
Left common carotid artery
Internal thoracic artery
Arch of aorta
Right phrenic nerve
Left phrenic nerve
Superior vena cava
Pectoralis major muscle
Paratracheal nodes
Anterior segmental bronchus
Left pulmonary artery, anterior segmental artery
Pectoralis minor muscle
Left lung, superior lobe
Azygos vein
Trachea
Intercostal nerve
Intrasegmental bronchus
Serratus anterior muscle
Long thoracic nerve
Long thoracic nerve
Right lung, superior lobe
Esophagus
External intercostal muscle
Thoracodorsal artery
Right vagus nerve [X]
Teres major muscle
Subscapularis muscle
Left vagus nerve [X]
Azygos vein
Scapula
Infraspinatus muscle
Oblique fissure
Oblique fissure
4th rib
Left lung, inferior lobe
Sympathetic trunk
Thoracic aorta
4th thoracic vertebra
Vertebromediastinal recess
Trapezius muscle
Thoracic duct

Figure 170.2 Horizontal Section through the Thorax at the Level of the Fourth Thoracic Vertebra (Caudal View)

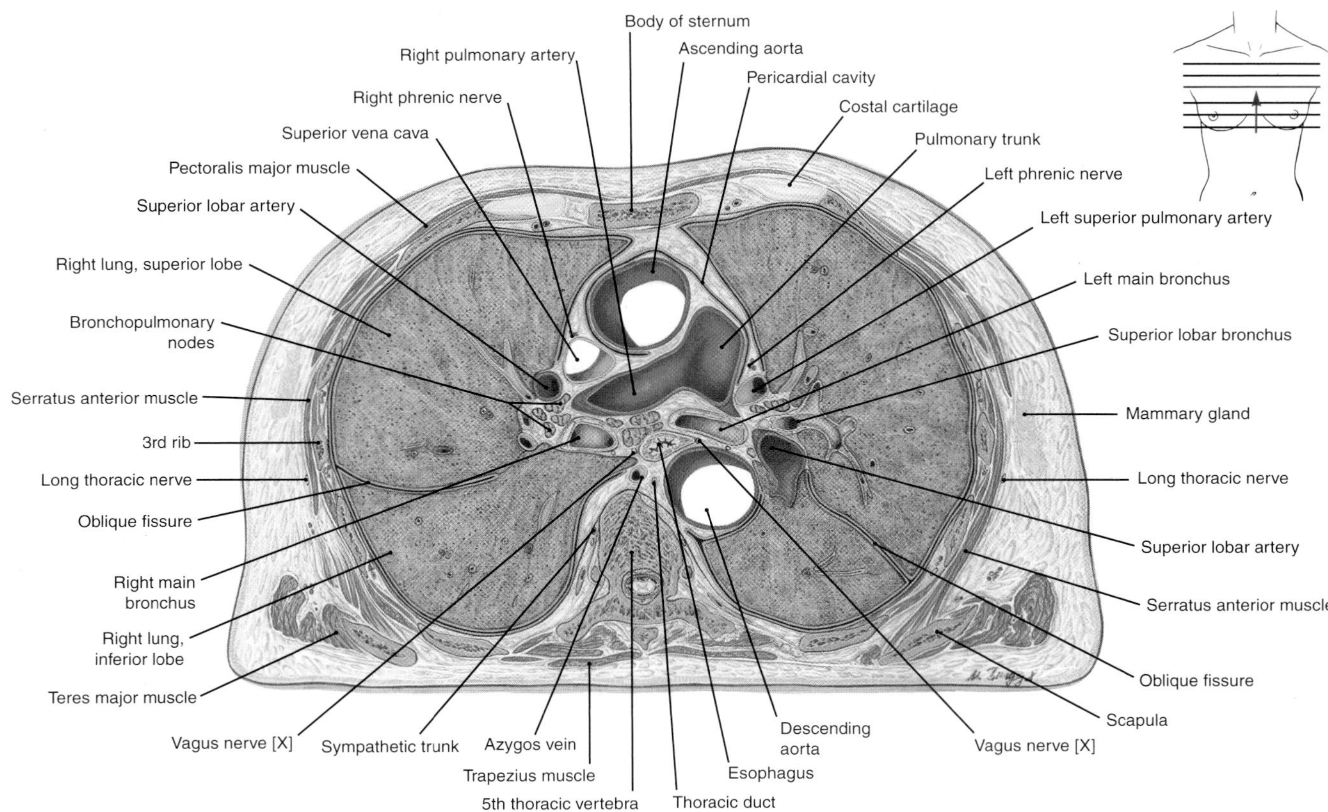
Body of sternum
Right pulmonary artery
Ascending aorta
Pericardial cavity
Right phrenic nerve
Costal cartilage
Superior vena cava
Pulmonary trunk
Pectoralis major muscle
Left phrenic nerve
Superior lobar artery
Left superior pulmonary artery
Right lung, superior lobe
Left main bronchus
Bronchopulmonary nodes
Superior lobar bronchus
Serratus anterior muscle
Mammary gland
3rd rib
Long thoracic nerve
Long thoracic nerve
Oblique fissure
Superior lobar artery
Right main bronchus
Serratus anterior muscle
Right lung, inferior lobe
Oblique fissure
Teres major muscle
Scapula
Vagus nerve [X]
Sympathetic trunk
Azygos vein
Descending aorta
Vagus nerve [X]
Trapezius muscle
Esophagus
5th thoracic vertebra
Thoracic duct

Figure 171.1 Horizontal Section through the Thorax at the Bifurcation of the Pulmonary Trunk (Caudal View)

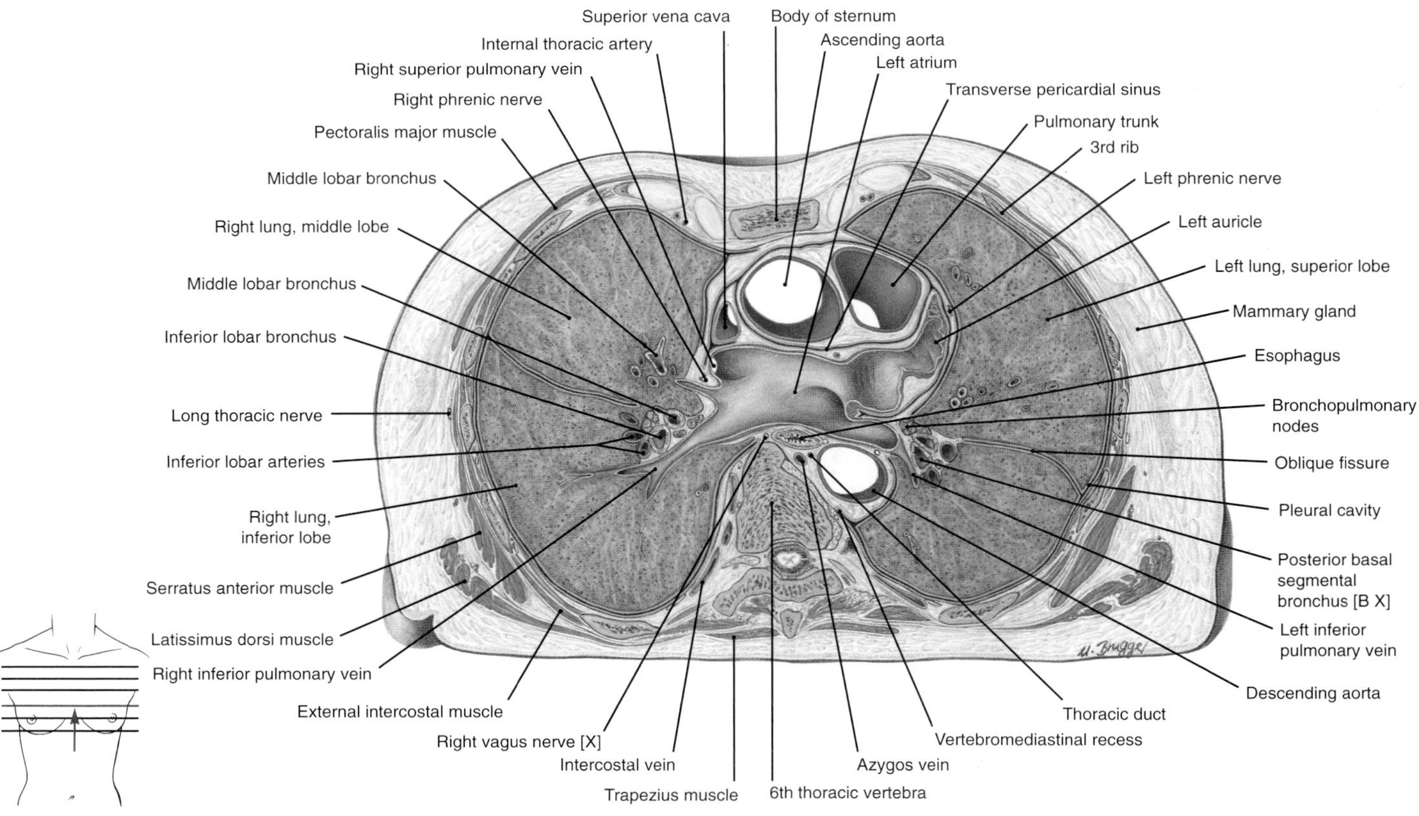
Superior vena cava
Body of sternum
Internal thoracic artery
Ascending aorta
Right superior pulmonary vein
Left atrium
Right phrenic nerve
Transverse pericardial sinus
Pectoralis major muscle
Pulmonary trunk
3rd rib
Middle lobar bronchus
Left phrenic nerve
Right lung, middle lobe
Left auricle
Left lung, superior lobe
Middle lobar bronchus
Mammary gland
Inferior lobar bronchus
Esophagus
Long thoracic nerve
Bronchopulmonary nodes
Inferior lobar arteries
Oblique fissure
Right lung, inferior lobe
Pleural cavity
Serratus anterior muscle
Posterior basal segmental bronchus [B X]
Latissimus dorsi muscle
Left inferior pulmonary vein
Right inferior pulmonary vein
Descending aorta
External intercostal muscle
Thoracic duct
Right vagus nerve [X]
Vertebromediastinal recess
Intercostal vein
Azygos vein
Trapezius muscle
6th thoracic vertebra

Figure 171.2 Horizontal Section through the Thorax at the Level of the Left Atrium (Caudal View)

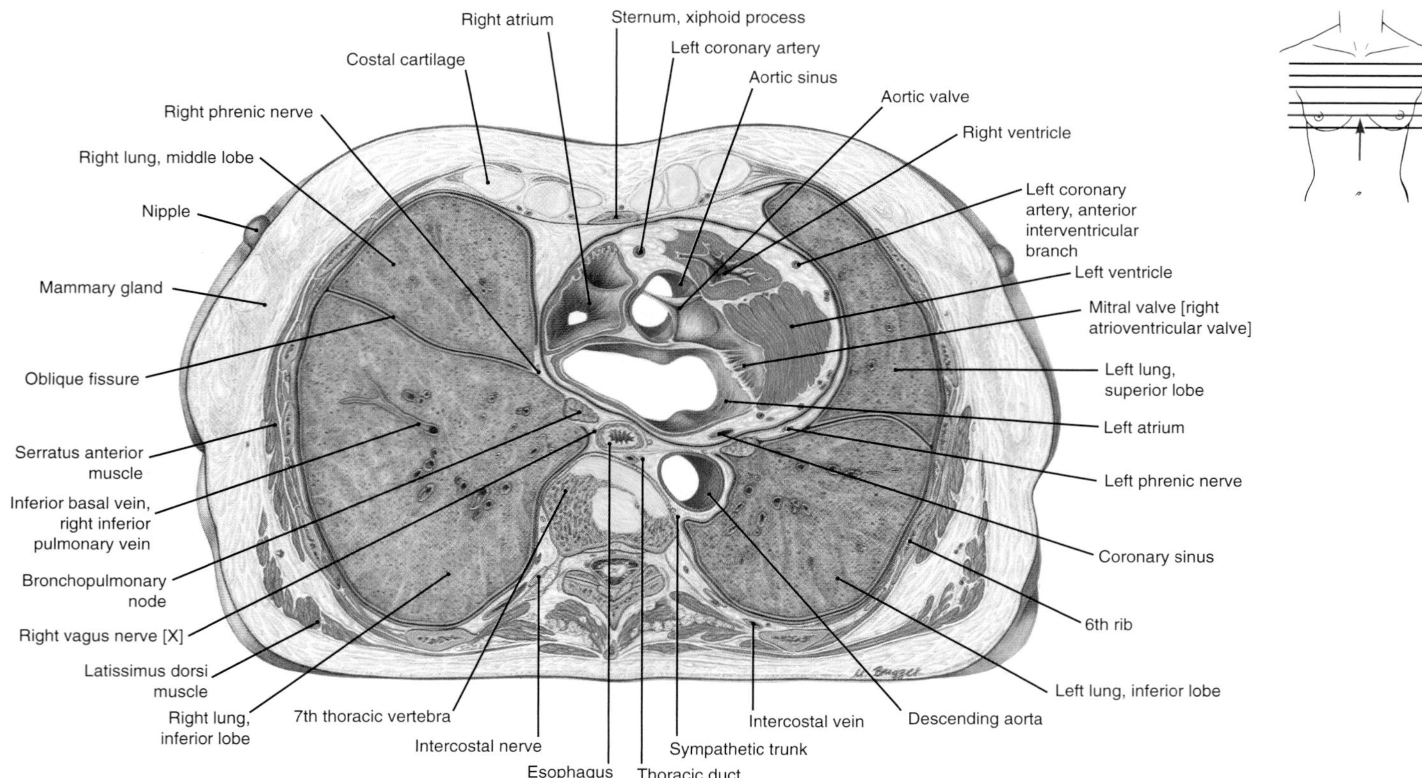
Right atrium
Sternum, xiphoid process
Left coronary artery
Costal cartilage
Aortic sinus
Aortic valve
Right phrenic nerve
Right ventricle
Right lung, middle lobe
Nipple
Left coronary artery, anterior interventricular branch
Mammary gland
Left ventricle
Mitral valve [right atrioventricular valve]
Oblique fissure
Left lung, superior lobe
Left atrium
Serratus anterior muscle
Left phrenic nerve
Inferior basal vein, right inferior pulmonary vein
Coronary sinus
Bronchopulmonary node
Right vagus nerve [X]
6th rib
Latissimus dorsi muscle
Left lung, inferior lobe
Right lung, inferior lobe
7th thoracic vertebra
Intercostal vein
Descending aorta
Intercostal nerve
Sympathetic trunk
Esophagus
Thoracic duct

Figure 172.1 Horizontal Section through the Thorax at the Level of the Seventh Thoracic Vertebra (Caudal View)

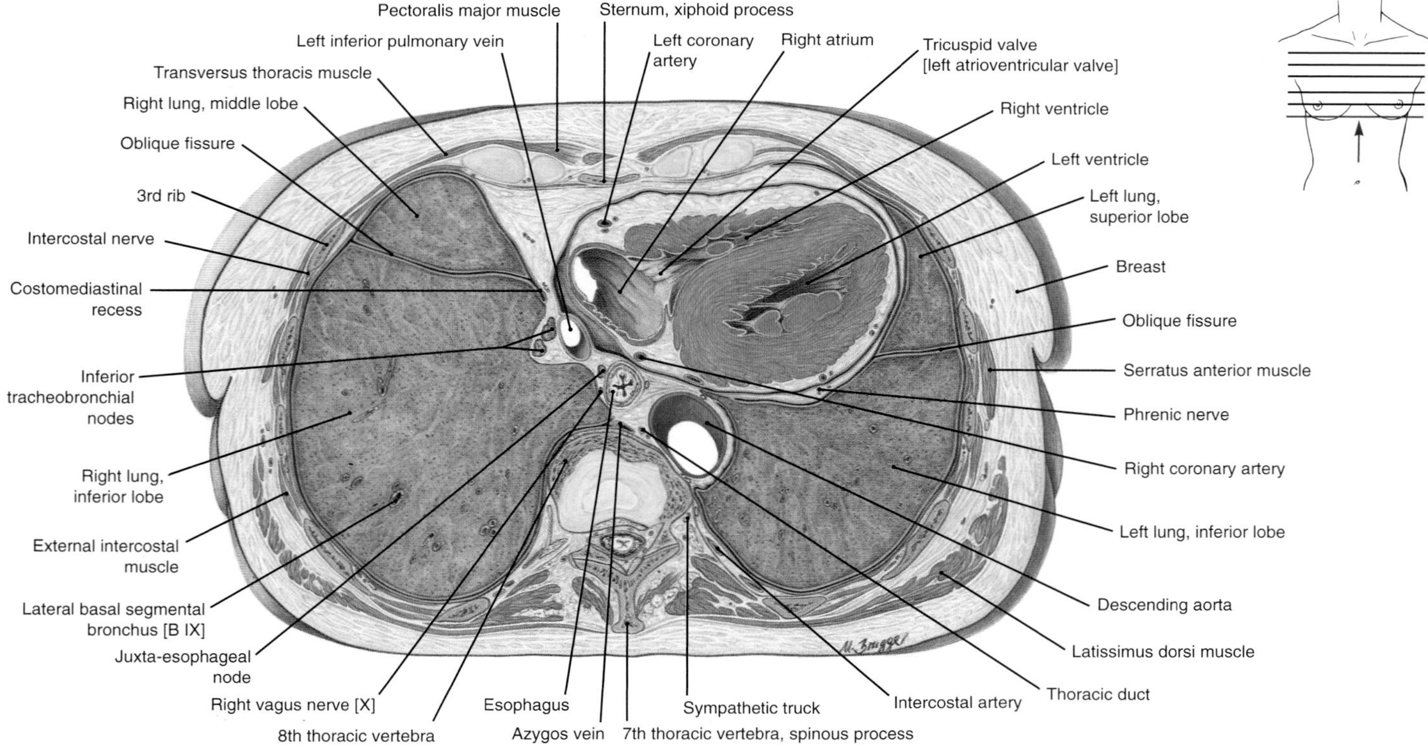
Pectoralis major muscle
Sternum, xiphoid process
Left inferior pulmonary vein
Left coronary artery
Right atrium
Tricuspid valve [left atrioventricular valve]
Transversus thoracis muscle
Right lung, middle lobe
Right ventricle
Oblique fissure
Left ventricle
3rd rib
Left lung, superior lobe
Intercostal nerve
Breast
Costomediastinal recess
Oblique fissure
Serratus anterior muscle
Inferior tracheobronchial nodes
Phrenic nerve
Right coronary artery
Right lung, inferior lobe
Left lung, inferior lobe
External intercostal muscle
Descending aorta
Lateral basal segmental bronchus [B IX]
Latissimus dorsi muscle
Juxta-esophageal node
Thoracic duct
Right vagus nerve [X]
Esophagus
Sympathetic truck
Intercostal artery
8th thoracic vertebra
Azygos vein
7th thoracic vertebra, spinous process

Figure 172.2 Horizontal Section through the Thorax at the Level of the Eighth Thoracic Vertebra (Caudal View)

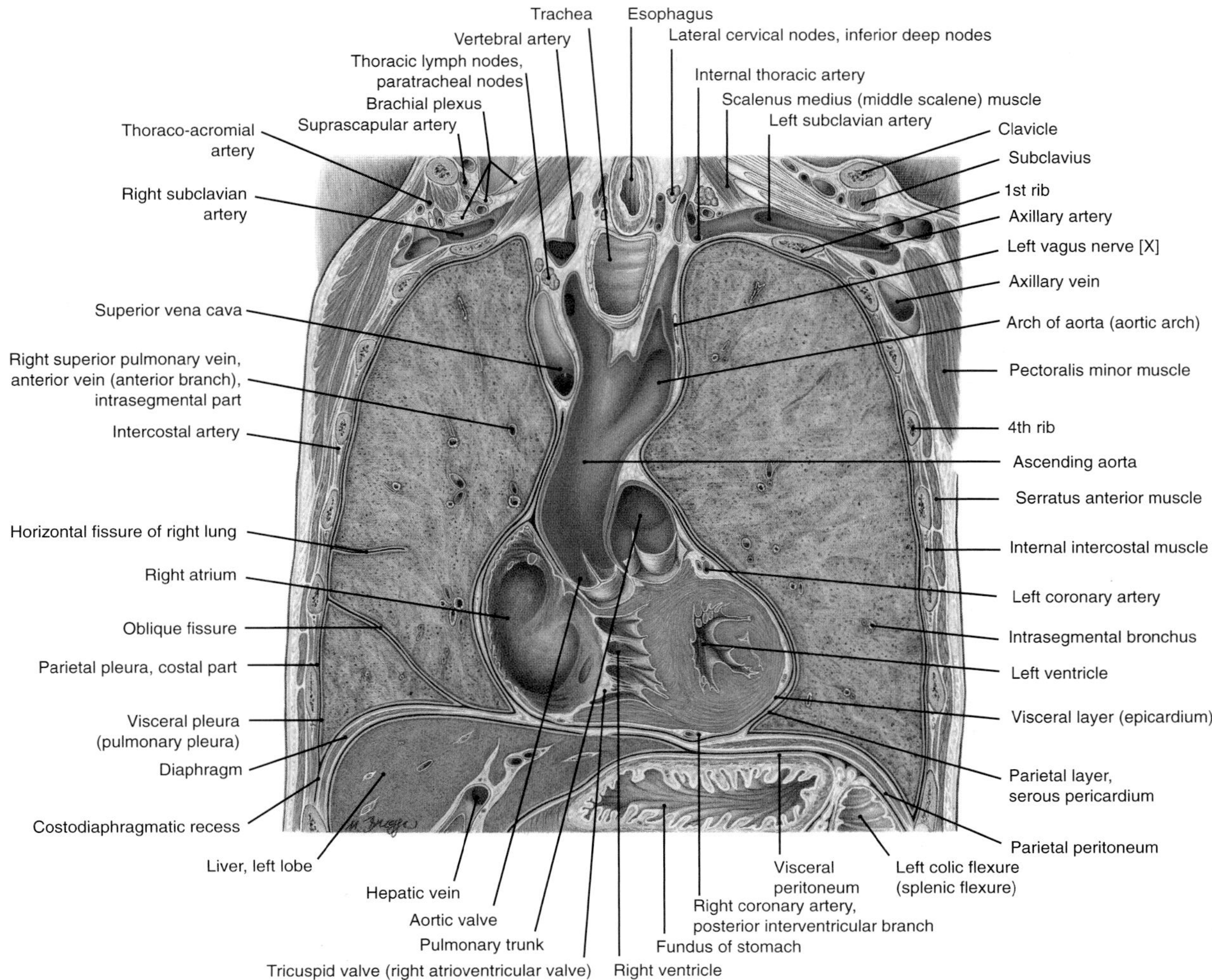
Trachea
Esophagus
Vertebral artery
Lateral cervical nodes, inferior deep nodes
Thoracic lymph nodes, paratracheal nodes
Internal thoracic artery
Brachial plexus
Scalenus medius (middle scalene) muscle
Suprascapular artery
Left subclavian artery
Thoraco-acromial artery
Clavicle
Subclavius
Right subclavian artery
1st rib
Axillary artery
Left vagus nerve [X]
Axillary vein
Superior vena cava
Arch of aorta (aortic arch)
Right superior pulmonary vein, anterior vein (anterior branch), intrasegmental part
Pectoralis minor muscle
Intercostal artery
4th rib
Ascending aorta
Serratus anterior muscle
Horizontal fissure of right lung
Internal intercostal muscle
Right atrium
Left coronary artery
Oblique fissure
Intrasegmental bronchus
Parietal pleura, costal part
Left ventricle
Visceral pleura (pulmonary pleura)
Visceral layer (epicardium)
Diaphragm
Parietal layer, serous pericardium
Costodiaphragmatic recess
Parietal peritoneum
Liver, left lobe
Visceral peritoneum
Left colic flexure (splenic flexure)
Hepatic vein
Right coronary artery, posterior interventricular branch
Aortic valve
Pulmonary trunk
Fundus of stomach
Tricuspid valve (right atrioventricular valve)
Right ventricle

Figure 173.1 Frontal Section through the Thoracic Cavity (Anterior View)

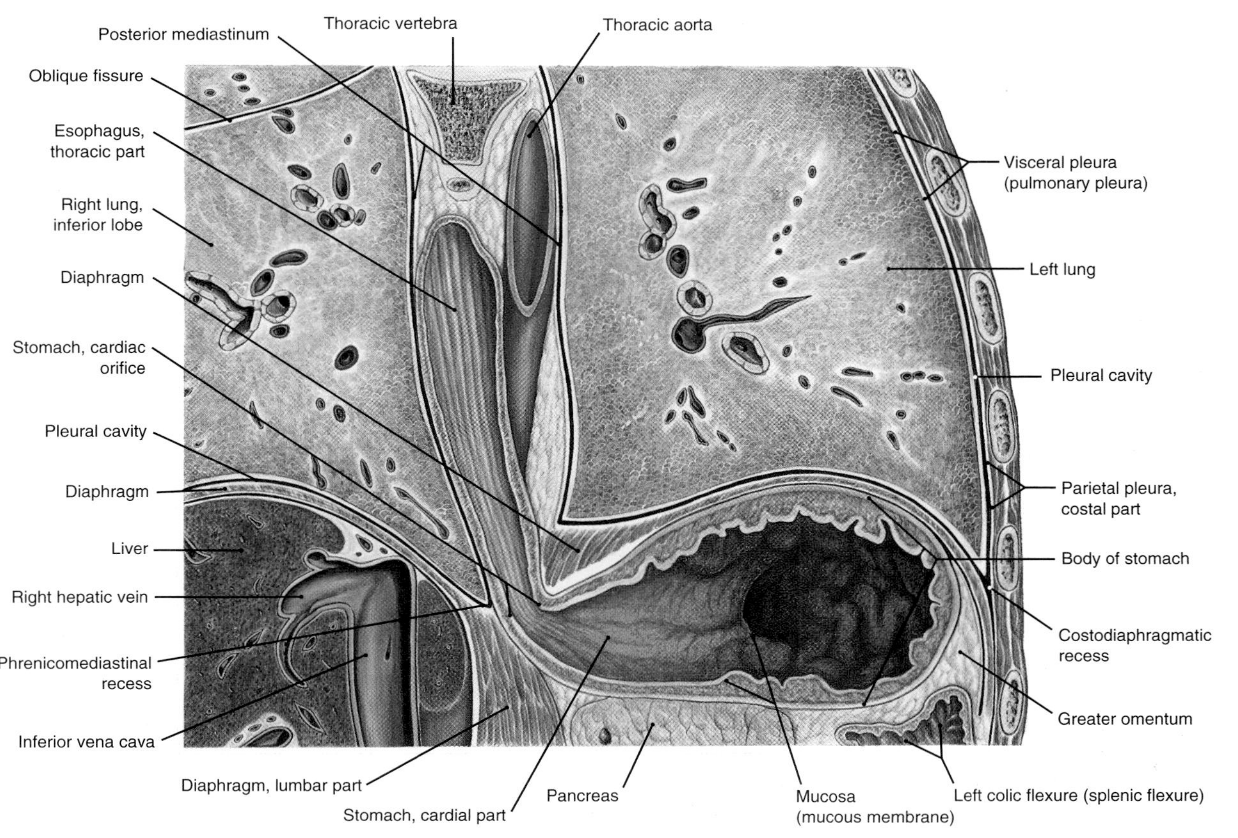
Posterior mediastinum
Thoracic vertebra
Thoracic aorta
Oblique fissure
Esophagus, thoracic part
Visceral pleura (pulmonary pleura)
Right lung, inferior lobe
Left lung
Diaphragm
Stomach, cardiac orifice
Pleural cavity
Pleural cavity
Diaphragm
Parietal pleura, costal part
Liver
Body of stomach
Right hepatic vein
Costodiaphragmatic recess
Phrenicomediastinal recess
Inferior vena cava
Greater omentum
Diaphragm, lumbar part
Pancreas
Mucosa (mucous membrane)
Left colic flexure (splenic flexure)
Stomach, cardial part

Figure 173.2 Frontal Section through the Lower Left Thorax and Upper Left Abdomen (Anterior View)

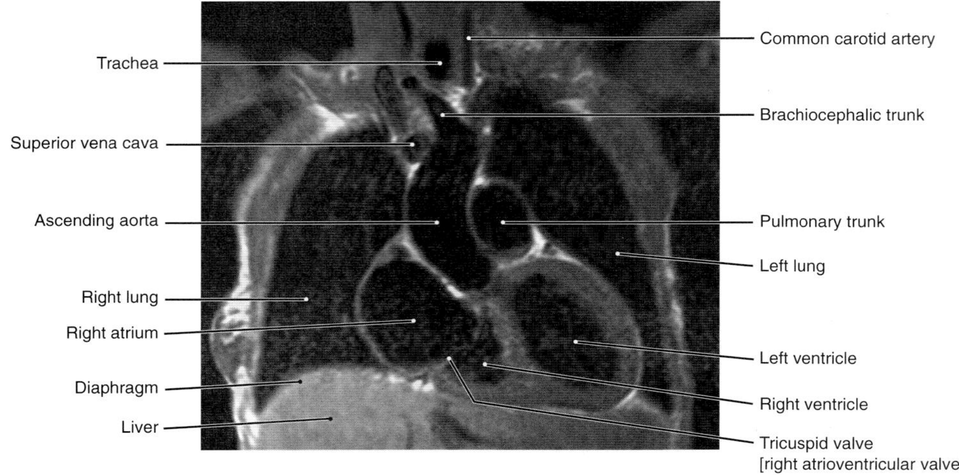

Trachea
Superior vena cava
Ascending aorta
Right lung
Right atrium
Diaphragm
Liver
Common carotid artery
Brachiocephalic trunk
Pulmonary trunk
Left lung
Left ventricle
Right ventricle
Tricuspid valve
[right atrioventricular valve]

Figure 174.1 Magnetic Resonance Image: Frontal Section of the Thorax at the Level of the Superior Vena Cava

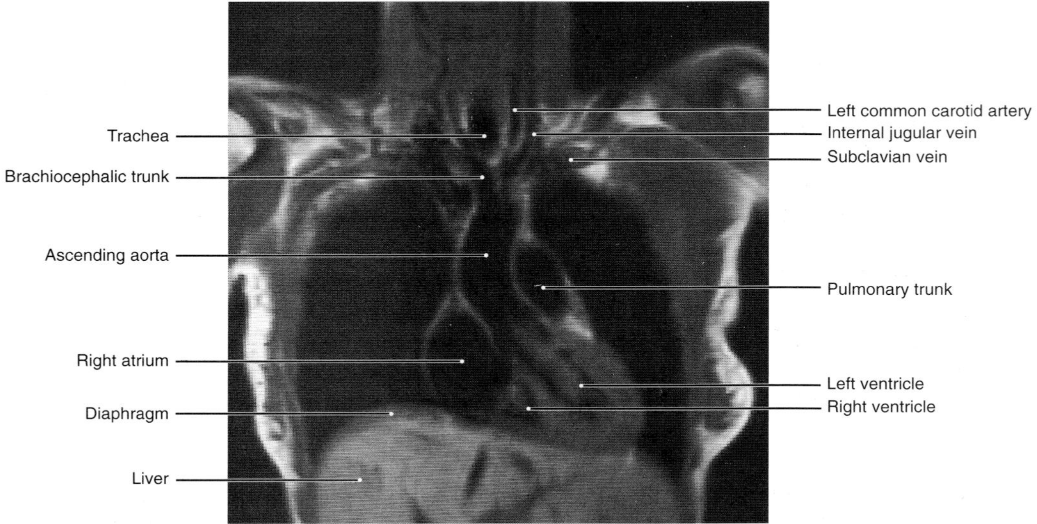

Trachea
Brachiocephalic trunk
Ascending aorta
Right atrium
Diaphragm
Liver
Left common carotid artery
Internal jugular vein
Subclavian vein
Pulmonary trunk
Left ventricle
Right ventricle

Figure 174.2 Magnetic Resonance Image: Frontal Section of the Thorax at the Level of the Ascending Aorta

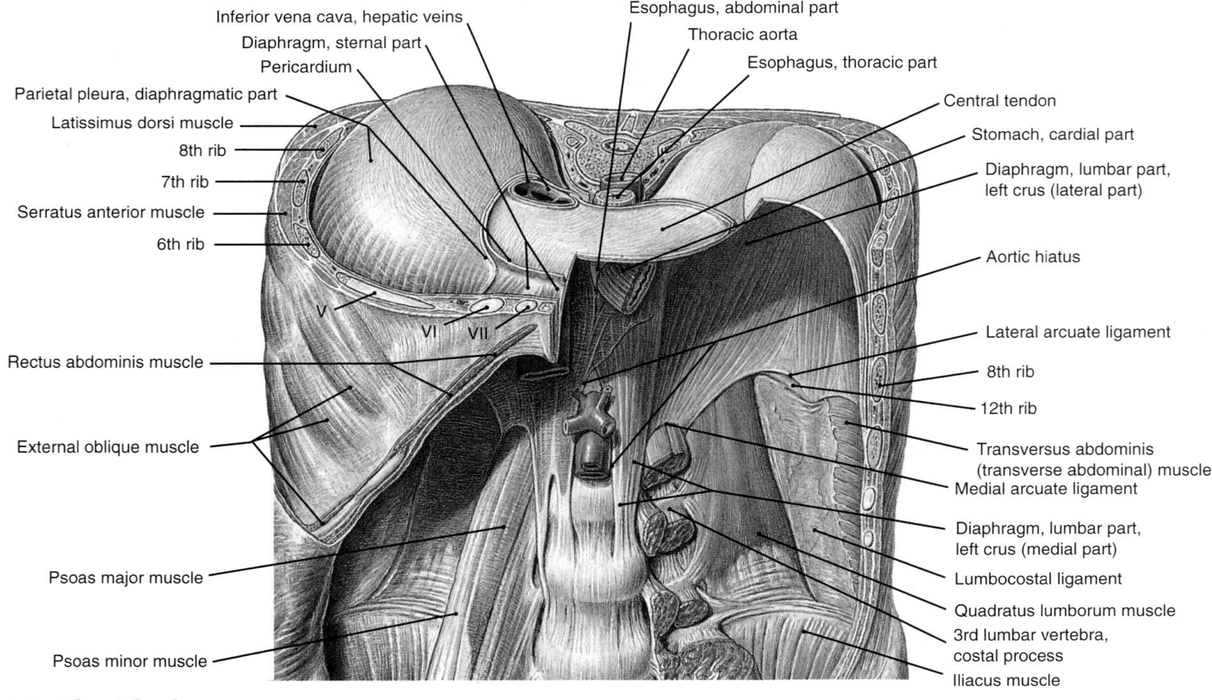

Inferior vena cava, hepatic veins
Diaphragm, sternal part
Pericardium
Parietal pleura, diaphragmatic part
Latissimus dorsi muscle
8th rib
7th rib
Serratus anterior muscle
6th rib
V
VI
VII
Rectus abdominis muscle
External oblique muscle
Psoas major muscle
Psoas minor muscle
Esophagus, abdominal part
Thoracic aorta
Esophagus, thoracic part
Central tendon
Stomach, cardial part
Diaphragm, lumbar part,
left crus (lateral part)
Aortic hiatus
Lateral arcuate ligament
8th rib
12th rib
Transversus abdominis
(transverse abdominal) muscle
Medial arcuate ligament
Diaphragm, lumbar part,
left crus (medial part)
Lumbocostal ligament
Quadratus lumborum muscle
3rd lumbar vertebra,
costal process
Iliacus muscle

Figure 174.3 The Diaphragm

NOTE the inferior vena cava (**vena caval orifice: level of T8**), the esophagus (**esophageal hiatus: level of T10**), and the aorta (**aortic hiatus: at the level of L1**).

THE ABDOMEN

3

PLATES

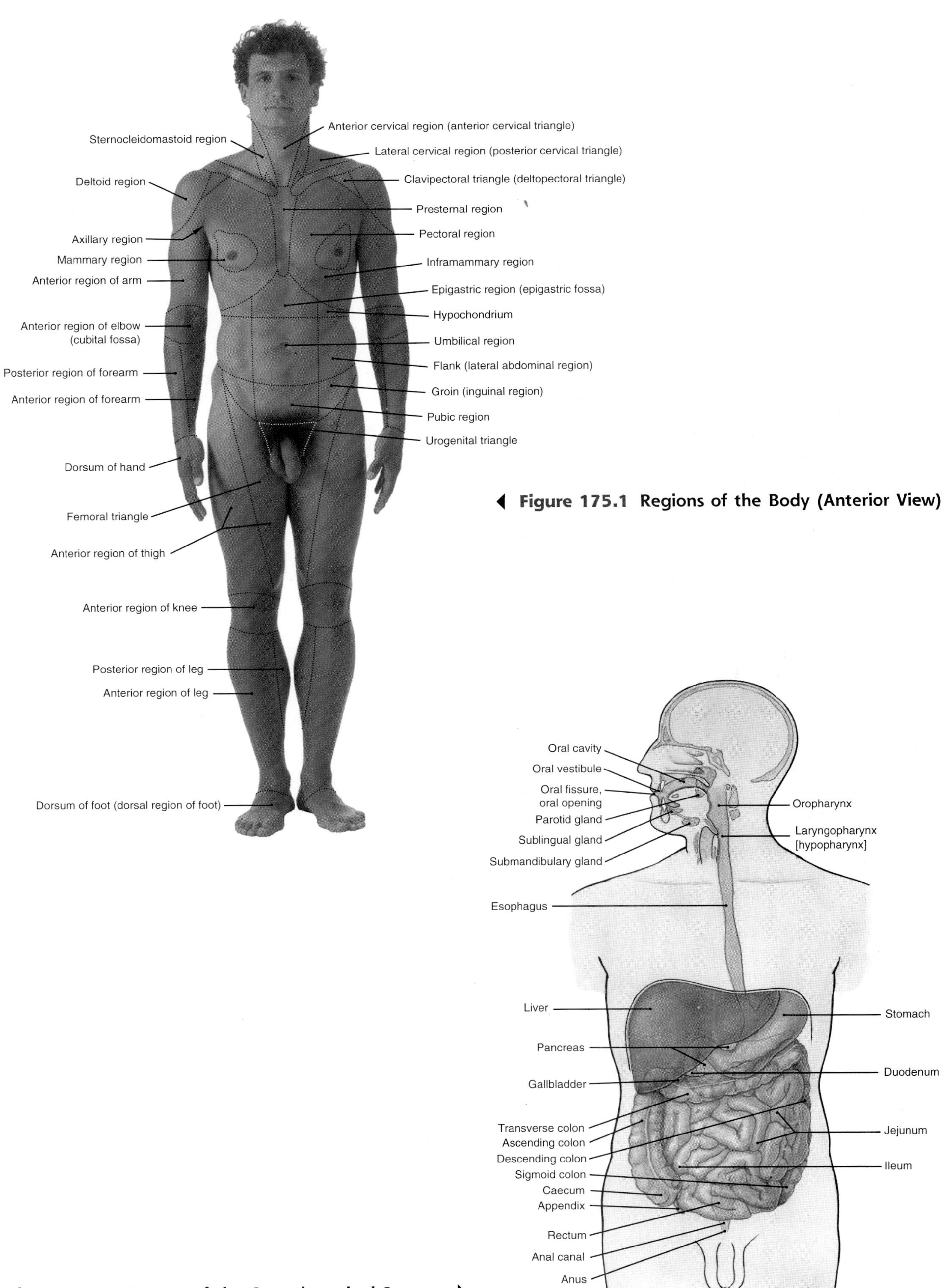
Sternocleidomastoid region
Anterior cervical region (anterior cervical triangle)
Lateral cervical region (posterior cervical triangle)
Deltoid region
Clavipectoral triangle (deltopectoral triangle)
Presternal region
Axillary region
Pectoral region
Mammary region
Inframammary region
Anterior region of arm
Epigastric region (epigastric fossa)
Hypochondrium
Anterior region of elbow (cubital fossa)
Umbilical region
Posterior region of forearm
Flank (lateral abdominal region)
Anterior region of forearm
Groin (inguinal region)
Pubic region
Urogenital triangle
Dorsum of hand
Femoral triangle
Anterior region of thigh
Anterior region of knee
Posterior region of leg
Anterior region of leg
Dorsum of foot (dorsal region of foot)
Oral cavity
Oral vestibule
Oral fissure, oral opening
Parotid gland
Sublingual gland
Submandibulary gland
Oropharynx
Laryngopharynx [hypopharynx]
Esophagus
Liver
Stomach
Pancreas
Duodenum
Gallbladder
Transverse colon
Ascending colon
Descending colon
Sigmoid colon
Caecum
Appendix
Jejunum
Ileum
Rectum
Anal canal
Anus

Figure 175.1 Regions of the Body (Anterior View)

Figure 175.2 Organs of the Gastrointestinal System

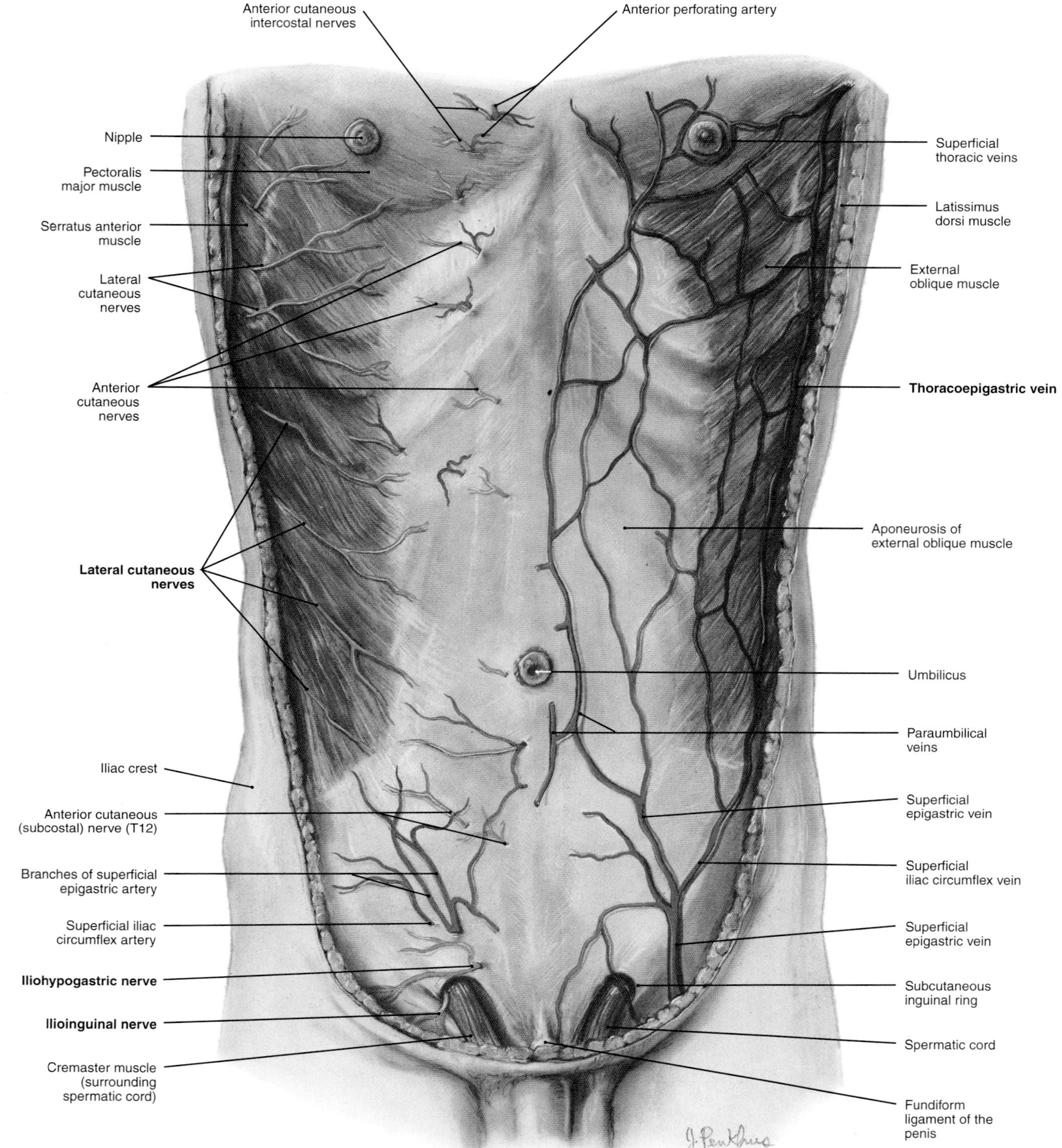
Anterior cutaneous intercostal nerves
Anterior perforating artery
Nipple
Pectoralis major muscle
Serratus anterior muscle
Lateral cutaneous nerves
Anterior cutaneous nerves
Lateral cutaneous nerves
Iliac crest
Anterior cutaneous (subcostal) nerve (T12)
Branches of superficial epigastric artery
Superficial iliac circumflex artery
Iliohypogastric nerve
Ilioinguinal nerve
Cremaster muscle (surrounding spermatic cord)
Superficial thoracic veins
Latissimus dorsi muscle
External oblique muscle
Thoracoepigastric vein
Aponeurosis of external oblique muscle
Umbilicus
Paraumbilical veins
Superficial epigastric vein
Superficial iliac circumflex vein
Superficial epigastric vein
Subcutaneous inguinal ring
Spermatic cord
Fundiform ligament of the penis

Figure 176 Superficial Nerves and Vessels of the Anterior Abdominal Wall

NOTE: (1) The distribution of the superficial vessels and cutaneous nerves upon the removal of the skin and fascia from the lower thoracic and anterior abdominal wall.

(2) The intercostal nerves supply the abdominal surface with lateral and anterior cutaneous branches.

(3) The ilioinguinal and iliohypogastric branches of the first lumbar nerve become superficial in the region of the **superficial inguinal ring.**

(4) The branches of the **superficial epigastric artery** (which arises from the femoral artery) ascending toward the umbilicus from the inguinal region.

(5) The **thoracoepigastric vein** serves as a means of communication between the femoral vein and the axillary vein. In cases of portal vein obstruction, these superficial veins become greatly enlarged (varicosed), a condition called caput medusae.

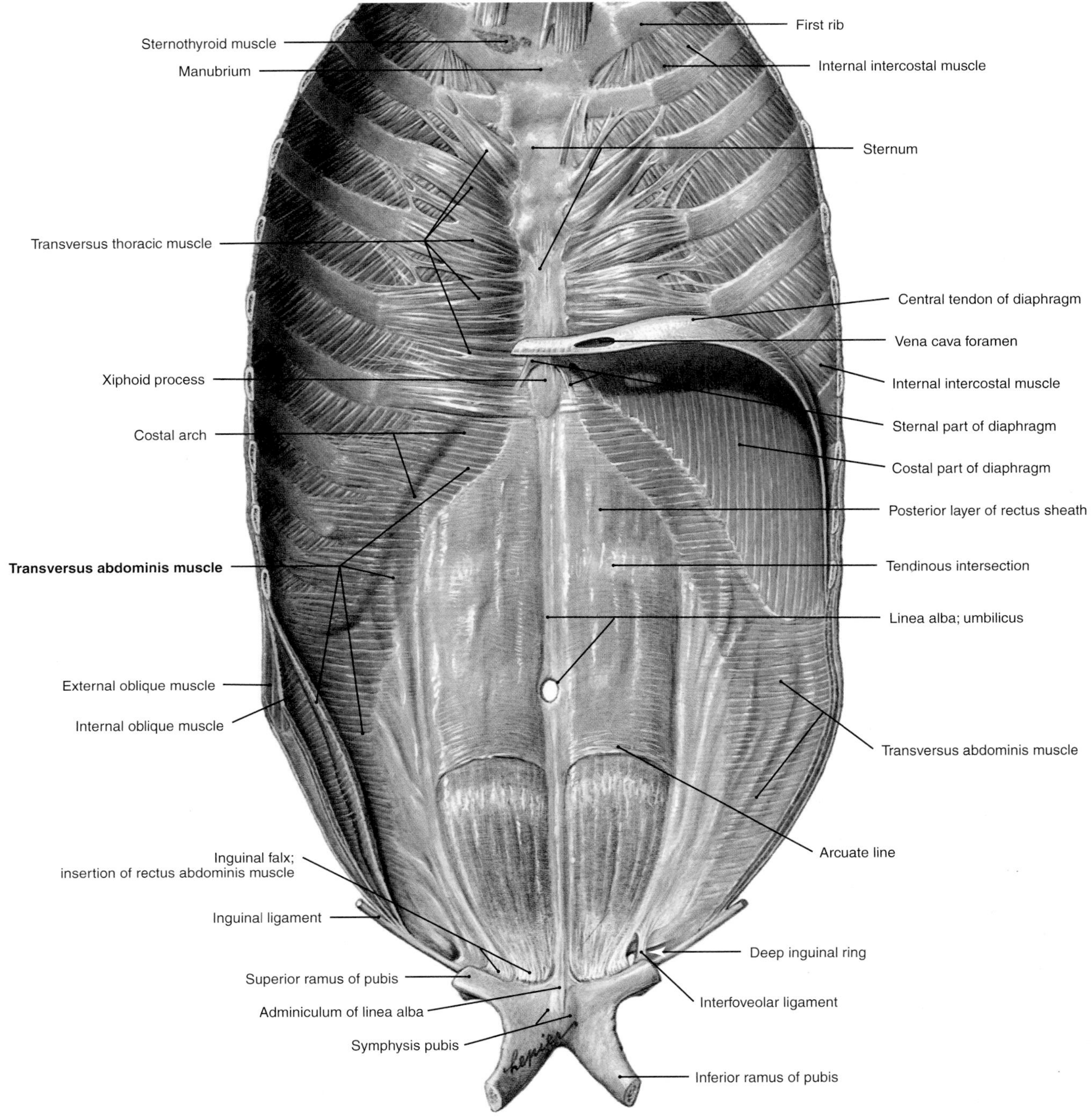
Sternothyroid muscle
Manubrium
First rib
Internal intercostal muscle
Sternum
Transversus thoracic muscle
Central tendon of diaphragm
Vena cava foramen
Internal intercostal muscle
Xiphoid process
Sternal part of diaphragm
Costal arch
Costal part of diaphragm
Posterior layer of rectus sheath
Transversus abdominis muscle
Tendinous intersection
Linea alba; umbilicus
External oblique muscle
Internal oblique muscle
Transversus abdominis muscle
Arcuate line
Inguinal falx;
insertion of rectus abdominis muscle
Inguinal ligament
Deep inguinal ring
Superior ramus of pubis
Interfoveolar ligament
Adminiculum of linea alba
Symphysis pubis
Inferior ramus of pubis

Figure 177 Inner Aspect of the Anterior Thoracic and Abdominal Wall

NOTE: (1) This posterior view of the anterior abdominal and thoracic wall shows to good advantage inferiorly the posterior layer of the rectus sheath and the relationship of the **arcuate line** to the umbilicus. Also note the transversus thoracis muscle on the inner surface of the rib cage.

(2) The opening of the **deep inguinal** (abdominal) **ring** and the **interfoveolar ligament,** a fibrous band that forms the medial edge of the deep inguinal ring and then courses superiorly and medially.

(3) The breadth of the transversus abdominis muscle, which lies adjacent to the next inner layer, the transversalis fascia (not shown).

(4) The transversus thoracis lies in the same plane as the transversus abdominis below. It arises on the inner surface of the sternum and the third to sixth costal cartilages. Its fibers course laterally and upward and insert on the costal cartilages of the second to sixth ribs, acting as depressors of the ribs.

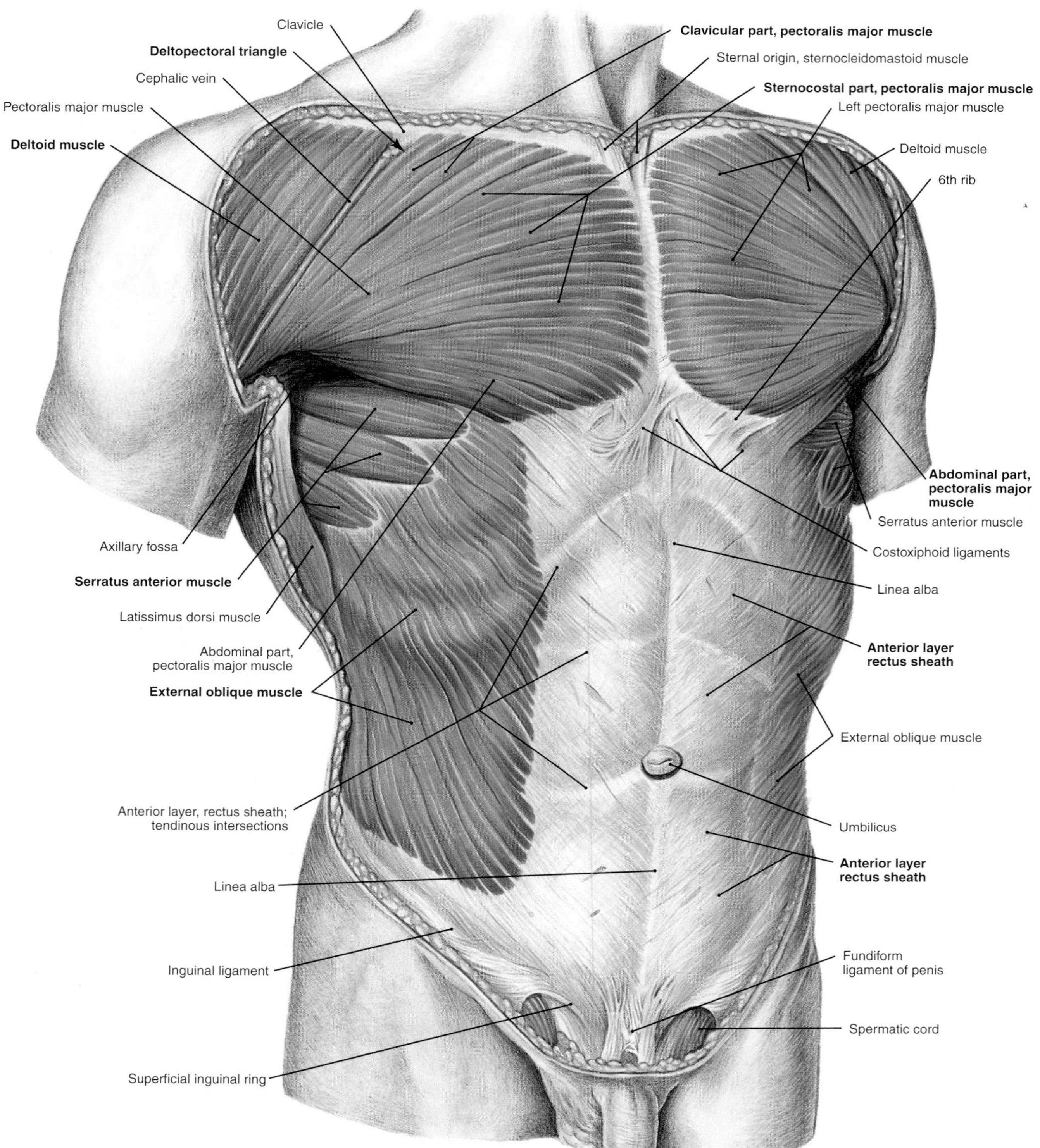
Clavicle
Deltopectoral triangle
Cephalic vein
Pectoralis major muscle
Deltoid muscle
Clavicular part, pectoralis major muscle
Sternal origin, sternocleidomastoid muscle
Sternocostal part, pectoralis major muscle
Left pectoralis major muscle
Deltoid muscle
6th rib
Abdominal part, pectoralis major muscle
Serratus anterior muscle
Costoxiphoid ligaments
Linea alba
Anterior layer rectus sheath
External oblique muscle
Umbilicus
Anterior layer rectus sheath
Fundiform ligament of penis
Spermatic cord
Axillary fossa
Serratus anterior muscle
Latissimus dorsi muscle
Abdominal part, pectoralis major muscle
External oblique muscle
Anterior layer, rectus sheath; tendinous intersections
Linea alba
Inguinal ligament
Superficial inguinal ring

Figure 178 Superficial Musculature of the Anterior Abdominal and Thoracic Wall

NOTE: (1) The first layer of muscles on the anterior abdominal wall consists of the **external oblique muscle** and its broad flat aponeurosis. Medially, this aponeurosis helps form the sheath of the rectus abdominis muscle and inferiorly, it becomes the **inguinal ligament.**

(2) The external oblique arises by means of seven or eight fleshy slips from the outer surfaces of the lower seven ribs, thereby interdigitating with the fleshy origin of the **serratus anterior muscle.**

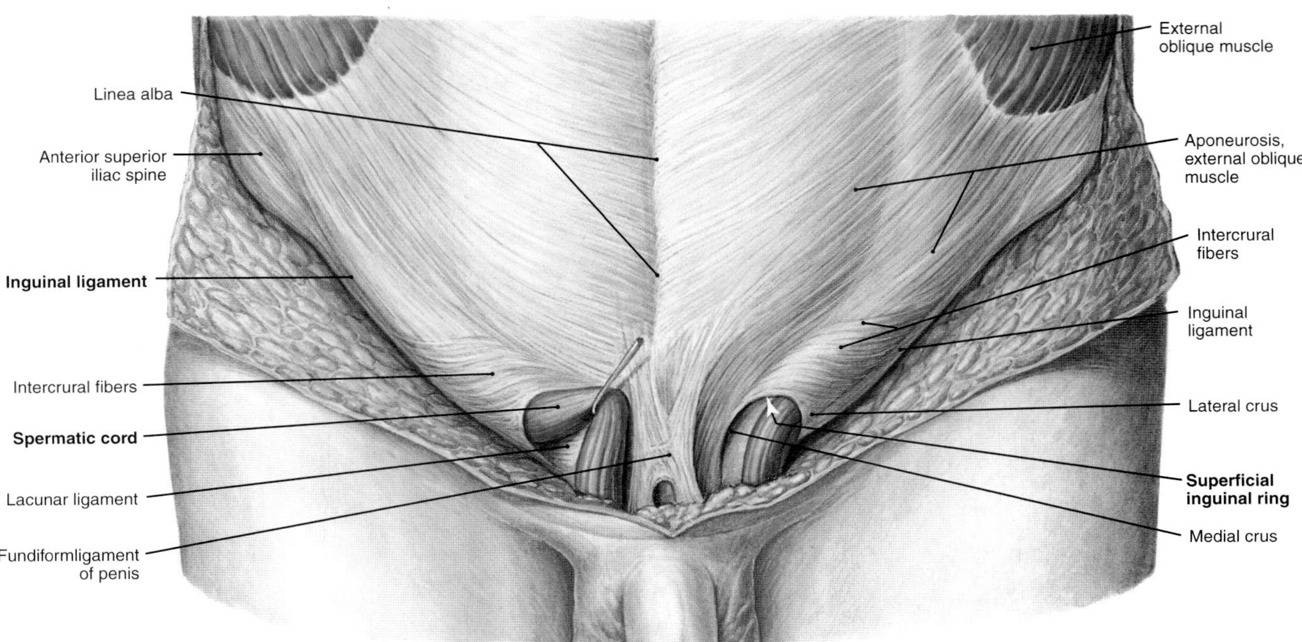
Linea alba
Anterior superior iliac spine
Inguinal ligament
Intercrural fibers
Spermatic cord
Lacunar ligament
Fundiformligament of penis
External oblique muscle
Aponeurosis, external oblique muscle
Intercrural fibers
Inguinal ligament
Lateral crus
Superficial inguinal ring
Medial crus

Figure 179.1 Superficial Inguinal Ring and Spermatic Cord

NOTE: (1) The superficial inguinal ring transmits the **spermatic cord** in the male and the **round ligament of the uterus** in the female. In this dissection, the right spermatic cord has been lifted to show the border of the ring as well as the **lacunar ligament.**

(2) The tendinous fibers of the aponeurosis are continuous with the fleshy fibers of the external oblique. They are directed inferomedially and decussate across the linea alba.

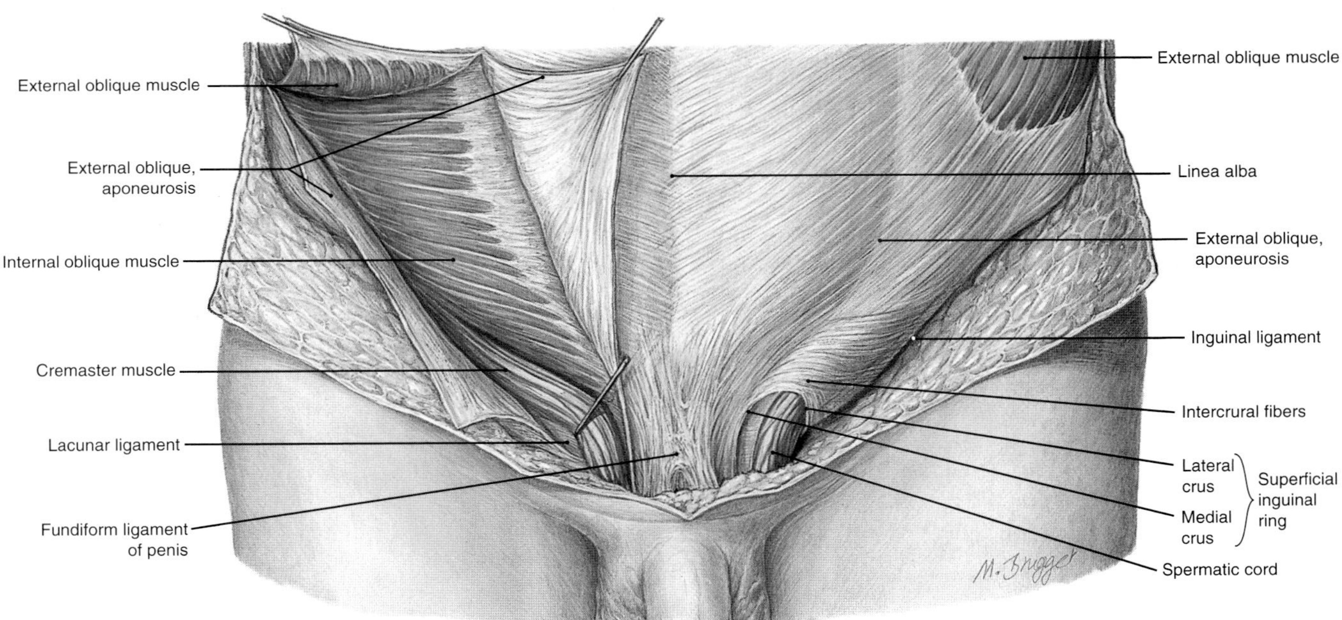
External oblique muscle
External oblique, aponeurosis
Internal oblique muscle
Cremaster muscle
Lacunar ligament
Fundiform ligament of penis
External oblique muscle
Linea alba
External oblique, aponeurosis
Inguinal ligament
Intercrural fibers
Lateral crus
Medial crus
Superficial inguinal ring
Spermatic cord

Figure 179.2 Right Internal Oblique Muscle (Inferior Part) and the Superficial Inguinal Ring

NOTE: (1) The aponeurosis of the external oblique muscle (reader's left) has been severed and lifted to show the inferior part of the internal oblique muscle.

(2) The right superficial inguinal ring has been opened and the right spermatic cord has been hooked and lifted.

(3) The superficial inguinal ring is a slit-like opening in the external oblique muscle. Observe how **the intercrural fibers** strengthen the lateral aspect of the superficial ring by extending between the **medial and lateral crura.**

(4) The **inguinal ligament** extends between the anterior superior iliac spine and the pubic tubercle. This ligament is formed by the lowermost fibers of the external oblique aponeurosis and **lends** support to the inferior part of the anterior abdominal wall.

(5) The fundiform ligament of the penis extends downward from the aponeurosis of the external oblique muscle.

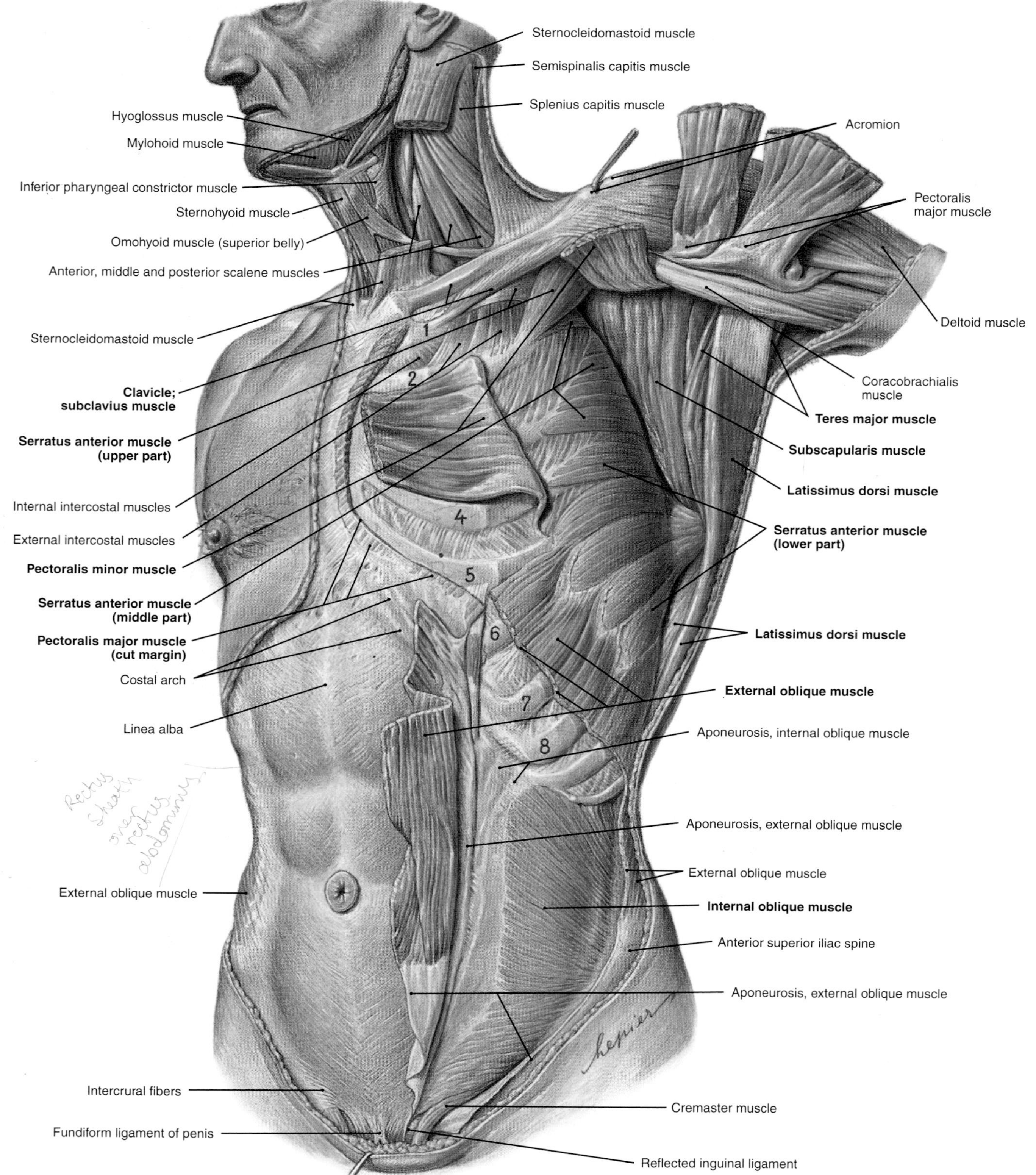
Sternocleidomastoid muscle
Semispinalis capitis muscle
Splenius capitis muscle
Acromion
Pectoralis major muscle
Deltoid muscle
Coracobrachialis muscle
Teres major muscle
Subscapularis muscle
Latissimus dorsi muscle
Serratus anterior muscle (lower part)
Latissimus dorsi muscle
External oblique muscle
Aponeurosis, internal oblique muscle
Aponeurosis, external oblique muscle
External oblique muscle
Internal oblique muscle
Anterior superior iliac spine
Aponeurosis, external oblique muscle
Cremaster muscle
Reflected inguinal ligament
Hyoglossus muscle
Mylohoid muscle
Inferior pharyngeal constrictor muscle
Sternohyoid muscle
Omohyoid muscle (superior belly)
Anterior, middle and posterior scalene muscles
Sternocleidomastoid muscle
Clavicle; subclavius muscle
Serratus anterior muscle (upper part)
Internal intercostal muscles
External intercostal muscles
Pectoralis minor muscle
Serratus anterior muscle (middle part)
Pectoralis major muscle (cut margin)
Costal arch
Linea alba
External oblique muscle
Intercrural fibers
Fundiform ligament of penis
1
2
4
5
6
7
8

Figure 180 Deeper Layers of the Musculature of the Trunk, Axilla, and Neck

NOTE: (1) The pectoralis major and minor muscles have been reflected to expose the underlying digitations of the serratus anterior muscle, which attaches to the upper nine ribs.

(2) The external oblique muscle and the lower lateral part of its aponeurosis have been severed in a semicircular manner near their origin to reveal the underlying internal oblique muscle, which comprises the second layer of anterior abdominal wall muscles.

(3) The muscle fibers of the external oblique course inferomedially (or in the same direction as you would put your hands in your side pockets), whereas **most** of the fibers of the internal oblique course in the opposite direction at a 90-degree angle.

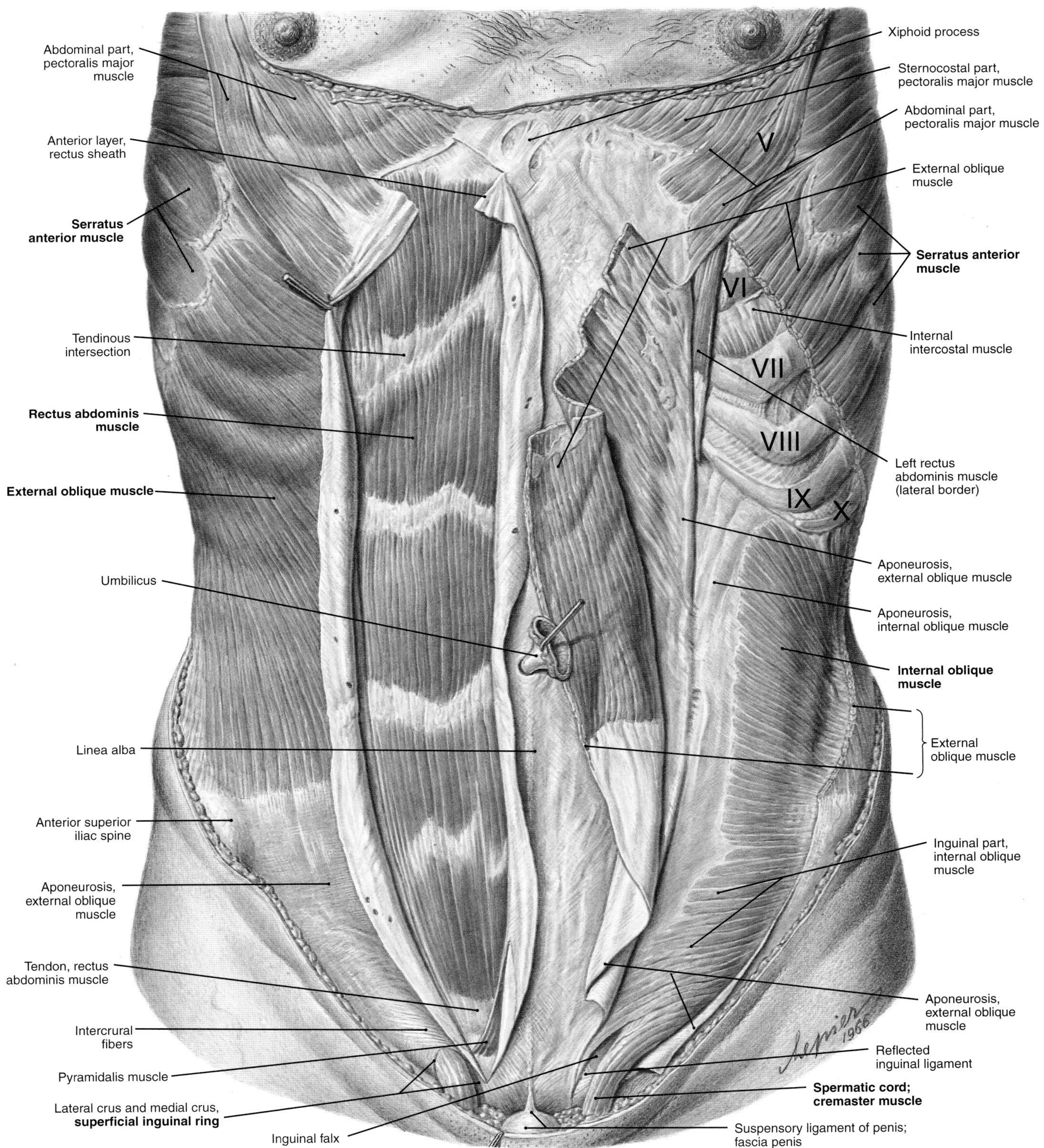

Abdominal part, pectoralis major muscle
Anterior layer, rectus sheath
Serratus anterior muscle
Tendinous intersection
Rectus abdominis muscle
External oblique muscle
Umbilicus
Linea alba
Anterior superior iliac spine
Aponeurosis, external oblique muscle
Tendon, rectus abdominis muscle
Intercrural fibers
Pyramidalis muscle
Lateral crus and medial crus, superficial inguinal ring
Inguinal falx
Xiphoid process
Sternocostal part, pectoralis major muscle
Abdominal part, pectoralis major muscle
External oblique muscle
Serratus anterior muscle
Internal intercostal muscle
Left rectus abdominis muscle (lateral border)
Aponeurosis, external oblique muscle
Aponeurosis, internal oblique muscle
Internal oblique muscle
External oblique muscle
Inguinal part, internal oblique muscle
Aponeurosis, external oblique muscle
Reflected inguinal ligament
Spermatic cord; cremaster muscle
Suspensory ligament of penis; fascia penis
V
VI
VII
VIII
IX
X

Figure 181 Anterior Abdominal Wall: Rectus Abdominis and Internal Oblique Muscles

Muscle	Origin	Insertion	Innervation	Action
External Oblique	Fleshy slips from the outer surface of the lower eight ribs (ribs 5 to 12)	Outer lip of the iliac crest; aponeurosis of external oblique, which ends in a midline raphe, the **linea alba**	Lower seven thoracic nerves (T6–T12)	Compresses the abdominal viscera; **both muscles**: flex the trunk forward; **each muscle**: bends the trunk to that side and rotates the front of the abdomen to the **opposite** side

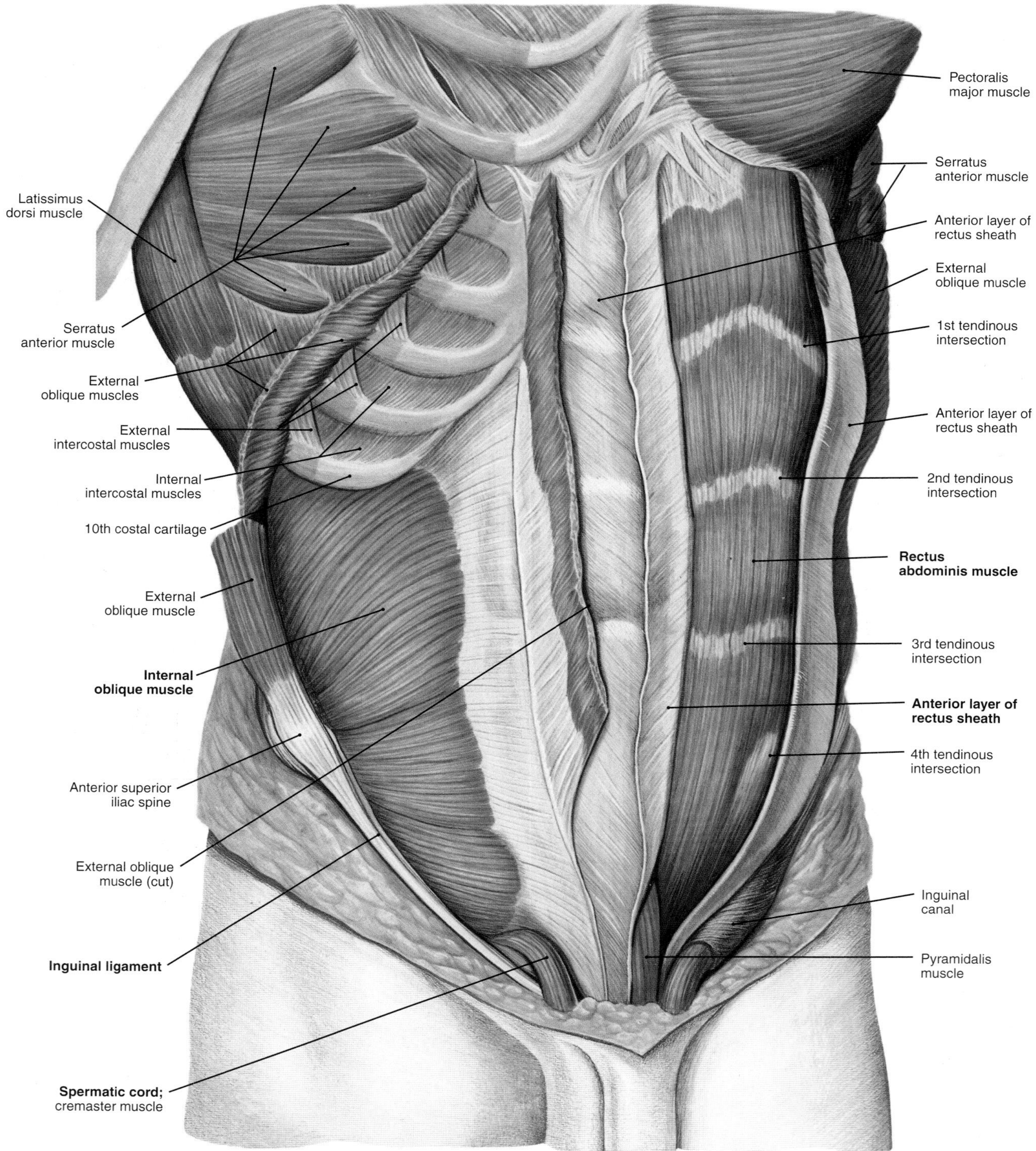
Pectoralis major muscle
Serratus anterior muscle
Anterior layer of rectus sheath
External oblique muscle
1st tendinous intersection
Anterior layer of rectus sheath
2nd tendinous intersection
Rectus abdominis muscle
3rd tendinous intersection
Anterior layer of rectus sheath
4th tendinous intersection
Inguinal canal
Pyramidalis muscle
Latissimus dorsi muscle
Serratus anterior muscle
External oblique muscles
External intercostal muscles
Internal intercostal muscles
10th costal cartilage
External oblique muscle
Internal oblique muscle
Anterior superior iliac spine
External oblique muscle (cut)
Inguinal ligament
Spermatic cord; cremaster muscle

Figure 182 Middle Layer of Abdominal Musculature: Internal Oblique Muscle

Muscle	Origin	Insertion	Innervation	Action
Internal Oblique	Lateral two-thirds of inguinal ligament; the middle lip of the iliac crest; the thoracolumbar fascia	Inferior border of the lower three or four ribs; the**linea alba**; aponeurosis fuses with that of the external oblique tohelp form the rectus sheath	Lower five thoracic nerves and the first lumbar nerve (T8–L1)	Compresses the abdominal viscera; **both muscles:** flex the trunk forward; **each muscle:** bends the trunk to that side but rotates the front of the abdomen toward the **same** side

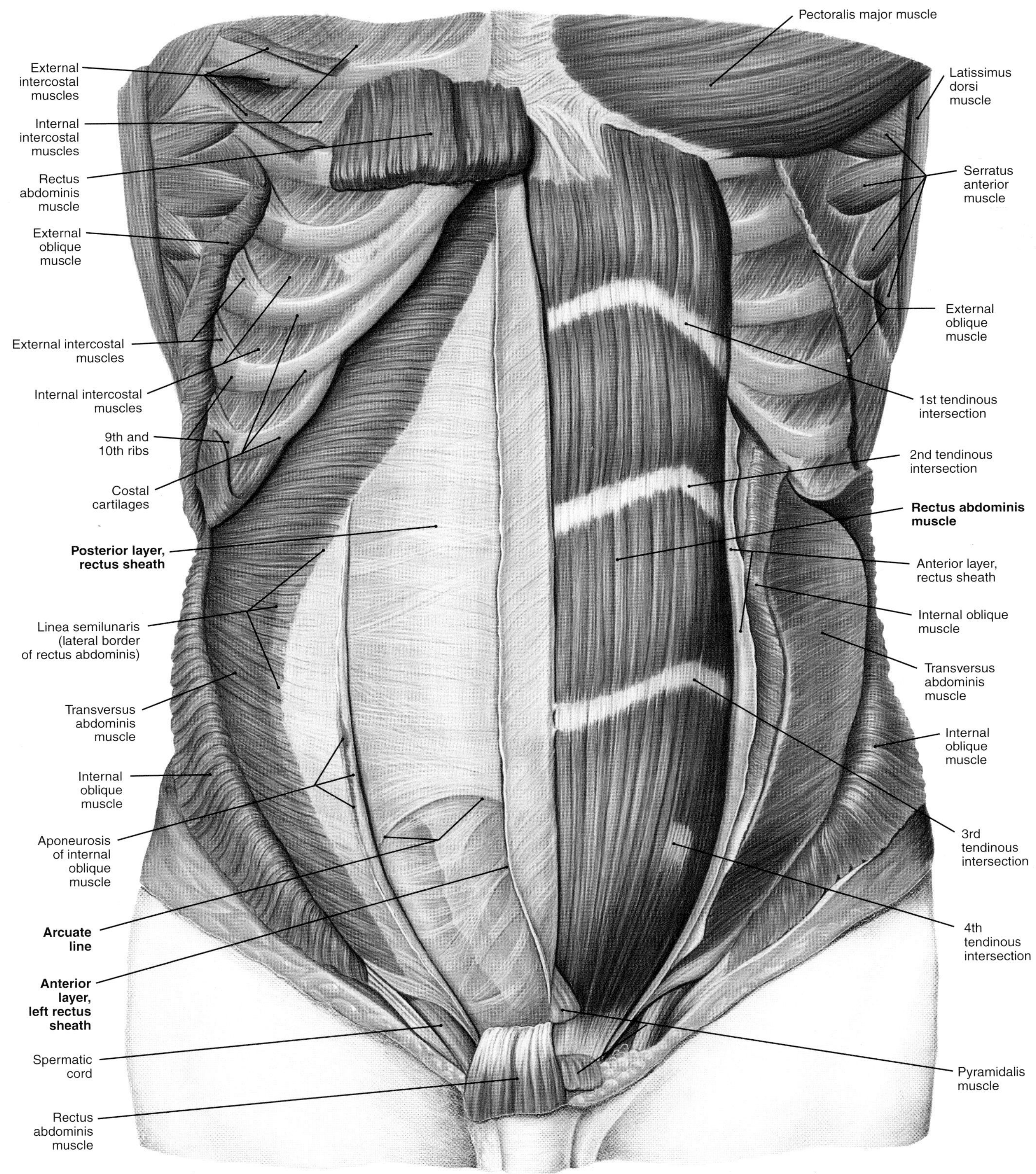
External intercostal muscles
Internal intercostal muscles
Rectus abdominis muscle
External oblique muscle
External intercostal muscles
Internal intercostal muscles
9th and 10th ribs
Costal cartilages
Posterior layer, rectus sheath
Linea semilunaris (lateral border of rectus abdominis)
Transversus abdominis muscle
Internal oblique muscle
Aponeurosis of internal oblique muscle
Arcuate line
Anterior layer, left rectus sheath
Spermatic cord
Rectus abdominis muscle
Pectoralis major muscle
Latissimus dorsi muscle
Serratus anterior muscle
External oblique muscle
1st tendinous intersection
2nd tendinous intersection
Rectus abdominis muscle
Anterior layer, rectus sheath
Internal oblique muscle
Transversus abdominis muscle
Internal oblique muscle
3rd tendinous intersection
4th tendinous intersection
Pyramidalis muscle

Figure 183 Deep Layer of Abdominal Musculature: Transversus Abdominis Muscle

Muscle	Origin	Insertion	Innervation	Action
Transversus abdominis	Lateral third of inguinal ligament and inner lip of iliac crest; thoracolumbar fascia; inner surface of lower six ribs	Ends in an aponeurosis; **upper fibers:** to linea alba, help form posterior layer of rectus sheath; **lower fibers:** attach to pubis to form **conjoined tendon**	Lower six thoracic and first lumbar nerves (T7–L1)	Tenses abdominal wall; compresses abdominal contents

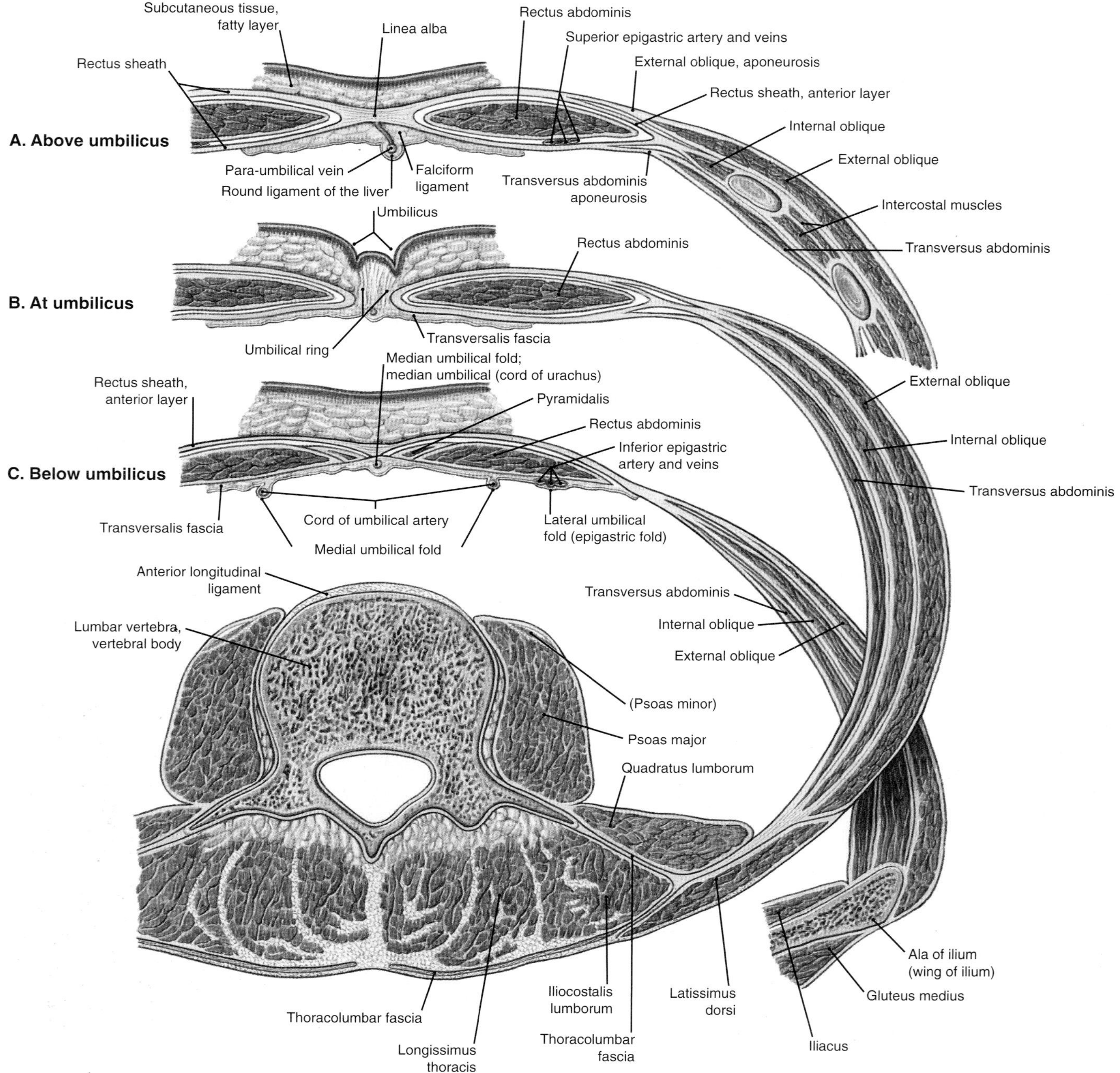
Subcutaneous tissue, fatty layer
Linea alba
Rectus abdominis
Superior epigastric artery and veins
External oblique, aponeurosis
Rectus sheath
Rectus sheath, anterior layer
Internal oblique
A. Above umbilicus
External oblique
Para-umbilical vein
Round ligament of the liver
Falciform ligament
Transversus abdominis aponeurosis
Intercostal muscles
Umbilicus
Transversus abdominis
Rectus abdominis
B. At umbilicus
Transversalis fascia
Umbilical ring
Median umbilical fold; median umbilical (cord of urachus)
Rectus sheath, anterior layer
External oblique
Pyramidalis
Rectus abdominis
Inferior epigastric artery and veins
Internal oblique
C. Below umbilicus
Transversus abdominis
Transversalis fascia
Cord of umbilical artery
Medial umbilical fold
Lateral umbilical fold (epigastric fold)
Anterior longitudinal ligament
Transversus abdominis
Lumbar vertebra, vertebral body
Internal oblique
External oblique
(Psoas minor)
Psoas major
Quadratus lumborum
Ala of ilium (wing of ilium)
Gluteus medius
Iliocostalis lumborum
Latissimus dorsi
Thoracolumbar fascia
Longissimus thoracis
Thoracolumbar fascia
Iliacus

Figure 184 Transverse Sections of the Abdomen at Three Different Levels

NOTE: (1) In **A**, the section is above the umbilicus; in **B**, the section is at the level of the umbilicus; in **C**, the section is below the umbilicus and below the arcuate line. Observe that in **C** only the **transversalis fascia** is found deep to the rectus abdominis muscle and that the posterior layer of the rectus sheath is absent.

(2) The complete transaction seen at the bottom of the figure is continuous with the lateral and anterior muscles at the level of the umbilicus (**B**).

(3) The differences in the sheath of the rectus abdominis (see Figs. 186.1 and 186.2).

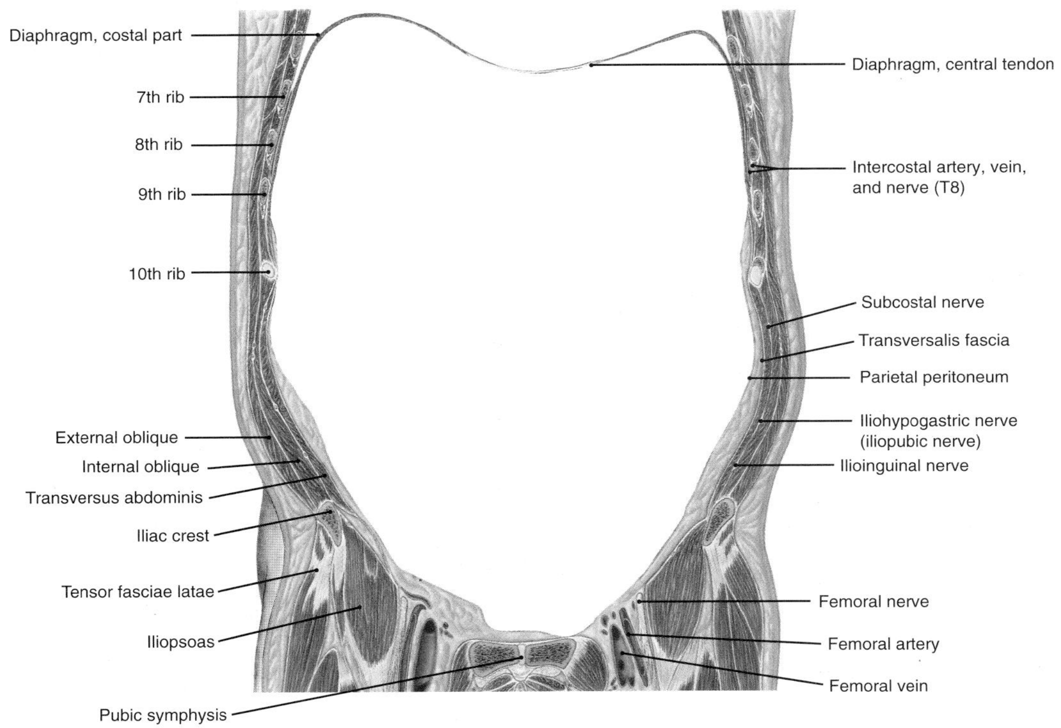
Diaphragm, costal part
7th rib
8th rib
9th rib
10th rib
External oblique
Internal oblique
Transversus abdominis
Iliac crest
Tensor fasciae latae
Iliopsoas
Pubic symphysis
Diaphragm, central tendon
Intercostal artery, vein, and nerve (T8)
Subcostal nerve
Transversalis fascia
Parietal peritoneum
Iliohypogastric nerve (iliopubic nerve)
Ilioinguinal nerve
Femoral nerve
Femoral artery
Femoral vein

Figure 185.1 Frontal Section of the Abdomen through the Iliac Crest and Symphysis Pubis

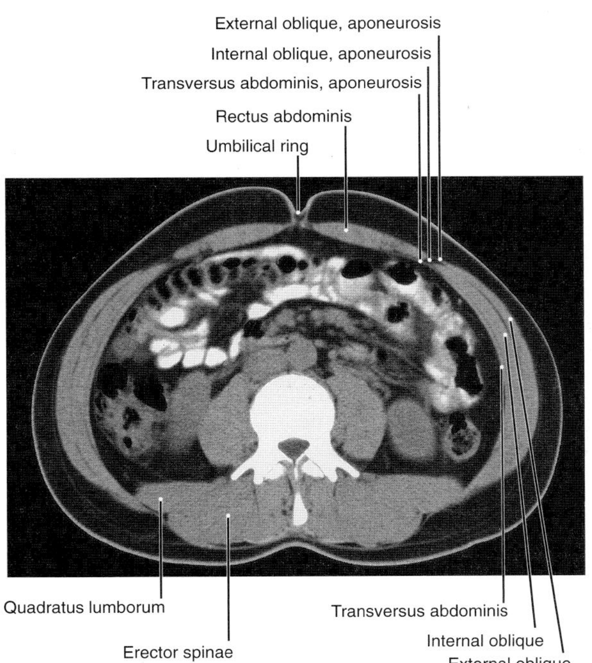
External oblique, aponeurosis
Internal oblique, aponeurosis
Transversus abdominis, aponeurosis
Rectus abdominis
Umbilical ring
Quadratus lumborum
Erector spinae
Transversus abdominis
Internal oblique
External oblique

Figure 185.2 Computed Tomographic Section of the Muscles of the Abdomen at the Level of the Umbilicus

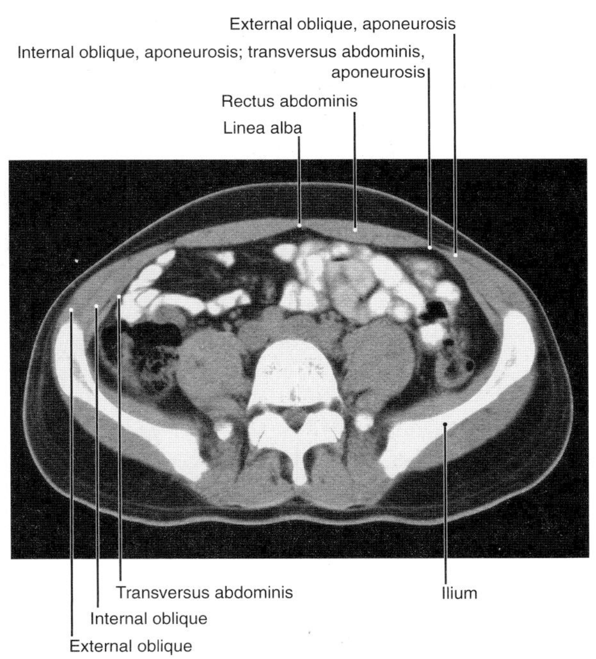
External oblique, aponeurosis
Internal oblique, aponeurosis; transversus abdominis, aponeurosis
Rectus abdominis
Linea alba
Transversus abdominis
Internal oblique
External oblique
Ilium

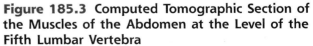

Figure 185.3 Computed Tomographic Section of the Muscles of the Abdomen at the Level of the Fifth Lumbar Vertebra

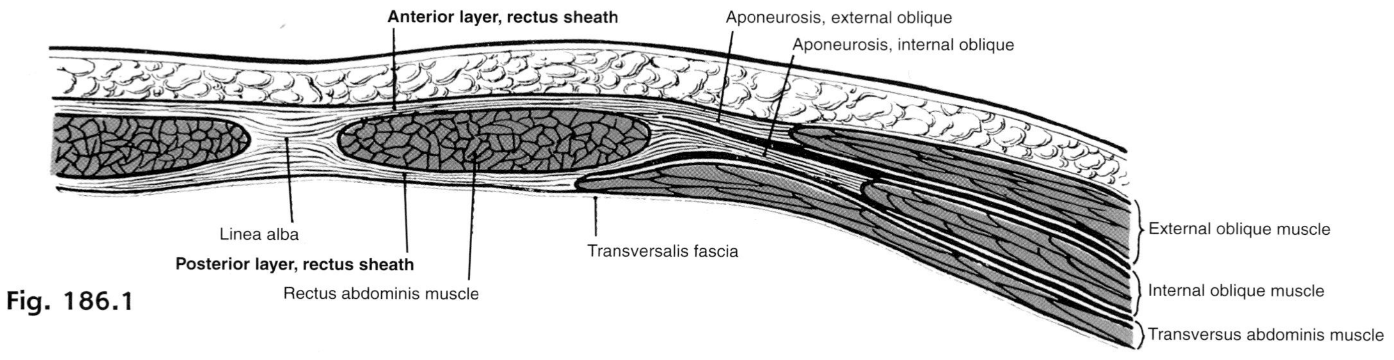
Anterior layer, rectus sheath
Aponeurosis, external oblique
Aponeurosis, internal oblique
Linea alba
Posterior layer, rectus sheath
Rectus abdominis muscle
Transversalis fascia
External oblique muscle
Internal oblique muscle
Transversus abdominis muscle

Fig. 186.1

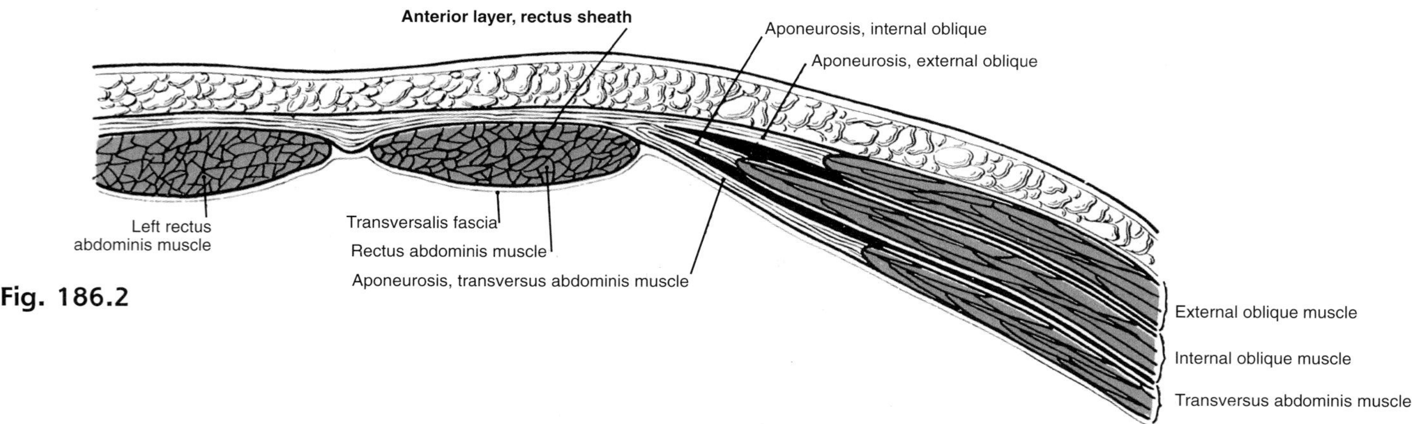
Anterior layer, rectus sheath
Aponeurosis, internal oblique
Aponeurosis, external oblique
Left rectus abdominis muscle
Transversalis fascia
Rectus abdominis muscle
Aponeurosis, transversus abdominis muscle
External oblique muscle
Internal oblique muscle
Transversus abdominis muscle

Fig. 186.2

Figures 186.1, 186.2 Transverse Sections of the Anterior Abdominal Wall: Above the Umbilicus and below the Arcuate Line

NOTE: (1) The sheath of the rectus abdominis is formed by the aponeurosis of the external oblique, internal oblique, and transversus abdominis muscles.

(2) The upper two-thirds of the sheath encloses the rectus muscle both anteriorly and posteriorly. To accomplish this, the internal oblique aponeurosis splits. Part of the internal oblique aponeurosis joins the aponeurosis of the external oblique to form the **anterior layer,** while the other portion joins the aponeurosis of the transversus abdominis to form the **posterior layer** (Fig. 186.1).

(3) The lower third of the sheath, located below the arcuate line, is deficient posteriorly, since the aponeuroses of all three muscles pass anterior to the rectus abdominis muscle (Fig. 186.2).

(4) Deep to the sheath and transversus muscle is located the **transversalis fascia,** interposed between the peritoneum and the anterior wall structures.

Muscle	Origin	Insertion	Innervation	Action
Rectus abdominis	Fifth, sixth, and seventh costal cartilages; costoxiphoid ligaments and xiphoid process	Crest of pubis and pubic tubercle; front of symphysis pubis	Lower seven thoracic nerves (T6–T12)	Flexes vertebral column; tenses anterior abdominal wall; compresses abdominal contents
Cremaster	Midway along the inguinal ligament as a continuation of internal oblique muscle	Onto tubercles and crest of pubis and sheath of rectus abdominis muscle (forms loops over spermatic cord that reach as far as testis)	Genital branch of genitofemoral nerve (L1, L2)	Pulls the testis upward toward the superficial inguinal ring
Pyramidalis	Anterior surface of pubis and anterior pubic ligament	Into **linea alba** between umbilicus and symphysis pubis (muscle variable in size; average, 6 to 7 cm in length)	12th thoracic nerve (T12)	Tenses **linea alba**

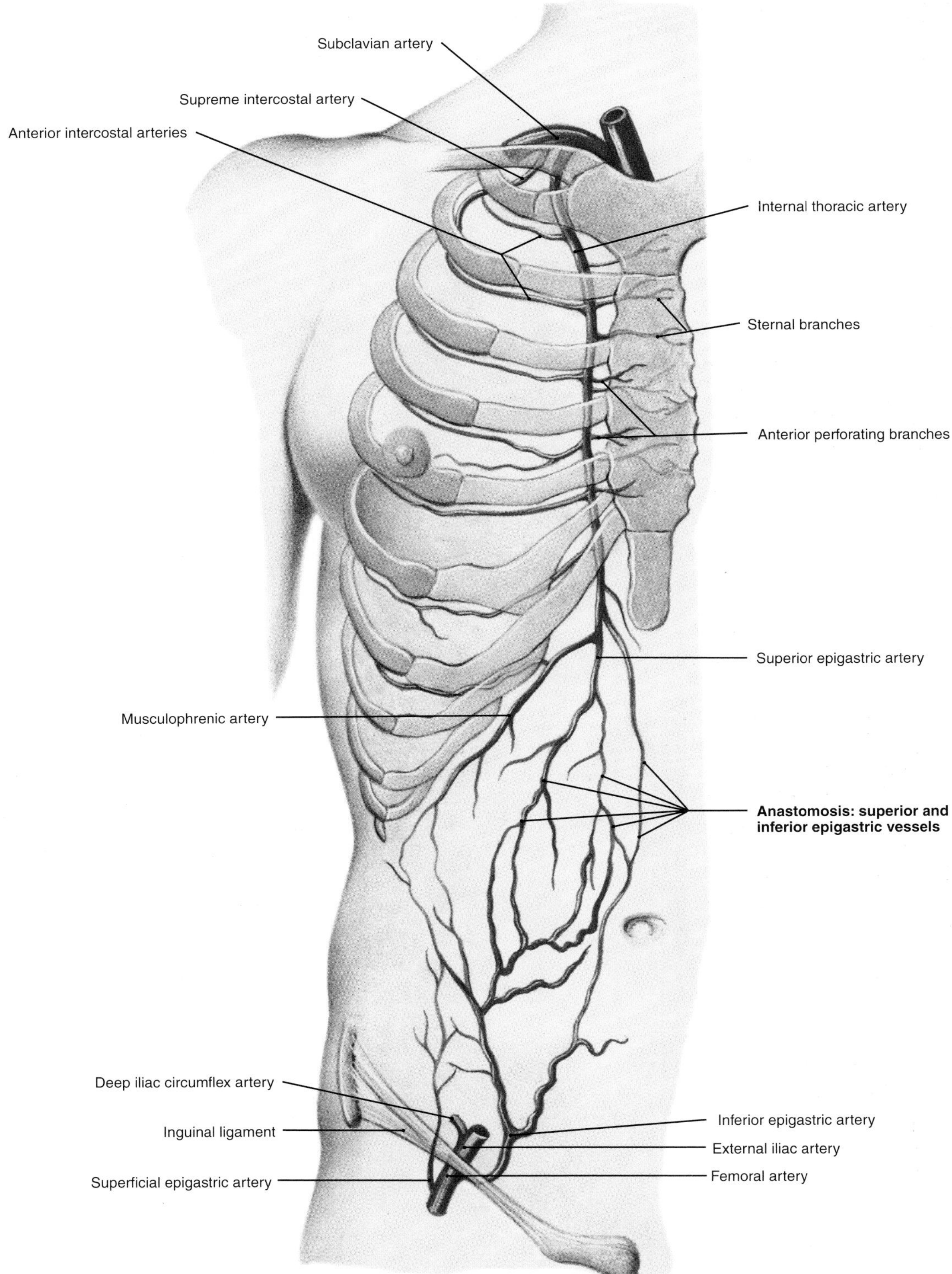
Subclavian artery
Supreme intercostal artery
Anterior intercostal arteries
Internal thoracic artery
Sternal branches
Anterior perforating branches
Superior epigastric artery
Musculophrenic artery
Anastomosis: superior and inferior epigastric vessels
Deep iliac circumflex artery
Inguinal ligament
Superficial epigastric artery
Inferior epigastric artery
External iliac artery
Femoral artery

Figure 187 Schematic Diagram of the Epigastric Anastomosis

NOTE: (1) The **internal thoracic artery** arises from the subclavian artery and descends behind the ribs parallel to the sternum.

(2) Below the sternum, the internal thoracic artery terminates by dividing into the **musculophrenic** and **superior epigastric arteries.**

(3) The musculophrenic artery courses laterally adjacent to the costal margin and helps supply the diaphragm, while the superior epigastric artery descends within the rectus sheath, where it enters the substance of the rectus abdominis muscle.

(4) The inferior epigastric artery is a branch of the external iliac artery. It ascends and enters the rectus sheath at the arcuate line and also ramifies within the rectus abdominis muscle, where it anastomoses with the superior epigastric. This anastomosis forms a functional interconnection between arteries that serve the upper and lower limbs.

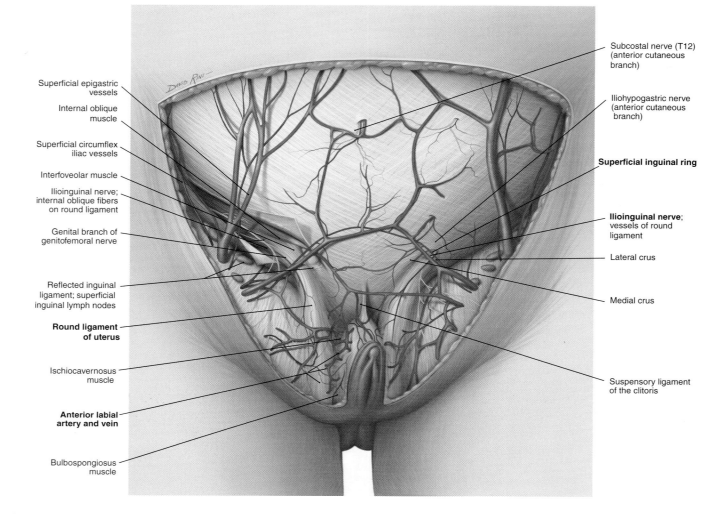
Superficial epigastric vessels
Internal oblique muscle
Superficial circumflex iliac vessels
Interfoveolar muscle
Ilioinguinal nerve; internal oblique fibers on round ligament
Genital branch of genitofemoral nerve
Reflected inguinal ligament; superficial inguinal lymph nodes
Round ligament of uterus
Ischiocavernosus muscle
Anterior labial artery and vein
Bulbospongiosus muscle
Subcostal nerve (T12) (anterior cutaneous branch)
Iliohypogastric nerve (anterior cutaneous branch)
Superficial inguinal ring
Ilioinguinal nerve; vessels of round ligament
Lateral crus
Medial crus
Suspensory ligament of the clitoris

Figure 188 Inguinal Region of the Anterior Abdominal Wall in the Female: Aponeurosis of the External Oblique

NOTE: (1) The skin and superficial fascia have been reflected from the inguinal region, exposing the aponeurosis of the external oblique muscle, the superficial inguinal ring, the superficial vessels and nerves of the lower abdominal wall, and the muscles and nerves of the clitoris.

(2) The **superficial inguinal ring** is an opening in the aponeurosis of the external oblique muscle. On the specimen's left (reader's right) the ring has been opened to reveal the lower course of the round ligament and the ilioinguinal nerve.

(3) The iliohypogastric nerve (branch of L1) as it penetrates the aponeurosis to become a sensory nerve after supplying motor fibers to the underlying musculature.

(4) Of the superficial vessels, observe the **superficial external pudendal** (labeled in Fig. 264), the **superficial iliac circumflex** and **superficial epigastric.** The latter vessels ascend within the superficial fascia between its superficial fatty (Camper's) and deep (Scarpa's) layers.

(5) The **superficial dorsal vein of the clitoris,** which may drain into either the left or right superficial external pudendal vein.

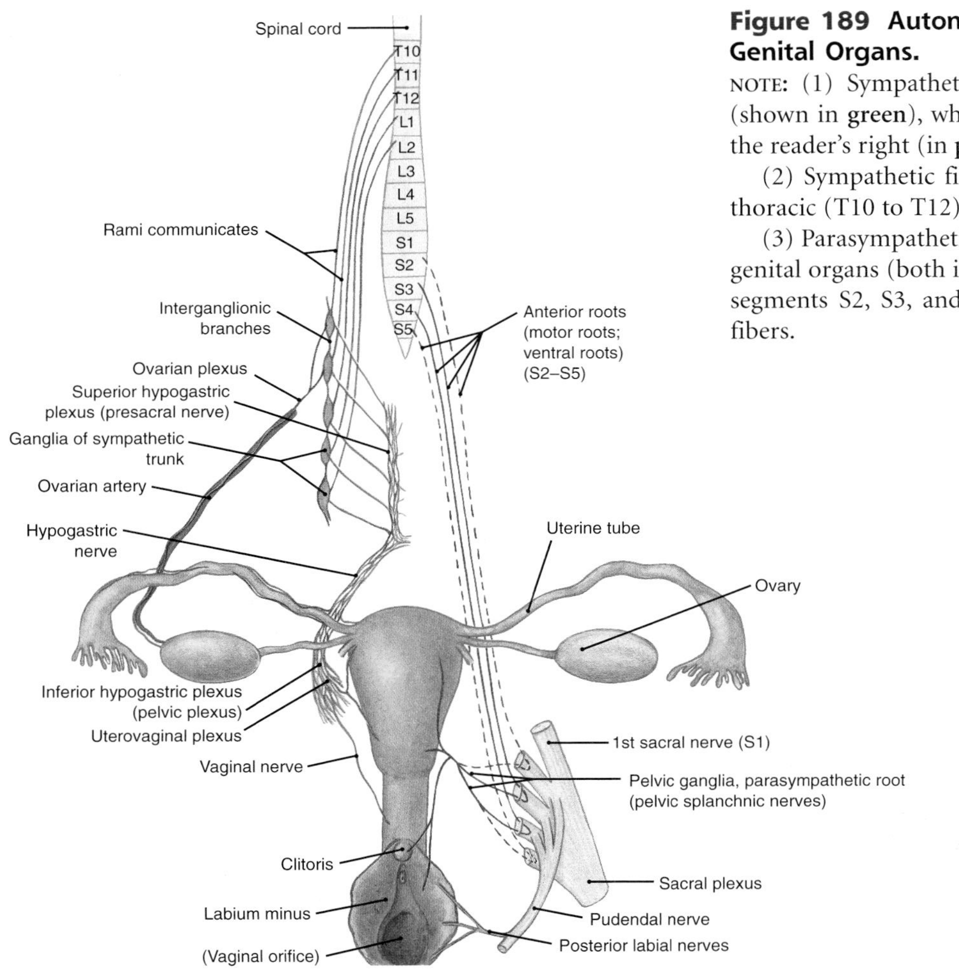
Spinal cord
T10
T11
T12
L1
L2
L3
L4
L5
S1
S2
S3
S4
S5
Rami communicates
Interganglionic branches
Ovarian plexus
Superior hypogastric plexus (presacral nerve)
Ganglia of sympathetic trunk
Ovarian artery
Hypogastric nerve
Anterior roots (motor roots; ventral roots) (S2–S5)
Uterine tube
Ovary
Inferior hypogastric plexus (pelvic plexus)
Uterovaginal plexus
Vaginal nerve
1st sacral nerve (S1)
Pelvic ganglia, parasympathetic root (pelvic splanchnic nerves)
Clitoris
Sacral plexus
Labium minus
Pudendal nerve
(Vaginal orifice)
Posterior labial nerves

Figure 189 Autonomic Innervation of the Female Genital Organs.

NOTE: (1) Sympathetic fibers are indicated on the reader's left (shown in **green**), while the parasympathetic fibers are shown on the reader's right (in **purple**).

(2) Sympathetic fibers descend into the pelvis from the lower thoracic (T10 to T12) and the upper lumbar (L1 to L3) segments.

(3) Parasympathetic preganglionic fibers that supply the female genital organs (both internal and external) are derived from sacral segments S2, S3, and S4. At times S1 and/or S5 also contribute fibers.

INNERVATION OF FEMALE GENITAL ORGANS (BOTH INTERNAL AND EXTERNAL)

	Origin	Course	Organ	Function
Parasympathetic part	Spinal cord, sacral part (S1) **S2**, **S3**, **S4**, (S5)	Pelvic ganglia, parasympathetic root [pelvic splanchnic nerves]	Uterine tube Uterus	Vasodilatation Vasodilatation
		↓ Cavernous nerves of clitoris	Vagina Clitoris	Production of fluid (transudate) Erection
Sympathetic part	Spinal cord, thoracic part **(T10 to T12)** Spinal cord, lumbar part **(L1 to L2 or L3)**	Superior mesenteric plexus ↓ Ovarian plexus	Ovary	Vasoconstriction
		↓ Renal plexus Sympathetic trunk ↓ Superior hypogastric plexus ↓ Hypogastric nerve ↓ Inferior hypogastric plexus ↓ Uterovaginal plexus	Uterine tube Uterus Vagina	Contraction
Somatic efferent **Somatic afferent**		Pudendal nerve Dorsal nerve of clitoris	Clitoris	
		Posterior labial nerves	Labia majora Ischiocavernosus Bulbospongiosus	Contraction

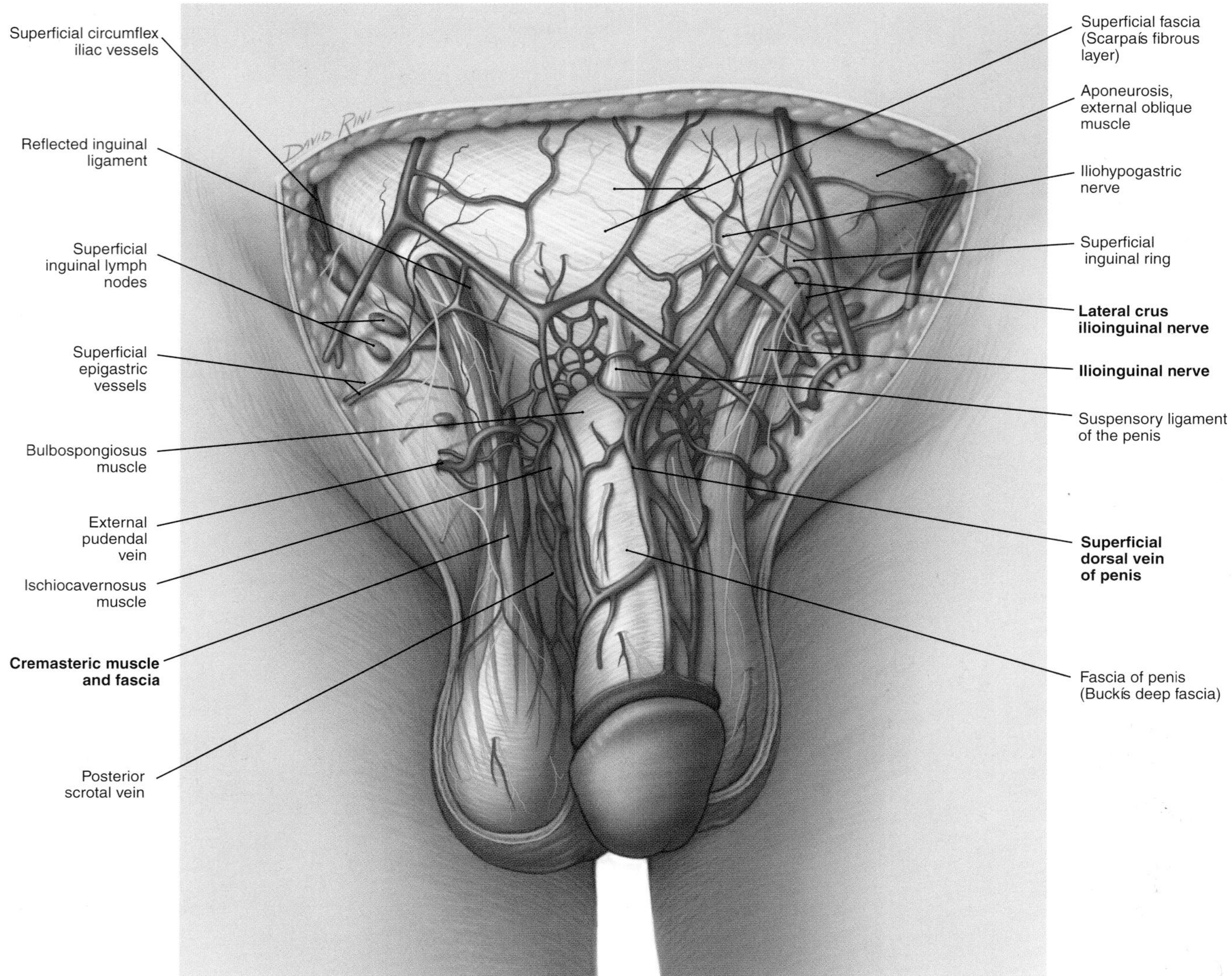
Superficial circumflex iliac vessels
Reflected inguinal ligament
Superficial inguinal lymph nodes
Superficial epigastric vessels
Bulbospongiosus muscle
External pudendal vein
Ischiocavernosus muscle
Cremasteric muscle and fascia
Posterior scrotal vein
Superficial fascia (Scarpa's fibrous layer)
Aponeurosis, external oblique muscle
Iliohypogastric nerve
Superficial inguinal ring
Lateral crus ilioinguinal nerve
Ilioinguinal nerve
Suspensory ligament of the penis
Superficial dorsal vein of penis
Fascia of penis (Buck's deep fascia)

Figure 190 Inguinal Region of the Anterior Abdominal Wall in the Male: Superficial Inguinal Rings and the Cremaster Muscle

NOTE: (1) On the specimen's right (reader's left), the skin and superficial fatty layer (Camper's) has been removed, while on the left side the skin, fatty layer, and superficial fibrous layer (Scarpa's) have been resected, revealing the aponeurosis of the external oblique muscle.

(2) The superficial inguinal rings have been exposed and the scrotal sacs opened. Observe the course of the **spermatic cord** from the scrotum to the superficial inguinal ring and the cremaster muscle and fascia surrounding the spermatic cord on the left.

(3) The **iliohypogastric nerve** penetrates the aponeurosis of the external oblique just above the superficial inguinal ring, and the **ilioinguinal nerve** emerges from the ring to supply the inguinal region and then continues as the **anterior scrotal nerve.**

(4) The external spermatic fascia (not labeled) covering the spermatic cord is seen on the right, while the cremasteric fascia and cremaster muscle are seen on the left after removal of the external spermatic fascia.

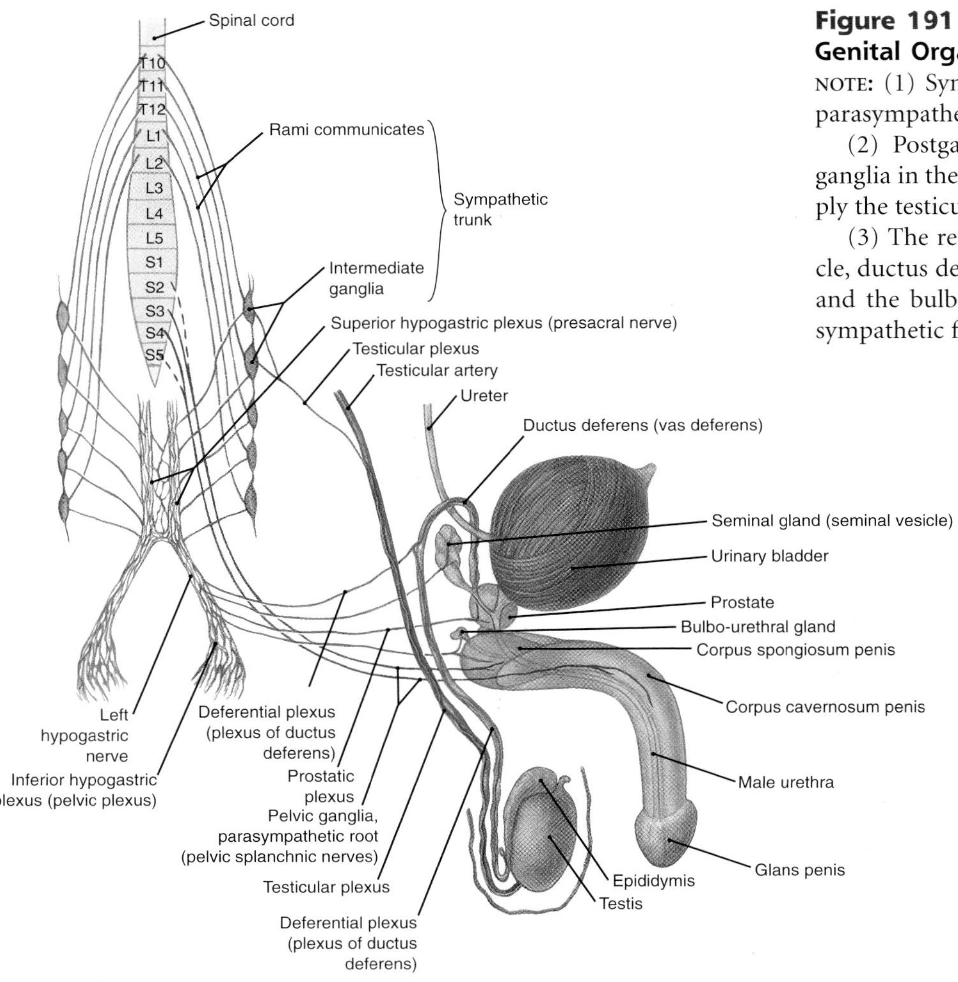

Spinal cord
T10
T11
T12
L1
L2
L3
L4
L5
S1
S2
S3
S4
S5
Rami communicates
Sympathetic trunk
Intermediate ganglia
Superior hypogastric plexus (presacral nerve)
Testicular plexus
Testicular artery
Ureter
Ductus deferens (vas deferens)
Seminal gland (seminal vesicle)
Urinary bladder
Prostate
Bulbo-urethral gland
Corpus spongiosum penis
Corpus cavernosum penis
Male urethra
Glans penis
Epididymis
Testis
Left hypogastric nerve
Inferior hypogastric plexus (pelvic plexus)
Deferential plexus (plexus of ductus deferens)
Prostatic plexus
Pelvic ganglia, parasympathetic root (pelvic splanchnic nerves)
Testicular plexus
Deferential plexus (plexus of ductus deferens)

Figure 191 Autonomic Innervation of the Male Genital Organs

NOTE: (1) Sympathetic fibers are shown in **green,** while parasympathetic fibers are shown in **purple.**

(2) Postganglionic sympathetic fibers derived from ganglia in the sympathetic chain in the sacral region supply the testicular artery and testis.

(3) The remaining male genital organs (seminal vesicle, ductus deferens, prostate gland, bulbourethral gland, and the bulb of the penis) receive their postganglionic sympathetic fibers from the hypogastric plexus.

INNERVATION OF MALE GENITALS

	Origin	Course	Organ	Function
Parasympathetic part	Spinal cord, sacral part (S1) **S2**, **S3**, **S4**, (S5)	Pelvic ganglia, parasympathetic root [pelvic splanchnic nerves]	Penis Corpora cavernosa and spongiosum	Vasodilatation Erection
Sympathetic part	Spinal cord, thoracic part (T10–T12) Spinal cord, lumbar part (L1–L2)	Superior and inferior mesenteric plexus ↓ Sympathetic trunk ↓ Testicular plexus ↓ Superior hypogastric plexus ↓ Hypogastric nerve ↓ Inferior hypogastric plexus	Testis Bulbo-urethral gland Ductus deferens [vas deferens] Seminal gland [seminal vesicle] Prostate	Regulation of blood flow Secretion Contraction, transportation of sperm into urethra Ejaculation into urethra
Somatic efferent **Somatic afferent**	Spinal cord, sacral part (S2–S4)	Pudendal nerve Posterior scrotal nerves Dorsal nerve of penis	(Sphincter of bladder) Ischiocavernosus Bulbospongiosus Skin of scrotum Skin of penis	Closure of bladder prevents retrograde ejaculation into the bladder Expulsion of ejaculate from urethra

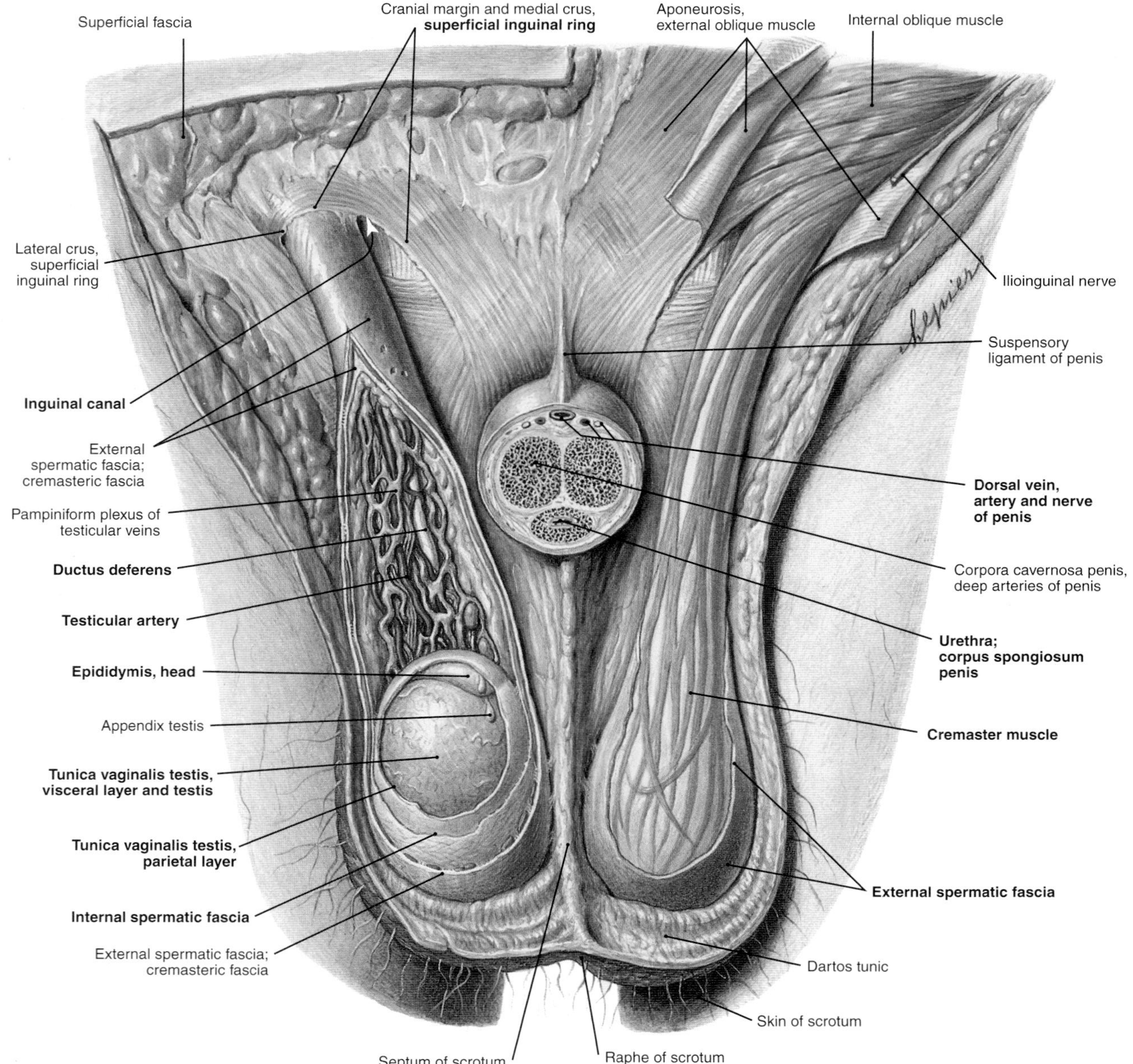
Superficial fascia
Cranial margin and medial crus, superficial inguinal ring
Aponeurosis, external oblique muscle
Internal oblique muscle
Lateral crus, superficial inguinal ring
Ilioinguinal nerve
Suspensory ligament of penis
Inguinal canal
External spermatic fascia; cremasteric fascia
Dorsal vein, artery and nerve of penis
Pampiniform plexus of testicular veins
Corpora cavernosa penis, deep arteries of penis
Ductus deferens
Testicular artery
Urethra; corpus spongiosum penis
Epididymis, head
Appendix testis
Cremaster muscle
Tunica vaginalis testis, visceral layer and testis
Tunica vaginalis testis, parietal layer
External spermatic fascia
Internal spermatic fascia
External spermatic fascia; cremasteric fascia
Dartos tunic
Skin of scrotum
Septum of scrotum
Raphe of scrotum

Figure 192 Spermatic Cord, Testis, Scrotum, and Cross Section of the Penis (Anterior View)

NOTE: (1) The **cremaster muscle** descends within the spermatic cord to the testis. It represents a continuation of muscle fibers of the internal oblique muscle of the anterior abdominal wall.

(2) The **testicular vessels** and **ductus deferens** within the spermatic cord. Observe the covering layers of the right testis, the innermost one of which is the **visceral layer of the tunica vaginalis testis.**

(3) Venous blood from the **pampiniform plexus of veins** ascends in the testicular vein. On the right side this vein drains into the inferior vena cava, while on the left side it drains into the left renal vein. If the veins of the left scrotum become varicosed, it may indicate a problem with the left kidney or in the left pelvis along the course of the vein. This could be due to a renal tumor.

(4) The cremaster muscle is responsible for elevating the testis in the scrotal sac when the testicular environment is especially cold (as in a cold shower). It also elevates if the skin of the upper medial thigh is stimulated. This reaction is due to the so-called cremasteric reflex.

Figure 193.1 Right Testis and Epididymis (Anterior View)
NOTE: The testis is suspended by its efferent duct system, which consists of the head, body, and tail of the epididymis, and this convoluted organ eventually leads to the ductus deferens (see Fig. 194.1).

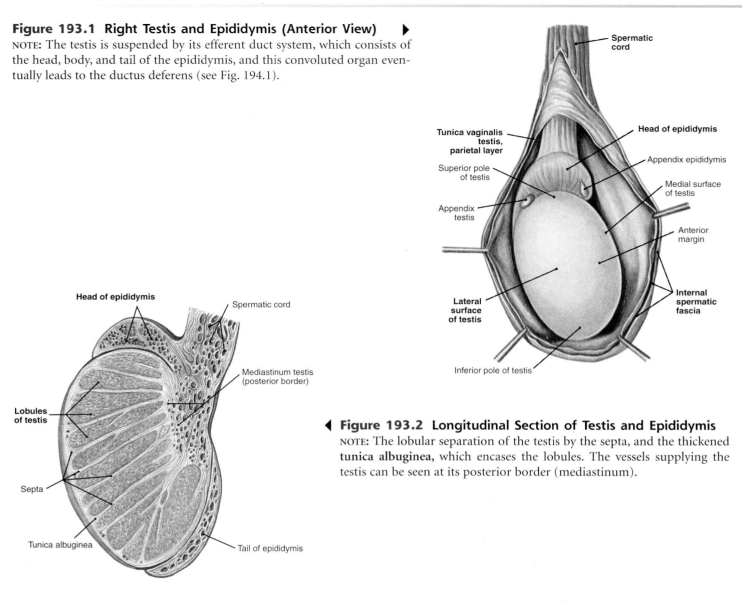

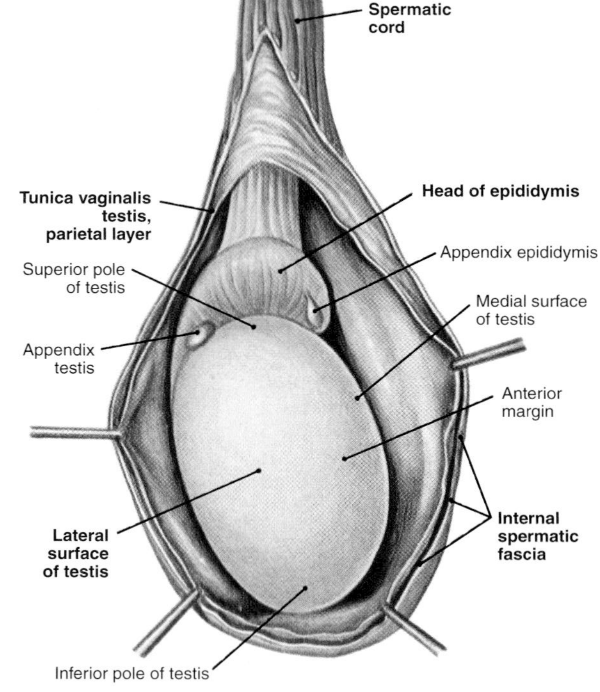
Spermatic cord
Tunica vaginalis testis, parietal layer
Head of epididymis
Superior pole of testis
Appendix epididymis
Medial surface of testis
Appendix testis
Anterior margin
Internal spermatic fascia
Lateral surface of testis
Inferior pole of testis

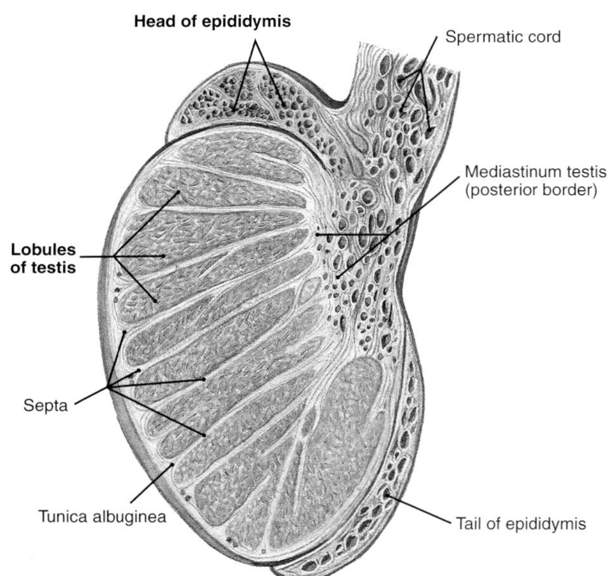
Head of epididymis
Spermatic cord
Mediastinum testis (posterior border)
Lobules of testis
Septa
Tunica albuginea
Tail of epididymis

Figure 193.2 Longitudinal Section of Testis and Epididymis
NOTE: The lobular separation of the testis by the septa, and the thickened **tunica albuginea,** which encases the lobules. The vessels supplying the testis can be seen at its posterior border (mediastinum).

Figure 193.3 Right Testis and Epididymis (Lateral View)
NOTE: The coverings of the testis represent evaginations of the layers forming the anterior abdominal wall. These evaginations precede the testis during its descent in the latter half of gestation. The comparable layers are as follows:

Anterior Abdominal Wall	Coverings of Testis
1. Skin	1. Skin } Scrotum
2. Superficial fascia	2. Dartos tunic } Scrotum
3. External oblique	3. External spermatic fascia
4. } Internal oblique	4. } Cremaster muscle and
5. } Transversus abdominis	5. } Cremasteric fascia
6. Transversalis fascia	6. Internal spermatic fascia
7. Extraperitoneal fat	7. Fatty layer
8. Peritoneum	8. Processus vaginalis

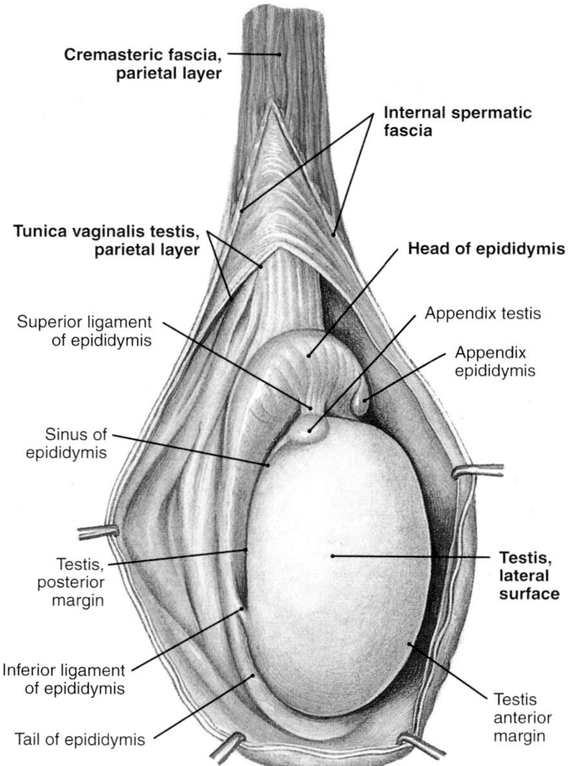
Cremasteric fascia, parietal layer
Internal spermatic fascia
Tunica vaginalis testis, parietal layer
Head of epididymis
Superior ligament of epididymis
Appendix testis
Appendix epididymis
Sinus of epididymis
Testis, posterior margin
Testis, lateral surface
Inferior ligament of epididymis
Testis anterior margin
Tail of epididymis

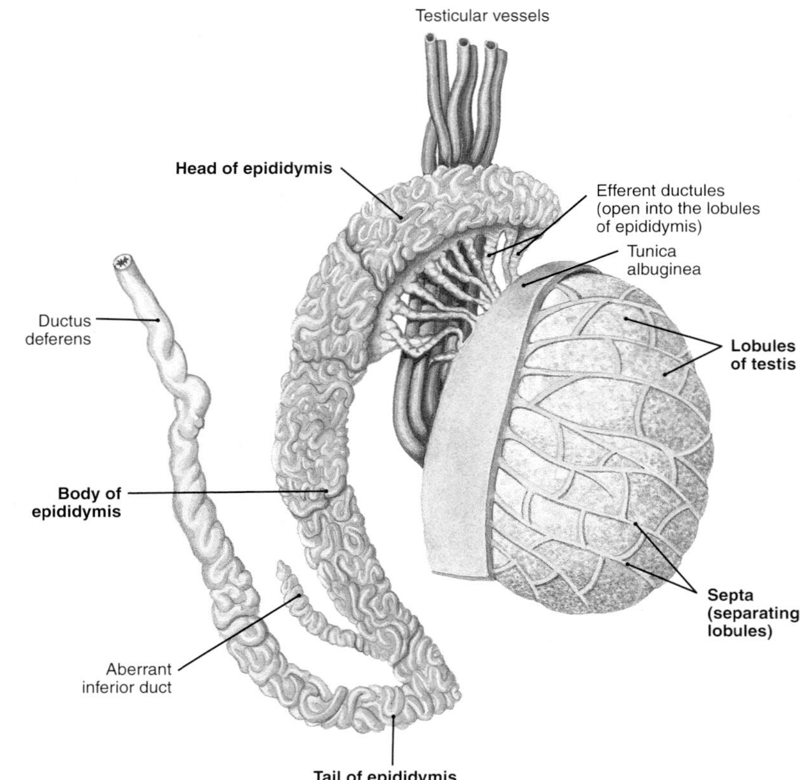
Testicular vessels
Head of epididymis
Efferent ductules (open into the lobules of epididymis)
Tunica albuginea
Ductus deferens
Lobules of testis
Body of epididymis
Septa (separating lobules)
Aberrant inferior duct
Tail of epididymis

Figure 194.1 Testis, Epididymis, and the Beginning of the Ductus Deferens

NOTE: (1) With the tunica vaginalis and tunica albuginea removed, the testicular lobule, separated by septa and containing the seminiferous tubules are exposed.

(2) From the lobules a group of 8 to 10 fine efferent ductules open into the **head of the epididymis.** Observe the highly convoluted nature of the epididymis. The head of the epididymis leads into the **body** and **tail,** which becomes the **ductus deferens.**

(3) The **testicular artery** (from the aorta) courses with the spermatic cord and the **pampiniform plexus** of veins.

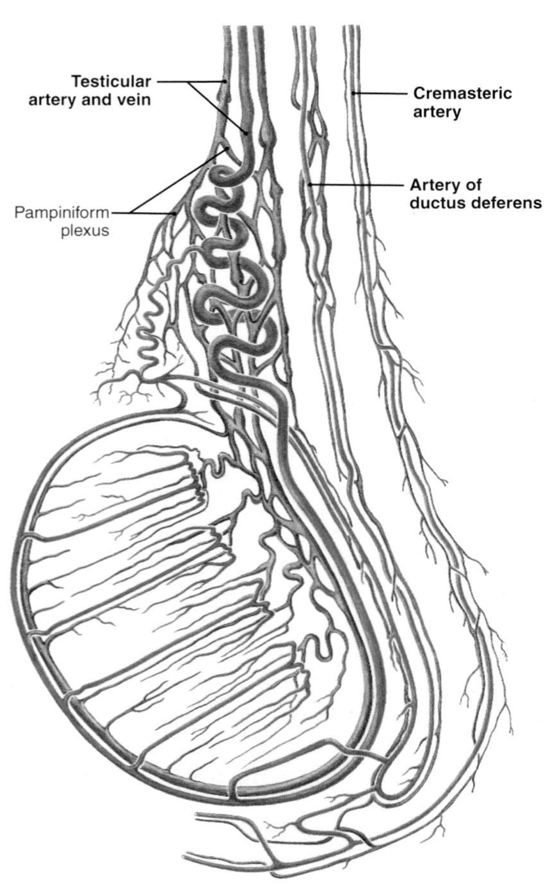
Testicular artery and vein
Cremasteric artery
Artery of ductus deferens
Pampiniform plexus

Figure 194.2 Schematic Representation of the Blood Supply of the Testis and Epididymis

(1) The testis and epididymis are served by the **testicular artery** (from the aorta), the **artery of the ductus deferens** (usually from the superior vesical artery). and the **cremasteric artery** (from the inferior epigastric artery).

(2) The **pampiniform plexus** of veins drains into the testicular vein, which on the left side flows into the left renal vein, and on the right side opens into the inferior vena cava.

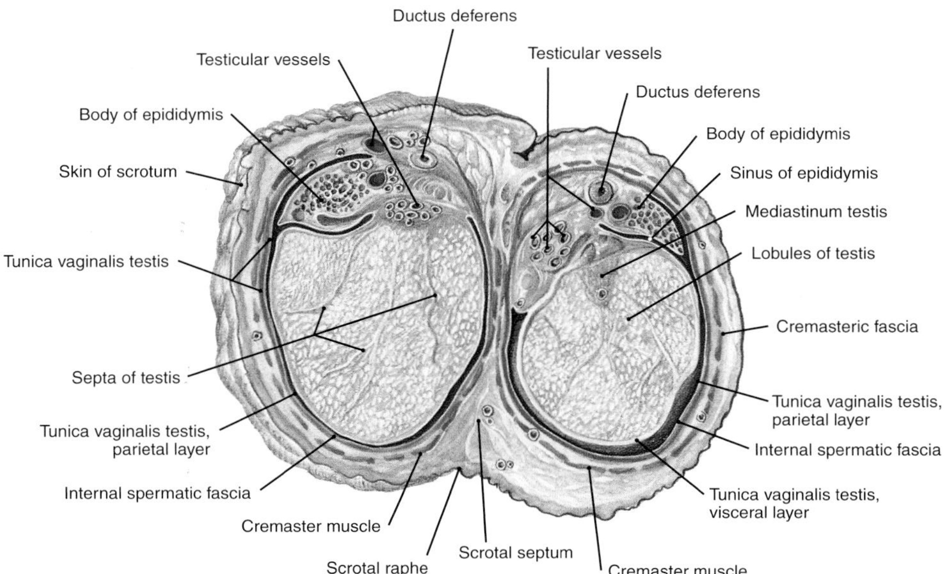
Ductus deferens
Testicular vessels
Testicular vessels
Ductus deferens
Body of epididymis
Body of epididymis
Skin of scrotum
Sinus of epididymis
Mediastinum testis
Tunica vaginalis testis
Lobules of testis
Cremasteric fascia
Septa of testis
Tunica vaginalis testis, parietal layer
Tunica vaginalis testis, parietal layer
Internal spermatic fascia
Internal spermatic fascia
Tunica vaginalis testis, visceral layer
Cremaster muscle
Scrotal septum
Scrotal raphe
Cremaster muscle

Figure 195.1 Cross Section of Testis and Scrotum

NOTE: (1) The scrotum is divided by the median raphe and septum into two lateral compartments, each surrounding an ovoid-shaped testis. The two scrotal compartments normally do not communicate.

(2) The **tunica vaginalis testis** consists of a **visceral layer** closely adherent to the testis and a **parietal layer,** which lines the inner surface of the internal spermatic fascia in the scrotum. A serous cavity or potential space between these two layers is a site where fluid might collect to form a **hydrocele.** These may be acquired or congenital.

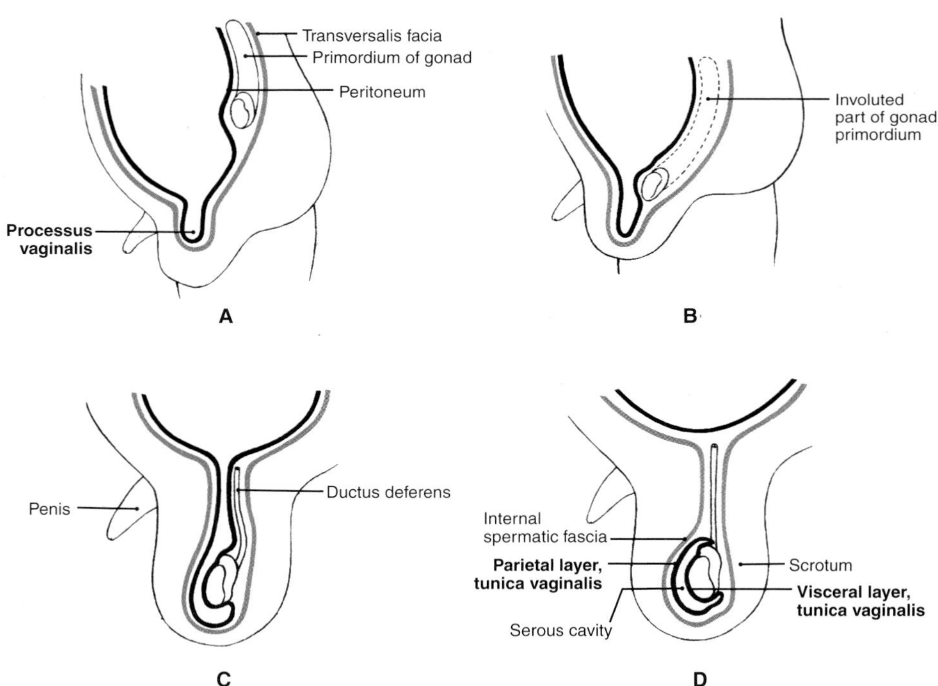
Transversalis facia
Primordium of gonad
Peritoneum
Involuted part of gonad primordium
Processus vaginalis
A
B
Penis
Ductus deferens
Internal spermatic fascia
Parietal layer, tunica vaginalis
Scrotum
Visceral layer, tunica vaginalis
Serous cavity
C
D

Figure 195.2 Diagrammatic Representation of Four Stages in the Descent of the Testis

NOTE: (1) (**A**) The testes commence development on the posterior wall of the fetus; (**B**) during the second trimester they attach to the posterior wall of the lower trunk at the boundary between the abdomen and pelvis in what is often called the "false pelvis.".

(2) During the latter half of the seventh month of gestation, the testes begin their descent into the scrotum (**B** and **C**); this is normally completed by the ninth month (**D**).

(3) Attached to the peritoneum, each testis carries with it a peritoneal sac that surrounds the organ in the scrotum as the **parietal and visceral layers of the tunica vaginalis.** The peritoneum lining the inguinal canal then fuses, closing off its communication with the abdominal cavity.

(4) When this fusion does not occur, the pathway may be used by a loop of intestine to enter the scrotum, forming **an indirect or congenital hernia.**

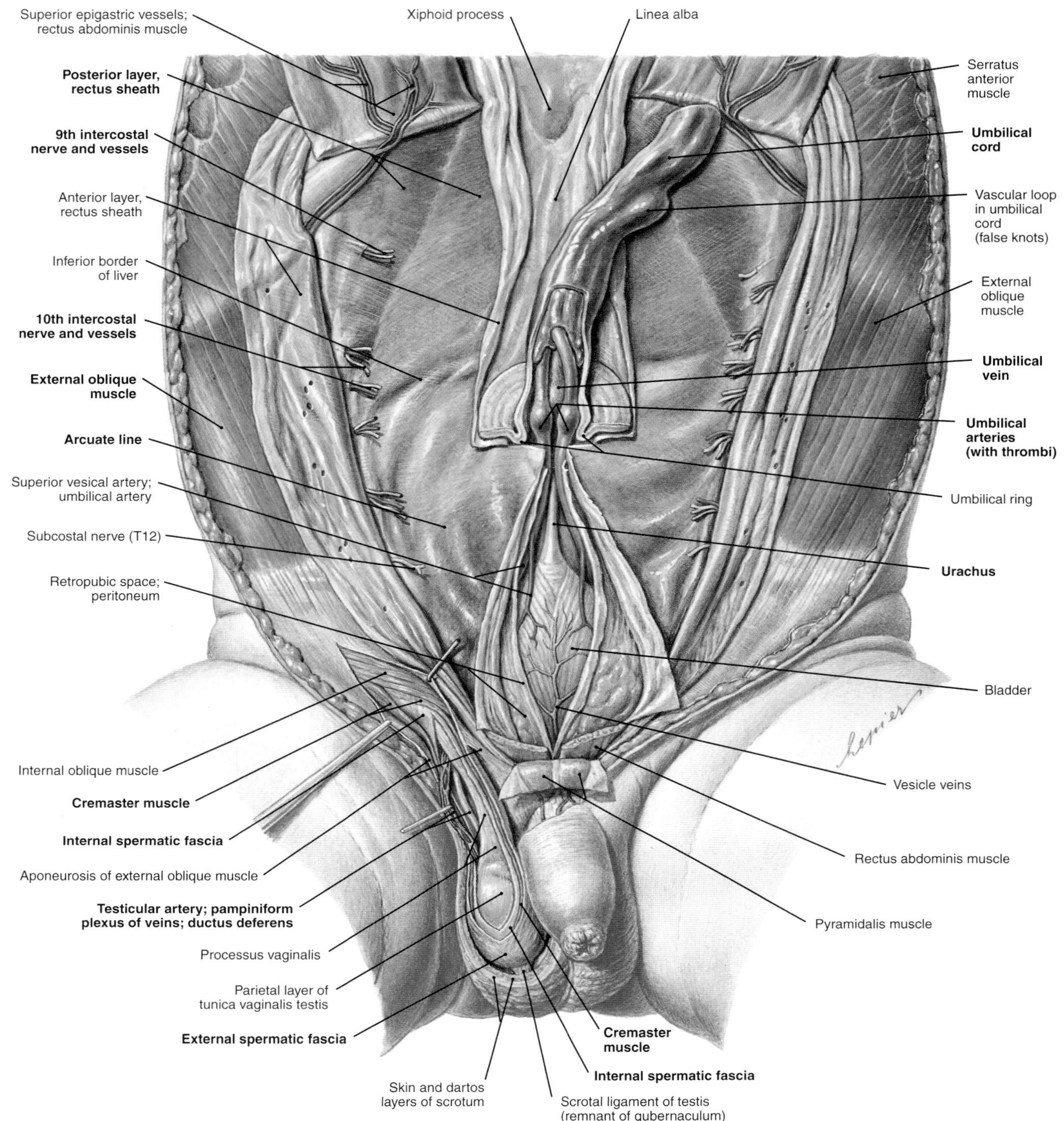
Superior epigastric vessels; rectus abdominis muscle
Xiphoid process
Linea alba
Posterior layer, rectus sheath
Serratus anterior muscle
9th intercostal nerve and vessels
Umbilical cord
Anterior layer, rectus sheath
Vascular loop in umbilical cord (false knots)
Inferior border of liver
External oblique muscle
10th intercostal nerve and vessels
Umbilical vein
External oblique muscle
Umbilical arteries (with thrombi)
Arcuate line
Superior vesical artery; umbilical artery
Umbilical ring
Subcostal nerve (T12)
Urachus
Retropubic space; peritoneum
Bladder
Internal oblique muscle
Vesicle veins
Cremaster muscle
Internal spermatic fascia
Rectus abdominis muscle
Aponeurosis of external oblique muscle
Testicular artery; pampiniform plexus of veins; ductus deferens
Pyramidalis muscle
Processus vaginalis
Parietal layer of tunica vaginalis testis
External spermatic fascia
Cremaster muscle
Internal spermatic fascia
Skin and dartos layers of scrotum
Scrotal ligament of testis (remnant of gubernaculum)

Figure 196 Deep Dissection of the Anterior Abdominal Wall and the Umbilical Region in the Newborn

NOTE: (1) The anterior layer of the rectus sheath is reflected laterally, and the two rectus abdominis muscles have been cut near the symphysis pubis and turned upward (almost out of view). This exposes the posterior layer of the rectus sheath and the **arcuate line.**

(2) An incision has been made in the midline between the umbilicus and the public symphysis exposing the **bladder, urachus,** the **umbilical arteries,** and the **umbilical vein.**

(3) The anterior aspect of the right spermatic cord and scrotal sac have been opened to show the ductus deferens and the **tunica vaginalis testis** surrounding the testis.

(4) The severed umbilical cord, usually 1 to 2 cm in diameter and about 50 cm, or 20 in., long. It contains the two umbilical arteries and the umbilical vein surrounded by a mucoid form of connective tissue called Wharton's jelly.

(5) At times, the umbilical vessels form harmless loops in the umbilical cord called "false knots." More rarely, looping of the cord may be of functional significance and such "true knots" may alter the circulation to and from the fetus.

(6) The bulges in the umbilical arteries. These are in situ blood clots that occlude the arteries, but which are probably postmortem phenomena in this dissection.

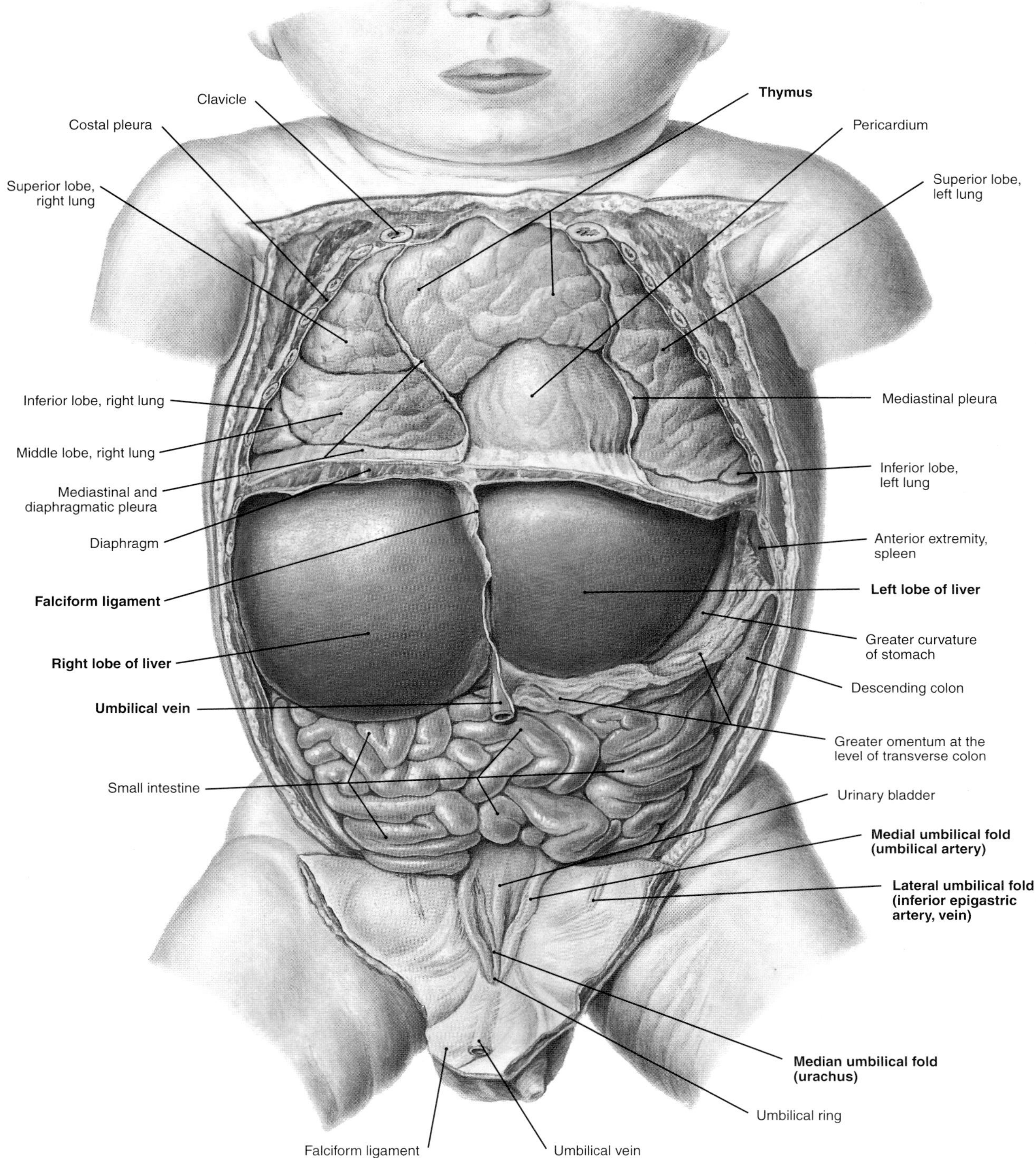
Clavicle
Costal pleura
Superior lobe, right lung
Thymus
Pericardium
Superior lobe, left lung
Inferior lobe, right lung
Middle lobe, right lung
Mediastinal and diaphragmatic pleura
Diaphragm
Falciform ligament
Right lobe of liver
Umbilical vein
Small intestine
Mediastinal pleura
Inferior lobe, left lung
Anterior extremity, spleen
Left lobe of liver
Greater curvature of stomach
Descending colon
Greater omentum at the level of transverse colon
Urinary bladder
Medial umbilical fold (umbilical artery)
Lateral umbilical fold (inferior epigastric artery, vein)
Median umbilical fold (urachus)
Umbilical ring
Falciform ligament
Umbilical vein

Figure 197 Abdominal and Thoracic Viscera Observed in Situ in the Newborn Child

NOTE: (1) The anterior body wall has been removed in this newborn child, uncovering the viscera. Observe the umbilical ligaments on the inner surface of the lower wall.

(2) The average newborn child weighs about 3300 g (7 lb) and measures about 50 cm (20 in.) from the top of the head to the sole of the foot. The umbilicus is located about 1.5 cm below the midpoint of this crown-to-heel length.

(3) The transverse diameter of the abdomen in the newborn is greatest above the umbilicus, due to the inordinate proportion of the abdomen occupied by the liver. The average weight of the liver in the neonate is about 120 g (4% of the body weight). In the adult the liver weighs 12 to 13 times that at birth (but only 2.5 to 3.5% of the body weight).

(4) The truncated shape of the thorax and the large thymus, weighing about 10 g at birth (0.42% of body weight at birth compared with 0.03 to 0.05% in the adult).

(5) The facts above are taken from: Crelin ES. Functional anatomy of the newborn, New Haven, CT: Yale University Press, 1973, which is an excellent short monograph (87 pages).

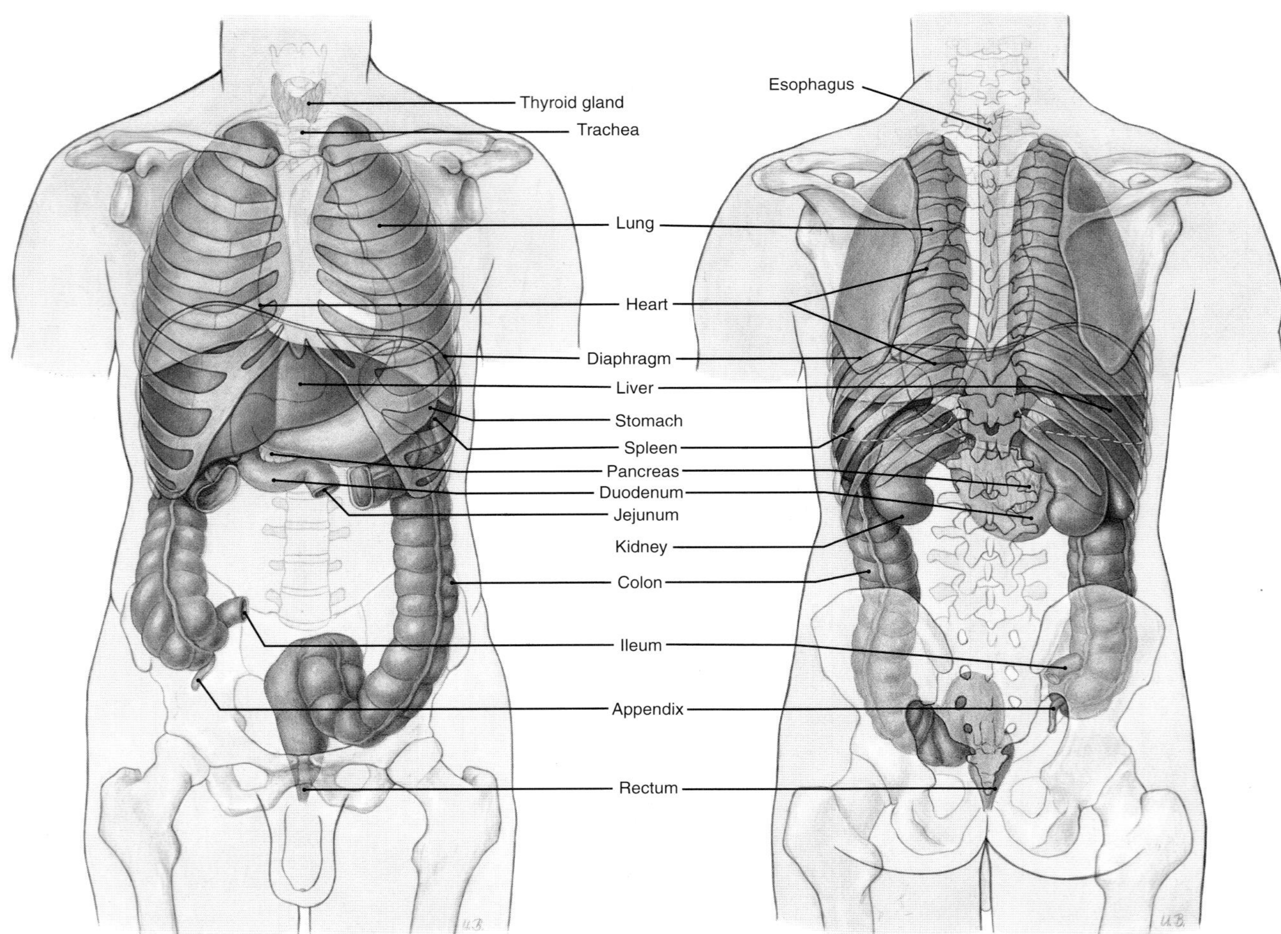
Thyroid gland
Trachea
Esophagus
Lung
Heart
Diaphragm
Liver
Stomach
Spleen
Pancreas
Duodenum
Jejunum
Kidney
Colon
Ileum
Appendix
Rectum

Figure 198.1 Surface Projection of Thoracic and Abdominal Organs (Anterior View)

Figure 198.2 Surface Projection of Thoracic and Abdominal Organs (Posterior View)

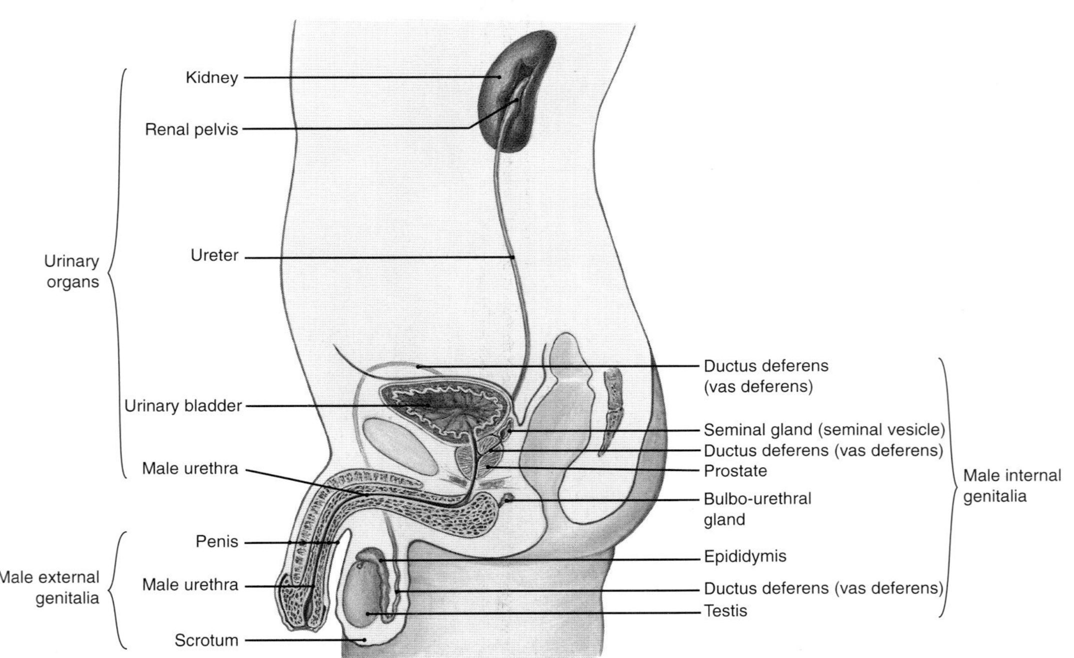
Kidney
Renal pelvis
Urinary organs
Ureter
Urinary bladder
Male urethra
Penis
Male external genitalia
Male urethra
Scrotum
Ductus deferens (vas deferens)
Seminal gland (seminal vesicle)
Ductus deferens (vas deferens)
Prostate
Bulbo-urethral gland
Male internal genitalia
Epididymis
Ductus deferens (vas deferens)
Testis

Figure 198.3 Surface Projection of Male Urogenital Organs (Left Lateral View)

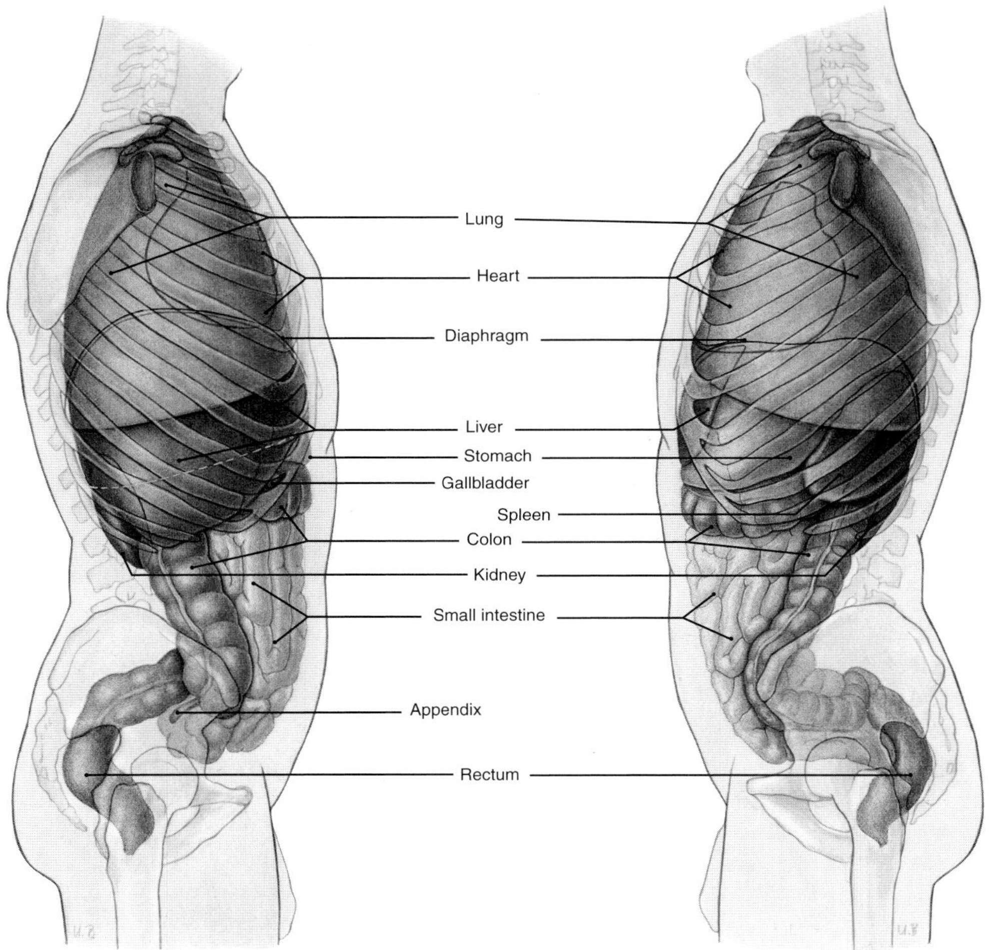
Lung
Heart
Diaphragm
Liver
Stomach
Gallbladder
Spleen
Colon
Kidney
Small intestine
Appendix
Rectum

Figure 199.1 Surface Projection of Thoracic and Abdominal Organs (Right Lateral View)

Figure 199.2 Surface Projection of Thoracic and Abdominal Organs (Left Lateral View)

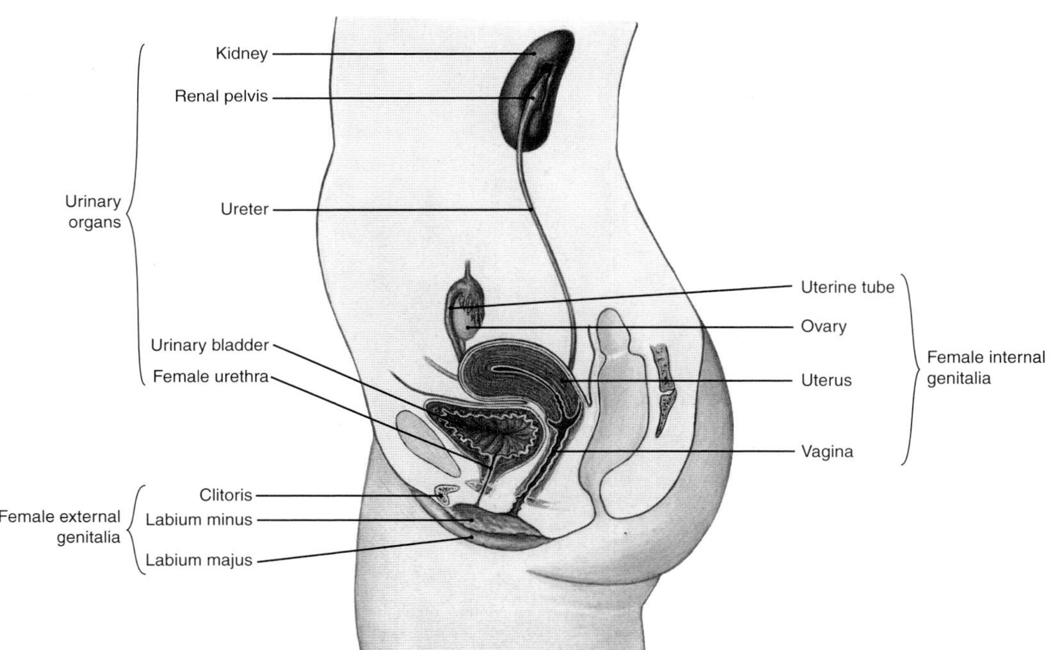
Kidney
Renal pelvis
Urinary organs
Ureter
Urinary bladder
Female urethra
Clitoris
Female external genitalia
Labium minus
Labium majus
Uterine tube
Ovary
Uterus
Vagina
Female internal genitalia

Figure 199.3 Surface Projection of Female Urogenital Organs (Left Lateral View)

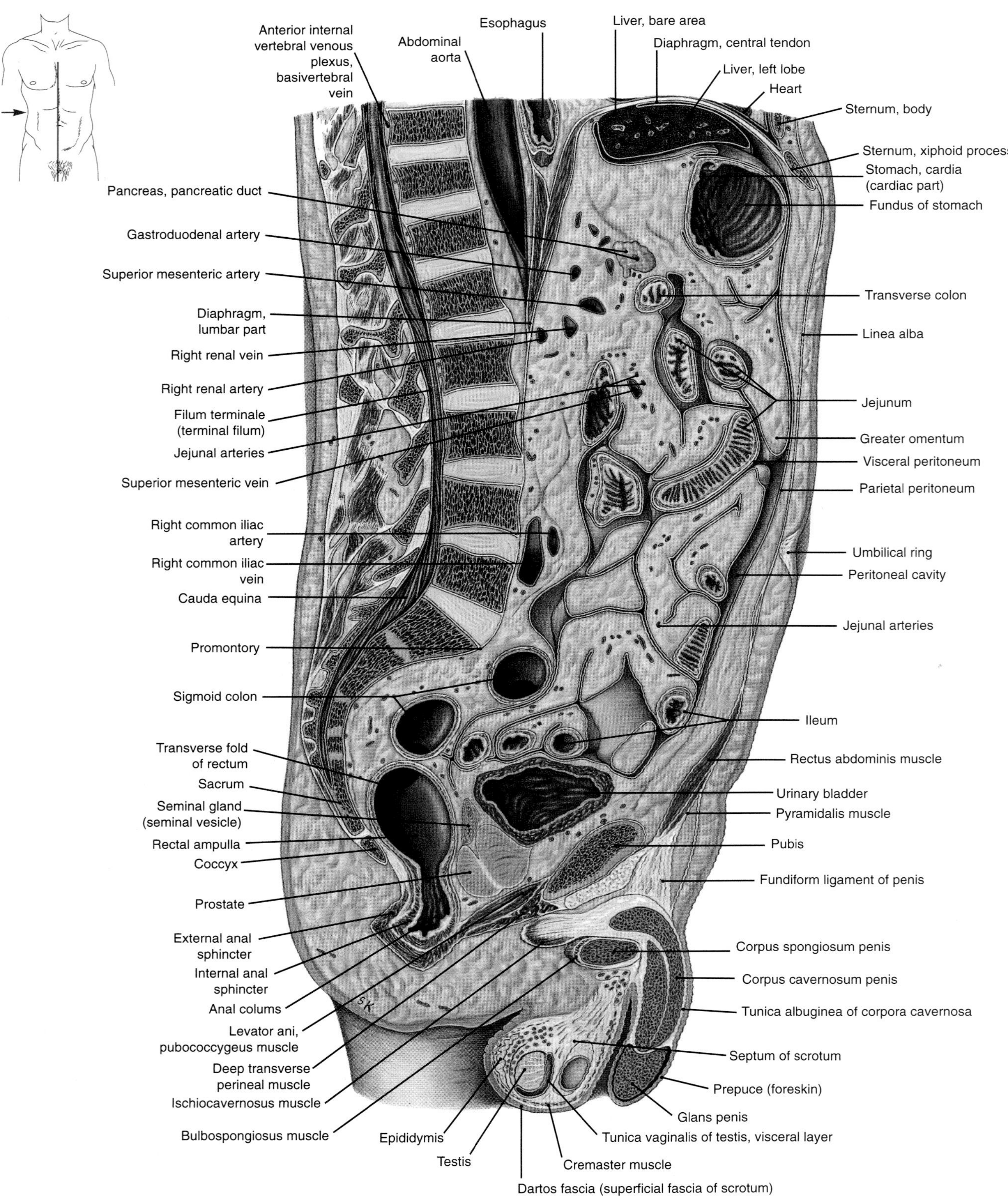

Anterior internal vertebral venous plexus, basivertebral vein
Abdominal aorta
Esophagus
Liver, bare area
Diaphragm, central tendon
Liver, left lobe
Heart
Sternum, body
Sternum, xiphoid process
Stomach, cardia (cardiac part)
Fundus of stomach
Pancreas, pancreatic duct
Gastroduodenal artery
Superior mesenteric artery
Diaphragm, lumbar part
Right renal vein
Right renal artery
Filum terminale (terminal filum)
Jejunal arteries
Superior mesenteric vein
Transverse colon
Linea alba
Jejunum
Greater omentum
Visceral peritoneum
Parietal peritoneum
Right common iliac artery
Right common iliac vein
Cauda equina
Umbilical ring
Peritoneal cavity
Jejunal arteries
Promontory
Sigmoid colon
Ileum
Transverse fold of rectum
Sacrum
Seminal gland (seminal vesicle)
Rectal ampulla
Coccyx
Rectus abdominis muscle
Urinary bladder
Pyramidalis muscle
Pubis
Fundiform ligament of penis
Prostate
External anal sphincter
Internal anal sphincter
Anal colums
Levator ani, pubococcygeus muscle
Deep transverse perineal muscle
Ischiocavernosus muscle
Bulbospongiosus muscle
Corpus spongiosum penis
Corpus cavernosum penis
Tunica albuginea of corpora cavernosa
Septum of scrotum
Prepuce (foreskin)
Glans penis
Tunica vaginalis of testis, visceral layer
Epididymis
Testis
Cremaster muscle
Dartos fascia (superficial fascia of scrotum)

Figure 200 Median Sagittal Section of the Male Abdomen and Pelvis

NOTE: (1) This figure is viewed from the right lateral aspect. Observe, however, that the external genitalia and anterior aspect of the pelvis are sectioned to the left of the median plane.

(2) The **filum terminale** and **cauda equina** within the central canal of the vertebral column. Observe also the seminal vesicle and prostate gland on the posterior aspect of the urinary bladder.

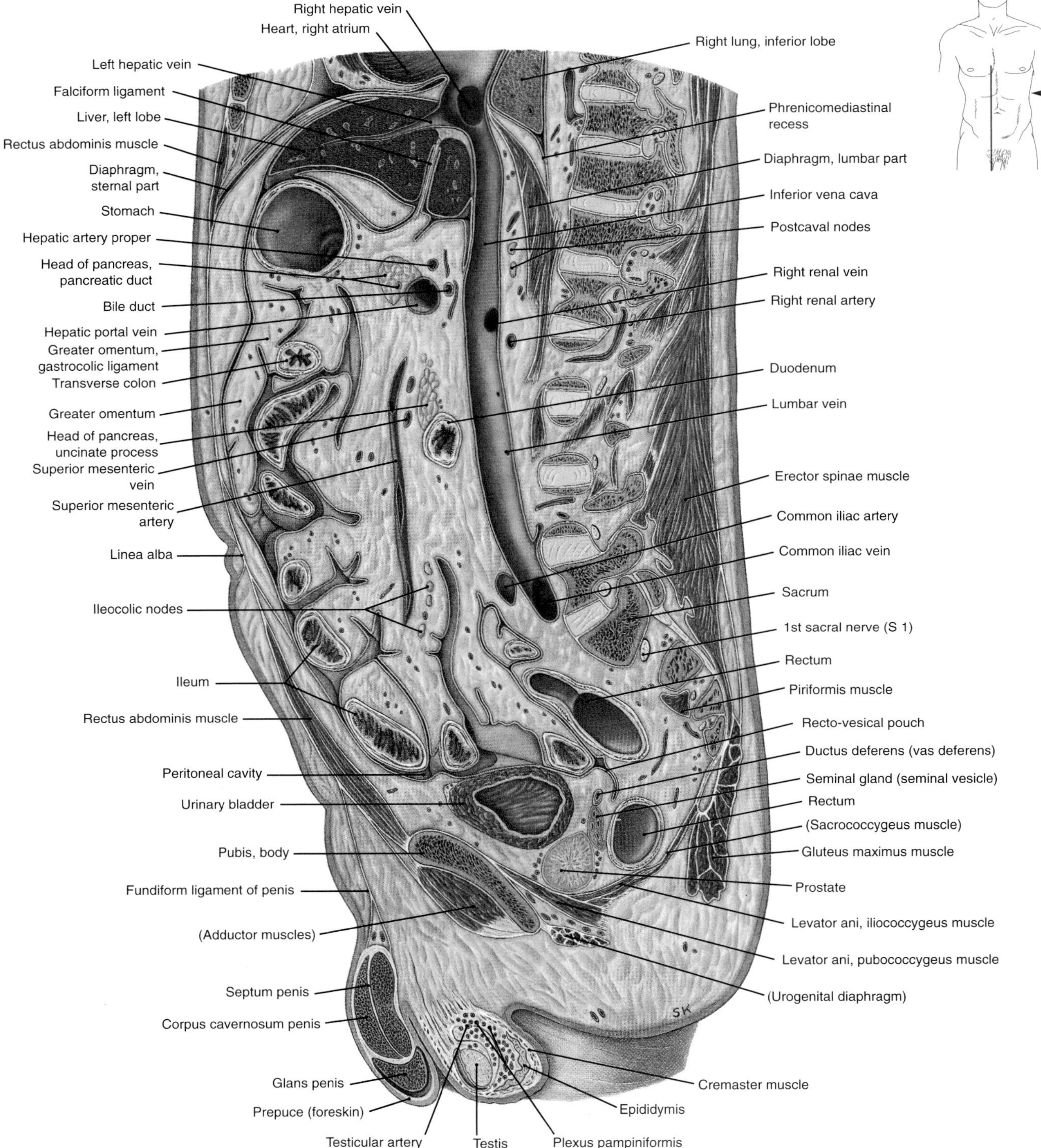
Right hepatic vein
Heart, right atrium
Left hepatic vein
Falciform ligament
Liver, left lobe
Rectus abdominis muscle
Diaphragm, sternal part
Stomach
Hepatic artery proper
Head of pancreas, pancreatic duct
Bile duct
Hepatic portal vein
Greater omentum, gastrocolic ligament
Transverse colon
Greater omentum
Head of pancreas, uncinate process
Superior mesenteric vein
Superior mesenteric artery
Linea alba
Ileocolic nodes
Ileum
Rectus abdominis muscle
Peritoneal cavity
Urinary bladder
Pubis, body
Fundiform ligament of penis
(Adductor muscles)
Septum penis
Corpus cavernosum penis
Glans penis
Prepuce (foreskin)
Testicular artery
Testis
Plexus pampiniformis
Epididymis
Cremaster muscle
(Urogenital diaphragm)
Levator ani, pubococcygeus muscle
Levator ani, iliococcygeus muscle
Prostate
Gluteus maximus muscle
(Sacrococcygeus muscle)
Rectum
Seminal gland (seminal vesicle)
Ductus deferens (vas deferens)
Recto-vesical pouch
Piriformis muscle
Rectum
1st sacral nerve (S 1)
Sacrum
Common iliac vein
Common iliac artery
Erector spinae muscle
Lumbar vein
Duodenum
Right renal artery
Right renal vein
Postcaval nodes
Inferior vena cava
Diaphragm, lumbar part
Phrenicomediastinal recess
Right lung, inferior lobe
SK

Figure 201 Paramedian Section of the Male Abdomen and Pelvis

NOTE: (1) This section bisects the inferior vena cava longitudinally as that vessel ascends along the posterior abdominal wall. Thus, this section was made to the right of the midline, and it is viewed from the left side.

(2) The head and the uncinate process of the pancreas, the hepatic artery and the portal vein, all right-sided structures.

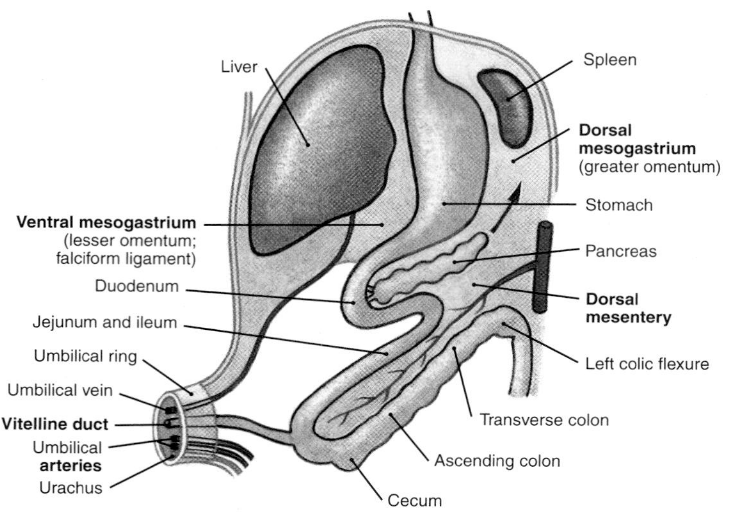

Liver
Spleen
Dorsal mesogastrium (greater omentum)
Stomach
Pancreas
Dorsal mesentery
Left colic flexure
Ventral mesogastrium (lesser omentum; falciform ligament)
Duodenum
Jejunum and ileum
Umbilical ring
Umbilical vein
Vitelline duct
Umbilical arteries
Urachus
Transverse colon
Ascending colon
Cecum

Figure 202.1 Developing Gastrointestinal Organs and Their Mesenteries

NOTE: (1) As the primitive gastrointestinal tube develops within the abdominal celom, it is suspended from the body wall by primitive peritoneal reflections, both ventrally and dorsally. The early peritoneal attachments to the expanding stomach are called the ventral mesogastrium and dorsal mesogastrium, whereas the dorsal mesentery develops on the posterior aspect of the primitive small and large intestine.

(2) The embryonic liver develops into the ventral mesogastrium, thereby dividing this ventral peritoneal attachment into:

(a) A portion between the anterior body wall and the liver, which eventually becomes the falciform ligament, and

(b) A portion between the liver and the stomach, which becomes the lesser omentum.

(3) On the dorsal aspect:

(a) The pancreas develops in relation to the primitive duodenum, both of which lose their mesenteries during gut rotation to become retroperitoneal.

(b) The dorsal mesogastrium, attaching along the greater curvature of the stomach and rotating with the stomach, becomes the greater omentum. This eventually encases the transverse colon.

(c) The dorsal mesentery remains attached to the small intestine, while the ascending and descending colon become displaced to the right and left side, respectively, becoming adherent to the posterior body wall.

(d) The sigmoid colon usually retains its mesentery, while that of the rectum becomes obliterated.

(4) Near the cecal end of the small intestine, the developing gastrointestinal canal communicates with the vitelline duct. Before birth, this duct usually becomes resorbed; when it persists (3% of cases), it results in a diverticulum of the ileum called Meckel's diverticulum.

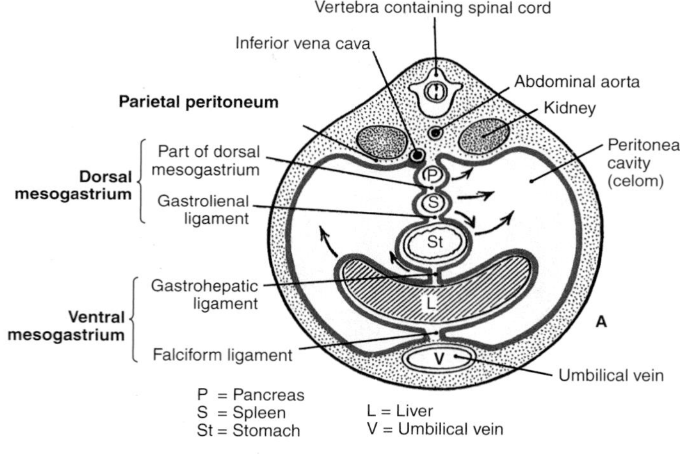

Vertebra containing spinal cord
Inferior vena cava
Abdominal aorta
Kidney
Parietal peritoneum
Dorsal mesogastrium
Part of dorsal mesogastrium
Gastrolienal ligament
Peritoneal cavity (celom)
Ventral mesogastrium
Gastrohepatic ligament
Falciform ligament
Umbilical vein
A
P
S
St
L
V
P = Pancreas
S = Spleen
St = Stomach
L = Liver
V = Umbilical vein

Figure 202.2A Cross-Sectional Diagram of Development of Mesogastria: Early Stage (about 6 weeks)

NOTE: (1) The primitive peritoneal reflections are indicated in red. The arrows show the direction of growth and movement by the various organs shown in Fig. 203.1B.

(2) At this early stage, the peritoneum completely surrounds the organs in the upper abdominal region (visceral peritoneum) and attaches peripherally to the body wall (parietal peritoneum). Attaching along the posterior border of the stomach, the dorsal mesogastrium then surrounds the spleen and pancreas. Anterior to the stomach, the liver becomes interposed between the stomach and the anterior body wall. This forms the gastrohepatic ligament (also called the lesser omentum) between the lesser curvature of the stomach and the liver, and the falciform ligament between the liver and the anterior body wall.

Vertebra with spinal cord
Abdominal aorta
Inferior vena cava
Dorsal mesogastrium
Kidney
Dorsal mesogastrium
Pancreas
Spleen
Dorsal mesogastrium (gastrolienal ligament)
Omental bursa
Stomach
Liver
Celom (peritoneal cavity)
Gastrohepatic ligament (porta hepatis)
B
V
Celom (peritoneal cavity)
Falciform ligament
Umbilical vein

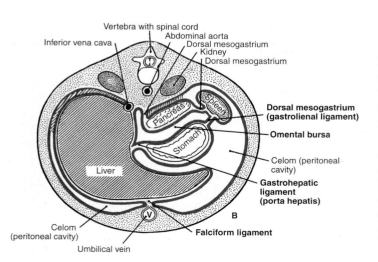

Figure 202.2B Cross-Sectional Diagram of Development of Mesogastria: Late Fetal Stage

NOTE: (1) With the rotation of the organs (in the direction of the arrows in Fig. 202.2A), the liver grows into the celomic cavity toward the right and contacts the inferior vena cava, while the stomach rotates such that its dorsal mesogastrium (greater curvature) is shifted to the left.

(2) The reflection of dorsal mesogastrium between the stomach and spleen becomes established as the gastrolienal ligament, while one layer of mesogastrium surrounding the pancreas and duodenum fuses to the posterior body wall. This fixates these two organs with a layer of peritoneum on their anterior surface, causing them to become retroperitoneal. The omental bursa also develops posterior to the stomach and anterior to the pancreas.

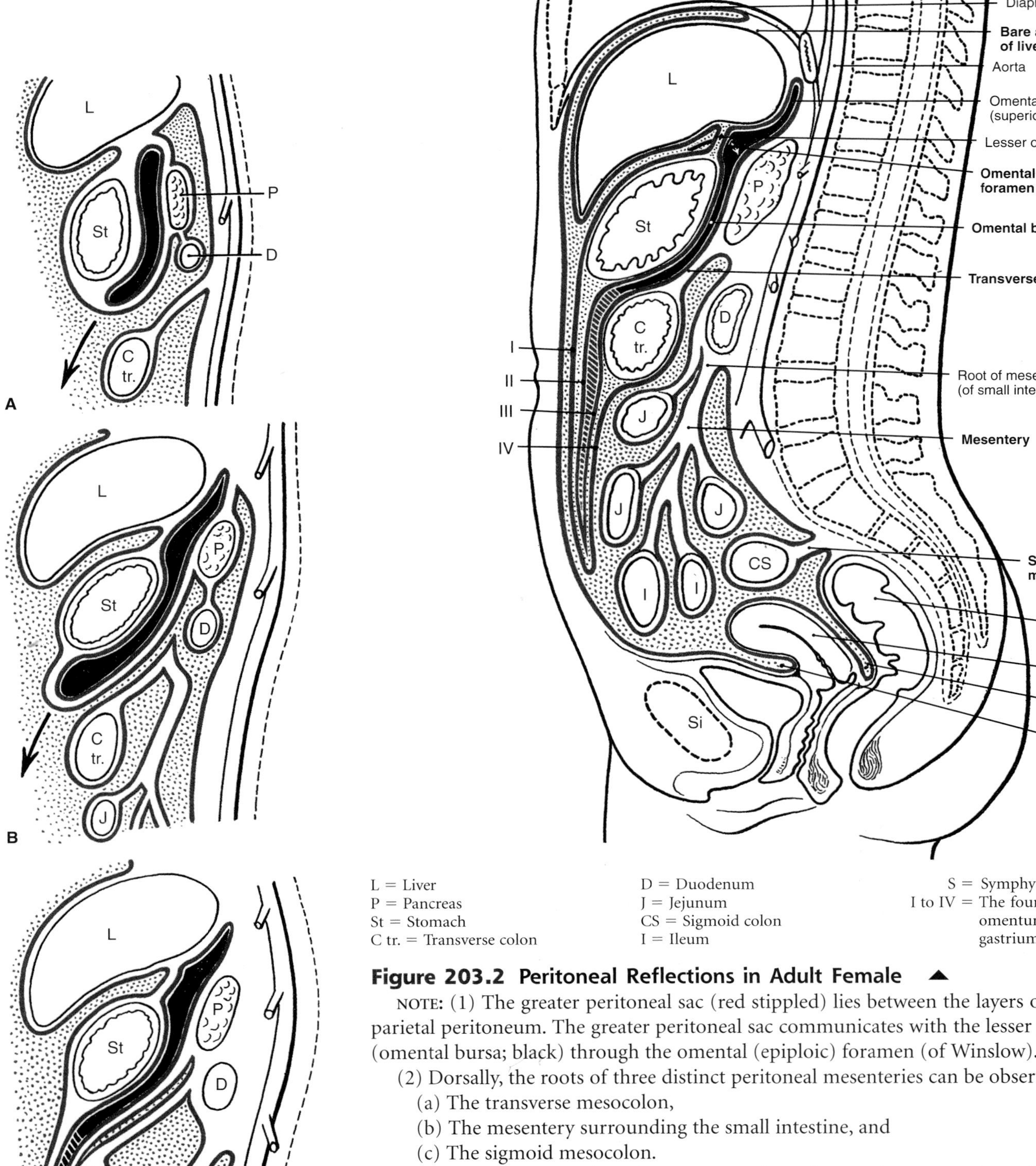
L
St
P
D
C tr.
A
B
J
C
Diaphragm
Bare area of liver
Aorta
Omental bursa (superior recess)
Lesser omentum
Omental (epiploic) foramen (arrow)
Omental bursa
Transverse mesocolon
Root of mesentery (of small intestine)
Mesentery
I
II
III
IV
CS
Sigmoid mesocolon
Rectum
Uterus
Rectouterine pouch (Douglas)
Vesicouterine pouch
Si

L = Liver
P = Pancreas
St = Stomach
C tr. = Transverse colon
D = Duodenum
J = Jejunum
CS = Sigmoid colon
I = Ileum
S = Symphysis pubis
I to IV = The four layers of greater omentum (dorsal mesogastrium)

Figure 203.2 Peritoneal Reflections in Adult Female ▲

NOTE: (1) The greater peritoneal sac (red stippled) lies between the layers of visceral and parietal peritoneum. The greater peritoneal sac communicates with the lesser peritoneal sac (omental bursa; black) through the omental (epiploic) foramen (of Winslow).

(2) Dorsally, the roots of three distinct peritoneal mesenteries can be observed:

(a) The transverse mesocolon,

(b) The mesentery surrounding the small intestine, and

(c) The sigmoid mesocolon.

(3) Behind the stomach and transverse colon, observe the retroperitoneal pancreas and duodenum. A portion of the liver is not surrounded by peritoneum (bare area of the liver) and lies adjacent to the diaphragm.

Figure 203.1A, B, C: Stages in the Development of the Omental Bursa (Sagittal Diagrams)

NOTE: (1) At 4 weeks, the dorsal border of the stomach grows faster than the ventral border, assisting in rotation of the stomach on its long axis. The greater curvature and its dorsal mesogastrium become directed to the left, whereas the lesser curvature and the ventral mesogastrium are directed to the right.

(2) By 8 weeks (**A**), the omental bursa (black) forms behind the stomach between the two leaves of dorsal mesogastrium. The pancreas and duodenum are still surrounded by dorsal mesentery. As gut rotation continues, the dorsal mesogastrium extends inferiorly (**B**, arrow) to form the greater omentum, which becomes a double reflection (four leaves) of the dorsal mesogastrium "trapping" the cavity of the omental bursa between the second and third leaves.

(3) Continued development (**C**) results in a further descent of the greater omentum over the abdominal viscera and a fusion (cross-hatched) of the second and third leaves inferiorly.

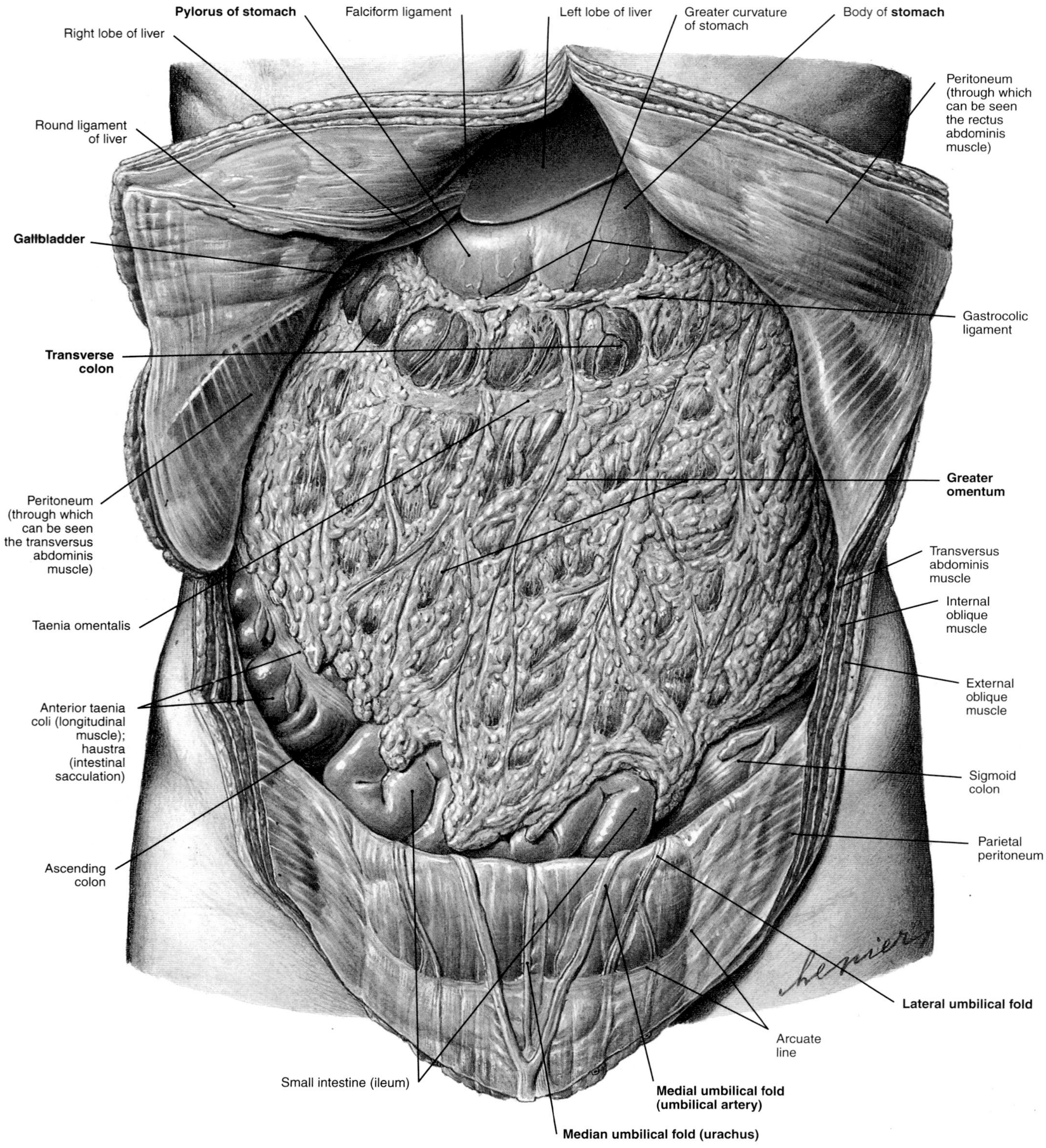

Pylorus of stomach
Falciform ligament
Left lobe of liver
Greater curvature of stomach
Body of stomach
Right lobe of liver
Peritoneum (through which can be seen the rectus abdominis muscle)
Round ligament of liver
Gallbladder
Gastrocolic ligament
Transverse colon
Greater omentum
Peritoneum (through which can be seen the transversus abdominis muscle)
Transversus abdominis muscle
Taenia omentalis
Internal oblique muscle
External oblique muscle
Anterior taenia coli (longitudinal muscle); haustra (intestinal sacculation)
Sigmoid colon
Parietal peritoneum
Ascending colon
Lateral umbilical fold
Arcuate line
Small intestine (ileum)
Medial umbilical fold (umbilical artery)
Median umbilical fold (urachus)

Figure 204 Abdominal Cavity, Viscera Left Intact

NOTE: (1) The **greater omentum**. It attaches along the greater curvature of the stomach, covers the intestines like an apron, and extends inferiorly almost to the pelvis.

(2) The **falciform ligament,** a remnant of the ventral mesogastrium, extends between the liver and the anterior body wall and separates the left and right lobes of the liver. The **round ligament** is the remnant of the obliterated umbilical vein.

(3) On the inner surface of the anterior abdominal wall, identify the following folds:

(a) **Median umbilical fold**: remnant of the urachus, which extended between the bladder and the umbilicus in the fetus.

(b) **Medial umbilical folds**: the obliterated umbilical arteries, which were the continuation of the superior vesical arteries to the umbilicus in the fetus.

(c) **Lateral umbilical folds**: a fold of peritoneum over the inferior epigastric vessels.

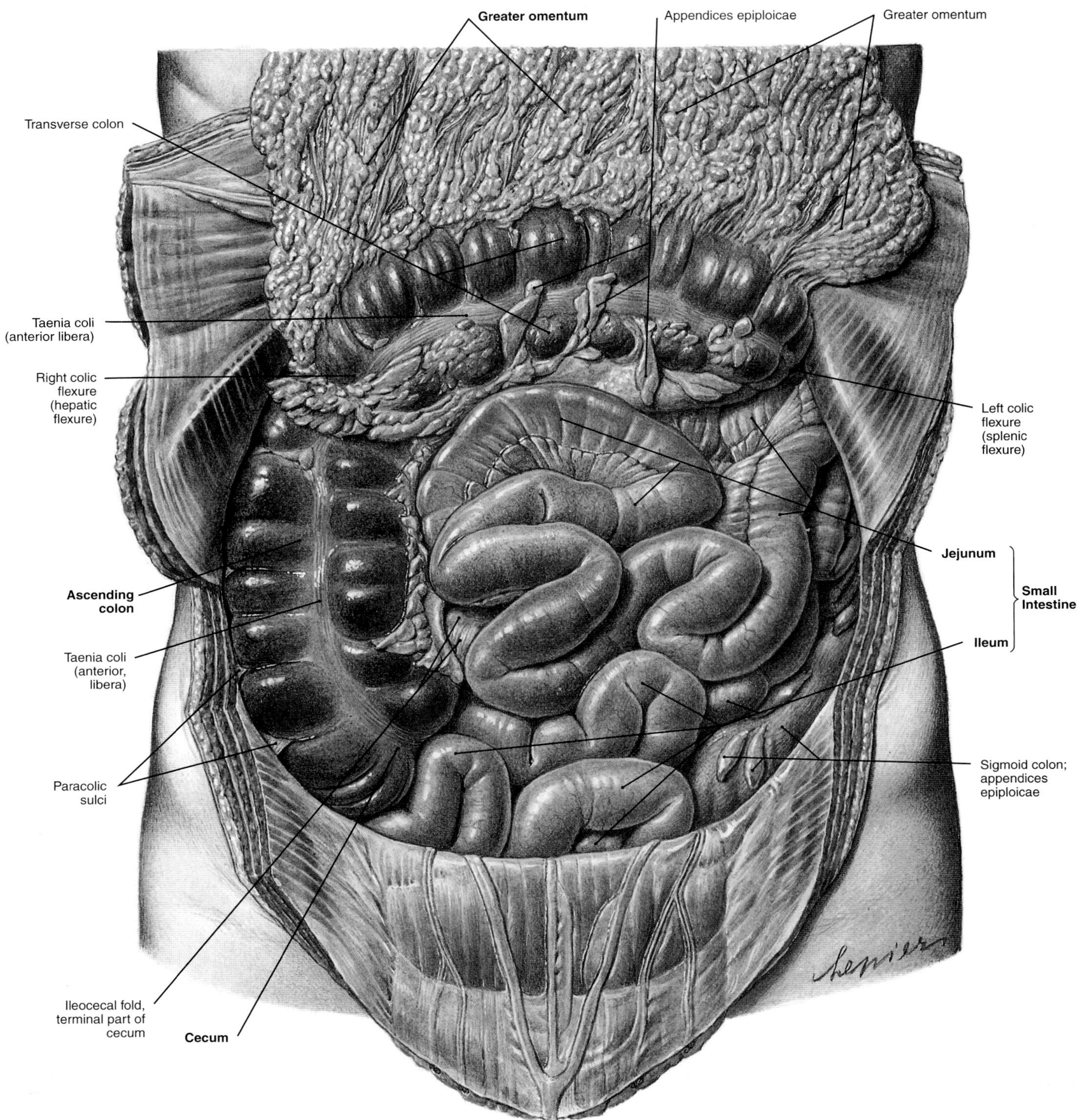
Greater omentum
Appendices epiploicae
Greater omentum
Transverse colon
Taenia coli
(anterior libera)
Right colic
flexure
(hepatic
flexure)
Left colic
flexure
(splenic
flexure)
Jejunum
Small
Intestine
Ileum
Ascending
colon
Taenia coli
(anterior,
libera)
Paracolic
sulci
Sigmoid colon;
appendices
epiploicae
Ileocecal fold,
terminal part of
cecum
Cecum

Figure 205 Abdominal Cavity, Ascending Colon, and Transverse Colon and Its Mesocolon

NOTE: (1) With the greater omentum reflected upward, the transverse colon is crossing the abdominal cavity from right to left in continuity with the ascending colon on the right and the descending colon on the left.

(2) Longitudinal muscles called **taeniae,** along the outer surface of the colon. These muscles are shorter than the other coats of the large intestine causing sacculations, which are called **haustrae.**

(3) Smooth irregular fatty masses called **appendices epiploicae** are suspended from the large intestine. These assist in the identification of the large gut.

(4) Below the mesocolon (inframesocolic) can be seen the small intestine, which consists of three portions: the **duodenum, jejunum,** and **ileum.** The outer wall of the small intestine is smooth and glistening and is not sacculated.

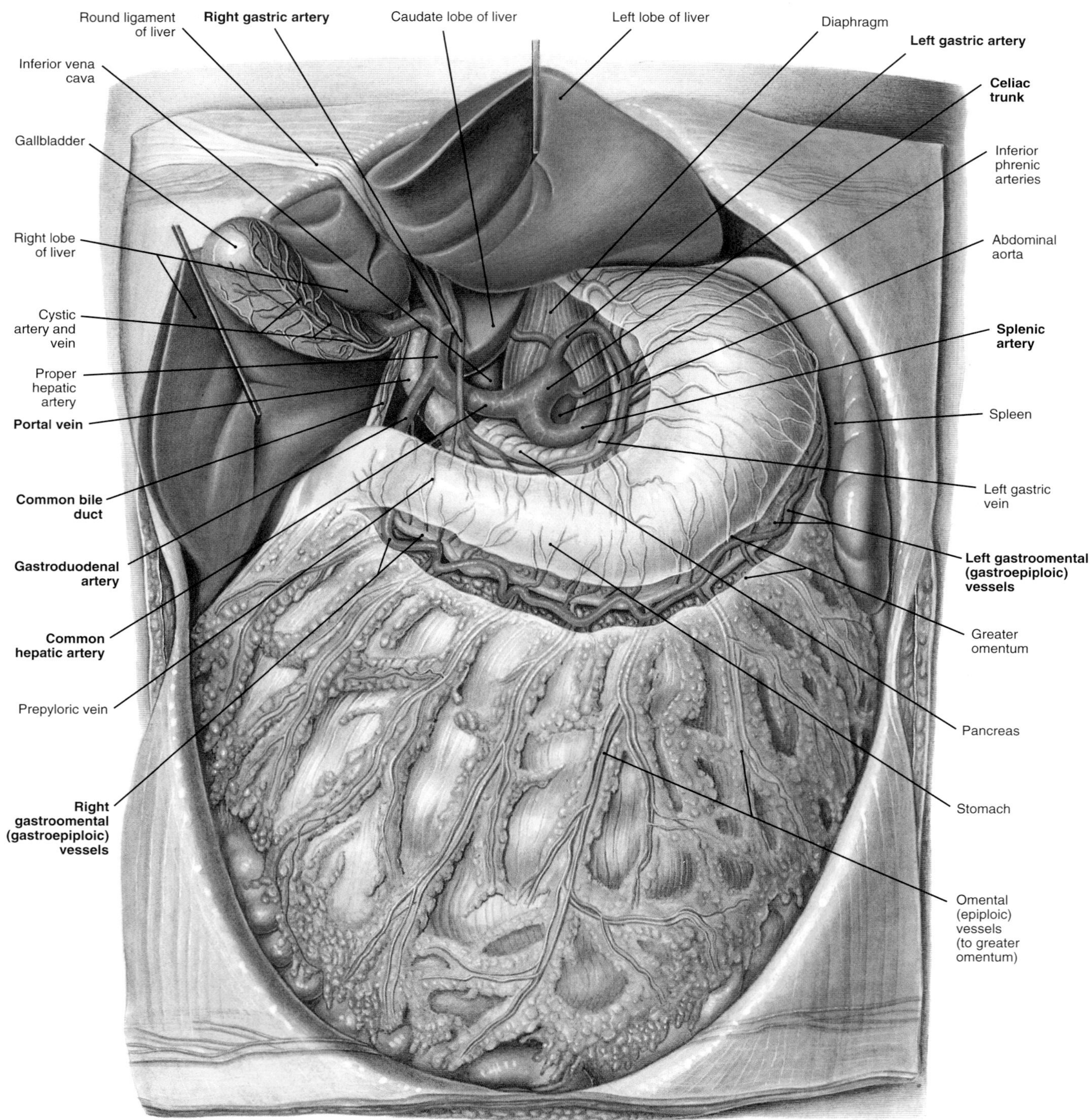
Round ligament of liver
Right gastric artery
Caudate lobe of liver
Left lobe of liver
Diaphragm
Left gastric artery
Celiac trunk
Inferior vena cava
Gallbladder
Inferior phrenic arteries
Right lobe of liver
Abdominal aorta
Cystic artery and vein
Splenic artery
Proper hepatic artery
Portal vein
Spleen
Common bile duct
Left gastric vein
Gastroduodenal artery
Left gastroomental (gastroepiploic) vessels
Common hepatic artery
Greater omentum
Prepyloric vein
Pancreas
Right gastroomental (gastroepiploic) vessels
Stomach
Omental (epiploic) vessels (to greater omentum)

Figure 206 Abdominal Cavity (3): Celiac Trunk and Its Branches

NOTE: (1) The lobes of the liver have been elevated and the lesser omentum has been removed between the lesser curvature of the stomach and the liver to reveal the **celiac trunk** (located anterior to the T12 vertebra) and its branches. These are:

(a) The **left gastric artery**, which courses along the lesser curvature of the stomach and anastomoses with the right gastric artery, a branch of the hepatic artery.

(b) The **splenic artery**, which courses to the left toward the hilum of the spleen, and

(c) The **hepatic artery**, which courses to the right and gives off the gastroduodenal artery before dividing to enter the lobes of the liver.

(2) The **gastroduodenal artery** gives rise to the **right gastroomental(gastroepiploic) artery,** which follows along the greater curvature of the stomach to anastomose with the **left gastroomental (gastroepiploic) branch** of the splenic artery.

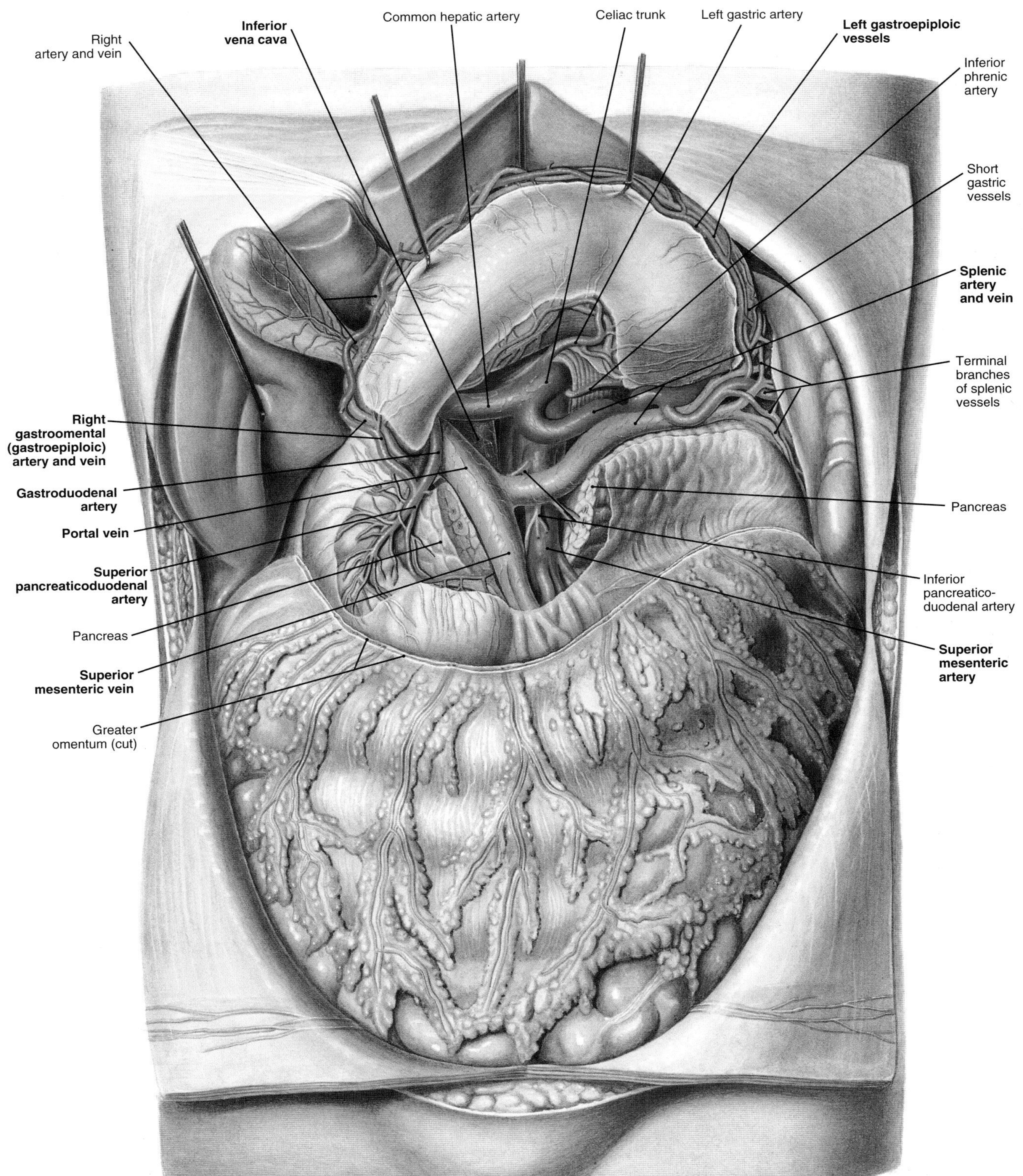
Right
artery and vein
Inferior
vena cava
Common hepatic artery
Celiac trunk
Left gastric artery
Left gastroepiploic
vessels
Inferior
phrenic
artery
Short
gastric
vessels
Splenic
artery
and vein
Terminal
branches
of splenic
vessels
Right
gastroomental
(gastroepiploic)
artery and vein
Gastroduodenal
artery
Portal vein
Superior
pancreaticoduodenal
artery
Pancreas
Superior
mesenteric vein
Greater
omentum (cut)
Pancreas
Inferior
pancreaticoduodenal artery
Superior
mesenteric
artery

Figure 207 Abdominal Cavity (4): Splenic Vessels and Formation of the Portal Vein

NOTE: (1) The greater omentum has been cut along the greater curvature of the stomach. The stomach is lifted to expose its posterior surface and the underlying pancreas, duodenum, and blood vessels. A part of the pancreas has been removed to reveal the **portal vein** formed by the junction of the **splenic and superior mesenteric veins.**

(2) The tortuous **splenic artery** in its course to the splenic hilum, and the **gastroduodenal artery,** behind the pyloric end of the stomach dividing into **right gastroomental** and **superior pancreaticoduodenal arteries.**

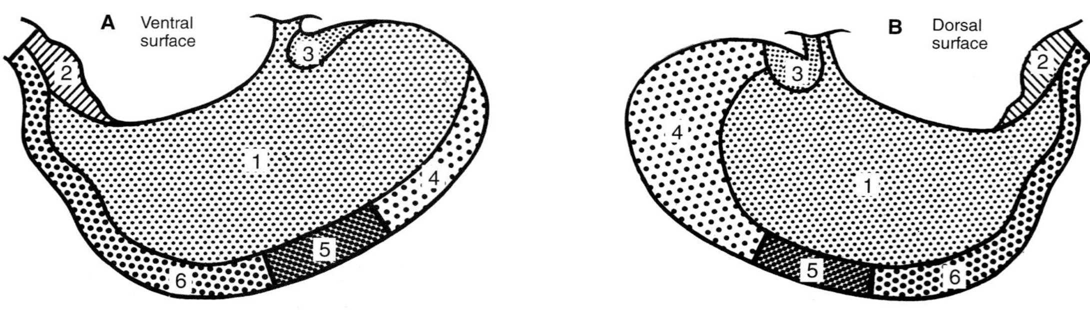
A Ventral surface
B Dorsal surface
1
2
3
4
5
6

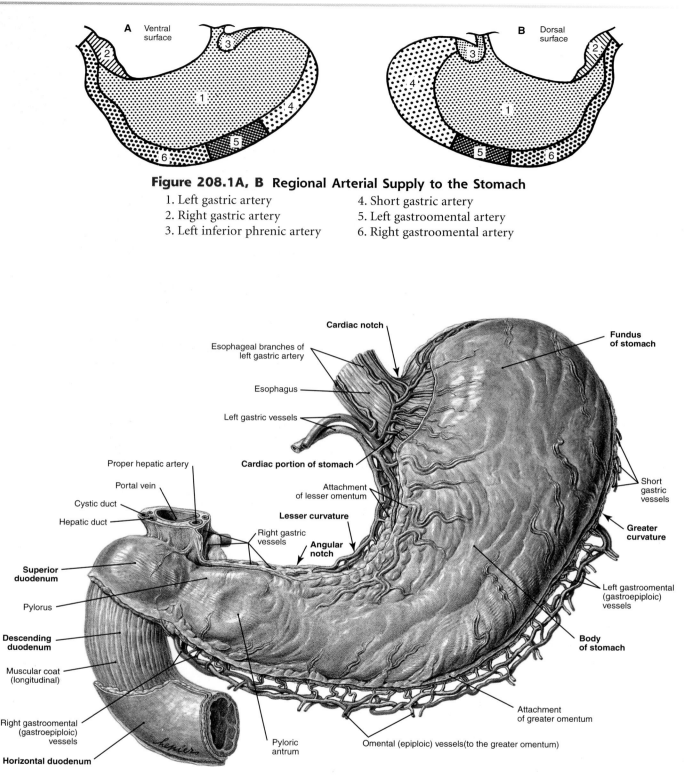

Figure 208.1A, B Regional Arterial Supply to the Stomach

1. Left gastric artery
2. Right gastric artery
3. Left inferior phrenic artery
4. Short gastric artery
5. Left gastroomental artery
6. Right gastroomental artery

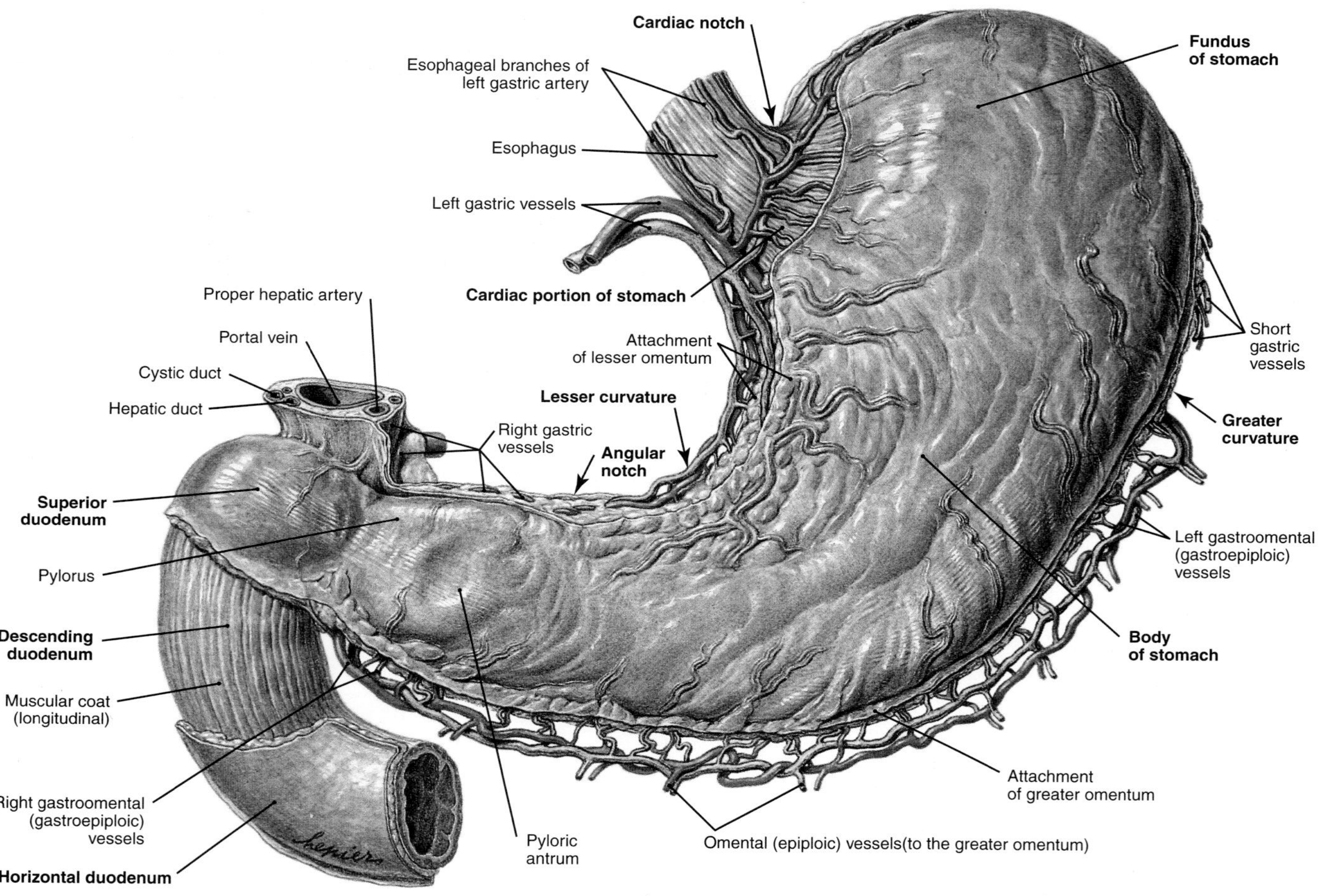
Cardiac notch
Fundus of stomach
Esophageal branches of left gastric artery
Esophagus
Left gastric vessels
Proper hepatic artery
Cardiac portion of stomach
Portal vein
Attachment of lesser omentum
Cystic duct
Short gastric vessels
Hepatic duct
Lesser curvature
Right gastric vessels
Angular notch
Greater curvature
Superior duodenum
Left gastroomental (gastroepiploic) vessels
Pylorus
Descending duodenum
Body of stomach
Muscular coat (longitudinal)
Attachment of greater omentum
Right gastroomental (gastroepiploic) vessels
Pyloric antrum
Omental (epiploic) vessels(to the greater omentum)
Horizontal duodenum

Figure 208.2 Anterior View of Stomach

NOTE: (1) The stomach is a dilated muscular sac situated in the gastrointestinal tract between the esophagus (cardiac end) and duodenum (pyloric end). It consists of an upper portion called the **fundus,** a middle portion, the **body,** and a tapering lower part, the **pyloric region.**

(2) Although the shape of the stomach varies, it presents two curvatures as borders. The **greater curvature** is directed toward the left and to it is attached the **greater omentum.** This border forms an acute angle with the esophagus called the **cardiac notch.**

(3) The **lesser curvature** constitutes the right border of the stomach and along this edge the **lesser omentum** is attached.

(4) The blood vessels supplying the stomach include:

(a) The **left and right gastric arteries** along the lesser curvature,

(b) The **left and right (gastroepiploic) arteries** along the greater curvature, and

(c) The **short gastric branches** of the **splenic artery.** Observe that the **esophageal branches** of the left **gastric artery** supply the cardiac end of the stomach.

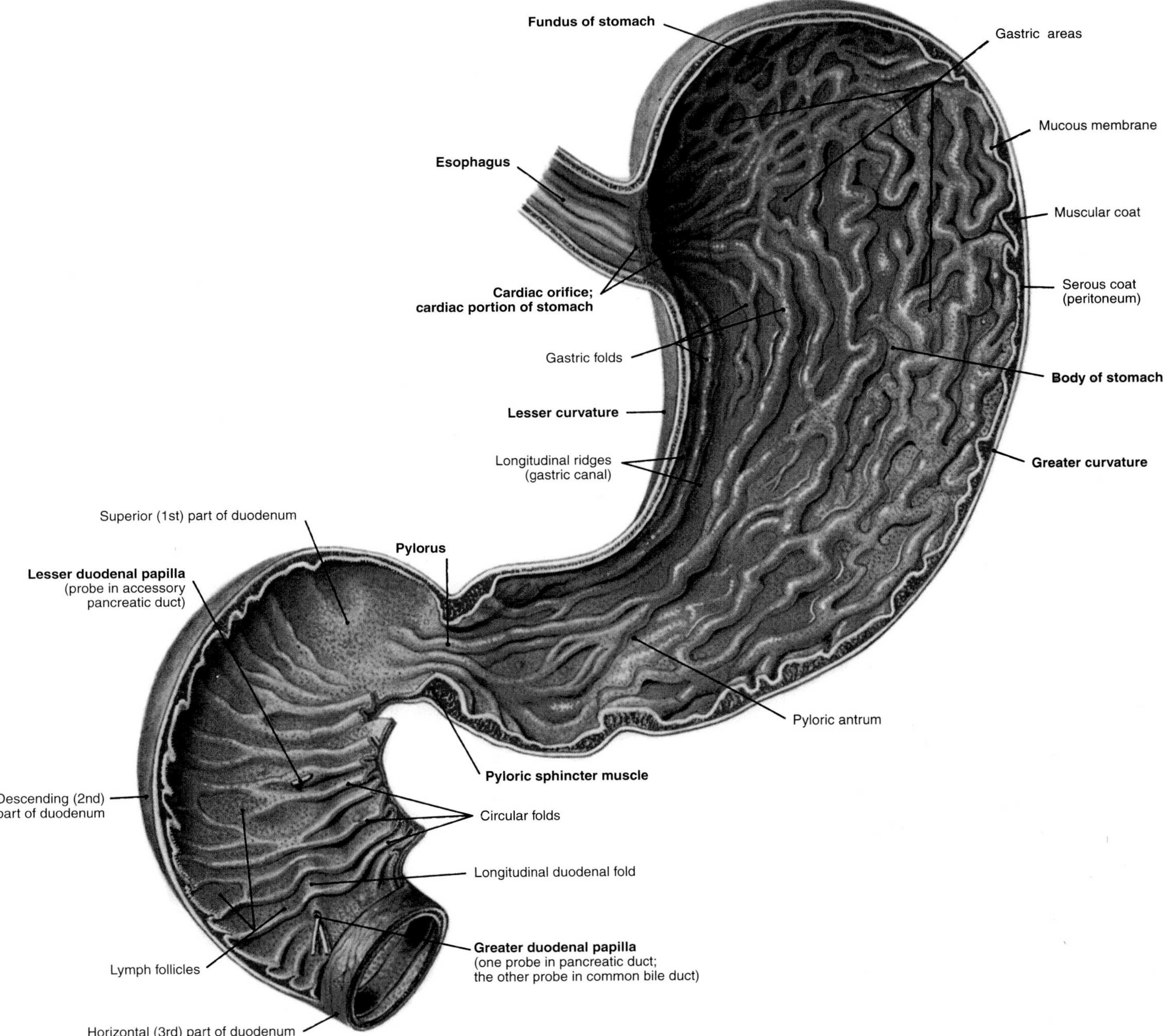
Fundus of stomach
Gastric areas
Mucous membrane
Esophagus
Muscular coat
Cardiac orifice;
cardiac portion of stomach
Serous coat
(peritoneum)
Gastric folds
Body of stomach
Lesser curvature
Longitudinal ridges
(gastric canal)
Greater curvature
Superior (1st) part of duodenum
Pylorus
Lesser duodenal papilla
(probe in accessory
pancreatic duct)
Pyloric antrum
Pyloric sphincter muscle
Descending (2nd)
part of duodenum
Circular folds
Longitudinal duodenal fold
Greater duodenal papilla
(one probe in pancreatic duct;
the other probe in common bile duct)
Lymph follicles
Horizontal (3rd) part of duodenum

Figure 209 Interior of the Stomach and Upper Duodenum

NOTE: (1) The mucosal lining of the stomach shows a series of longitudinally oriented gastric folds or empty rugae, which tend to disappear when the stomach is full and distended. These folds are more regular along the lesser curvature and form the grooved gastric canal. Food does not travel along this canal (magenstrasse).

(2) The surface of the first part of the duodenum is smooth, but the circular ridges characteristic of the small intestine commence in the second, or descending, portion of the duodenum.

(3) A circular muscle, the **pyloric sphincter**, guards the pyloric junction of the stomach with the duodenum. It diminishes the lumen of the gastrointestinal tract at this point. The pylorus is to the right of midline at the level of the first lumbar vertebra.

(4) The openings in the wall of the duodenum. The **greater duodenal papilla** serves as the site of the openings of both the common bile duct and the main pancreatic duct. The accessory pancreatic duct opens 2 cm more proximally through the lesser duodenal papilla.

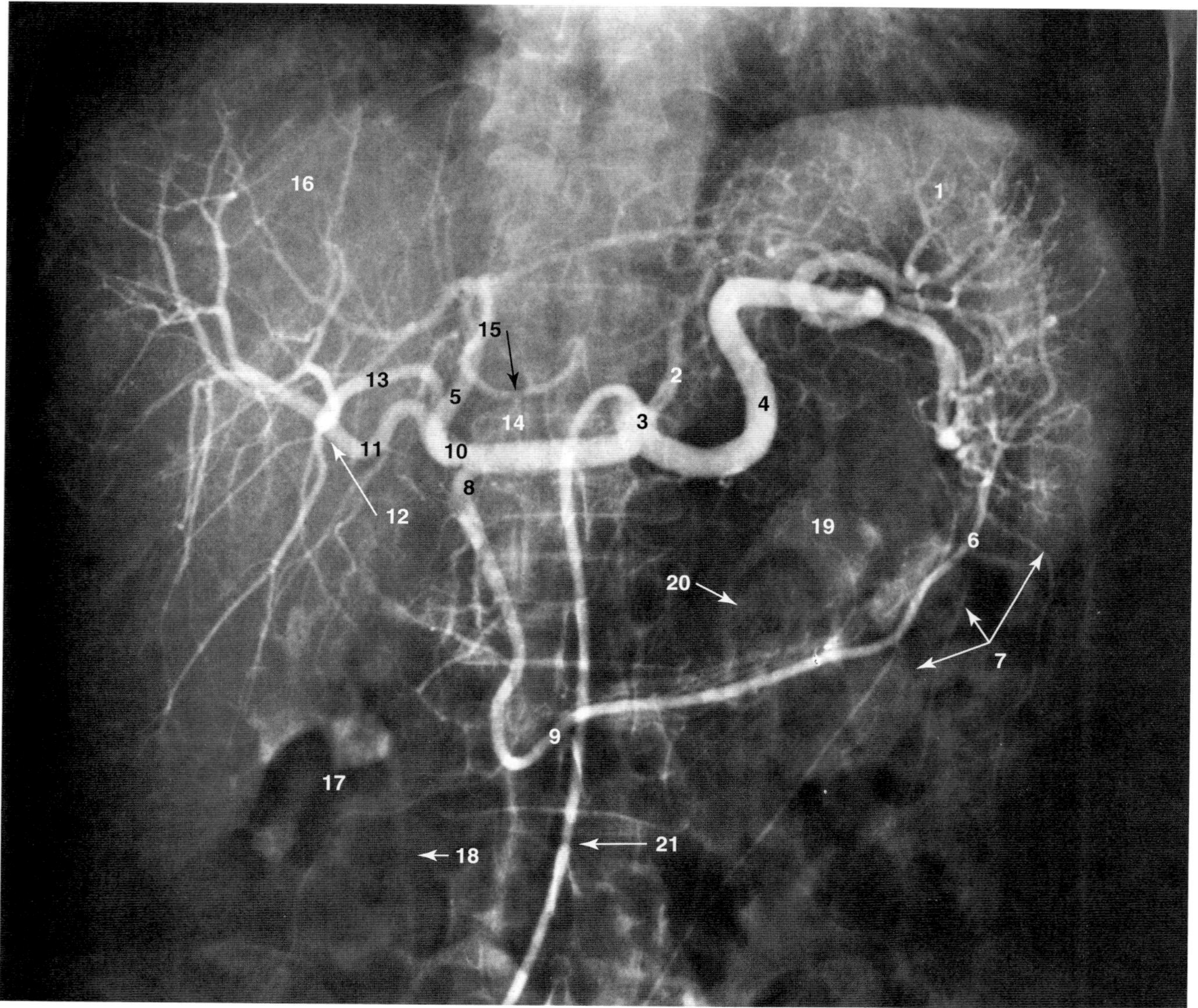
16
1
15
13
5
2
14
3
4
11
10
8
12
19
6
20
7
9
17
18
21

Figure 210 Celiac Trunk Arteriogram

NOTE: (1) This figure is a negative print from a radiograph of the upper abdomen after injection of a contrast medium through a catheter (21, arrow) in the abdominal aorta directed upward to the point where the **celiac trunk** (3) branches from the aorta.

(2) The three primary vessels arising from the celiac trunk (3) are the **left gastric artery** (2), the **splenic artery** (4), directed toward the spleen (1), and the **common hepatic artery** (5), which courses directly to the right toward the liver (16).

(3) The **left gastroomental (gastroepiploic) artery** arises from one of the lower hilar branches of the splenic artery. As it courses along the greater curvature to anastomose with the **right gastroomental (gastroepiploic)**, the **left gastroomental (gastroepiploic)** gives rise to **omental (epiploic) arteries** (7, arrows) which descend to supply the greater omentum. The right gastroomental (gastroepiploic) (9) arises from the **gastroduodenal artery** (8), which courses downward from the **common hepatic artery** (5).

(4) Beyond the origin of the gastroduodenal artery (8) the common hepatic artery (5) is called the **proper hepatic artery** (10).

(5) The proper hepatic artery (10) divides into the **right hepatic artery** (11), from which branches the **cystic artery** (12) to the gallbladder, the **middle hepatic artery** (13), and the **left hepatic artery** (14, arrow). The hepatic vessels supply the liver.

(6) From the right hepatic artery (14) in this individual branches the **right gastric artery** (15, arrow). Just as frequently, the right gastric artery arises from the common hepatic (5). The right gastric artery courses along the lesser curvature of the stomach to anastomose with the **left gastric** (2).

(7) The right renal pelvis (17) and the right ureter (18, arrow) can be seen inferiorly. Because of the liver, these structures on the right side are significantly lower than the left renal pelvis (19) and the origin of the left ureter (20, arrow).

(From Wicke, 4th ed.)

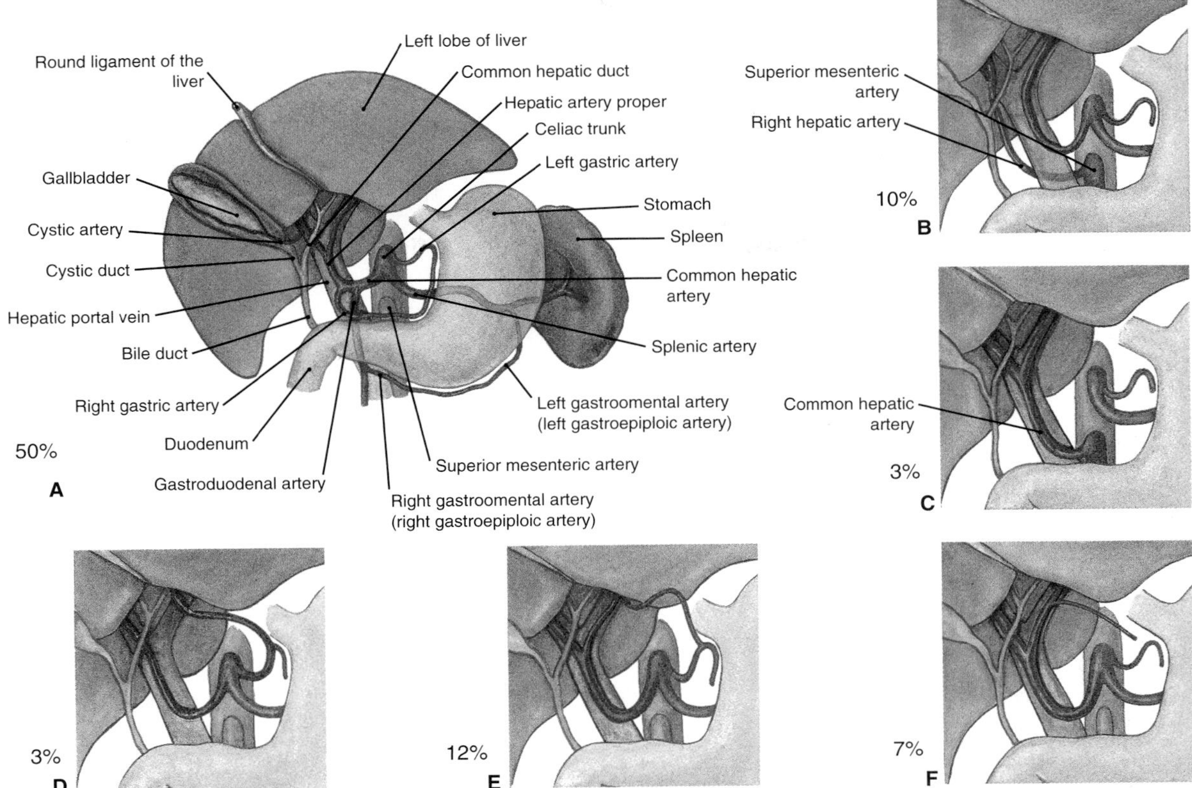

Round ligament of the liver
Left lobe of liver
Common hepatic duct
Hepatic artery proper
Celiac trunk
Left gastric artery
Gallbladder
Stomach
Spleen
Cystic artery
Cystic duct
Common hepatic artery
Hepatic portal vein
Bile duct
Splenic artery
Right gastric artery
Left gastroomental artery
(left gastroepiploic artery)
50%
A
Duodenum
Gastroduodenal artery
Superior mesenteric artery
Right gastroomental artery
(right gastroepiploic artery)
Superior mesenteric artery
Right hepatic artery
10%
B
Common hepatic artery
3%
C
3%
D
12%
E
7%
F

Figure 211.1A–F Variations in the Blood Supply to the Liver

A: Normal pattern as shown in most diagrams.
B: Superior mesenteric artery helping to supply the liver.
C: Common hepatic artery arising from the superior mesenteric artery.
D: Left gastric artery supplying the left lobe of the liver.
E: Branch of the left gastric artery helping to supply the left lobe of the liver (with the left branch of the hepatic artery).
F: An accessory branch from the proper hepatic artery supplying the lesser curvature of the stomach.
(In 25% of cases, the superior mesenteric artery participates in the arterial supply to the liver.)

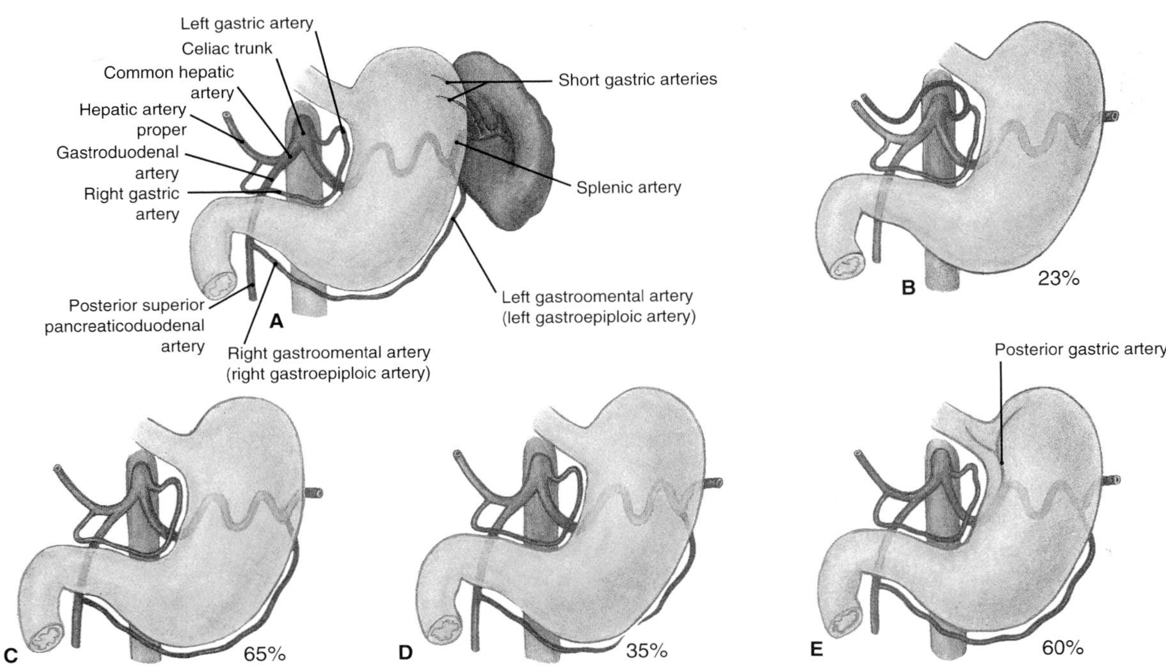

Left gastric artery
Celiac trunk
Common hepatic artery
Hepatic artery proper
Gastroduodenal artery
Right gastric artery
Short gastric arteries
Splenic artery
Posterior superior pancreaticoduodenal artery
A
Right gastroomental artery
(right gastroepiploic artery)
Left gastroomental artery
(left gastroepiploic artery)
B
23%
Posterior gastric artery
C
65%
D
35%
E
60%

Figure 211.2A–E Variations in the Arterial Blood Supply to the Stomach

A: Normal pattern as shown in most diagrams.
B: Left gastric artery participating in the supply of the left lobe of the liver.
C: Anastomosis between the right and left gastroomental (gastroepiploic) arteries along the greater curvature.
D: No anastomosis between the right and left gastroomental (gastroepiploic) arteries along the greater curvature.
E: An accessory posterior gastric artery (from the splenic) that helps to supply the posterior surface of the stomach.

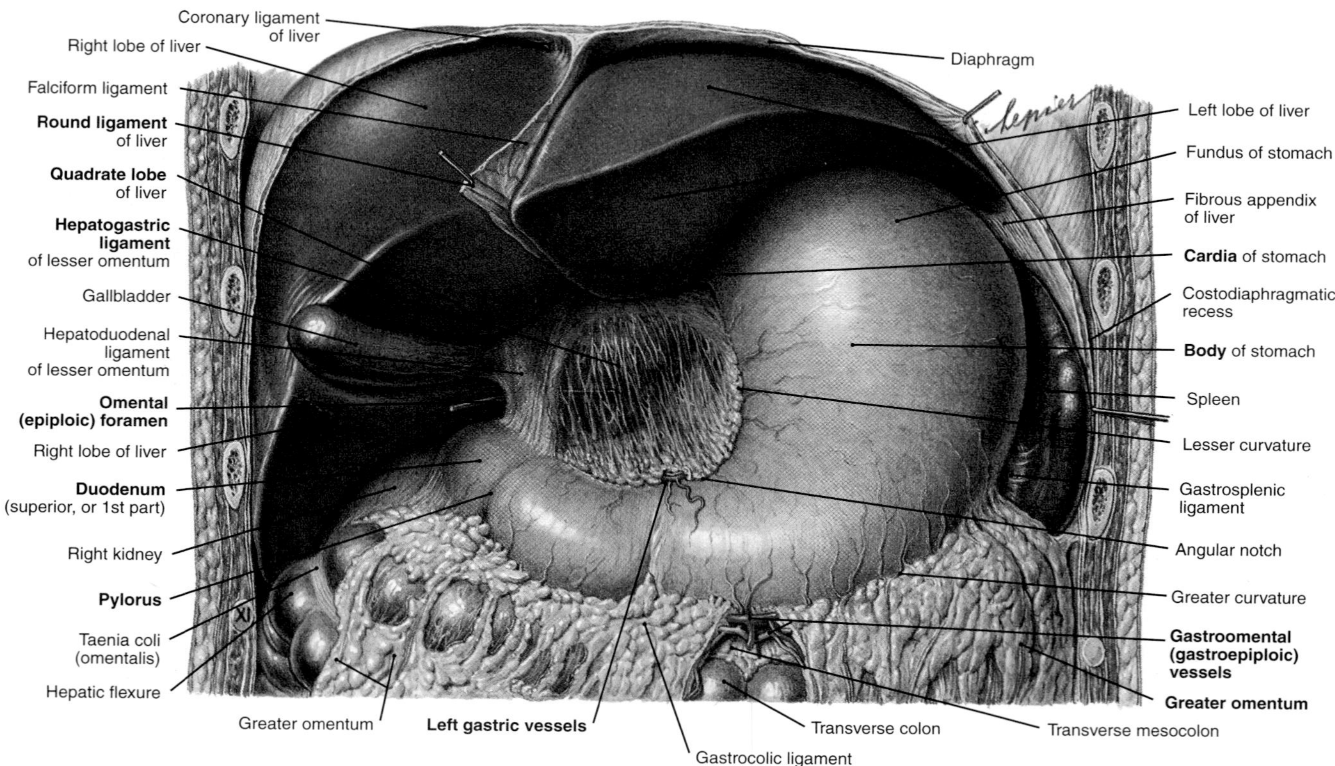
Coronary ligament of liver
Right lobe of liver
Falciform ligament
Round ligament of liver
Quadrate lobe of liver
Hepatogastric ligament of lesser omentum
Gallbladder
Hepatoduodenal ligament of lesser omentum
Omental (epiploic) foramen
Right lobe of liver
Duodenum (superior, or 1st part)
Right kidney
Pylorus
Taenia coli (omentalis)
Hepatic flexure
Greater omentum
Left gastric vessels
Gastrocolic ligament
Transverse colon
Transverse mesocolon
Diaphragm
Left lobe of liver
Fundus of stomach
Fibrous appendix of liver
Cardia of stomach
Costodiaphragmatic recess
Body of stomach
Spleen
Lesser curvature
Gastrosplenic ligament
Angular notch
Greater curvature
Gastroomental (gastroepiploic) vessels
Greater omentum
XI

Figure 212.1 Lesser Omentum, Stomach, Liver, and Spleen

NOTE: (1) The liver is elevated and a probe inserted through the **omental (epiploic) foramen** into the vestibule of the **omental bursa.** By way of this opening, the greater peritoneal sac communicates with the lesser peritoneal sac (omental bursa). The **lesser omentum** consists of the **hepatogastric** and **hepatoduodenal ligaments.**

(2) The omental (epiploic) foramen is situated just below the liver and readily admits two fingers. It is bound **superiorly** by the caudate lobe of the liver, **inferiorly** by the superior part of the duodenum, **posteriorly** by the inferior vena cava, and **anteriorly** by the lesser omentum, which ensheathes the hepatic artery, portal vein, and bile ducts at the **porta hepatis.**

(3) The greater omentum extends along the greater curvature from spleen to duodenum.

(4) The gallbladder is situated between the right and quadrate lobes of the liver and projects just beyond the inferior border of the liver, thereby coming into contact directly with the anterior abdominal wall at this site.

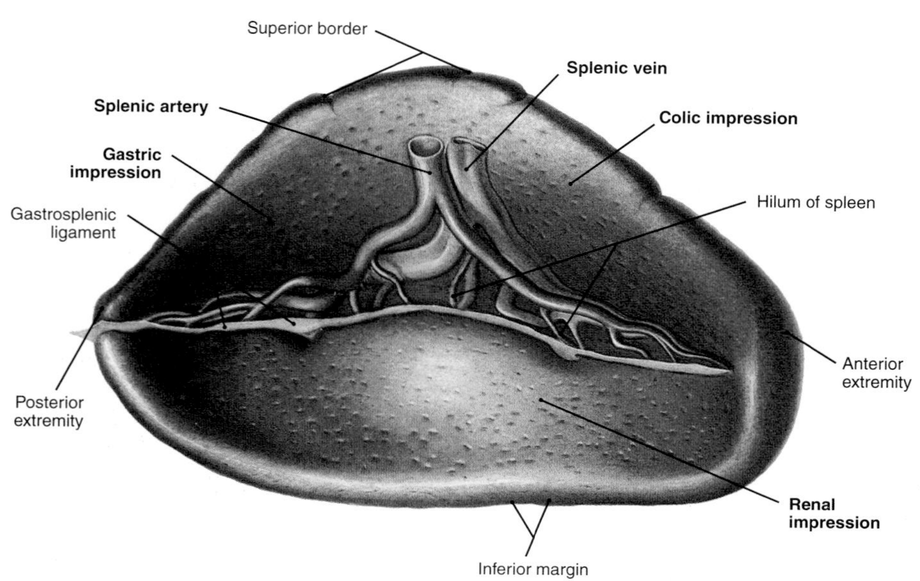
Superior border
Splenic artery
Gastric impression
Gastrosplenic ligament
Posterior extremity
Splenic vein
Colic impression
Hilum of spleen
Anterior extremity
Renal impression
Inferior margin

Figure 212.2 Spleen (Visceral Surface)

NOTE: The spleen is situated in the left hypochondriac region between the fundus of the stomach and the diaphragm. Its visceral surface shows the gastric and renal impressions that conform to the shapes of the stomach and left kidney. In addition, the left colic flexure, the tail of the pancreas, and the left adrenal gland, which overlies the left kidney, are related to this visceral surface.

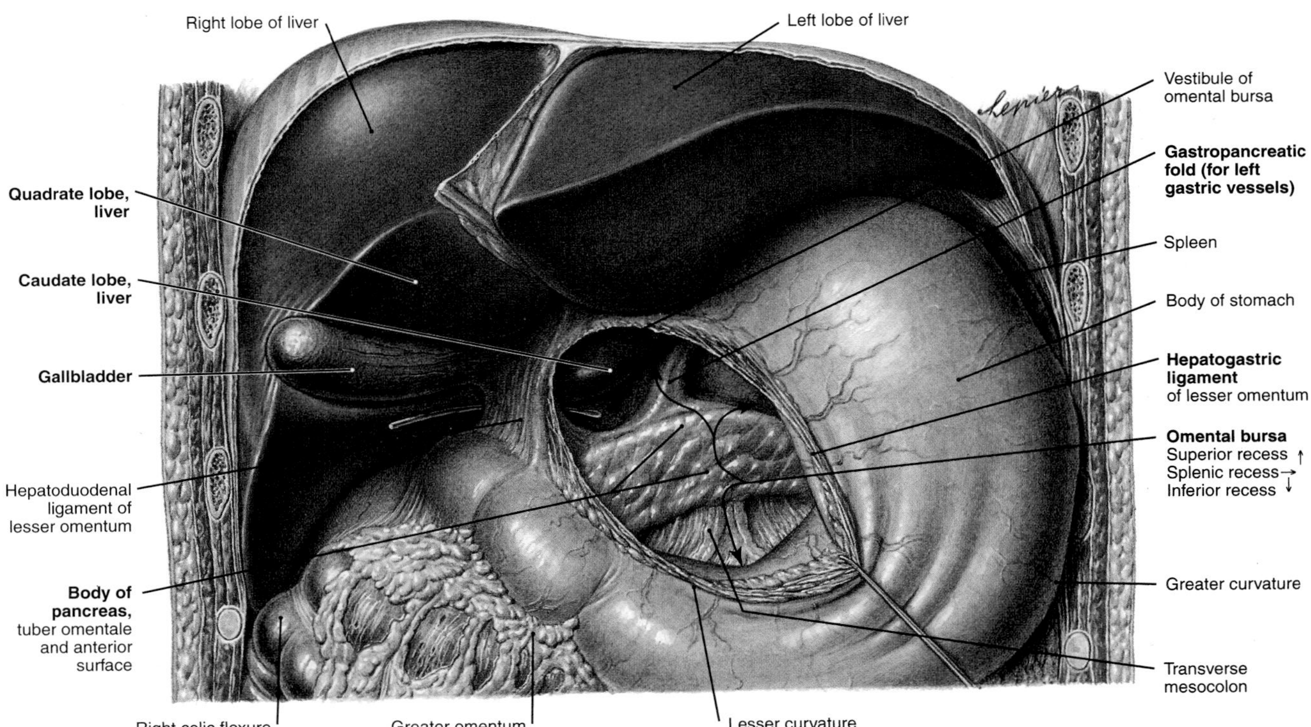
Right lobe of liver
Left lobe of liver
Vestibule of omental bursa
Gastropancreatic fold (for left gastric vessels)
Spleen
Body of stomach
Hepatogastric ligament of lesser omentum
Omental bursa
Superior recess
Splenic recess
Inferior recess
Greater curvature
Transverse mesocolon
Quadrate lobe, liver
Caudate lobe, liver
Gallbladder
Hepatoduodenal ligament of lesser omentum
Body of pancreas, tuber omentale and anterior surface
Right colic flexure
Greater omentum
Lesser curvature

Figure 213.1 Omental Bursa, Caudate Lobe of Liver, and Body of Pancreas

NOTE: (1) With the liver elevated and the lesser curvature of the stomach pulled to the left, the exposure obtained by opening the omental bursa through the hepatogastric part of the lesser omentum has been enlarged. The superior, splenic, and inferior recesses of this bursa are indicated by arrows.

(2) The portion of the omental bursa adjacent to the omental (epiploic) foramen is called the **vestibule.** Observe the **gastropancreatic fold,** which crosses the dorsal wall of the bursa. This fold is a reflection of peritoneum covering the left gastric artery coursing from the celiac trunk to its destination, the lesser curvature of the stomach.

(3) Exposure of the omental bursa reveals the **caudate lobe** of the liver situated on the dorsal surface of the **right lobe.** Also seen is the anterior surface of the body of the pancreas coursing transversely behind the stomach.

(4) The **left lobe** of the liver overlies the lesser curvature, the fundus, and part of the body of the stomach. The **caudate lobe** behind the porta hepatis and the **quadrate lobe,** located between the fossa of the gall bladder and the round ligament, come into contact with

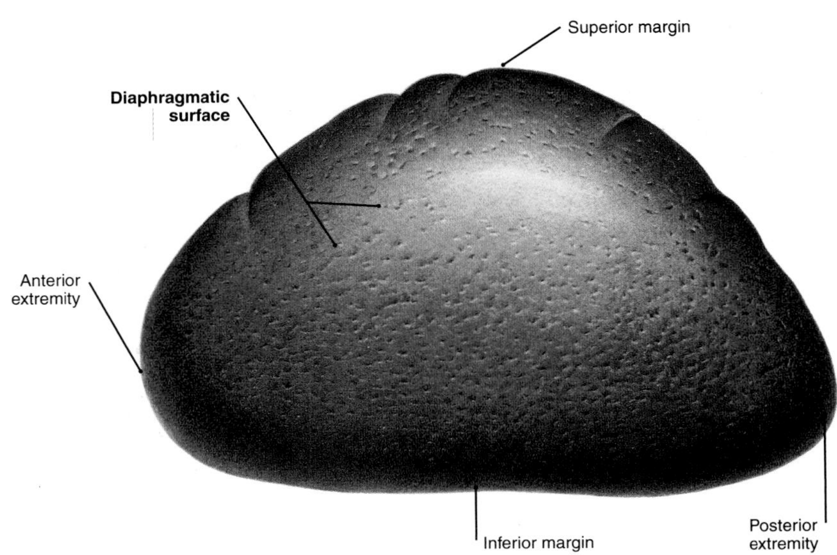
Superior margin
Diaphragmatic surface
Anterior extremity
Inferior margin
Posterior extremity

Figure 213.2 Spleen (Diaphragmatic Surface)

NOTE: The diaphragmatic surface of the spleen is directed posterolaterally. The normal spleen may vary in weight from 100 to 400 g. Its proximity to the 9th, 10th, and 11th ribs makes it vulnerable to rib fractures in this region.

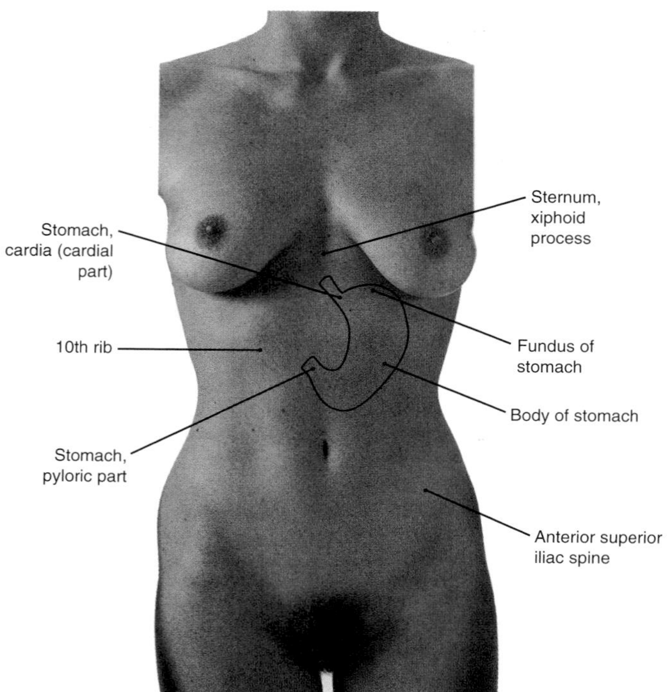
Stomach, cardia (cardial part)
Sternum, xiphoid process
10th rib
Fundus of stomach
Body of stomach
Stomach, pyloric part
Anterior superior iliac spine

Figure 214.1 Surface Projection of "Normal" Stomach

NOTE: (1) In this figure the person is standing upright.

(2) The shape and positioning of the stomach are often altered by changes in its content and by organs surrounding the stomach.

(3) The adult stomach has a capacity of about 1500 ml, while at birth it is only about 30 ml.

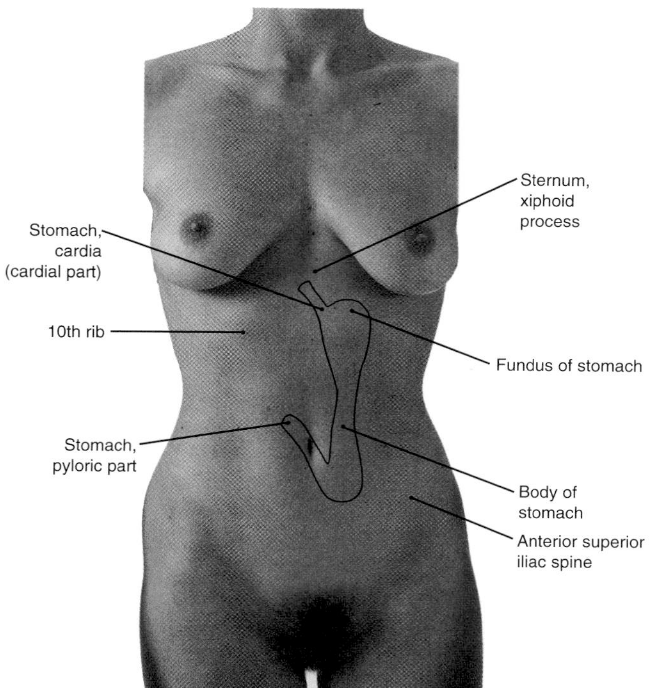
Stomach, cardia (cardial part)
Sternum, xiphoid process
10th rib
Fundus of stomach
Stomach, pyloric part
Body of stomach
Anterior superior iliac spine

Figure 214.2 Surface Projection of a "Normal Fishhook" Stomach

NOTE: (1) In this figure the person is standing upright;

(2) A "long stomach" of the type shown here can extend as far inferiorly as the upper pelvis (see radiograph in Fig. 214.3)

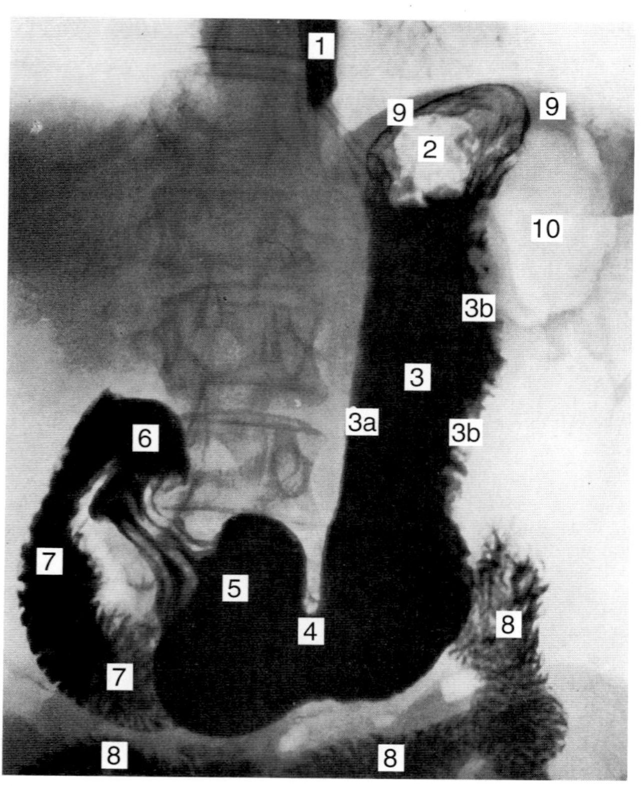
1
9
9
2
10
3b
3
3a
3b
6
7
5
4
8
7
8
8

Figure 214.3 Radiograph of the Lower Esophagus, Stomach, Duodenum, and Proximal Jejunum

NOTE: This is a normal "J-shaped" or "fishhook" stomach. The cardiac and pyloric ends of the stomach are more securely attached to the posterior body wall, whereas the body and pyloric parts are more mobile. Frequently in the upright position, the greater curvature hangs as low as the brim of the pelvis.

1. Esophagus
2. Stomach fundus (air bubble)
3. Body of stomach
3a. Lesser curvature
3b. Greater curvature
4. Peristaltic constriction at angular notch
5. Pyloric antrum (expanded)
6. Bulb of superior duodenum (first part)
7. Descending duodenum (second part)
8. Jejunum
9. Left dome of diaphragm
10. Gas in left colic flexure

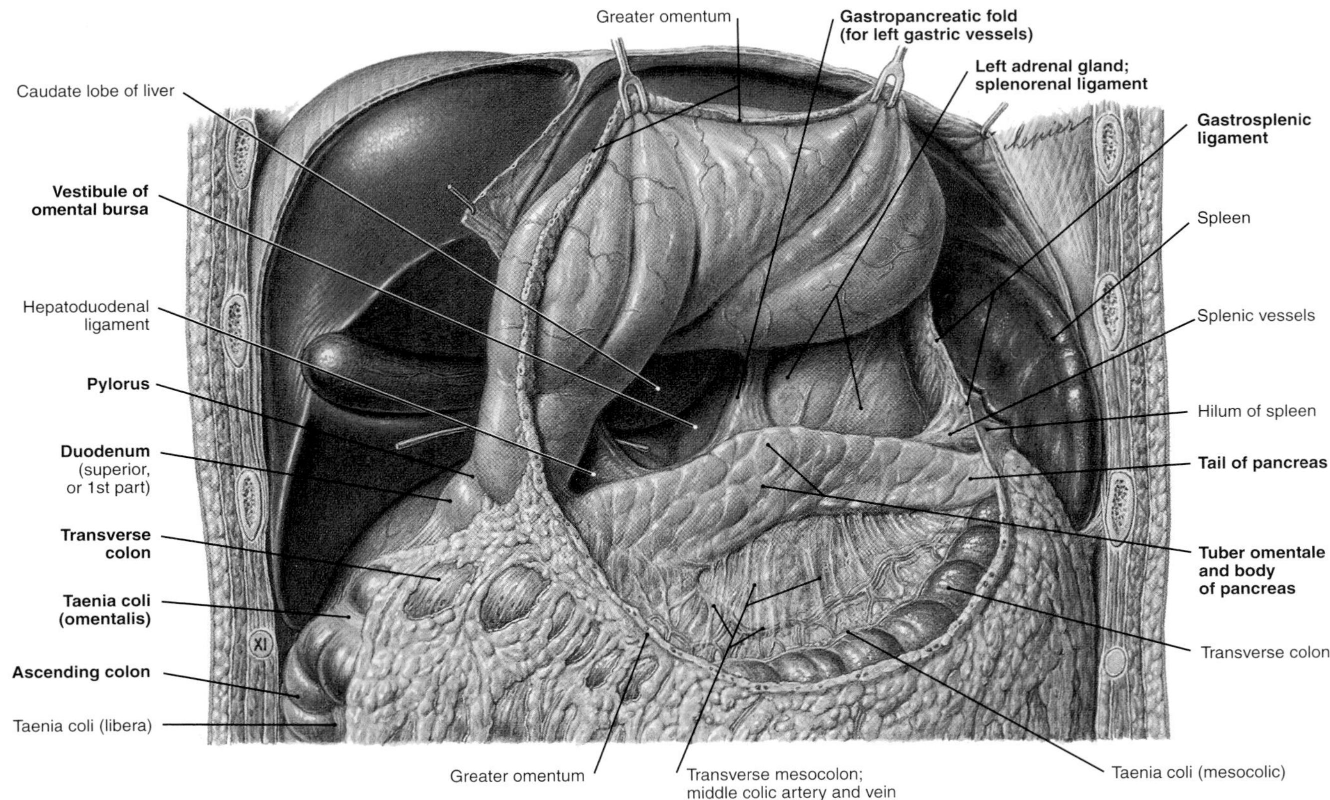
Greater omentum
Gastropancreatic fold
(for left gastric vessels)
Left adrenal gland;
splenorenal ligament
Caudate lobe of liver
Gastrosplenic
ligament
Vestibule of
omental bursa
Spleen
Hepatoduodenal
ligament
Splenic vessels
Pylorus
Hilum of spleen
Duodenum
(superior,
or 1st part)
Tail of pancreas
Transverse
colon
Tuber omentale
and body
of pancreas
Taenia coli
(omentalis)
Transverse colon
Ascending colon
Taenia coli (libera)
Greater omentum
Transverse mesocolon;
middle colic artery and vein
Taenia coli (mesocolic)

Figure 215.1 Omental Bursa and Structures in the Stomach Bed
NOTE that the greater omentum has been cut along the entire greater curvature of the stomach, and the organ has been lifted to expose the omental bursa. Note also that the **gastrosplenic** and **splenorenal** ligaments have been cut, and that the tail of the pancreas is oriented toward the hilum of the spleen.

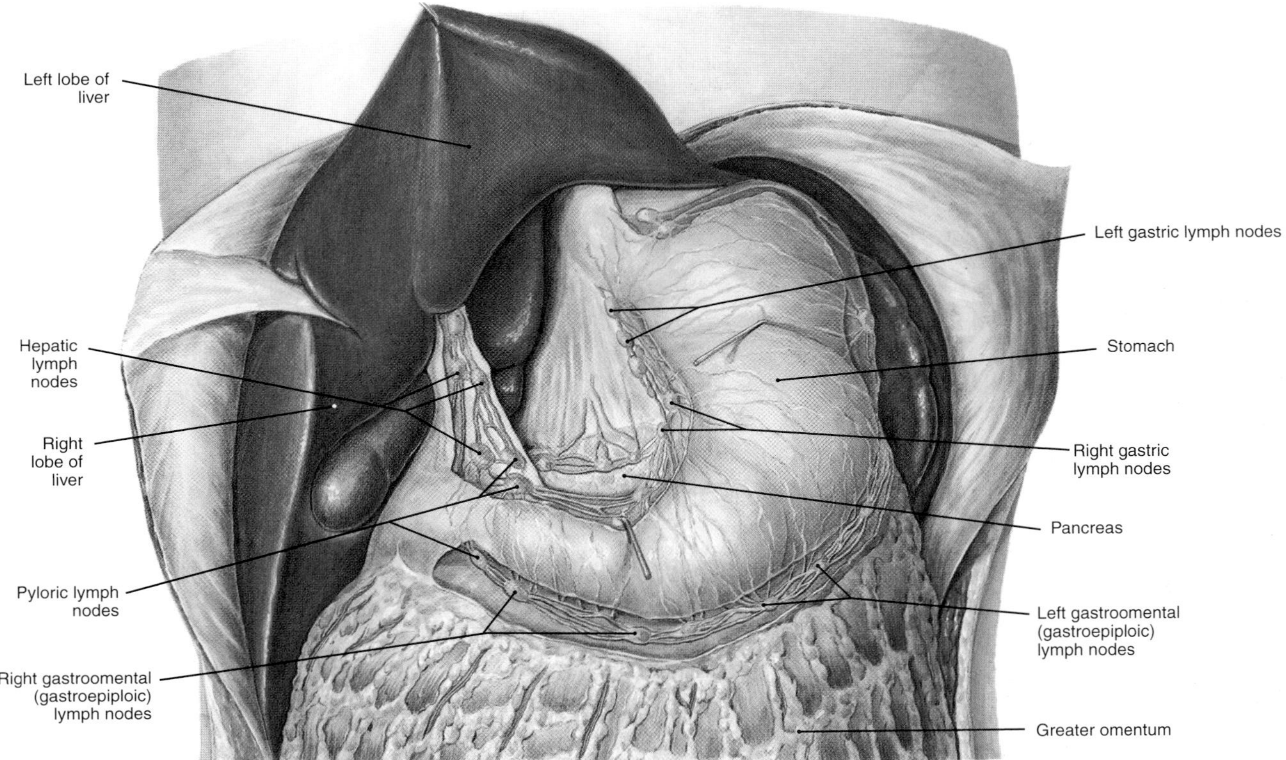
Left lobe of
liver
Left gastric lymph nodes
Stomach
Hepatic
lymph
nodes
Right
lobe of
liver
Right gastric
lymph nodes
Pancreas
Pyloric lymph
nodes
Left gastroomental
(gastroepiploic)
lymph nodes
Right gastroomental
(gastroepiploic)
lymph nodes
Greater omentum

Figure 215.2 Lymph Vessels and Nodes of the Stomach, Porta Hepatis, and Pancreas
NOTE that lymph nodes lie along the greater and lesser curvatures of the stomach with the gastroomental (gastroepiploic) and left gastric vessels. Those in the porta hepatis follow the branches of the hepatic artery and posterior to the stomach the pancreatic nodes are located along the splenic vessels. Most of these nodes drain to the **preaortic nodes.**

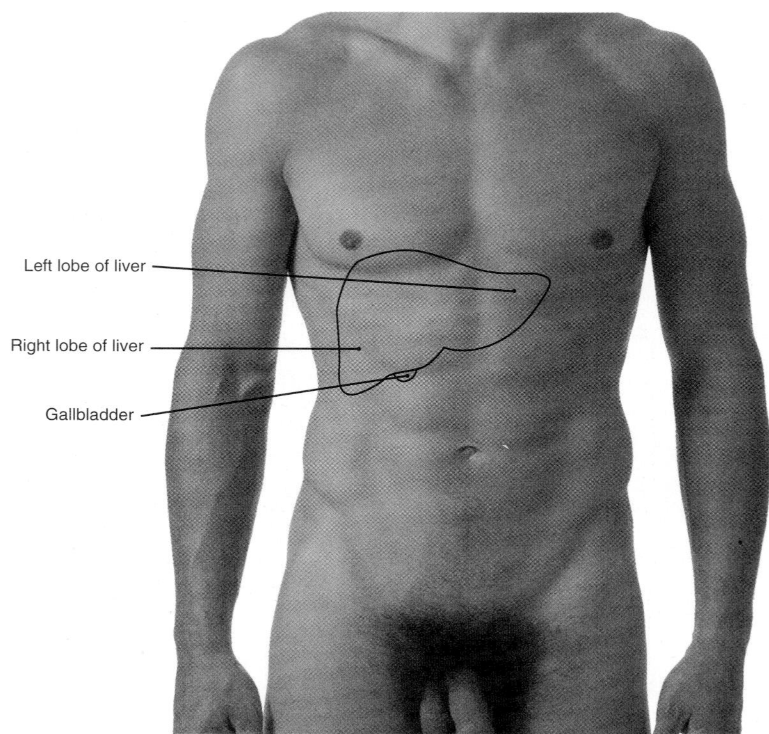
Left lobe of liver
Right lobe of liver
Gallbladder

Figure 216.1 Surface Projection of the Liver during the Midrespiratory Phase

NOTE: (1) The position of the healthy liver is related to the various phases of the respiratory cycle. This figure demonstrates the position of the liver between inspiration and expiration (midrespiratory phase).

(2) During inspiration, the diaphragm descends and pushes the liver inferiorly. During expiration, the diaphragm elevates and with it also the liver. The dome of the right lobe of the liver during expiration rises to the level of the right fifth rib.

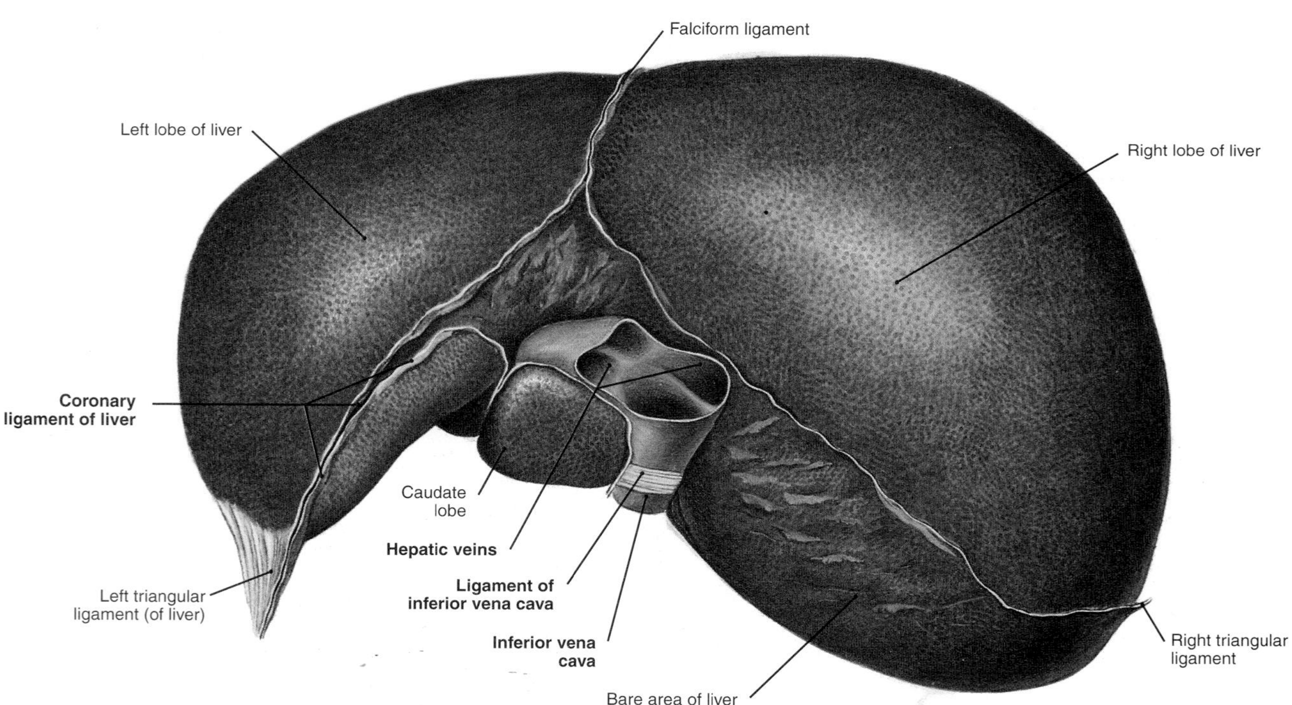
Falciform ligament
Left lobe of liver
Right lobe of liver
Coronary ligament of liver
Caudate lobe
Hepatic veins
Left triangular ligament (of liver)
Ligament of inferior vena cava
Inferior vena cava
Right triangular ligament
Bare area of liver

Figure 216.2 Dorsocranial View of the Liver

NOTE: (1) The visceral peritoneum closely adheres to the surface of the liver and is called the **coronary ligament.** Between its two leaves a portion of the liver, called the **bare area,** is devoid of peritoneum and is in contact with the abdominal surface of the diaphragm.

(2) The **hepatic veins** converge superiorly to empty into the superior vena cava.

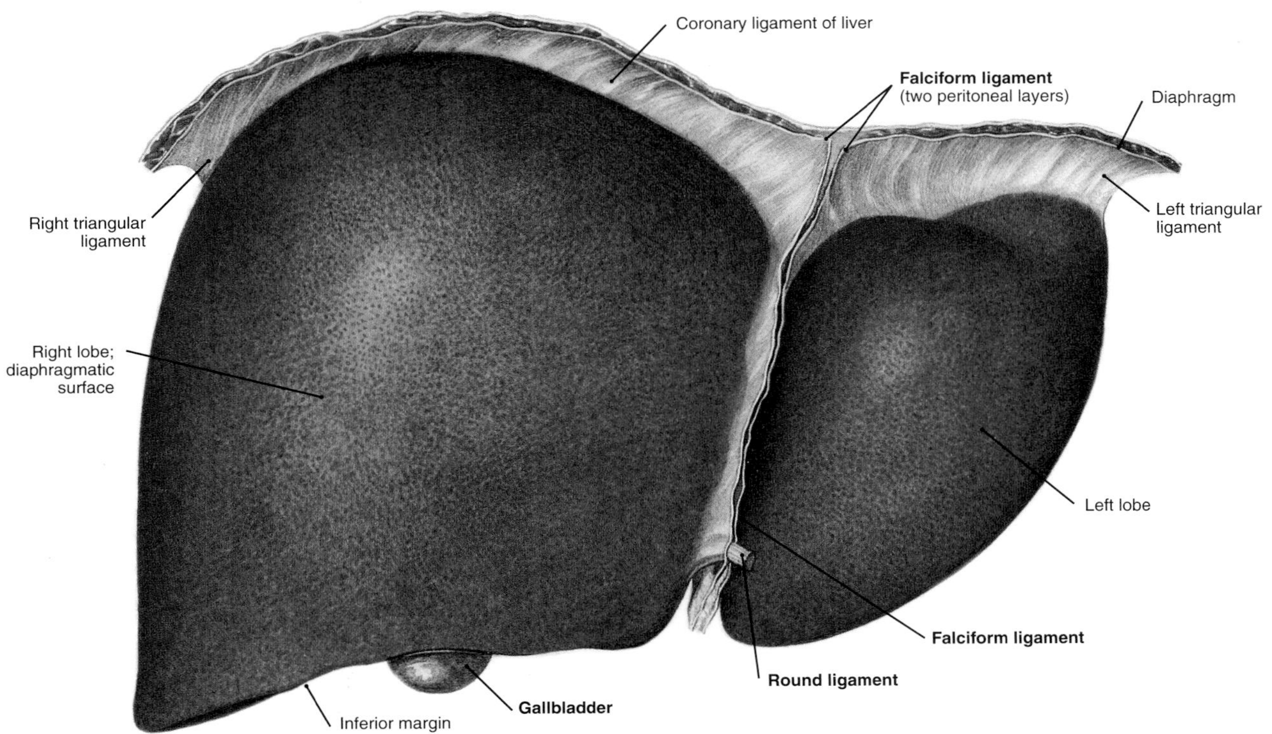
Coronary ligament of liver
Falciform ligament
(two peritoneal layers)
Diaphragm
Right triangular ligament
Left triangular ligament
Right lobe; diaphragmatic surface
Left lobe
Falciform ligament
Round ligament
Gallbladder
Inferior margin

Figure 217.1 Anterior Surface of the Liver (with Diaphragmatic Attachment)

NOTE: The **falciform ligament** separates the right and left lobes of the liver. It contains a fibrous cord, the **round ligament of the liver,** which was the **umbilical vein** during fetal life. Observe also the fundus of the gall bladder below the inferior margin of the liver.

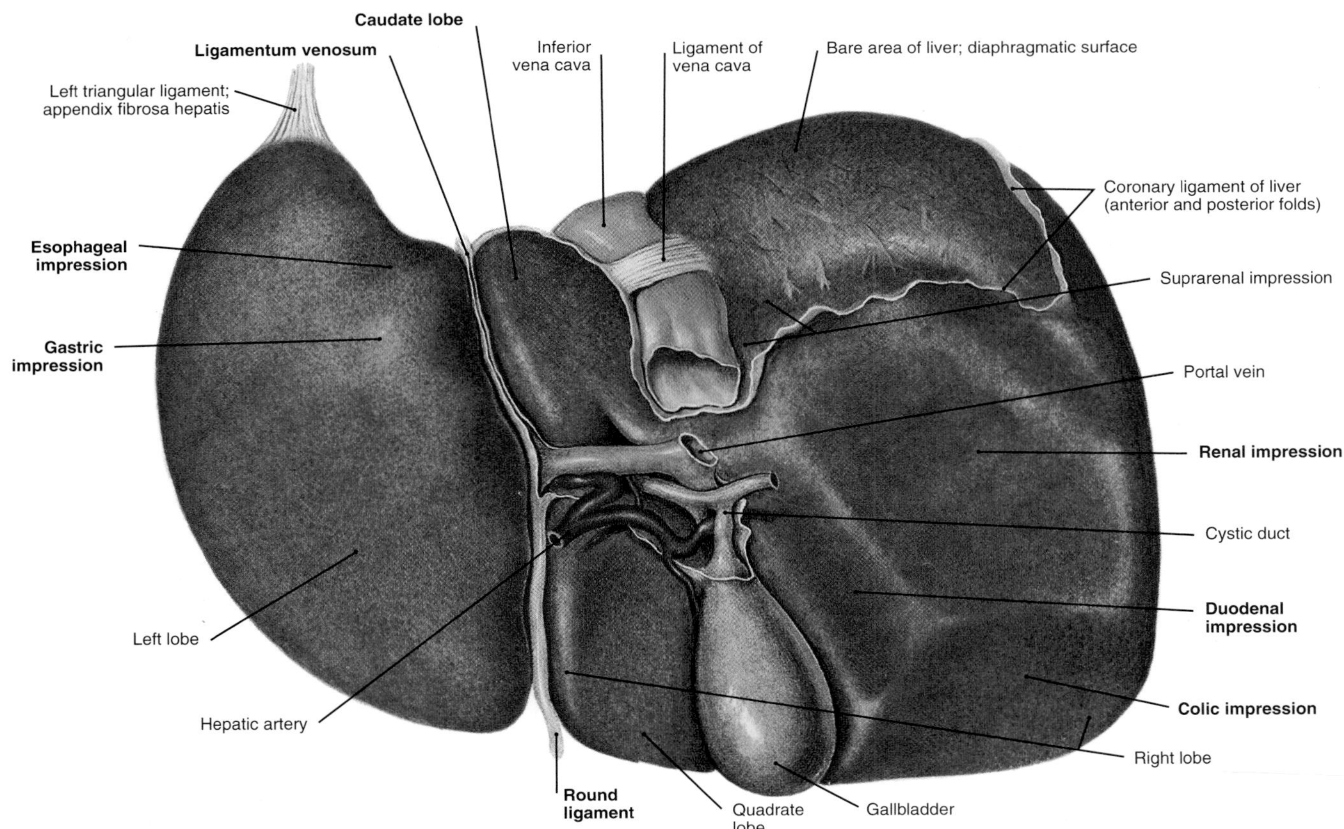
Caudate lobe
Ligamentum venosum
Inferior vena cava
Ligament of vena cava
Bare area of liver; diaphragmatic surface
Left triangular ligament; appendix fibrosa hepatis
Coronary ligament of liver
(anterior and posterior folds)
Esophageal impression
Suprarenal impression
Gastric impression
Portal vein
Renal impression
Cystic duct
Duodenal impression
Left lobe
Colic impression
Hepatic artery
Right lobe
Round ligament
Quadrate lobe
Gallbladder

Figure 217.2 Posterior (Visceral) Surface of the Liver and the Gallbladder

NOTE the impressions made by the abdominal organs on the ventral surface of the liver, and the inferior vena cava, which separates the **caudate** and **right lobes.** The gallbladder, portal vein, hepatic artery, and common bile duct bound the **quadrate lobe,** and the **ligamentum venosus** (ductus venosus) extends from the **round ligament** (umbilical vein).

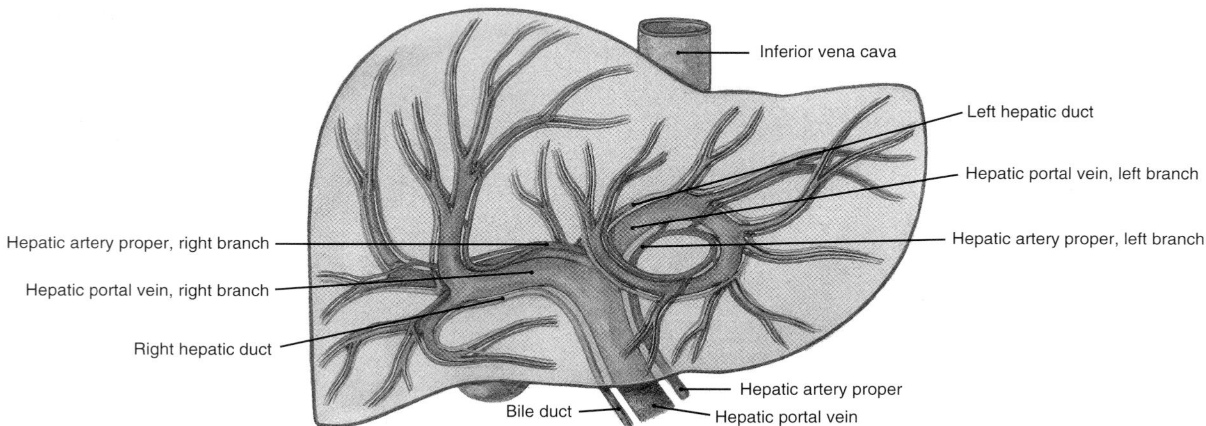
Inferior vena cava
Left hepatic duct
Hepatic portal vein, left branch
Hepatic artery proper, left branch
Hepatic artery proper, right branch
Hepatic portal vein, right branch
Right hepatic duct
Hepatic artery proper
Bile duct
Hepatic portal vein

Figure 218.1 Branching of the Portal Vein, Hepatic Artery, and Bile Duct

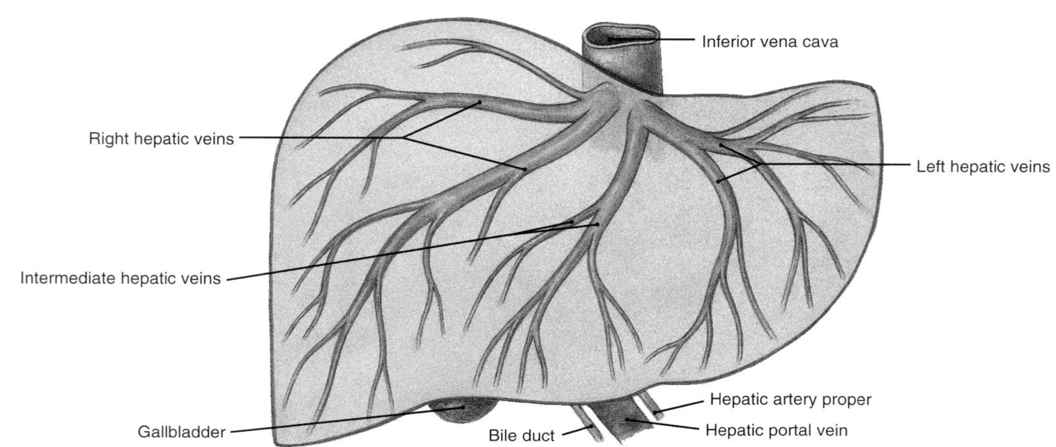
Inferior vena cava
Right hepatic veins
Left hepatic veins
Intermediate hepatic veins
Hepatic artery proper
Gallbladder
Bile duct
Hepatic portal vein

Figure 218.2 Draining Pattern of the Hepatic Veins

Figures 218.1 and 218.2 Branching Patterns of the Portal Vein, Hepatic Artery, and Tributaries of the Hepatic Vein

NOTE: (1) The portal vein and hepatic artery branch in such a way that results in segmental regions of the liver that receive their own arterial and venous branches.

(2) The portal vein and hepatic artery and veins divide the organ functionally and anatomically into a right and a left liver.

(3) The branching of these vessels forms the basis of the segmental anatomy of the liver, which is extremely important surgically, since they allow segmental resection of the liver when appropriate.

(4) The portal vein initially divides into right and left branches, as does the hepatic artery. The main fissure of this division is along a line that "passes from the tip of the gallbladder to the site where the falciform ligament disappears posteriorly" (from Launois B, and Jamieson GG (eds). Surgical anatomy of the liver and associated structures. In: Modern operative techniques in liver surgery. Edinburgh: Churchill Livingstone, 1993.)

(5) There are eight liver **segments.** The right and left livers each divide into sectors that then divide into segments (four on the left and four on the right). Each segment receives a branch of the portal vein and the hepatic artery and drains into its own segmental hepatic vein.

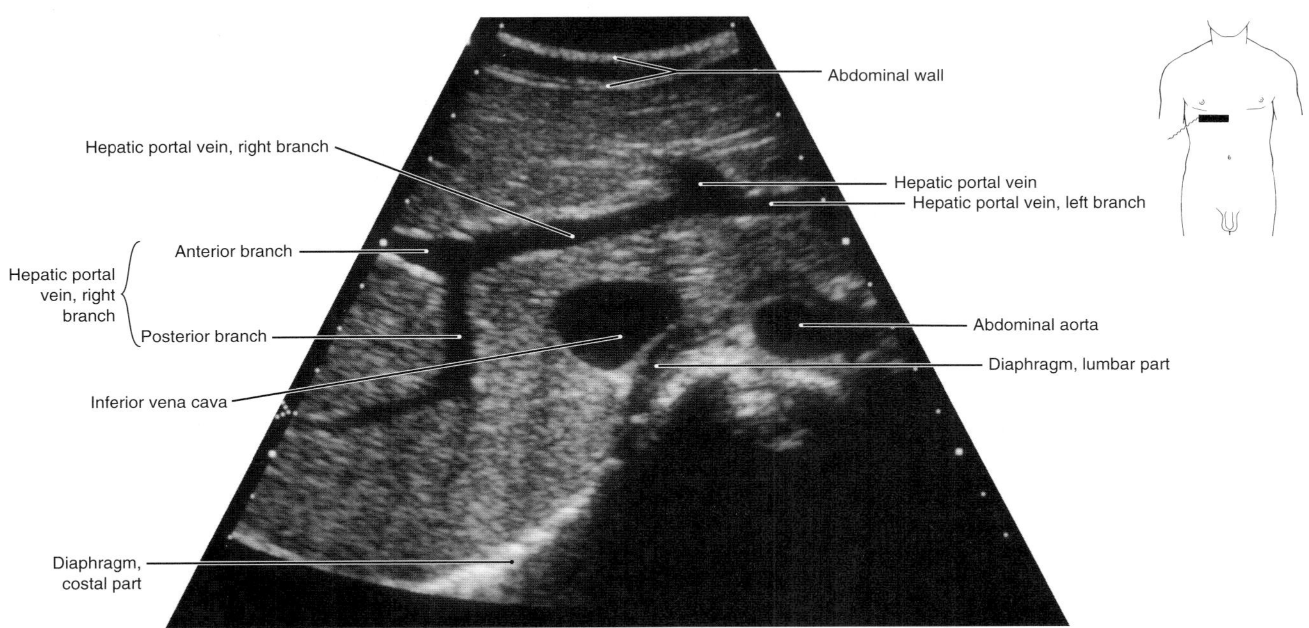
Abdominal wall
Hepatic portal vein, right branch
Hepatic portal vein
Hepatic portal vein, left branch
Hepatic portal vein, right branch
Anterior branch
Posterior branch
Abdominal aorta
Diaphragm, lumbar part
Inferior vena cava
Diaphragm, costal part

Figure 219.1 Ultrasound Scan of Openings of the Hepatic Veins into the Inferior Vena Cava (Inferior Aspect)

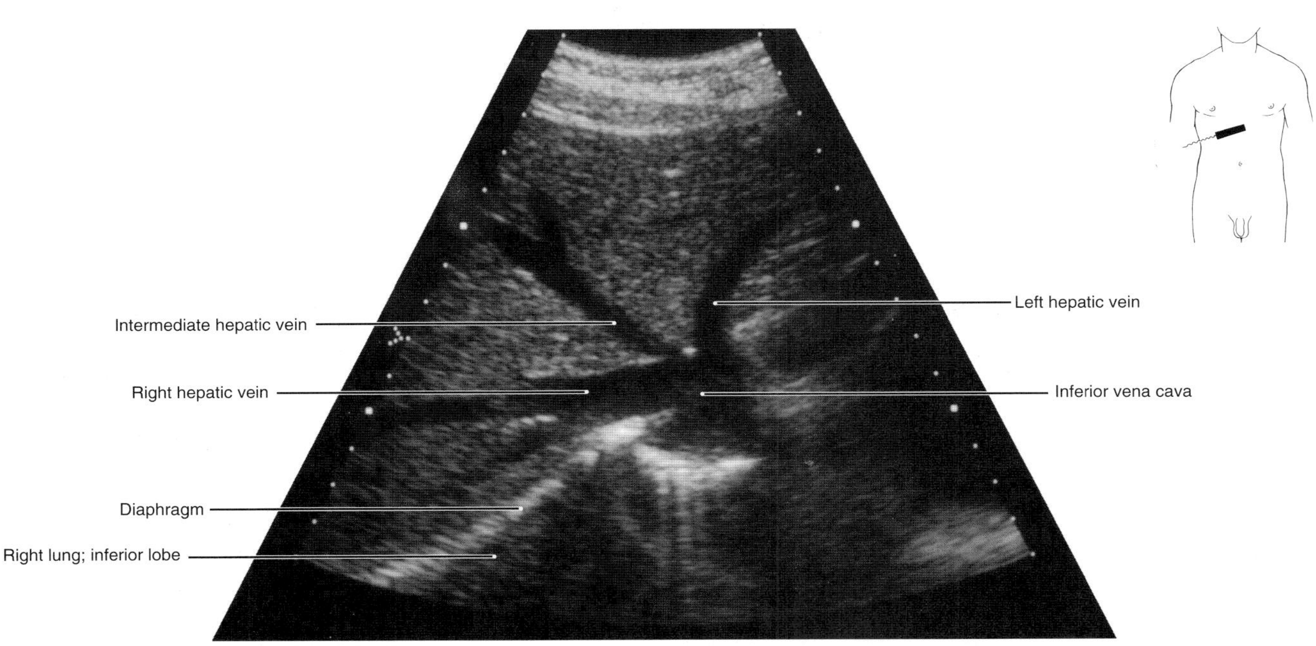
Left hepatic vein
Intermediate hepatic vein
Right hepatic vein
Inferior vena cava
Diaphragm
Right lung; inferior lobe

Figure 219.2 Ultrasound Scan of the Portal Vein and its Division into Right and Left Branches

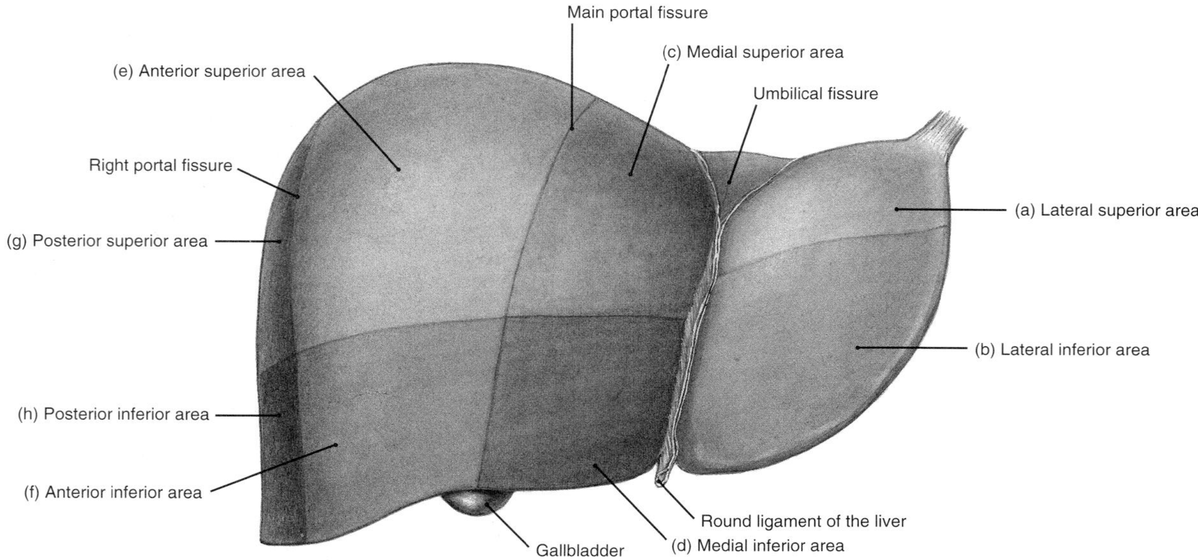
Main portal fissure
(c) Medial superior area
(e) Anterior superior area
Umbilical fissure
Right portal fissure
(a) Lateral superior area
(g) Posterior superior area
(b) Lateral inferior area
(h) Posterior inferior area
(f) Anterior inferior area
Round ligament of the liver
Gallbladder
(d) Medial inferior area

Figure 220.1 Segments of the Liver: Anterior (Diaphragmatic) Surface

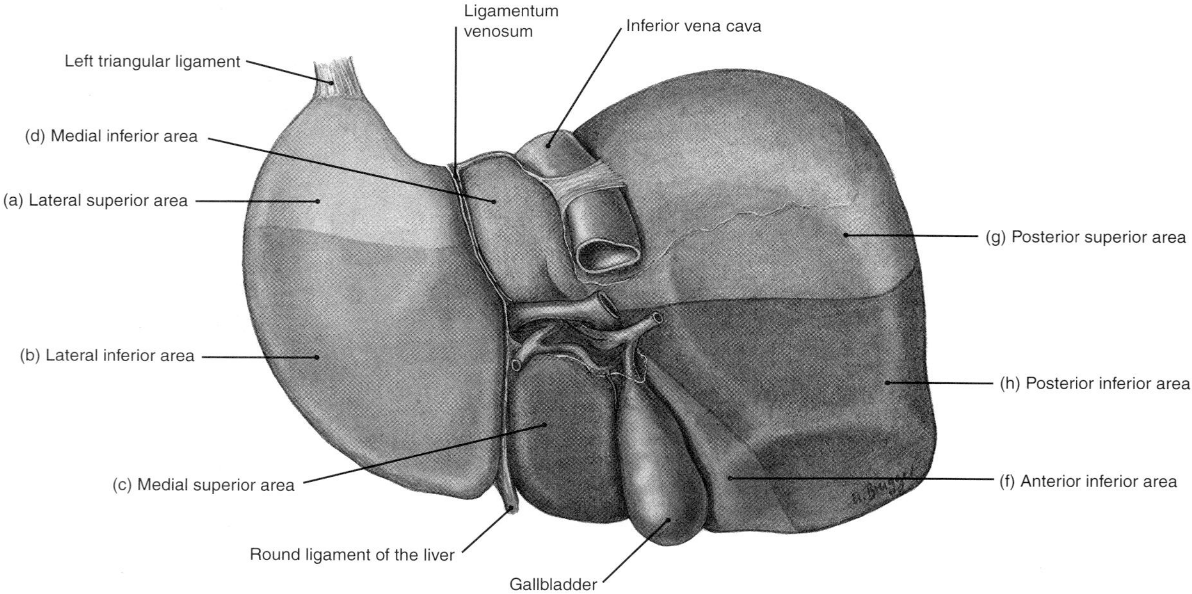
Ligamentum venosum
Inferior vena cava
Left triangular ligament
(d) Medial inferior area
(a) Lateral superior area
(g) Posterior superior area
(b) Lateral inferior area
(h) Posterior inferior area
(f) Anterior inferior area
(c) Medial superior area
Round ligament of the liver
Gallbladder

Figure 220.2 Segments of the Liver: Posterior (Visceral) Surface

NOTE: (1) Topographically, there are four lobes of the liver: the right and left lobes (separated by the falciform ligament) and the **caudate** and **quadrate** lobes (best seen on the visceral surface).

(2) The caudate lobe is located between the **ligamentum venosum** and the **inferior vena cava** and the quadrate lobe lies between the **gallbladder** and the **round ligament of the liver** (see Fig. 220.1).

(3) Of considerable surgical importance is the division of the liver into **hepatic divisions and segments.** These have been determined in relationship to the divisions of the hepatic artery and the accompanying branching of the hepatic ducts and portal vein.

(4) There are **four hepatic divisions: anterior, posterior, medial,** and **lateral.** Each of these is divided into **superior** and **inferior areas,** making a total of **eight hepatic segments.** These are the

(a) Lateral superior segment
(b) Lateral inferior segment
(c) Medial superior segment
(d) Medial inferior segment
(e) Anterior superior segment
(f) Anterior inferior segment
(g) Posterior superior segment
(h) Posterior inferior segment

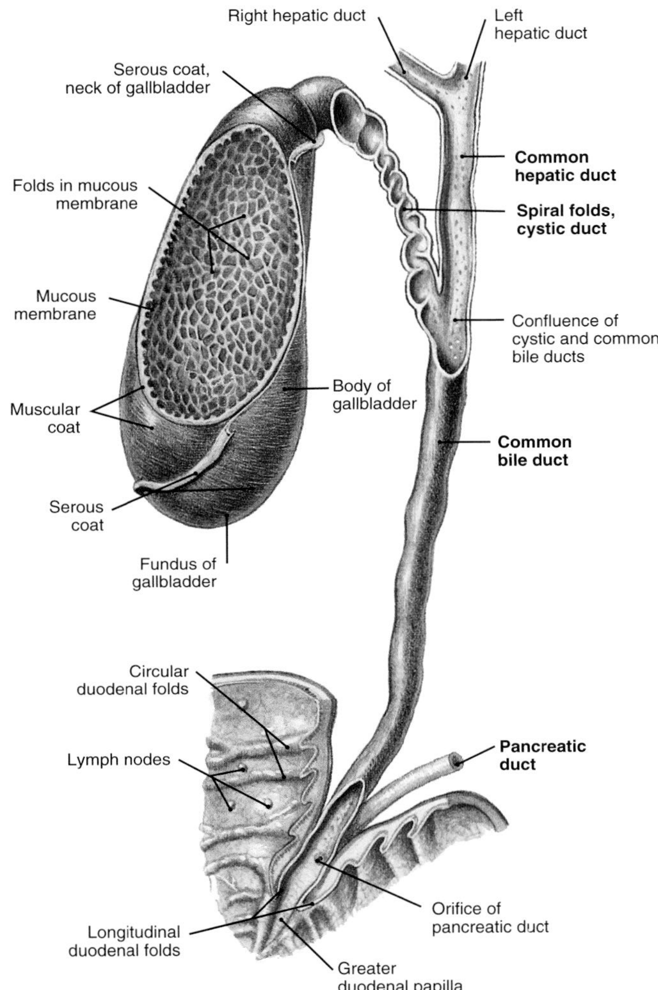
Right hepatic duct
Left hepatic duct
Serous coat, neck of gallbladder
Folds in mucous membrane
Common hepatic duct
Spiral folds, cystic duct
Mucous membrane
Confluence of cystic and common bile ducts
Muscular coat
Body of gallbladder
Common bile duct
Serous coat
Fundus of gallbladder
Circular duodenal folds
Lymph nodes
Pancreatic duct
Longitudinal duodenal folds
Orifice of pancreatic duct
Greater duodenal papilla

Figure 221.1 Gallbladder and Biliary Duct System

NOTE: (1) The wall of the gallbladder has been opened to reveal the meshwork characteristic of the surface of the mucosal layer. The pear-shaped gallbladder stores bile, which reaches it from the liver. Its capacity is about 35 ml.

(2) The spiral nature of the **cystic duct,** which emerges from the neck of the gallbladder. Normally, the cystic duct measures about 1½ in. in length and joins the **common hepatic duct** (which also is about 1½ in. long) to form the **common bile duct.**

(3) The common bile duct descends about 3 in. to open into the second or descending portion of the duodenum.

(4) At its point of entrance into the duodenum (greater duodenal papilla), the common bile duct is joined by the **main pancreatic duct** (duct of Wirsung).

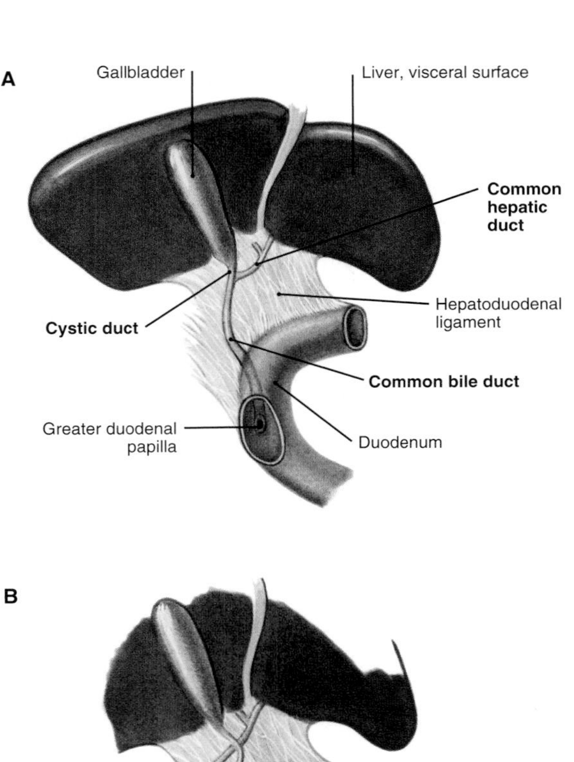
A
Gallbladder
Liver, visceral surface
Common hepatic duct
Hepatoduodenal ligament
Cystic duct
Common bile duct
Greater duodenal papilla
Duodenum

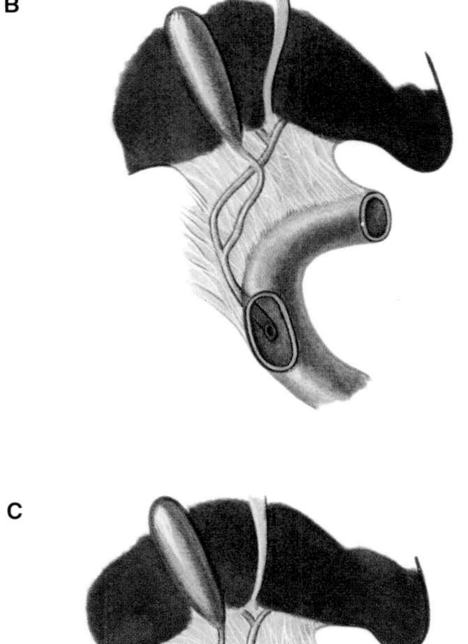
B

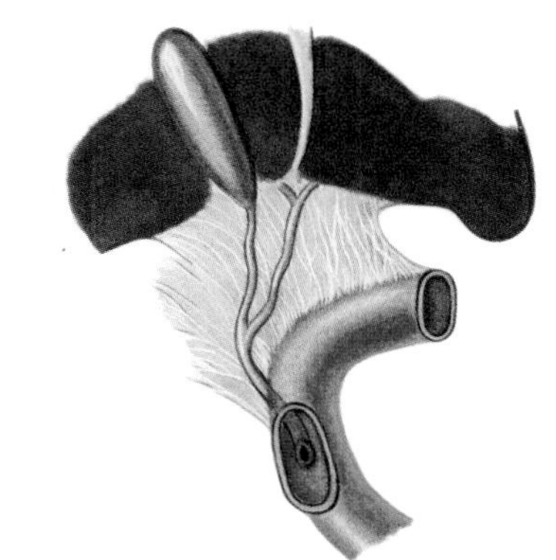
C

Figure 221.2A, B, C Variations in the Union of the Cystic and Common Hepatic Ducts

NOTE: Usually the cystic duct lies to the right of the common hepatic duct at a point just superior to the level of the first part of the duodenum. Variations in this schema occur as indicated in the following three examples:

A: The union of the cystic and common hepatic ducts occurs close to the liver, resulting in short cystic and common hepatic ducts and a long common bile duct.

B: The cystic duct crosses to the left of the common hepatic duct and joins the hepatic duct low, resulting in a short common bile duct.

C: The cystic duct remains to the right of the common hepatic duct but still joins it close to the site of penetration of the duodenum, again resulting in a short common bile duct.

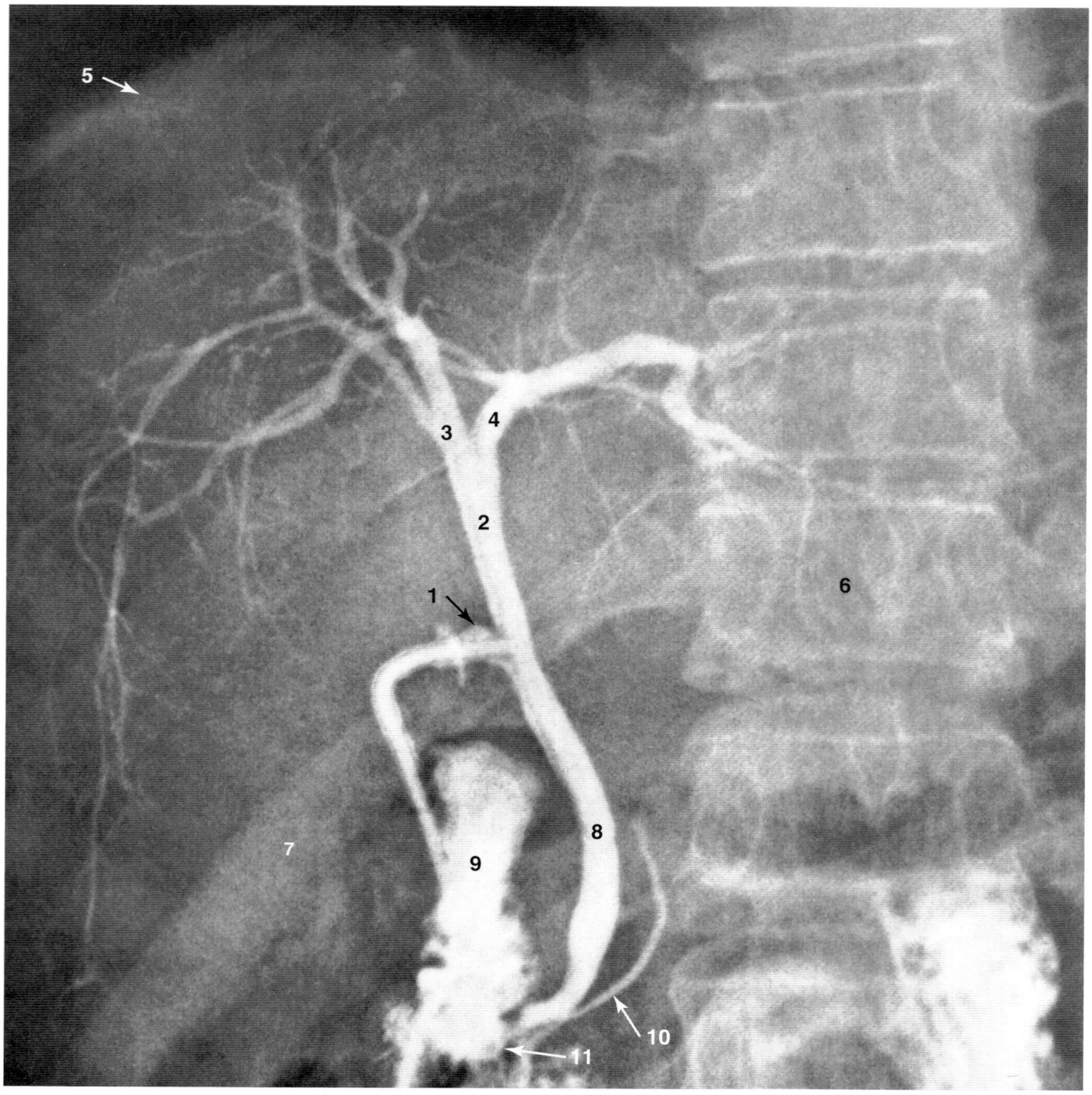

Figure 222.1 Intraoperative Cholangiogram: Radiograph of Biliary Duct System

NOTE: The gallbladder has been removed and a catheter and tube have been inserted through the stump of the cystic duct (1) into the common hepatic duct (2) and contrast medium injected into the biliary system. Other structures are numbered as follows:

3. Right hepatic duct
4. Left hepatic duct
5. Diaphragm
6. 11th thoracic vertebra
7. 11th rib
8. Common bile duct
9. Duodenum (second, descending part)
10. Main pancreatic duct
11. Greater duodenal papilla

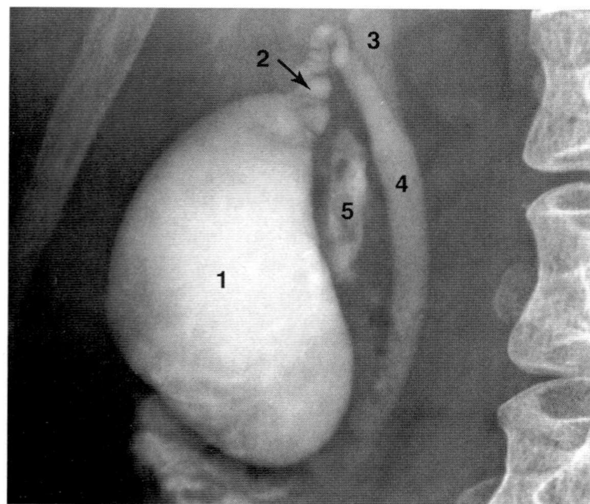
3
2
4
5
1

Figure 222.2 Radiograph of Gallbladder and Biliary Ducts

1. Body of the gallbladder
2. Cystic duct with spiral valves
3. Common hepatic duct
4. Union of common hepatic and cystic ducts to form common bile duct
5. Contrast medium in duodenum

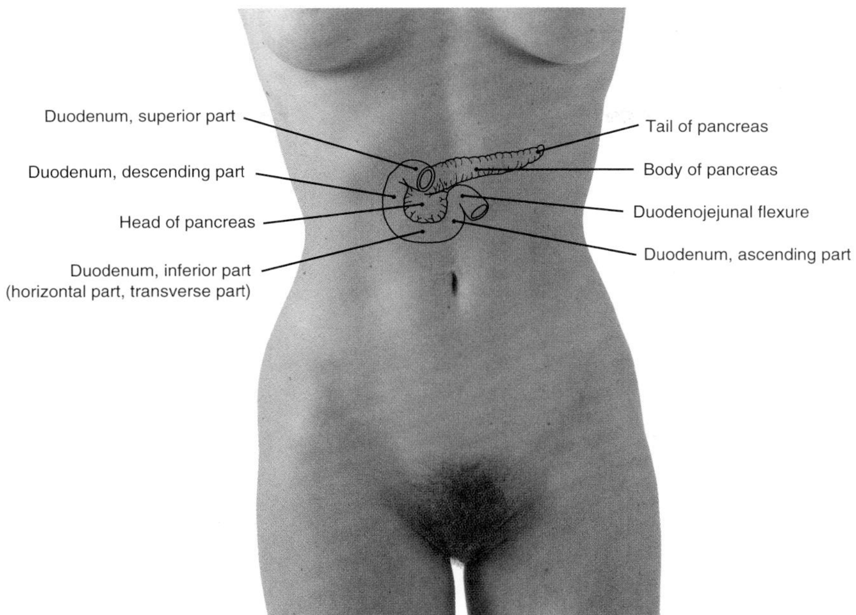
Duodenum, superior part
Duodenum, descending part
Head of pancreas
Duodenum, inferior part (horizontal part, transverse part)
Tail of pancreas
Body of pancreas
Duodenojejunal flexure
Duodenum, ascending part

Figure 223.1 Surface Projection of the Duodenum and Pancreas

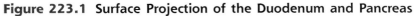

Common hepatic artery
Gastric (coronary) vein
Inferior vena cava
Aorta
Right hepatic artery
Aortic hiatus
Portal vein
Left gastric artery
Left suprarenal gland
Diaphragm
Right suprarenal gland
Splenic artery and vein
Hepatic duct
Left kidney
Cystic duct
Gastroduodenal artery
Tail of pancreas
Right kidney
Superior mesenteric artery and vein
Celiac trunk
Gastroduodenal vein
Renal artery
Head of pancreas
Renal vein
Descending (2nd) part of duodenum
Renal pelvis
Middle colic vessels
Duodenal suspensory ligament (ligament of Treitz)
Right colic artery and vein
Horizontal (3rd) part of duodenum
Jejunum
Quadratus lumborum muscle
Left ureter
Psoas major muscle
Right ureter
Inferior mesenteric vein
Right testicular artery and vein (♀ rt. ovarian a.v.)
Inferior mesenteric artery
Small intestinal vessels

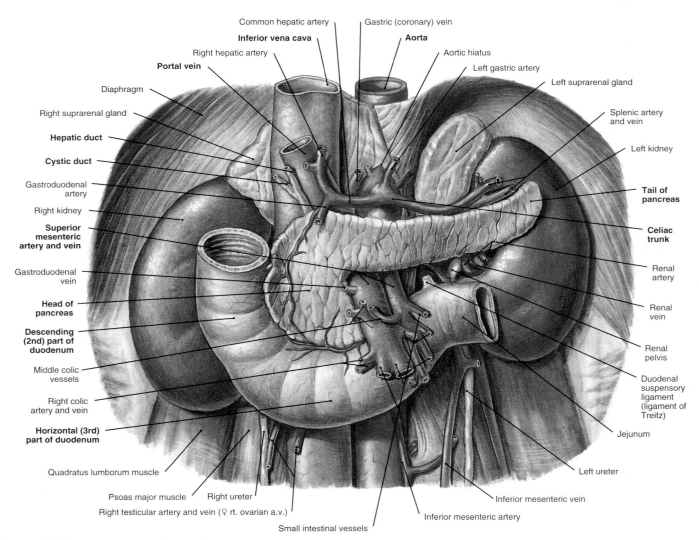

Figure 223.2 Pancreas and Duodenum

NOTE: (1) The **head** of the pancreas lies to the right of the midline and is in contact with the inferior vena cava and the common bile duct dorsally and the transverse colon (not shown) ventrally.

(2) The **body** of the pancreas crosses the midline at the L1 level, and it is in contact posteriorly with the aorta, the superior mesenteric vessels, the left kidney, and the left adrenal gland.

(3) The **tail** of the pancreas is in contact with the spleen laterally, the left kidney posteriorly, and the splenic flexure of the colon anteriorly.

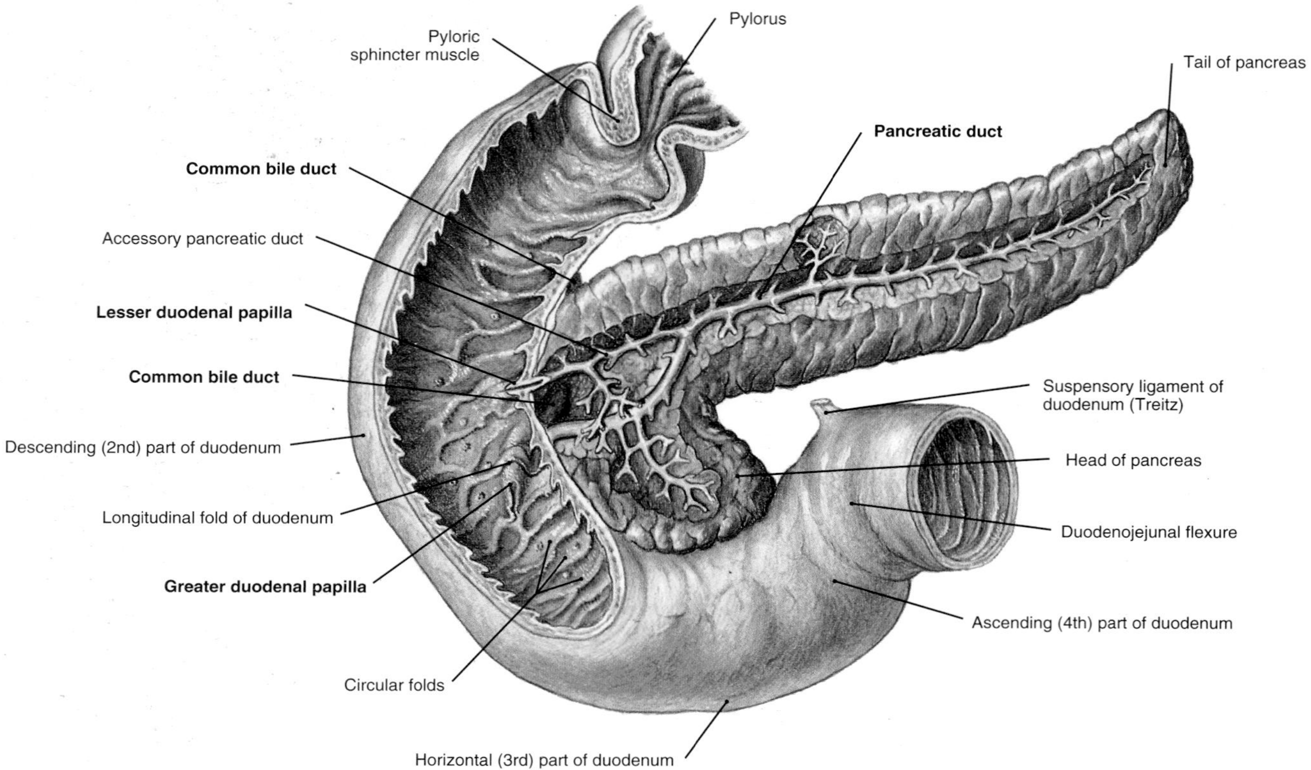
Pyloric sphincter muscle
Pylorus
Tail of pancreas
Pancreatic duct
Common bile duct
Accessory pancreatic duct
Lesser duodenal papilla
Common bile duct
Suspensory ligament of duodenum (Treitz)
Descending (2nd) part of duodenum
Head of pancreas
Duodenojejunal flexure
Longitudinal fold of duodenum
Greater duodenal papilla
Ascending (4th) part of duodenum
Circular folds
Horizontal (3rd) part of duodenum

Figure 224.1 Pancreatic Duct System

NOTE: (1) The main pancreatic duct system has been dissected in this specimen. Observe how the accessory pancreatic duct extends straight into the duodenum through the lesser duodenal papilla. The main pancreatic duct, however, bends caudally to drain most of the head of the pancreas and then opens into the greater duodenal papilla with the common bile duct.

(2) From the pylorus to the duodenojejunal flexure, the duodenum measures about 10 in. At its termination, a suspensory ligament (of Treitz) marks the commencement of the jejunum. Here the small intestine becomes surrounded by peritoneum and is suspended from the posterior abdominal wall by the mesentery of the small intestine.

(3) The duodenum and pancreas are both retroperitoneal structures.

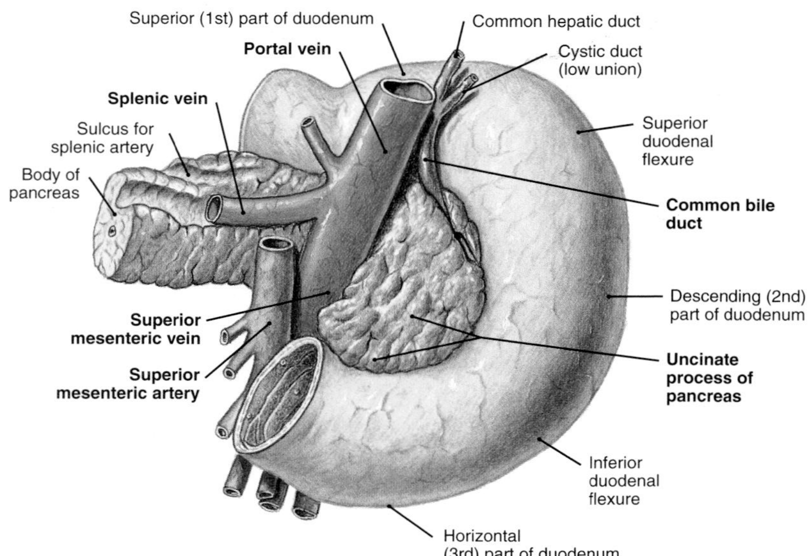
Superior (1st) part of duodenum
Common hepatic duct
Portal vein
Cystic duct (low union)
Splenic vein
Sulcus for splenic artery
Superior duodenal flexure
Body of pancreas
Common bile duct
Descending (2nd) part of duodenum
Superior mesenteric vein
Uncinate process of pancreas
Superior mesenteric artery
Inferior duodenal flexure
Horizontal (3rd) part of duodenum

Figure 224.2 Head of Pancreas and Duodenum (Dorsal View)

NOTE: (1) This posterior view of the pancreatic head and its **uncinate process** shows the **common bile duct** embedded in the pancreas as the duct descends adjacent to the duodenum.

(2) Observe the **portal vein** as it ascends to the liver coursing posterior to the pancreatic head. Realize that the portal vein is the continuation superiorly beyond the junction of the **splenic vein** and the **superior mesenteric vein.**

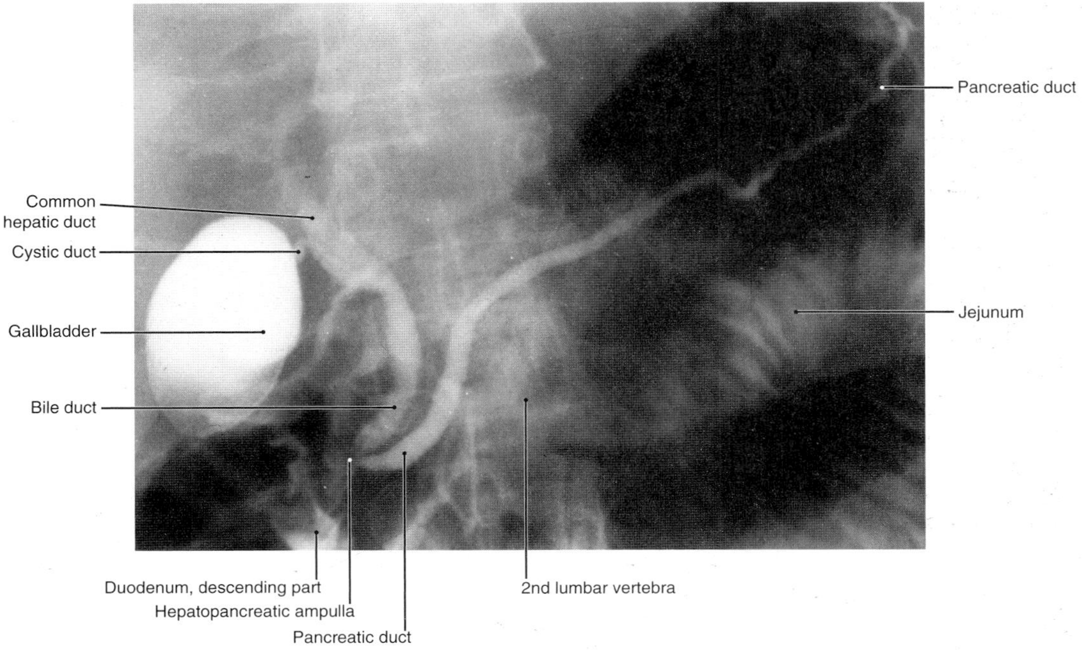
Pancreatic duct
Common hepatic duct
Cystic duct
Gallbladder
Jejunum
Bile duct
Duodenum, descending part
Hepatopancreatic ampulla
Pancreatic duct
2nd lumbar vertebra

Figure 225.1 Pancreatic Duct, Common Bile Duct, and Gallbladder

NOTE: (1) This radiograph was taken following the injection of a contrast medium through a cannula placed in the common duct formed by junction of the main pancreatic duct and the common bile duct along the second part of the duodenum.

(2) The pancreatic duct is visible throughout its extent (i.e., from the splenic hilum to the hepatopancreatic ampulla). Also visible are the common hepatic duct and the common bile duct along with the gallbladder and a short part of the cystic duct.

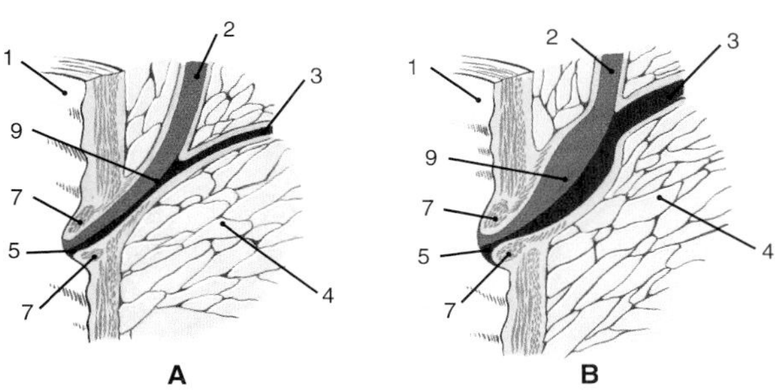
A
B

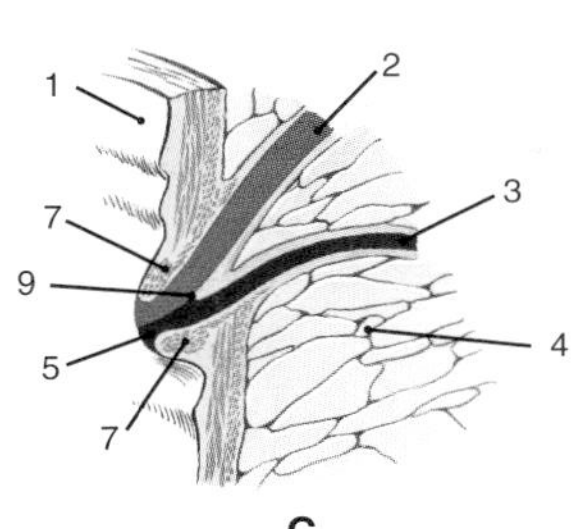
C

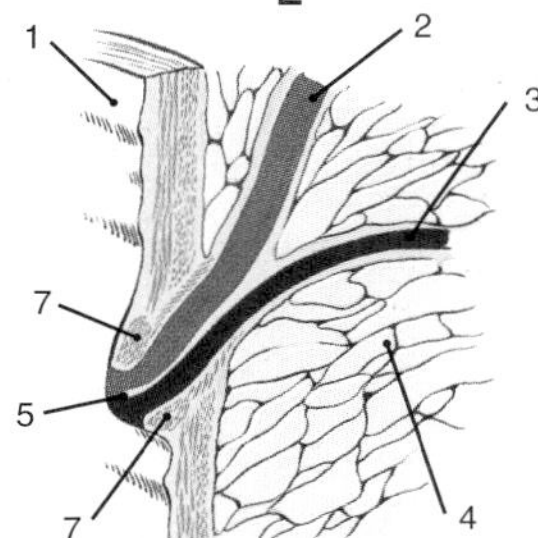
E

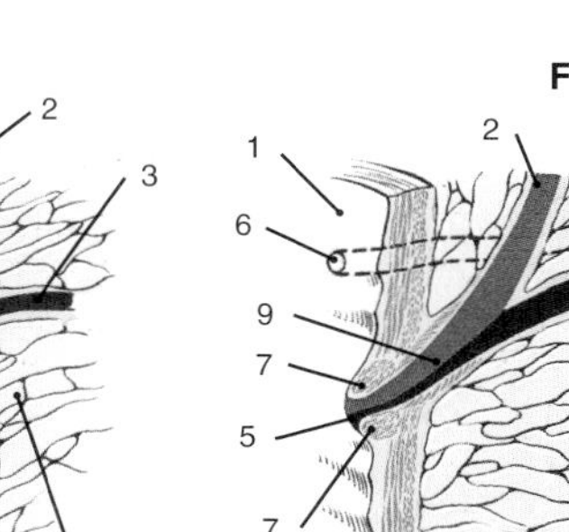
F

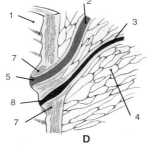

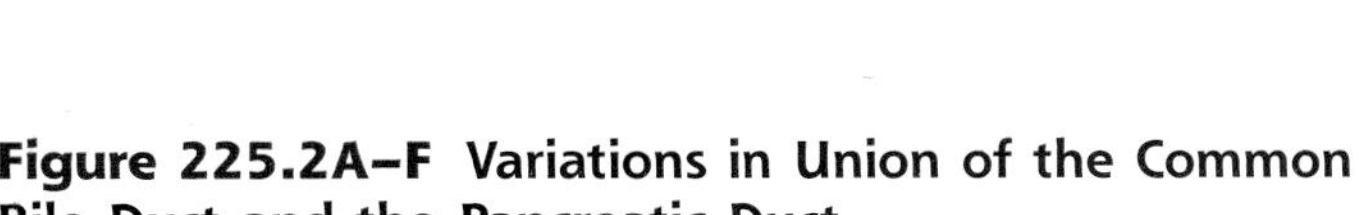

Figure 225.2A–F Variations in Union of the Common Bile Duct and the Pancreatic Duct

A: Pancreatic and common bile ducts join early, resulting in a long hepatopancreatic duct.

B: A long hepatopancreatic duct is modified by an expanded ampulla.

C: Pancreatic and common bile ducts join very close to the greater duodenal papilla, resulting in a short hepatopancreatic duct.

D: Both pancreatic and common bile ducts open separately on a somewhat larger duodenal papilla.

E: Pancreatic and common bile ducts drain through a single opening, but the ducts are separated by a septum.

F: Long hepatopancreatic duct along with a well-developed accessory pancreatic duct, which opens through the lesser duodenal papilla.

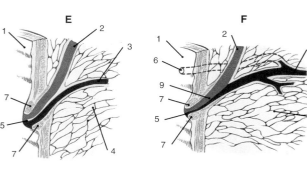

1. Duodenum
2. Common bile duct
3. Pancreatic duct (Wirsung)
4. Pancreas
5. Greater duodenal papilla
6. Accessory pancreatic duct (Santorini, in F)
7. Sphincter (Oddi) at duodenal papilla
8. Pancreatic duct separate opening
9. Hepatopancreatic duct

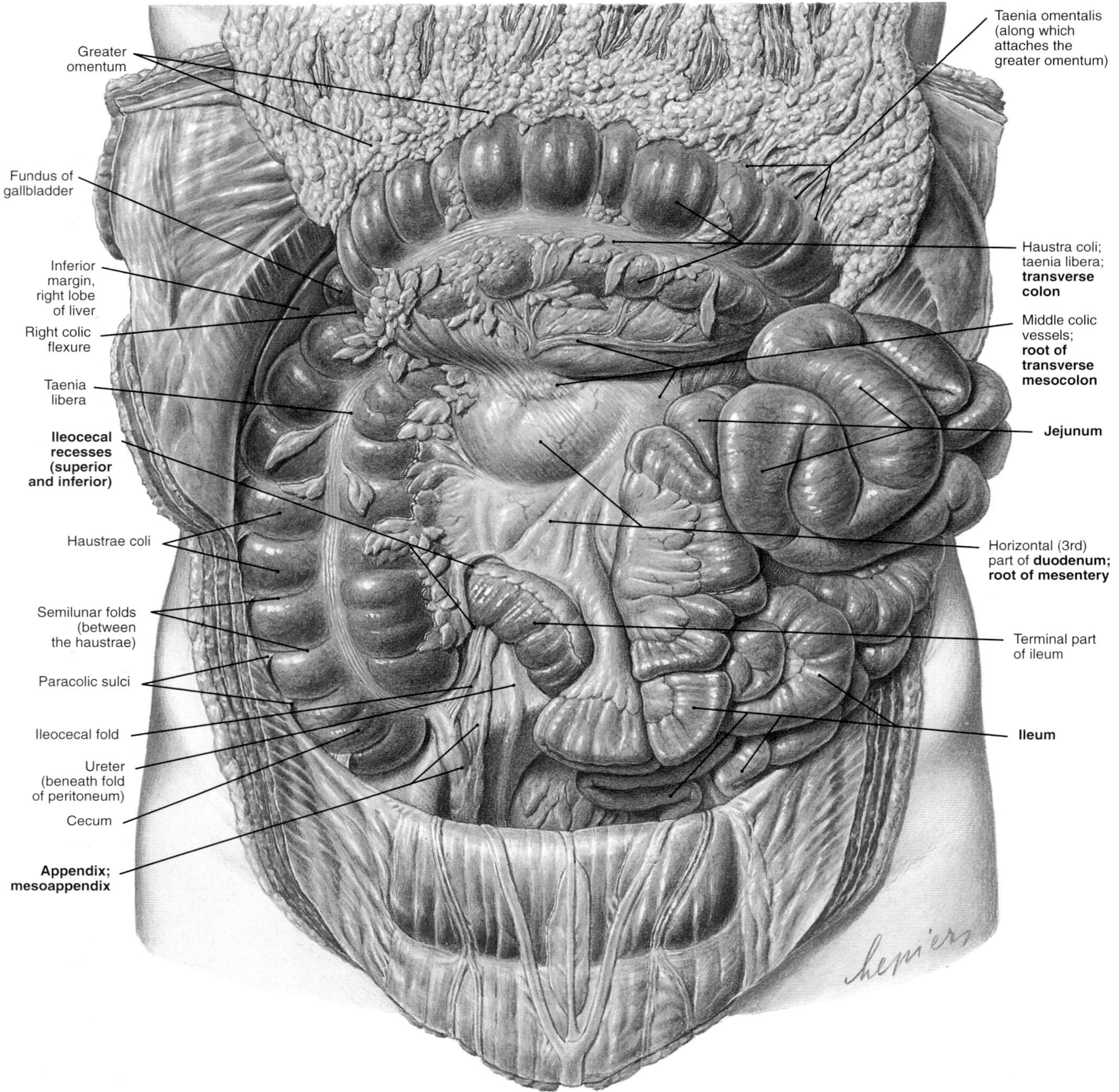
Greater omentum
Taenia omentalis (along which attaches the greater omentum)
Fundus of gallbladder
Inferior margin, right lobe of liver
Right colic flexure
Taenia libera
Ileocecal recesses (superior and inferior)
Haustrae coli
Semilunar folds (between the haustrae)
Paracolic sulci
Ileocecal fold
Ureter (beneath fold of peritoneum)
Cecum
Appendix; mesoappendix
Haustra coli; taenia libera; transverse colon
Middle colic vessels; root of transverse mesocolon
Jejunum
Horizontal (3rd) part of duodenum; root of mesentery
Terminal part of ileum
Ileum

Figure 226 Abdominal Cavity: Jejunum, Ileum, and Ascending and Transverse Colons

NOTE: (1)The greater omentum has been reflected superiorly, and the jejunum and ileum have been pulled to the left to expose the **root of the mesentery of the small intestine.**

(2) The horizontal (third) part of the duodenum, which is retroperitoneal and is covered by the smooth and glistening peritoneum.

(3) The junction of the distal portion of the ileum with the cecum. At this **ileocecal junction** the **ileocecal fold,** the **appendix,** and the **mesoappendix** can be identified. The appendix may extend cranially behind the cecum, toward the left and behind the ileum, or as demonstrated here, inferiorly over the pelvic brim.

(4) The transverse colon and the small intestine beyond the duodenal junction are more mobile than most other organs because they are attached to the transverse mesocolon and the mesentery.

(5) The retroperitoneal position of the **right ureter** as it descends over the pelvic brim on its course toward the urinary bladder in the pelvis.

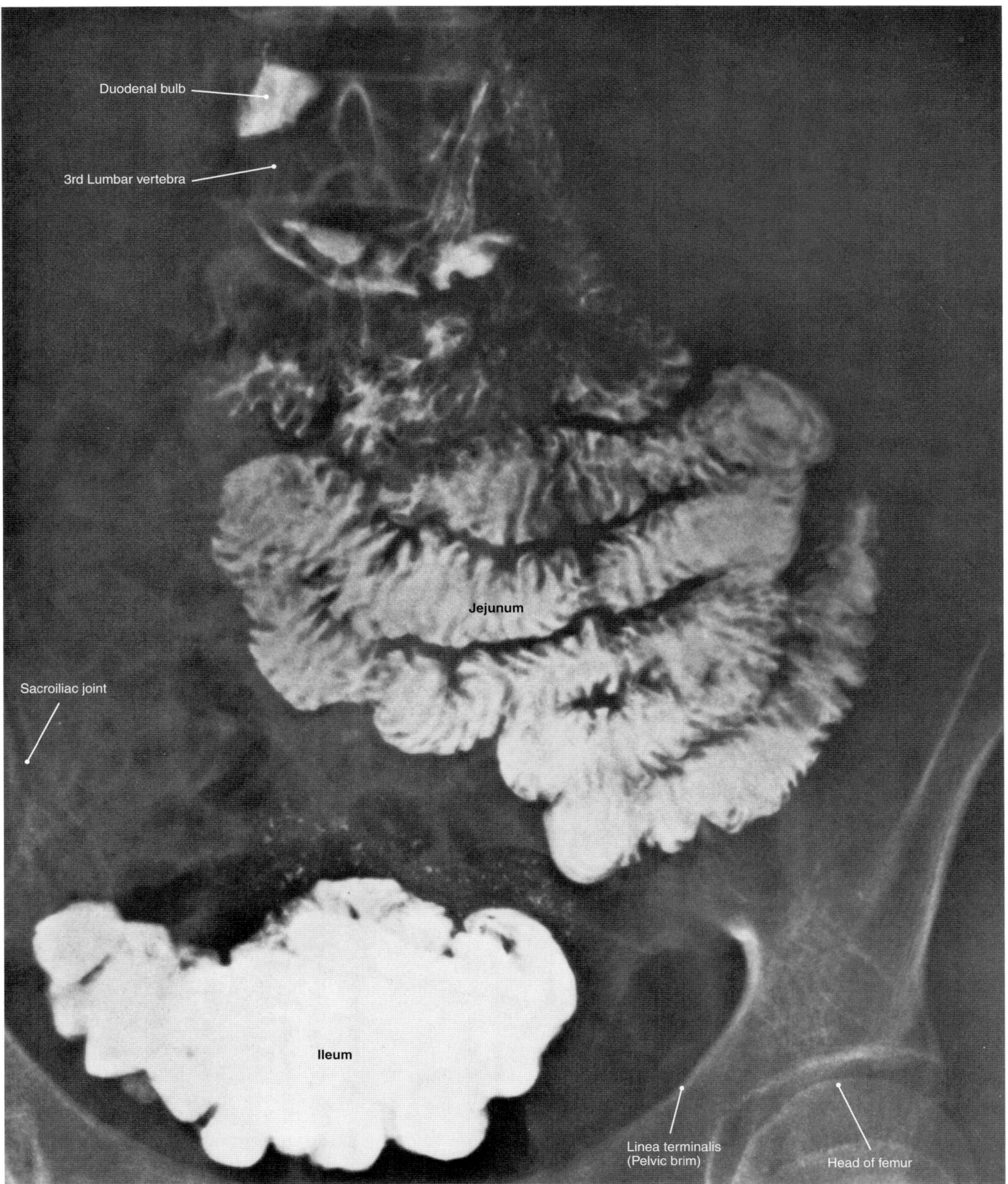
Duodenal bulb
3rd Lumbar vertebra
Jejunum
Sacroiliac joint
Ileum
Linea terminalis
(Pelvic brim)
Head of femur

Figure 227 Jejunum and Ileum Filled with a Contrast Medium

NOTE: (1) The **jejunum** and **ileum** extend between the duodenojejunal junction and the ileocecal valve. This part of the small intestine is completely covered with peritoneum and can be seen to be arranged in a series of coils;

(2) The jejunum is about $1\frac{1}{2}$ in. in diameter and about two-fifths of the small intestine beyond the duodenum, while the ileum is the distal three-fifths and is slightly smaller in diameter.

(From Wicke, 4th ed.)

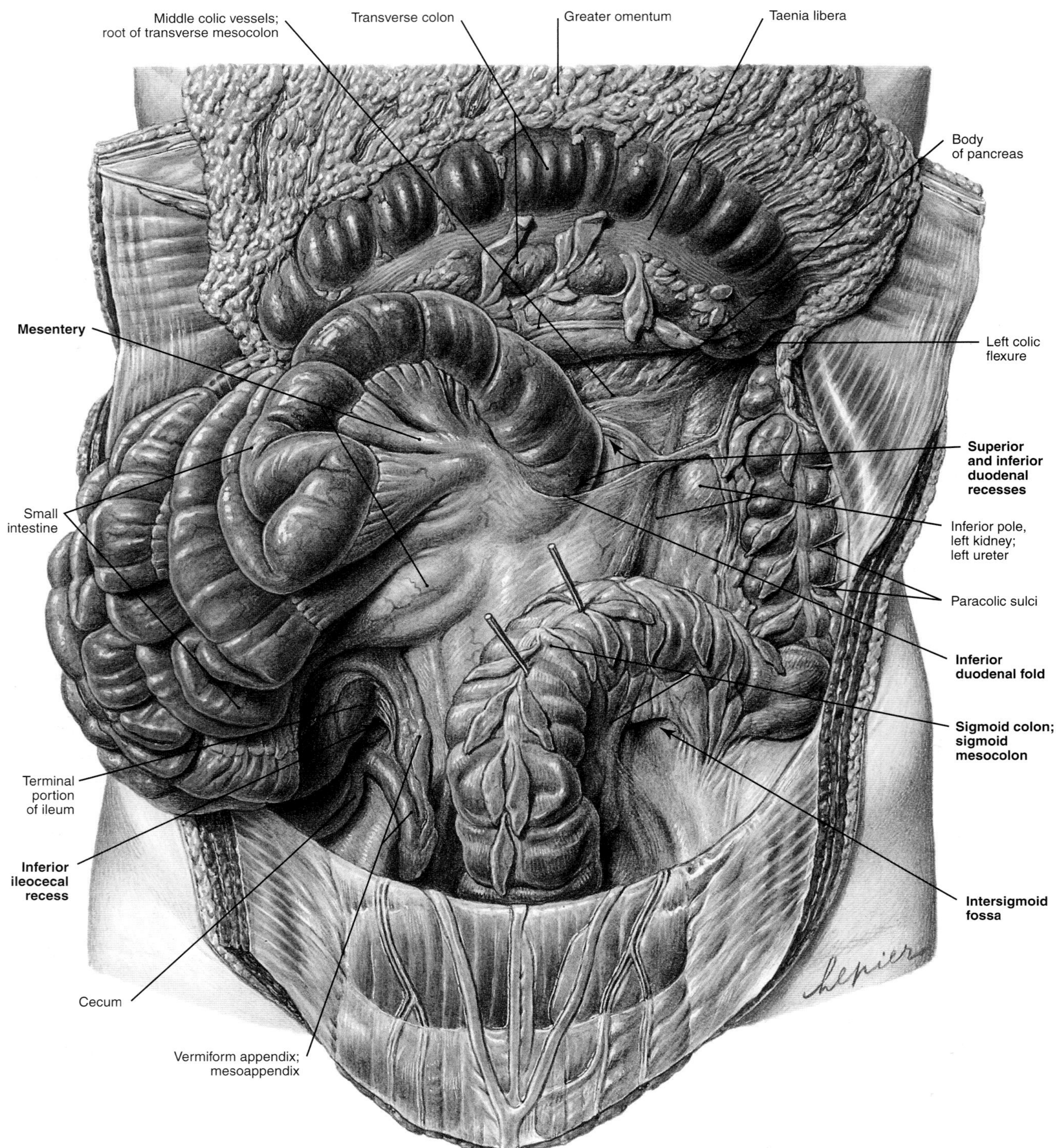
Middle colic vessels;
root of transverse mesocolon
Transverse colon
Greater omentum
Taenia libera
Body
of pancreas
Mesentery
Left colic
flexure
Superior
and inferior
duodenal
recesses
Small
intestine
Inferior pole,
left kidney;
left ureter
Paracolic sulci
Inferior
duodenal fold
Sigmoid colon;
sigmoid
mesocolon
Terminal
portion
of ileum
Inferior
ileocecal
recess
Intersigmoid
fossa
Cecum
Vermiform appendix;
mesoappendix

Figure 228 Abdominal Cavity: Descending and Sigmoid Colon and the Duodenojejunal Junction

NOTE: (1) The transverse colon and greater omentum have been reflected upward and the jejunum and ileum have been pulled to the right to reveal the **duodenojejunal junction** and the **descending** and **sigmoid colon.**

(2) At the duodenojejunal junction the small intestine acquires a mesentery. At this site, there are frequently found duodenal fossae or recesses located in relationship to the junction. Among these, the **superior** and **inferior duodenal recesses** are found in more than 50% of cases. These are of importance because they represent possible sites of herniation.

(3) The sigmoid colon is mobile (because of its mesocolic attachment), whereas the descending colon is fixed to the posterior wall of the abdomen.

(4) The **intersigmoid fossa** is located behind the sigmoid mesocolon and between that mesocolon and the peritoneum reflected over the external iliac vessels.

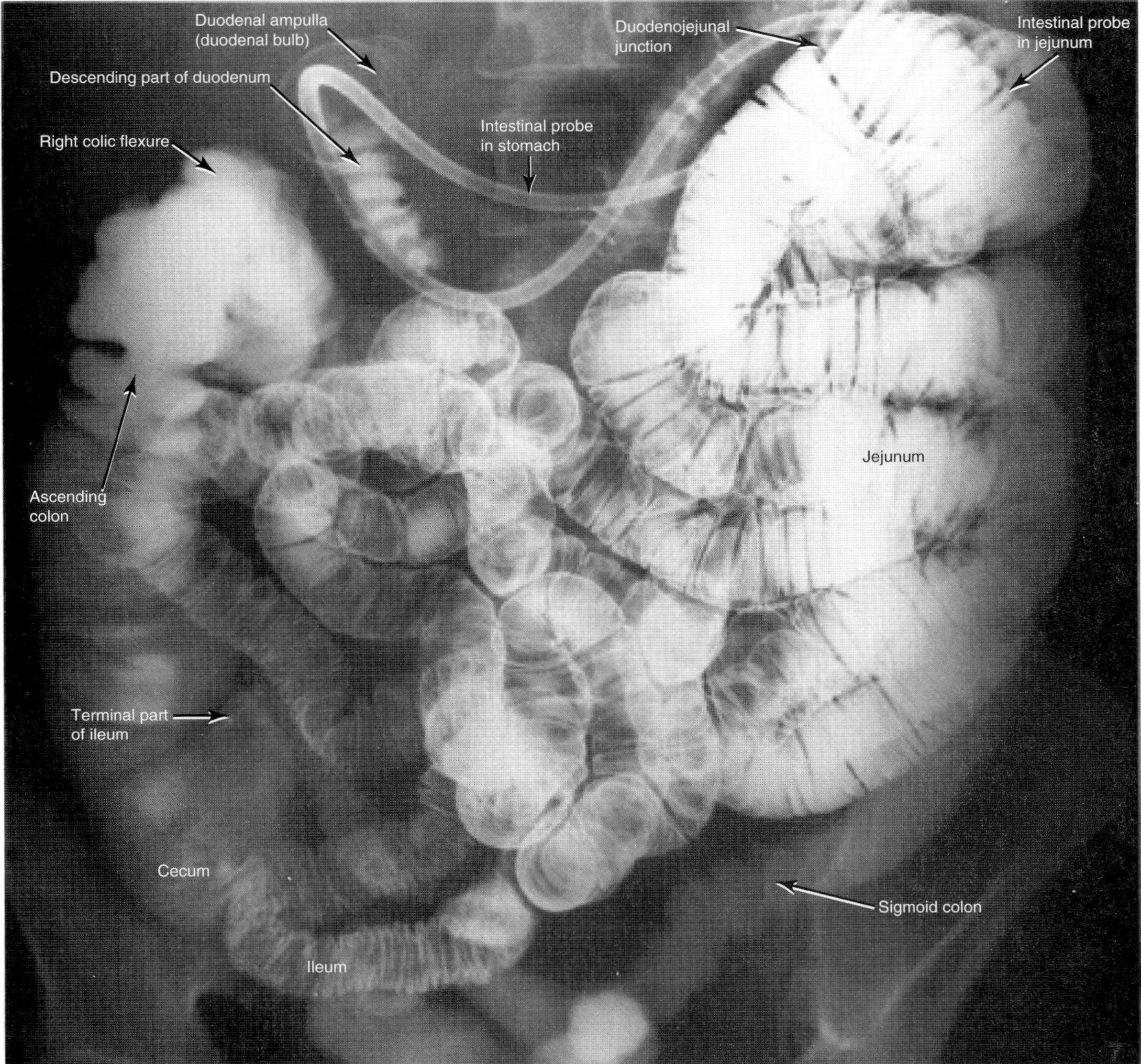
Duodenal ampulla
(duodenal bulb)
Duodenojejunal
junction
Intestinal probe
in jejunum
Descending part of duodenum
Right colic flexure
Intestinal probe
in stomach
Jejunum
Ascending
colon
Terminal part
of ileum
Cecum
Sigmoid colon
Ileum

Figure 229 Radiograph of the Jejunum, Ileum, Cecum, and Ascending Colon

NOTE: (1) This radiograph of the small bowel was obtained following an injection of a contrast medium into the gastrointestinal tract (enteroclysis). The intestinal probe in this case was introduced through the stomach and duodenum to the jejunum.

(2) The cecum, ascending colon, right colic flexure, and sigmoid colon are also recognizable.

(3) Some of the medium had entered the descending part of the duodenum also to be visualized.

(From Wicke, 4th ed.)

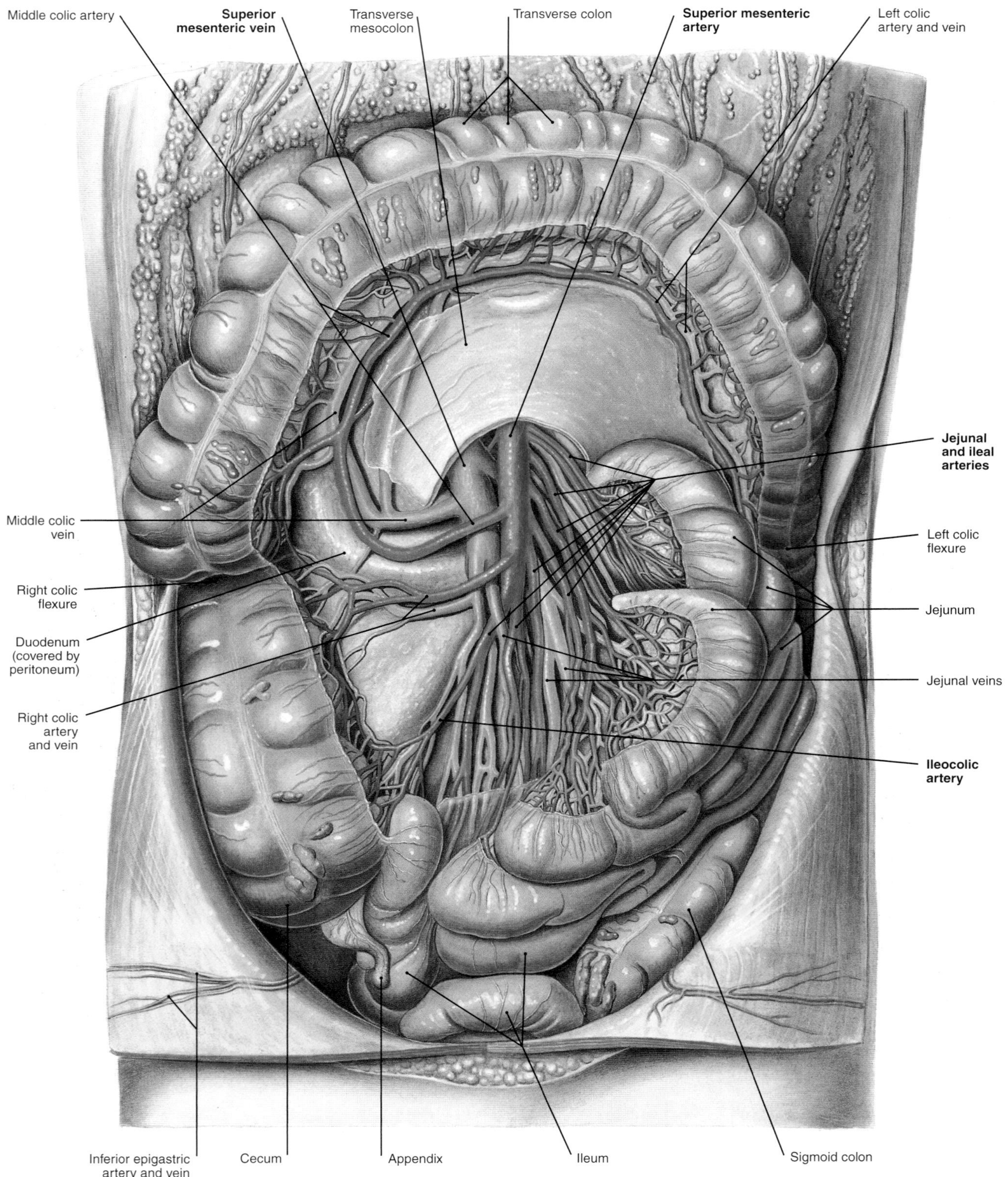
Middle colic artery
Superior mesenteric vein
Transverse mesocolon
Transverse colon
Superior mesenteric artery
Left colic artery and vein
Jejunal and ileal arteries
Middle colic vein
Left colic flexure
Right colic flexure
Jejunum
Duodenum (covered by peritoneum)
Jejunal veins
Right colic artery and vein
Ileocolic artery
Inferior epigastric artery and vein
Cecum
Appendix
Ileum
Sigmoid colon

Figure 230 Abdominal Cavity: Superior Mesenteric Vessels and Branches

NOTE: (1) The small intestine is pushed to the left and the loops of bowel have been dissected to expose the branches of the superior mesenteric vessels.

(2) The **jejunal and ileal arteries** branch from the left side of the mesenteric artery. There are about 15 of these vessels.

(3) Branching from the right side of the superior mesenteric artery are the **ileocolic, right colic**, and **middle colic arteries.** These vessels form rich anastomoses.

(4) The small intestine measures about 22 ft in length, commencing at the pyloric end of the stomach and extending to the ileocecal junction, where the large intestine starts.

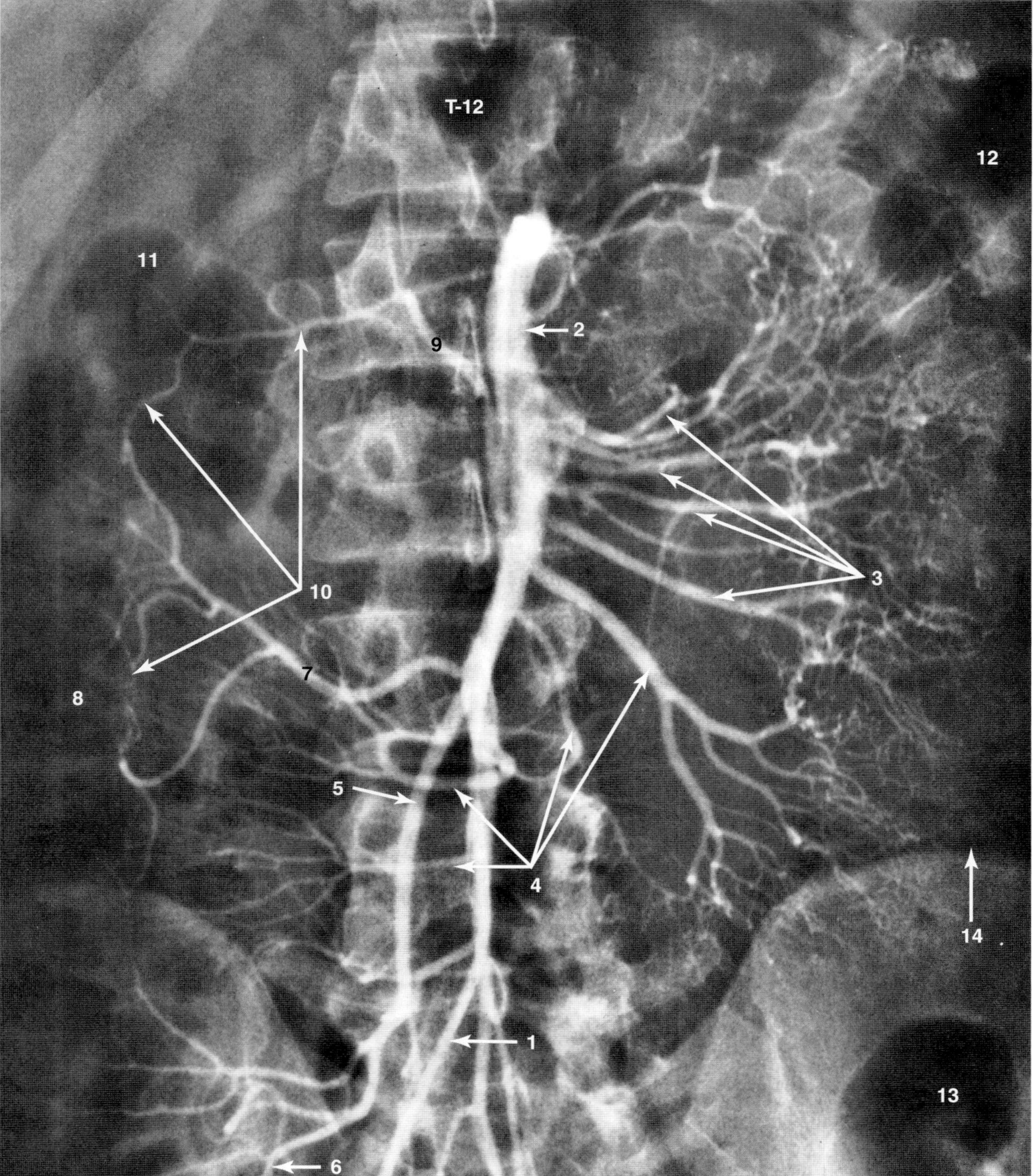
T-12
12
11
2
9
3
10
7
8
5
4
14
1
13
6

Figure 231 Superior Mesenteric Arteriogram

NOTE: (1) A catheter (1) has been inserted into the common iliac artery and through the abdominal aorta to the point of branching of the superior mesenteric artery (2). Contrast medium was injected to visualize the principal branches of that vessel. The original radiograph is shown as a negative print.

(2) The jejunal (3) and ileal (4) arteries branching as a sequence of vessels (about 15 in number), which supply all of the small intestine beyond the duodenum.

(3) The ileocolic artery (5) and its appendicular branch (6), the right colic (7) and middle colic (9) arteries, which supply the cecum, ascending colon (8), and transverse colon. Anastomoses among these vessels along the margin of the colon contribute to the formation of the marginal artery (10).

(4) Other structures can be identified. These include the right colic flexure (11), the left colic flexure (12), the sigmoid colon (13), the body of the T12 vertebra, and the iliac crest (14).

(From Wicke, 3rd ed.)

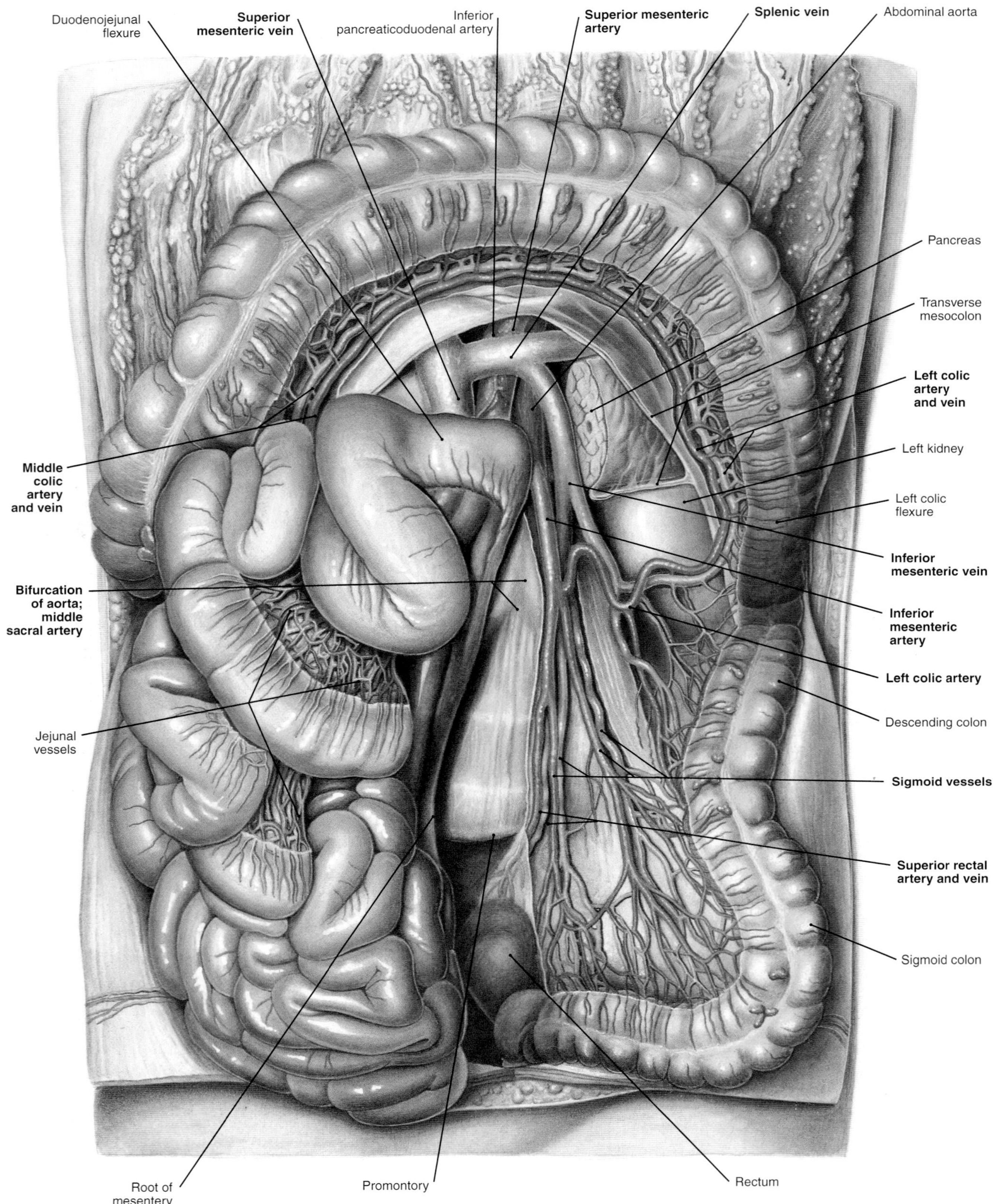
Duodenojejunal flexure
Superior mesenteric vein
Inferior pancreaticoduodenal artery
Superior mesenteric artery
Splenic vein
Abdominal aorta
Pancreas
Transverse mesocolon
Left colic artery and vein
Left kidney
Left colic flexure
Inferior mesenteric vein
Inferior mesenteric artery
Left colic artery
Descending colon
Sigmoid vessels
Superior rectal artery and vein
Sigmoid colon
Rectum
Promontory
Root of mesentery
Jejunal vessels
Bifurcation of aorta; middle sacral artery
Middle colic artery and vein

Figure 232 Abdominal Cavity: Inferior Mesenteric Vessels and Branches

NOTE: (1) The small intestine has been pushed to the right and parts of the pancreas and transverse mesocolon have been removed to expose the origin of the superior mesenteric artery from the aorta and the drainage of the superior mesenteric vein into the splenic vein.

(2) The inferior mesenteric artery supplies the descending colon via the **left colic artery** and the sigmoid colon and rectum via the **sigmoid** and **superior rectal arteries.**

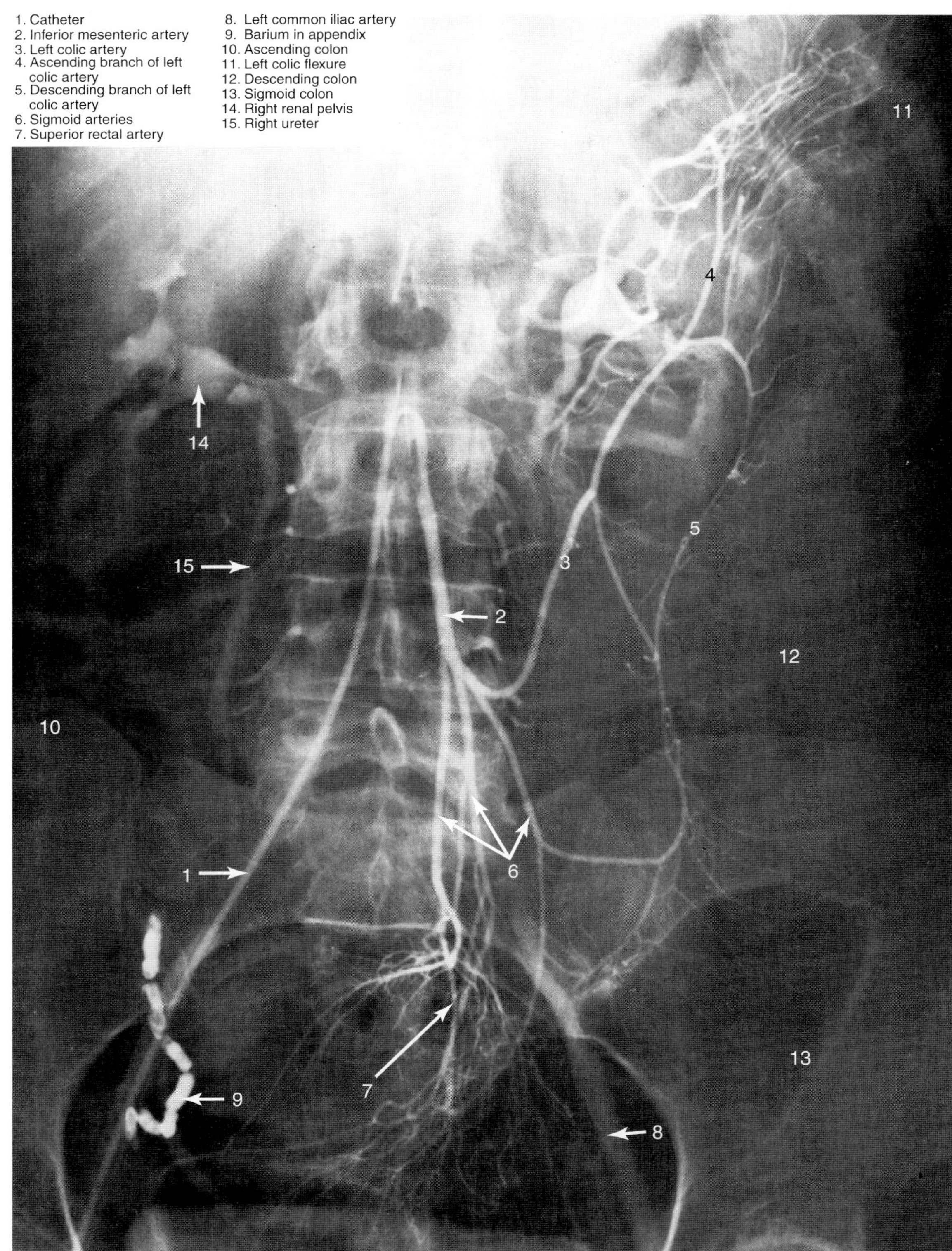
1. Catheter
2. Inferior mesenteric artery
3. Left colic artery
4. Ascending branch of left colic artery
5. Descending branch of left colic artery
6. Sigmoid arteries
7. Superior rectal artery
8. Left common iliac artery
9. Barium in appendix
10. Ascending colon
11. Left colic flexure
12. Descending colon
13. Sigmoid colon
14. Right renal pelvis
15. Right ureter
11
4
14
5
15
3
2
12
10
6
1
13
9
7
8

Figure 233 Inferior Mesenteric Arteriogram

NOTE: (1) A catheter (1) was inserted through the right internal iliac artery and directed upward into the abdominal aorta to the origin of the **inferior mesenteric artery.** Contrast medium was injected into that artery to demonstrate its field of distribution.

(2) The branches of the inferior mesenteric artery shown above are normal. The **left colic artery** (3) shows both an ascending (4) and a descending (5) branch.

(3) Several **sigmoid arteries** (5) supply the sigmoid colon (13), and these anastomose above with branches of the left colic artery (3) and below with the **superior rectal artery** (7).

(From Wicke, 3rd ed.)

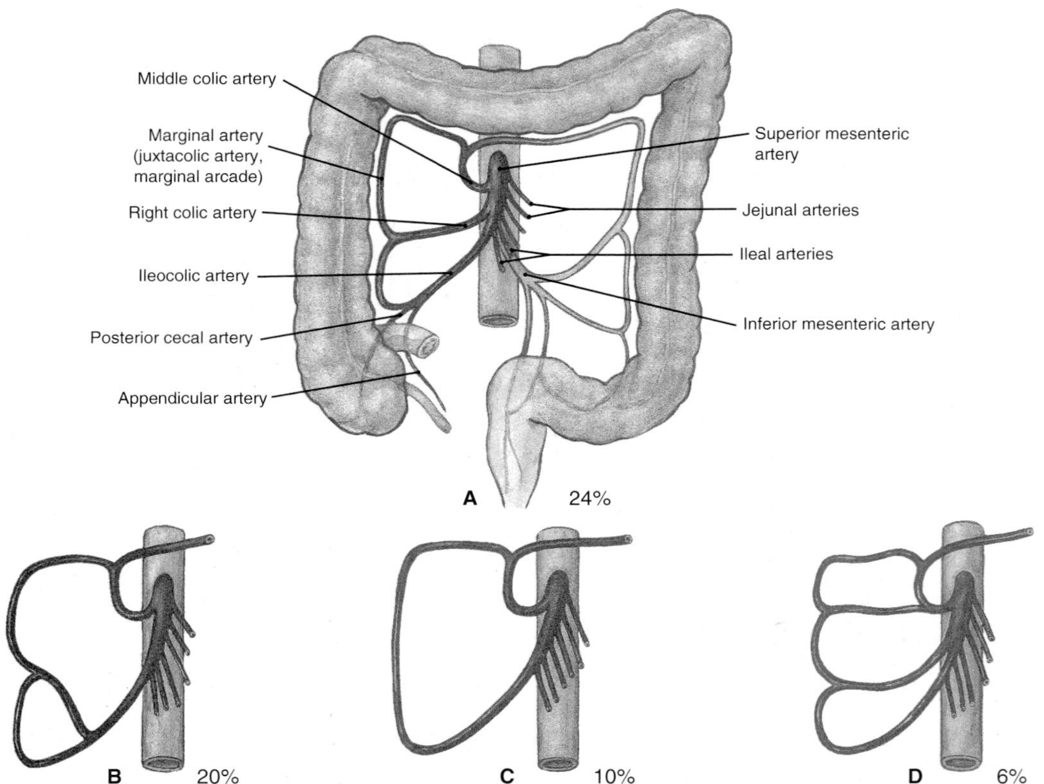
Middle colic artery
Marginal artery (juxtacolic artery, marginal arcade)
Right colic artery
Ileocolic artery
Posterior cecal artery
Appendicular artery
Superior mesenteric artery
Jejunal arteries
Ileal arteries
Inferior mesenteric artery
A 24%
B 20%
C 10%
D 6%

Figure 234.1 Variations in the Branching of the Superior Mesenteric Artery

NOTE: (1) Normal pattern: ascending and transverse colon supplied by three branches.
(2) Formation of an ileocolic and right colic trunk.
(3) Only two branches with the right colic artery absent.
(4) Two right colic arteries.

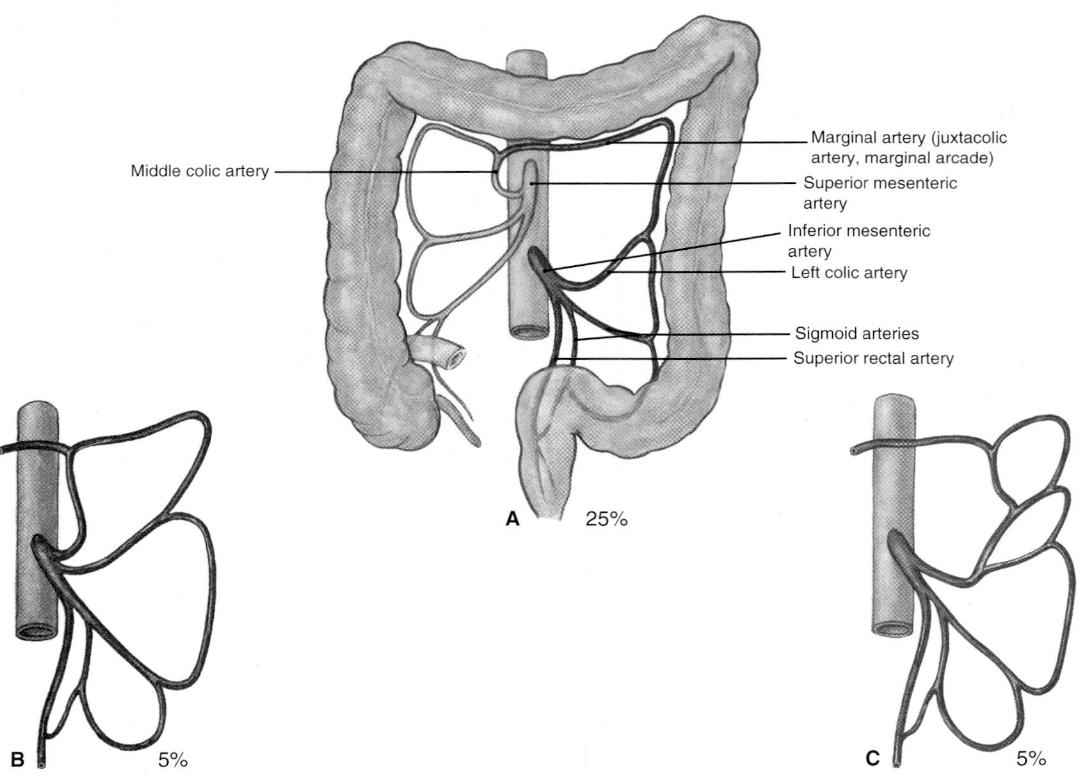
Middle colic artery
Marginal artery (juxtacolic artery, marginal arcade)
Superior mesenteric artery
Inferior mesenteric artery
Left colic artery
Sigmoid arteries
Superior rectal artery
A 25%
B 5%
C 5%

Figure 234.2 Variations in the Branching of the Inferior Mesenteric Artery

NOTE: (1) Single trunk that divides into three branches (for descending colon, sigmoid colon and rectum);
(2) An accessory middle colic artery branching from the inferior mesenteric;
(3) An accessory middle colic artery from the left colic artery. (For "normal pattern" see Fig. 232.)

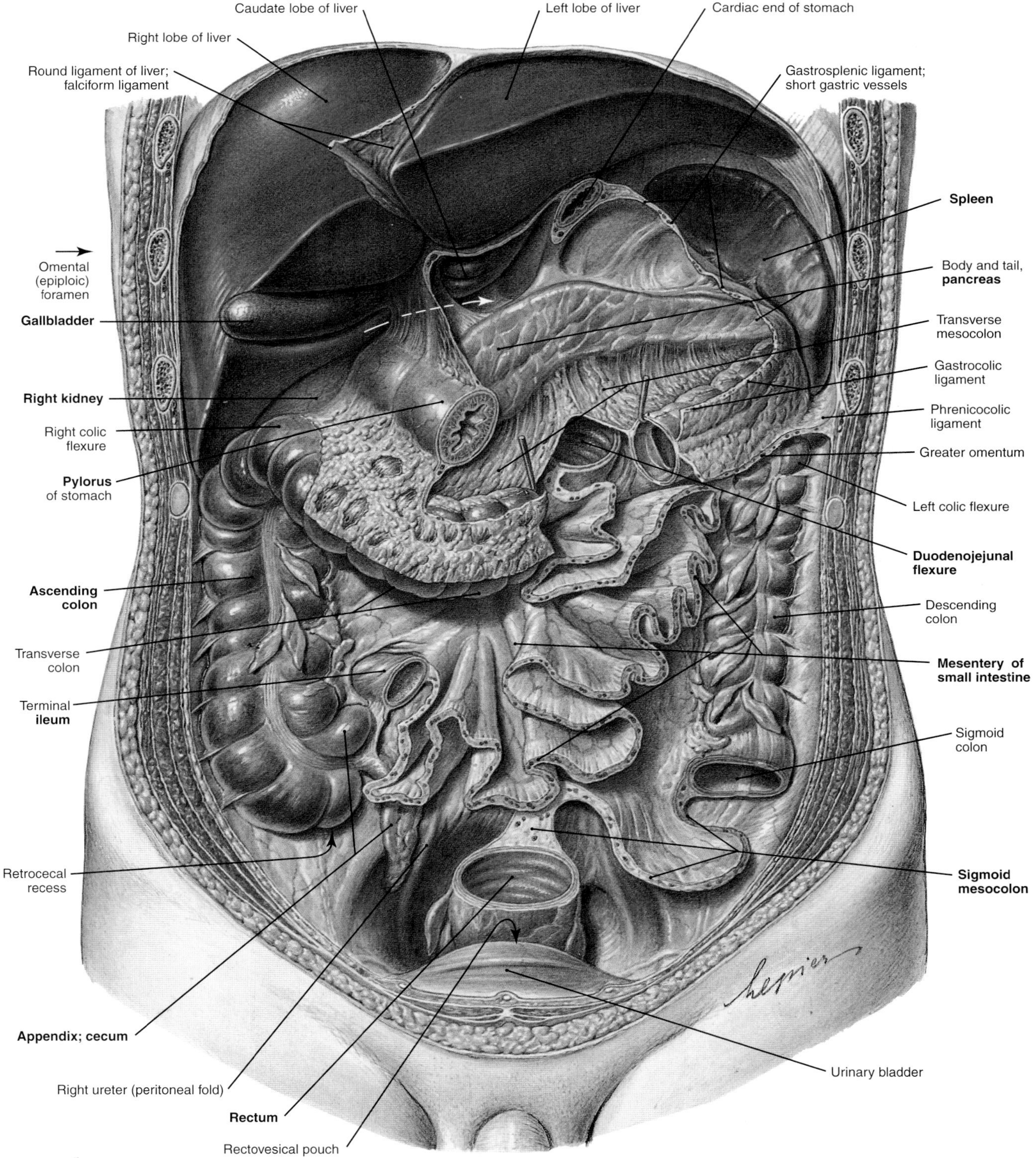
Caudate lobe of liver
Left lobe of liver
Cardiac end of stomach
Right lobe of liver
Round ligament of liver; falciform ligament
Gastrosplenic ligament; short gastric vessels
Spleen
Omental (epiploic) foramen
Body and tail, pancreas
Gallbladder
Transverse mesocolon
Gastrocolic ligament
Right kidney
Phrenicocolic ligament
Right colic flexure
Greater omentum
Pylorus of stomach
Left colic flexure
Duodenojejunal flexure
Ascending colon
Descending colon
Transverse colon
Mesentery of small intestine
Terminal ileum
Sigmoid colon
Retrocecal recess
Sigmoid mesocolon
Appendix; cecum
Urinary bladder
Right ureter (peritoneal fold)
Rectum
Rectovesical pouch

Figure 235 Abdominal Cavity: Large Intestine and Mesenteries

NOTE: (1) The stomach was cut just proximal to the pylorus and removed, the small intestine was severed at the duodenojejunal junction and at the distal ileum and also removed (by cutting the mesentery). A part of the transverse colon was resected along the greater omentum, and the sigmoid colon was removed to reveal its mesocolon.

(2) The **mesentery of the small intestine** extends obliquely across the posterior abdominal wall from the **duodenojejunal junction** to the **ileocecal junction.** In this 6 or 7 in., the mesenteric folds accommodate all of the loops of jejunum and ileum.

(3) The **ascending colon** and **descending colon** are fused to the posterior abdominal wall, whereas the **transverse colon** and **sigmoid colon** are suspended by their respective mesocolons.

(4) Vessels and nerves supplying the small intestine course between the layers of the mesentery to achieve the organ.

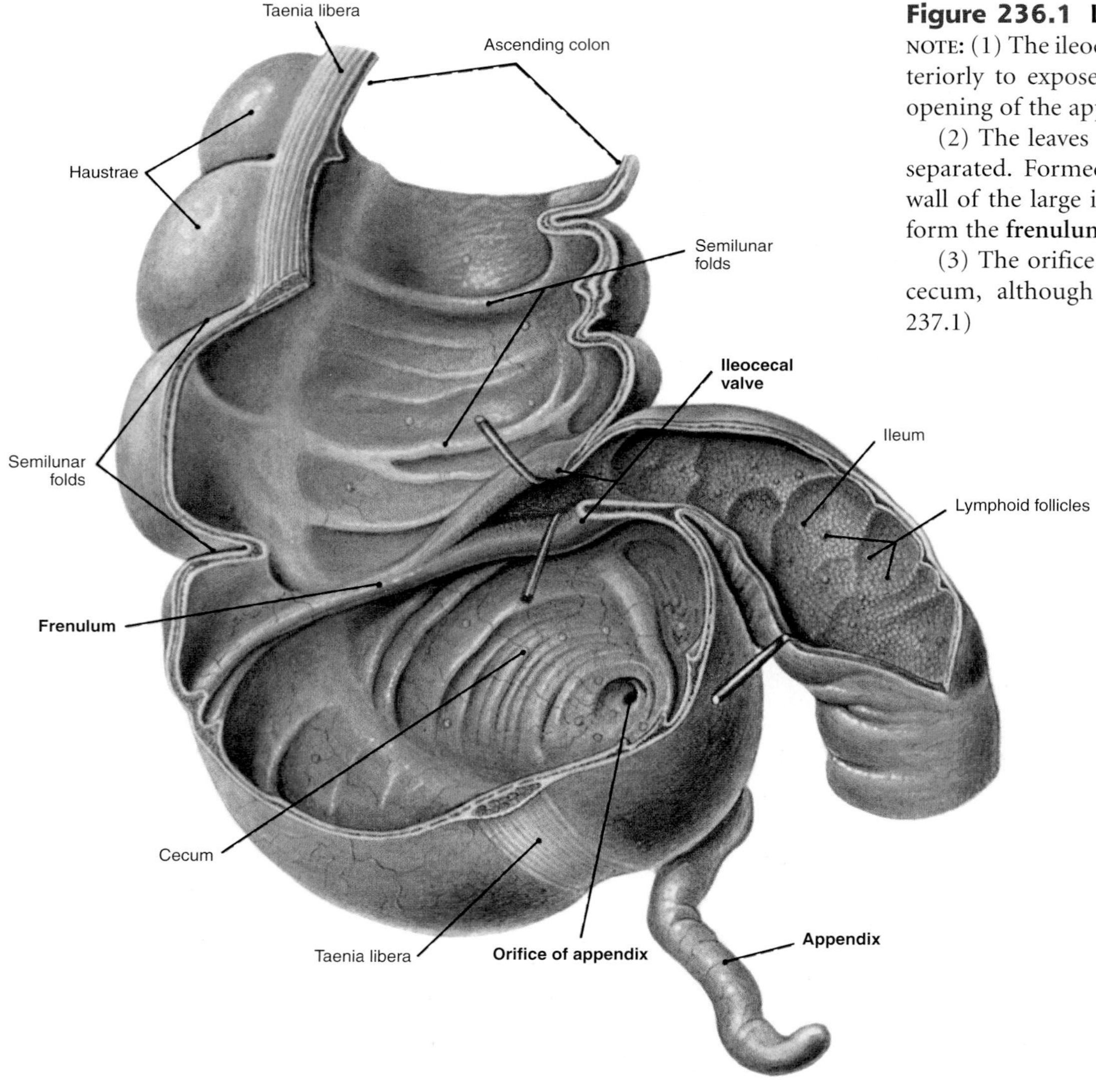
Taenia libera
Ascending colon
Haustrae
Semilunar folds
Ileocecal valve
Ileum
Lymphoid follicles
Semilunar folds
Frenulum
Cecum
Taenia libera
Orifice of appendix
Appendix

Figure 236.1 Ileocecal Junction

NOTE: (1) The ileocecal region has been opened anteriorly to expose the ileocecal junction and the opening of the appendix.

(2) The leaves of the **ileocecal valve** have been separated. Formed by two reflected folds of the wall of the large intestine, the folds then unite to form the **frenulum.**

(3) The orifice of the **appendix** opens into the cecum, although its direction varies (see Fig. 237.1)

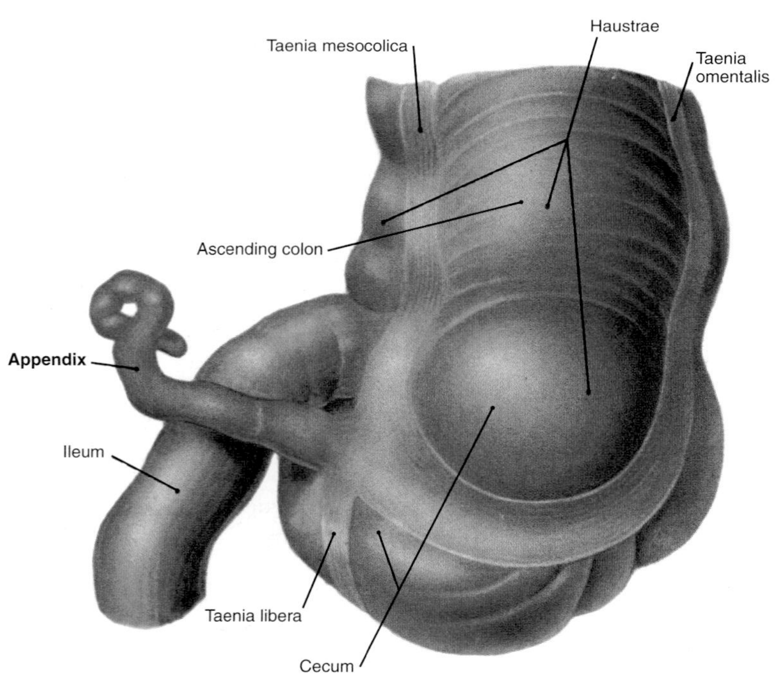
Taenia mesocolica
Haustrae
Taenia omentalis
Ascending colon
Appendix
Ileum
Taenia libera
Cecum

Figure 236.2 Dorsal View of the Cecum and Appendix

NOTE: (1) The attachments of the ileum and appendix to the cecum are clearly visualized with the peritoneum stripped away.

(2) The **taeniae coli** (three) are strips of longitudinal smooth muscle. The **taenia libera** is located anterior on the cecum, the **taenia mesocolica** is situated posteromedially, whereas the **taenia omentalis** is located posterolaterally on the cecum.

(3) The three taeniae come together at the origin of the appendix on the cecum.

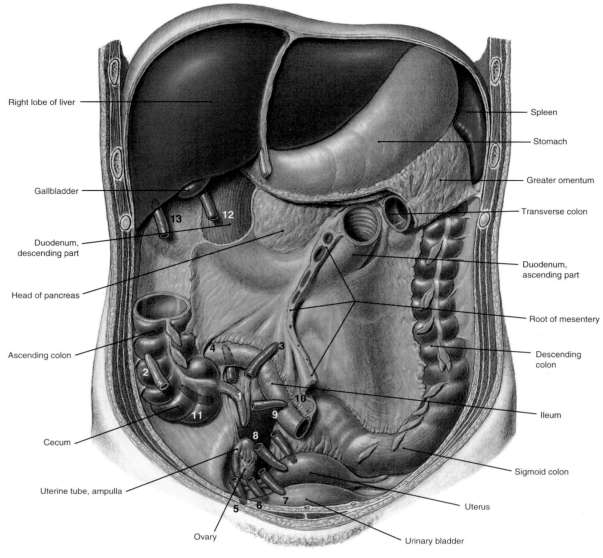

Right lobe of liver
Gallbladder
Duodenum, descending part
Head of pancreas
Ascending colon
Cecum
Uterine tube, ampulla
Ovary
Spleen
Stomach
Greater omentum
Transverse colon
Duodenum, ascending part
Root of mesentery
Descending colon
Ileum
Sigmoid colon
Uterus
Urinary bladder
1
2
3
4
5
6
7
8
9
10
11
12
13

1. Over the pelvic brim
2. Anterolaterally
3. Toward the root of the mesentery
4. Dorsal to the terminal ileum
5. Toward the deep inguinal ring
6. In the uterovesical pouch
7. Anterior to the bladder
8. On the uterus or uterine tube
9. In the rectouterine pouch
10. Medially, anterior to the ileum
11. Behind the cecum
12. Toward the gallbladder
13. Toward the liver

Figure 237.1 Variations in the Location of the Appendix
NOTE that at least 13 sites for the appendix have been reported, most common are #11, 1, 3, 10, and 4, respectively.

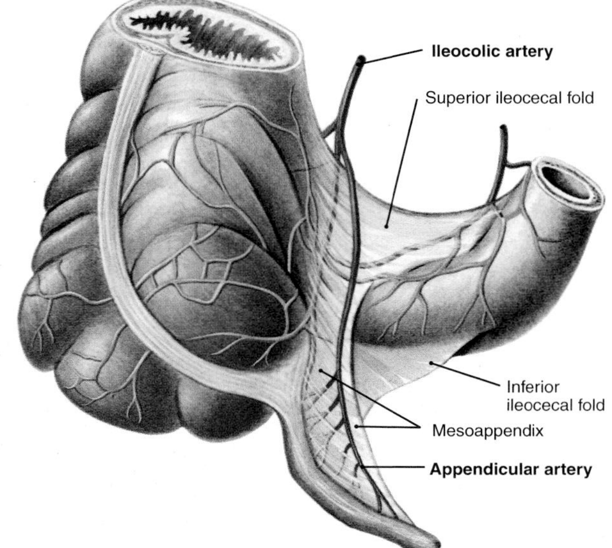
Ileocolic artery
Superior ileocecal fold
Inferior ileocecal fold
Mesoappendix
Appendicular artery

Figure 237.2 Blood Supply to the Vermiform Appendix
NOTE: The appendix usually receives its vascular supply by way of the **appendicular artery**, a branch of the ileocolic artery, and it descends either anterior to the ileocecal junction (as shown) or behind it.

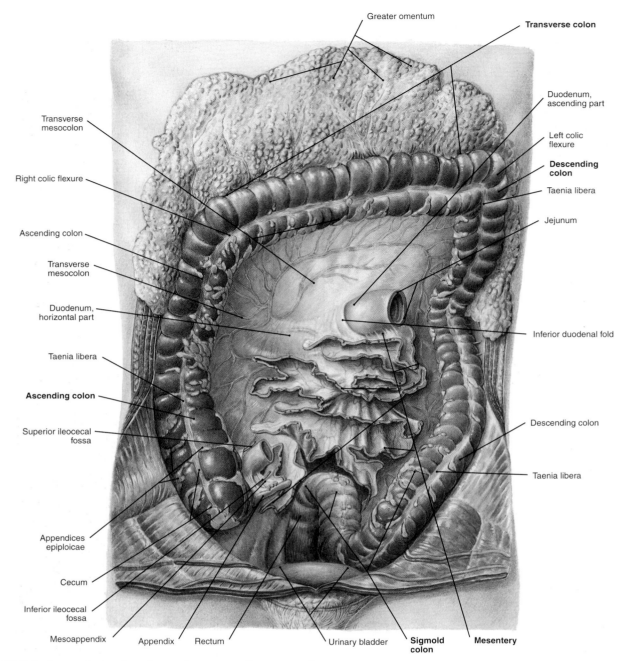

Greater omentum
Transverse colon
Transverse mesocolon
Duodenum, ascending part
Left colic flexure
Descending colon
Right colic flexure
Taenia libera
Jejunum
Ascending colon
Transverse mesocolon
Duodenum, horizontal part
Inferior duodenal fold
Taenia libera
Ascending colon
Superior ileocecal fossa
Descending colon
Taenia libera
Appendices epiploicae
Cecum
Inferior ileocecal fossa
Mesoappendix
Appendix
Rectum
Urinary bladder
Sigmoid colon
Mesentery

Figure 238.1 Large Intestine from Cecum to Rectum

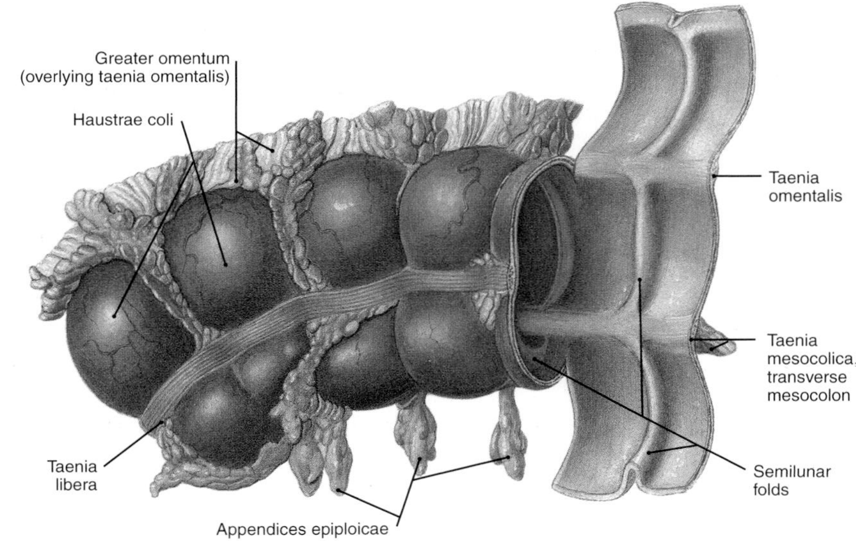
Greater omentum (overlying taenia omentalis)
Haustrae coli
Taenia omentalis
Taenia mesocolica, transverse mesocolon
Semilunar folds
Taenia libera
Appendices epiploicae

Figure 238.2 Segment of Transverse Colon

NOTE: (1) A cut was made along the **taenia libera** at the right of this segment of transverse colon, and its wall opened to show its inner surface.

(2) The greater omentum attaches along the **taenia omentalis**, the transverse mesocolon attaches along the **taenia mesocolica**, whereas the **taenia libera** is free from such attachments.

(3) The large intestine is about 5 ft long and its diameter (1.5 to 3 in.) varies, being widest at the cecum, then narrowing, and dilating again at the rectal ampulla.

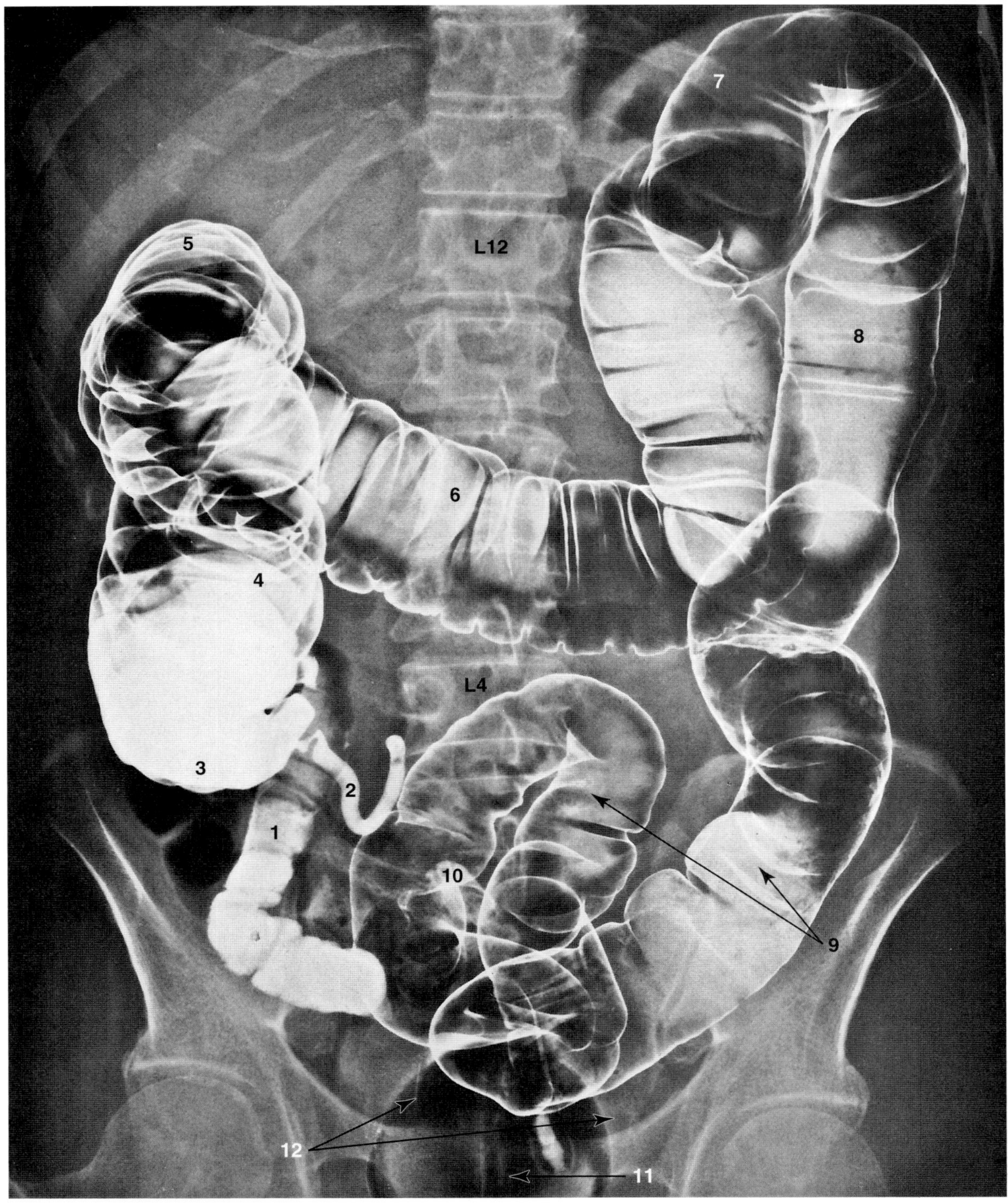
7
5
L12
8
6
4
L4
3
2
1
10
9
12
11

Figure 239 Radiographic Anatomy of the Large Intestine (Double Contrast)

NOTE: (1) In this patient, barium sulfate was administered as an enema and the mixture was then expelled and the colon insufflated with air (barium–air double contrast method).

(2) The cecum (3) is usually located in the iliac fossa of the lower right quadrant, and it forms a cul-de-sac that opens into the ascending colon (4). The terminal ileum (1) most often joins the cecum on its medial or posterior surface. The appendix (2) extends from the cecum about 2 cm below the ileocecal opening. The right colic flexure (5) continues to the left to become the transverse colon (6).

(3) The transverse colon, suspended by its mesentery, crosses the abdomen. It turns inferiorly at the left colic flexure (7) as the descending colon (8).

(4) The descending colon becomes the sigmoid colon (9) at the inlet to the lesser pelvis. With its mesentery, the sigmoid colon leads into the rectum (10), within the true pelvis.

(5) The locations of the T12 and L4 vertebrae, the symphysis pubis (11), and an air-filled balloon (12).

(From Wicke, 3rd ed.)

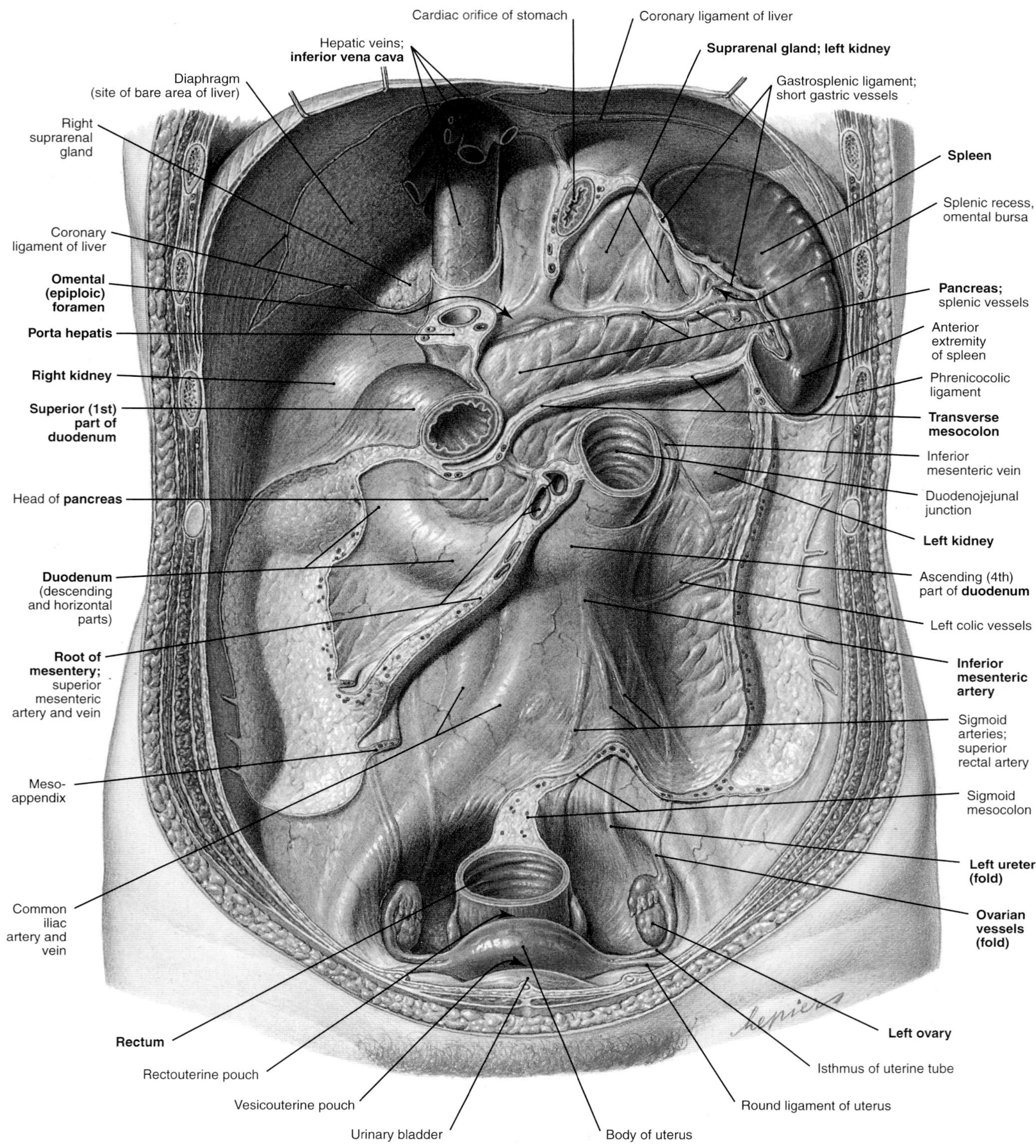
Cardiac orifice of stomach
Coronary ligament of liver
Hepatic veins; inferior vena cava
Suprarenal gland; left kidney
Diaphragm (site of bare area of liver)
Gastrosplenic ligament; short gastric vessels
Right suprarenal gland
Spleen
Splenic recess, omental bursa
Coronary ligament of liver
Omental (epiploic) foramen
Pancreas; splenic vessels
Porta hepatis
Anterior extremity of spleen
Right kidney
Phrenicocolic ligament
Superior (1st) part of duodenum
Transverse mesocolon
Inferior mesenteric vein
Duodenojejunal junction
Head of pancreas
Left kidney
Duodenum (descending and horizontal parts)
Ascending (4th) part of duodenum
Left colic vessels
Root of mesentery; superior mesenteric artery and vein
Inferior mesenteric artery
Sigmoid arteries; superior rectal artery
Meso-appendix
Sigmoid mesocolon
Left ureter (fold)
Common iliac artery and vein
Ovarian vessels (fold)
Left ovary
Rectum
Isthmus of uterine tube
Rectouterine pouch
Round ligament of uterus
Vesicouterine pouch
Urinary bladder
Body of uterus

Figure 240 Abdominal Cavity; Posterior Abdominal Peritoneum (Female)

NOTE: (1) The stomach and the intestines (except for the duodenum and rectum) have been removed and their mesenteries cut close to their roots on the posterior abdominal wall. The liver and gallbladder were also removed, but the spleen and the retroperitoneal organs (duodenum, pancreas, adrenal glands, kidneys and ureters, aorta, and inferior vena cava) are intact.

(2) The ascending and descending portions of the large intestine are fused to the posterior abdominal wall with peritoneum covering their anterior surfaces.

(3) The course of the ureters and ovarian vessels descending over the pelvic brim. Observe the ovaries, uterine tubes, and uterus located in the pelvis and their relationship to the rectum and bladder.

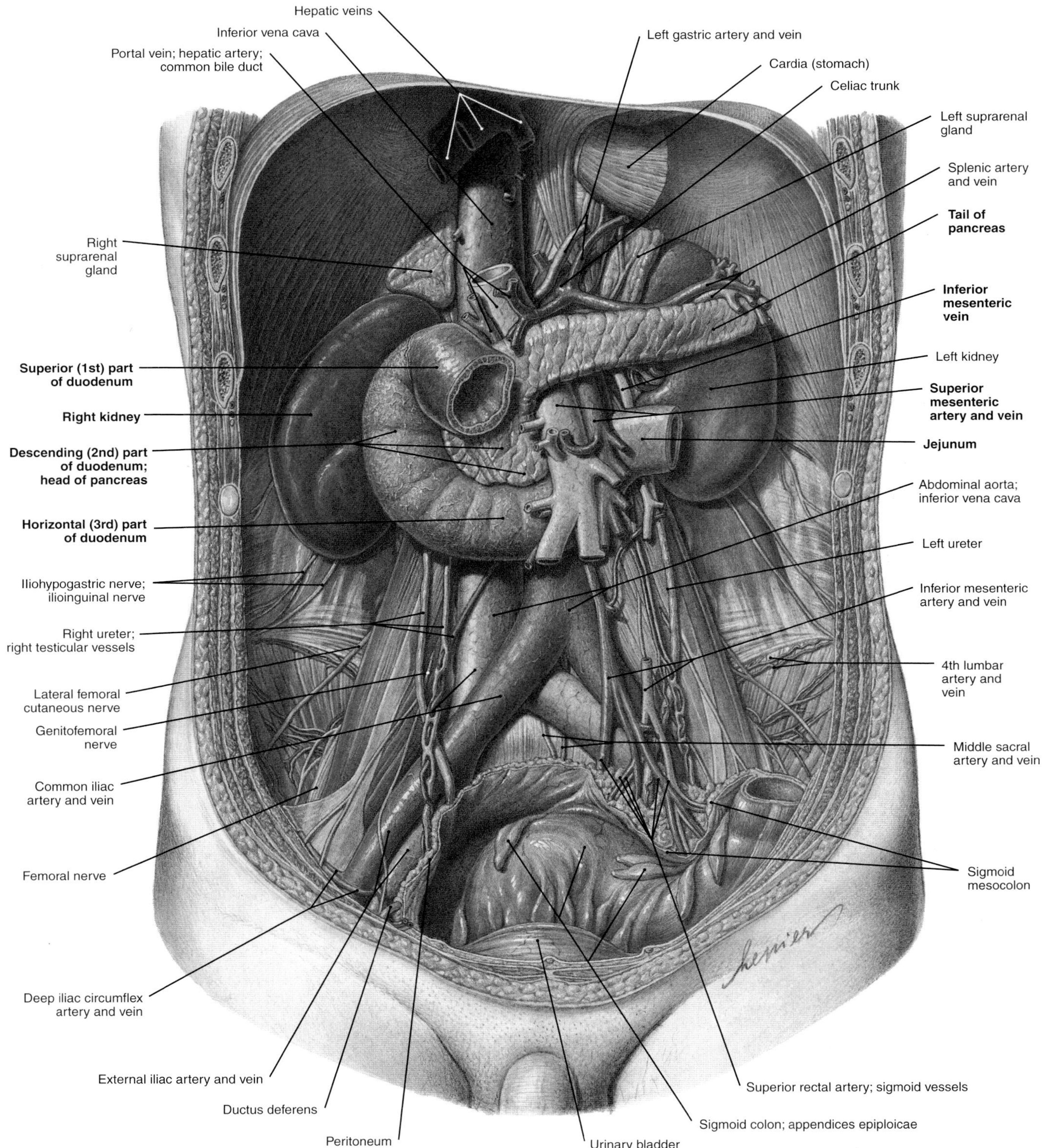
Hepatic veins
Inferior vena cava
Portal vein; hepatic artery; common bile duct
Left gastric artery and vein
Cardia (stomach)
Celiac trunk
Left suprarenal gland
Splenic artery and vein
Tail of pancreas
Right suprarenal gland
Inferior mesenteric vein
Left kidney
Superior (1st) part of duodenum
Right kidney
Superior mesenteric artery and vein
Jejunum
Descending (2nd) part of duodenum; head of pancreas
Abdominal aorta; inferior vena cava
Horizontal (3rd) part of duodenum
Left ureter
Iliohypogastric nerve; ilioinguinal nerve
Inferior mesenteric artery and vein
Right ureter; right testicular vessels
4th lumbar artery and vein
Lateral femoral cutaneous nerve
Genitofemoral nerve
Middle sacral artery and vein
Common iliac artery and vein
Sigmoid mesocolon
Femoral nerve
Deep iliac circumflex artery and vein
External iliac artery and vein
Superior rectal artery; sigmoid vessels
Ductus deferens
Sigmoid colon; appendices epiploicae
Peritoneum
Urinary bladder

Figure 241 Abdominal Cavity: Retroperitoneal Organs (Male)

NOTE: (1) The curvature of the duodenum lies ventral to the hilum of the right kidney, and the duodenojejunal junction is ventral to the lower medial border of the left kidney. The right kidney is slightly lower than the left.

(2) The head of the pancreas lies anterior to the inferior vena cava and within the curve of the duodenum. An extension of the pancreatic head, the uncinate process (see Fig 224.2) lies behind the root of the superior mesenteric vessels.

(3) Upon crossing the midline at the L1 level, the posterior surface of the body and tail of the pancreas is in contact with the middle third of the left kidney.

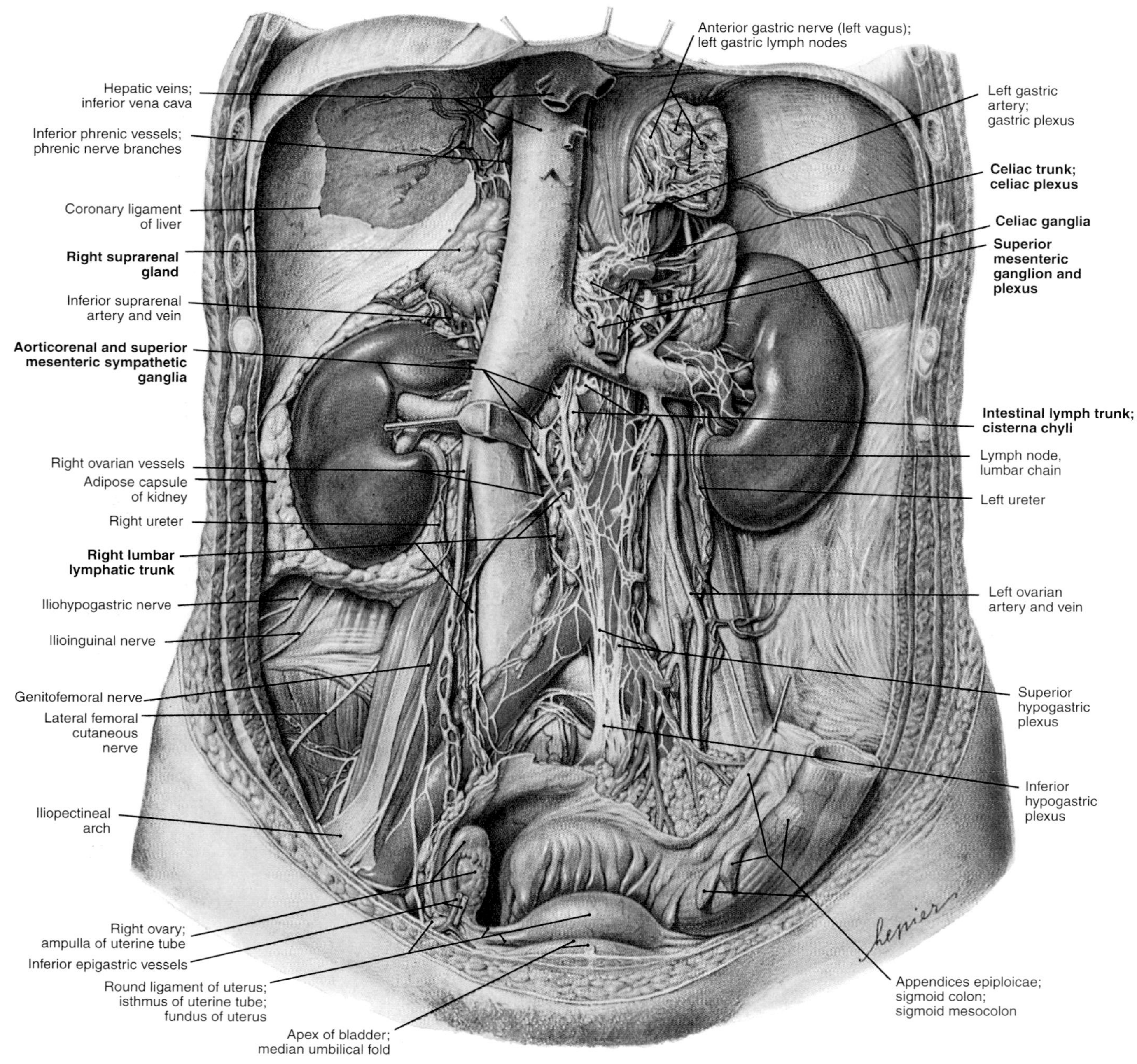
Anterior gastric nerve (left vagus); left gastric lymph nodes
Hepatic veins; inferior vena cava
Inferior phrenic vessels; phrenic nerve branches
Coronary ligament of liver
Right suprarenal gland
Inferior suprarenal artery and vein
Aorticorenal and superior mesenteric sympathetic ganglia
Right ovarian vessels
Adipose capsule of kidney
Right ureter
Right lumbar lymphatic trunk
Iliohypogastric nerve
Ilioinguinal nerve
Genitofemoral nerve
Lateral femoral cutaneous nerve
Iliopectineal arch
Right ovary; ampulla of uterine tube
Inferior epigastric vessels
Round ligament of uterus; isthmus of uterine tube; fundus of uterus
Apex of bladder; median umbilical fold
Left gastric artery; gastric plexus
Celiac trunk; celiac plexus
Celiac ganglia
Superior mesenteric ganglion and plexus
Intestinal lymph trunk; cisterna chyli
Lymph node, lumbar chain
Left ureter
Left ovarian artery and vein
Superior hypogastric plexus
Inferior hypogastric plexus
Appendices epiploicae; sigmoid colon; sigmoid mesocolon

Figure 242 Abdominal Cavity: Lymphatics and Nerves of the Posterior Abdominal Wall

NOTE: (1) Lymphatic channels draining the pelvic organs and the structures of the posterior abdominal wall course along iliac nodes to the right and left chains of lumbar nodes, which parallel the aorta.

(2) The lumbar lymphatic trunks are joined by intestinal trunks draining the gastrointestinal organs to form the cisterna chyli.

(3) The complexity of the sympathetic ganglia and autonomic plexuses found in relationship to the abdominal aorta and its branches.

(4) The **superior hypogastric plexus** contains autonomic nerve fibers along with visceral afferent fibers. The autonomic fibers include **postganglionic sympathetic fibers descending** from ganglia in the abdomen to supply pelvic organs and **preganglionic parasympathetic fibers** from S2, S3, and S4 **ascending** to the abdomen to supply innervation of the large intestine beyond the transverse colon, where the vagal fibers cease.

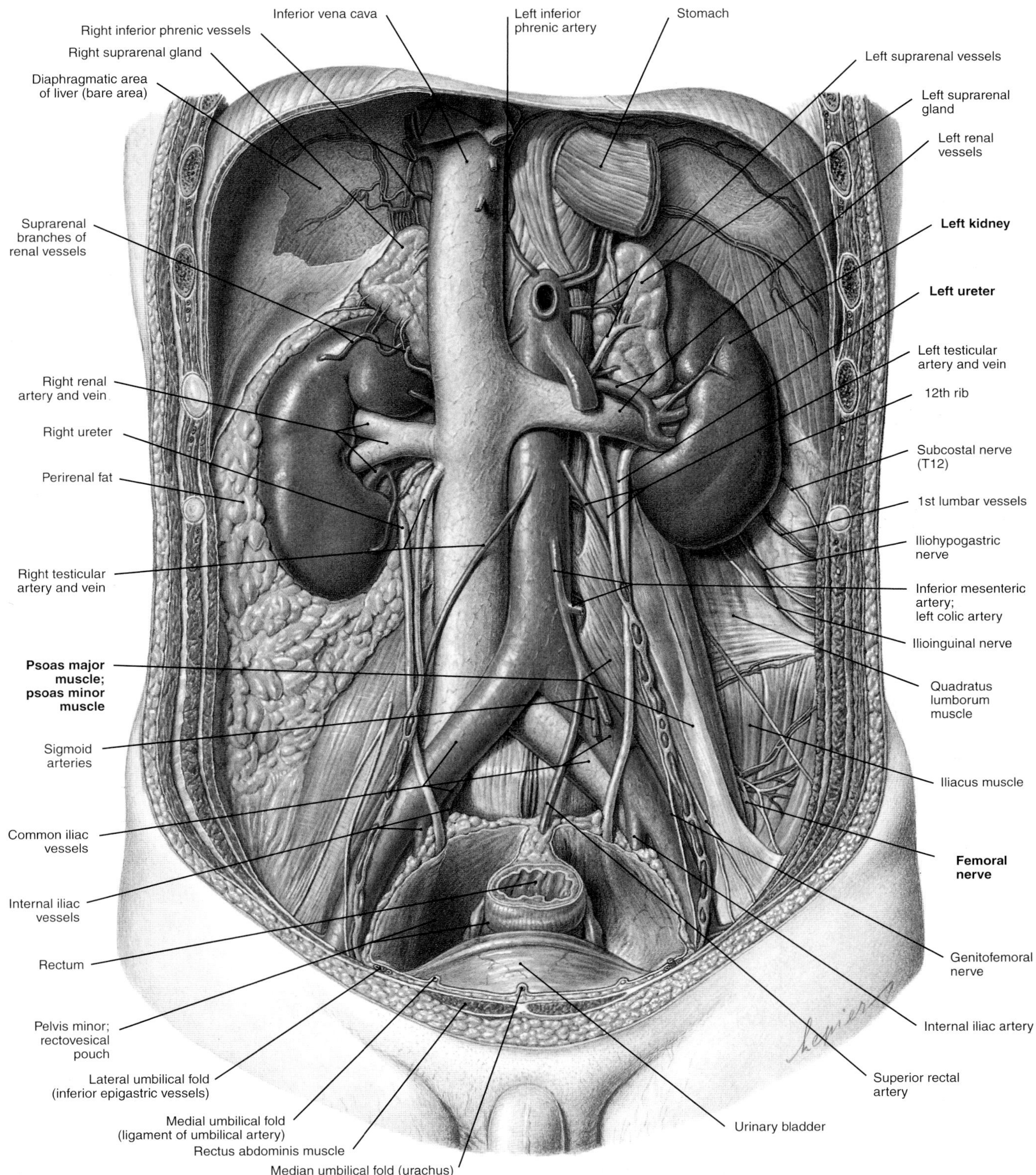
Inferior vena cava
Left inferior phrenic artery
Stomach
Right inferior phrenic vessels
Right suprarenal gland
Diaphragmatic area of liver (bare area)
Left suprarenal vessels
Left suprarenal gland
Left renal vessels
Suprarenal branches of renal vessels
Left kidney
Left ureter
Left testicular artery and vein
Right renal artery and vein
12th rib
Right ureter
Subcostal nerve (T12)
Perirenal fat
1st lumbar vessels
Iliohypogastric nerve
Right testicular artery and vein
Inferior mesenteric artery; left colic artery
Ilioinguinal nerve
Psoas major muscle; psoas minor muscle
Quadratus lumborum muscle
Sigmoid arteries
Iliacus muscle
Common iliac vessels
Femoral nerve
Internal iliac vessels
Rectum
Genitofemoral nerve
Pelvis minor; rectovesical pouch
Internal iliac artery
Lateral umbilical fold (inferior epigastric vessels)
Superior rectal artery
Medial umbilical fold (ligament of umbilical artery)
Urinary bladder
Rectus abdominis muscle
Median umbilical fold (urachus)

Figure 243 Abdominal Cavity: Posterior Abdominal Wall

NOTE: (1) The kidneys, ureters, suprarenal glands, and great vessels and their branches in the posterior abdominal wall.

(2) The kidneys extend between T12 and L3, and the ureters course inferiorly over the pelvic brim near the iliac bifurcation to terminate in the bladder.

(3) The suprarenal glands capping the upper pole of each kidney. These are highly vascular and vital organs of internal secretion (endocrine).

(4) The aorta enters the abdomen through the aortic hiatus (T12), and the inferior vena cava lies to the right of the vertebral column.

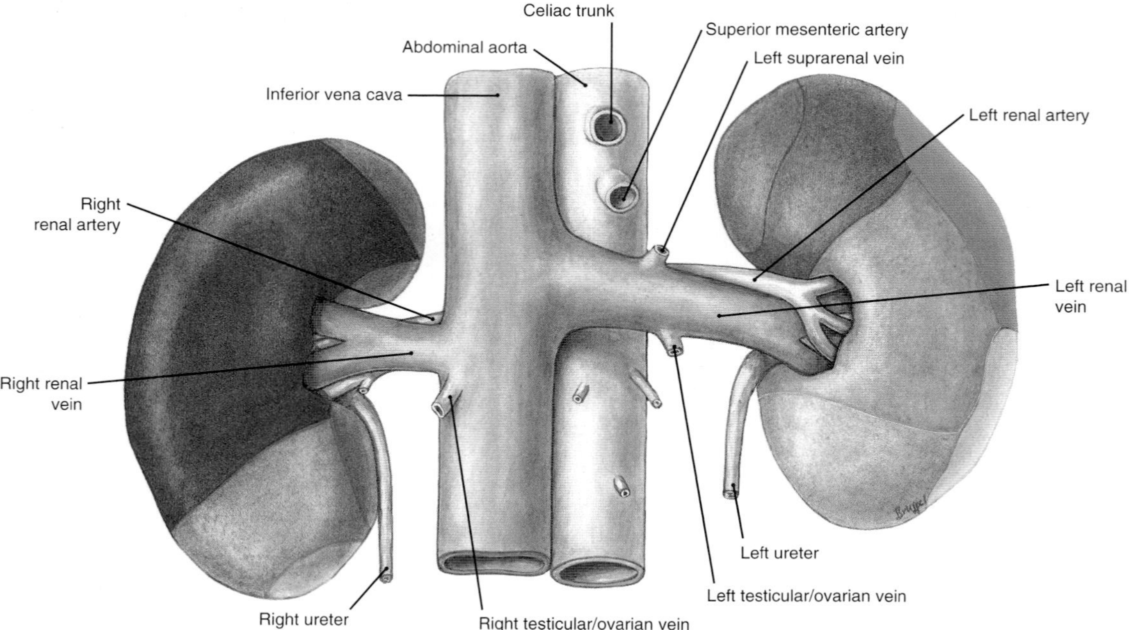

Celiac trunk
Superior mesenteric artery
Abdominal aorta
Left suprarenal vein
Inferior vena cava
Left renal artery
Right renal artery
Left renal vein
Right renal vein
Left ureter
Left testicular/ovarian vein
Right ureter
Right testicular/ovarian vein

Figure 244.1 Anterior Surface Contact Relationships of the Kidneys

NOTE: (1) The relationships of abdominal organs to the anterior surface of the kidneys are characterized either by a peritoneal reflection (**serosal**) intervening between the overlying organ and the kidney or a direct contact between the kidney and the overlying organ (**fibrous**).

(2) The structures in contact with the anterior surface of the **right kidney** are the right suprarenal gland, hepatorenal ligament, duodenum (second part), liver, right colic flexure and transverse colon, and a small area of the jejunum.

(3) The structures in contact with the anterior surface of the **left kidney** are the left suprarenal gland, stomach, spleen, pancreas, jejunum, and left colic flexure. (see **Color Code** below)

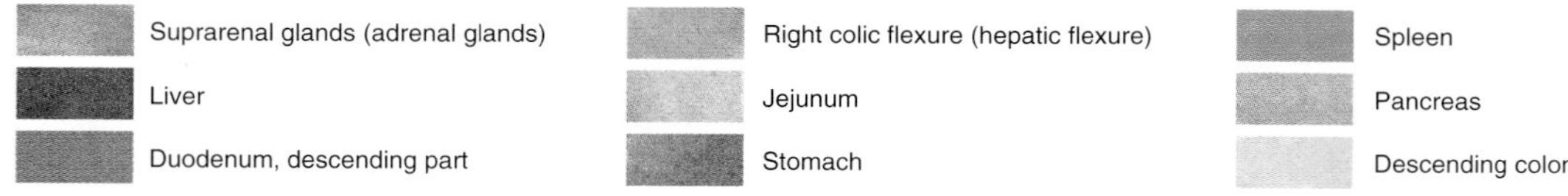

Suprarenal glands (adrenal glands)
Liver
Duodenum, descending part
Right colic flexure (hepatic flexure)
Jejunum
Stomach
Spleen
Pancreas
Descending colon

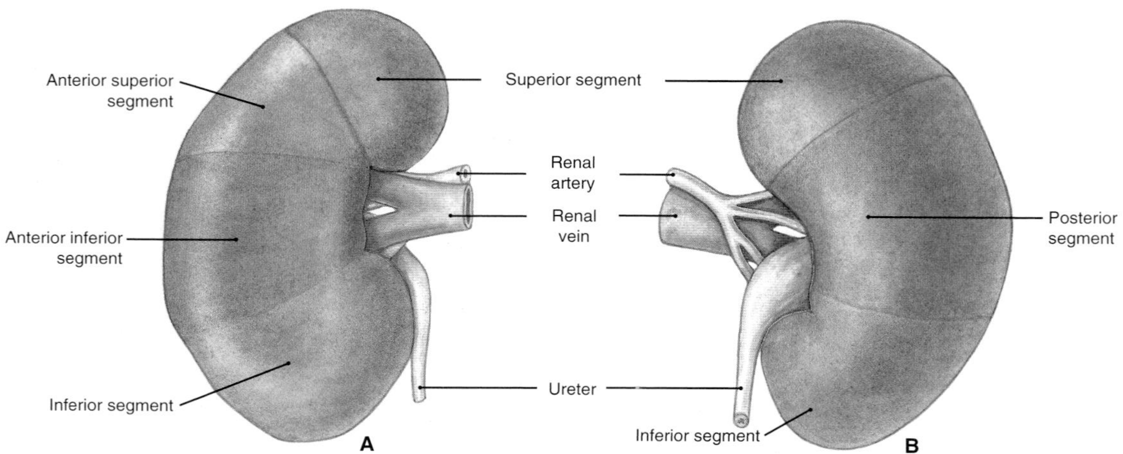

Anterior superior segment
Superior segment
Renal artery
Renal vein
Anterior inferior segment
Posterior segment
Inferior segment
Ureter
Inferior segment
A
B

Figure 244.2 Segments of the Right Kidney

NOTE: A: Anterior surface of the renal segments.

B: Posterior surface of the renal segments.

Each segment has the same color on both anterior (A) and posterior (B) views of this right kidney.

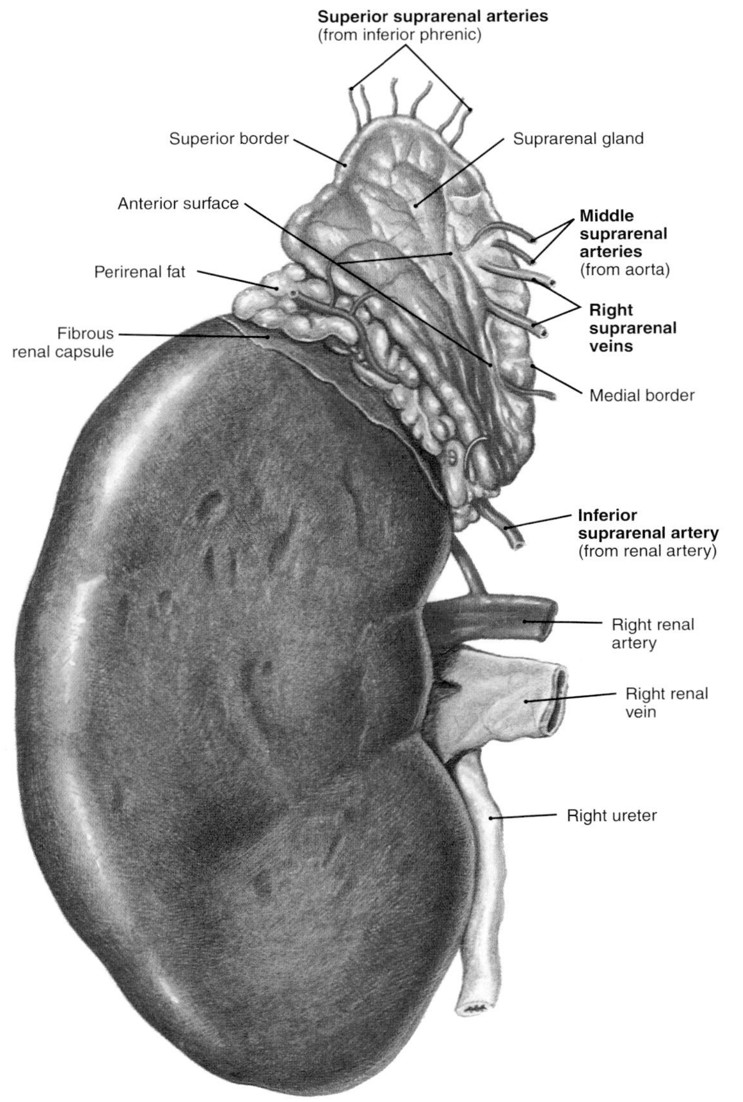
Superior suprarenal arteries
(from inferior phrenic)
Superior border
Suprarenal gland
Anterior surface
Middle
suprarenal
arteries
(from aorta)
Perirenal fat
Right
suprarenal
veins
Fibrous
renal capsule
Medial border
Inferior
suprarenal artery
(from renal artery)
Right renal
artery
Right renal
vein
Right ureter

◀ Figure 245.1 Right Kidney and Suprarenal Gland

NOTE: (1) The suprarenal or adrenal gland is an endocrine gland whose secretions are vital for life. The glands are located in the posterior abdominal region and situated adjacent to the superior poles of the kidneys.

(2) The **right suprarenal gland** is pyramidal in shape, and its anterior surface lies behind the inferior vena cava and adjacent to the right lobe of the liver. Its posterior surface is in contact with the diaphragm and the right kidney.

(3) The suprarenal glands are highly vascular and receive arterial blood from branches directly off the aorta and others from the inferior phrenic and renal arteries. Venous blood is drained by a single vein or by a pair of veins that, on the right side, flow directly into the inferior vena cava, and on the left, into the renal vein.

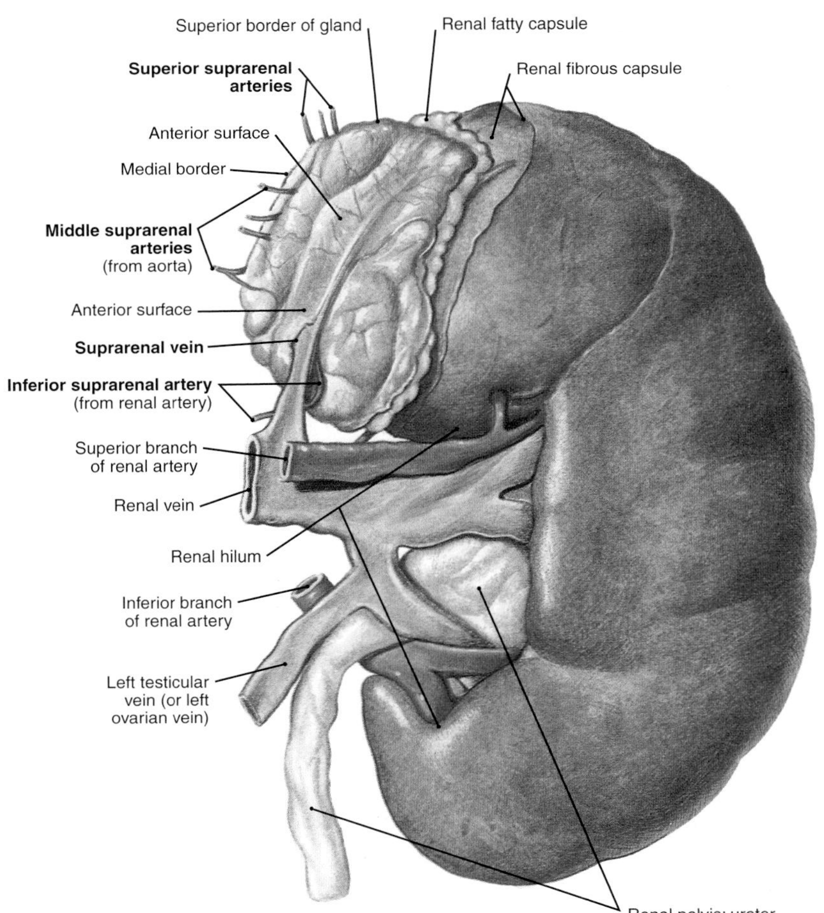
Superior border of gland
Renal fatty capsule
Superior suprarenal
arteries
Renal fibrous capsule
Anterior surface
Medial border
Middle suprarenal
arteries
(from aorta)
Anterior surface
Suprarenal vein
Inferior suprarenal artery
(from renal artery)
Superior branch
of renal artery
Renal vein
Renal hilum
Inferior branch
of renal artery
Left testicular
vein (or left
ovarian vein)
Renal pelvis; ureter

Figure 245.2 Left Kidney and Suprarenal Gland ▶

NOTE: (1) The **left suprarenal gland** is oriented onto the medial surface of the upper pole of the left kidney. It presents a crescentic shape with its concave surface adjacent to the kidney. Its anterior surface lies behind the cardiac end of the stomach and pancreas (behind the omental bursa), whereas its posterior surface rests on the crus of the diaphragm.

(2) The combined weight of the two glands averages about 10 g. The glands are each surrounded by an investing fibrous capsule, around which is a certain amount of areolar tissue.

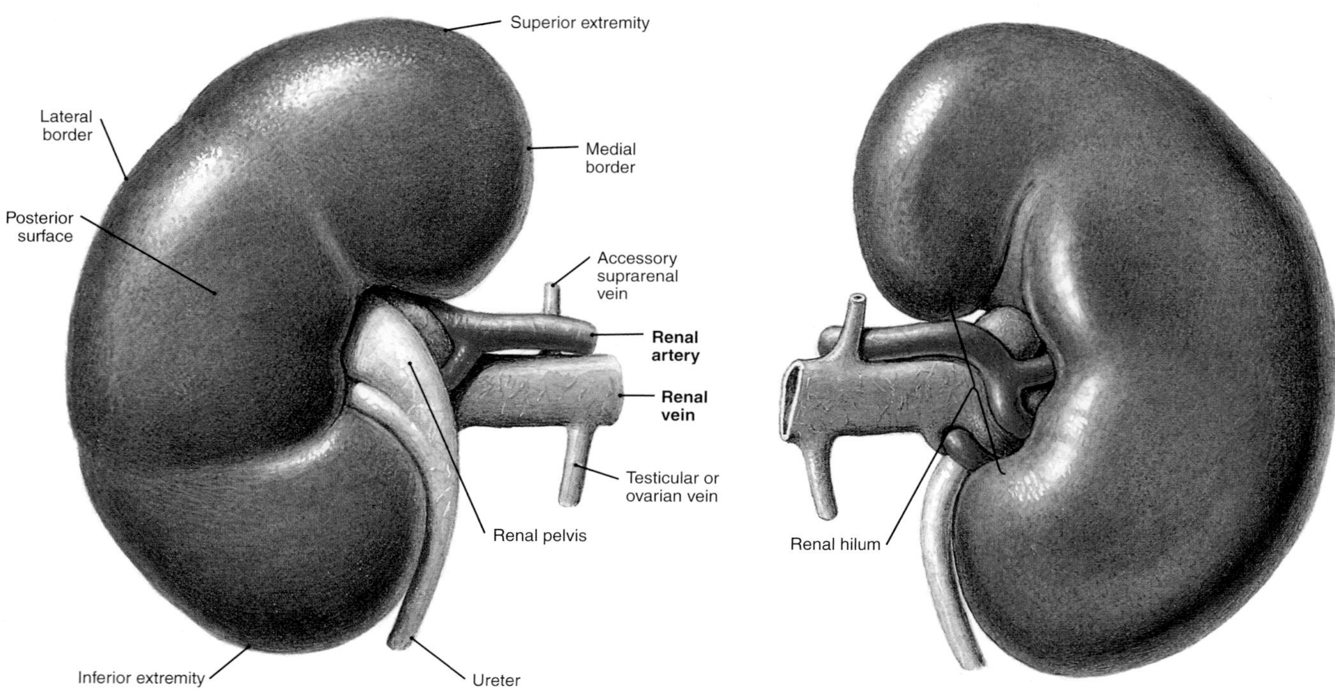
Superior extremity
Lateral border
Medial border
Posterior surface
Accessory suprarenal vein
Renal artery
Renal vein
Testicular or ovarian vein
Renal pelvis
Renal hilum
Inferior extremity
Ureter

Figure 246.1 Left Kidney (Dorsal View) **Figure 246.2 Left Kidney (Ventral View)**

NOTE: (1) The kidneys are paired, bean-shaped organs, and normally weigh about 125 to 150 g each. Their lateral borders are convex and their medial borders concave, the latter being interrupted by the renal vessels and the ureter.

(2) The **ureter** is the most posterior structure at the hilum (see Fig. 246.1). The **renal vein** is the most anterior structure at the hilum, but the **renal artery** frequently divides into anterior and posterior branches (or divisions), and the anterior branch often enters the kidney ventral to the renal vein, as shown in Figure 246.2.

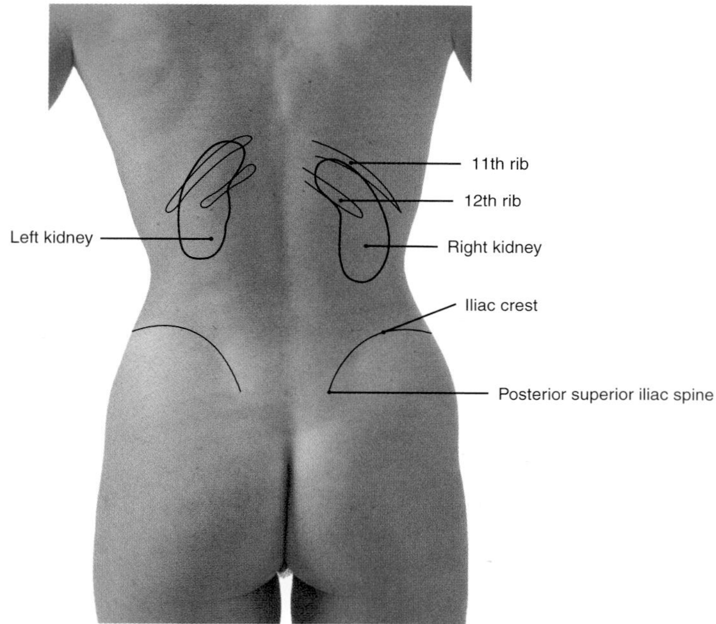
11th rib
12th rib
Left kidney
Right kidney
Iliac crest
Posterior superior iliac spine

Figure 246.3 Surface Anatomy of the Back, Showing the Projection of the Kidney

NOTE: (1) The right kidney is more caudal than the left. Note that the large right lobe of the liver lies just superior to the right kidney.

(2) The inferior poles of the two kidneys are oriented more laterally than the superior poles. Observe the relationship of the kidneys to the 11th and 12th ribs on the two sides.

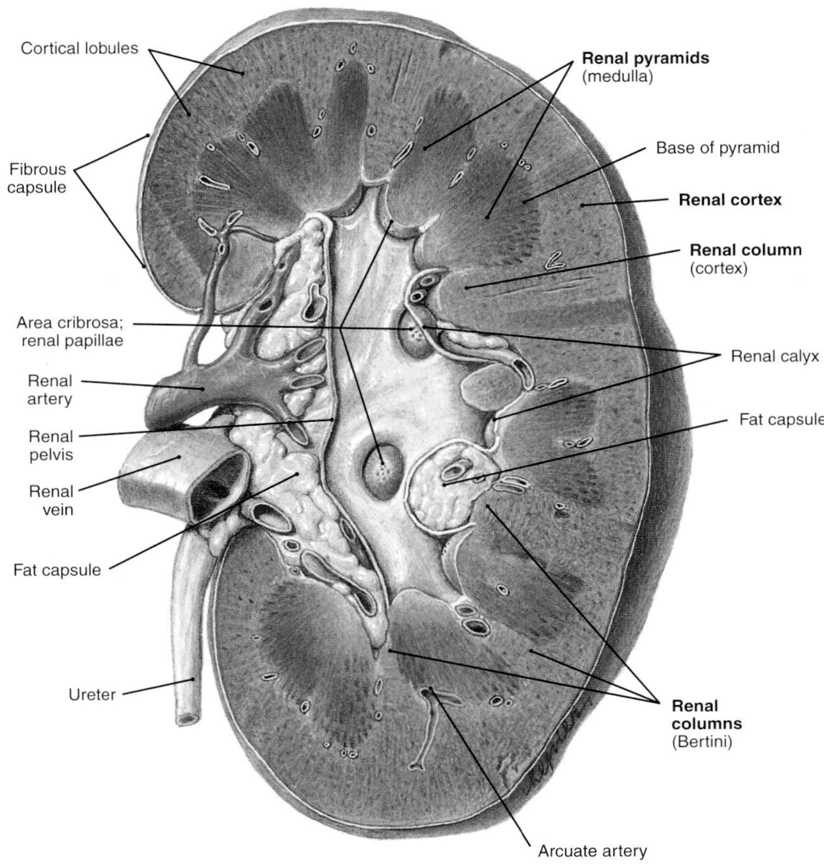

Cortical lobules
Fibrous capsule
Area cribrosa; renal papillae
Renal artery
Renal pelvis
Renal vein
Fat capsule
Ureter
Renal pyramids (medulla)
Base of pyramid
Renal cortex
Renal column (cortex)
Renal calyx
Fat capsule
Renal columns (Bertini)
Arcuate artery

Figure 247.1 Left Kidney: Frontal Section through Renal Vessels

NOTE: (1) The **cortex** of the kidney consists of an outer layer of somewhat lighter and granular-looking tissue, which is also seen to dip as **renal columns** (of Bertini) toward the pelvis of the kidney, thereby separating the conical **renal pyramids** of the **medulla.**

(2) Within the cortex are found the tufted glomeruli and convoluted tubules, whereas the renal pyramids principally contain the loops of Henle and the collecting tubes.

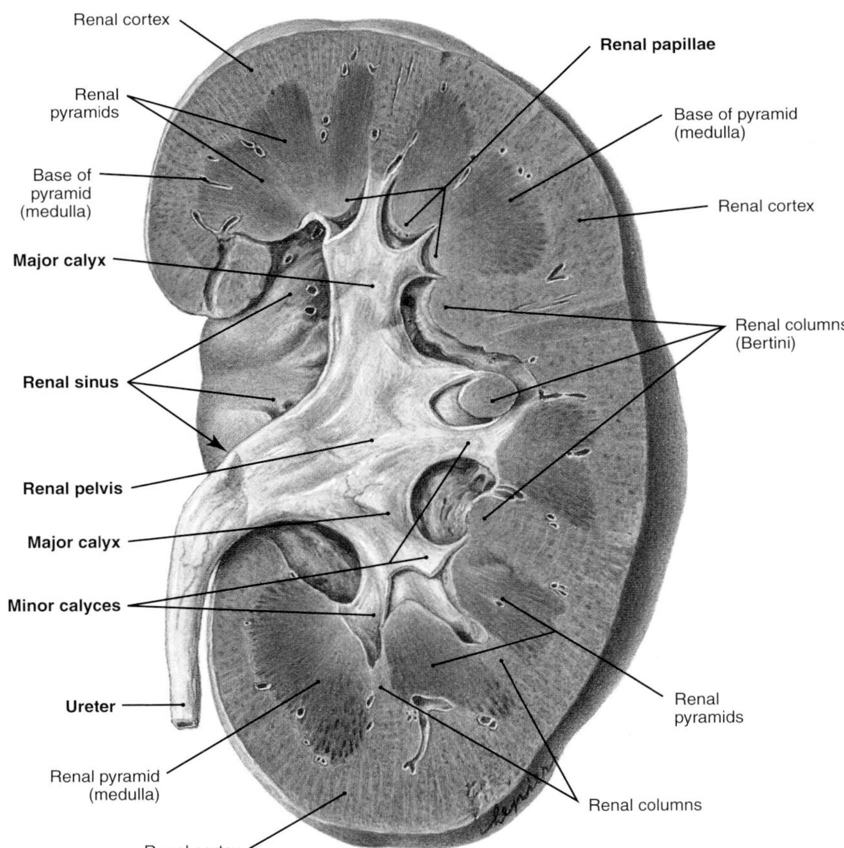

Renal cortex
Renal pyramids
Base of pyramid (medulla)
Major calyx
Renal sinus
Renal pelvis
Major calyx
Minor calyces
Ureter
Renal pyramid (medulla)
Renal cortex
Renal papillae
Base of pyramid (medulla)
Renal cortex
Renal columns (Bertini)
Renal pyramids
Renal columns

Figure 247.2 Left Kidney: Frontal Section through Renal Pelvis

NOTE: (1) This frontal section cuts through the renal pelvis and ureter. The **renal papillae** are cupped by small collecting tubes, the **minor calyces.**

(2) Several minor calyces unite to form a **major calyx,** whereas the **renal pelvis** is formed by the union of two or three major calyces. Leading from the renal pelvis is the somewhat more narrowed **ureter.**

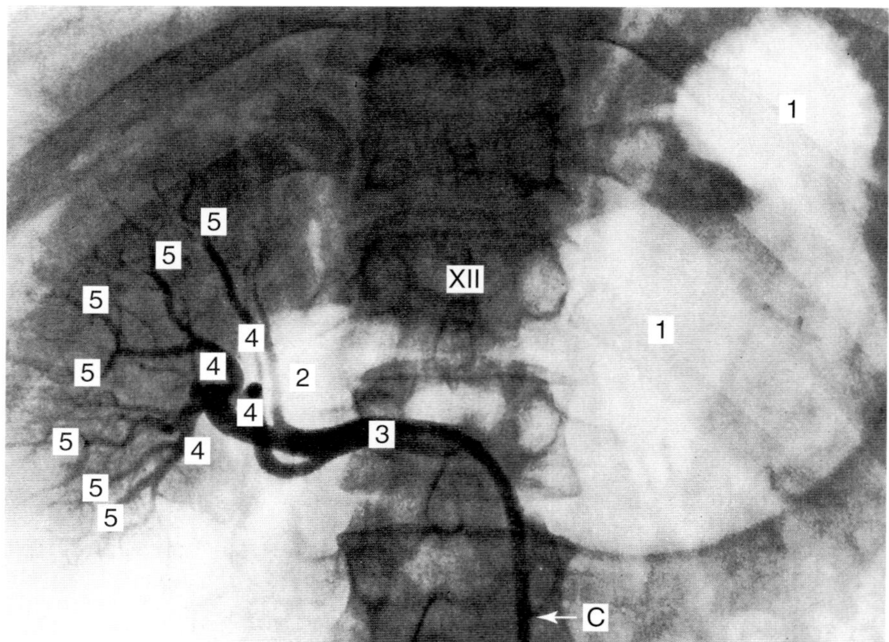
1
5
5
XII
5
4
1
5
4
2
4
3
5
4
5
5
C
1. Stomach
2. Superior (first) part of duodenum
3. Right renal artery
4. Interlobar arteries
5. Interlobular arteries
C. Catheter
XII. 12th thoracic vertebra

Figure 248.1 Arteriogram of Right Renal Artery and Its Branches

NOTE: (1) An arterial catheter (C) has been inserted into the femoral artery and passed through the abdominal aorta and then the **right renal artery.** Observe the division of the renal artery successively into **interlobar arteries.**

(2) As the interlobar arteries reach the junction of the renal cortex and medulla, they arch over the bases of the pyramids, forming **arcuate arteries** (not numbered in this figure). From the arcuate arteries branch a series of **interlobular arteries** (5), which extend through the afferent arterioles entering the renal glomeruli.

(3) The stomach (1) and superior part of the duodenum (2), which are filled with air.

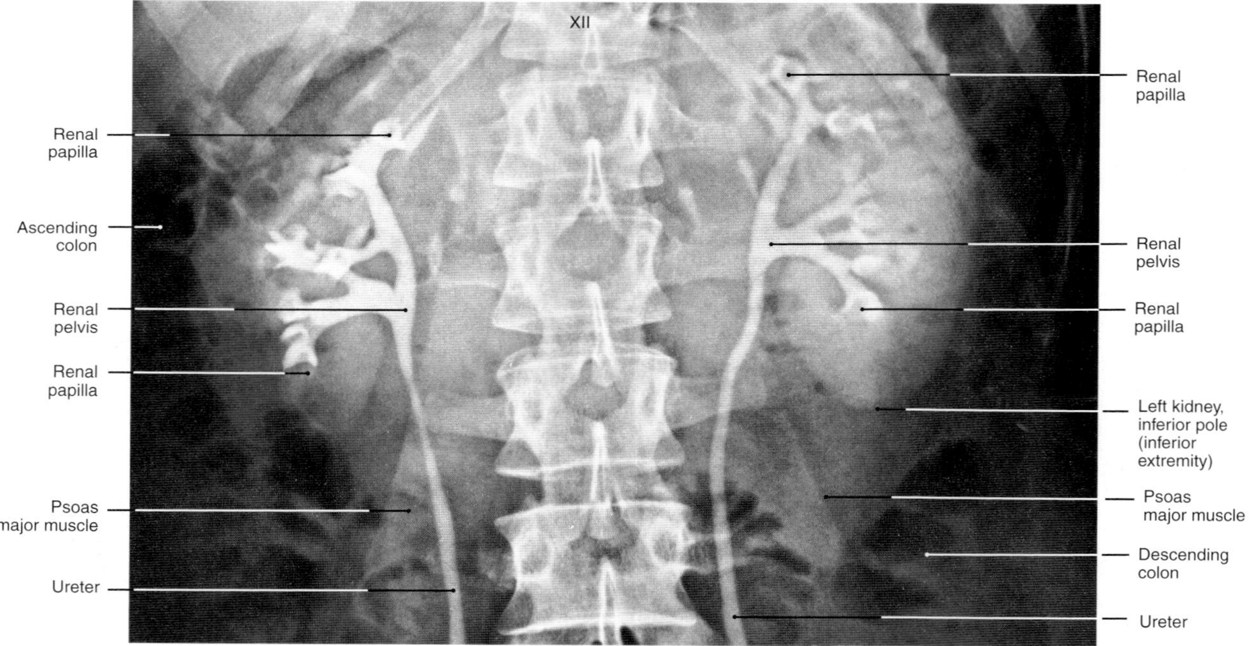
XII
Renal papilla
Ascending colon
Renal pelvis
Renal papilla
Psoas major muscle
Ureter
Renal papilla
Renal pelvis
Renal papilla
Left kidney, inferior pole (inferior extremity)
Psoas major muscle
Descending colon
Ureter

Figure 248.2 Retrograde Pyelogram

NOTE: (1) A radiopaque substance has been introduced into each ureter and forced into the renal pelvis, major calyces, and minor calyces of each side. Observe that into the minor calyces project the renal papillae, resulting in radiolucent invaginations into the radiopaque minor calyces.

(2) The shadow of the superior extremity of the left kidney extending to top of the body of the T12 vertebra, while the right kidney is somewhat more inferior.

(3) The lateral margins of the psoas major muscles. The ureters course toward the pelvis along their anterior surfaces.

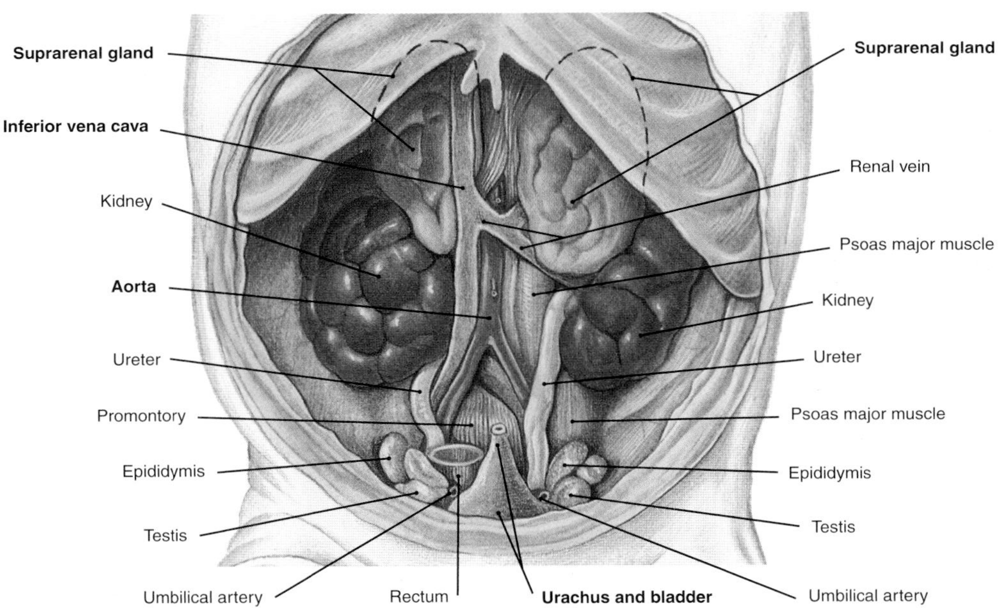
Suprarenal gland
Inferior vena cava
Kidney
Aorta
Ureter
Promontory
Epididymis
Testis
Umbilical artery
Rectum
Urachus and bladder
Suprarenal gland
Renal vein
Psoas major muscle
Kidney
Ureter
Psoas major muscle
Epididymis
Testis
Umbilical artery

Figure 249.1 Posterior Abdominal Wall in 5-Month Fetus

NOTE: (1) The kidneys and adrenal glands in a 5-month fetus. The upper abdominal organs and the intestines have been removed. The part of the suprarenal glands lying behind the costal margin is indicated by dashed lines.

(2) The **lobulated** appearance of the **fetal kidneys.** Even at birth this lobulation is obvious, but as maturation proceeds the surface slowly becomes smooth.

(3) The large **suprarenal glands** and the enlarged and tortuous **ureters.** The testes and epididymis are still located in the lesser pelvis adjacent to the point at which the abdominal inguinal ring will form the entrance to the inguinal canal.

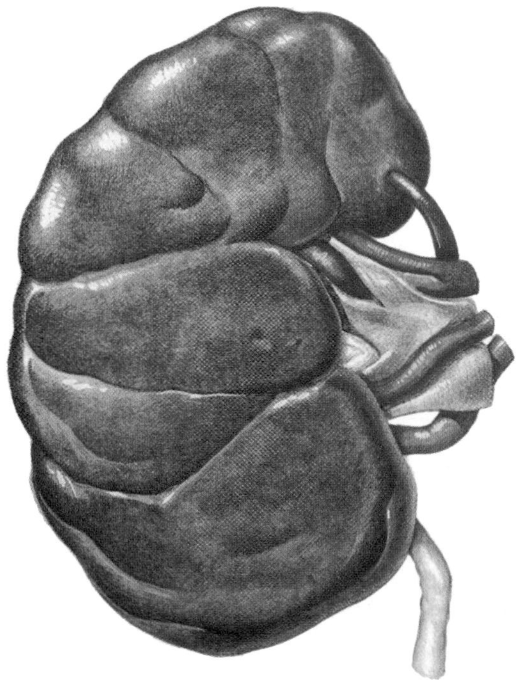

Figure 249.2 Fetal Lobulation May Persist in the Adult Kidney

NOTE: The kidney of the fetus is divided into small lobules that are separated by interlacing grooves on the renal surface. This lobulation usually disappears during the first postnatal year but may persist in the adult but with **no functional impairment.**

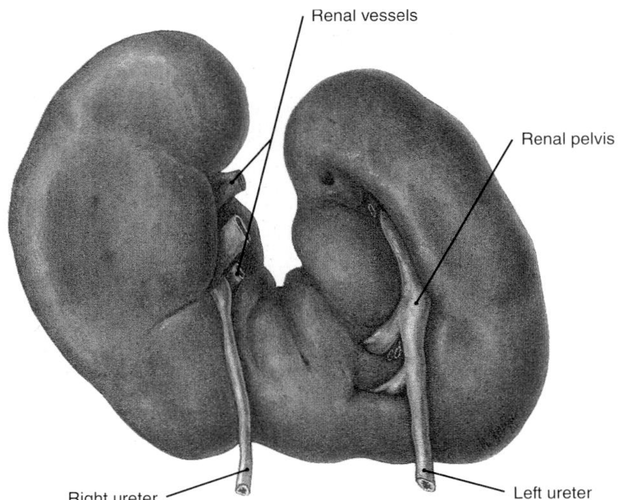
Renal vessels
Renal pelvis
Right ureter
Left ureter

Figure 249.3 Horseshoe Kidney (Anterior View)

NOTE: (1) **Horseshoe kidney** is a common anomaly (1 in 500 persons) in which the lower poles of the kidneys are fused.

(2) The fusion crosses the midline and is often found at the level of the aortic bifurcation. The ureters in the horseshoe kidney lie ventral to the renal vessels.

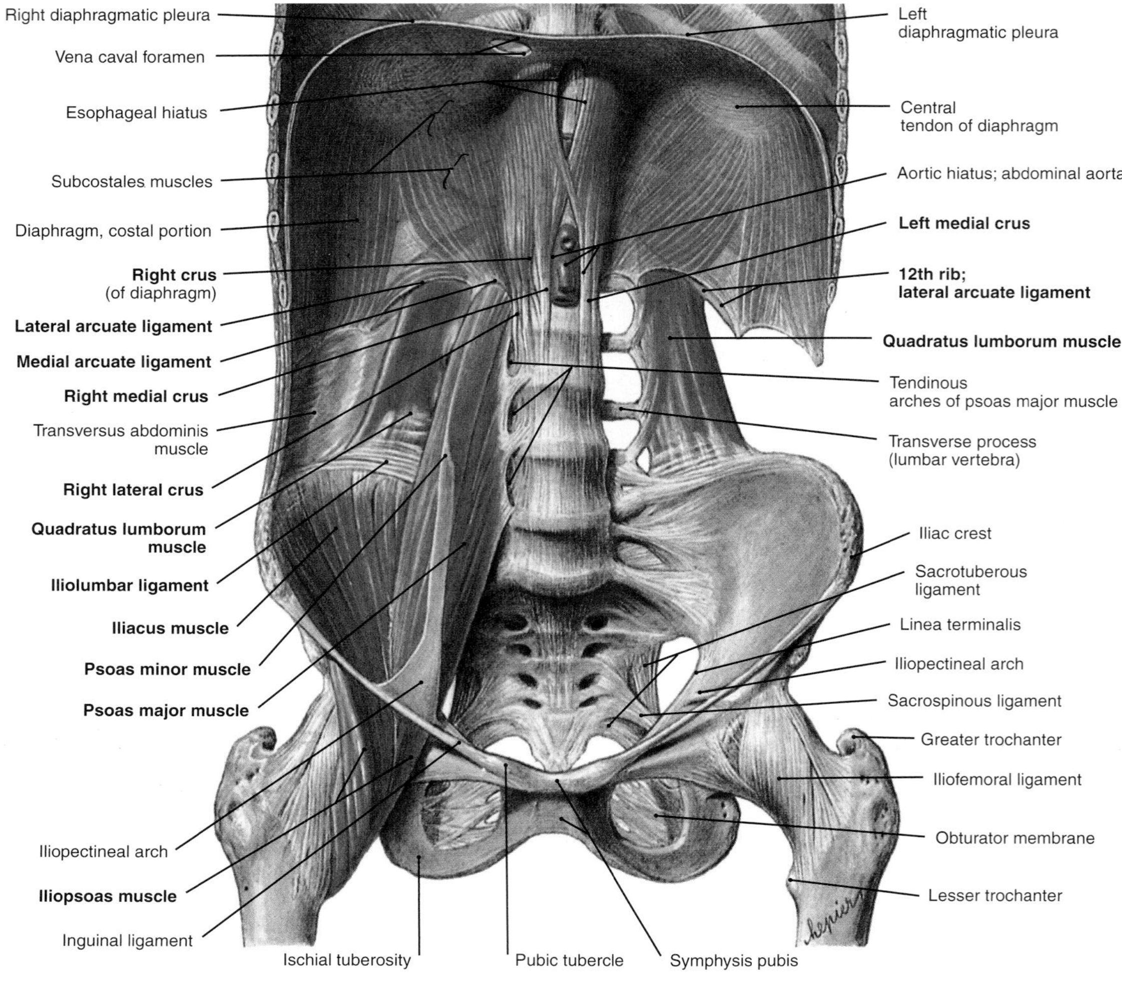
Right diaphragmatic pleura
Vena caval foramen
Esophageal hiatus
Subcostales muscles
Diaphragm, costal portion
Right crus (of diaphragm)
Lateral arcuate ligament
Medial arcuate ligament
Right medial crus
Transversus abdominis muscle
Right lateral crus
Quadratus lumborum muscle
Iliolumbar ligament
Iliacus muscle
Psoas minor muscle
Psoas major muscle
Iliopectineal arch
Iliopsoas muscle
Inguinal ligament
Ischial tuberosity
Pubic tubercle
Symphysis pubis
Left diaphragmatic pleura
Central tendon of diaphragm
Aortic hiatus; abdominal aorta
Left medial crus
12th rib; lateral arcuate ligament
Quadratus lumborum muscle
Tendinous arches of psoas major muscle
Transverse process (lumbar vertebra)
Iliac crest
Sacrotuberous ligament
Linea terminalis
Iliopectineal arch
Sacrospinous ligament
Greater trochanter
Iliofemoral ligament
Obturator membrane
Lesser trochanter

Figure 250.1 Diaphragm and Posterior Abdominal Wall Muscles

NOTE: (1) The posterior attachments of the **diaphragm**:

(a) The **right and left crura** arising from the bodies of the upper three or four lumbar vertebrae.

(b) The **right and left medial arcuate ligaments** (thickenings in the psoas fascia).

(c) The **lateral arcuate ligaments** along the 12th rib overlying the quadratus lumborum muscle.

(2) The **psoas major** and **minor muscles** that descend from the lumbar vertebrae and join the iliacus.

(3) The **quadratus lumborum** between the 12th rib, the transverse processes of the lumbar vertebrae, and the iliac crest.

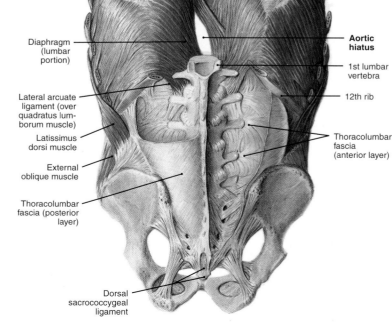

Central tendon
Diaphragm (lumbar portion)
Lateral arcuate ligament (over quadratus lumborum muscle)
Latissimus dorsi muscle
External oblique muscle
Thoracolumbar fascia (posterior layer)
Dorsal sacrococcygeal ligament
Vena caval foramen
Esophageal hiatus
Aortic hiatus
1st lumbar vertebra
12th rib
Thoracolumbar fascia (anterior layer)

Figure 250.2 Posterior View of Diaphragm

NOTE: (1) The posterior half of the bony thorax was removed to show the diaphragm from behind.

(2) The muscle fibers of the diaphragm converge to insert into a central tendon. The right dome of the diaphragm is higher than the left.

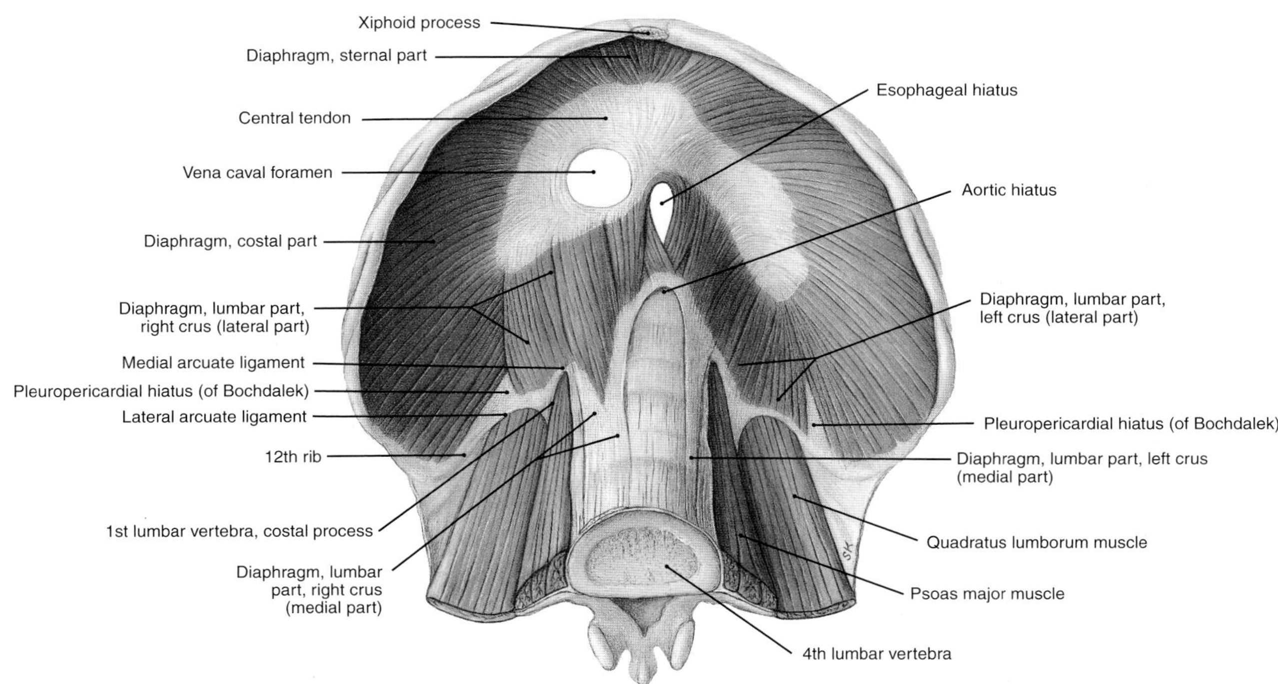
Xiphoid process
Diaphragm, sternal part
Central tendon
Vena caval foramen
Diaphragm, costal part
Diaphragm, lumbar part, right crus (lateral part)
Medial arcuate ligament
Pleuropericardial hiatus (of Bochdalek)
Lateral arcuate ligament
12th rib
1st lumbar vertebra, costal process
Diaphragm, lumbar part, right crus (medial part)
Esophageal hiatus
Aortic hiatus
Diaphragm, lumbar part, left crus (lateral part)
Pleuropericardial hiatus (of Bochdalek)
Diaphragm, lumbar part, left crus (medial part)
Quadratus lumborum muscle
Psoas major muscle
4th lumbar vertebra

Figure 251 Diaphragm (from below) and Arcuate Ligaments

NOTE: (1) The muscle fibers of the diaphragm arise from the xiphoid process, the inner surface of the ribs, the medial and lateral arcuate ligaments and the bodies of the upper lumbar vertebrae (crura).

(2) From all of these origins the fibers converge to insert into the central tendon of the diaphragm.

(3) Its three large apertures transmit the inferior vena cava (T8), the esophagus (T10), and the aorta (T12). Two smaller apertures in the crura transmit the greater and lesser splanchnic nerves.

Muscle	Origin	Insertion	Innervation	Action
Diaphragm	**Sternal part:** Dorsum of xiphoid process. **Costal part:** Inner surfaces of cartilages and adjacent parts of lower six ribs. **Lumbar part:** Medial and lateral arcuate ligaments; crura from bodies of upper two or three lumbar vertebrae.	Central tendon of diaphragm	Phrenic nerve C3, C4, C5	Active during inspiration; assists in increasing intraabdominal pressure
Quadratus Lumborum	Iliolumbar ligament and the adjacent iliac crest	Medial half of the 12th rib and into the transverse processes of upper four lumbar vertebrae	Branches from T12, L1, L2, L3 (L4) nerves	Flexes vertebral column to the same side; fixes 12th rib in breathing; both muscles together extend lumbar vertebrae
Psoas Major	Transverse process and body of T12 and upper four lumbar vertebrae; intervertebral disks between T12 and L5	Lesser trochanter of femur (also receives the fibers of iliacus muscle)	Branches from upper four lumbar nerves	Powerful flexor of thigh at hip; when femurs are fixed, they flex the trunk, as in sitting up from a supine position
Psoas Minor (muscle present in about 40% of cadavers)	Lateral surface of bodies of T12 and L1 vertebrae	Pectineal line and iliopectineal eminence and the iliac fascia (often merges with psoas major tendon)	Branch from L1 nerve	Weak flexor of the thigh at the hip joint
Iliacus	Iliac fossa; anterior inferior iliac spine	Lesser trochanter of femur in common with tendon of psoas major muscle	Femoral nerve (L2, L3)	Powerful flexor of thigh at the hip joint

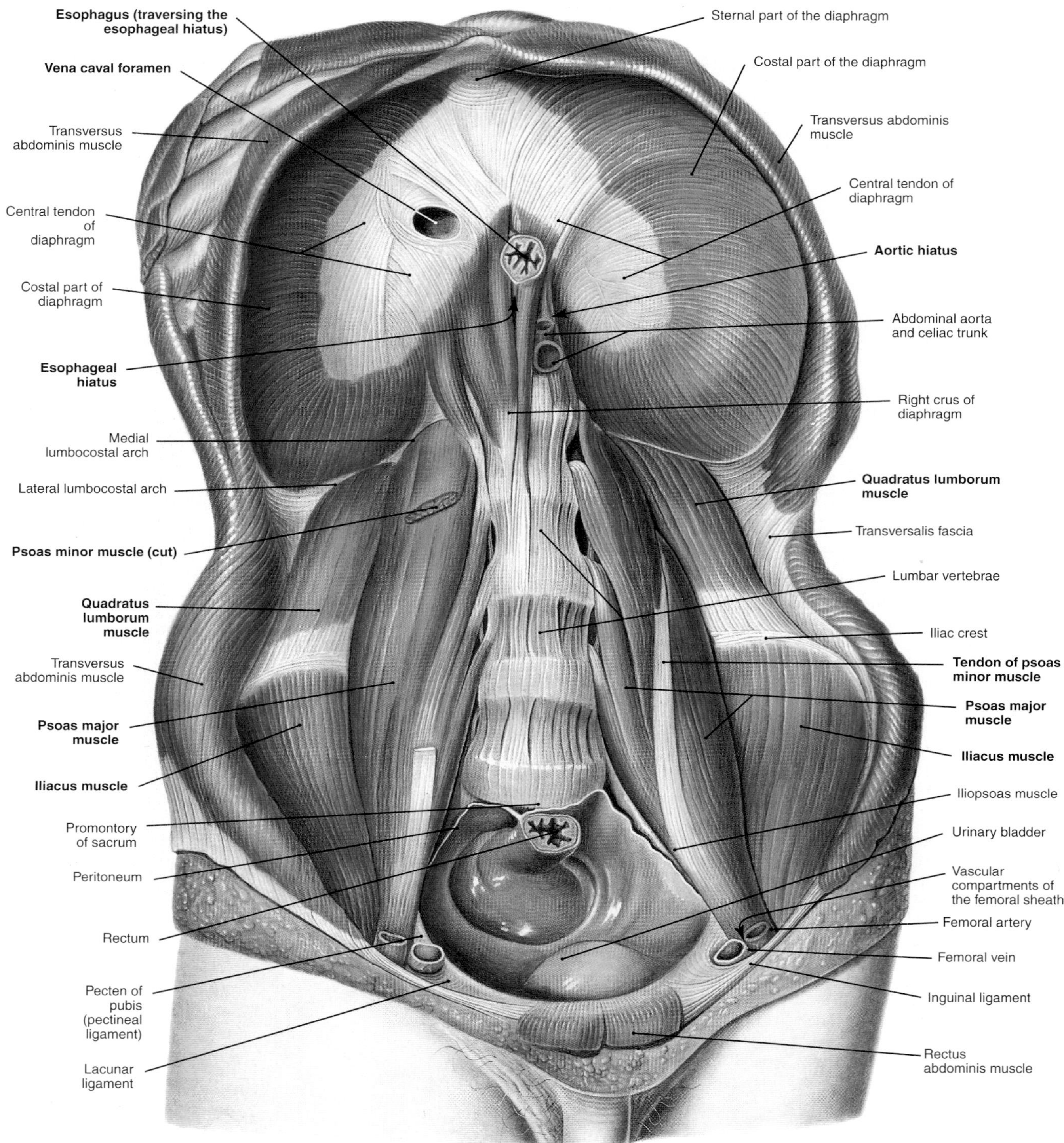
Esophagus (traversing the esophageal hiatus)
Vena caval foramen
Transversus abdominis muscle
Central tendon of diaphragm
Costal part of diaphragm
Esophageal hiatus
Medial lumbocostal arch
Lateral lumbocostal arch
Psoas minor muscle (cut)
Quadratus lumborum muscle
Transversus abdominis muscle
Psoas major muscle
Iliacus muscle
Promontory of sacrum
Peritoneum
Rectum
Pecten of pubis (pectineal ligament)
Lacunar ligament
Sternal part of the diaphragm
Costal part of the diaphragm
Transversus abdominis muscle
Central tendon of diaphragm
Aortic hiatus
Abdominal aorta and celiac trunk
Right crus of diaphragm
Quadratus lumborum muscle
Transversalis fascia
Lumbar vertebrae
Iliac crest
Tendon of psoas minor muscle
Psoas major muscle
Iliacus muscle
Iliopsoas muscle
Urinary bladder
Vascular compartments of the femoral sheath
Femoral artery
Femoral vein
Inguinal ligament
Rectus abdominis muscle

Figure 252 Psoas Minor, Psoas Major, Iliacus, and Quadratus Lumborum Muscles and Diaphragm

NOTE: (1) The **psoas minor muscle** lies anterior to the psoas major, and it merges with the lower part of the psoas major above the inguinal ligament.

(2) The **psoas major muscle** descends deep to the inguinal ligament and is joined by the iliacus muscle.

(3) The **iliacus muscle** arises from the iliac fossa, converges with the psoas major, and their joint tendon inserts onto the lesser trochanter of the femur.

(4) The **quadratus lumborum muscle** is a four-sided muscle on the dorsal wall of the abdomen, and it is located between the 12th rib, the iliac crest, and the transverse processes of the upper four lumbar vertebrae.

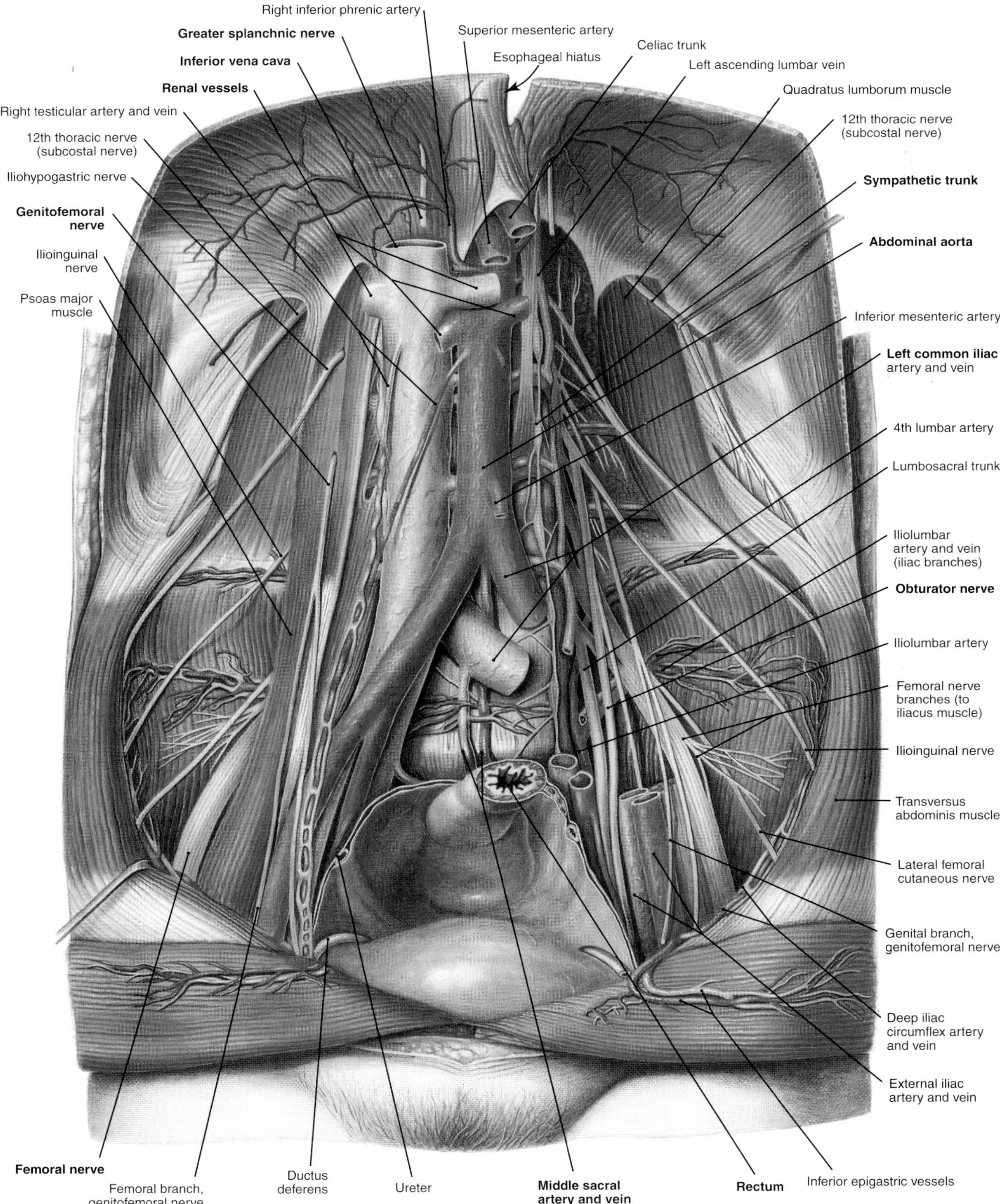
Right inferior phrenic artery
Greater splanchnic nerve
Superior mesenteric artery
Celiac trunk
Inferior vena cava
Esophageal hiatus
Left ascending lumbar vein
Renal vessels
Quadratus lumborum muscle
Right testicular artery and vein
12th thoracic nerve (subcostal nerve)
12th thoracic nerve (subcostal nerve)
Iliohypogastric nerve
Sympathetic trunk
Genitofemoral nerve
Abdominal aorta
Ilioinguinal nerve
Psoas major muscle
Inferior mesenteric artery
Left common iliac artery and vein
4th lumbar artery
Lumbosacral trunk
Iliolumbar artery and vein (iliac branches)
Obturator nerve
Iliolumbar artery
Femoral nerve branches (to iliacus muscle)
Ilioinguinal nerve
Transversus abdominis muscle
Lateral femoral cutaneous nerve
Genital branch, genitofemoral nerve
Deep iliac circumflex artery and vein
External iliac artery and vein
Femoral nerve
Femoral branch, genitofemoral nerve
Ductus deferens
Ureter
Middle sacral artery and vein
Rectum
Inferior epigastric vessels

Figure 253 Posterior Abdominal Vessels and Nerves

NOTE: (1) The abdominal organs and the left psoas muscle have been removed. See the **greater splanchnic nerves** enter the abdomen through the diaphragmatic crura. Identify the **inferior phrenic arteries** and the **abdominal sympathetic chain**.

(2) The **testicular arteries** arising from the aorta below the renal arteries. Inferiorly, the testicular artery and vein join the **ductus deferens** to enter the inguinal canal through the abdominal inguinal ring just lateral to the inferior epigastric vessels. Observe the **middle sacral vessels** descending into the pelvis in the midline.

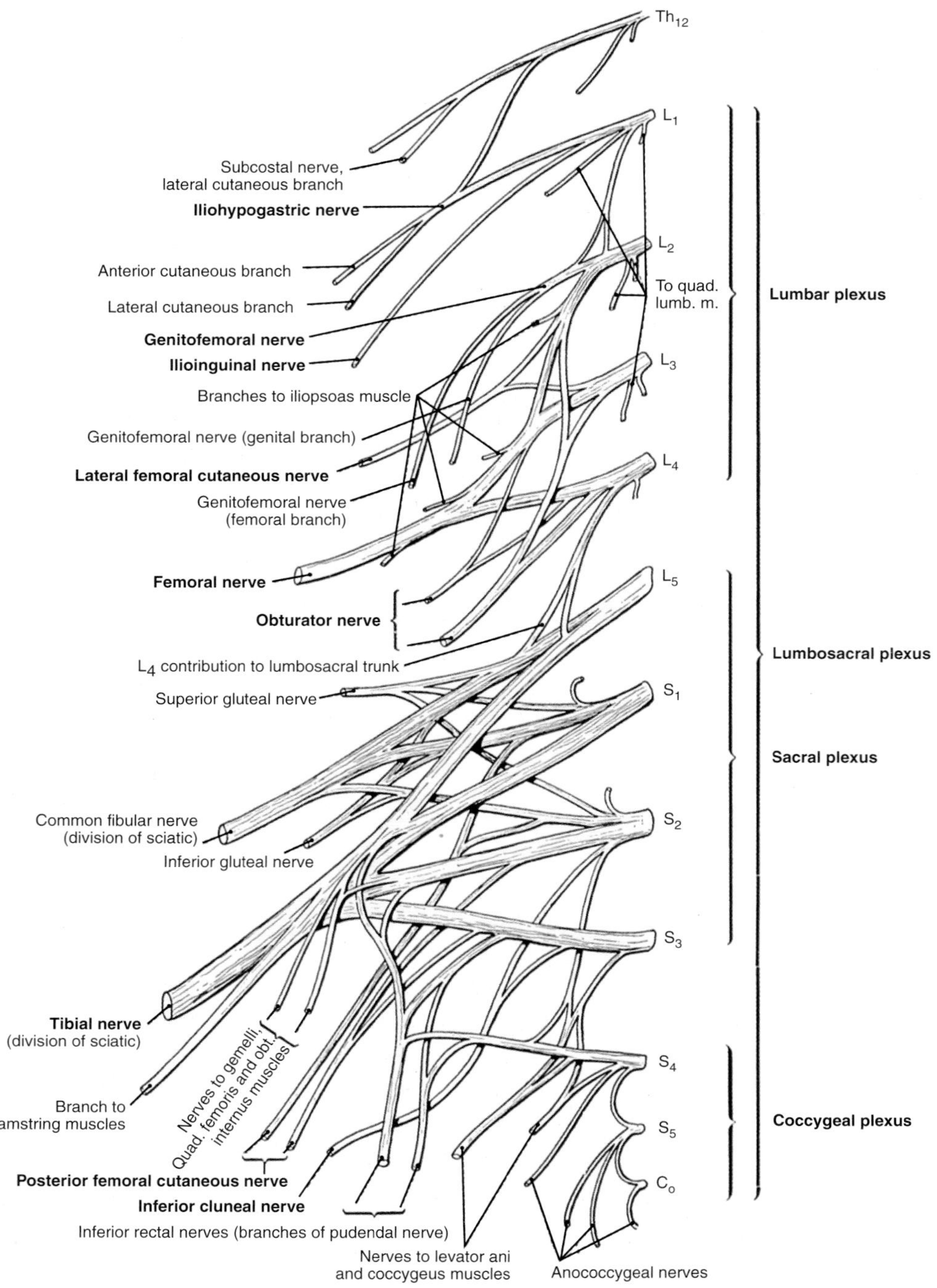
Th12
L1
L2
L3
L4
L5
S1
S2
S3
S4
S5
Co
Subcostal nerve, lateral cutaneous branch
Iliohypogastric nerve
Anterior cutaneous branch
Lateral cutaneous branch
Genitofemoral nerve
Ilioinguinal nerve
Branches to iliopsoas muscle
Genitofemoral nerve (genital branch)
Lateral femoral cutaneous nerve
Genitofemoral nerve (femoral branch)
Femoral nerve
Obturator nerve
L4 contribution to lumbosacral trunk
Superior gluteal nerve
Common fibular nerve (division of sciatic)
Inferior gluteal nerve
Tibial nerve (division of sciatic)
Branch to hamstring muscles
Nerves to gemelli, Quad. femoris and obt. internus muscles
Posterior femoral cutaneous nerve
Inferior cluneal nerve
Inferior rectal nerves (branches of pudendal nerve)
Nerves to levator ani and coccygeus muscles
Anococcygeal nerves
To quad. lumb. m.
Lumbar plexus
Lumbosacral plexus
Sacral plexus
Coccygeal plexus

Figure 254 Diagram of the Lumbar, Sacral, Pudendal, and Coccygeal Nerve Plexuses

NOTE: (1) The **subcostal** (T12) and **L1 nerves** are distributed mainly to the lower abdominal wall, and L1 divides into the **ilioinguinal** and **iliohypogastric nerves.**

(2) **L2, L3,** and **L4** are the principal segments forming the **lumbar plexus. L1** contributes some fibers to the **genitofemoral nerve.** From these segments are derived the:

(a) **Genitofemoral nerve** (L1, L2)
(b) **Lateral femoral cutaneous nerve** (L2, L3)
(c) **Obturator nerve** (L2, L3, L4)
(d) **Femoral nerve** (L2, L3, L4)

(3) **L5, S1, S2,** and **S3** with some contribution from **L4** form the **sacral plexus.** From these segments are derived:

(a) **Superior gluteal nerve** (L4, L5, S1)
(b) **Inferior gluteal nerve** (L5, S1, S2)
(c) **Posterior femoral cutaneous nerve** (S1, S2, S3)
(d) **Sciatic nerve:**
common fibular nerve (L4, L5, S1, S2)
tibial nerve (L4, L5, S1, S2, S3)

(4) **S2, S3,** and **S4** also contribute to the **pudendal nerve,** which is the main sensory and motor nerve of the perineum.

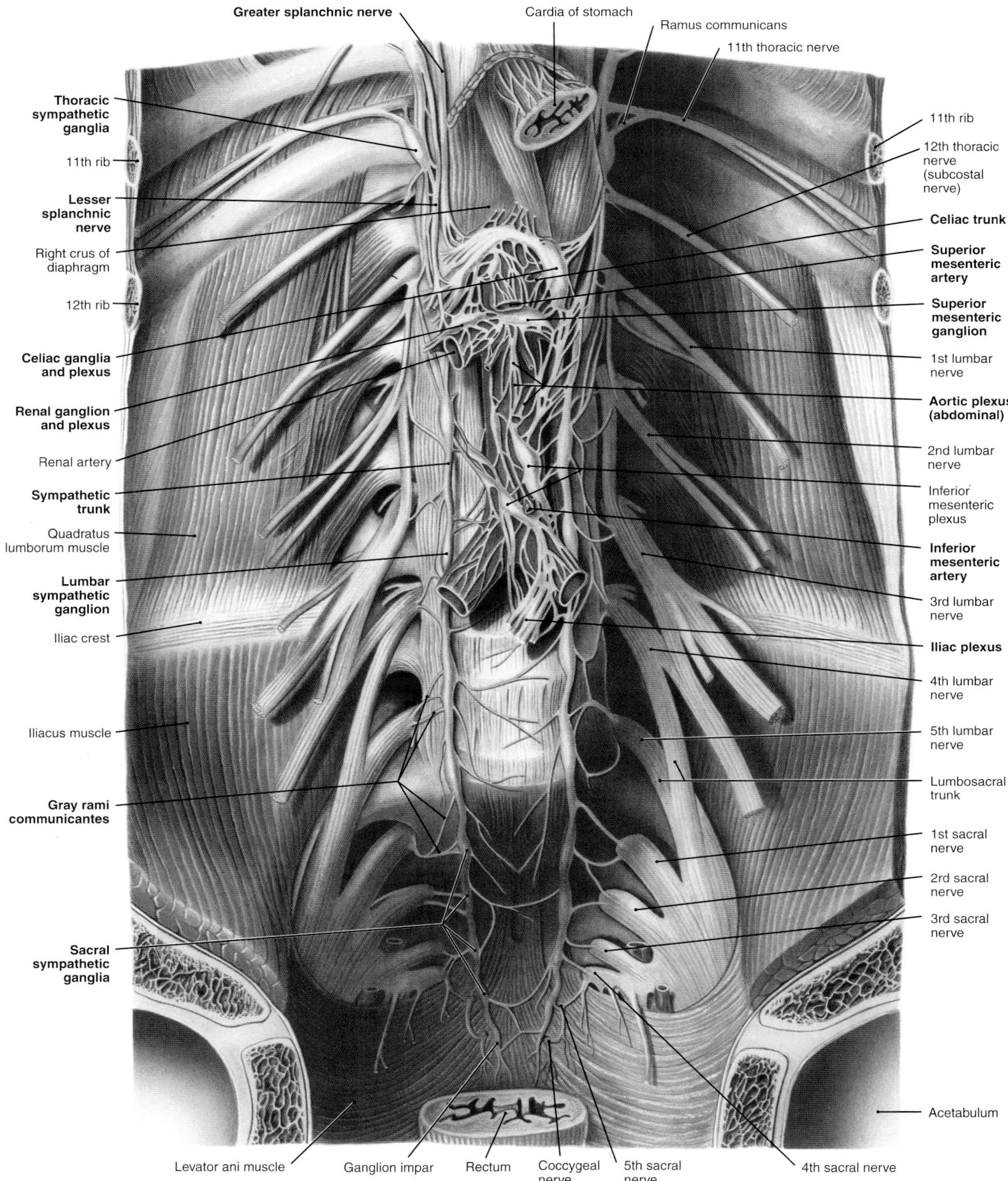
Greater splanchnic nerve
Cardia of stomach
Ramus communicans
11th thoracic nerve
Thoracic sympathetic ganglia
11th rib
Lesser splanchnic nerve
Right crus of diaphragm
12th rib
Celiac ganglia and plexus
Renal ganglion and plexus
Renal artery
Sympathetic trunk
Quadratus lumborum muscle
Lumbar sympathetic ganglion
Iliac crest
Iliacus muscle
Gray rami communicantes
Sacral sympathetic ganglia
11th rib
12th thoracic nerve (subcostal nerve)
Celiac trunk
Superior mesenteric artery
Superior mesenteric ganglion
1st lumbar nerve
Aortic plexus (abdominal)
2nd lumbar nerve
Inferior mesenteric plexus
Inferior mesenteric artery
3rd lumbar nerve
Iliac plexus
4th lumbar nerve
5th lumbar nerve
Lumbosacral trunk
1st sacral nerve
2rd sacral nerve
3rd sacral nerve
Acetabulum
Levator ani muscle
Ganglion impar
Rectum
Coccygeal nerve
5th sacral nerve
4th sacral nerve

Figure 255 Lumbar Sympathetic Trunk and Abdominal Autonomic Ganglia

NOTE: (1) The two sympathetic chains of ganglia descending from the thorax through the abdomen and into the pelvis; observe the plexuses and their associated ganglia, which overlie the major arteries branching from the aorta.

(2) The **celiac plexuses** and the **superior mesenteric, inferior mesenteric, renal, aortic,** and **iliac plexuses** form dense networks of autonomic fibers from which many of the abdominal and pelvic viscera receive sympathetic innervation.

(3) The **splanchnic nerves** (containing preganglionic sympathetic fibers) join the upper abdominal ganglia, where their fibers synapse with postganglionic neurons.

(4) Below L2 only **gray rami** connect the ganglia of the sympathetic chain with the segmental nerves, since preganglionic fibers do not emerge from the spinal cord below L2.

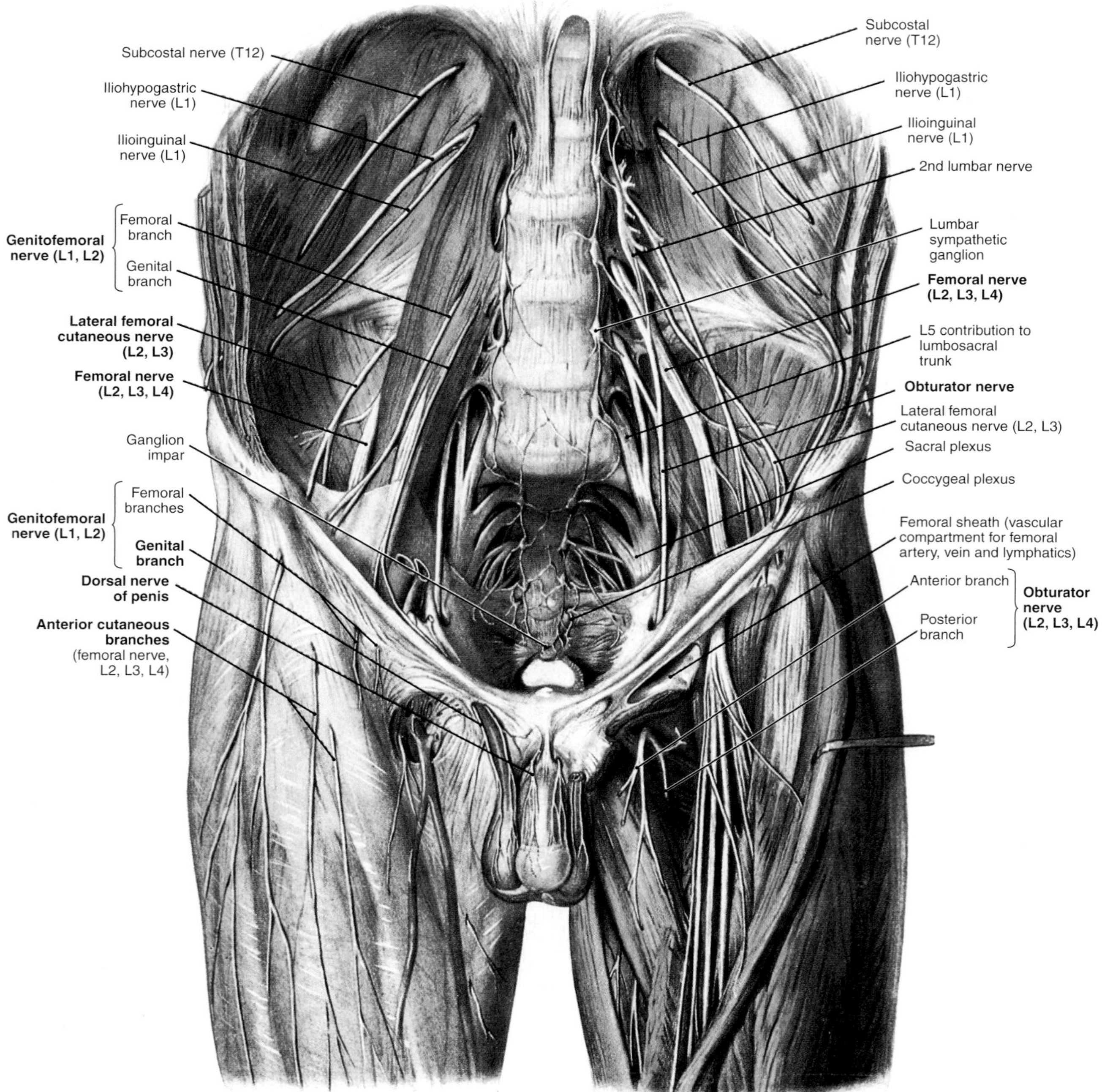

Subcostal nerve (T12)
Iliohypogastric nerve (L1)
Ilioinguinal nerve (L1)
Genitofemoral nerve (L1, L2)
Femoral branch
Genital branch
Lateral femoral cutaneous nerve (L2, L3)
Femoral nerve (L2, L3, L4)
Ganglion impar
Genitofemoral nerve (L1, L2)
Femoral branches
Genital branch
Dorsal nerve of penis
Anterior cutaneous branches (femoral nerve, L2, L3, L4)
Subcostal nerve (T12)
Iliohypogastric nerve (L1)
Ilioinguinal nerve (L1)
2nd lumbar nerve
Lumbar sympathetic ganglion
Femoral nerve (L2, L3, L4)
L5 contribution to lumbosacral trunk
Obturator nerve
Lateral femoral cutaneous nerve (L2, L3)
Sacral plexus
Coccygeal plexus
Femoral sheath (vascular compartment for femoral artery, vein and lymphatics)
Anterior branch
Posterior branch
Obturator nerve (L2, L3, L4)

Figure 256 Lumbosacral Plexus: Posterior Abdominal Wall and Anterior Thigh

NOTE: (1) On the left side, the psoas muscles have been removed to reveal the **lumbar plexus** more completely. The lumbar nerves emerge from the spinal cord and descend along the posterior abdominal wall within the substance of the psoas muscles. The **12th thoracic** (subcostal) **nerve** courses around the abdominal wall below the 12th rib.

(2) The **first lumbar nerve** divides into **iliohypogastric** and **ilioinguinal branches.** The ilioinguinal nerve descends obliquely toward the iliac crest and penetrates the transversus and internal oblique muscles to join the spermatic cord, becoming cutaneous at the superficial inguinal ring.

(3) The **genitofemoral nerve** courses superficially on the surface of the psoas major muscle. It divides into a **genital branch** (which supplies the cremaster muscle and the skin of the scrotum) and a **femoral branch** (which is sensory to the upper anterior thigh).

(4) The **femoral** and **obturator nerves** derived from the posterior and anterior divisions of **L2, L3,** and **L4,** respectively descend to innervate the anterior and medial groups of the femoral muscles.

(5) The femoral nerve enters the thigh beneath the inguinal ligament and divides into both sensory and motor branches, whereas the obturator nerve courses more medially through the obturator foramen to innervate the adductor muscle group.

(6) **L4** and **L5** nerve roots (**lumbosacral trunk**) join with the upper three sacral nerves to form the **sacral plexus,** from which is derived, among other nerves, the large **sciatic nerve,** which reaches the gluteal region through the greater sciatic foramen.

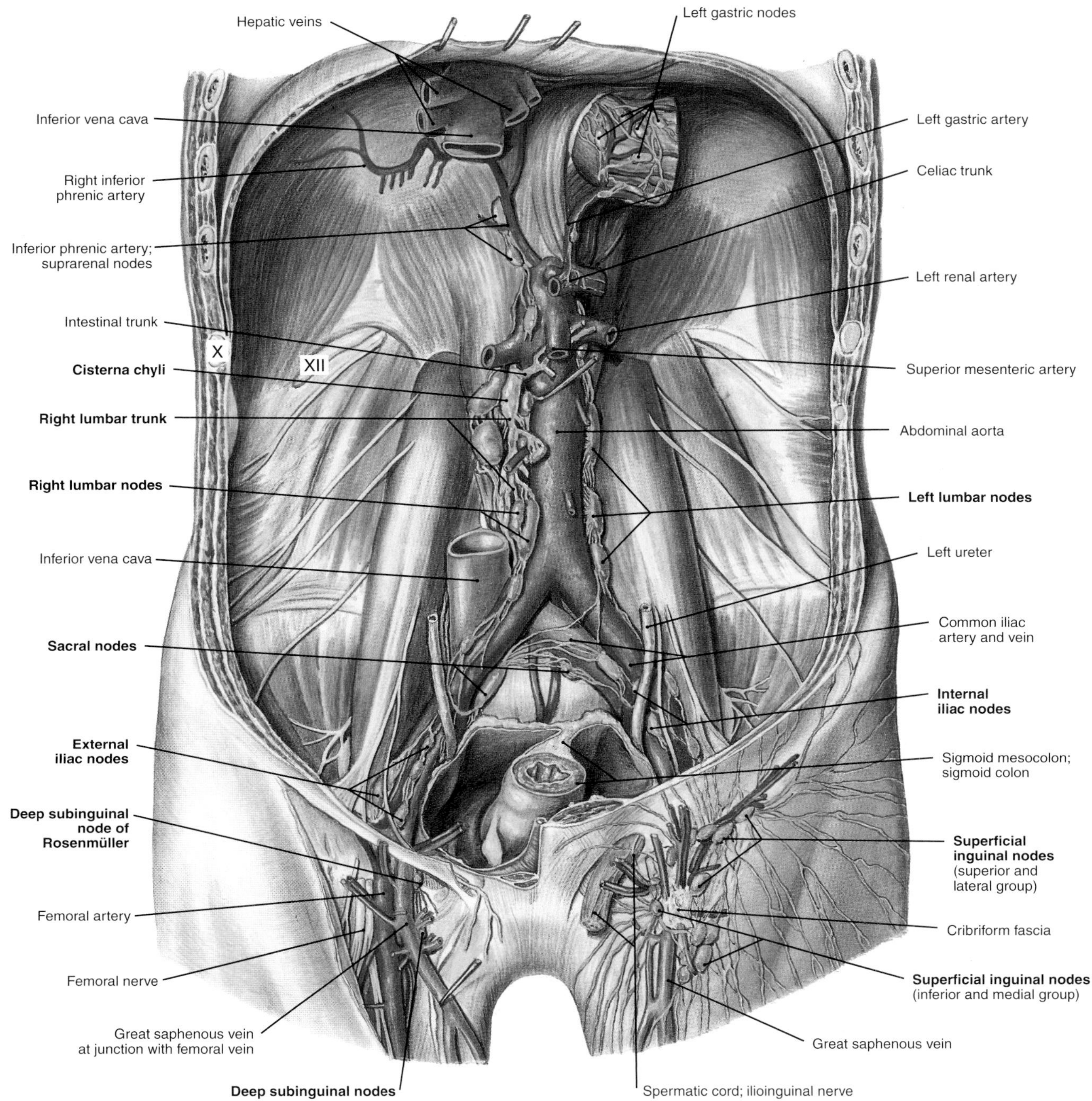

Hepatic veins
Left gastric nodes
Inferior vena cava
Left gastric artery
Right inferior phrenic artery
Celiac trunk
Inferior phrenic artery; suprarenal nodes
Left renal artery
Intestinal trunk
X
XII
Cisterna chyli
Superior mesenteric artery
Right lumbar trunk
Abdominal aorta
Right lumbar nodes
Left lumbar nodes
Inferior vena cava
Left ureter
Common iliac artery and vein
Sacral nodes
Internal iliac nodes
External iliac nodes
Sigmoid mesocolon; sigmoid colon
Deep subinguinal node of Rosenmüller
Superficial inguinal nodes (superior and lateral group)
Femoral artery
Cribriform fascia
Femoral nerve
Superficial inguinal nodes (inferior and medial group)
Great saphenous vein at junction with femoral vein
Great saphenous vein
Deep subinguinal nodes
Spermatic cord; ilioinguinal nerve

Figure 257 Inguinal, Pelvic, and Lumbar (Aortic) Lymph Nodes

NOTE: (1) Chains of lymph nodes and lymphatic vessels lie along the paths of major blood vessels from the inguinal region to the diaphragm. The **superficial inguinal nodes** lie just distal to the inguinal ligament within the superficial fascia.

(2) There are 10 to 20 superficial inguinal nodes, and they receive drainage from the genitalia, perineum, gluteal region, and anterior abdominal wall. More deeply, **subinguinal nodes** drain the lower extremity, one of which lies in the femoral ring (Rosenmüller's or Cloquet's node).

(3) Within the pelvis, visceral lymph nodes lie close to the organs that they drain and they channel lymph along the paths of major blood vessels, such as the **external, internal,** and **common iliac nodes** located along these vessels in the pelvis.

(4) On the posterior abdominal wall are located the **right** and **left lumbar** chains coursing along the abdominal aorta, while **preaortic nodes** are arranged around the roots of the major unpaired aortic branches, forming the **celiac** and **superior** and **inferior mesenteric nodes.**

(5) At the level of the L2 vertebra, there is a confluence of lymph channels that forms a dilated sac, the **cisterna chyli.** This is located somewhat posterior and to the right of the aorta, and it marks the commencement of the **thoracic duct.**

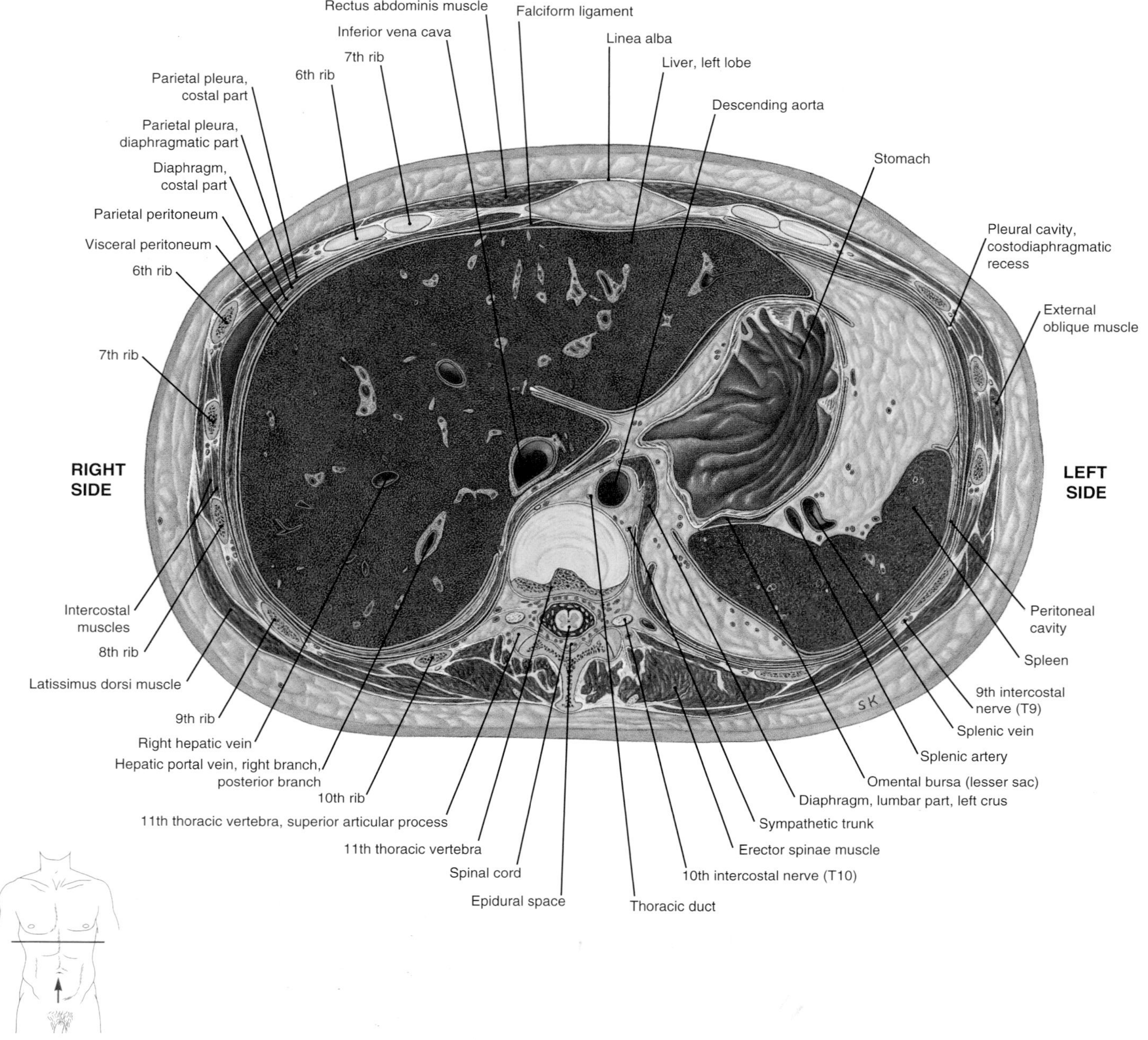
Rectus abdominis muscle
Falciform ligament
Inferior vena cava
Linea alba
7th rib
Liver, left lobe
Parietal pleura, costal part
6th rib
Descending aorta
Parietal pleura, diaphragmatic part
Stomach
Diaphragm, costal part
Parietal peritoneum
Pleural cavity, costodiaphragmatic recess
Visceral peritoneum
6th rib
External oblique muscle
7th rib
RIGHT SIDE
LEFT SIDE
Intercostal muscles
Peritoneal cavity
8th rib
Spleen
Latissimus dorsi muscle
9th intercostal nerve (T9)
9th rib
Splenic vein
Right hepatic vein
Splenic artery
Hepatic portal vein, right branch, posterior branch
Omental bursa (lesser sac)
10th rib
Diaphragm, lumbar part, left crus
11th thoracic vertebra, superior articular process
Sympathetic trunk
11th thoracic vertebra
Erector spinae muscle
Spinal cord
10th intercostal nerve (T10)
Epidural space
Thoracic duct

Figure 258 Transverse Section of the Abdomen at the Level of T11 (Caudal Aspect)

NOTE: (1) The aorta is seen to the left of the bodies of the thoracic vertebrae above the diaphragm. Observe the thoracic duct slightly to the right of the aorta.

(2) Below the diaphragm, the liver is mostly to the right and the spleen is to the left of the midline. Observe the location of the inferior vena cava posterior to the liver and to the right of the midline.

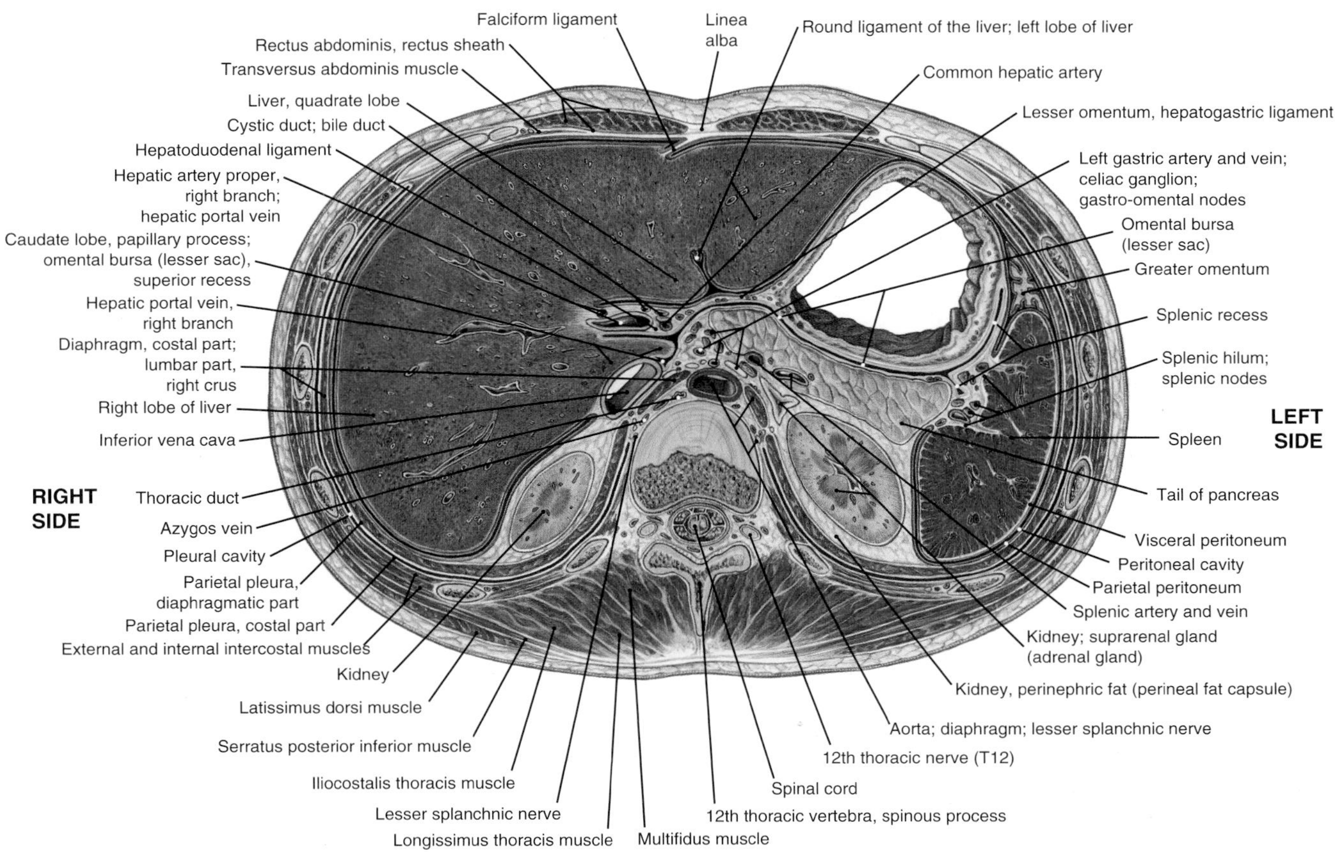

Falciform ligament
Linea alba
Round ligament of the liver; left lobe of liver
Rectus abdominis, rectus sheath
Transversus abdominis muscle
Common hepatic artery
Liver, quadrate lobe
Cystic duct; bile duct
Lesser omentum, hepatogastric ligament
Hepatoduodenal ligament
Hepatic artery proper, right branch; hepatic portal vein
Left gastric artery and vein; celiac ganglion; gastro-omental nodes
Caudate lobe, papillary process; omental bursa (lesser sac), superior recess
Omental bursa (lesser sac)
Greater omentum
Hepatic portal vein, right branch
Splenic recess
Diaphragm, costal part; lumbar part, right crus
Splenic hilum; splenic nodes
Right lobe of liver
Inferior vena cava
Spleen
LEFT SIDE
RIGHT SIDE
Thoracic duct
Tail of pancreas
Azygos vein
Visceral peritoneum
Pleural cavity
Peritoneal cavity
Parietal pleura, diaphragmatic part
Parietal peritoneum
Parietal pleura, costal part
Splenic artery and vein
External and internal intercostal muscles
Kidney; suprarenal gland (adrenal gland)
Kidney
Kidney, perinephric fat (perineal fat capsule)
Latissimus dorsi muscle
Aorta; diaphragm; lesser splanchnic nerve
Serratus posterior inferior muscle
12th thoracic nerve (T12)
Iliocostalis thoracis muscle
Spinal cord
Lesser splanchnic nerve
12th thoracic vertebra, spinous process
Longissimus thoracis muscle
Multifidus muscle

Figure 259.1 Transverse Section of the Abdomen between T12 and L1 (Caudal Aspect)

NOTE: (1) Both the parietal and the visceral layers of the peritoneum of the greater peritoneal sac (cavity) are shown in blue, while surrounding the lesser sac, the peritoneum is shown in blue-green.

(2) The kidneys, located anterior to the posterior abdominal wall, have been sectioned transversely. Observe also the perirenal fat surrounding them.

(3) The abdominal aorta is near or at the midline and the inferior vena cava to the right of the midline.

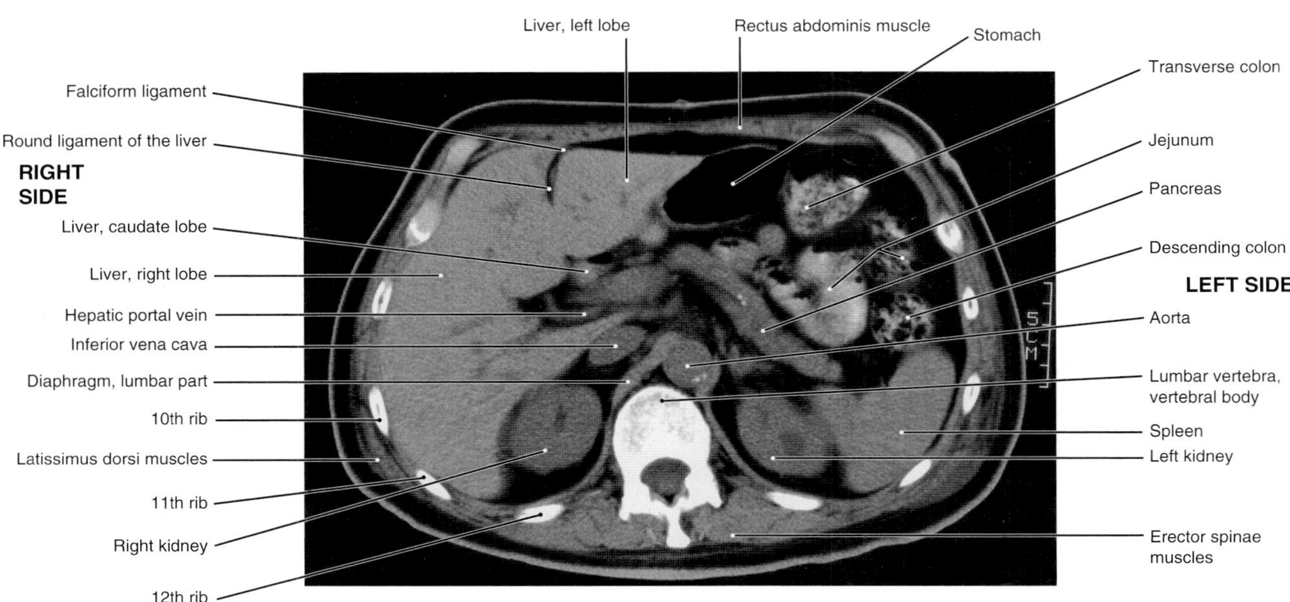

Liver, left lobe
Rectus abdominis muscle
Stomach
Transverse colon
Falciform ligament
Round ligament of the liver
Jejunum
RIGHT SIDE
Pancreas
Liver, caudate lobe
Descending colon
Liver, right lobe
LEFT SIDE
Hepatic portal vein
Aorta
Inferior vena cava
Diaphragm, lumbar part
Lumbar vertebra, vertebral body
10th rib
Spleen
Latissimus dorsi muscles
Left kidney
11th rib
Right kidney
Erector spinae muscles
12th rib
5 CM

Figure 259.2 Computed Tomographic Transverse Section of the Abdomen at L1 (Caudal Aspect)

Liver, left lobe
Stomach
Gallbladder
Hepatic portal vein
Splenic vein
9th rib
Round ligament of the liver
Transverse colon
8th rib
Rectus abdominis muscle
Parietal peritoneum
Superior mesenteric artery
Peritoneal cavity
Pancreas
Diaphragm, costal part
Costodiaphragmatic recess
Pancreatic node
Parietal pleura, diaphragmatic part
Jejunum
Parietal pleura, costal part
8th rib
9th rib
Liver, right lobe
Descending colon
10th rib
Renal artery
RIGHT SIDE
LEFT SIDE
11th rib
Latissimus dorsi muscle
Inferior vena cava
Renal pelvis
Diaphragm, lumbar part
12th rib
Renal medulla
Minor calyx
Sympathetic trunk
Kidney
Renal sinus
Erector spinae muscles
1st lumbar vertebra
Renal cortex
Cauda equina
Renal vein
Inferior mesenteric artery
Abdominal aorta

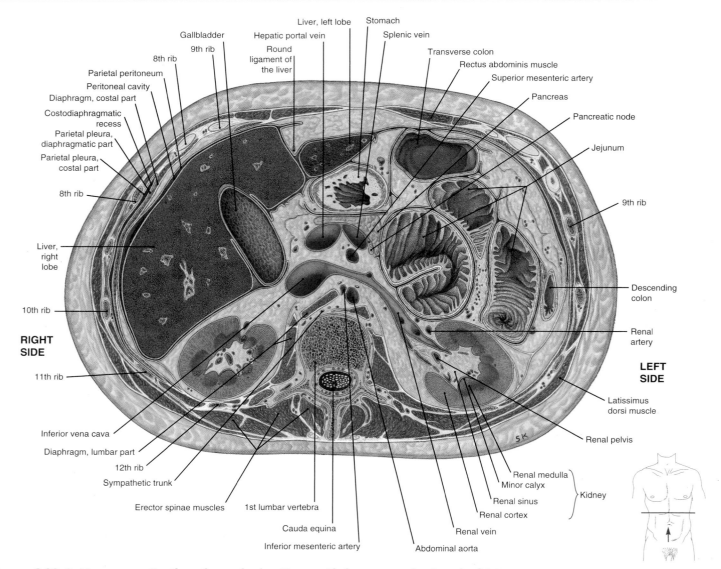

Figure 260.1 Transverse Section through the Upper Abdomen at the Level of L1

NOTE: (1) This section goes through the hilum of the left kidney and shows the left renal vein crossing the vertebral column to then enter the inferior vena cava.

(2) The loops of jejunum on the left and the pancreas forming a bed for the posterior aspect of the stomach.

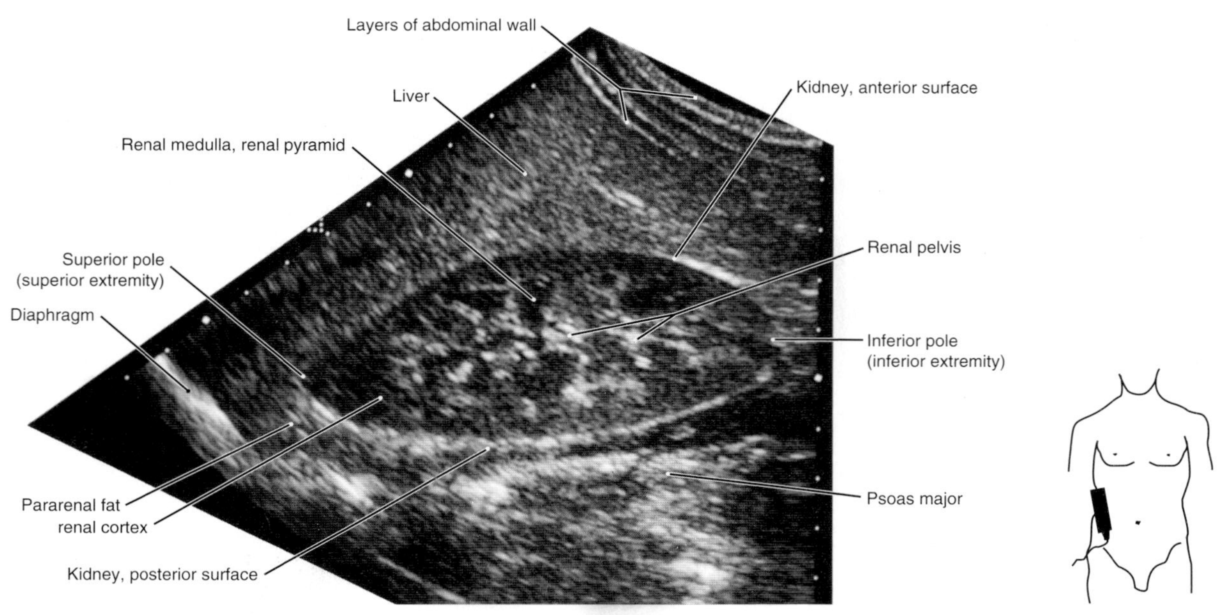
Layers of abdominal wall
Liver
Kidney, anterior surface
Renal medulla, renal pyramid
Renal pelvis
Superior pole
(superior extremity)
Diaphragm
Inferior pole
(inferior extremity)
Psoas major
Pararenal fat
renal cortex
Kidney, posterior surface

Figure 260.2 Ultrasound Scan of the Right Kidney

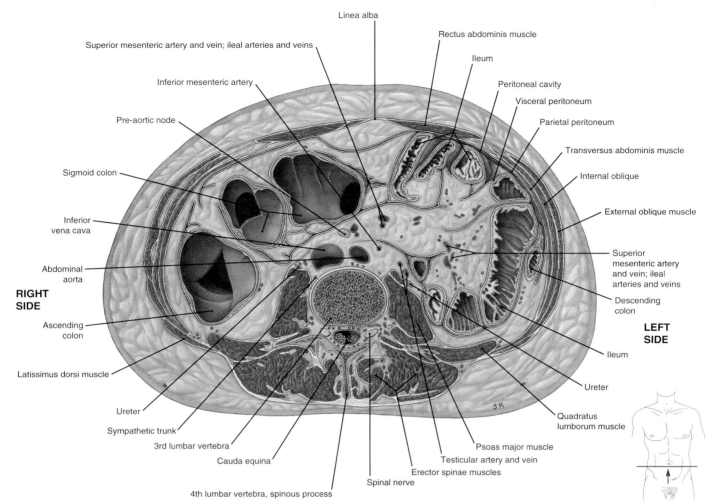

Linea alba
Rectus abdominis muscle
Superior mesenteric artery and vein; ileal arteries and veins
Ileum
Inferior mesenteric artery
Peritoneal cavity
Visceral peritoneum
Pre-aortic node
Parietal peritoneum
Transversus abdominis muscle
Sigmoid colon
Internal oblique
External oblique muscle
Inferior vena cava
Superior mesenteric artery and vein; ileal arteries and veins
Abdominal aorta
RIGHT SIDE
Descending colon
Ascending colon
LEFT SIDE
Ileum
Latissimus dorsi muscle
Ureter
Ureter
Quadratus lumborum muscle
Sympathetic trunk
3rd lumbar vertebra
Psoas major muscle
Cauda equina
Testicular artery and vein
Erector spinae muscles
Spinal nerve
4th lumbar vertebra, spinous process

Figure 261.1 Transverse Section of the Abdomen at the Level of L3 (Caudal Aspect)

NOTE: (1) This section is through the lower abdomen and visualized from the caudal aspect.

(2) A loop of sigmoid colon extends far superiorly in the abdomen, and two parts of it are sectioned in this specimen.

(3) The inferior vena cava to the right of the midline and the aorta directly anterior to the body of the L3 vertebra.

(4) The spinal cord at this level shows the cauda equina. These are the roots of the lower lumbar and sacral nerves.

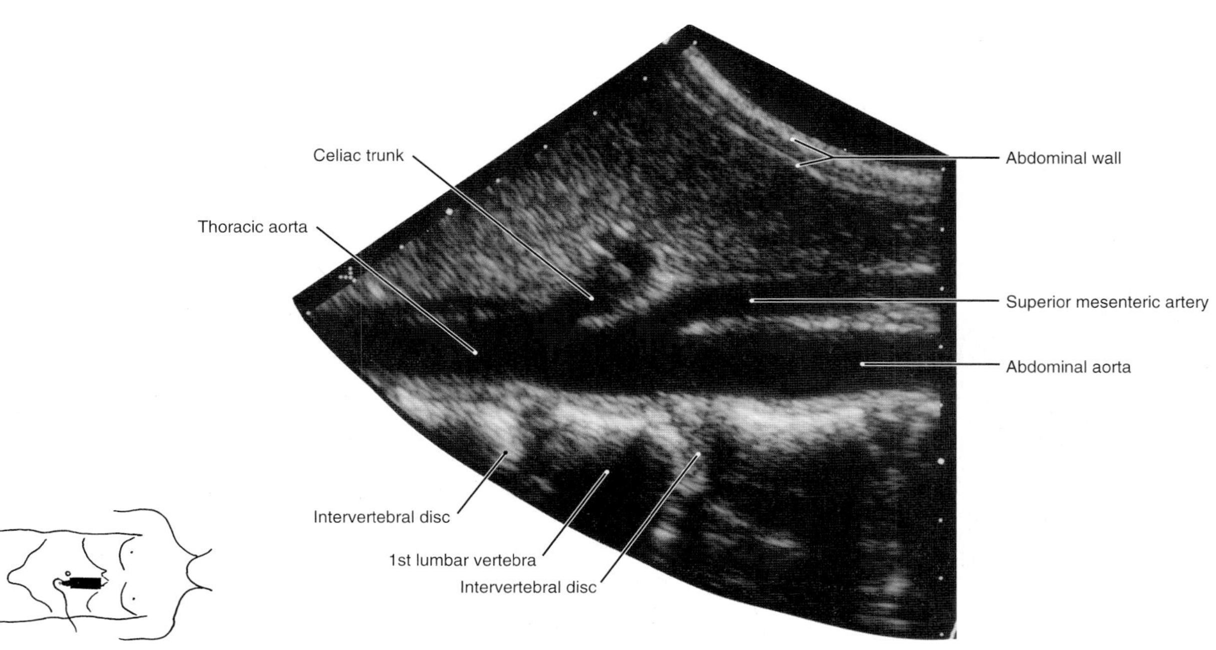
Celiac trunk
Abdominal wall
Thoracic aorta
Superior mesenteric artery
Abdominal aorta
Intervertebral disc
1st lumbar vertebra
Intervertebral disc

Figure 261.2 Ultrasound Scan of the Abdominal Aorta and Its Celiac Trunk and Superior Mesenteric Branches

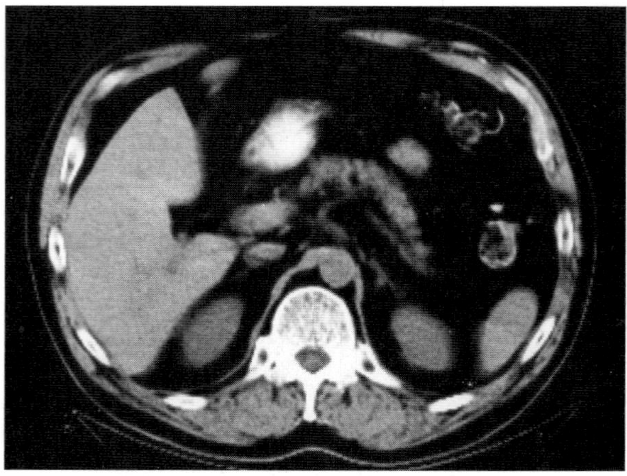

Figure 262.1A CT Scan, Abdomen (about L1)
CT scan of the upper abdominal organs at the level of the superior pole of the kidney.

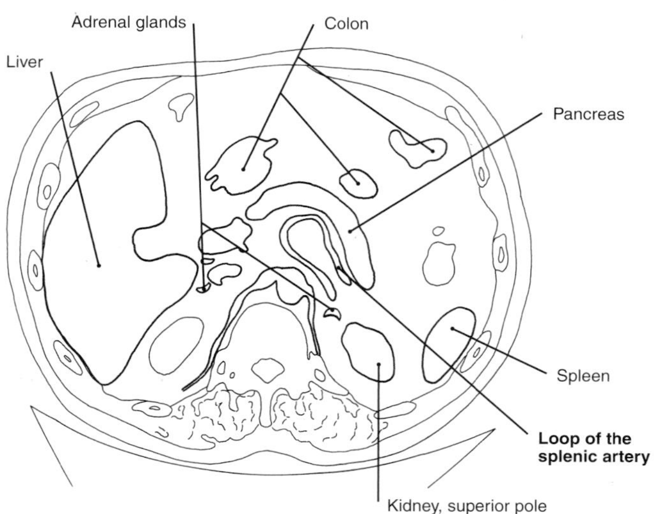
Adrenal glands
Colon
Liver
Pancreas
Spleen
Loop of the splenic artery
Kidney, superior pole

Figure 262.1B Outline Diagram for Figure 262.1A.

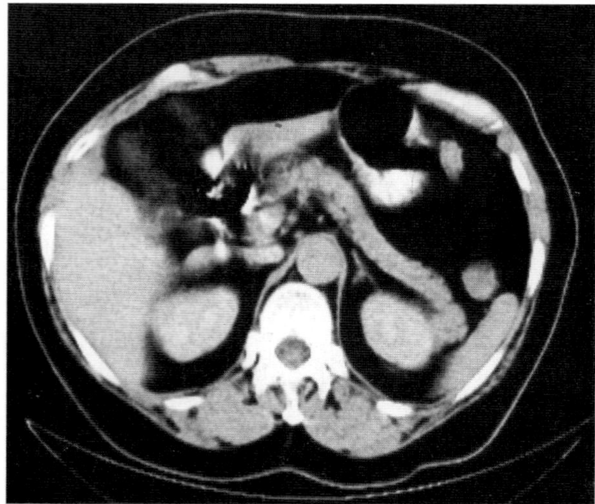

Figure 262.2A CT Scan, Abdomen (L1 to L2)
CT scan of the upper abdominal organs at the level of the body of the pancreas.

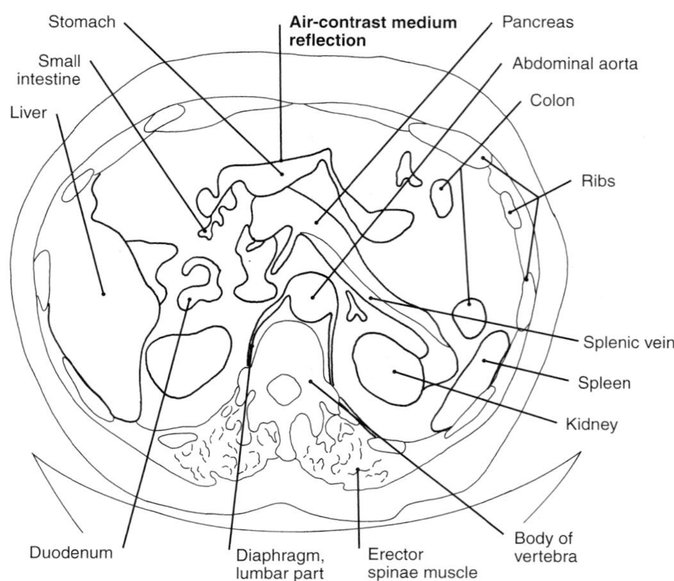
Stomach
Air-contrast medium reflection
Pancreas
Small intestine
Abdominal aorta
Liver
Colon
Ribs
Splenic vein
Spleen
Kidney
Body of vertebra
Duodenum
Diaphragm, lumbar part
Erector spinae muscle

Figure 262.2B Outline Diagram for Figure 262.2A.

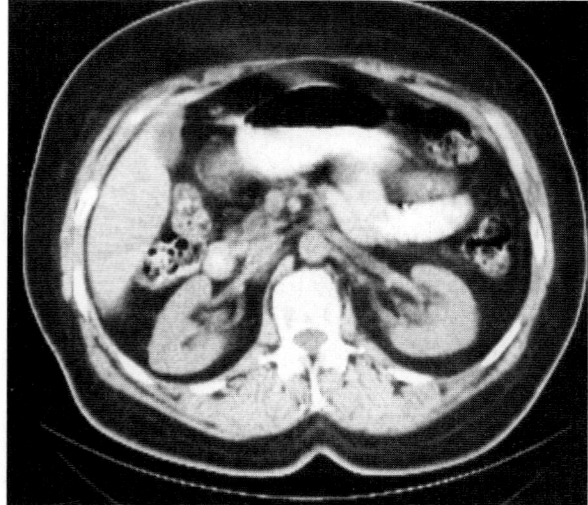

Figure 262.3A CT Scan, Abdomen (about L2)
CT scan of the upper abdominal organs at the level of the renal vessels.

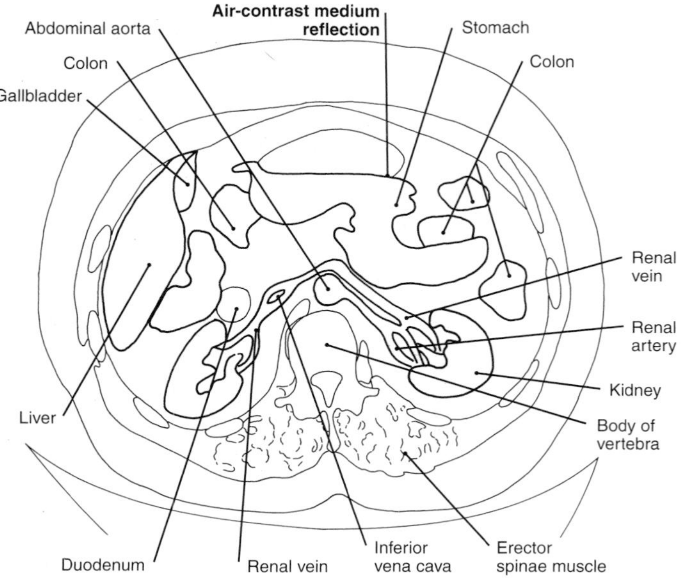
Abdominal aorta
Air-contrast medium reflection
Stomach
Colon
Colon
Gallbladder
Renal vein
Renal artery
Kidney
Body of vertebra
Liver
Duodenum
Renal vein
Inferior vena cava
Erector spinae muscle

Figure 262.3B Outline Diagram for Figure 262.3A.

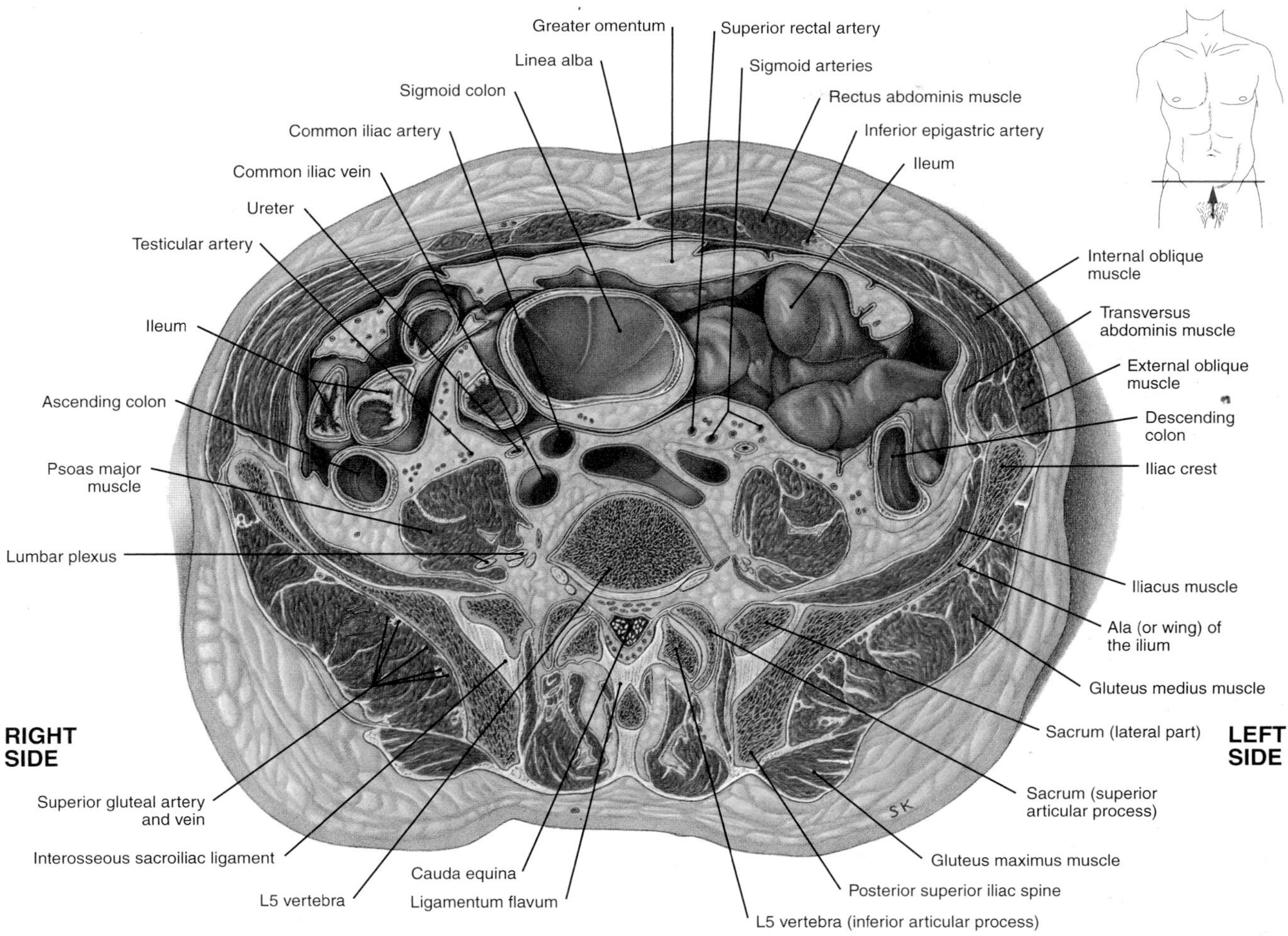
Greater omentum
Superior rectal artery
Linea alba
Sigmoid arteries
Sigmoid colon
Rectus abdominis muscle
Common iliac artery
Inferior epigastric artery
Common iliac vein
Ileum
Ureter
Testicular artery
Internal oblique muscle
Ileum
Transversus abdominis muscle
External oblique muscle
Ascending colon
Descending colon
Psoas major muscle
Iliac crest
Lumbar plexus
Iliacus muscle
Ala (or wing) of the ilium
Gluteus medius muscle
RIGHT SIDE
Sacrum (lateral part)
LEFT SIDE
Superior gluteal artery and vein
Sacrum (superior articular process)
Interosseous sacroiliac ligament
Gluteus maximus muscle
Cauda equina
Posterior superior iliac spine
L5 vertebra
Ligamentum flavum
L5 vertebra (inferior articular process)

Figure 263.1 Transverse Section through the Abdomen at the Fifth Lumbar Level (Sacroiliac Joint)

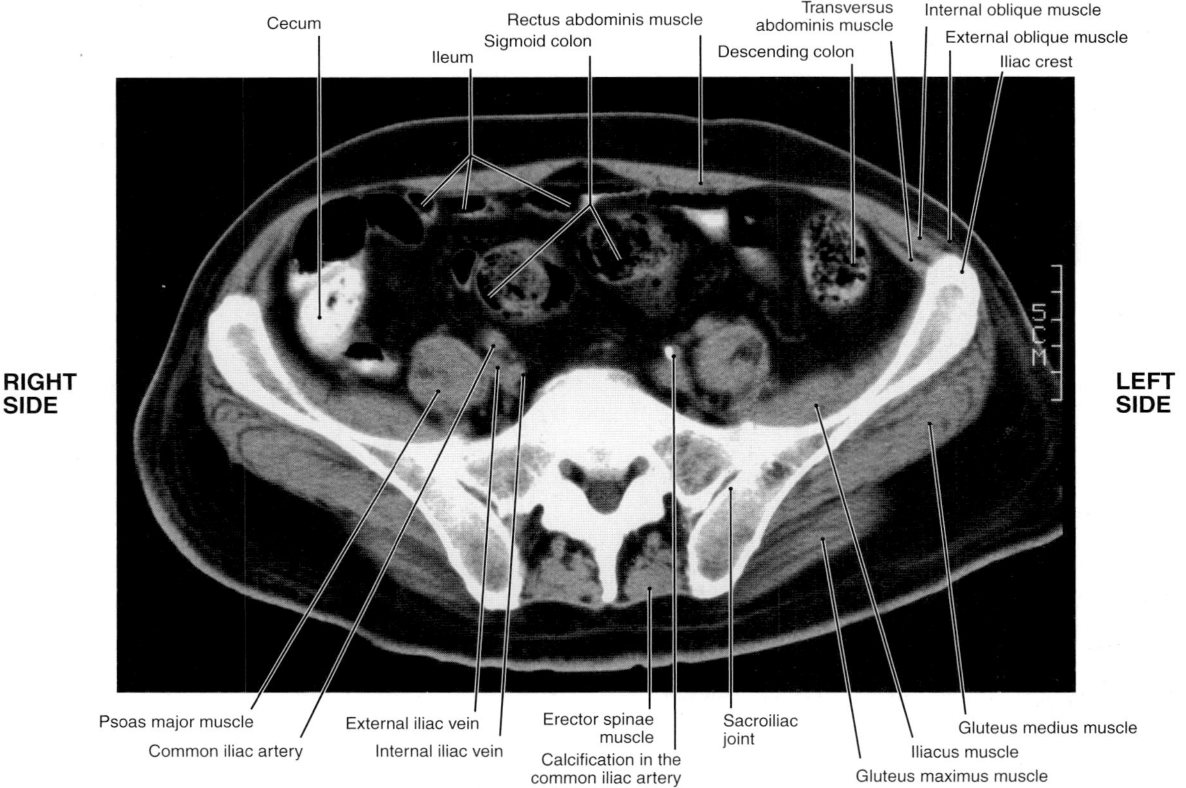
Cecum
Rectus abdominis muscle
Transversus abdominis muscle
Internal oblique muscle
Sigmoid colon
External oblique muscle
Ileum
Descending colon
Iliac crest
5 CM
RIGHT SIDE
LEFT SIDE
Psoas major muscle
External iliac vein
Erector spinae muscle
Sacroiliac joint
Gluteus medius muscle
Common iliac artery
Internal iliac vein
Calcification in the common iliac artery
Iliacus muscle
Gluteus maximus muscle

Figure 263.2 Computerized Tomographic (CT) Scan at the Fifth Lumbar Level (Sacroiliac Joint)

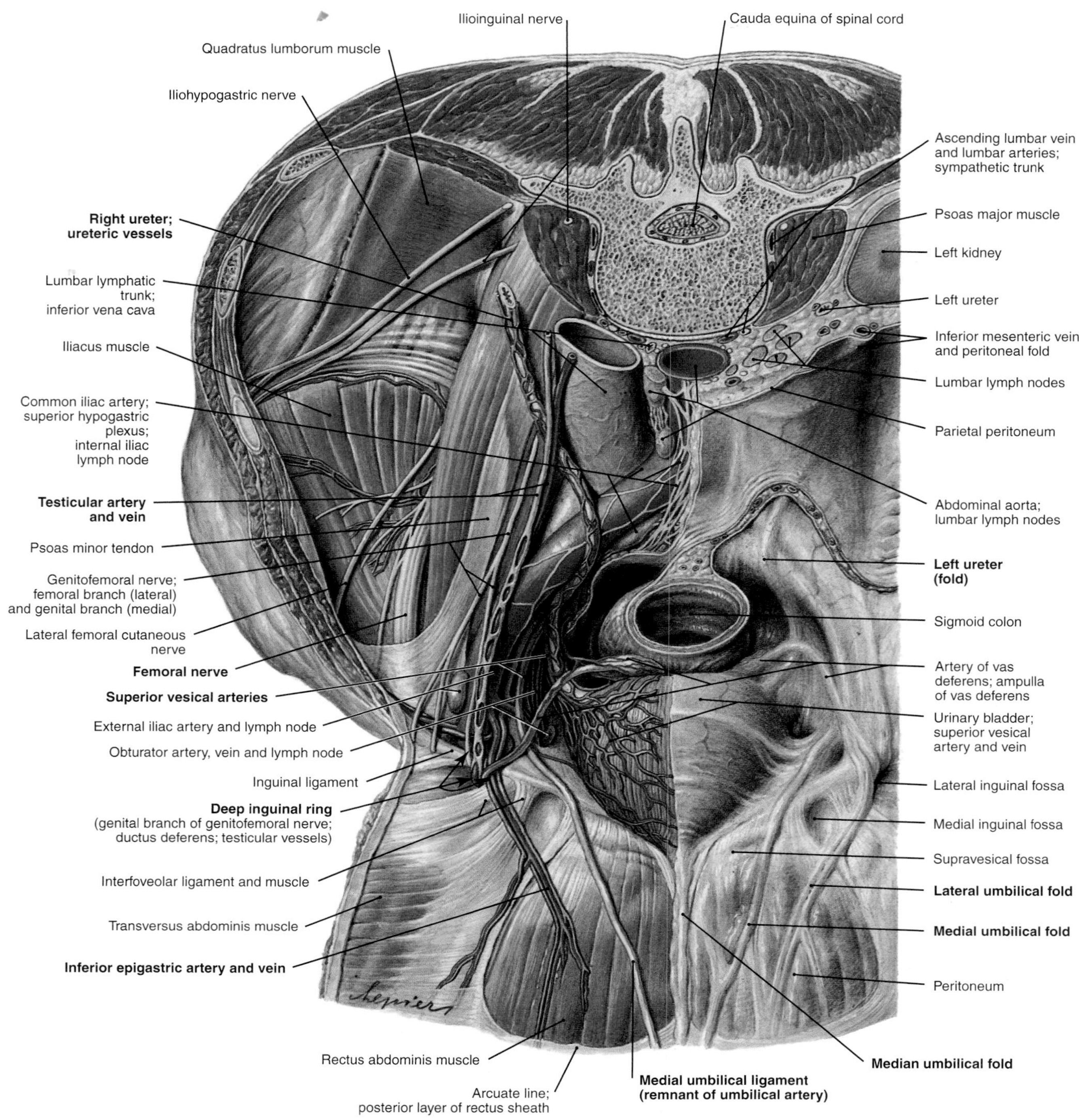
Ilioinguinal nerve
Cauda equina of spinal cord
Quadratus lumborum muscle
Iliohypogastric nerve
Ascending lumbar vein and lumbar arteries; sympathetic trunk
Right ureter; ureteric vessels
Psoas major muscle
Left kidney
Lumbar lymphatic trunk; inferior vena cava
Left ureter
Iliacus muscle
Inferior mesenteric vein and peritoneal fold
Lumbar lymph nodes
Common iliac artery; superior hypogastric plexus; internal iliac lymph node
Parietal peritoneum
Testicular artery and vein
Abdominal aorta; lumbar lymph nodes
Psoas minor tendon
Left ureter (fold)
Genitofemoral nerve; femoral branch (lateral) and genital branch (medial)
Sigmoid colon
Lateral femoral cutaneous nerve
Femoral nerve
Artery of vas deferens; ampulla of vas deferens
Superior vesical arteries
External iliac artery and lymph node
Urinary bladder; superior vesical artery and vein
Obturator artery, vein and lymph node
Inguinal ligament
Lateral inguinal fossa
Deep inguinal ring (genital branch of genitofemoral nerve; ductus deferens; testicular vessels)
Medial inguinal fossa
Supravesical fossa
Interfoveolar ligament and muscle
Lateral umbilical fold
Transversus abdominis muscle
Medial umbilical fold
Inferior epigastric artery and vein
Peritoneum
Rectus abdominis muscle
Median umbilical fold
Medial umbilical ligament (remnant of umbilical artery)
Arcuate line; posterior layer of rectus sheath

Figure 264 Vessels and Nerves of the Inferior Abdomen and Pelvis

NOTE: (1) The entire anterior abdominal wall has been opened and reflected downward, thereby exposing its inner (posterior) surface. The body has been transected through the lumbar region just below the third lumbar vertebra, and the peritoneum has been stripped away on the right side but left intact on the left.

(2) This dissection shows the intact male pelvic viscera viewed from above. Observe the course of the **ureters** as they cross the pelvic brim anterior to the **common iliac arteries.** The ureter surrounded by blood vessels is seen to course medially toward the bladder, whereas the **ductus deferens** (on its path to the seminal vesicle) courses ventral to the ureter.

(3) The convergence of the **testicular vessels, ductus deferens,** and **genital branch** of the **genitofemoral nerve** at the abdominal inguinal ring to help form the **spermatic cord.**

(4) The origins within the pelvis of the umbilical ligaments and folds:

(a) The **median umbilical fold** extending from the bladder to the umbilicus (**urachus**).

(b) The **medial umbilical fold** formed by a peritoneal reflection over the obliterated umbilical artery.

(c) The **lateral umbilical fold** formed by peritoneum covering the inferior epigastric vessels.

THE PELVIS AND PERINEUM

4

PLATES

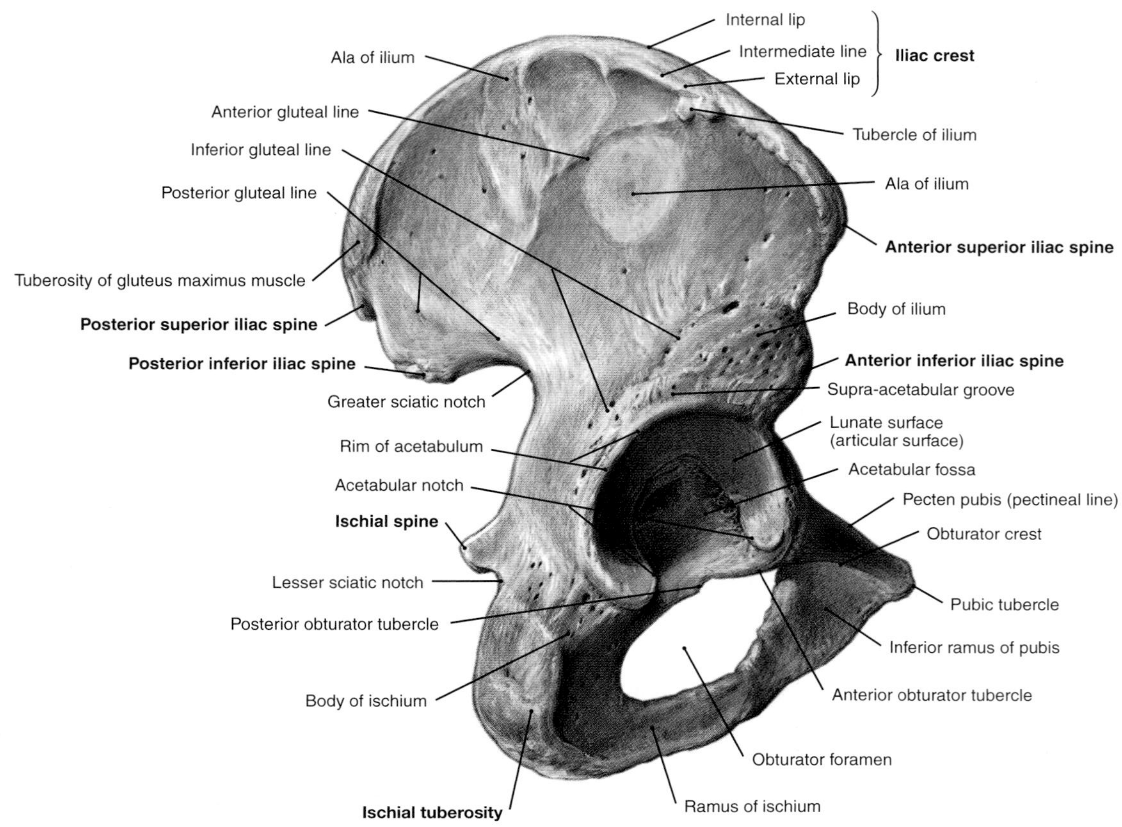
Internal lip
Intermediate line
External lip
Iliac crest
Ala of ilium
Anterior gluteal line
Inferior gluteal line
Posterior gluteal line
Tubercle of ilium
Ala of ilium
Anterior superior iliac spine
Tuberosity of gluteus maximus muscle
Posterior superior iliac spine
Posterior inferior iliac spine
Body of ilium
Anterior inferior iliac spine
Supra-acetabular groove
Greater sciatic notch
Rim of acetabulum
Lunate surface
(articular surface)
Acetabular notch
Acetabular fossa
Pecten pubis (pectineal line)
Ischial spine
Obturator crest
Lesser sciatic notch
Pubic tubercle
Posterior obturator tubercle
Inferior ramus of pubis
Body of ischium
Anterior obturator tubercle
Obturator foramen
Ischial tuberosity
Ramus of ischium

Figure 265.1 Lateral View of the Adult Right Hip Bone

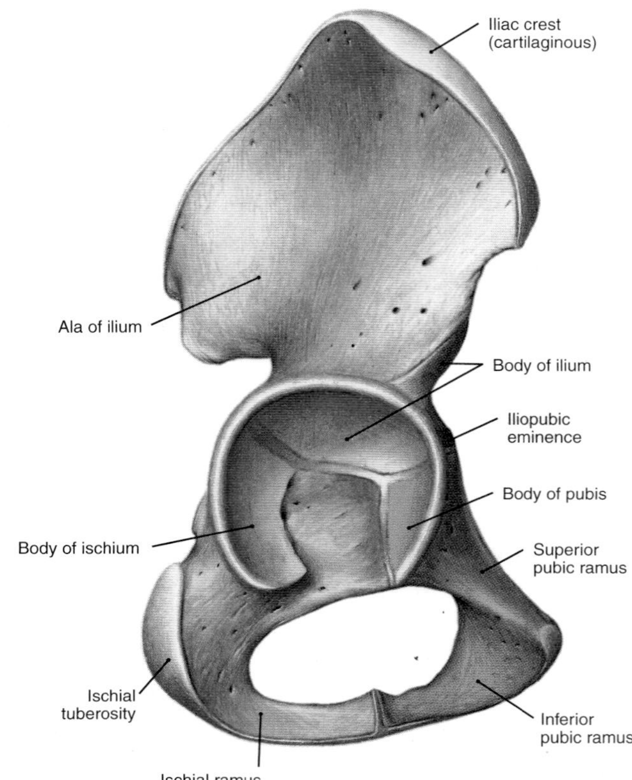
Iliac crest
(cartilaginous)
Ala of ilium
Body of ilium
Iliopubic
eminence
Body of pubis
Body of ischium
Superior
pubic ramus
Ischial
tuberosity
Inferior
pubic ramus
Ischial ramus

Figure 265.2: Hip Bone of 5-Year-Old Child (Lateral View)

NOTE: The hipbone is formed by a fusion of the **ilium** (yellow), **ischium** (green), and **pubis** (orange). Although ossification of the inferior pubic ramus occurs during the 7th or 8th year, complete fusion of the three bones at the **acetabulum** occurs sometime between the 15th and 20th years.

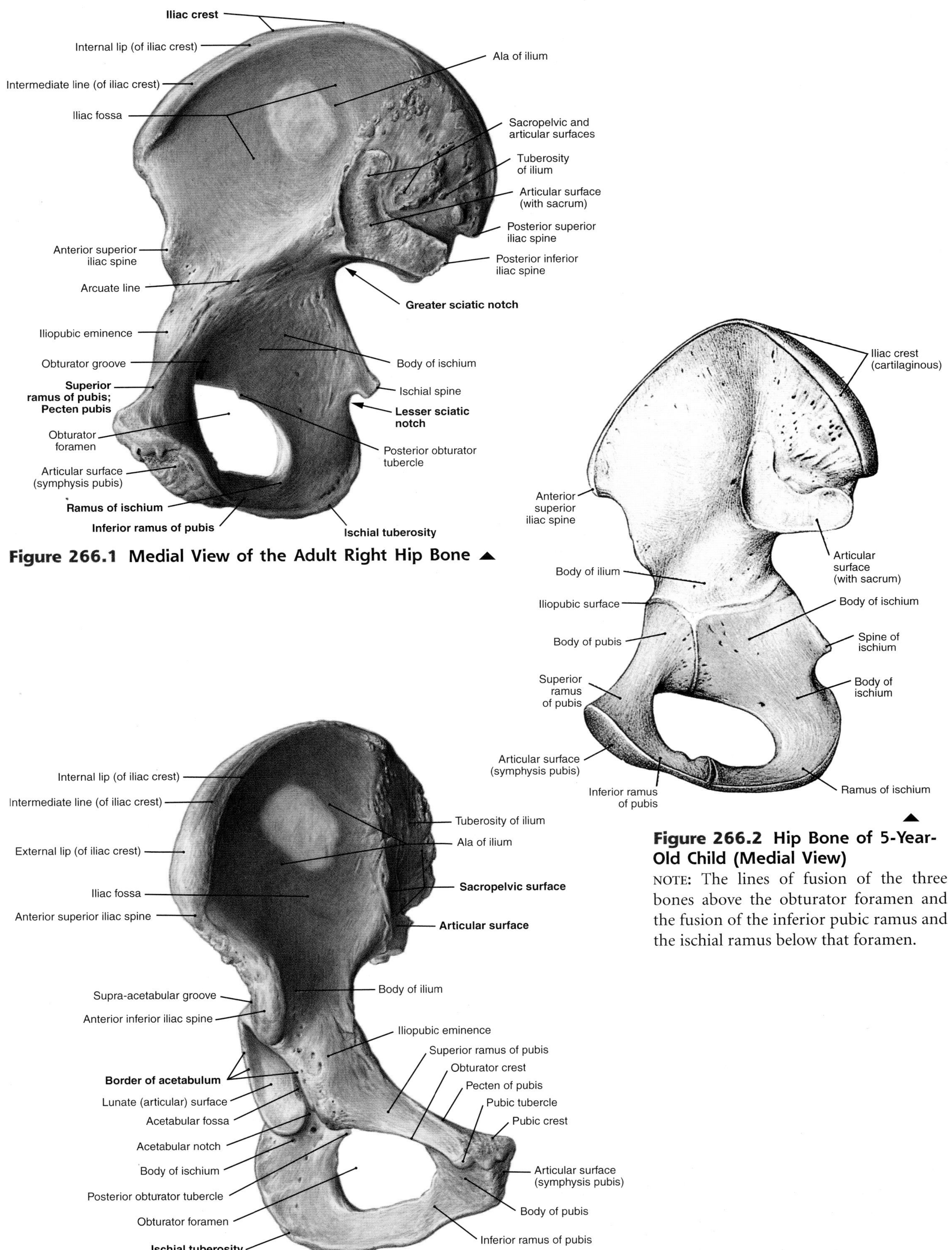
Iliac crest
Internal lip (of iliac crest)
Ala of ilium
Intermediate line (of iliac crest)
Iliac fossa
Sacropelvic and articular surfaces
Tuberosity of ilium
Articular surface (with sacrum)
Posterior superior iliac spine
Anterior superior iliac spine
Posterior inferior iliac spine
Arcuate line
Greater sciatic notch
Iliopubic eminence
Body of ischium
Obturator groove
Superior ramus of pubis; Pecten pubis
Ischial spine
Lesser sciatic notch
Obturator foramen
Posterior obturator tubercle
Articular surface (symphysis pubis)
Ramus of ischium
Inferior ramus of pubis
Ischial tuberosity

Figure 266.1 Medial View of the Adult Right Hip Bone ▲

Iliac crest (cartilaginous)
Anterior superior iliac spine
Articular surface (with sacrum)
Body of ilium
Iliopubic surface
Body of ischium
Body of pubis
Spine of ischium
Superior ramus of pubis
Body of ischium
Articular surface (symphysis pubis)
Inferior ramus of pubis
Ramus of ischium

Figure 266.2 Hip Bone of 5-Year-Old Child (Medial View) ▲

NOTE: The lines of fusion of the three bones above the obturator foramen and the fusion of the inferior pubic ramus and the ischial ramus below that foramen.

Internal lip (of iliac crest)
Intermediate line (of iliac crest)
Tuberosity of ilium
Ala of ilium
External lip (of iliac crest)
Sacropelvic surface
Iliac fossa
Anterior superior iliac spine
Articular surface
Supra-acetabular groove
Body of ilium
Anterior inferior iliac spine
Iliopubic eminence
Superior ramus of pubis
Obturator crest
Border of acetabulum
Pecten of pubis
Lunate (articular) surface
Pubic tubercle
Acetabular fossa
Pubic crest
Acetabular notch
Body of ischium
Articular surface (symphysis pubis)
Posterior obturator tubercle
Body of pubis
Obturator foramen
Inferior ramus of pubis
Ischial tuberosity

Figure 266.3 Anterior View of the Adult Right Hip Bone

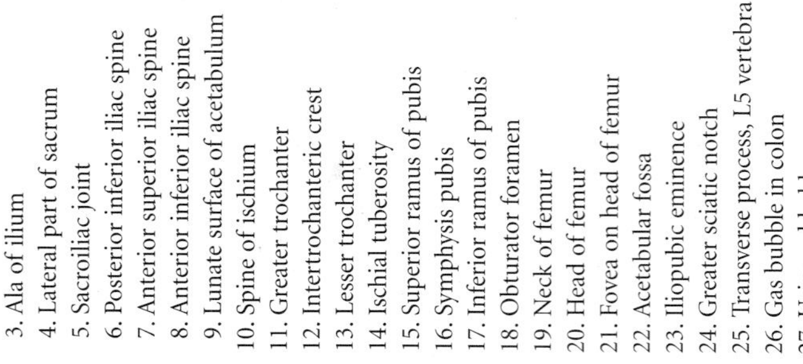

1. Iliac crest
2. Gas bubble in colon
3. Ala of ilium
4. Lateral part of sacrum
5. Sacroiliac joint
6. Posterior inferior iliac spine
7. Anterior superior iliac spine
8. Anterior inferior iliac spine
9. Lunate surface of acetabulum
10. Spine of ischium
11. Greater trochanter
12. Intertrochanteric crest
13. Lesser trochanter
14. Ischial tuberosity
15. Superior ramus of pubis
16. Symphysis pubis
17. Inferior ramus of pubis
18. Obturator foramen
19. Neck of femur
20. Head of femur
21. Fovea on head of femur
22. Acetabular fossa
23. Iliopubic eminence
24. Greater sciatic notch
25. Transverse process, L5 vertebra
26. Gas bubble in colon
27. Urinary bladder

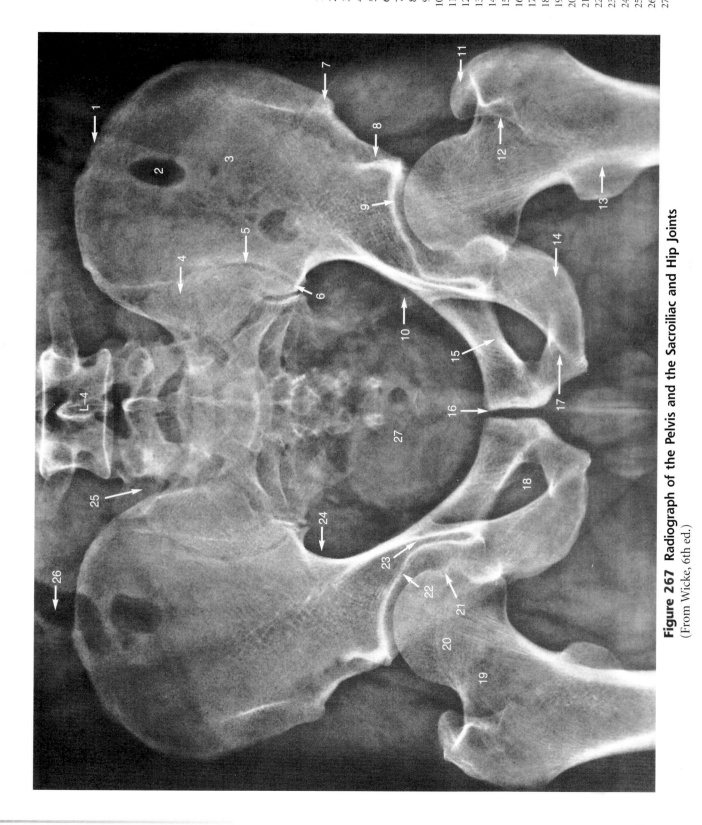

Figure 267 Radiograph of the Pelvis and the Sacroiliac and Hip Joints
(From Wicke, 6th ed.)

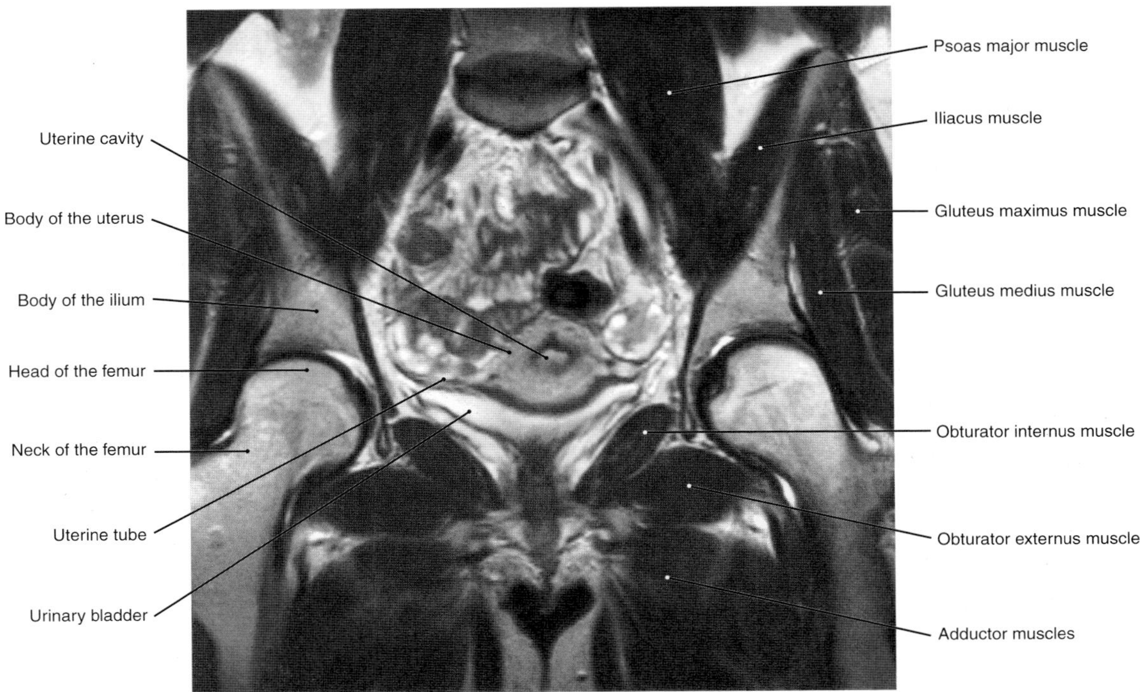
Psoas major muscle
Iliacus muscle
Uterine cavity
Body of the uterus
Gluteus maximus muscle
Body of the ilium
Gluteus medius muscle
Head of the femur
Obturator internus muscle
Neck of the femur
Uterine tube
Obturator externus muscle
Urinary bladder
Adductor muscles

Figure 268.1 Frontal Section; Magnetic Resonance Tomograph of Female Pelvis (Anterior View)

NOTE: (1) This magnetic resonance tomograph is in the frontal plane and goes through both hip joints.

(2) The flattened bladder and the anteverted uterus that angles forward over the superior surface of the bladder. Observe also the body of the uterus, the uterine cavity, and the uterine tube.

(3) The neck and head of the femur projecting into the acetabular fossa.

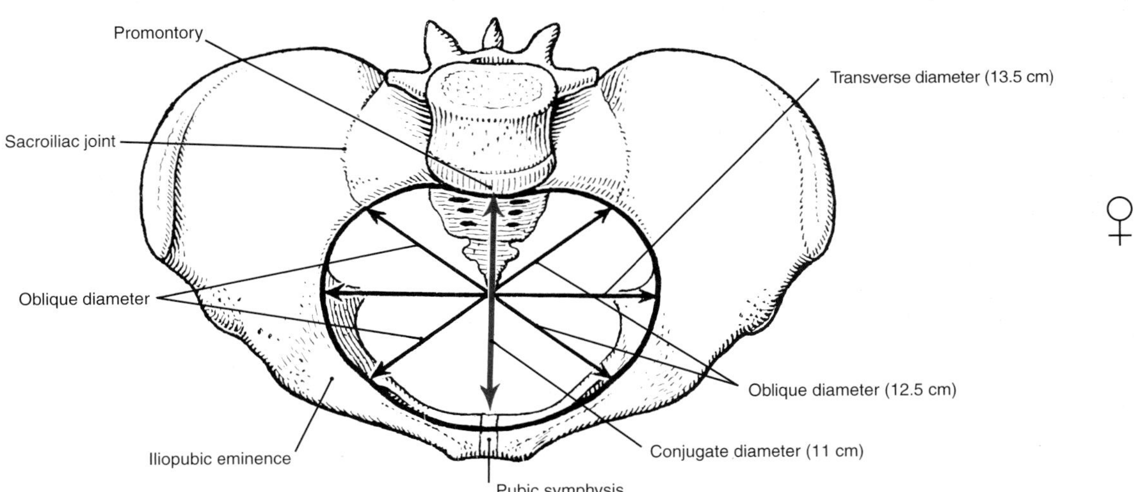
Promontory
Transverse diameter (13.5 cm)
Sacroiliac joint
Oblique diameter
Oblique diameter (12.5 cm)
Iliopubic eminence
Conjugate diameter (11 cm)
Pubic symphysis

♀

Figure 268.2 Diagram of Female Pelvis Showing Conjugate, Transverse, and Oblique Diameters

NOTE the following differences between the female and male pelvis:

(1) The **cavity of the true pelvis** in women is more shallow and wider than that in men.

(2) The **superior aperture** is oval or rounded in females, but heart-shaped in males.

(3) The **inferior aperture** is comparatively larger in females, and the female coccyx is more movable than in males. (Continued in Fig. 269.2 notes.)

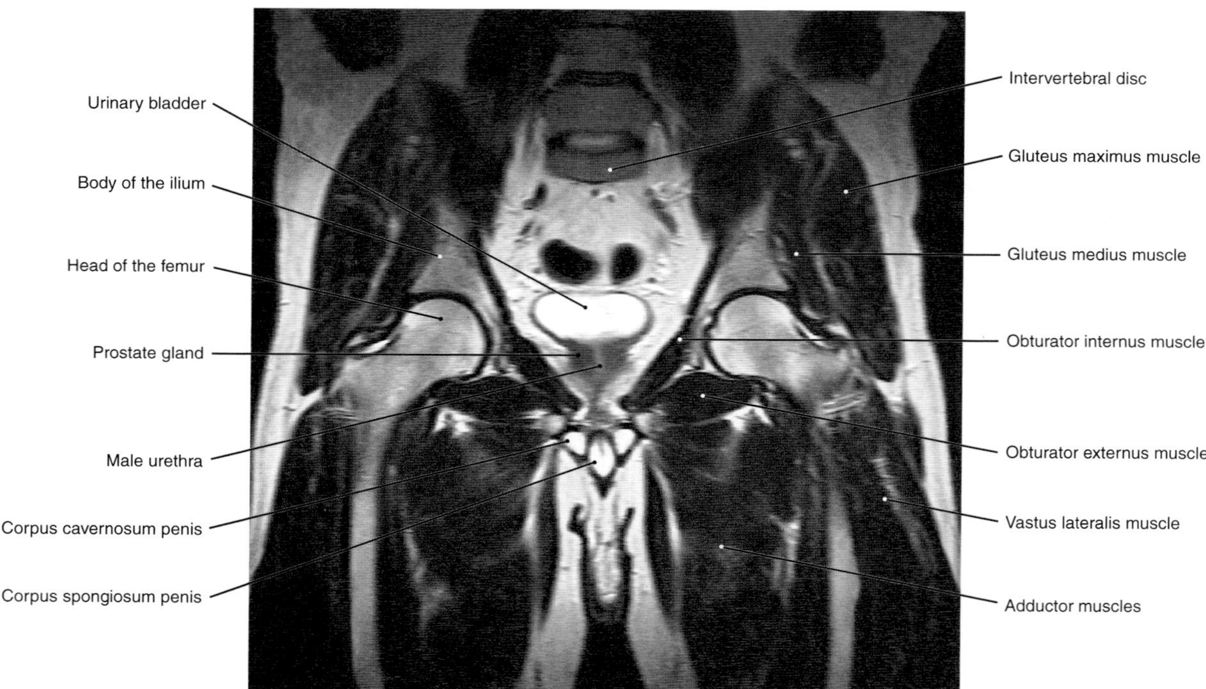
Urinary bladder
Body of the ilium
Head of the femur
Prostate gland
Male urethra
Corpus cavernosum penis
Corpus spongiosum penis
Intervertebral disc
Gluteus maximus muscle
Gluteus medius muscle
Obturator internus muscle
Obturator externus muscle
Vastus lateralis muscle
Adductor muscles

Figure 269.1 Frontal Section; Magnetic Resonance Tomograph of Male Pelvis (Anterior View)
NOTE: (1) This magnetic resonance tomograph is in the frontal plane and passes through both hip joints.

(2) The male bladder and urethra. Also note the corpus cavernosa penis on the two sides and the corpus spongiosum penis between them.

♂

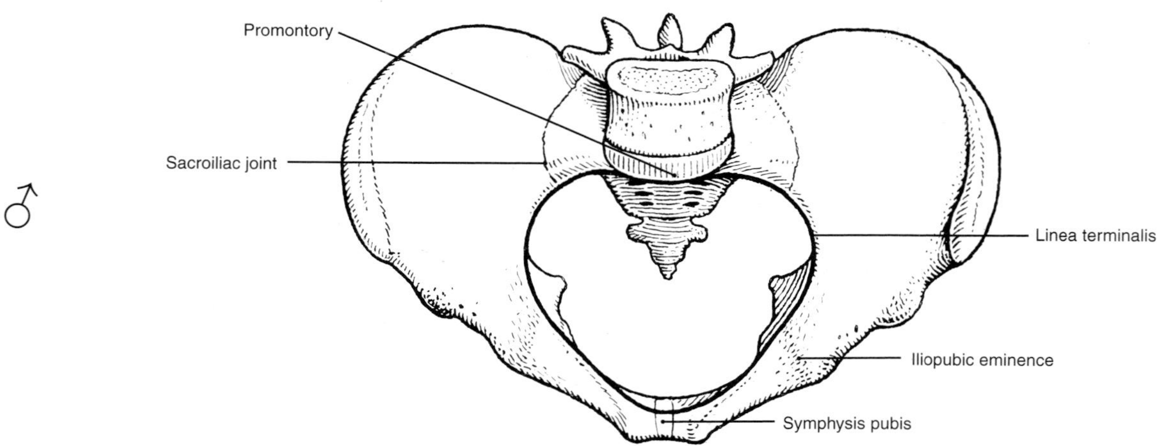
Promontory
Sacroiliac joint
Linea terminalis
Iliopubic eminence
Symphysis pubis

Figure 269.2 Diagram of the Male Pelvis
Differences between the female and male pelvis (continued):

(4) The **pubic arch** (**subpubic angle**) is greater in females and, therefore, the **ischial tuberosities** are farther apart than in males.
(5) The **obturator foramen** is usually oval in shape in women but more rounded in men.
(6) The female **pelvic bones** are more delicate and lighter than the male pelvic bones.
(7) The **sacrum** is shorter and wider in females, and it is usually less curved than in males.
(8) The **ischial spines** project less in females, and the **sciatic notches** are usually wider and more shallow than in males.

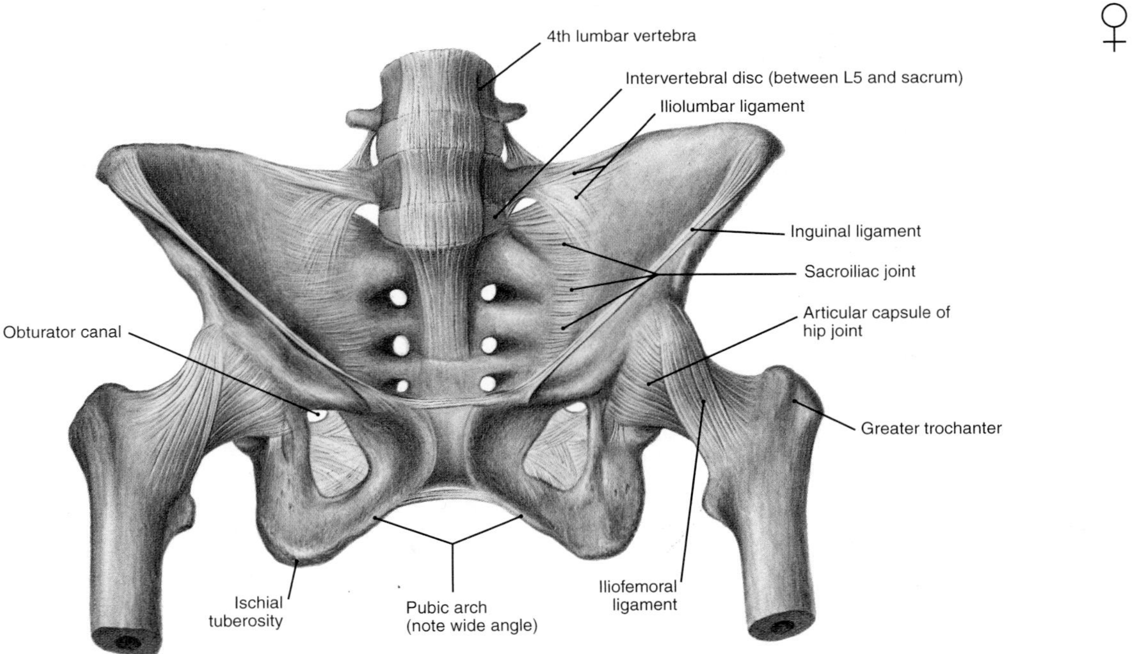

♀
4th lumbar vertebra
Intervertebral disc (between L5 and sacrum)
Iliolumbar ligament
Inguinal ligament
Sacroiliac joint
Articular capsule of hip joint
Obturator canal
Greater trochanter
Ischial tuberosity
Pubic arch (note wide angle)
Iliofemoral ligament

Figure 270.1 Female Pelvis and Ligaments: Articulations of the Pelvic Girdle and Hip Joints (Anteroinferior View)

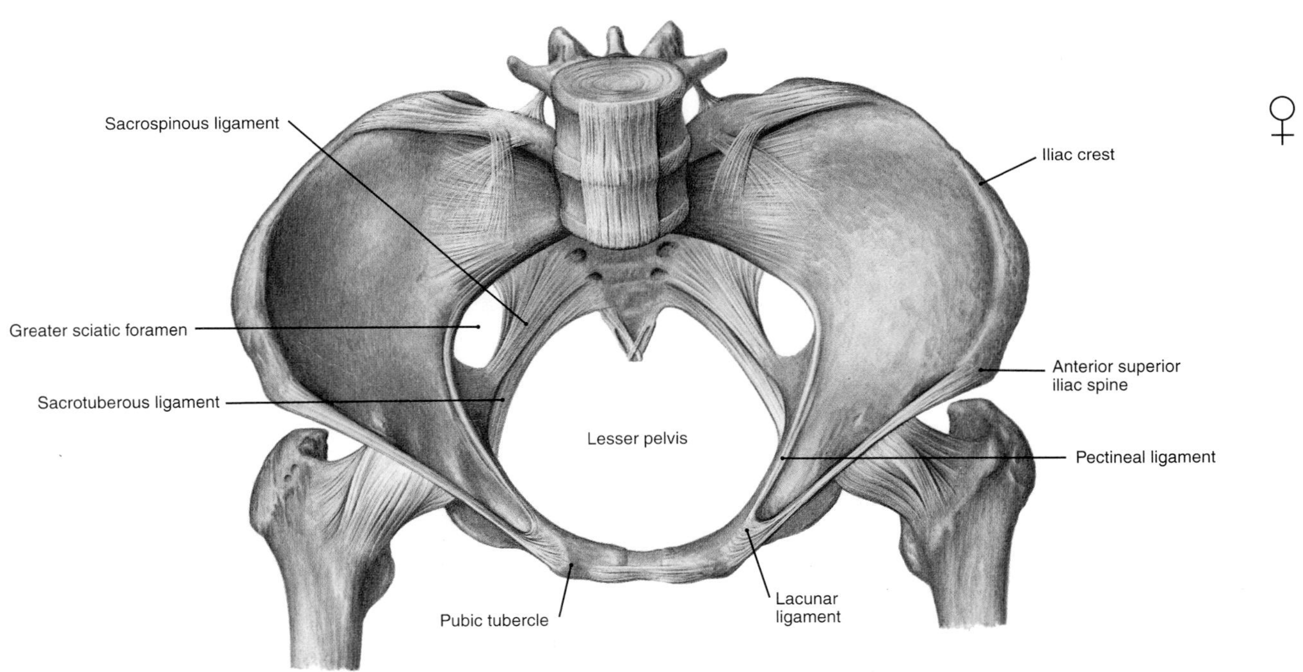

♀
Sacrospinous ligament
Iliac crest
Greater sciatic foramen
Anterior superior iliac spine
Sacrotuberous ligament
Lesser pelvis
Pectineal ligament
Pubic tubercle
Lacunar ligament

Figure 270.2 Female Pelvis and Ligaments Viewed from Above

NOTE: (1) The forward inclination of the pelvis shown here corresponds to the position of the pelvis while the person is standing upright.

(2) In addition to having wider diameters both at the pelvic inlet and outlet, the female lesser pelvis is more circular in shape than that in the male (compare with Fig. 271.2).

(3) The larger capacity of the lesser or true pelvis in the female, and the fact that the female hormones of pregnancy tend to relax the pelvic ligaments, serve to facilitate the function of child-bearing.

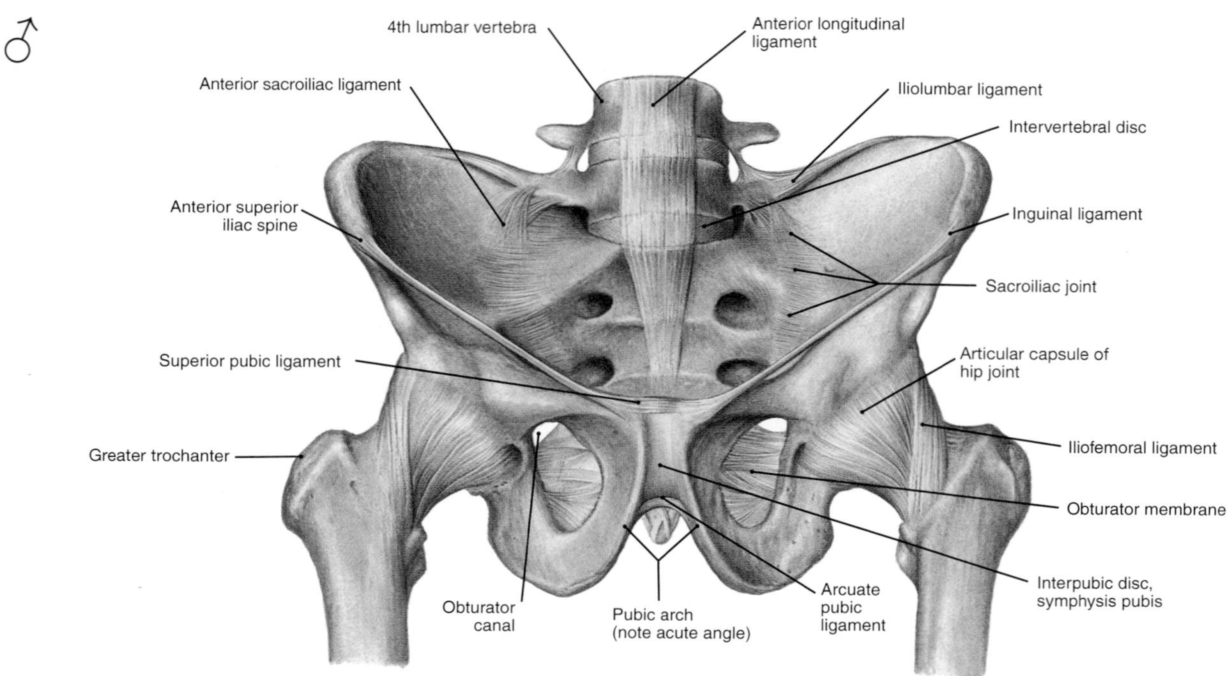
4th lumbar vertebra
Anterior longitudinal ligament
Anterior sacroiliac ligament
Iliolumbar ligament
Intervertebral disc
Anterior superior iliac spine
Inguinal ligament
Sacroiliac joint
Superior pubic ligament
Articular capsule of hip joint
Greater trochanter
Iliofemoral ligament
Obturator membrane
Interpubic disc, symphysis pubis
Obturator canal
Pubic arch (note acute angle)
Arcuate pubic ligament

Figure 271.1 Male Pelvis and Associated Ligaments (Anterior Aspect)

NOTE: (1) The pelvis is formed by the articulations of the left and right hip bones anteriorly at the **symphysis pubis** and posteriorly with the sacrum, coccyx, and fifth lumbar vertebra of the vertebral column.

(2) The articulations inferiorly of the pelvis with the two femora allow the weight of the head, trunk, and upper extremities to be transmitted to the lower limbs, thereby maintaining the upright posture characteristic of the human.

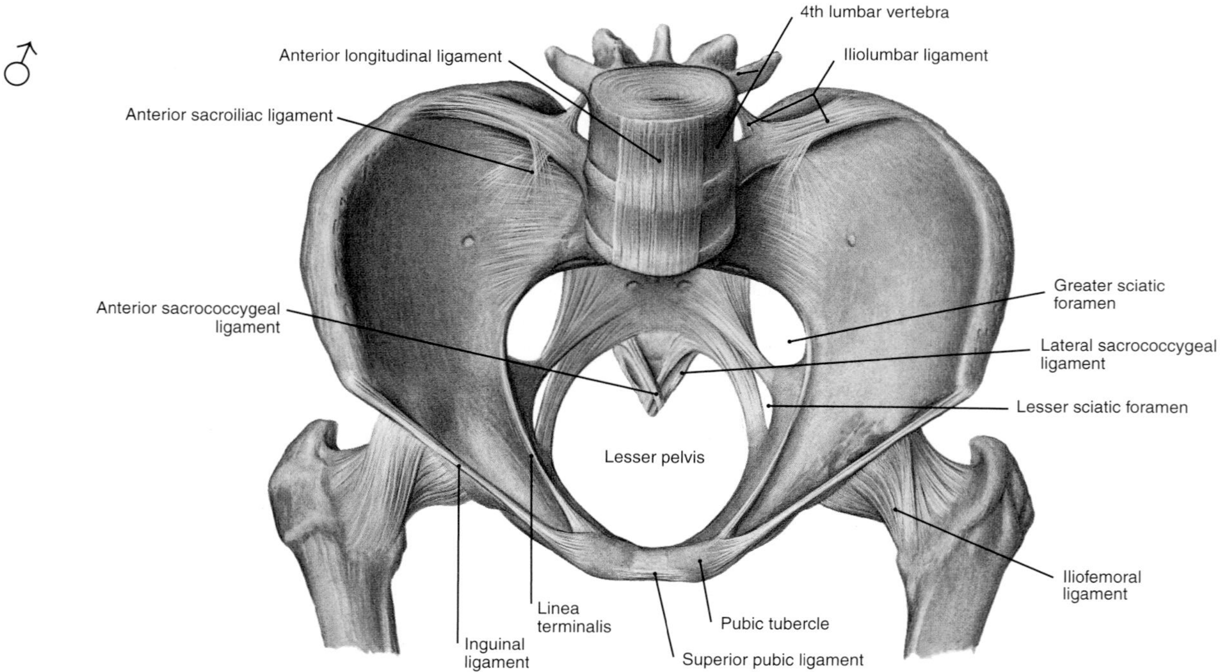
4th lumbar vertebra
Anterior longitudinal ligament
Iliolumbar ligament
Anterior sacroiliac ligament
Anterior sacrococcygeal ligament
Greater sciatic foramen
Lateral sacrococcygeal ligament
Lesser sciatic foramen
Lesser pelvis
Iliofemoral ligament
Linea terminalis
Pubic tubercle
Inguinal ligament
Superior pubic ligament

Figure 271.2 Male Pelvis and Ligaments Viewed from Above

NOTE: The size of the **pelvic inlet** (superior aperture of the **lesser pelvis**) and **inferior outlet** of the male pelvis is smaller than that in the female (see Fig. 270.2). Thus, the **lesser pelvis** is deeper and more narrow in the male, and its cavity has a smaller capacity than that seen in the female. In the male, the pelvic bones are thicker and heavier, and generally, the **major pelvis** (above the pelvic brim) is larger than that in the female.

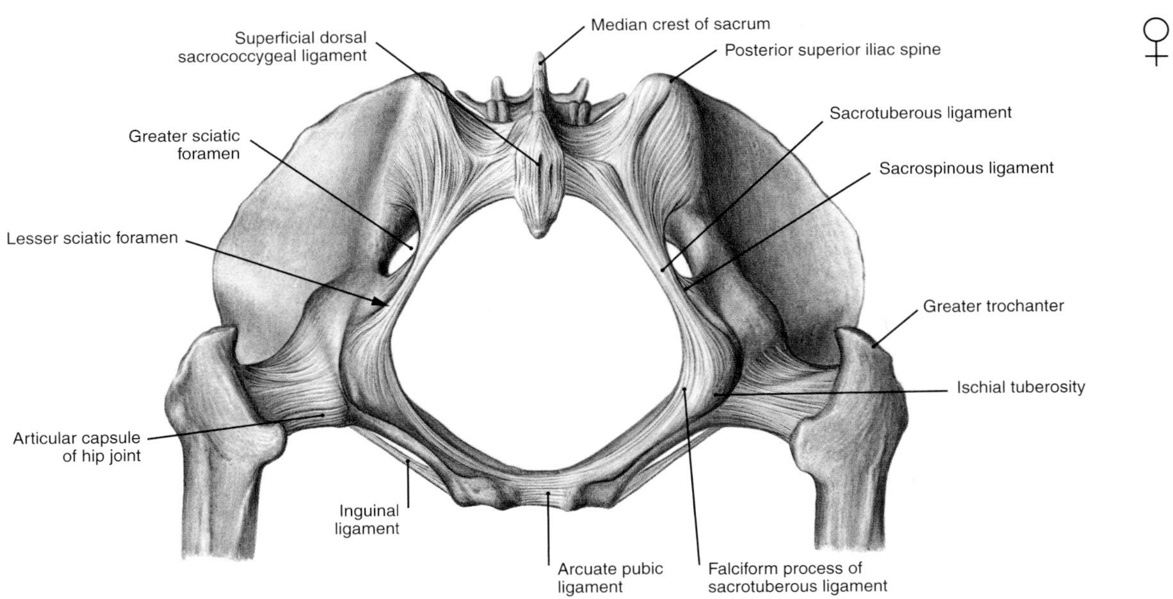
Superficial dorsal sacrococcygeal ligament
Median crest of sacrum
Posterior superior iliac spine
Sacrotuberous ligament
Greater sciatic foramen
Sacrospinous ligament
Lesser sciatic foramen
Greater trochanter
Ischial tuberosity
Articular capsule of hip joint
Inguinal ligament
Arcuate pubic ligament
Falciform process of sacrotuberous ligament

Figure 272.1 Female Pelvic Outlet Showing the Pelvic Ligaments and Viewed from Below

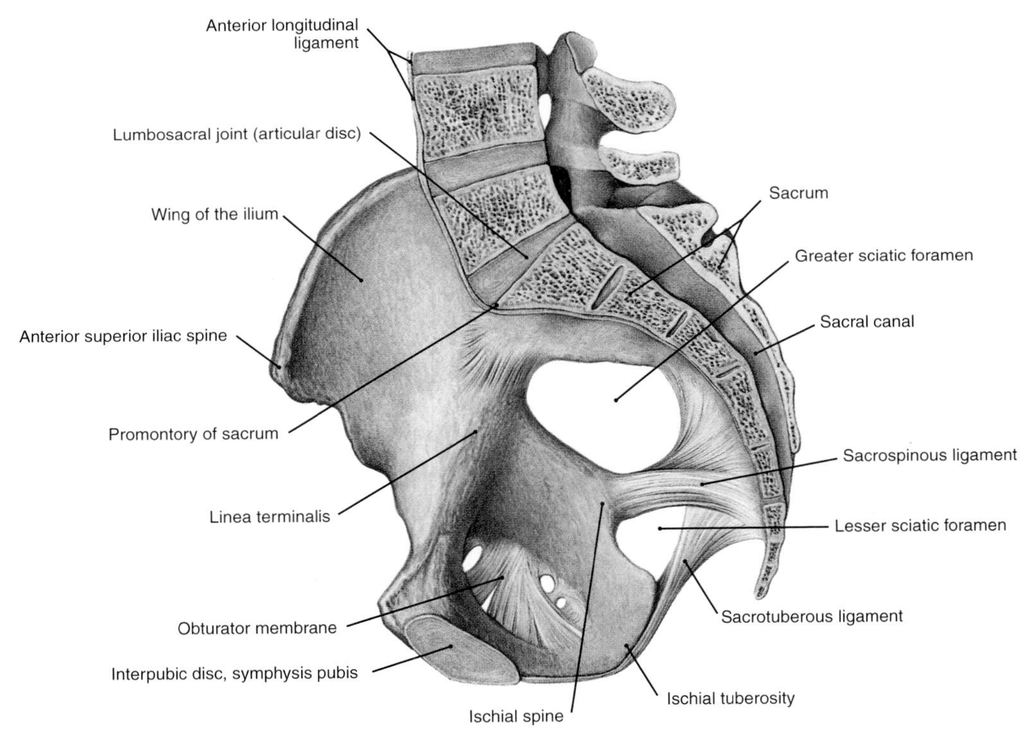
Anterior longitudinal ligament
Lumbosacral joint (articular disc)
Wing of the ilium
Sacrum
Greater sciatic foramen
Sacral canal
Anterior superior iliac spine
Promontory of sacrum
Sacrospinous ligament
Linea terminalis
Lesser sciatic foramen
Sacrotuberous ligament
Obturator membrane
Interpubic disc, symphysis pubis
Ischial tuberosity
Ischial spine

Figure 272.2 Articulations and Ligaments of the Female Hemisected Pelvis

NOTE: (1) The **sacrospinous ligament** courses between the **sacrum** and the **ischial spine** and forms the lower border of the **greater sciatic foramen.**

(2) The **lesser sciatic foramen** is bounded above by the **sacrospinous ligament** and below by the **sacrotuberous ligament.** The latter extends between the **sacrum** and the **ischial tuberosity.**

(3) These two foramina allow the emergence of muscles, nerves, and arteries from the pelvis to the gluteal region and the entrance of veins from the gluteal region to the pelvis.

(4) Because the sacrum lies beneath the remainder of the vertebral column, considerable weight is transmitted to it from above. This tends to rotate the upper end of the sacrum forward and downward and its lower end and the coccyx backward and upward. The sacrotuberous and sacrospinous ligaments add stability to the sacroiliac joint by resisting these forces.

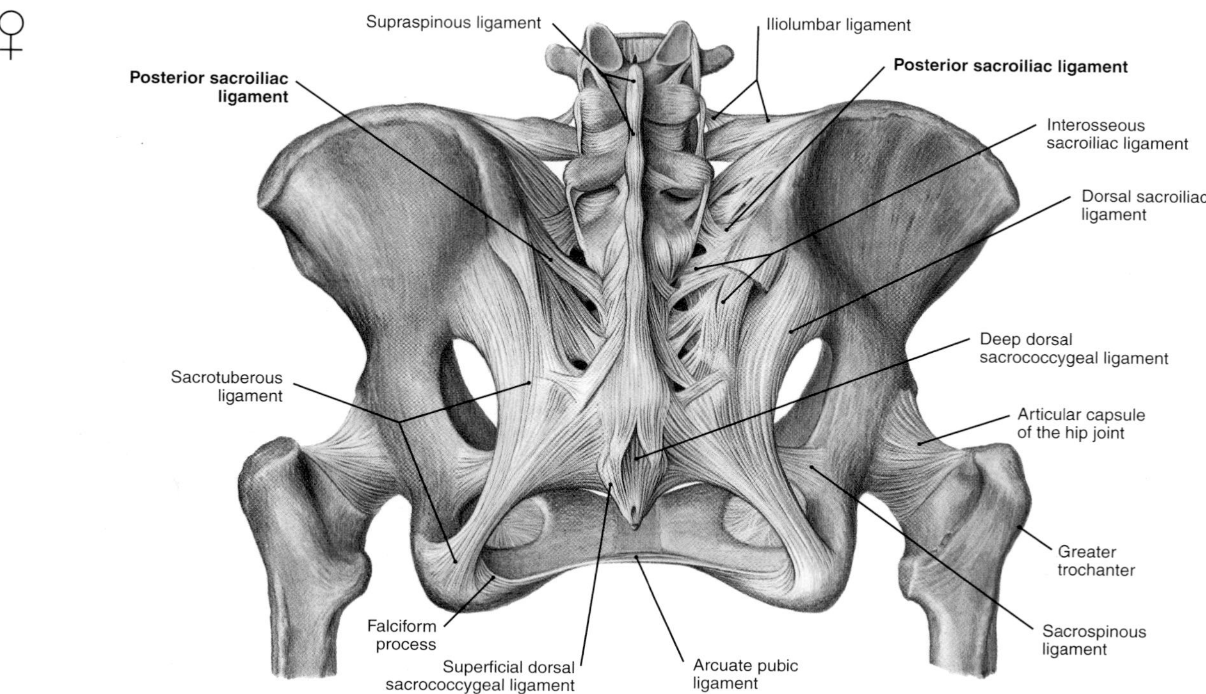
♀
Supraspinous ligament
Iliolumbar ligament
Posterior sacroiliac ligament
Posterior sacroiliac ligament
Interosseous sacroiliac ligament
Dorsal sacroiliac ligament
Deep dorsal sacrococcygeal ligament
Sacrotuberous ligament
Articular capsule of the hip joint
Greater trochanter
Sacrospinous ligament
Falciform process
Superficial dorsal sacrococcygeal ligament
Arcuate pubic ligament

Figure 273.1 Female Pelvis with Joints and Ligaments (Posterior Aspect)

NOTE: (1) Broad ligamentous bands articulate the two hip bones posteriorly with the sacrum and coccyx. Observe the strong **posterior (dorsal) sacroiliac ligament.**

(2) The posterior sacroiliac ligament is composed of short **transverse fibers** that interconnect the ilium with the upper part of the lateral crest of the sacrum, whereas the longer **vertical fibers** attach the third and fourth transverse tubercles of the sacrum to the superior and inferior posterior iliac spines, many blending with fibers of the sacrotuberous ligament.

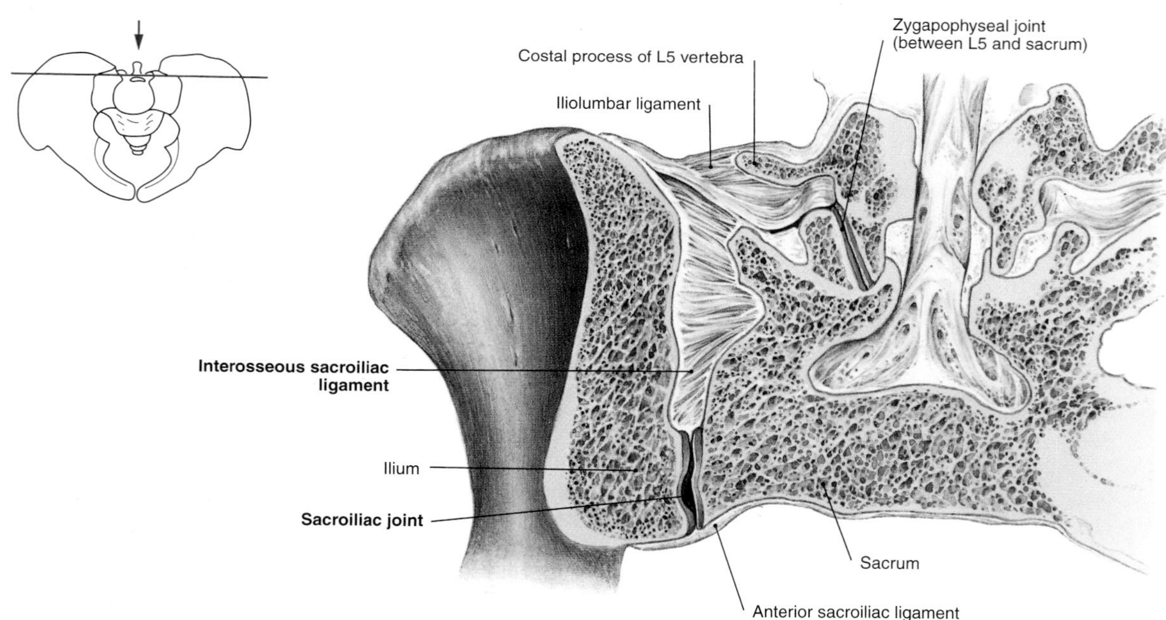
Zygapophyseal joint (between L5 and sacrum)
Costal process of L5 vertebra
Iliolumbar ligament
Interosseous sacroiliac ligament
Ilium
Sacroiliac joint
Sacrum
Anterior sacroiliac ligament

Figure 273.2 Frontal Section through the Sacroiliac Joint

NOTE: (1) The **sacroiliac joint** is a synovial joint connecting the **auricular surface** of the sacrum with the reciprocally curved **auricular surface** of the ilium.

(2) This joint is bound by the **anterior** and **interosseous sacroiliac ligaments** (shown in this figure) as well as the **posterior** (dorsal) **sacroiliac ligament** (shown in Fig. 273.1).

(3) The interosseous sacroiliac ligament is the strongest ligament between the sacrum and ilium, and it stretches above and behind the synovial joint.

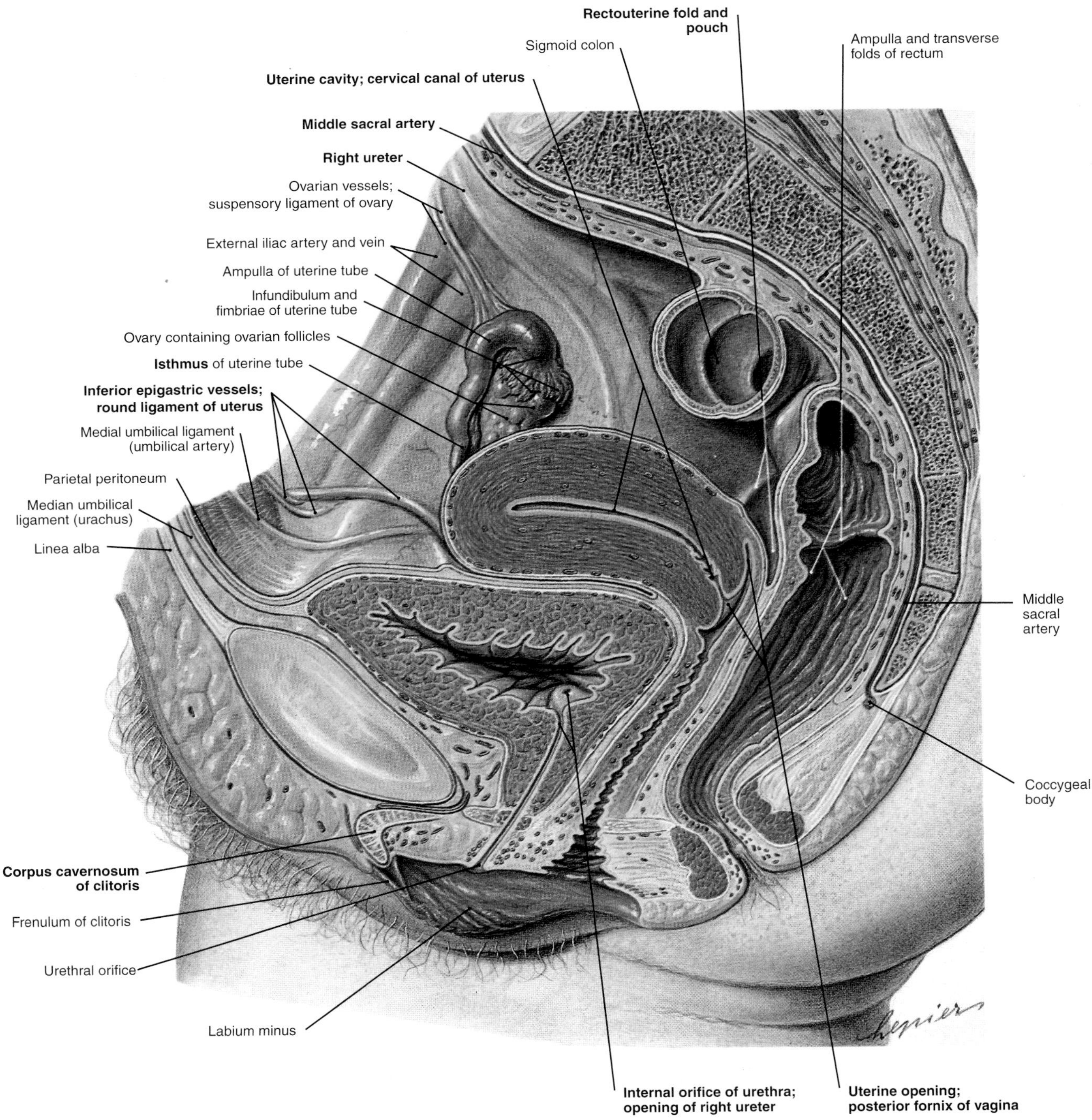
Rectouterine fold and pouch
Sigmoid colon
Ampulla and transverse folds of rectum
Uterine cavity; cervical canal of uterus
Middle sacral artery
Right ureter
Ovarian vessels; suspensory ligament of ovary
External iliac artery and vein
Ampulla of uterine tube
Infundibulum and fimbriae of uterine tube
Ovary containing ovarian follicles
Isthmus of uterine tube
Inferior epigastric vessels; round ligament of uterus
Medial umbilical ligament (umbilical artery)
Parietal peritoneum
Median umbilical ligament (urachus)
Linea alba
Middle sacral artery
Coccygeal body
Corpus cavernosum of clitoris
Frenulum of clitoris
Urethral orifice
Labium minus
Internal orifice of urethra; opening of right ureter
Uterine opening; posterior fornix of vagina

Figure 274 Adult Female Pelvis (Median Sagittal Section)

NOTE: (1) This medial view of the hemisected female pelvis shows the relationships of the **bladder, uterus, vagina, rectum, ovary,** and **uterine tube.** Observe the retropubic position of the empty bladder and the short course of the female urethra, leading from the bladder through the **urogenital diaphragm** to open in the midline, anterior to the vagina.

(2) The **posterior fornix** of the vagina reaches superiorly to lie in front of the **rectouterine pouch (of Douglas),** being separated from it only by the vaginal wall. Observe that the vagina and uterus are interposed between the bladder and rectum.

(3) The **round ligament of the uterus** is directed laterally and anteriorly to enter the deep inguinal ring, and note the course of the **inferior epigastric vessels** in relation to this ligament. Observe the **ovarian vessels** within the **suspensory ligament of the ovary** and the **ureter** along the posterolateral wall of the pelvis.

(4) Shown are the **large bowel** and the direct course of the **rectum** toward the **anal canal.** The peritoneum is reflected over the anterior surface of the rectum, thereby lining the rectouterine pouch.

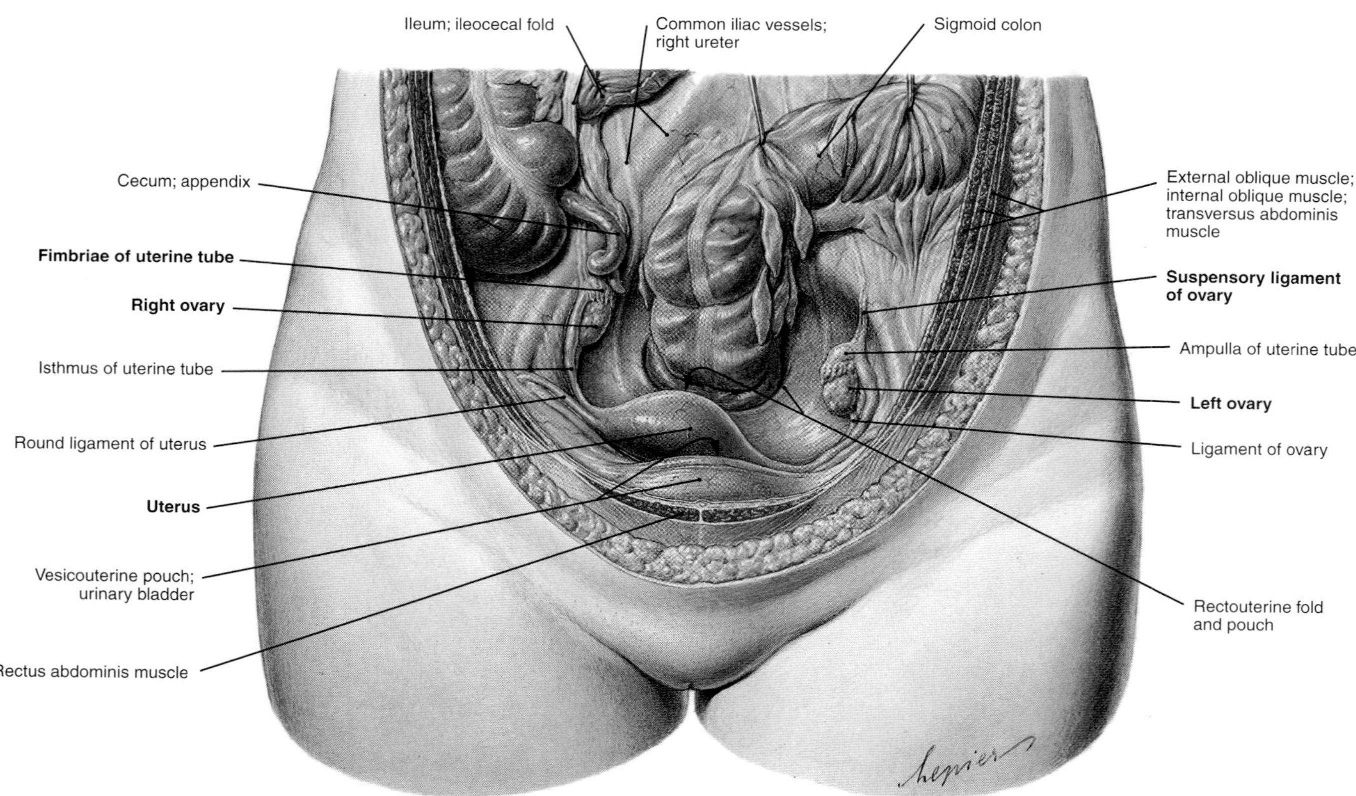
Ileum; ileocecal fold
Common iliac vessels; right ureter
Sigmoid colon
Cecum; appendix
Fimbriae of uterine tube
Right ovary
Isthmus of uterine tube
Round ligament of uterus
Uterus
Vesicouterine pouch; urinary bladder
Rectus abdominis muscle
External oblique muscle; internal oblique muscle; transversus abdominis muscle
Suspensory ligament of ovary
Ampulla of uterine tube
Left ovary
Ligament of ovary
Rectouterine fold and pouch

Figure 275.1 Pelvic Viscera of an Adult Female (Anterior View)

NOTE: (1) The ovaries are situated on the posterolateral aspect of the true pelvis on each side. Having descended from the posterior abdominal wall to their location just below the pelvic brim, the ovaries are held in position by peritoneal ligamentous attachments. The suspensory ligament of the ovary transmits the ovarian vessels and ovarian autonomic nerves.

(2) The uterus is positioned between the bladder and the rectum, and frequently it is located somewhat to one or the other side of the midline.

(3) The fimbriae of the uterine tubes extend from the ampullae of the tubes to encircle the upper medial surface of the ovaries. The uterine tubes vary from 3 to 6 in. in length, and they convey the ova to the uterus. It is within the uterine tube that fertilization of the ovum usually occurs.

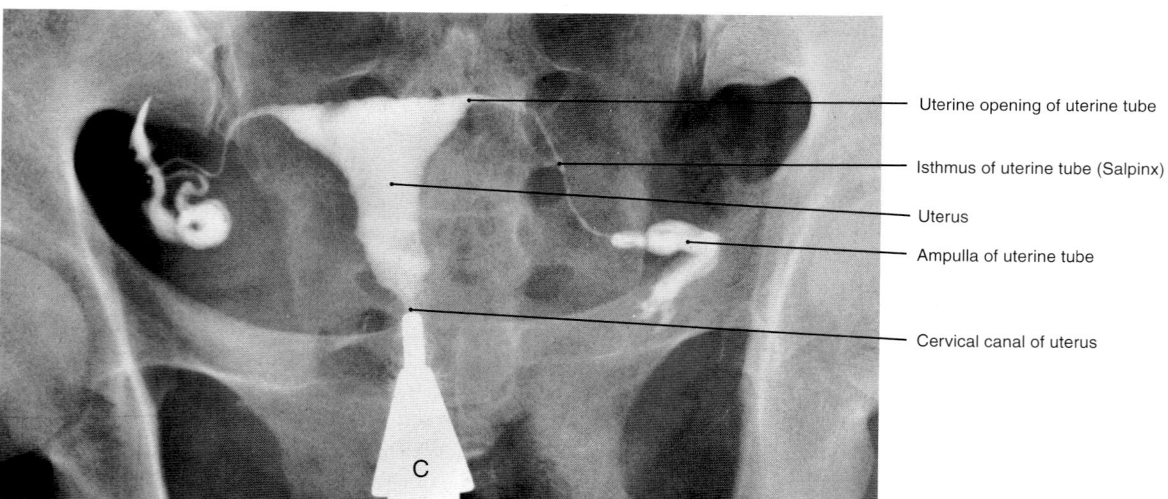
Uterine opening of uterine tube
Isthmus of uterine tube (Salpinx)
Uterus
Ampulla of uterine tube
Cervical canal of uterus
C

Figure 275.2 Uterosalpingogram

NOTE: (1) A cannula (C) was placed in the vagina, and radiopaque material was injected into the uterus and uterine tube. Observe the narrow lumen of the isthmus of the uterine tubes and how the tubes enlarge at the ampullae.

(2) On the specimen's left side (reader's right), even the fimbriated end of the tube is discernible, whereas on the specimen's right side (reader's left) a small portion of the radiopaque material has been forced into the pelvis through the opening in the uterine tube.

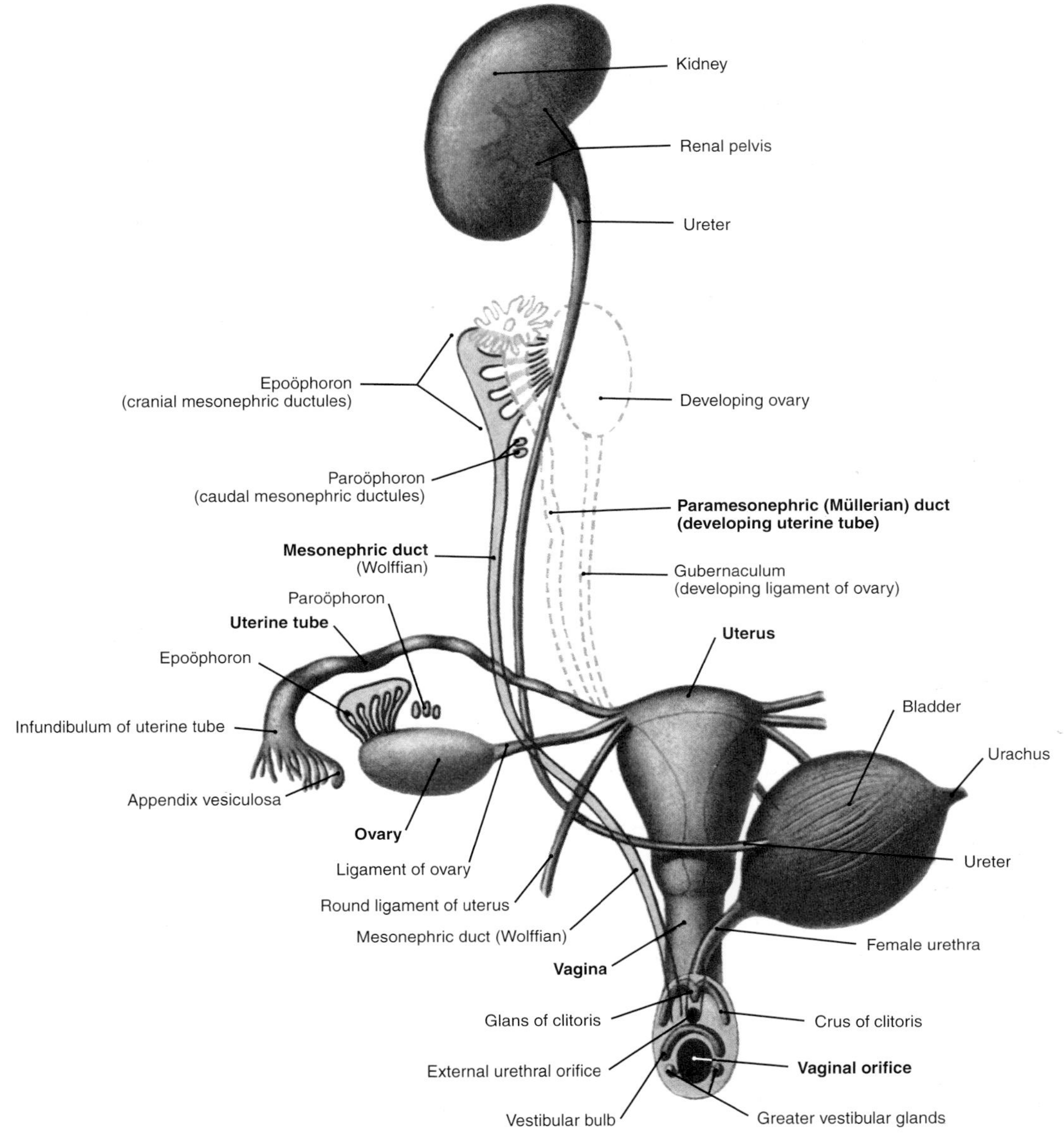
Kidney
Renal pelvis
Ureter
Epoöphoron
(cranial mesonephric ductules)
Developing ovary
Paroöphoron
(caudal mesonephric ductules)
Paramesonephric (Müllerian) duct
(developing uterine tube)
Mesonephric duct
(Wolffian)
Gubernaculum
(developing ligament of ovary)
Paroöphoron
Uterine tube
Uterus
Epoöphoron
Bladder
Infundibulum of uterine tube
Urachus
Appendix vesiculosa
Ovary
Ureter
Ligament of ovary
Round ligament of uterus
Mesonephric duct (Wolffian)
Female urethra
Vagina
Glans of clitoris
Crus of clitoris
External urethral orifice
Vaginal orifice
Vestibular bulb
Greater vestibular glands

Figure 276 Diagram of the Female Genitourinary Organs and Their Embryologic Precursors

NOTE: (1) This figure shows:

(a) All of the organs of the adult female genitourinary system (dark red-brown).

(b) The structures and relevant positions of the female genital organs (gonad and ligament of the ovary and uterine tube) prior to their descent into the pelvis (interrupted lines).

(c) The structures that become atrophic during development (pink with red outline).

(2) The urinary system of females (as in males) includes the kidney, which produces urine from the blood; and the ureter, which conveys the urine to the bladder, where it is stored. Leading from the bladder is the urethra, through which urine passes to the external urethral orifice during micturition.

(3) The adult female genital system includes the **ovary, uterine tube, uterus**, and **vagina,** plus the associated glands and external genital organs.

(4) At one time during development, structures capable of developing into both male and female genital systems existed. In the female, the Müllerian, or paramesonephric, duct becomes vestigial. Also, the developing gonads become ovaries, while their attachments become the ligaments of the ovaries.

(5) The ovaries produce ova that are discharged periodically between adolescence and menopause. The ova are captured by the uterine tube, where fertilization may occur. If this happens, the fertilized ovum is transported to the uterus, and about a week after fertilization, implantation occurs in the wall of the uterus.

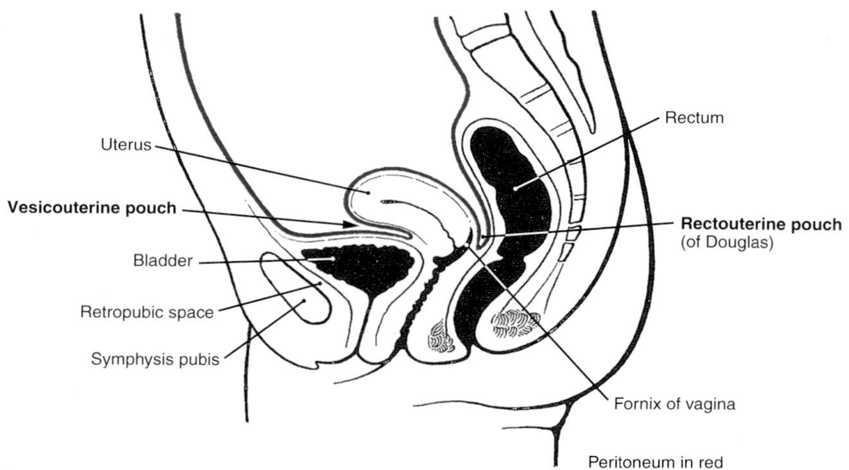
Uterus
Vesicouterine pouch
Bladder
Retropubic space
Symphysis pubis
Rectum
Rectouterine pouch
(of Douglas)
Fornix of vagina
Peritoneum in red

Figure 277.1 Diagram of Peritoneal Reflections over Female Pelvic Organs (Midsagittal Section)

NOTE: (1) The parietal peritoneum is reflected over the free abdominal surface of the pelvic organs. Observe that as the uterus and vagina are interposed between the bladder and rectum, peritoneal pouches are formed between the bladder and the uterus (vesicouterine) and between the rectum and the uterus (rectouterine pouch of Douglas).

(2) The **vesicouterine pouch** is shallow. The forward tilt, or inclination, of the uterus (anteversion) toward the superior surface of the bladder reduces the potential size of the vesicouterine pouch.

(3) The vesicouterine pouch does not extend as far inferiorly as the vagina, whereas the deeper **rectouterine pouch** dips to the level of the posterior fornix of the vagina. This important anatomical relationship stresses the fact that the posterior fornix is separated from the peritoneal cavity only by the thin vaginal wall and the peritoneum.

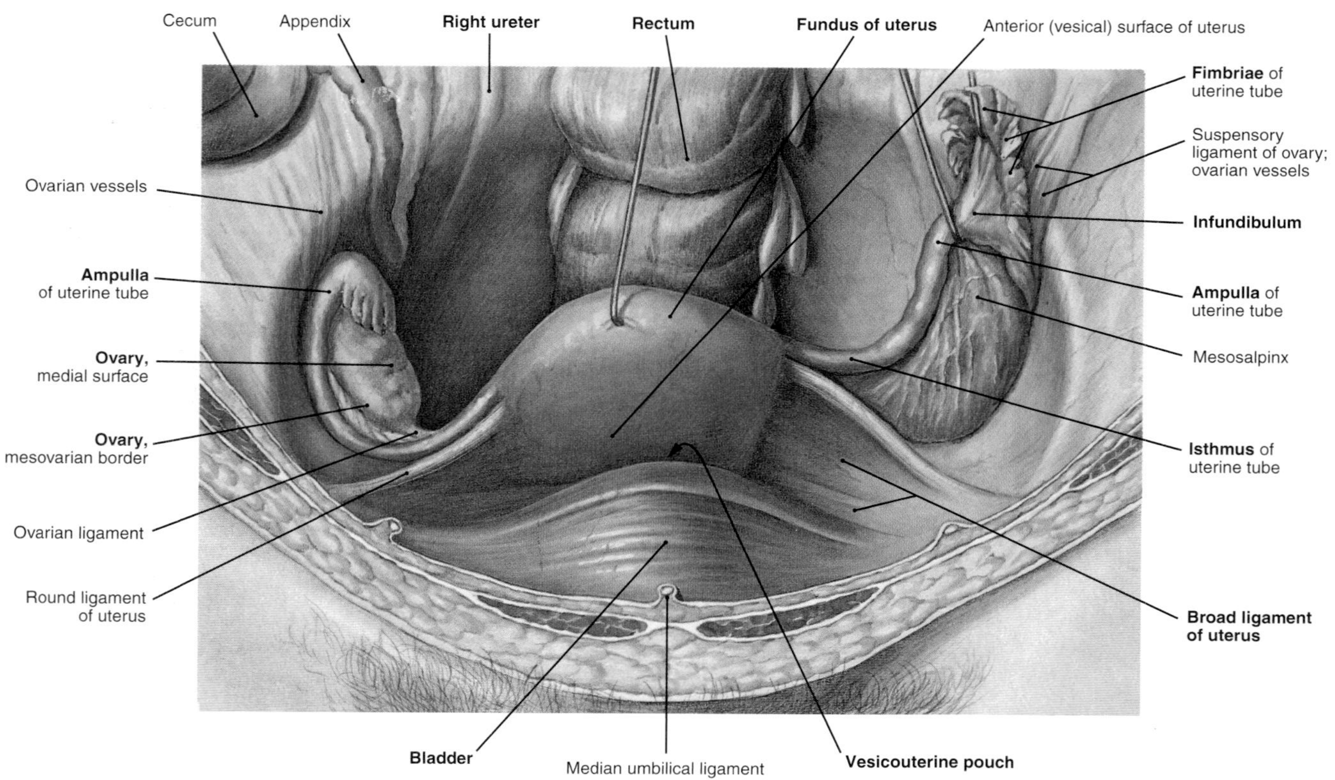
Cecum
Appendix
Right ureter
Rectum
Fundus of uterus
Anterior (vesical) surface of uterus
Fimbriae of uterine tube
Suspensory ligament of ovary; ovarian vessels
Infundibulum
Ampulla of uterine tube
Mesosalpinx
Isthmus of uterine tube
Broad ligament of uterus
Ovarian vessels
Ampulla of uterine tube
Ovary, medial surface
Ovary, mesovarian border
Ovarian ligament
Round ligament of uterus
Bladder
Median umbilical ligament
Vesicouterine pouch

Figure 277.2 Female Pelvic Organs (Anterosuperior View)

NOTE: The body of the uterus has been elevated, thereby exposing the **vesicouterine pouch** and demonstrating the **broad ligaments.**

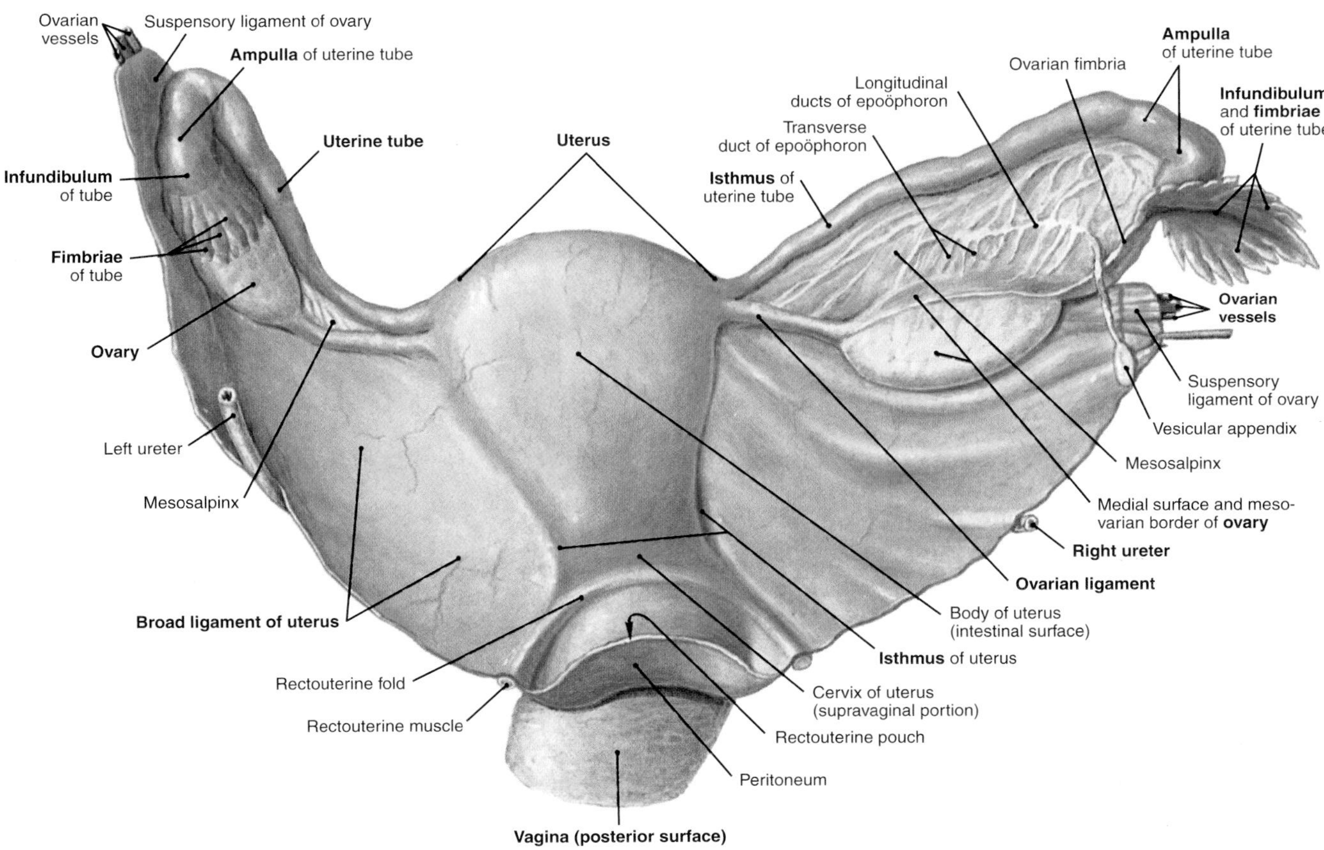
Ovarian vessels
Suspensory ligament of ovary
Ampulla of uterine tube
Infundibulum of tube
Fimbriae of tube
Ovary
Uterine tube
Uterus
Left ureter
Mesosalpinx
Broad ligament of uterus
Rectouterine fold
Rectouterine muscle
Vagina (posterior surface)
Peritoneum
Rectouterine pouch
Cervix of uterus (supravaginal portion)
Isthmus of uterus
Body of uterus (intestinal surface)
Ovarian ligament
Right ureter
Medial surface and meso-varian border of ovary
Mesosalpinx
Vesicular appendix
Suspensory ligament of ovary
Ovarian vessels
Infundibulum and fimbriae of uterine tube
Ampulla of uterine tube
Ovarian fimbria
Longitudinal ducts of epoöphoron
Transverse duct of epoöphoron
Isthmus of uterine tube

Figure 278.1 Pelvic Reproductive Organs of an Immature Girl (Posterior View)

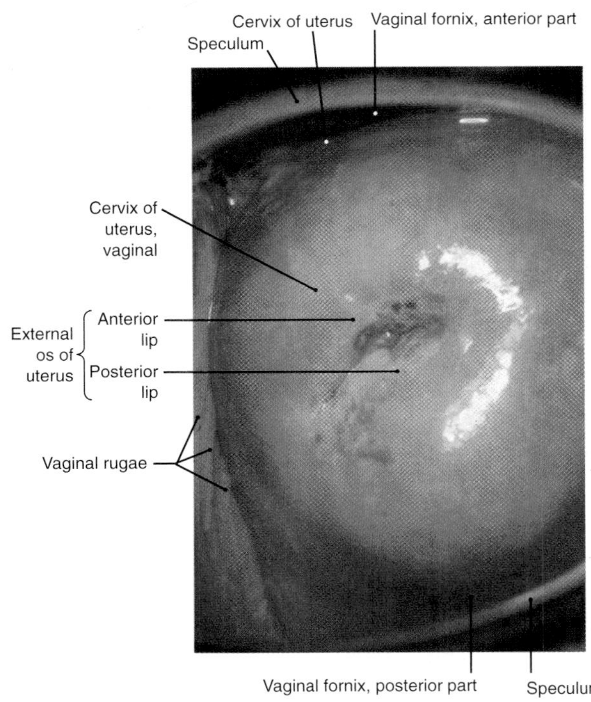
Cervix of uterus
Vaginal fornix, anterior part
Speculum
Cervix of uterus, vaginal
External os of uterus
Anterior lip
Posterior lip
Vaginal rugae
Vaginal fornix, posterior part
Speculum

Figure 278.2 Vaginal Surface of the Cervix in a Young Nulliparous Woman

NOTE that this young woman has never given birth to a child.

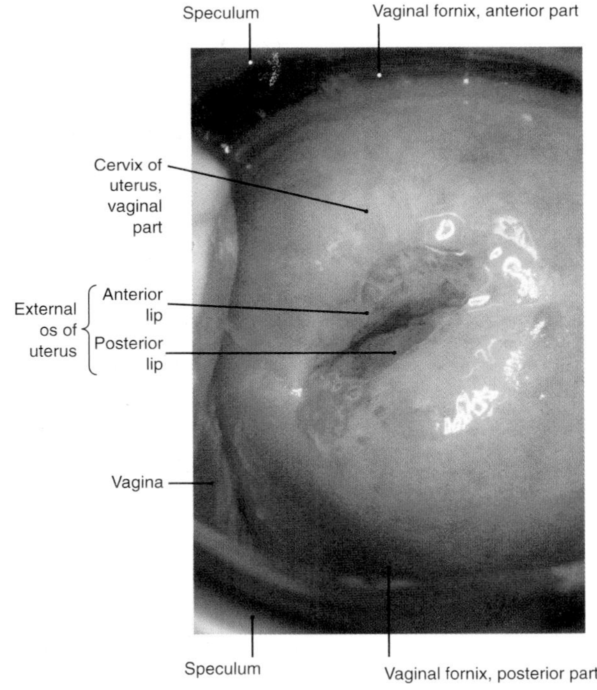
Speculum
Vaginal fornix, anterior part
Cervix of uterus, vaginal part
External os of uterus
Anterior lip
Posterior lip
Vagina
Speculum
Vaginal fornix, posterior part

Figure 278.3 Vaginal Surface of the Cervix in a Young Multiparous Woman

NOTE that this young woman has given birth to two children.

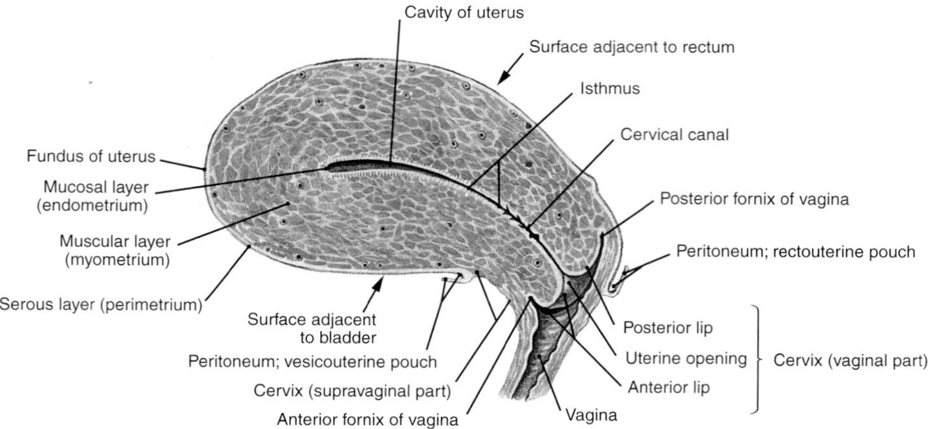
Cavity of uterus
Surface adjacent to rectum
Isthmus
Cervical canal
Fundus of uterus
Mucosal layer (endometrium)
Muscular layer (myometrium)
Serous layer (perimetrium)
Posterior fornix of vagina
Peritoneum; rectouterine pouch
Surface adjacent to bladder
Peritoneum; vesicouterine pouch
Cervix (supravaginal part)
Anterior fornix of vagina
Posterior lip
Uterine opening
Anterior lip
Cervix (vaginal part)
Vagina

Figure 279.1 Median Sagittal Section through the Uterus and Upper Vagina

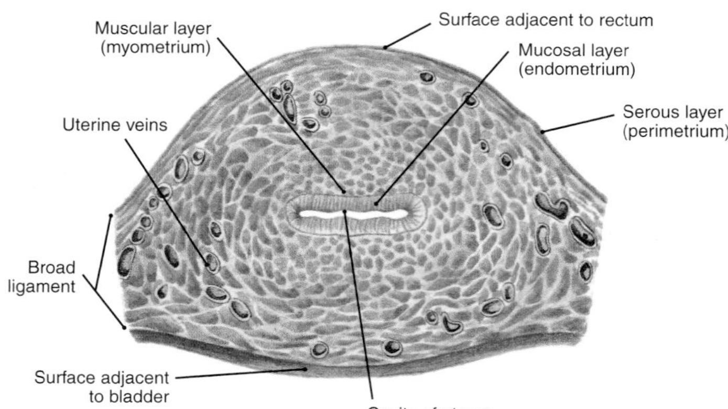
Muscular layer (myometrium)
Surface adjacent to rectum
Mucosal layer (endometrium)
Serous layer (perimetrium)
Uterine veins
Broad ligament
Surface adjacent to bladder
Cavity of uterus

Figure 279.2 Cross Section through the Body of the Uterus

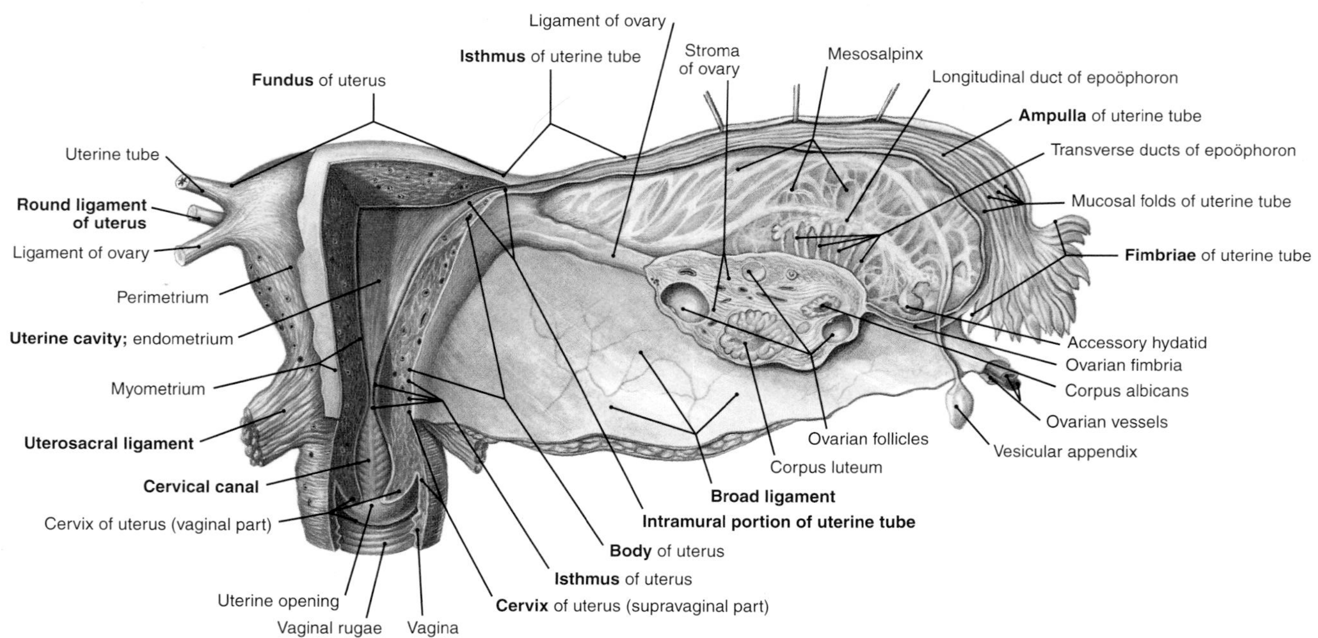
Ligament of ovary
Isthmus of uterine tube
Stroma of ovary
Mesosalpinx
Fundus of uterus
Longitudinal duct of epoöphoron
Ampulla of uterine tube
Uterine tube
Transverse ducts of epoöphoron
Round ligament of uterus
Mucosal folds of uterine tube
Ligament of ovary
Fimbriae of uterine tube
Perimetrium
Uterine cavity; endometrium
Accessory hydatid
Ovarian fimbria
Myometrium
Corpus albicans
Ovarian vessels
Uterosacral ligament
Ovarian follicles
Vesicular appendix
Corpus luteum
Cervical canal
Broad ligament
Intramural portion of uterine tube
Cervix of uterus (vaginal part)
Body of uterus
Isthmus of uterus
Uterine opening
Cervix of uterus (supravaginal part)
Vaginal rugae
Vagina

Figure 279.3 Frontal Section of Uterus, Uterine Tube, and Ovary

NOTE: (1) The vagina communicates with the pelvic cavity through the uterus and the uterine tube. The lumen of this pathway varies in diameter, and its most narrow sites are the isthmus of the uterus and the intrauterine (intramural) part of the uterine tube.

(2) The uterus consists of the **cervix** (vaginal and supravaginal portions), the **body** and the **fundus.** The cervix and the body are interconnected by the **isthmus.**

(3) The attachments of the uterus include:

(a) The **broad ligaments** that attach to the lateral margins of the uterus.

(b) The fibrous **round ligaments** and the **ligaments of the ovaries** attached just below the uterine tubes.

(c) The **uterosacral ligaments.**

(d) The **cardinal ligaments (of Mackenrodt)** that attach along the lateral border of the uterus and vagina. With the pelvic diaphragm, the cardinal ligaments offer important support to the uterus and vagina.

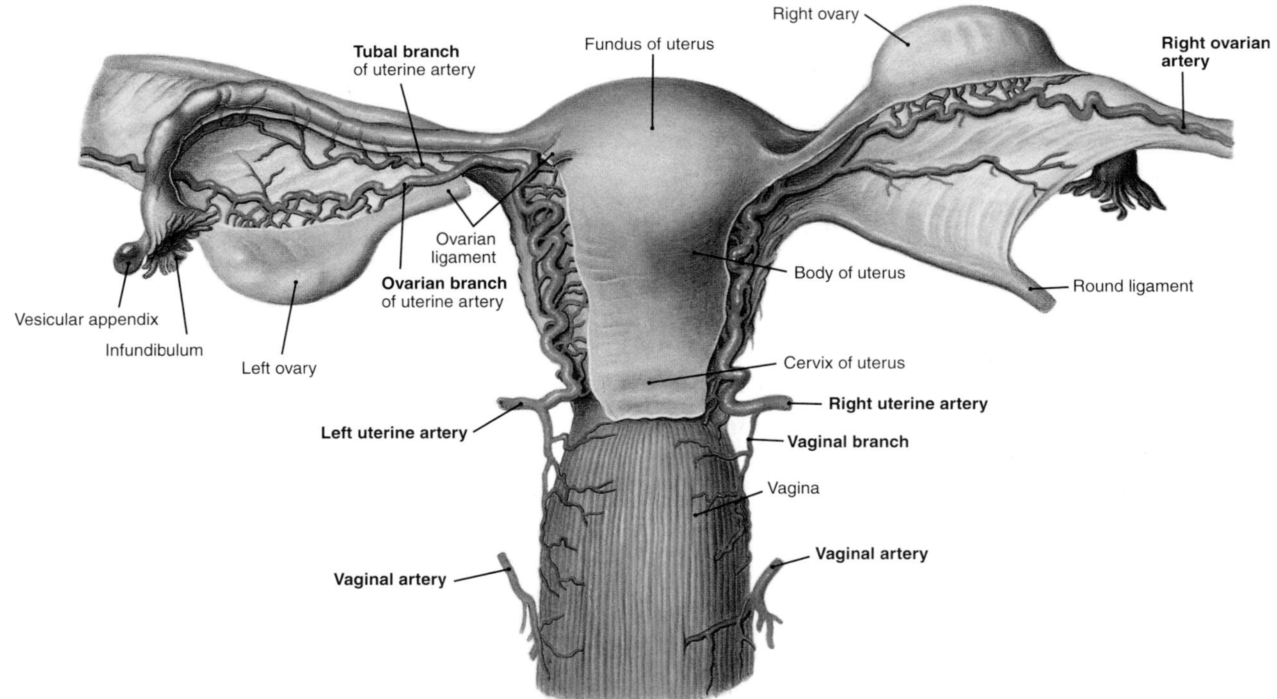
Right ovary
Fundus of uterus
Tubal branch of uterine artery
Right ovarian artery
Ovarian ligament
Ovarian branch of uterine artery
Body of uterus
Round ligament
Vesicular appendix
Infundibulum
Left ovary
Cervix of uterus
Right uterine artery
Left uterine artery
Vaginal branch
Vagina
Vaginal artery
Vaginal artery

Figure 280.1 Arterial Supply to Female Pelvic Genital Organs

NOTE: (1) The vessels supplying the female pelvic genital organs are the **uterine arteries** from the internal iliac and the **ovarian arteries** that stem from the aorta. They anastomose freely along both lateral borders of the uterus.

(2) The uterine artery also anastomoses with the arterial supply to the vagina. Often the **vaginal arteries** arise from the uterine arteries, but they may branch from the inferior vesical artery or even directly from the internal iliac artery.

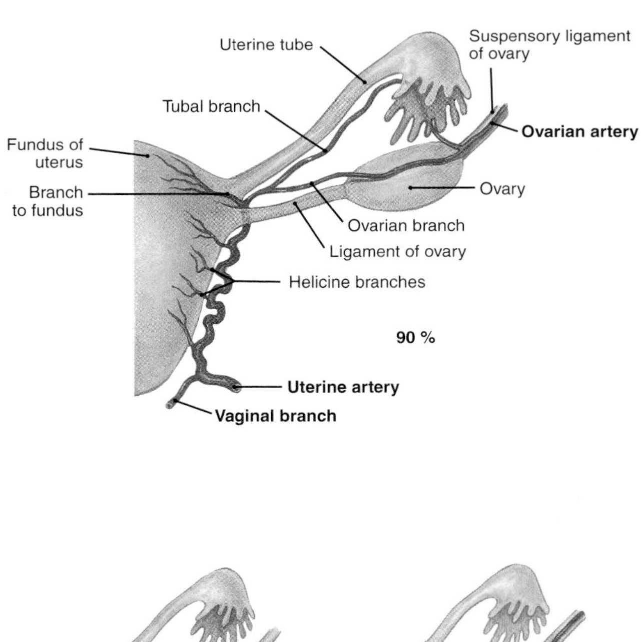
Uterine tube
Suspensory ligament of ovary
Tubal branch
Ovarian artery
Fundus of uterus
Branch to fundus
Ovary
Ovarian branch
Ligament of ovary
Helicine branches
90 %
Uterine artery
Vaginal branch

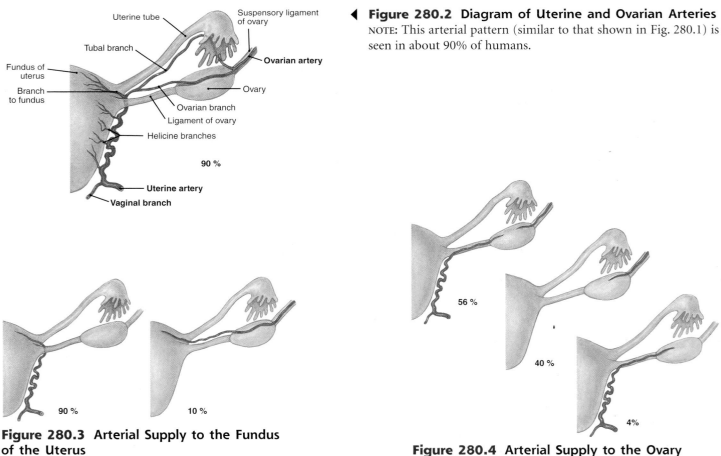

Figure 280.2 Diagram of Uterine and Ovarian Arteries

NOTE: This arterial pattern (similar to that shown in Fig. 280.1) is seen in about 90% of humans.

90 %

10 %

Figure 280.3 Arterial Supply to the Fundus of the Uterus

NOTE: In 90% of cases the fundus gets blood from the uterine artery, whereas in 10% it comes from the ovarian artery.

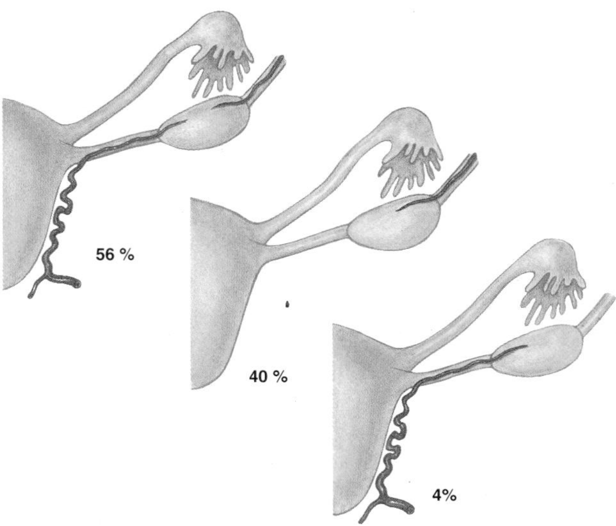
56 %
40 %
4%

Figure 280.4 Arterial Supply to the Ovary

NOTE: In 56% of cases, blood to the ovary comes from both the ovarian and uterine arteries, in 40% from the ovarian artery only, and in 4% from the uterine artery only.

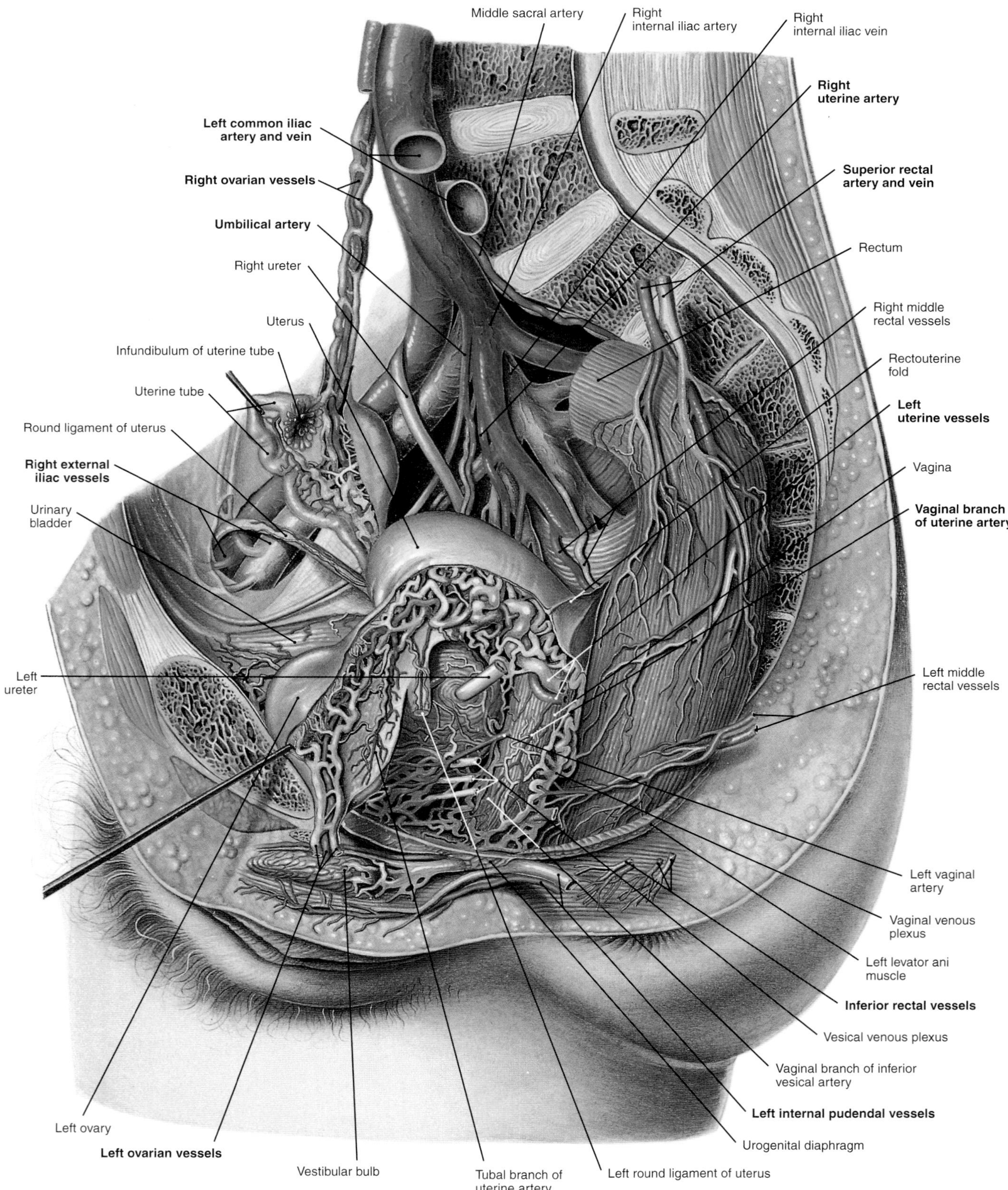
Middle sacral artery
Right internal iliac artery
Right internal iliac vein
Right uterine artery
Left common iliac artery and vein
Right ovarian vessels
Superior rectal artery and vein
Umbilical artery
Rectum
Right ureter
Right middle rectal vessels
Uterus
Infundibulum of uterine tube
Rectouterine fold
Uterine tube
Left uterine vessels
Round ligament of uterus
Vagina
Right external iliac vessels
Vaginal branch of uterine artery
Urinary bladder
Left ureter
Left middle rectal vessels
Left vaginal artery
Vaginal venous plexus
Left levator ani muscle
Inferior rectal vessels
Vesical venous plexus
Vaginal branch of inferior vesical artery
Left internal pudendal vessels
Left ovary
Urogenital diaphragm
Left ovarian vessels
Vestibular bulb
Tubal branch of uterine artery
Left round ligament of uterus

Figure 281 Blood Vessels of the Female Pelvis and Genital System

NOTE: (1) The left half of the pelvis has been removed to expose the pelvic organs and their dense plexuses of veins (**ovarian, vaginal, uterine,** and **vesical**), which accompany their respective arteries.

(2) With the exception of the **ovarian artery** (from the aorta) and the **superior rectal artery** (from the inferior mesenteric) all other arteries to the pelvic organs, perineum, and genital tract are derived from the **internal iliac artery** or its branches.

(3) The course of the **ureter** is a descending one, crossing the external iliac vessels over the pelvic brim. The ureter then courses **under the uterine vessels** before entering the bladder.

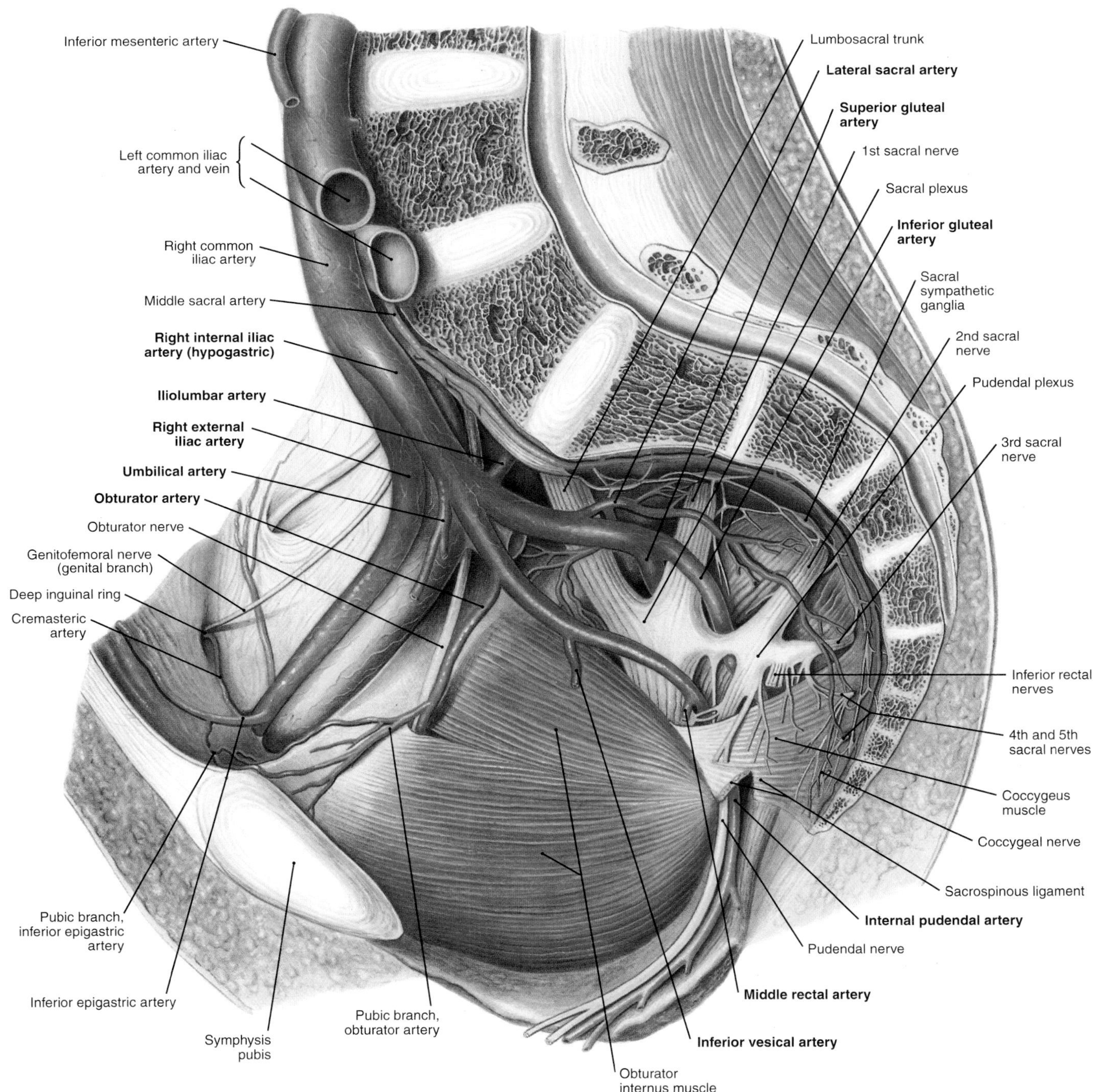

Inferior mesenteric artery
Left common iliac artery and vein
Right common iliac artery
Middle sacral artery
Right internal iliac artery (hypogastric)
Iliolumbar artery
Right external iliac artery
Umbilical artery
Obturator artery
Obturator nerve
Genitofemoral nerve (genital branch)
Deep inguinal ring
Cremasteric artery
Pubic branch, inferior epigastric artery
Inferior epigastric artery
Symphysis pubis
Pubic branch, obturator artery
Obturator internus muscle
Inferior vesical artery
Middle rectal artery
Pudendal nerve
Internal pudendal artery
Sacrospinous ligament
Coccygeal nerve
Coccygeus muscle
4th and 5th sacral nerves
Inferior rectal nerves
3rd sacral nerve
Pudendal plexus
2nd sacral nerve
Sacral sympathetic ganglia
Inferior gluteal artery
Sacral plexus
1st sacral nerve
Superior gluteal artery
Lateral sacral artery
Lumbosacral trunk

Figure 282 Blood Vessels and Nerves of the Pelvic Wall

NOTE: (1) This is a midsagittal view of the right pelvic wall seen from the left side with the pelvic viscera removed and the parietal blood vessels and nerves demonstrated.

(2) The principal arteries of the pelvic wall are derived from the internal iliac artery. Although the branches of this vessel are quite variable, it courses about 1½ in. toward the greater sciatic foramen before dividing, usually into **posterior** and **anterior divisions.**

(3) The posterior division vessels include (a) the **iliolumbar** (b) the **lateral sacral,** and (c) the **superior gluteal,** which leaves the pelvis superior to the piriformis.

(4) The anterior division usually gives rise to four visceral arteries (**umbilical, inferior vesical, middle rectal,** and **uterine** or **deferential**; see Fig. 281). Two parietal vessels from the anterior divisions are the obturator, which courses through the obturator canal to the medial thigh, and the **internal pudendal,** which leaves the pelvis through the greater sciatic foramen and crosses the ischial spine to enter the lesser sciatic foramen. It then courses toward the perineum by way of the **pudendal canal** to get to the perineum.

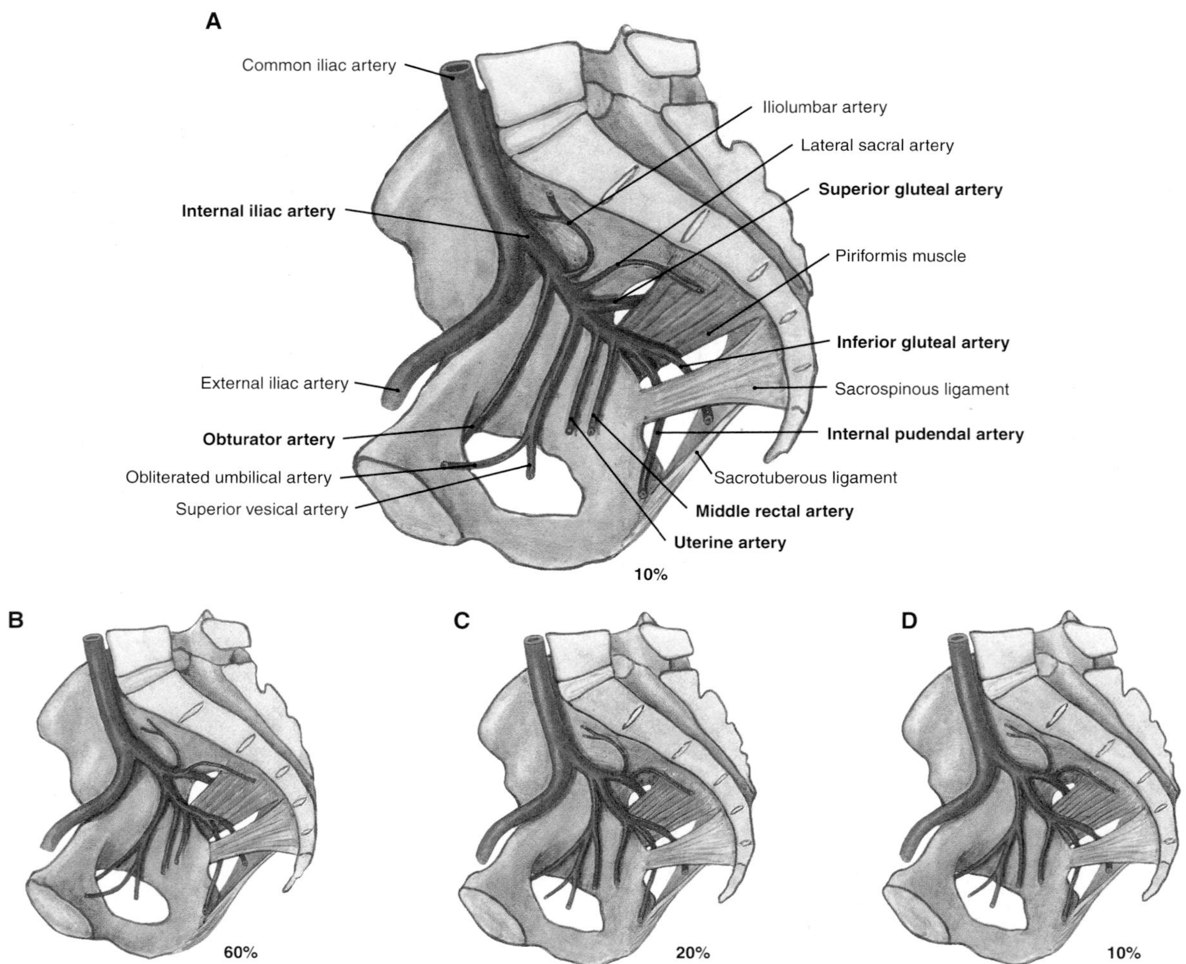
A
Common iliac artery
Iliolumbar artery
Lateral sacral artery
Superior gluteal artery
Internal iliac artery
Piriformis muscle
Inferior gluteal artery
External iliac artery
Sacrospinous ligament
Obturator artery
Internal pudendal artery
Obliterated umbilical artery
Sacrotuberous ligament
Superior vesical artery
Middle rectal artery
Uterine artery
10%
B
C
D
60%
20%
10%

Figure 283.1 Variations in the Divisions of the Internal Iliac Artery

NOTE: (1) In 10% of specimens (shown in **A**) the internal iliac artery itself gives off all branches.

(2) In 60% of specimens (shown in **B**) the internal iliac artery divides into two main branches—an anterior and a posterior trunk.

(3) In 20% of specimens (shown in **C**) the internal iliac artery divides into three branches.

(4) In 10% of specimens (shown in **D**) the internal iliac artery divides into more than three branches.

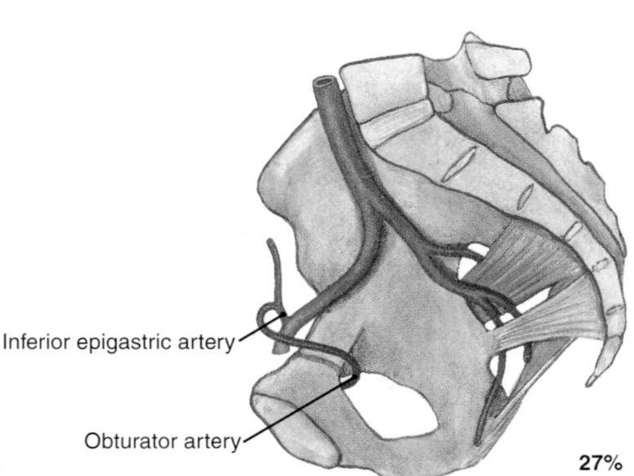
Inferior epigastric artery
Obturator artery
27%

Figure 283.2 Aberrant Origin of the Obturator Artery

NOTE: (1) The obturator artery arises from the internal iliac artery or one of its branches in nearly 70% of bodies, but in 27% of cases the obturator artery arises from the **inferior epigastric artery**, as shown in this figure.

(2) If the course of the aberrant obturator artery is lateral to the lacunar ligament, then repair of a femoral hernia is relatively safe, but if it curves along the free margin of the lacunar ligament, the vessel could easily be injured during hernia repair. (From Picks, J.W., Anson, B.J., and Ashley, F.H. *Am J Anat.* 70:317–344,1942.)

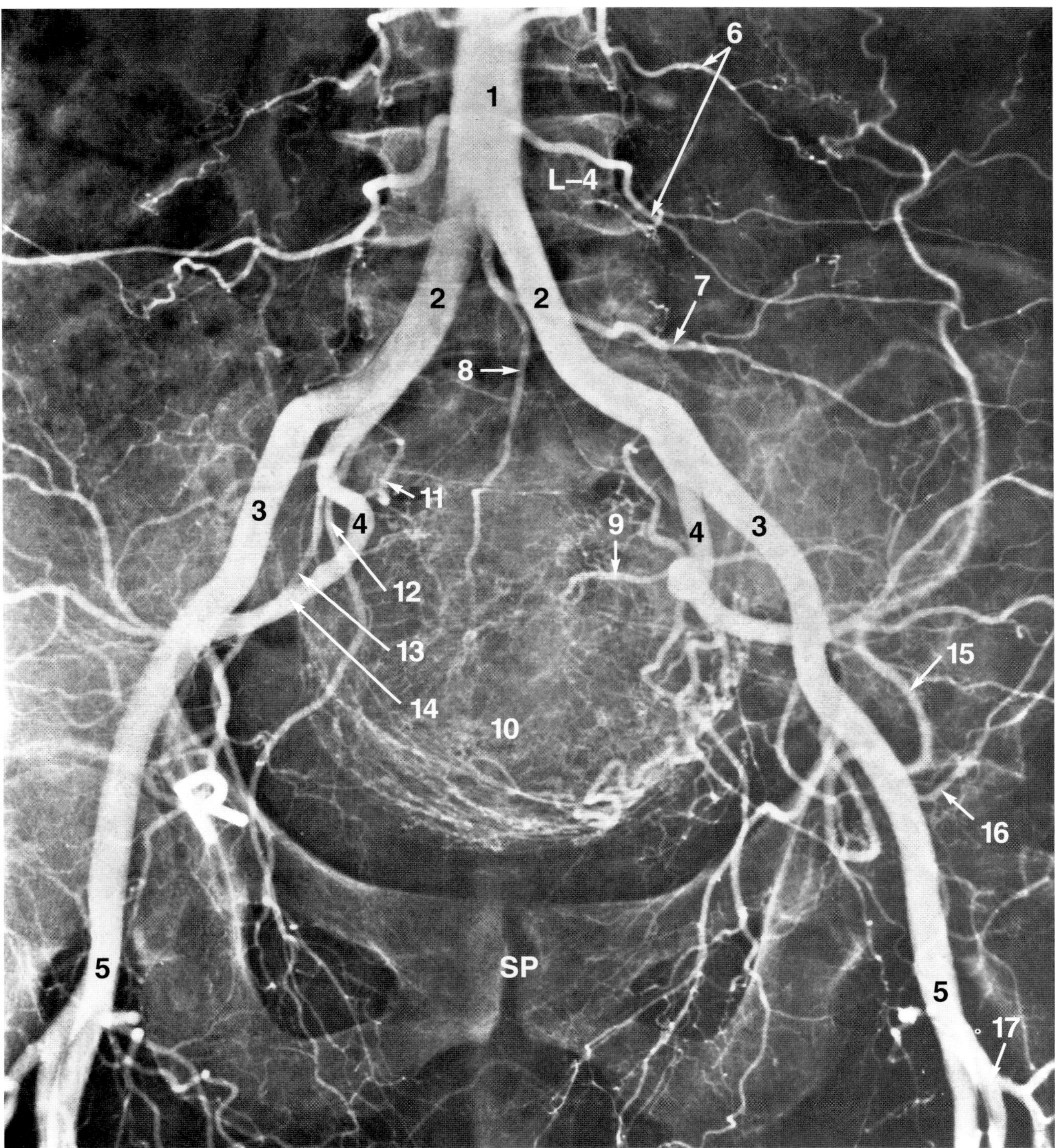

1
L–4
6
2
2
7
8
11
3
4
9
4
3
12
13
15
14
10
16
R
5
SP
5
17

Figure 284 Arteriogram of the Iliac Arteries and Their Branches in a Female

NOTE: The bifurcation of the aorta (1) into the two common iliac arteries (2) occurs at the lower border of the body of the L4 vertebra. The common iliac vessels branch into external (3) and internal (4) iliac arteries. The internal iliac artery (4) on each side serves a number of branches to the pelvis, perineum, and gluteal region, whereas the external iliac artery (3), after giving off the inferior epigastric (15) and deep circumflex iliac (16) arteries, becomes the femoral artery below the inguinal ligament.
(From Wicke, 6th ed.)

1. Abdominal aorta
2. Common iliac artery
3. External iliac artery
4. Internal iliac artery
5. Femoral artery
6. Lumbar arteries
7. Iliolumbar artery
8. Median sacral artery
9. Uterine artery
10. Uterus
11. Lateral sacral artery
12. Obturator artery
13. Internal pudendal artery
14. Superior gluteal artery
15. Inferior epigastric artery
16. Deep circumflex iliac artery
17. Deep femoral artery

SP = Symphysis pubis
L4 = 4th lumbar vertebra

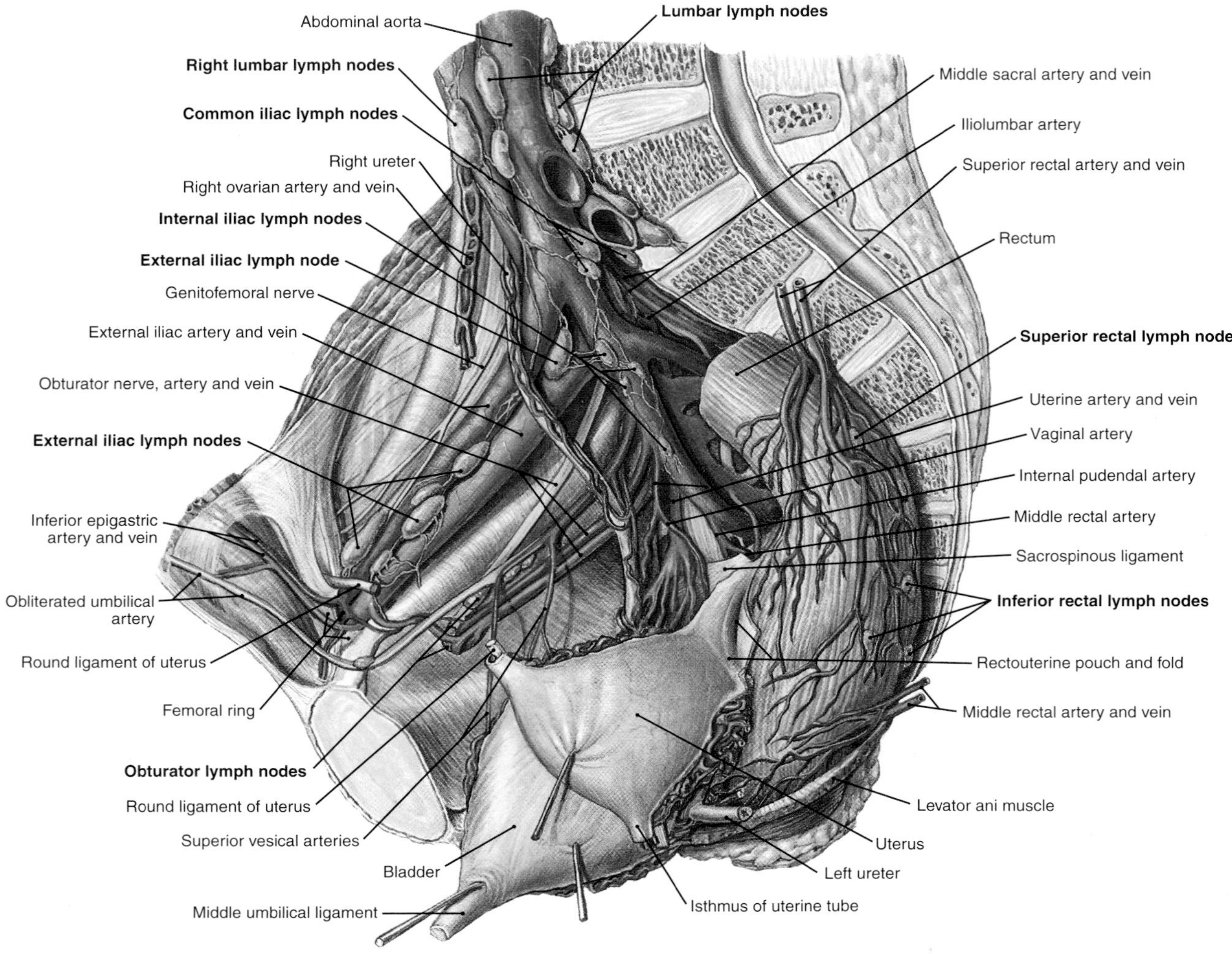
Abdominal aorta
Lumbar lymph nodes
Right lumbar lymph nodes
Common iliac lymph nodes
Right ureter
Right ovarian artery and vein
Internal iliac lymph nodes
External iliac lymph node
Genitofemoral nerve
External iliac artery and vein
Obturator nerve, artery and vein
External iliac lymph nodes
Inferior epigastric artery and vein
Obliterated umbilical artery
Round ligament of uterus
Femoral ring
Obturator lymph nodes
Round ligament of uterus
Superior vesical arteries
Bladder
Middle umbilical ligament
Isthmus of uterine tube
Left ureter
Uterus
Levator ani muscle
Middle rectal artery and vein
Rectouterine pouch and fold
Inferior rectal lymph nodes
Sacrospinous ligament
Middle rectal artery
Internal pudendal artery
Vaginal artery
Uterine artery and vein
Superior rectal lymph node
Rectum
Superior rectal artery and vein
Iliolumbar artery
Middle sacral artery and vein

Figure 285.1 Lymph Vessels and Nodes of the Female Pelvis ▲

NOTE: (1) The lymph nodes in the pelvis lie along the course of the major vessels. Lymphatic channels drain superiorly and posteriorly to right and left **lumbar nodes,** which lie bilaterally along the psoas major muscles on both sides of the aorta.

(2) Lymph from the bladder drains laterally to **external iliac** and **internal iliac nodes.** These nodes also receive lymph from the fundus, body and cervix of the uterus, and vagina in women and the prostate and seminal vesicles in men.

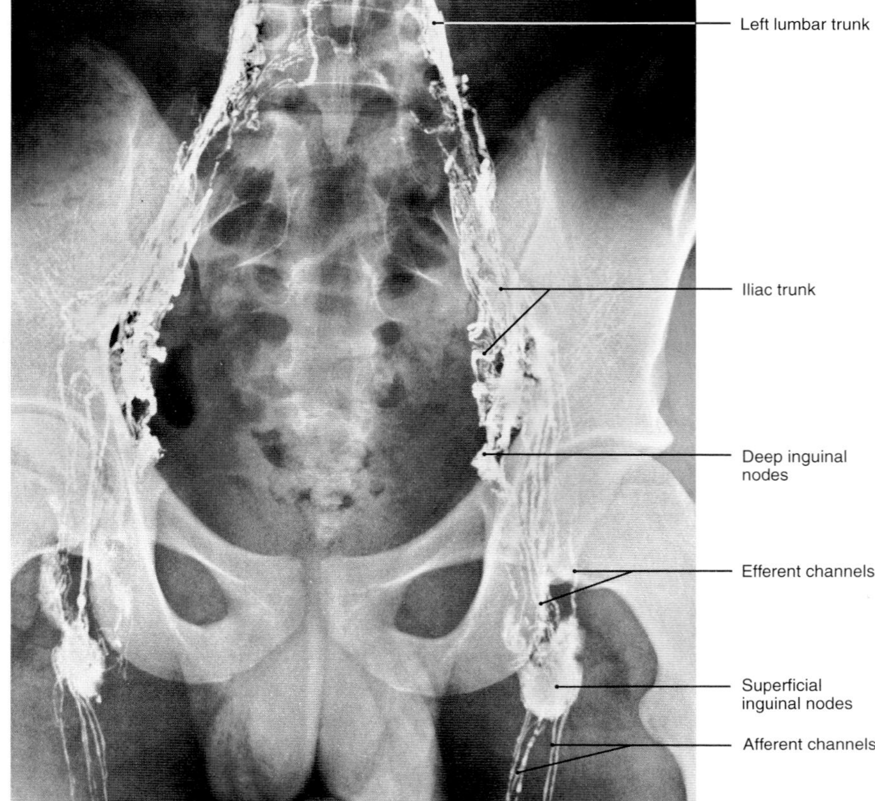
Left lumbar trunk
Iliac trunk
Deep inguinal nodes
Efferent channels
Superficial inguinal nodes
Afferent channels

Figure 285.2 Lymphograph of Pelvis and Lumbar Region ▶

NOTE: This lymphograph shows lymphatic channels along the femoral vessels (below) and their connections with iliac and lumbar lymph nodes (above).

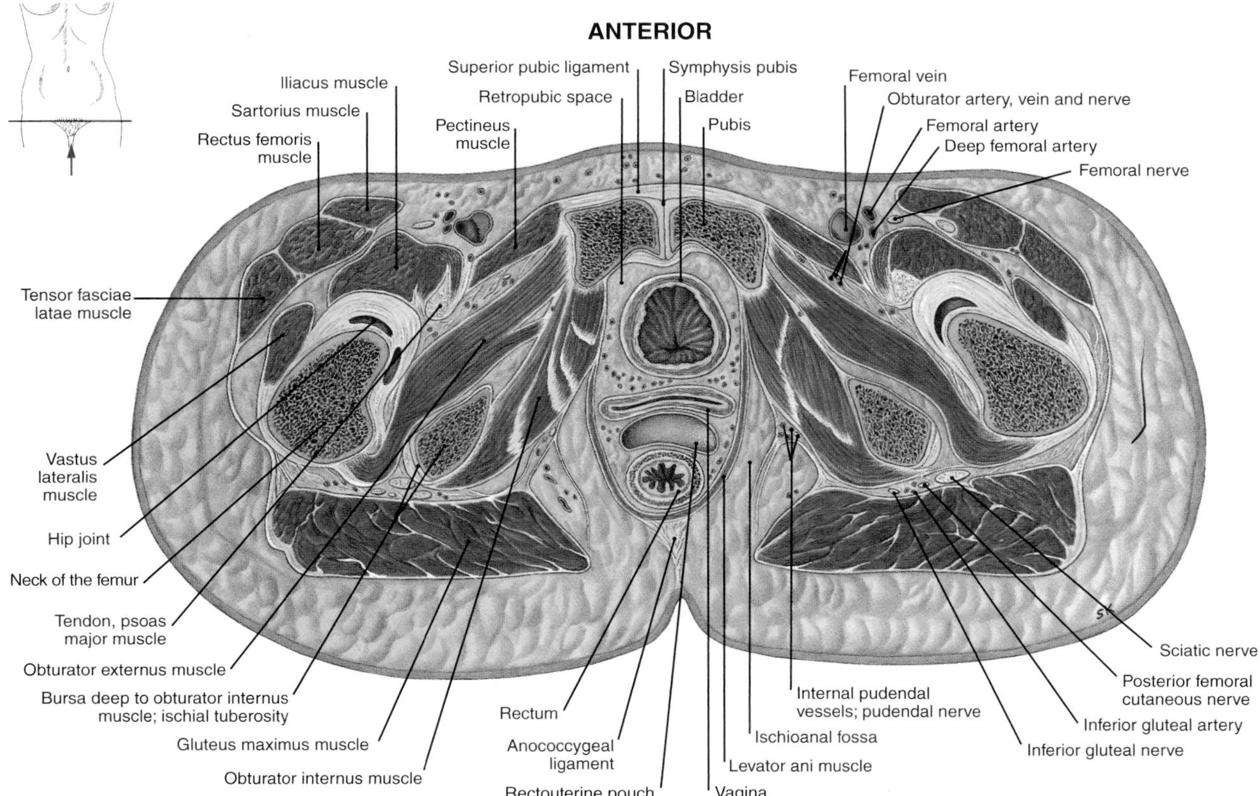
ANTERIOR
Iliacus muscle
Sartorius muscle
Rectus femoris muscle
Superior pubic ligament
Retropubic space
Pectineus muscle
Symphysis pubis
Bladder
Pubis
Femoral vein
Obturator artery, vein and nerve
Femoral artery
Deep femoral artery
Femoral nerve
Tensor fasciae latae muscle
Vastus lateralis muscle
Hip joint
Neck of the femur
Tendon, psoas major muscle
Obturator externus muscle
Bursa deep to obturator internus muscle; ischial tuberosity
Gluteus maximus muscle
Obturator internus muscle
Rectum
Anococcygeal ligament
Rectouterine pouch
Vagina
Levator ani muscle
Ischioanal fossa
Internal pudendal vessels; pudendal nerve
Inferior gluteal nerve
Inferior gluteal artery
Posterior femoral cutaneous nerve
Sciatic nerve

Figure 286.1 Cross Section of the Female Pelvis at the Level of the Symphysis Pubis

NOTE: The viscera medially and the **obturator internus muscle** laterally in the pelvis. Observe also the attachment of the **levator ani muscle** from the fascia overlying the obturator internus muscle and how the levator separates the pelvis from the perineum below. Compare this figure with Fig. 286.2.

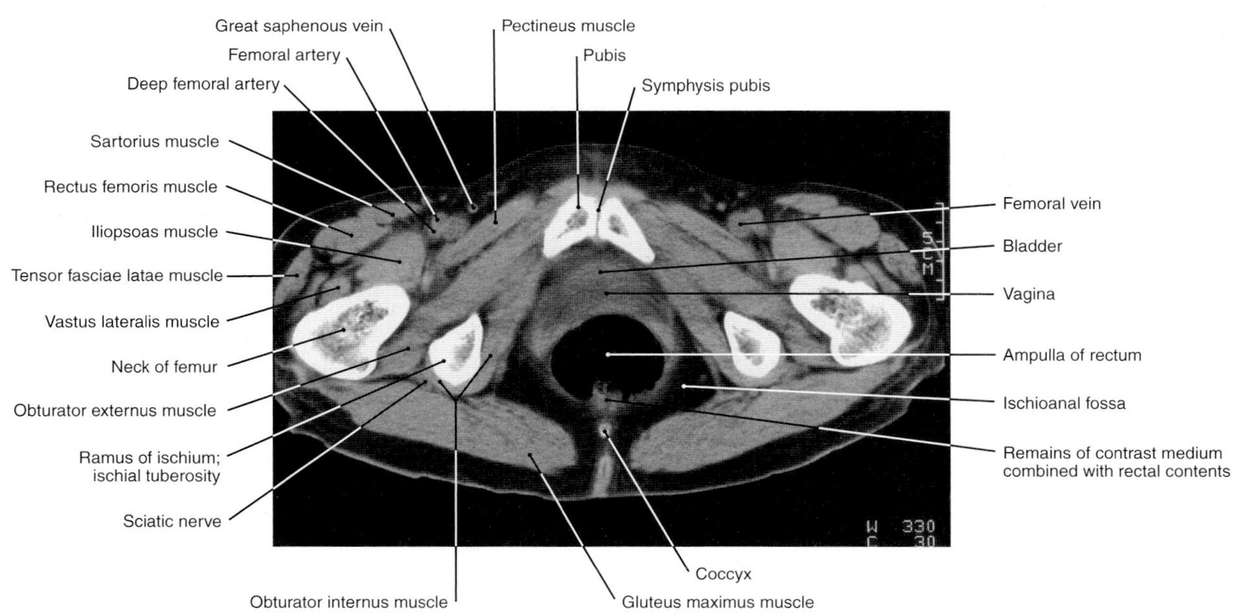
Great saphenous vein
Femoral artery
Deep femoral artery
Pectineus muscle
Pubis
Symphysis pubis
Sartorius muscle
Rectus femoris muscle
Iliopsoas muscle
Tensor fasciae latae muscle
Vastus lateralis muscle
Neck of femur
Obturator externus muscle
Ramus of ischium; ischial tuberosity
Sciatic nerve
Femoral vein
Bladder
Vagina
Ampulla of rectum
Ischioanal fossa
Remains of contrast medium combined with rectal contents
W 330
C 30
Obturator internus muscle
Coccyx
Gluteus maximus muscle

Figure 286.2 CT of the Female Pelvis Taken from Below

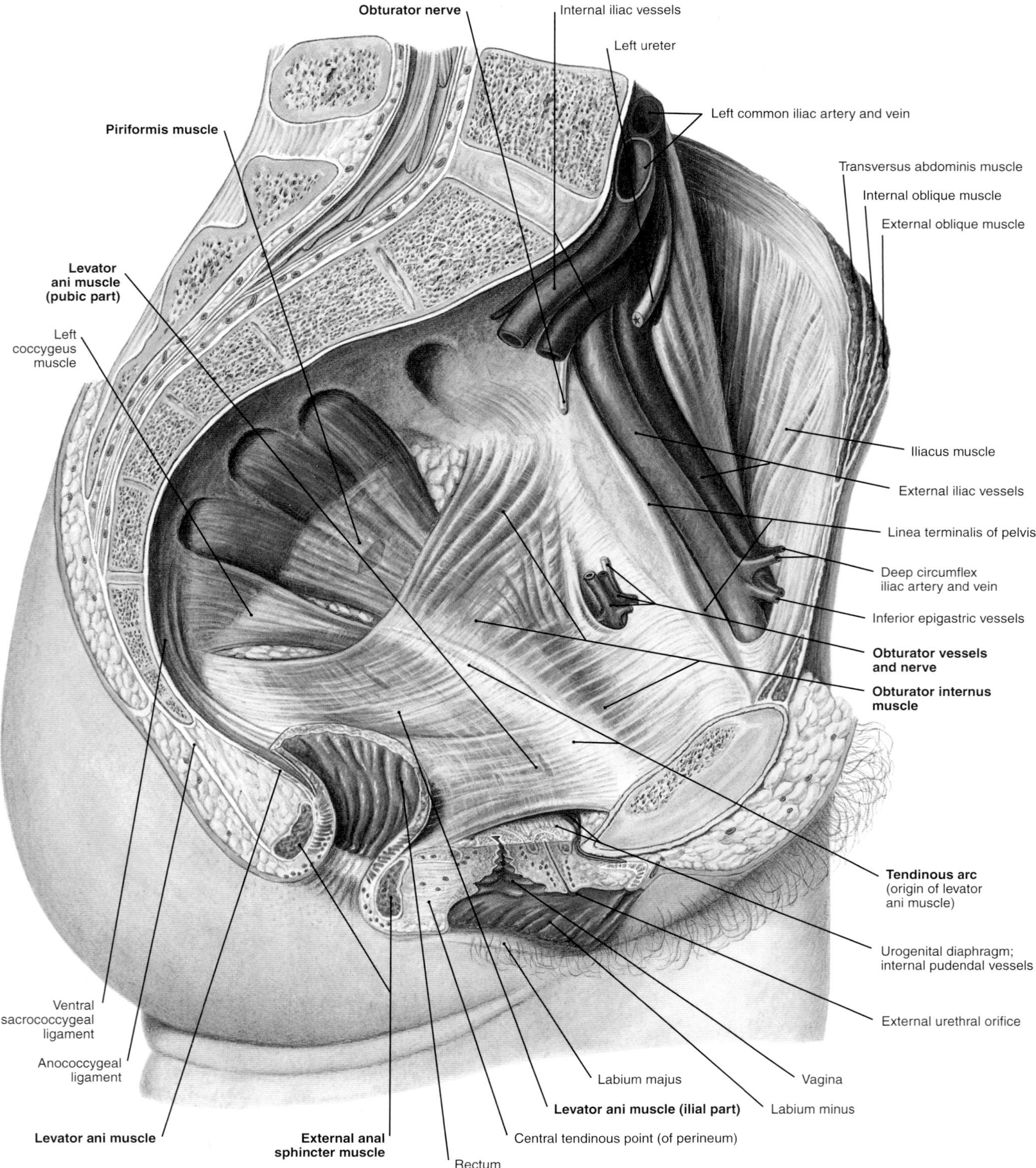
Obturator nerve
Internal iliac vessels
Left ureter
Left common iliac artery and vein
Piriformis muscle
Transversus abdominis muscle
Internal oblique muscle
External oblique muscle
Levator ani muscle (pubic part)
Left coccygeus muscle
Iliacus muscle
External iliac vessels
Linea terminalis of pelvis
Deep circumflex iliac artery and vein
Inferior epigastric vessels
Obturator vessels and nerve
Obturator internus muscle
Tendinous arc (origin of levator ani muscle)
Urogenital diaphragm; internal pudendal vessels
External urethral orifice
Ventral sacrococcygeal ligament
Anococcygeal ligament
Labium majus
Vagina
Levator ani muscle (ilial part)
Labium minus
Levator ani muscle
External anal sphincter muscle
Central tendinous point (of perineum)
Rectum

Figure 287 Muscles of the Lateral Wall and Floor of the Female Pelvis (Left Side)

NOTE: (1) The lateral wall of the true pelvis is covered by the piriformis and obturator internus muscles, whereas the floor is formed by the pubic and ischial parts of the levator ani muscle, and more posteriorly, by the coccygeus muscle.

(2) The **piriformis muscle** arises from the ventral surface of the second, third, and fourth sacral vertebrae, but it is studied with the gluteal muscles because its fibers converge and leave the pelvis through the greater sciatic foramen.

(3) The **obturator internus muscle** arises from the lateral and anterior wall of the true bony pelvis and it surrounds the obturator foramen (note obturator vessels and nerve). Its tendon passes out of the pelvis to the gluteal region through the lesser sciatic foramen.

(4) Both the **pubic** and **ischial** parts of the **levator ani muscle** arise from the tendinous arc of the obturator internus fascia.

Cauda equina
Erector spinae muscle
Common iliac artery
5th lumbar vertebra
Common iliac vein
Spinal nerve
Sympathetic trunk
Femoral nerve
Ureter
Psoas minor tendon
Ileum
Gluteus medius muscle
Psoas major muscle
Cecum
Iliacus muscle
Ilium
Transversus abdominis muscle
Sigmoid colon
Internal oblique muscle
Suspensory ligament of ovary
External oblique muscle
Uterine tube
Uterine tube, fimbriae
Round ligament of uterus
Fundus of uterus
Lateral umbilical fold
Ovary
Inferior epigastric artery
Urinary bladder
Rectus abdominis muscle
Linea alba
Median umbilical fold

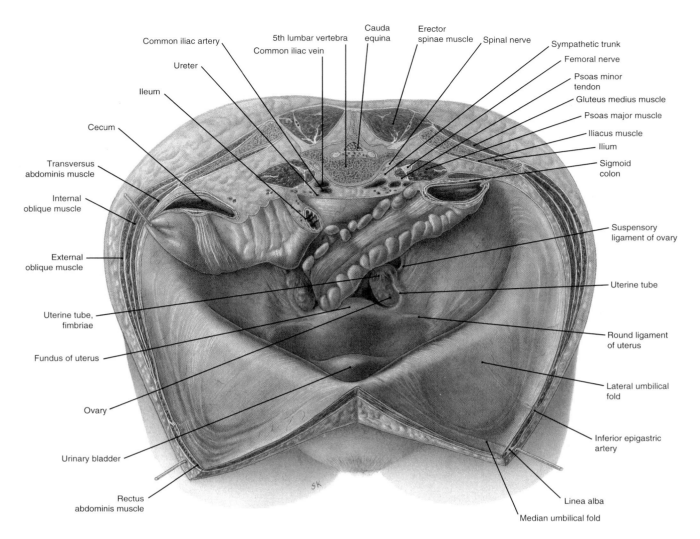

Figure 288.1 Superior View of Female Pelvic Organs at the Level of L5

NOTE: (1) The fundus of the uterus, uterine tube, ovary, round ligament, and the urinary bladder anterior to the uterus and bladder posterior to the uterus;

(2) The peritoneum overlies the pelvic organs. It descends anterior to the bladder and between the bladder and uterus and between the uterus and rectum.

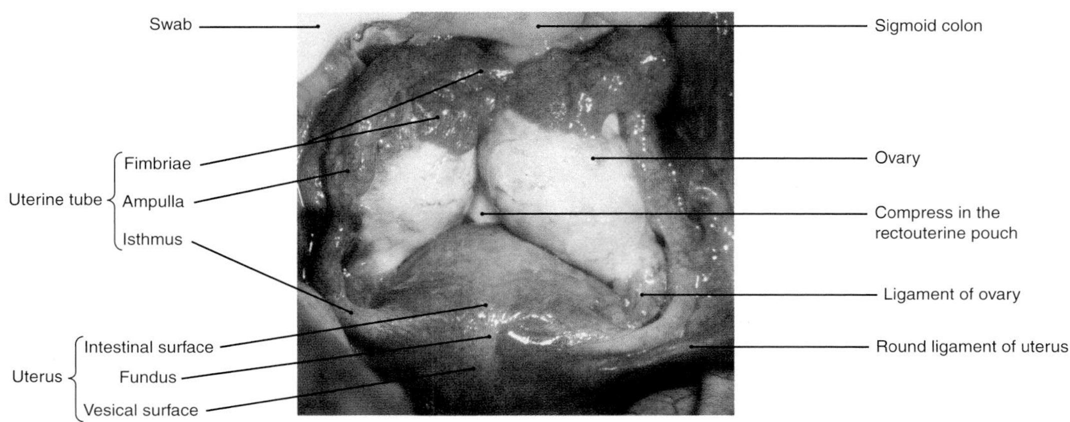
Swab
Sigmoid colon
Uterine tube
Fimbriae
Ampulla
Isthmus
Ovary
Compress in the rectouterine pouch
Ligament of ovary
Uterus
Intestinal surface
Fundus
Vesical surface
Round ligament of uterus

Figure 288.2 Surgical Exposure of the Internal Genitalia in a Young Female

NOTE: (1) The ovaries are displaced superomedially by compresses in the rectouterine pouch (of Douglas).

(2) The **fimbria, ampulla, and isthmus of the uterine tube.** On the right side, observe the **ligament of the ovary** and the **round ligament of the uterus.**

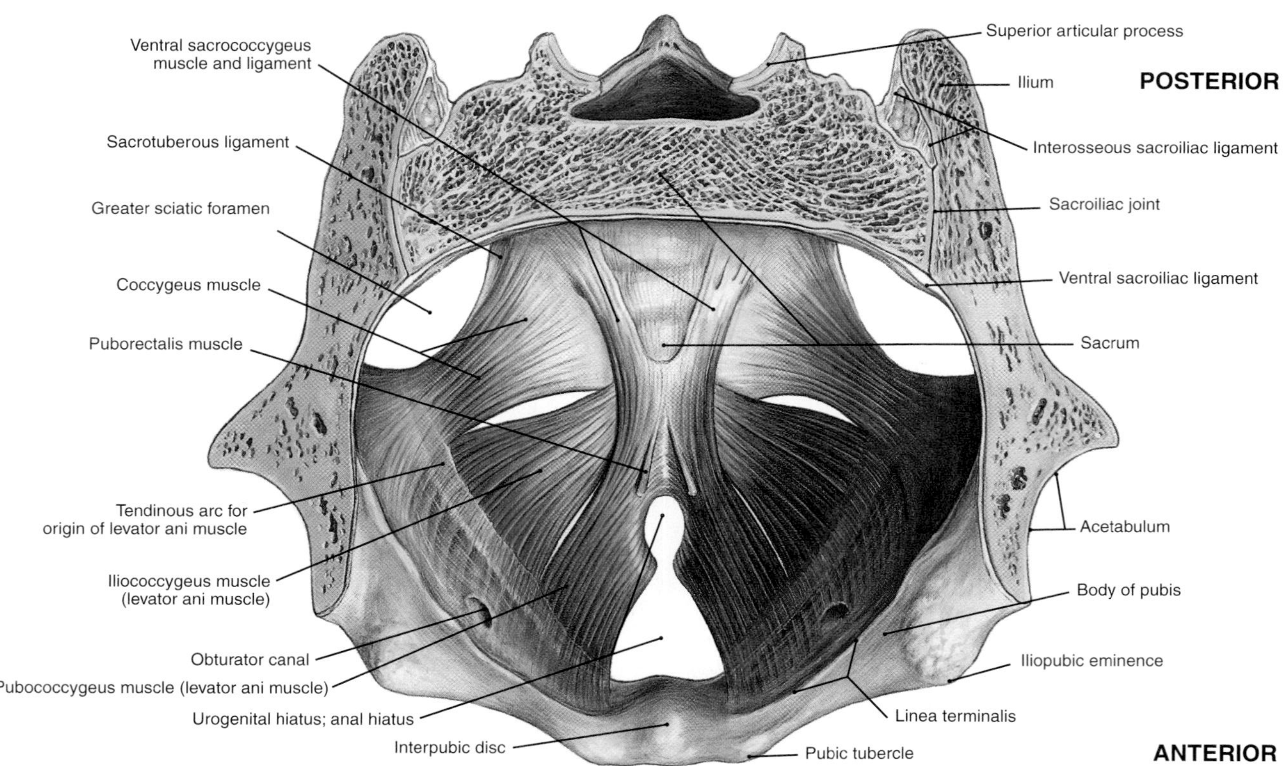
Ventral sacrococcygeus muscle and ligament
Sacrotuberous ligament
Greater sciatic foramen
Coccygeus muscle
Puborectalis muscle
Tendinous arc for origin of levator ani muscle
Iliococcygeus muscle (levator ani muscle)
Obturator canal
Pubococcygeus muscle (levator ani muscle)
Urogenital hiatus; anal hiatus
Interpubic disc
Superior articular process
Ilium
POSTERIOR
Interosseous sacroiliac ligament
Sacroiliac joint
Ventral sacroiliac ligament
Sacrum
Acetabulum
Body of pubis
Iliopubic eminence
Linea terminalis
Pubic tubercle
ANTERIOR

Figure 289.1 Muscular Floor of the Female Pelvis Viewed from Above

NOTE: (1) The muscular floor of the pelvis is formed anteriorly by the **pubococcygeus** and anterolaterally by the **iliococcygeus** portions of the **levator ani muscle** and posterolaterally by the **coccygeus muscle**, which lies above the sacrotuberous ligament.

(2) At the **urogenital hiatus** is located the **urogenital (UG) diaphragm,** which is formed by the deep transverse perineal muscles and the membranous sphincter of the urethra, which lie between two layers of fascia (see Fig. 296.2). The urethra and vagina penetrate through the UG diaphragm in the female.

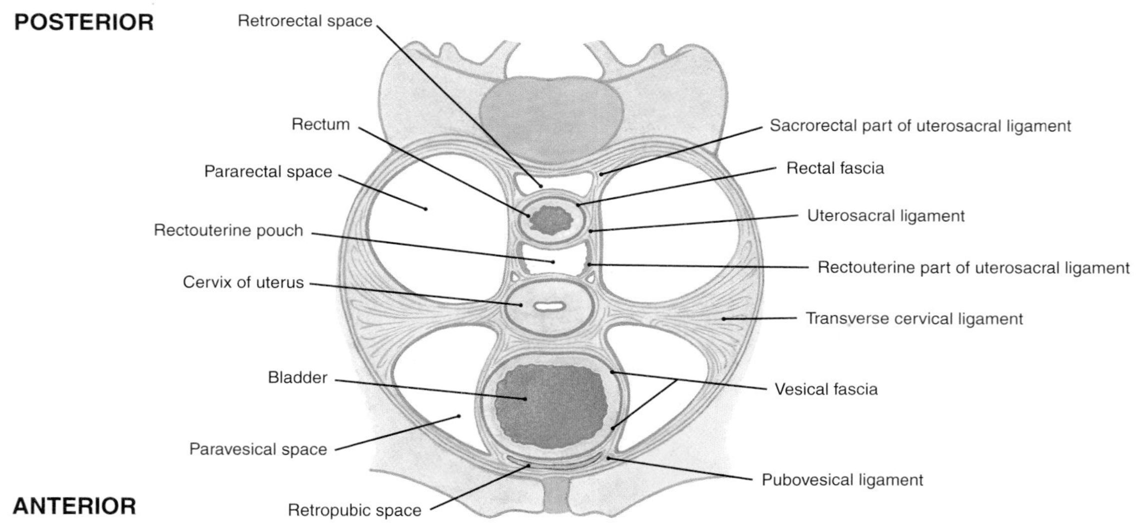
POSTERIOR
Retrorectal space
Rectum
Pararectal space
Rectouterine pouch
Cervix of uterus
Bladder
Paravesical space
Retropubic space
ANTERIOR
Sacrorectal part of uterosacral ligament
Rectal fascia
Uterosacral ligament
Rectouterine part of uterosacral ligament
Transverse cervical ligament
Vesical fascia
Pubovesical ligament

Figure 289.2 Uterine Ligaments at the Cervix Just above the Pelvic Floor (Diagram)

NOTE: (1) Just above the floor of the pelvis (formed by the levator ani and coccygeus muscles) is located the cervix of the uterus in women. Extending laterally from the uterine cervix and from the upper vagina to the fascia covering the levator ani muscles are the **transverse cervical ligaments** (also called **lateral cervical, cardinal,** or **Mackenrodt's ligaments**).

(2) The transverse cervical ligaments are located at the base of the broad ligaments and below the uterine vessels. Observe that the **uterosacral ligaments** also attach to the cervix and upper vagina, but course backward around the rectum to the front of the sacrum.

(3) The uterus is supported in position by (a) its attachment to the bladder and rectum, (b) the transverse cervical and uterosacral ligaments, and (c) the musculature that forms the pelvic floor and urogenital diaphragm.

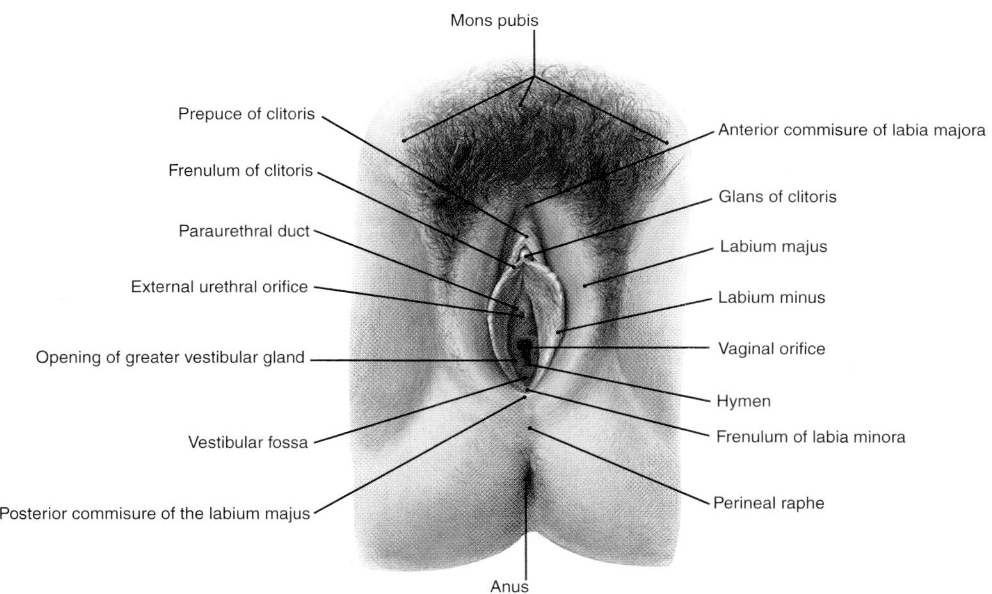
Mons pubis
Prepuce of clitoris
Anterior commisure of labia majora
Frenulum of clitoris
Glans of clitoris
Paraurethral duct
Labium majus
External urethral orifice
Labium minus
Opening of greater vestibular gland
Vaginal orifice
Hymen
Frenulum of labia minora
Vestibular fossa
Perineal raphe
Posterior commisure of the labium majus
Anus

Figure 290.1 External Genitalia of an 18-Year-Old Virgin

NOTE: (1) The female **external genitalia** are (a) the mons pubis, (b) the labia majora, (c) the labia minora, (d) the clitoris, and (e) the vestibule of the vagina. The **orifices** of the female perineum include the openings of the (a) urethra, (b) vagina, (c) ducts of the two greater vestibular glands, (d) small paraurethral ducts (of Skene), and (e) anus.

(2) The **mons pubis** is a rounded mound of skin and adipose tissue anterior to the symphysis pubis; in the adult it is covered with genital hair.

(3) The **labia majora** are two elongated folds of skin and fat extending from the mons pubis toward the anus. They vary in size and thickness depending on age and obesity, and their anterior ends receive the fibrous round ligaments of the uterus. The labia majora are the female structures homologous to the male scrotum.

(4) The **labia minora** are two thin folds of skin situated between the labia majora. They commence at the glans clitoris, and small extensions pass over the dorsum of the clitoris to form the **prepuce.** Posteriorly, they meet in the midline to form the **frenulum.**

(5) The **clitoris** is the homologue of the male penis. It is an erectile organ that measures one inch or less in length and consists of two corpora cavernosa attached by crura to the pubic rami. It is suspended by a fibrous ligament and capped by the **glans.**

(6) The **vestibule** of the vagina is the region between the two labia minora. Into it open the **urethra,** the **ducts of the greater vestibular glands,** and the **vagina.** In the virgin, the vaginal orifice is partially closed by a thin membrane, the **hymen,** which usually is ruptured at first copulation. Since its form and extent are quite variable, virginity cannot be absolutely determined by its absence.

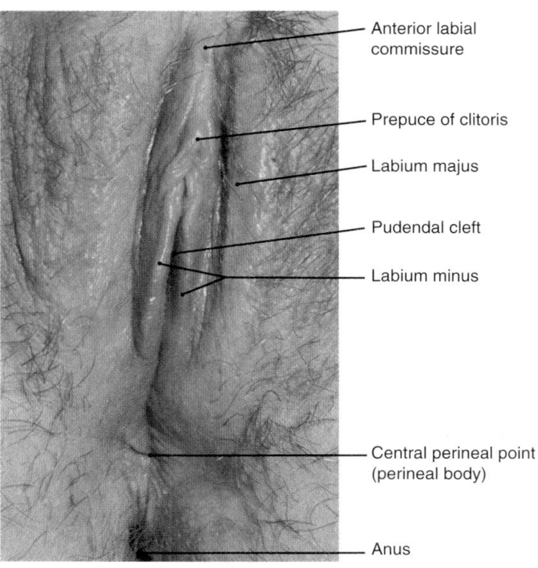
Anterior labial commissure
Prepuce of clitoris
Labium majus
Pudendal cleft
Labium minus
Central perineal point (perineal body)
Anus

Figure 290.2 Perineal Structures in a 26-Year-Old Woman

NOTE: In this photograph the labia minora are approximated so that the vaginal and urethral orifices are not visible.

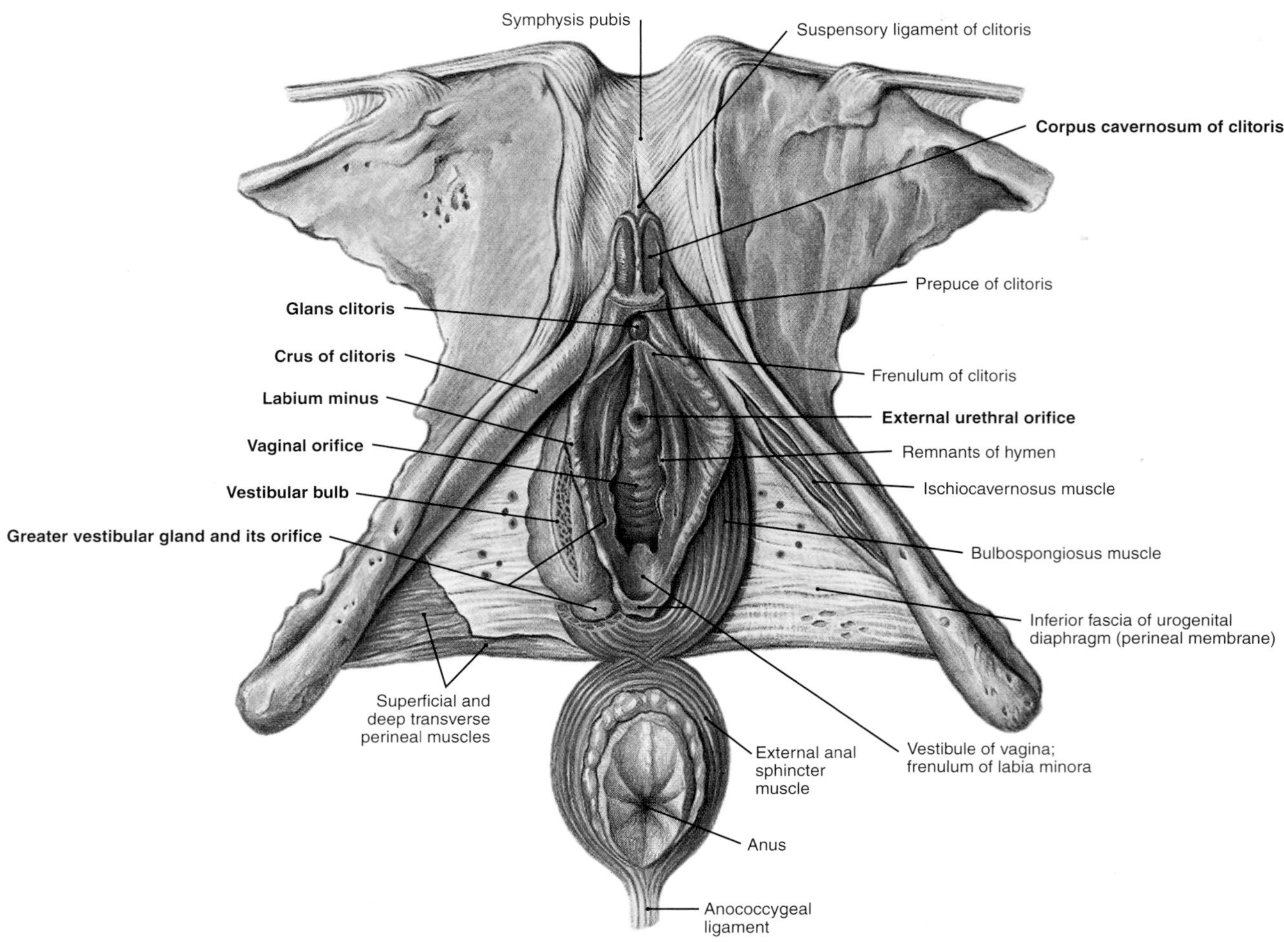
Symphysis pubis
Suspensory ligament of clitoris
Corpus cavernosum of clitoris
Prepuce of clitoris
Glans clitoris
Crus of clitoris
Frenulum of clitoris
Labium minus
External urethral orifice
Vaginal orifice
Remnants of hymen
Ischiocavernosus muscle
Vestibular bulb
Greater vestibular gland and its orifice
Bulbospongiosus muscle
Inferior fascia of urogenital diaphragm (perineal membrane)
Superficial and deep transverse perineal muscles
External anal sphincter muscle
Vestibule of vagina; frenulum of labia minora
Anus
Anococcygeal ligament

Figure 291.1 Dissected Female External Genitalia

NOTE: (1) The skin and fascia of the labia majora have been removed. Observe the **crura, body** and **glans clitoris**, the **vestibular bulbs,** and the location of the **greater vestibular glands.**

(2) Each crus of the clitoris is covered by an **ischiocavernosus muscle,** and the vestibular bulbs are surrounded by the **bulbospongiosus muscles.**

(3) The **greater vestibular glands** (of Bartholin) are found just behind the vestibular bulbs. During sexual stimulation, they secrete a viscous fluid that lubricates the vagina.

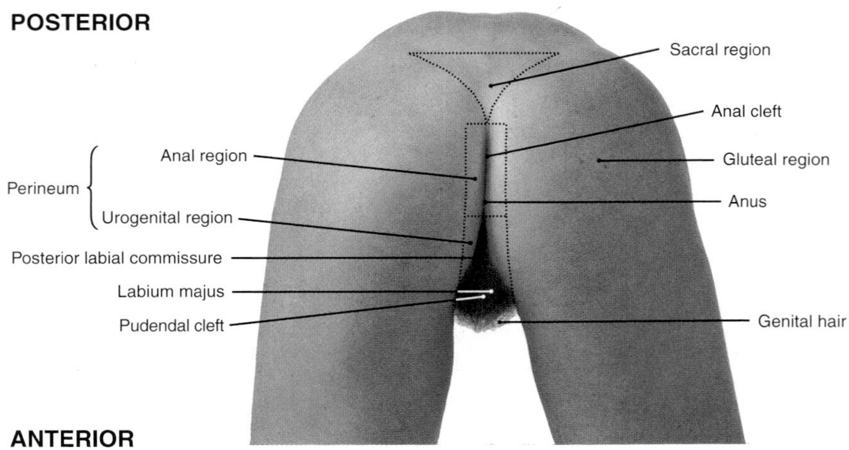
POSTERIOR
Sacral region
Anal cleft
Gluteal region
Anus
Perineum
Anal region
Urogenital region
Posterior labial commissure
Labium majus
Pudendal cleft
Genital hair
ANTERIOR

Figure 291.2 Surface Anatomy of the Female Sacral, Gluteal, and Perineal Regions (Posteroinferior View)

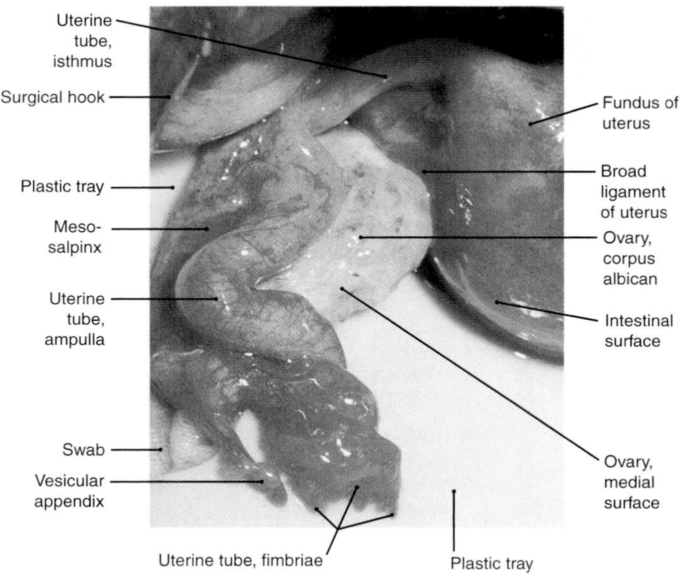

Uterine tube, isthmus
Surgical hook
Plastic tray
Meso-salpinx
Uterine tube, ampulla
Swab
Vesicular appendix
Uterine tube, fimbriae
Plastic tray
Ovary, medial surface
Intestinal surface
Ovary, corpus albican
Broad ligament of uterus
Fundus of uterus

Figure 292.1 Uterine Tube and Ovary
NOTE that this is a surgical exposure of the ovary, uterine tube, and its fimbriated opening.

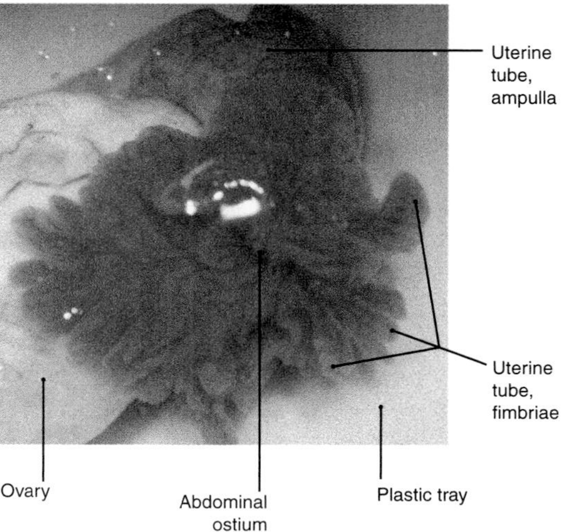

Uterine tube, ampulla
Uterine tube, fimbriae
Plastic tray
Abdominal ostium
Ovary

Figure 292.2 Abdominal Opening of the Uterine Tube
NOTE the fimbriated opening and ampulla of the uterine tube.

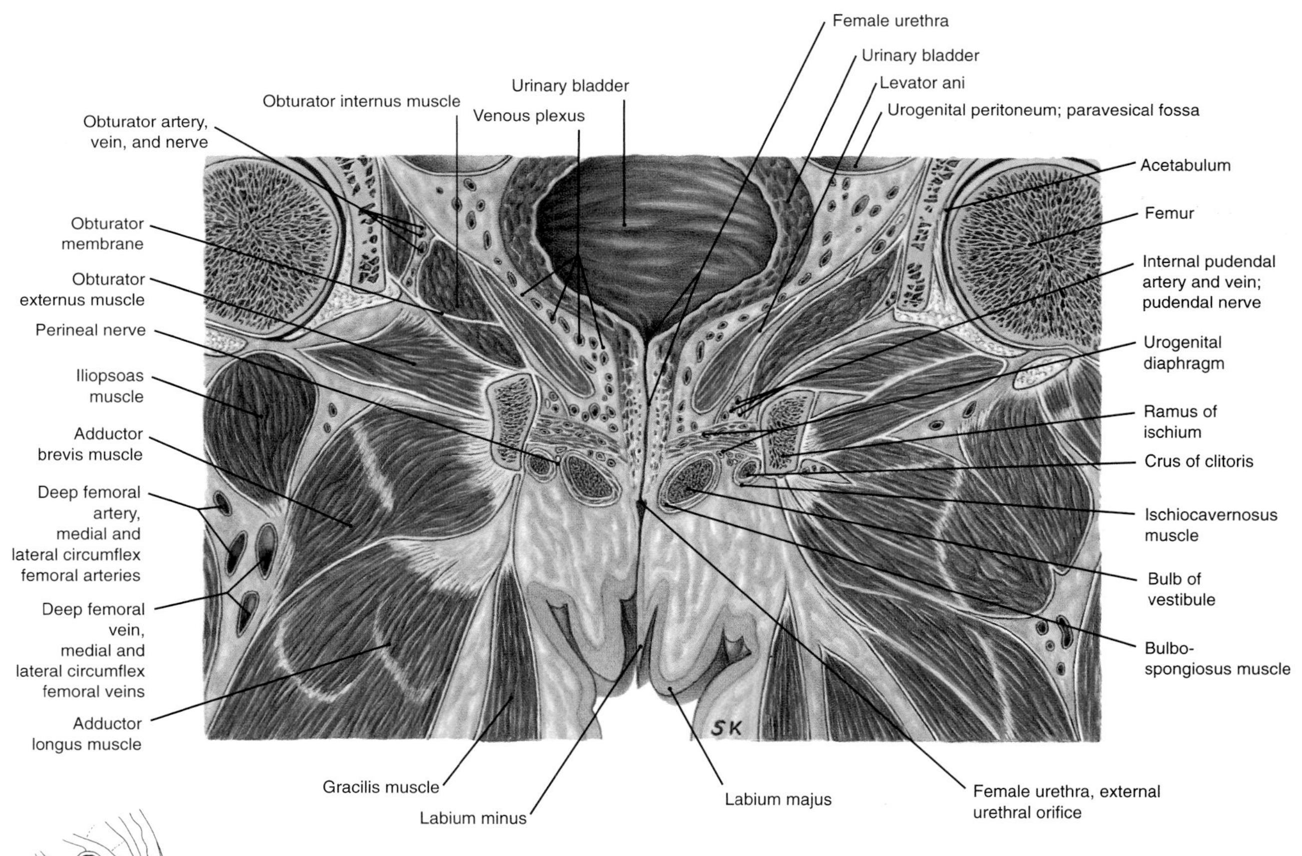

Female urethra
Urinary bladder
Levator ani
Urogenital peritoneum; paravesical fossa
Acetabulum
Femur
Internal pudendal artery and vein; pudendal nerve
Urogenital diaphragm
Ramus of ischium
Crus of clitoris
Ischiocavernosus muscle
Bulb of vestibule
Bulbo-spongiosus muscle
Female urethra, external urethral orifice
Labium majus
Labium minus
Gracilis muscle
Adductor longus muscle
Deep femoral vein, medial and lateral circumflex femoral veins
Deep femoral artery, medial and lateral circumflex femoral arteries
Adductor brevis muscle
Iliopsoas muscle
Perineal nerve
Obturator externus muscle
Obturator membrane
Obturator artery, vein, and nerve
Obturator internus muscle
Urinary bladder
Venous plexus
SK

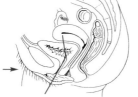

Figure 292.3 Oblique Section of the Female Pelvis (Anterior View)
NOTE that this section goes through the urinary bladder and urethra.

SUPERFICIAL MUSCLES OF THE UROGENITAL REGION

Muscle	Origin	Insertion	Innervation	Action
Superficial transverse perineal muscle (male and female)	Medial and anterior part of the ischial tuberosity	Into the perineal body (female) or central tendinous point (male) in front of the anus	Perineal branch of the pudendal nerve (S2, S3, S4)	Simultaneous contraction of the two muscles helps to fix the central tendinous point of the perineum.
Ischiocavernosus muscle (female)	Inner surface of the ischial tuberosity behind the crus clitoris and from the adjacent part of the ramus of the ischium	Fibers end in an aponeurosis, which inserts onto the sides and under the surface of the crus clitoris.	Perineal branch of the pudendal nerve (S2, S3, S4)	Compresses the crus clitoris, retarding the return of blood and thereby helping to maintain erection of the clitoris.
Ischiocavernosus muscle (male)	Inner surface of the ischial tuberosity behind the crus penis and from the ramus of the ischium on each side of the crus	Fibers end in an aponeurosis attached to the sides and under surface of the corpus cavernosum on each side as they join to form the body of the penis.	Perineal branch of the pudendal nerve (S2, S3, S4)	Compresses the crus penis and thereby helps to maintain erection.
Bulbospongiosus muscle (female)	Fibers attached posteriorly to the perineal body	Fibers pass anteriorly around the vagina and are inserted into the corpora cavernosa clitoris.	Perineal branch of the pudendal nerve (S2, S3, S4)	Decreases the orifice of the vagina; anterior fibers assist erection of the clitoris by compressing the deep dorsal vein of the clitoris.
Bulbospongiosus muscle (male)	From the central tendinous point and the ventral extension of the median raphe between the two bulbospongiosus muscles.	**Posterior fibers:** end in connective tissue of the fascia of UG diaphragm. **Middle fibers:** encircle the bulb of the penis and the corpus spongiosum. **Anterior fibers:** spread over the side of the corpus cavernosum and extend anteriorly as a tendinous expansion over the dorsal vessels.	Perineal branch of the pudendal nerve (S2, S3, S4)	Aids in emptying the urethra at end of urination; by compressing the dorsal vein, it also helps maintain penile erection; contracts during ejaculation.

Figure 293 Internal Anatomy of the Vaginal Wall

NOTE: (1) The uterus, external female genitalia, and opened vaginal wall are viewed from above.

(2) The vaginal rugae that characterize the inner vaginal wall. Note also the slit-like external os of the uterus and a mucous plug between its anterior and posterior lips.

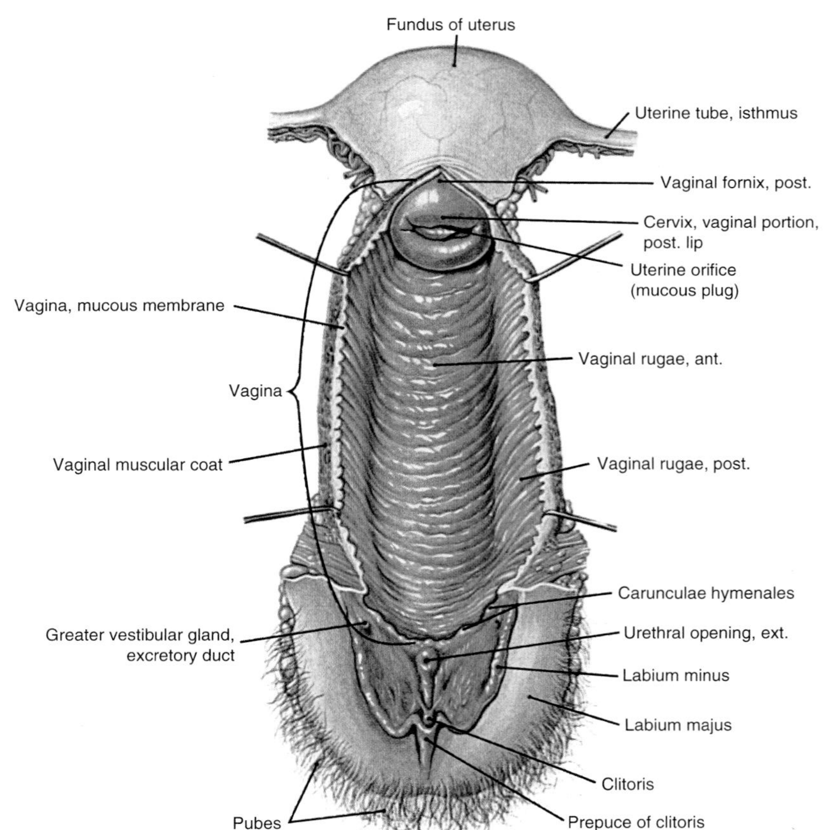
Fundus of uterus
Uterine tube, isthmus
Vaginal fornix, post.
Cervix, vaginal portion, post. lip
Uterine orifice (mucous plug)
Vagina, mucous membrane
Vaginal rugae, ant.
Vagina
Vaginal muscular coat
Vaginal rugae, post.
Carunculae hymenales
Greater vestibular gland, excretory duct
Urethral opening, ext.
Labium minus
Labium majus
Clitoris
Pubes
Prepuce of clitoris

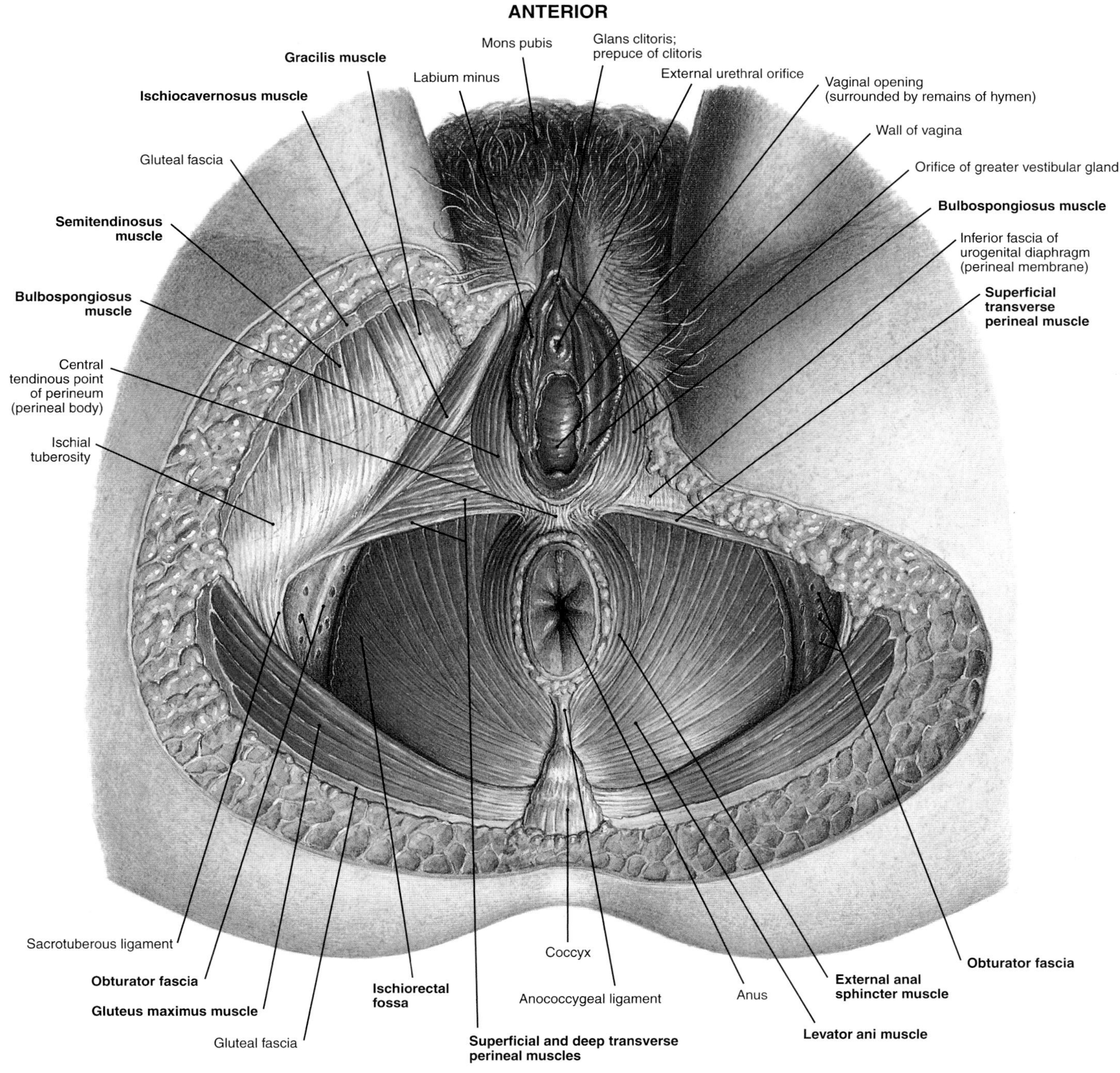
ANTERIOR
Mons pubis
Glans clitoris; prepuce of clitoris
Gracilis muscle
Labium minus
External urethral orifice
Ischiocavernosus muscle
Vaginal opening (surrounded by remains of hymen)
Wall of vagina
Gluteal fascia
Orifice of greater vestibular gland
Bulbospongiosus muscle
Semitendinosus muscle
Inferior fascia of urogenital diaphragm (perineal membrane)
Bulbospongiosus muscle
Superficial transverse perineal muscle
Central tendinous point of perineum (perineal body)
Ischial tuberosity
Sacrotuberous ligament
Coccyx
Obturator fascia
Obturator fascia
Ischiorectal fossa
External anal sphincter muscle
Anococcygeal ligament
Anus
Gluteus maximus muscle
Levator ani muscle
Gluteal fascia
Superficial and deep transverse perineal muscles
POSTERIOR

Figure 294 Muscles of the Female Perineum

NOTE: (1) The perineum is a diamond-shaped region located below the pelvis and separated from it by the muscular pelvic diaphragm. The perineum is bounded by the **symphysis pubis** anteriorly, the **coccyx** posteriorly and the two **ischial tuberosities** laterally. A line drawn across the perineum anterior to the anus between the two ischial tuberosities divides the perineum into an anterior **urogenital region** and a posterior **anal region.**

(2) The *urogenital region* contains the external genitalia and the associated muscles and glands. Often books refer to *superficial and deep perineal compartments* (spaces or pouches). The **superficial perineal compartment** lies superficial to the inferior layer of fascia of the urogenital diaphragm, and it contains the ischiocavernosus, bulbocavernosus, and superficial transverse perineal muscles and the perineal vessels and nerves. It is limited superficially by a layer of deep fascia (the external perineal fascia) just deep to **Colles' fascia.**

(3) The **deep perineal compartment** is the space enclosed between the two layers of the urogenital diaphragm. It contains the deep transverse perineal and urethral sphincter muscles and is traversed by the urethra and the vagina in the female.

(4) The *anal region* is situated posterior to the urogenital region; it contains the anus surrounded by the external anal sphincter muscle. A large portion of the anal region is occupied by the two fat-filled **ischiorectal fossae.**

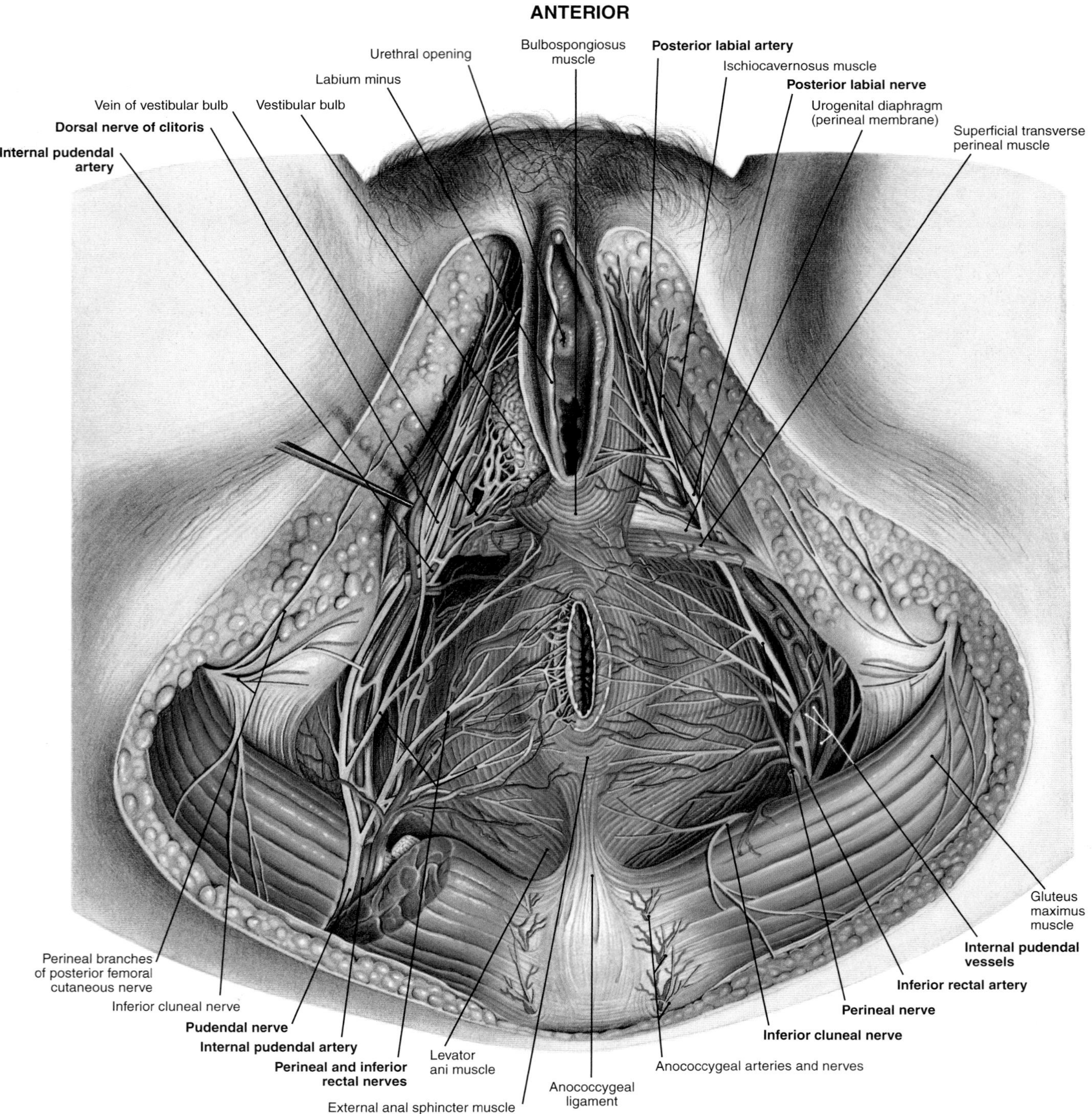
ANTERIOR
Urethral opening
Bulbospongiosus muscle
Posterior labial artery
Ischiocavernosus muscle
Labium minus
Posterior labial nerve
Vein of vestibular bulb
Vestibular bulb
Urogenital diaphragm (perineal membrane)
Dorsal nerve of clitoris
Superficial transverse perineal muscle
Internal pudendal artery
Gluteus maximus muscle
Internal pudendal vessels
Perineal branches of posterior femoral cutaneous nerve
Inferior rectal artery
Inferior cluneal nerve
Perineal nerve
Pudendal nerve
Inferior cluneal nerve
Internal pudendal artery
Levator ani muscle
Perineal and inferior rectal nerves
Anococcygeal arteries and nerves
Anococcygeal ligament
External anal sphincter muscle
POSTERIOR

Figure 295 Nerves and Blood Vessels of the Female Perineum

NOTE: (1) The branches of the **pudendal nerve** supply most of the perineal structures. This nerve arises from the second, third, and fourth sacral segments of the spinal cord. Within the pelvis it is joined by the **internal pudendal artery and vein.** The vessels and nerve leave the pelvis through the greater sciatic foramen along the lower border of the piriformis muscle, cross the ischial spine to reenter the pelvis through the lesser sciatic foramen.

(2) The pudendal structures reach the perineum by way of the **pudendal canal** (of Alcock) deep to the fascia of the obturator internus muscle. Their branches, the **inferior rectal vessels** and **nerves,** cross the ischiorectal fossa toward the midline to supply the levator ani and external anal sphincter muscles as well as other structures in the anal region.

(3) The pudendal vessels and nerve then continue anteriorly as the **perineal vessels** and **nerve** and enter the urogenital region by penetrating the urogenital diaphragm. They branch again into superficial and deep branches to supply structures in the superficial and deep compartments. The superficial branches supply the labia majora and the external genital structures, whereas the deep branches supply the muscles, vestibular bulb, and clitoris.

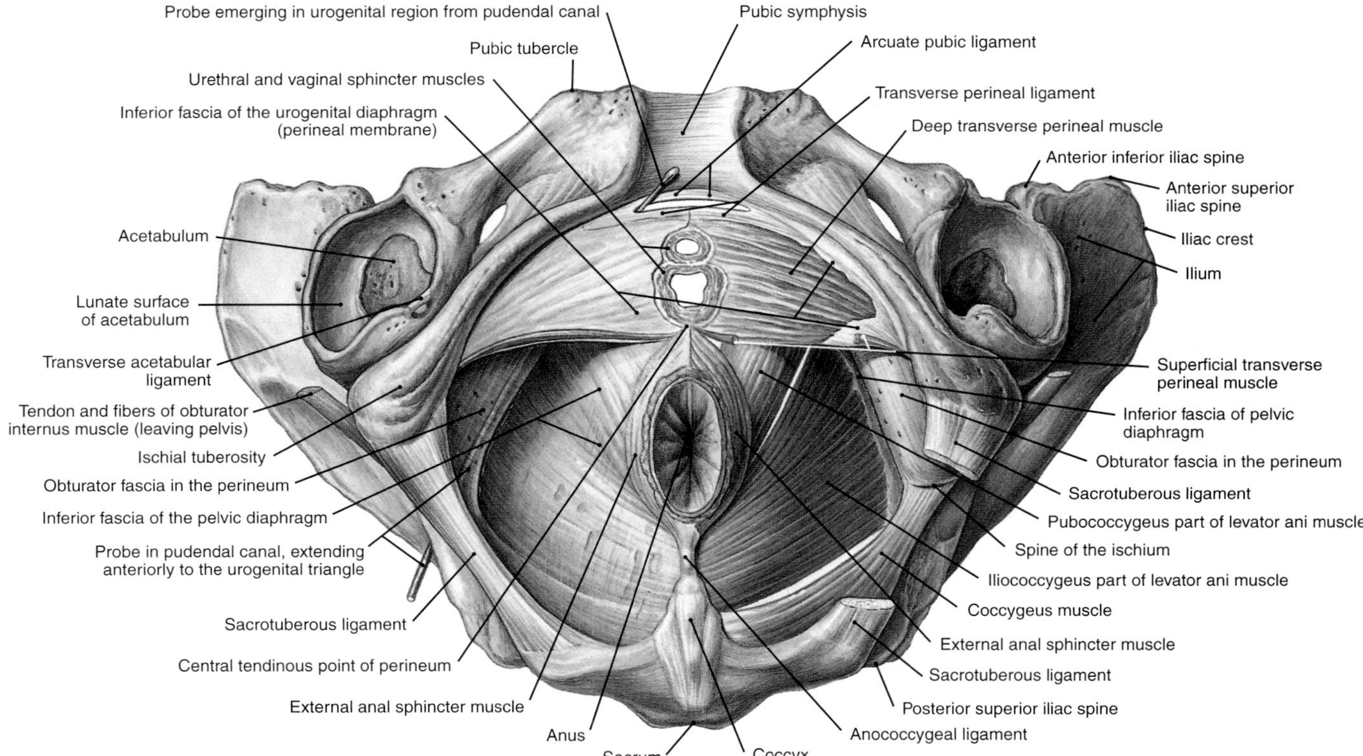

Probe emerging in urogenital region from pudendal canal
Pubic symphysis
Pubic tubercle
Arcuate pubic ligament
Urethral and vaginal sphincter muscles
Transverse perineal ligament
Inferior fascia of the urogenital diaphragm (perineal membrane)
Deep transverse perineal muscle
Anterior inferior iliac spine
Anterior superior iliac spine
Acetabulum
Iliac crest
Ilium
Lunate surface of acetabulum
Transverse acetabular ligament
Superficial transverse perineal muscle
Tendon and fibers of obturator internus muscle (leaving pelvis)
Inferior fascia of pelvic diaphragm
Ischial tuberosity
Obturator fascia in the perineum
Obturator fascia in the perineum
Sacrotuberous ligament
Inferior fascia of the pelvic diaphragm
Pubococcygeus part of levator ani muscle
Probe in pudendal canal, extending anteriorly to the urogenital triangle
Spine of the ischium
Iliococcygeus part of levator ani muscle
Coccygeus muscle
Sacrotuberous ligament
External anal sphincter muscle
Central tendinous point of perineum
Sacrotuberous ligament
External anal sphincter muscle
Posterior superior iliac spine
Anococcygeal ligament
Anus
Sacrum
Coccyx

Figure 296.1 Musculature of the Floor of the Female Pelvis, Viewed from the Inferior, or Perineal, Aspect

NOTE: (1) On the left side (reader's right) the inferior fascias of the pelvic and urogenital diaphragms have been removed.

(2) The musculature of the urogenital diaphragm completes the anterior part of the female pelvic floor but allows the urethra and vagina to traverse the urogenital hiatus.

(3) The **central point of the perineum** interposed in the midline between the urogenital diaphragm and the anterior end of the raphe formed by the two external anal sphincters.

(4) The anal hiatus is surrounded by the **pubococcygeus** parts of the levator ani muscles. These are reinforced above by the puborectalis muscle and below by the external sphincter. Observe that the **iliococcygeus** sweeps medially to the coccyx, but some fibers also insert into the short midline **anococcygeal raphe** and **ligament.**

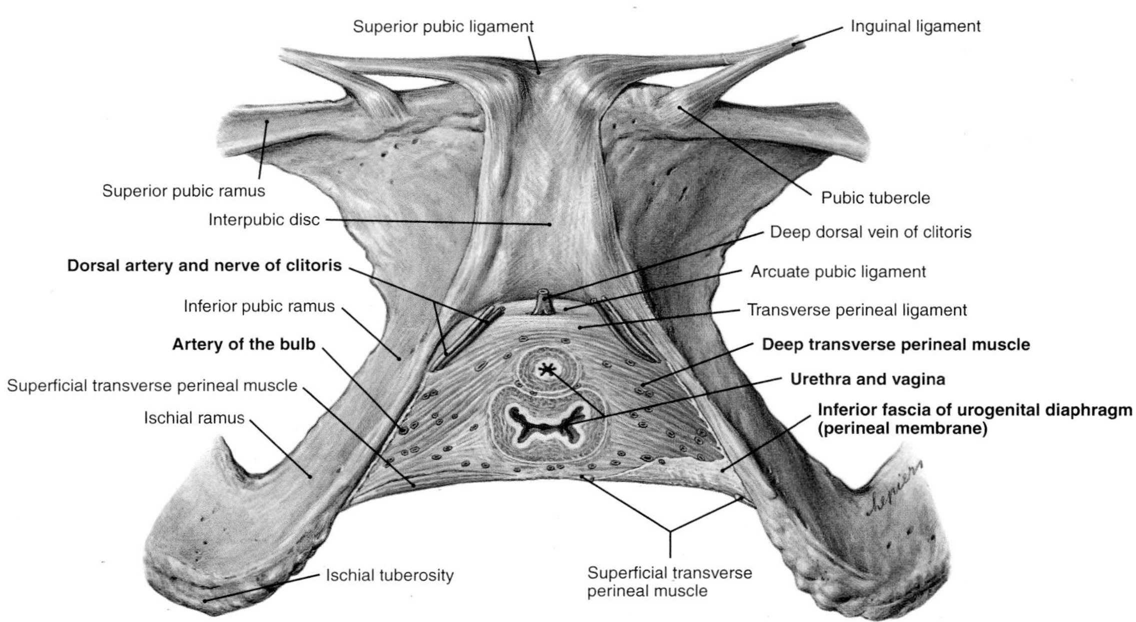

Superior pubic ligament
Inguinal ligament
Superior pubic ramus
Pubic tubercle
Interpubic disc
Deep dorsal vein of clitoris
Dorsal artery and nerve of clitoris
Arcuate pubic ligament
Inferior pubic ramus
Transverse perineal ligament
Artery of the bulb
Deep transverse perineal muscle
Superficial transverse perineal muscle
Urethra and vagina
Ischial ramus
Inferior fascia of urogenital diaphragm (perineal membrane)
Ischial tuberosity
Superficial transverse perineal muscle

Figure 296.2 Urogenital Diaphragm in the Female

NOTE: The female **urethra** and **vagina** both pass through the **urogenital diaphragm.** Observe the circular **sphincter** surrounding the membranous urethra and the **deep transverse perineal muscles** that are covered by deep fascia on both their superior and inferior surfaces.

MUSCLES RELATED TO THE PELVIC DIAPHRAGM

Muscle	Origin	Insertion	Innervation	Action
Levator ani consisting of: pubococcygeus iliococcygeus pubovaginalis levator of prostate puborectalis	From a tendinous arch (along the fascia of the obturator internus muscle). The arch extends from the symphysis pubis to the ischial spine.	Into the coccyx; the anococcygeal raphe and ligament; the external anal sphincter, central tendinous point of the perineum	Pudendal nerve (S3, S4, S5)	Supports and slightly raises the floor of the pelvis; it resists intraabdominal pressure, as in forced expiration.
Coccygeus	Spine of the ischium; sacrospinous ligament	Lateral margin of coccyx and sacrum	Pudendal plexus (S4, S5 nerves)	Draws coccyx forward during parturition or defecation. Supports pelvic floor.
External anal sphincter: Subcutaneous part (a band of fibers just deep to the skin)	Attached anteriorly to the perineal body or central tendinous point and posteriorly to the anococcygeal ligament		Pudendal nerve, rectal branch (S4)	Anal sphincter is in a state of tonic contraction; upon defecation the muscle relaxes.
Superficial part (lies deep to the subcutaneous part; main part of muscle)	From the anococcygeal ligament	Into the perineal body or central tendinous point		
Deep part (forms a complete sphincter of the anal canal	Fibers surround the anal canal and are applied closely to the internal anal sphincter.			

DEEP MUSCLES OF THE UROGENITAL REGION

Muscle	Origin	Insertion	Innervation	Action
Deep transverse perineal muscle (female)	Inferior ramus of the ischium	To the side of the vagina, meeting fibers of the muscle from the other side	Perineal branch of the pudendal nerve (S2, S3, S4)	Helps to fix the perineal body and assists the urethrovaginal sphincter.
Deep transverse perineal muscle (male)	Inferior ramus of the ischium	Fibers course to the median line, where they interlace in a tendinous raphe with fibers from the other side.	Perineal branch of the pudendal nerve (S2, S3, S4)	Helps to fix the perineal body and assists the urethral sphincter.
Urethrovaginal sphincter (female)	Inferior fibers: From the transverse perineal ligament. Superior fibers: From the inner surface of the pubic ramus.	Course backward on both sides of the urethra Encircle the lower end of the urethra	Perineal branch of the pudendal nerve (S2, 3, 4)	Acts as a voluntary constrictor of the urethra and vagina.
Sphincter of the urethra (male) (surrounds the membranous part of the urethra)	Superficial part: From the transverse perineal ligament. Deep part: From the ramus of the pubis.	Most fibers form a circular sphincter that invests the membranous urethra; some fibers join the perineal body.	Perineal branch of the pudendal nerve (S2, S3, S4)	Acts as the voluntary constrictor of the membranous urethra.

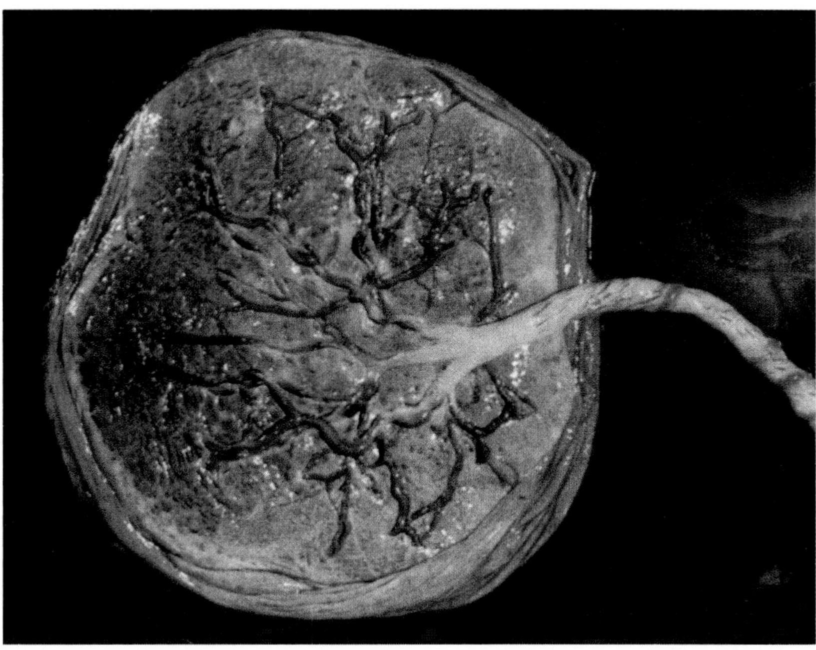

Figure 298.1 Placenta and Umbilical Cord Viewed from the Fetal Surface
NOTE that the fetal surface is smooth and glistening because of the amnion.

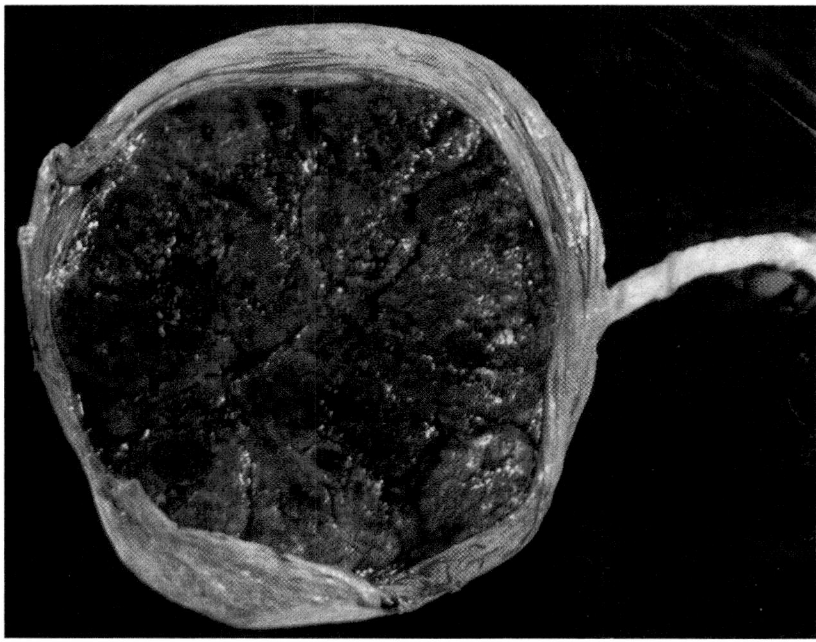

Figure 298.2 Placenta and Umbilical Cord Viewed from the Maternal Surface
NOTE that the maternal surface of the placenta is divided by grooves to form cotyledons, or lobules. There are 15 to 20 cotyledons in the normal human placenta and the surface color is red because of blood.

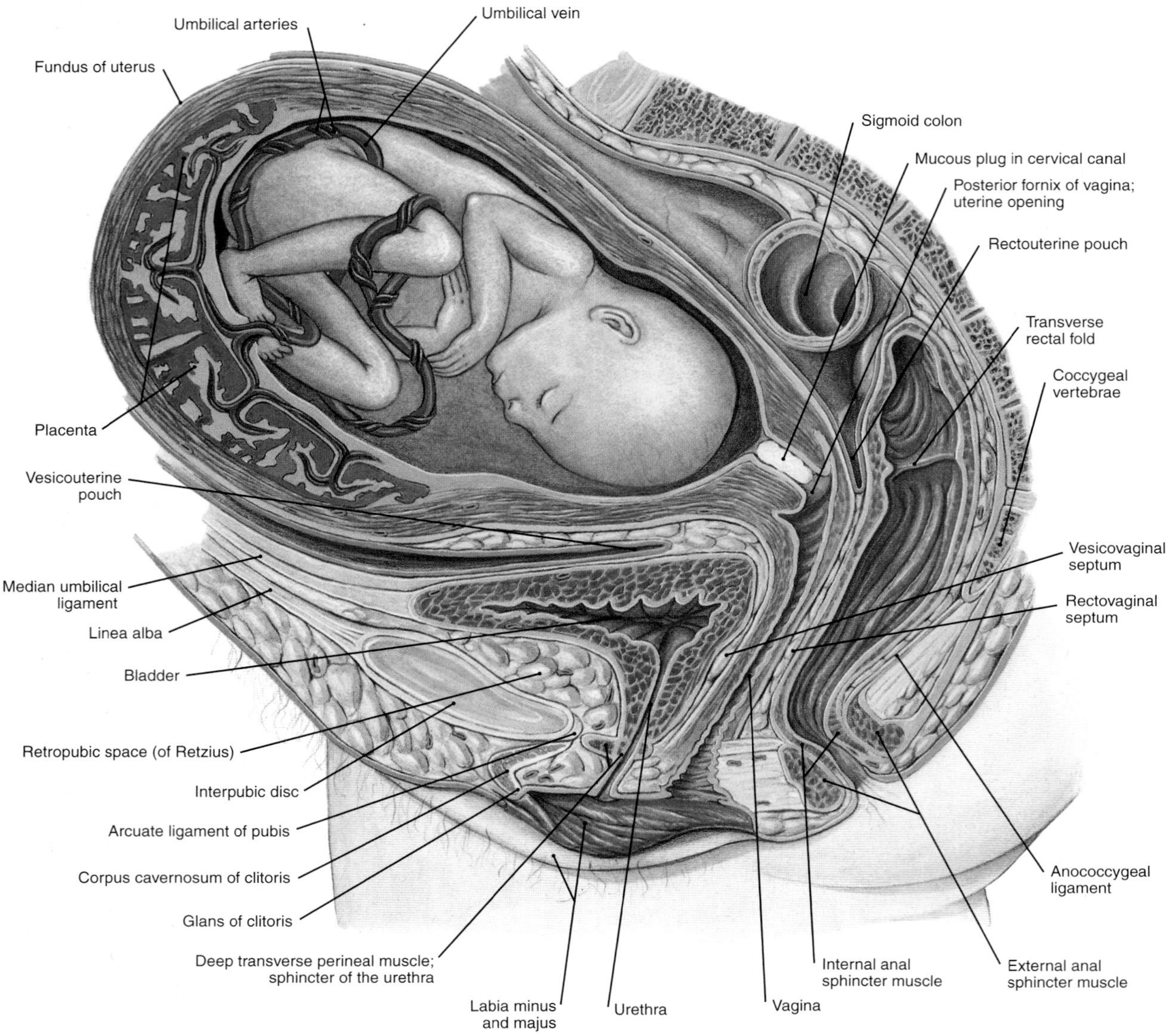

Umbilical arteries
Umbilical vein
Fundus of uterus
Sigmoid colon
Mucous plug in cervical canal
Posterior fornix of vagina; uterine opening
Rectouterine pouch
Transverse rectal fold
Coccygeal vertebrae
Placenta
Vesicouterine pouch
Median umbilical ligament
Linea alba
Bladder
Vesicovaginal septum
Rectovaginal septum
Retropubic space (of Retzius)
Interpubic disc
Arcuate ligament of pubis
Corpus cavernosum of clitoris
Glans of clitoris
Deep transverse perineal muscle; sphincter of the urethra
Labia minus and majus
Urethra
Vagina
Internal anal sphincter muscle
External anal sphincter muscle
Anococcygeal ligament

Figure 299.1 Pregnant Uterus Shortly before Birth, Right Half of Pelvis
NOTE: (1) The pelvis, including the uterus, has been hemisected, while the newborn fetus is shown intact.

(2) In this cephalic longitudinal presentation of the fetus, the placenta is oriented toward the maternal anterior abdominal wall, in contrast to the longitudinal presentation shown in Fig. 300, which shows the back **positioned to the left side of the pelvis.**

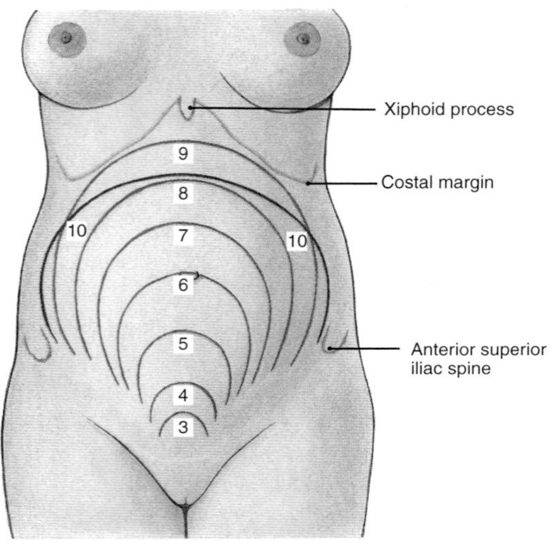
Xiphoid process
Costal margin
Anterior superior iliac spine
9
8
10
7
10
6
5
4
3

Figure 299.2 Diagrammatic Representation of Uterine Growth during Pregnancy (Anterior View)
NOTE: (1) Growth of the uterus is shown in 28-day **lunar months**, hence 10 months rather than 9 calendar months.

(2) By the end of the fourth lunar month, the uterus occupies most of the pelvis. Near the end of pregnancy, it occupies most of the abdomen and extends to the costal margin.

(3) During the last lunar month, the fetus (and fundus of the uterus) descends somewhat, in preparation for the birth process.

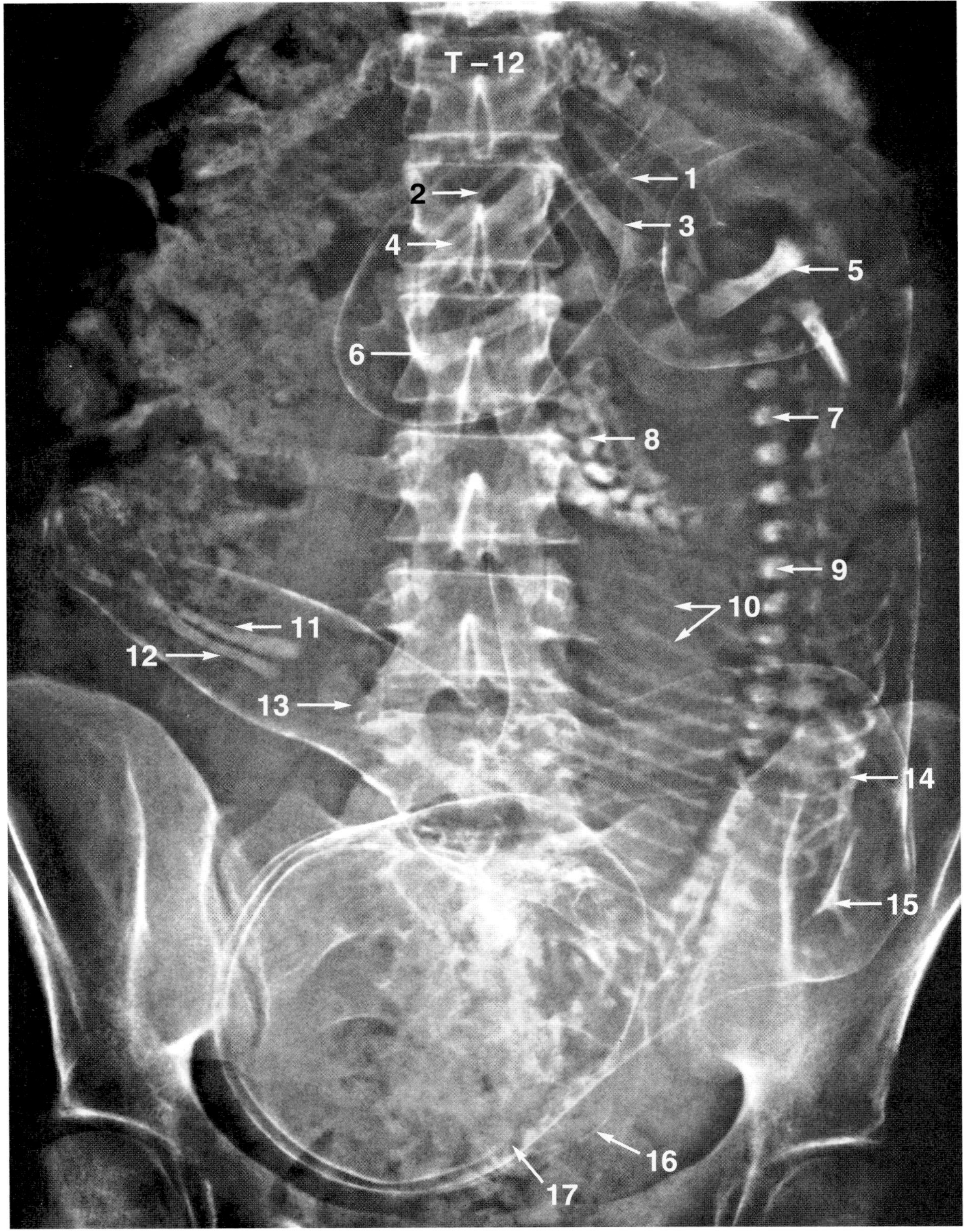
T-12
1
2
3
4
5
6
7
8
9
10
11
12
13
14
15
16
17

Figure 300 Fetal Roentgenogram

NOTE: The body contours of the near-term fetus in utero and a number of the ossifying bones. Observe that the uterus extends to the maternal T12 vertebral body level.

(From Wicke, 6th ed.)

1. Right fibula
2. Left fibula
3. Right tibia
4. Left tibia
5. Right femur
6. Left femur
7. L5 vertebra (fetal)
8. Small intestine (fetal)
9. L1 vertebra (fetal)
10. Ribs
11. Left ulna
12. Left radius
13. Left humerus
14. Right humerus
15. Right scapula
16. External ear
17. Fetal head

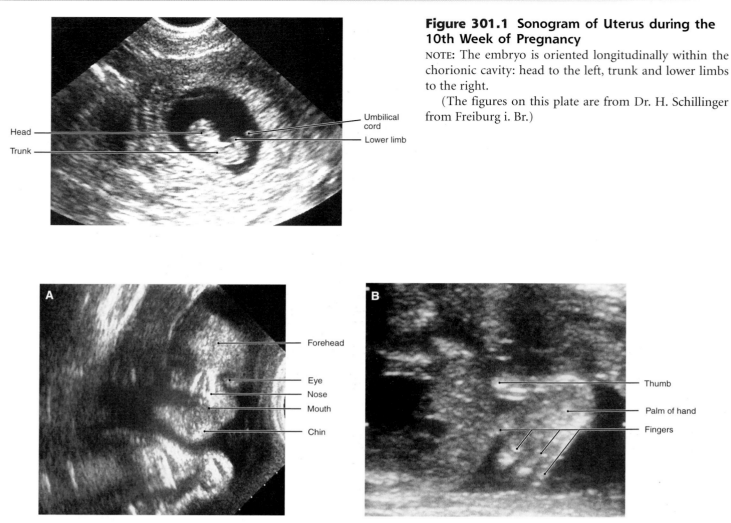

Head
Trunk
Umbilical cord
Lower limb

Figure 301.1 Sonogram of Uterus during the 10th Week of Pregnancy

NOTE: The embryo is oriented longitudinally within the chorionic cavity: head to the left, trunk and lower limbs to the right.

(The figures on this plate are from Dr. H. Schillinger from Freiburg i. Br.)

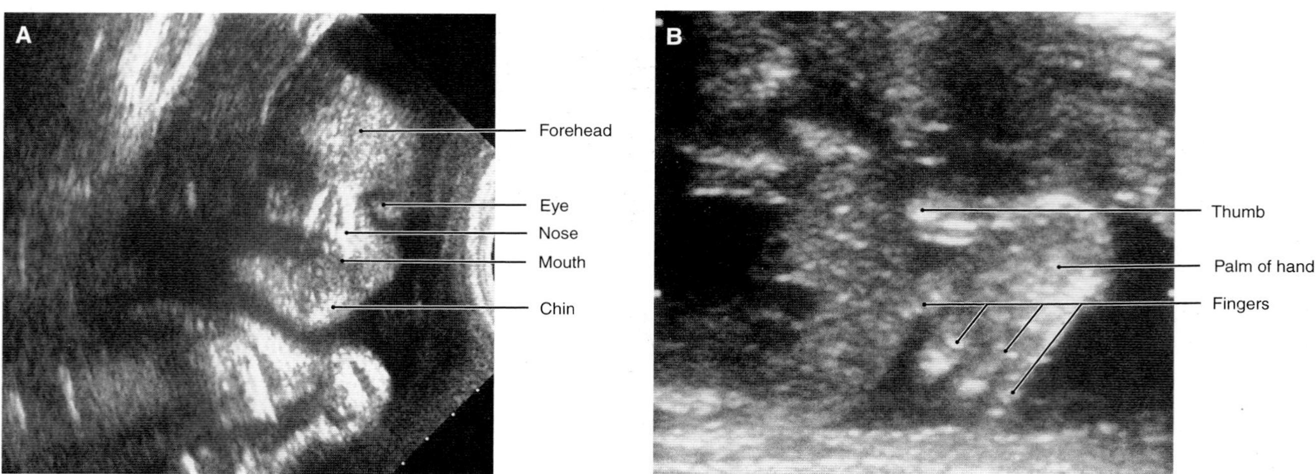
A
Forehead
Eye
Nose
Mouth
Chin
B
Thumb
Palm of hand
Fingers

Figure 301.2A and B Sonogram of Uterus during the 24th Week of Pregnancy

NOTE: (1) In A, a frontal section through the face shows the facial features of the fetus, presenting the fetal "portrait."

(2) In B, the sonogram shows the fetal hand, clearly demonstrating all of the fingers and the thumb.

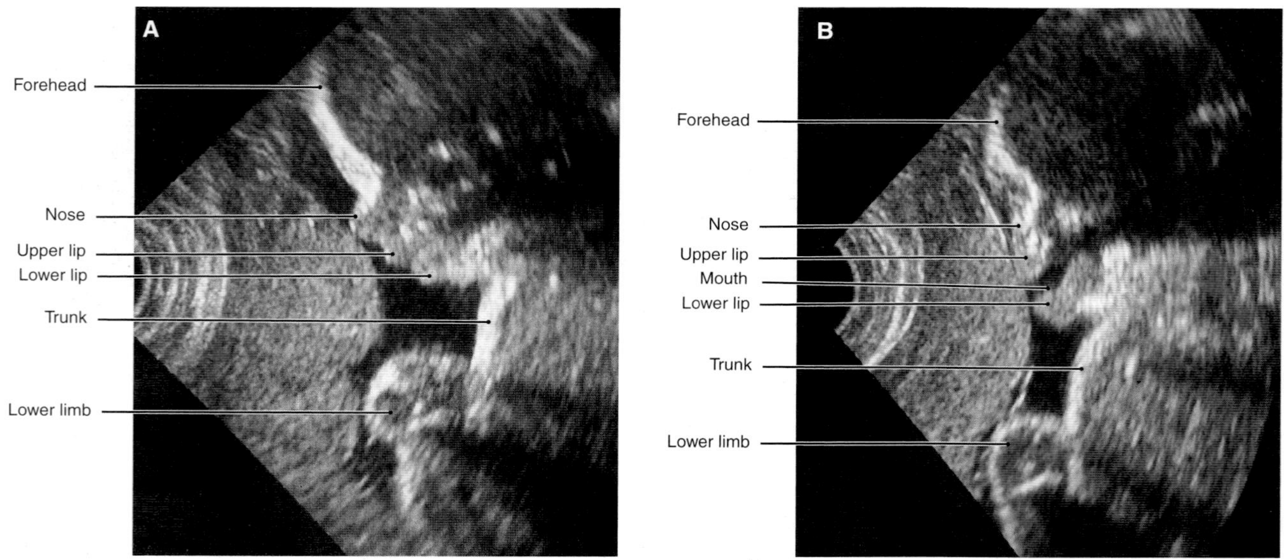
A
Forehead
Nose
Upper lip
Lower lip
Trunk
Lower limb
B
Forehead
Nose
Upper lip
Mouth
Lower lip
Trunk
Lower limb

Figure 301.3A and B Sonogram of Uterus during 28th Week of Pregnancy

NOTE: (1) In A, the longitudinal section shows the fetal head and body in profile.

(2) In B, the fetus has opened its mouth and expanded its trunk, indicating the sporadic diaphragmatic and swallowing movements that occur during the latter part of fetal life, when large amounts of amniotic fluid are ingested.

Ventral ramus, S2 nerve; spinal branch, lateral sacral vessels
Ventral ramus, S1 nerve; spinal branch, lateral sacral vessels
Ventral ramus, L5 nerve; lumbar artery and vein
External and internal iliac veins
Common iliac artery
Sigmoid mesocolon
Left ureter
Ductus deferens
Sigmoid colon; appendices epiploicae
Peritoneum over bladder
Urinary bladder
Rectus abdominis muscle
Pubis
Puboprostatic ligament (pubovesical ligament)
Spermatic cord
Ductus deferens
Cremaster muscle
Dartos layer (scrotum)
Crus penis; deep artery of penis
Ischiocavernosus muscle
Deep transverse perineal muscle; urogenital diaphragm
Urethral sphincter muscle
Prostate gland
Bulbourethral gland and duct
Bulbospongiosus muscle
Deep transverse perineal muscle
External anal sphincter muscle
Rectum, perineal flexure
Anococcygeal ligament
Levator ani muscle
Anococcygeal ligament
Seminal vesicle
Sacrococcygeal joint
Rectovesical pouch
Rectum, sacral flexure
Gluteus maximus muscle
Piriformis muscle
Parietal peritoneum
Sacrum

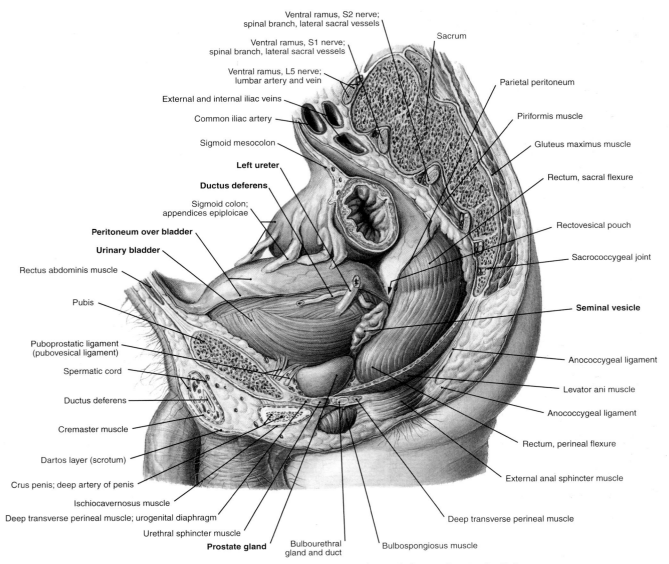

Figure 302.1 Male Pelvic Organs Viewed from the Left Side

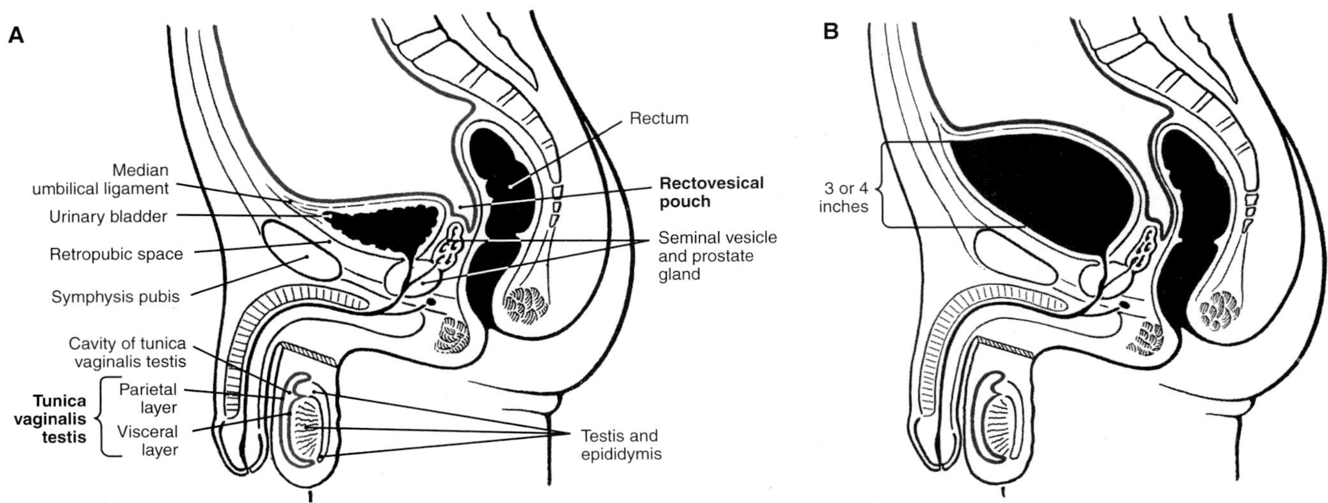
A
Median umbilical ligament
Urinary bladder
Retropubic space
Symphysis pubis
Cavity of tunica vaginalis testis
Tunica vaginalis testis
Parietal layer
Visceral layer
Rectum
Rectovesical pouch
Seminal vesicle and prostate gland
Testis and epididymis
B
3 or 4 inches

Figure 302.2A and B Peritoneal Reflection over the Pelvic Organs: Empty and Full Bladder

NOTE: (1) When the bladder is empty (**A**), the peritoneum extends down to the level of the symphysis pubis, but when the bladder is full (**B**), the peritoneum is elevated 3 or 4 in.

(2) The prostate and bladder may be reached **without entering the peritoneal cavity** anteriorly above the pubis and through the perineum by ascending in front of the rectum.

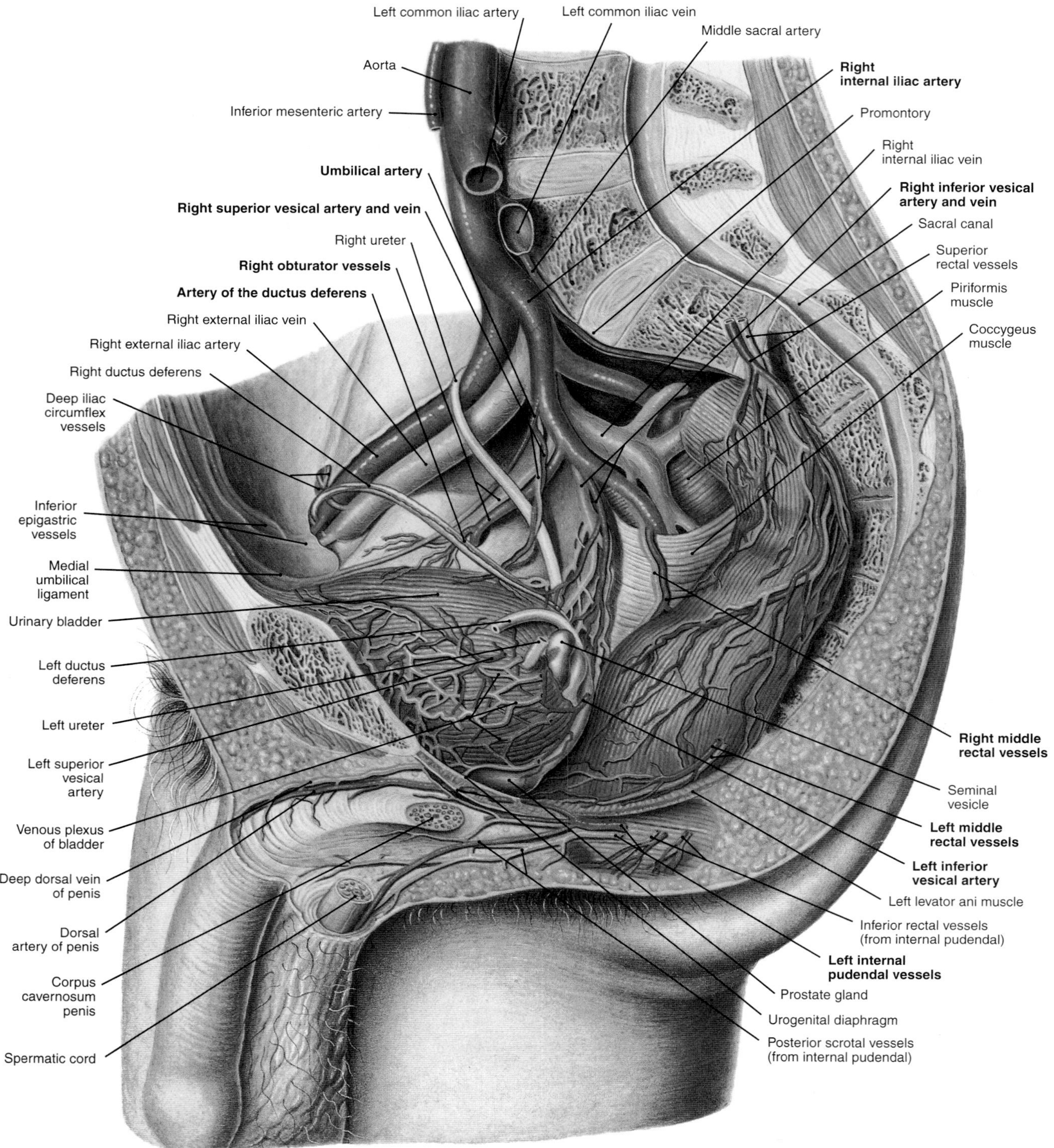
Left common iliac artery
Left common iliac vein
Middle sacral artery
Aorta
Inferior mesenteric artery
Umbilical artery
Right superior vesical artery and vein
Right ureter
Right obturator vessels
Artery of the ductus deferens
Right external iliac vein
Right external iliac artery
Right ductus deferens
Deep iliac circumflex vessels
Inferior epigastric vessels
Medial umbilical ligament
Urinary bladder
Left ductus deferens
Left ureter
Left superior vesical artery
Venous plexus of bladder
Deep dorsal vein of penis
Dorsal artery of penis
Corpus cavernosum penis
Spermatic cord
Right internal iliac artery
Promontory
Right internal iliac vein
Right inferior vesical artery and vein
Sacral canal
Superior rectal vessels
Piriformis muscle
Coccygeus muscle
Right middle rectal vessels
Seminal vesicle
Left middle rectal vessels
Left inferior vesical artery
Left levator ani muscle
Inferior rectal vessels (from internal pudendal)
Left internal pudendal vessels
Prostate gland
Urogenital diaphragm
Posterior scrotal vessels (from internal pudendal)

Figure 303 Blood Vessels of the Male Pelvis, Perineum, and External Genitalia

NOTE: (1) The aorta bifurcates into the **common iliac arteries,** which then divide into the **external** and **internal iliac arteries.** The external iliac becomes the principal arterial trunk of the lower extremity, whereas the internal iliac artery supplies the organs of the pelvis and perineum.

(2) The **visceral branches** of the internal iliac are: (a) the umbilical (from which is derived the superior vesical artery), (b) the inferior vesical, (c) the artery of the vas deferens (uterine artery in females), and (d) the middle rectal.

(3) The **parietal branches** include: (a) the iliolumbar, (b) lateral sacral, (c) superior gluteal, (d) inferior gluteal, (e) obturator, and (f) internal pudendal.

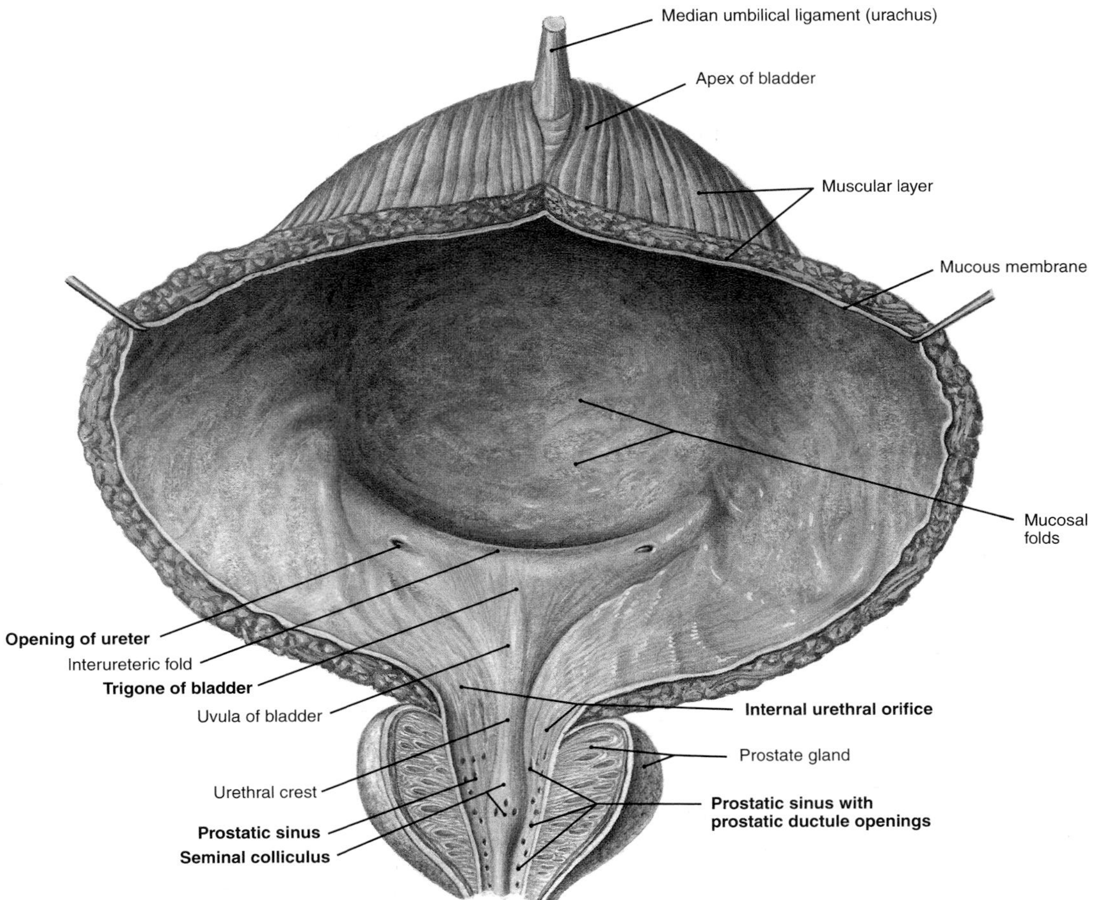
Median umbilical ligament (urachus)
Apex of bladder
Muscular layer
Mucous membrane
Mucosal folds
Opening of ureter
Interureteric fold
Trigone of bladder
Uvula of bladder
Internal urethral orifice
Prostate gland
Urethral crest
Prostatic sinus with prostatic ductule openings
Prostatic sinus
Seminal colliculus

Figure 304.1 Bladder and Prostatic Urethra Incised Anteriorly

NOTE: (1) The smooth triangular area at the base of the bladder called the **trigone,** which is bounded by the two orifices of the ureters and the opening of the prostatic urethra.

(2) The **seminal colliculus** is a mound on the posterior wall of the prostatic urethra, on both sides of which lie the **prostatic sinuses.** Into these open the ducts of the prostate gland. In the center of the colliculus is a small blind pouch, the **prostatic utricle;** on both sides of the utricle are the single orifices of the **ejaculatory ducts** (openings not labeled).

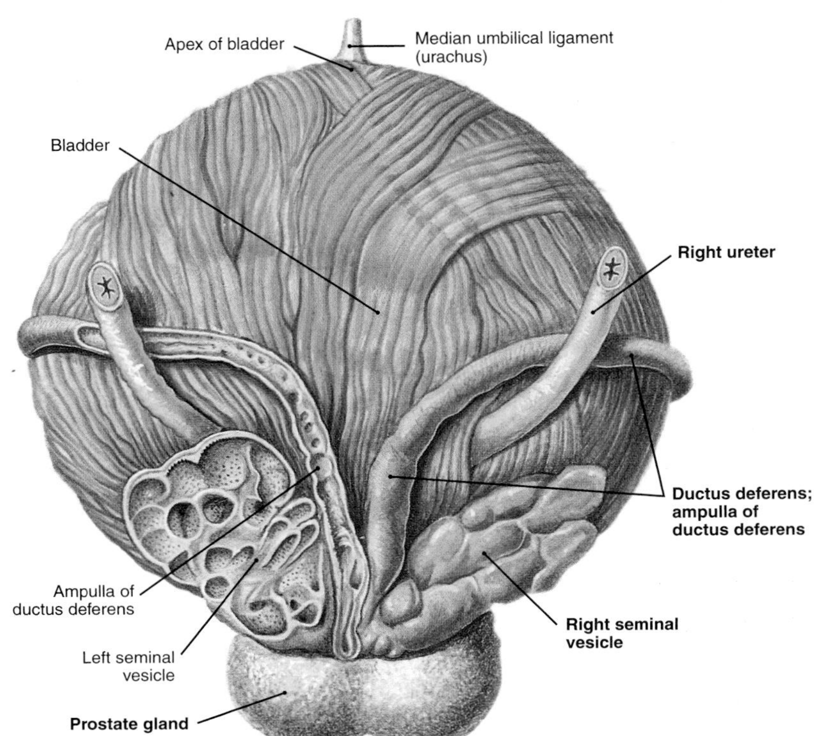
Apex of bladder
Median umbilical ligament (urachus)
Bladder
Right ureter
Ductus deferens; ampulla of ductus deferens
Ampulla of ductus deferens
Left seminal vesicle
Right seminal vesicle
Prostate gland

Figure 304.2 Posterior Surface of the Bladder: Seminal Vesicles, Ureters, and Deferent Ducts

NOTE: (1) The ureters, deferent ducts, seminal vesicles, and prostate gland are all in contact with the inferior aspect of the posterior surface of the bladder.

(2) The **ureters** penetrate the bladder diagonally at points about 2 in. apart. Upon entering the bladder, each ureter is crossed anteriorly by the ductus deferens.

(3) The deferent ducts join the ducts of the lobulated seminal vesicles to form the two ejaculatory ducts.

(4) The prostate hugs the bladder at its outlet, surrounding the prostatic urethra.

(5) All of these organs lie directly in front of the rectum and can be palpated during a rectal examination.

Base of bladder
Ductus deferens
Orifice of ureter
Seminal vesicle
Trigone of bladder
Internal urethral orifice
Ampulla of ductus deferens
Prostatic urethra
Prostate gland
Prostate gland
Ejaculatory duct
Membranous urethra

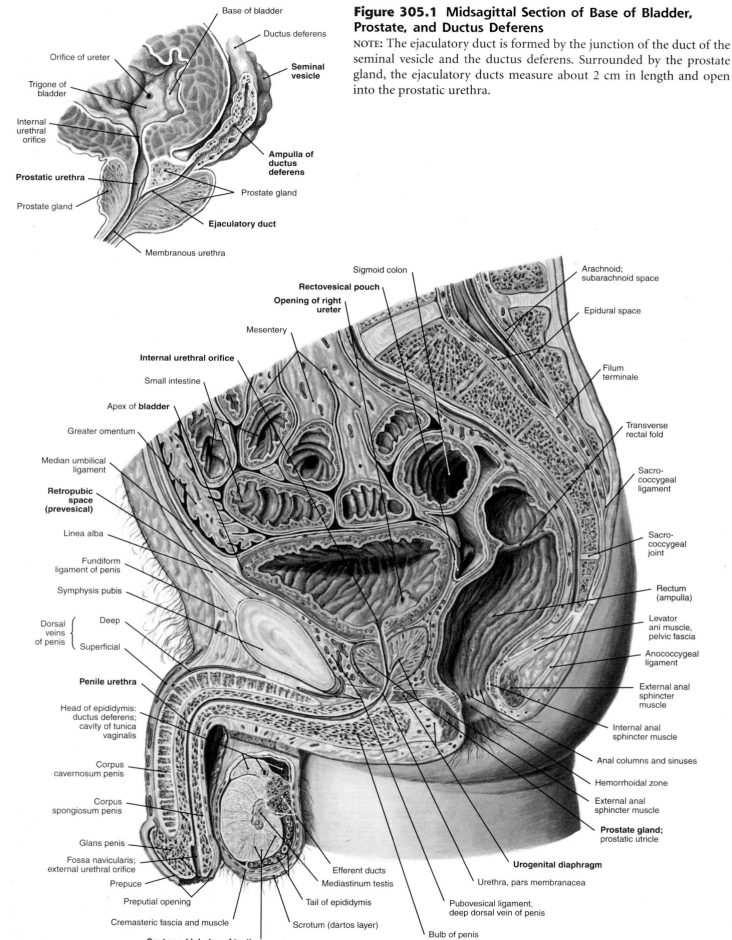

Figure 305.1 Midsagittal Section of Base of Bladder, Prostate, and Ductus Deferens

NOTE: The ejaculatory duct is formed by the junction of the duct of the seminal vesicle and the ductus deferens. Surrounded by the prostate gland, the ejaculatory ducts measure about 2 cm in length and open into the prostatic urethra.

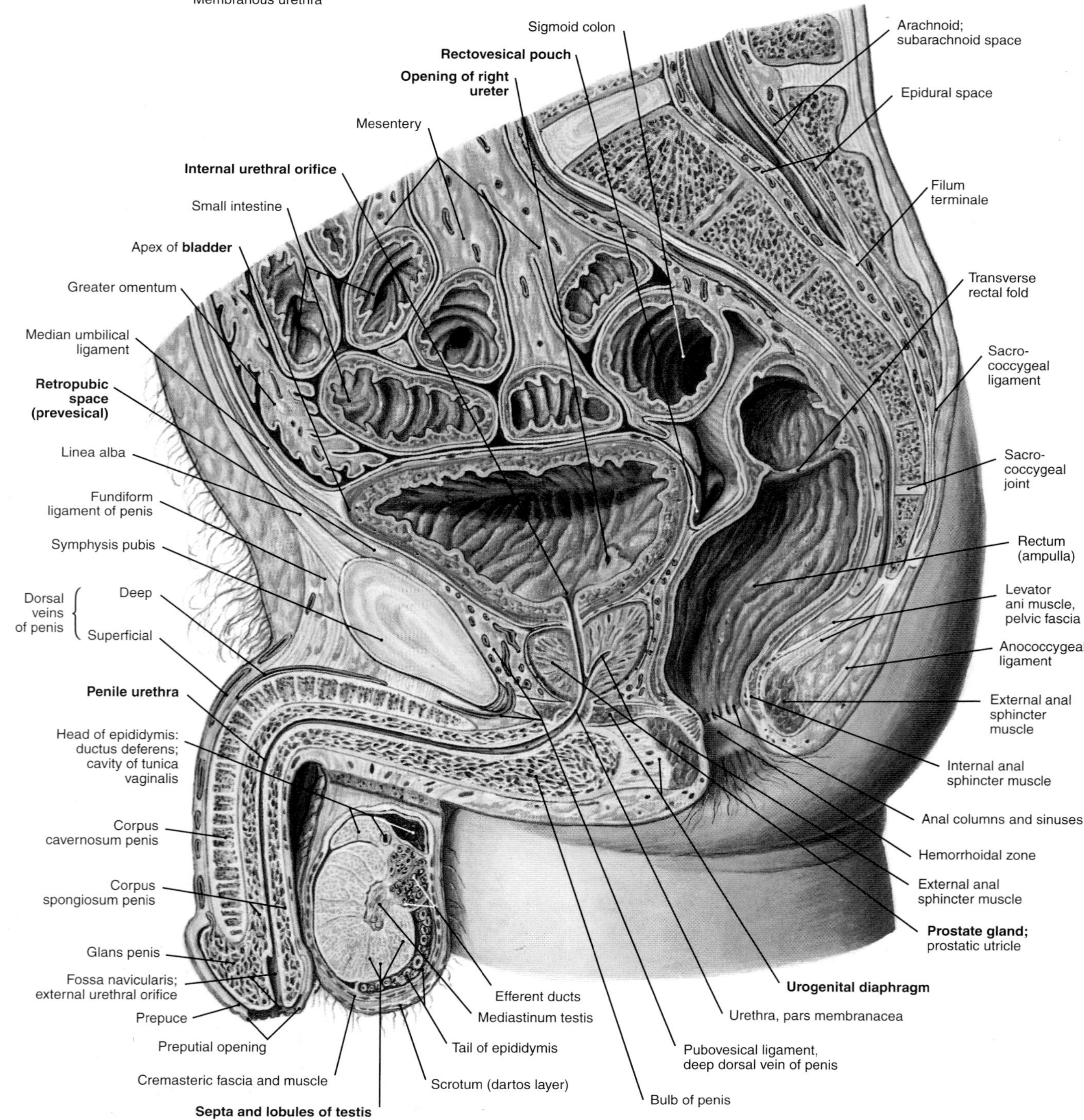
Sigmoid colon
Rectovesical pouch
Opening of right ureter
Mesentery
Internal urethral orifice
Small intestine
Apex of bladder
Greater omentum
Median umbilical ligament
Retropubic space (prevesical)
Linea alba
Fundiform ligament of penis
Symphysis pubis
Dorsal veins of penis
Deep
Superficial
Penile urethra
Head of epididymis: ductus deferens; cavity of tunica vaginalis
Corpus cavernosum penis
Corpus spongiosum penis
Glans penis
Fossa navicularis; external urethral orifice
Prepuce
Preputial opening
Cremasteric fascia and muscle
Septa and lobules of testis
Scrotum (dartos layer)
Tail of epididymis
Mediastinum testis
Efferent ducts
Bulb of penis
Pubovesical ligament, deep dorsal vein of penis
Urethra, pars membranacea
Urogenital diaphragm
Arachnoid; subarachnoid space
Epidural space
Filum terminale
Transverse rectal fold
Sacro-coccygeal ligament
Sacro-coccygeal joint
Rectum (ampulla)
Levator ani muscle, pelvic fascia
Anococcygeal ligament
External anal sphincter muscle
Internal anal sphincter muscle
Anal columns and sinuses
Hemorrhoidal zone
External anal sphincter muscle
Prostate gland; prostatic utricle

Figure 305.2 Median Sagittal Section of the Male Pelvis and Perineum Showing the Pelvic Viscera and the External Genitalia

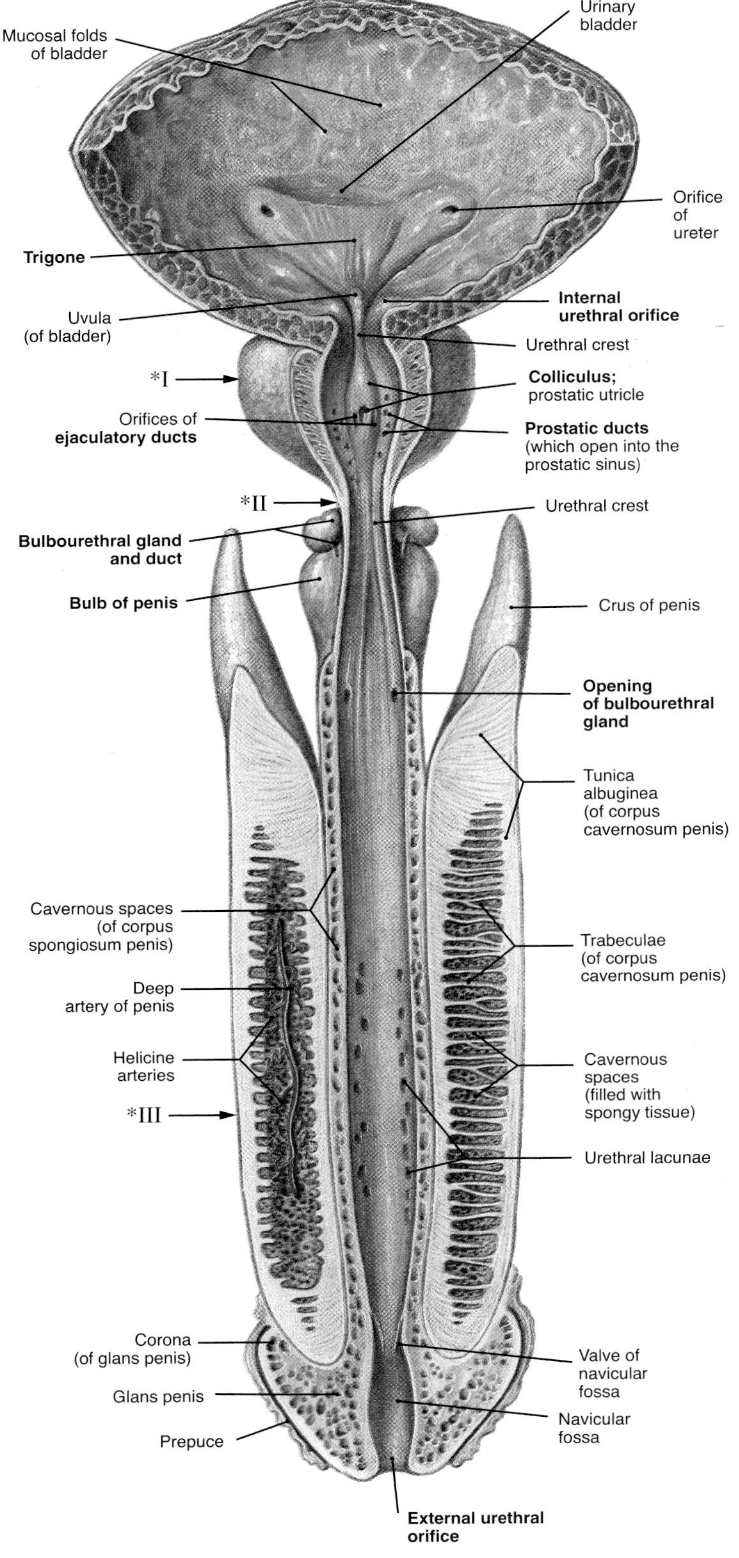
Mucosal folds of bladder
Urinary bladder
Orifice of ureter
Trigone
Uvula (of bladder)
Internal urethral orifice
Urethral crest
*I
Colliculus; prostatic utricle
Orifices of ejaculatory ducts
Prostatic ducts (which open into the prostatic sinus)
*II
Urethral crest
Bulbourethral gland and duct
Bulb of penis
Crus of penis
Opening of bulbourethral gland
Tunica albuginea (of corpus cavernosum penis)
Cavernous spaces (of corpus spongiosum penis)
Trabeculae (of corpus cavernosum penis)
Deep artery of penis
Helicine arteries
Cavernous spaces (filled with spongy tissue)
*III
Urethral lacunae
Corona (of glans penis)
Valve of navicular fossa
Glans penis
Navicular fossa
Prepuce
External urethral orifice

Figure 306.1 Male Urethra and Its Associated Orifices

NOTE: (1) The male urethra extends from the internal urethral orifice at the bladder to the external urethral orifice at the end of the glans penis. In males, it traverses the prostate gland, the urogenital diaphragm (membrane), and penis, and is, therefore, divided into **prostatic, membranous,** and **penile** parts.

(2) Before ejaculation, a viscous fluid from the **bulbourethral glands** (of Cowper) lubricates the urethra. These glands are located in the urogenital diaphragm, but their ducts open 1 in. distally in the penile urethra.

(3) The total urethra measures between 7 and 8 in. in length, the prostatic part about 1 1/2 in., the membranous part about 1/2 in., and the penile part 5 to 6 in. The **prostatic urethra** receives the secretions of the ejaculatory ducts along with those from the prostate. Enlargement of the prostate, often occurring in older men, tends to constrict the urethra at this site, resulting in difficulty in urination.

(4) The **membranous urethra** is short and narrow and it is completely surrounded by the circular fibers of the voluntary urethral sphincter muscle. Relaxation of this sphincter initiates urination, while its tonic contraction constricts the urethra and maintains urinary continence.

(5) The **penile urethra** is surrounded initially by the bulb of the penis and the bulbospongiosus muscle. It traverses the penile shaft within the corpus spongiosum penis. The internal surface of the distal half is marked by small recesses called the urethral lacunae.

* Parts of urethra
I = Prostatic part
II = Membranous part
III = Penile part

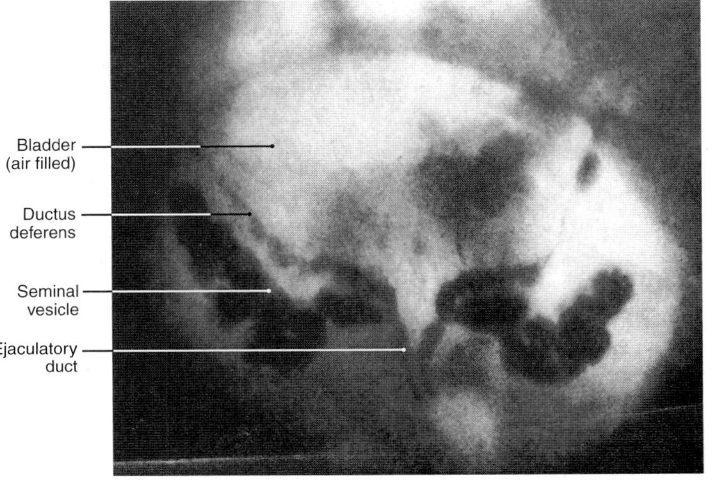
Bladder (air filled)
Ductus deferens
Seminal vesicle
Ejaculatory duct

Figure 306.2 Radiograph of Bladder, Seminal Vesicles, Deferent Ducts, and Ejaculatory Ducts

NOTE: The bladder has been filled with air and appears light, while the seminal vesicles, deferent ducts, and ejaculatory ducts stand out as dark because of an injected contrast medium.

Figure 307.1 Diagram of the Male Genitourinary System

NOTE: (1) This figure shows: (a) the organs of the adult male genitourinary system (dark red-brown), (b) the structures of the genital system prior to the descent of the testis (interrupted blue lines), and (c) those structures that partially or entirely became atrophic and disappeared during development (pink structures with red outlines).

(2) The **urinary system** includes the *kidneys,* which produce urine by filtration of the blood, the *ureters,* which convey urine to the *bladder,* where it is stored, and the *urethra,* through which urine is discharged.

(3) The adult male genital system includes the *testis,* where sperm are generated, the *epididymis* and *ductus deferens,* which transport sperm to the *ejaculatory duct,* where the *seminal vesicle* joins the genital system. The *prostate* and *bulbourethral glands,* along with the ejaculatory ducts, join the *urethra,* which then courses through the prostate and *penis.*

(4) Embryologically, structures capable of developing into either sex exist in all individuals. In the male the **mesonephric** (Wolffian) **duct** becomes the epididymis, ductus deferens, ejaculatory duct, and seminal vesicle along with the penis, while the **paramesonephric** (Müllerian) **duct** is suppressed.

(5) The testes are developed on the posterior abdominal wall, to which each is attached by a fibrous genital ligament called the **gubernaculum testis.** As development continues, each testis *migrates* from its site of formation, so that by the fifth month it lies adjacent to the abdominal inguinal ring. The gubernaculum is still attached to anterior abdominal wall tissue, which by this time has evaginated as the developing scrotum. The testes then commence their descent through the inguinal canal, so that by the eighth month they usually lie in the scrotum attached by a peritoneal reflection, the processus vaginalis testis, which becomes the **tunica vaginalis testis.**

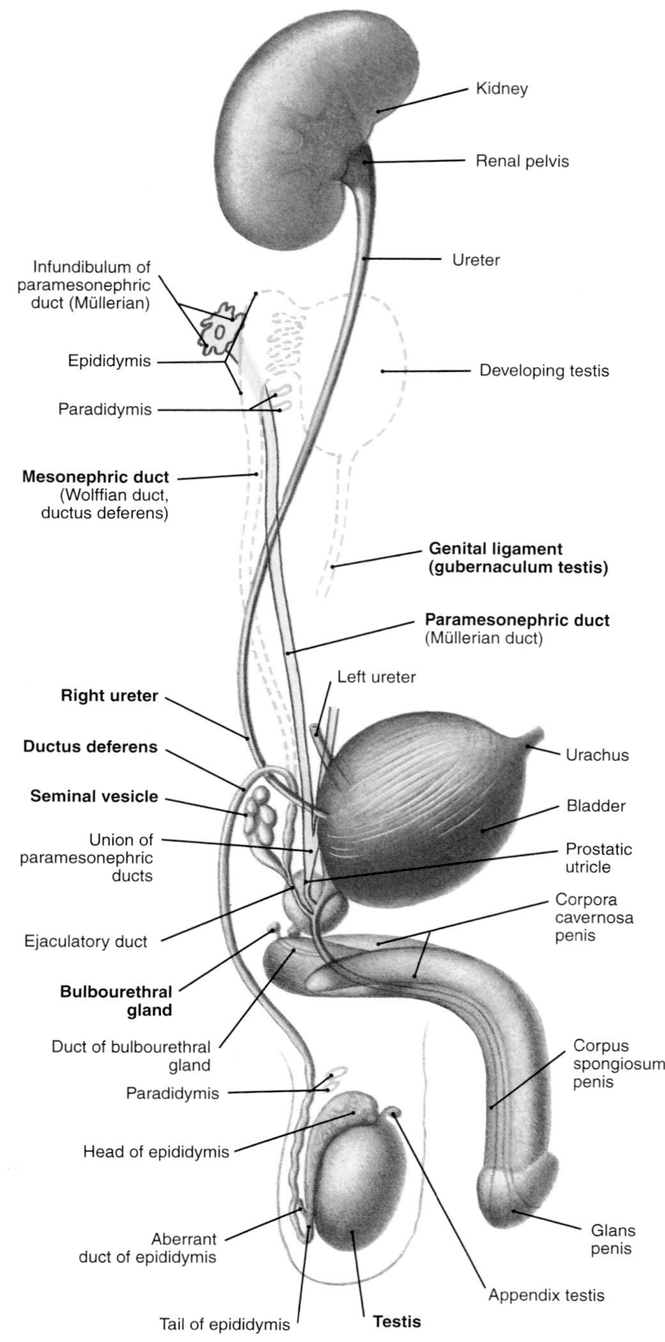
Kidney
Renal pelvis
Ureter
Infundibulum of paramesonephric duct (Müllerian)
Epididymis
Developing testis
Paradidymis
Mesonephric duct (Wolffian duct, ductus deferens)
Genital ligament (gubernaculum testis)
Paramesonephric duct (Müllerian duct)
Left ureter
Right ureter
Ductus deferens
Urachus
Seminal vesicle
Bladder
Union of paramesonephric ducts
Prostatic utricle
Corpora cavernosa penis
Ejaculatory duct
Bulbourethral gland
Duct of bulbourethral gland
Corpus spongiosum penis
Paradidymis
Head of epididymis
Aberrant duct of epididymis
Glans penis
Appendix testis
Tail of epididymis
Testis

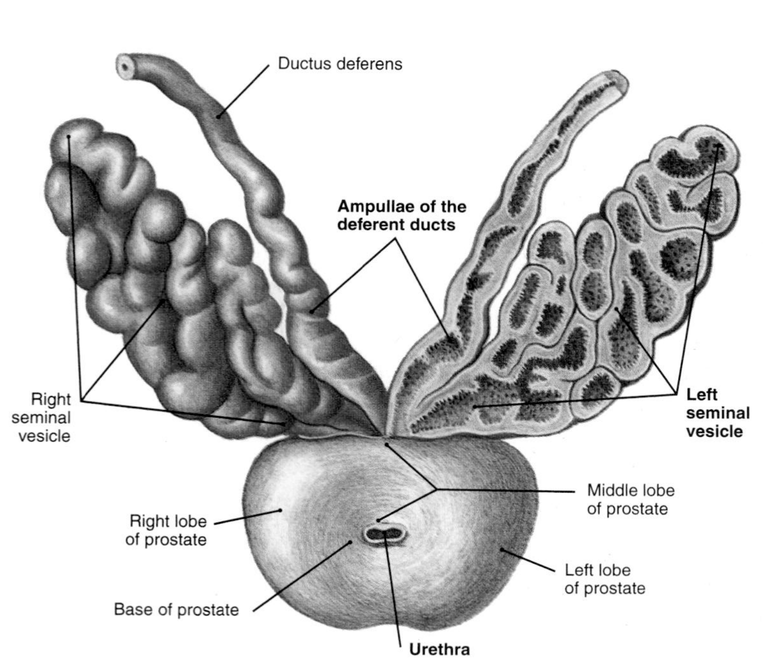
Ductus deferens
Ampullae of the deferent ducts
Right seminal vesicle
Left seminal vesicle
Middle lobe of prostate
Right lobe of prostate
Left lobe of prostate
Base of prostate
Urethra

Figure 307.2 Prostate Gland, Seminal Vesicles, and Ampullae of the Deferent Ducts (Superior View)

NOTE: (1) The left seminal vesicle and ductus deferens were cut longitudinally, while the urethra was cut transversely, distal to the bladder.

(2) The **prostate gland** is conical in shape and normally measures just over $1\frac{1}{2}$ in. across, 1 in. in thickness, and slightly longer than 1 in. vertically. In the young adult, it weighs about 25 g and is formed by two lateral lobes surrounding a middle lobe.

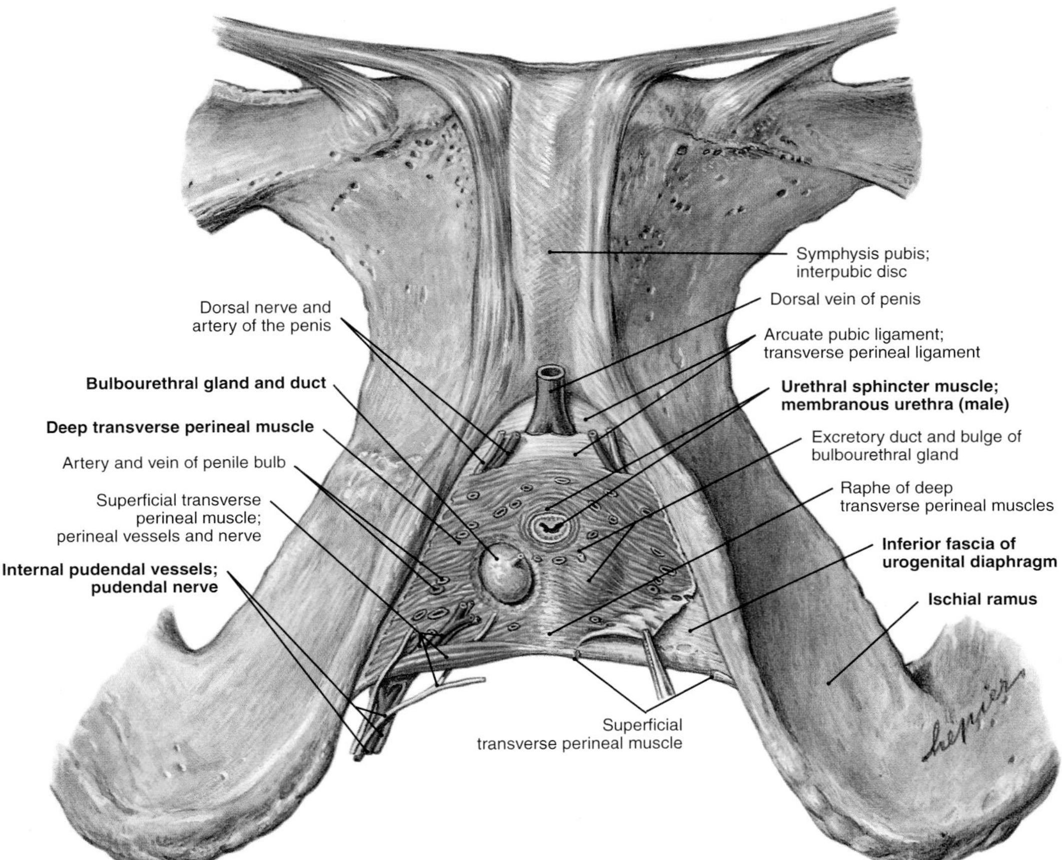
Symphysis pubis; interpubic disc
Dorsal vein of penis
Arcuate pubic ligament; transverse perineal ligament
Urethral sphincter muscle; membranous urethra (male)
Excretory duct and bulge of bulbourethral gland
Raphe of deep transverse perineal muscles
Inferior fascia of urogenital diaphragm
Ischial ramus
Dorsal nerve and artery of the penis
Bulbourethral gland and duct
Deep transverse perineal muscle
Artery and vein of penile bulb
Superficial transverse perineal muscle; perineal vessels and nerve
Internal pudendal vessels; pudendal nerve
Superficial transverse perineal muscle

Figure 308.1 Urogenital Diaphragm; Deep Transverse Perineal Muscle (Male)

NOTE: (1) The **deep transverse perineal muscle** stretches between the ischial rami and is covered by fascia on both its internal (pelvic or superior) surface and its external (perineal or inferior) surface. These two fascias and the muscle form the **urogenital diaphragm.**

(2) The region between the two fascias is often referred to as the **deep perineal compartment** (pouch, cleft, or space). In the male it contains: (a) the deep transverse perineal muscle, (b) the sphincter of the urethra, (c) the bulbourethral glands, (d) the membranous urethra, and (e) branches of the internal pudendal vessels and nerve.

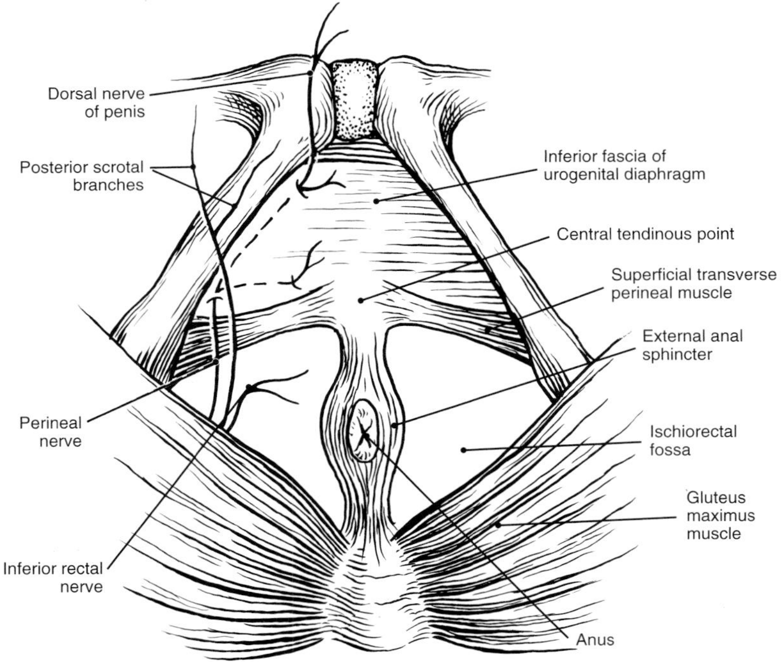
Dorsal nerve of penis
Posterior scrotal branches
Perineal nerve
Inferior rectal nerve
Inferior fascia of urogenital diaphragm
Central tendinous point
Superficial transverse perineal muscle
External anal sphincter
Ischiorectal fossa
Gluteus maximus muscle
Anus

Figure 308.2 Branches of the Pudendal Nerve in the Perineum

NOTE: (1) The perineal branches of the pudendal nerve emerge at the lateral aspect of the ischiorectal fossa.

(2) The inferior rectal nerve crosses the fossa to supply the levator ani and external anal sphincter muscles.

(3) The remaining branches course anteriorly into the urogenital triangle region and supply sensory innervation to all structures there and motor innervation to the urogenital muscles.

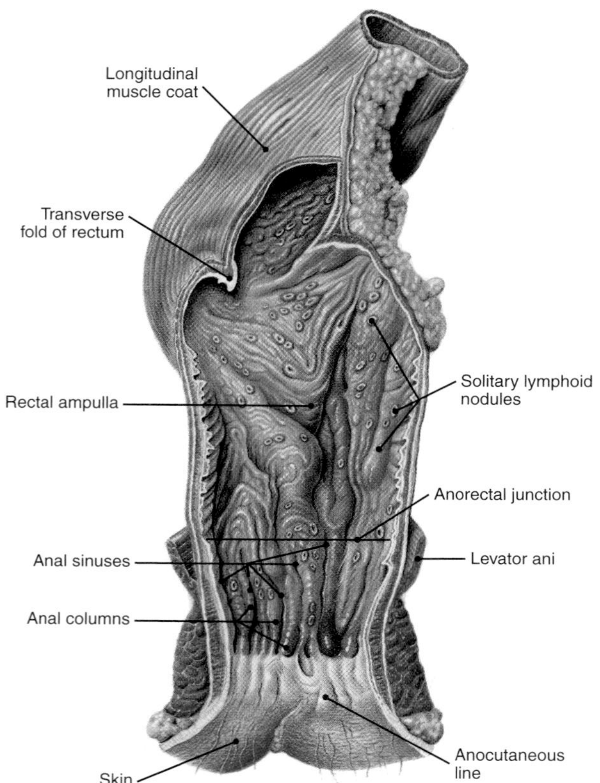
Longitudinal muscle coat
Transverse fold of rectum
Rectal ampulla
Solitary lymphoid nodules
Anorectal junction
Anal sinuses
Levator ani
Anal columns
Skin
Anocutaneous line

Figure 309.1 Inner Surface of the Rectum and Anal Canal

NOTE: (1) The sigmoid colon becomes the **rectum** at the level of the middle of the sacrum. The rectum, 5 in. in length, then becomes the **anal canal**, the terminal 1½ in. of the gastrointestinal tract. The rectum is dilated near its junction with the anal canal, giving rise to the **rectal ampulla.**

(2) The rectal mucosa is thrown into transverse folds, usually three in number, called **horizontal folds** or **valves of Houston.**

(3) Below the rectal ampulla is a series of vertical folds, called the **anal columns,** each containing an artery and a vein. Between the anal columns are the **anal sinuses.** If the veins in this region become varicosed, a condition called hemorrhoids, or piles, results.

(4) Distal to the anal columns is a zone, **Hilton's line,** where the epithelium changes from columnar to stratified squamous.

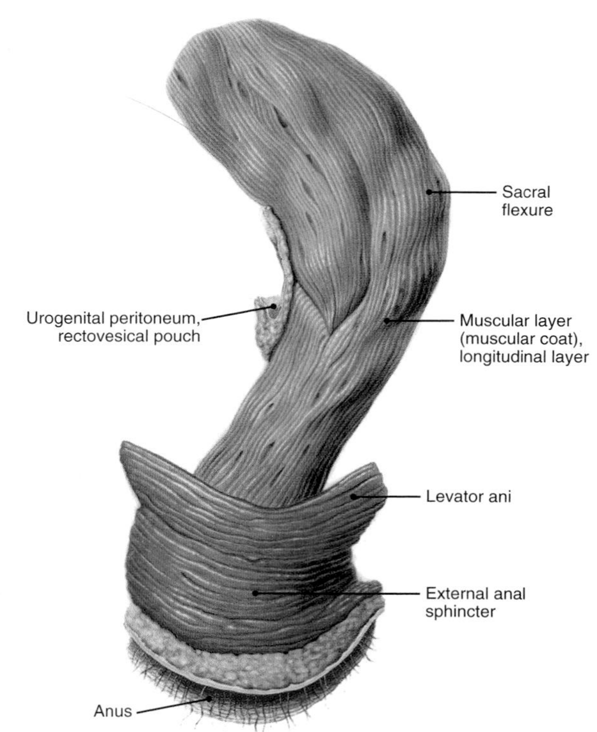
Sacral flexure
Urogenital peritoneum, rectovesical pouch
Muscular layer (muscular coat), longitudinal layer
Levator ani
External anal sphincter
Anus

Figure 309.2: External Surface of Rectum (Lateral View)

NOTE: (1) The rectum shows a dorsally directed **sacral flexure** proximally and a less pronounced **perineal flexure** distally. Peritoneum ensheathes the rectum ventrally almost as far as the ampulla (to the bladder in the male and the uterus in the female).

(2) The fibers of the **levator ani muscle** (which form the floor of the pelvis) surround the rectum and are continued distally as the **external anal sphincter muscle.**

(3) The **internal anal sphincter muscle** (seen in Figs. 309.1 and 309.3) is composed of smooth muscle and really represents a thickening of the muscular layer in the wall of the rectum.

Figure 309.3 Frontal Section through the Rectum (Diagrammatic)

NOTE: The **external anal sphincter** consists of **subcutaneous, superficial,** and **deep** parts (see Plate 297). Compare this diagram with Fig. 309.1.

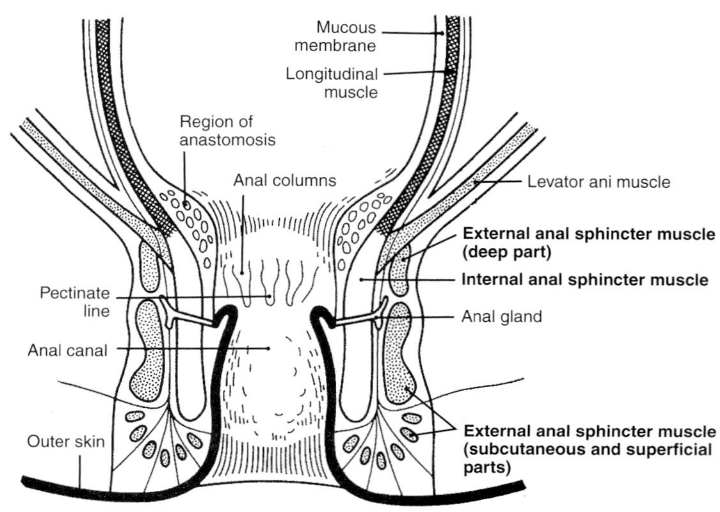
Mucous membrane
Longitudinal muscle
Region of anastomosis
Anal columns
Levator ani muscle
External anal sphincter muscle (deep part)
Internal anal sphincter muscle
Pectinate line
Anal gland
Anal canal
Outer skin
External anal sphincter muscle (subcutaneous and superficial parts)

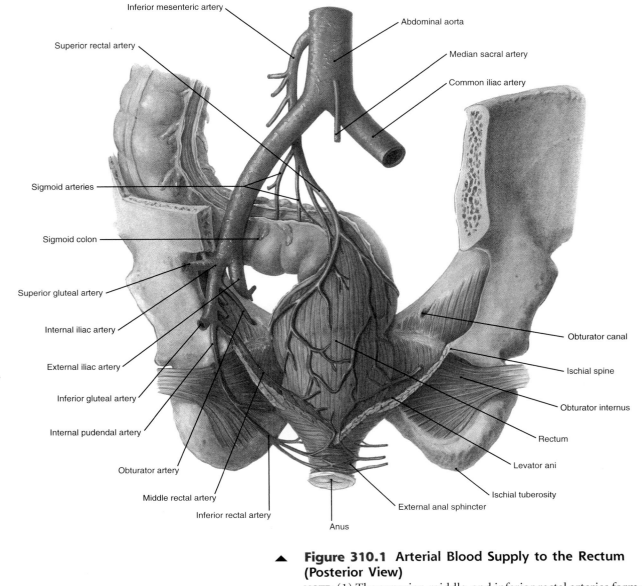

Inferior mesenteric artery
Superior rectal artery
Abdominal aorta
Median sacral artery
Common iliac artery
Sigmoid arteries
Sigmoid colon
Superior gluteal artery
Internal iliac artery
External iliac artery
Inferior gluteal artery
Internal pudendal artery
Obturator artery
Middle rectal artery
Inferior rectal artery
Anus
External anal sphincter
Ischial tuberosity
Levator ani
Rectum
Obturator internus
Ischial spine
Obturator canal

Figure 310.1 Arterial Blood Supply to the Rectum (Posterior View)

NOTE: (1) The superior, middle, and inferior rectal arteries form an anastomosis.

(2) The **superior** rectal artery has an **abdominal source,** the **middle** rectal artery has a **pelvic source,** and the **inferior** rectal artery has a **perineal source.**

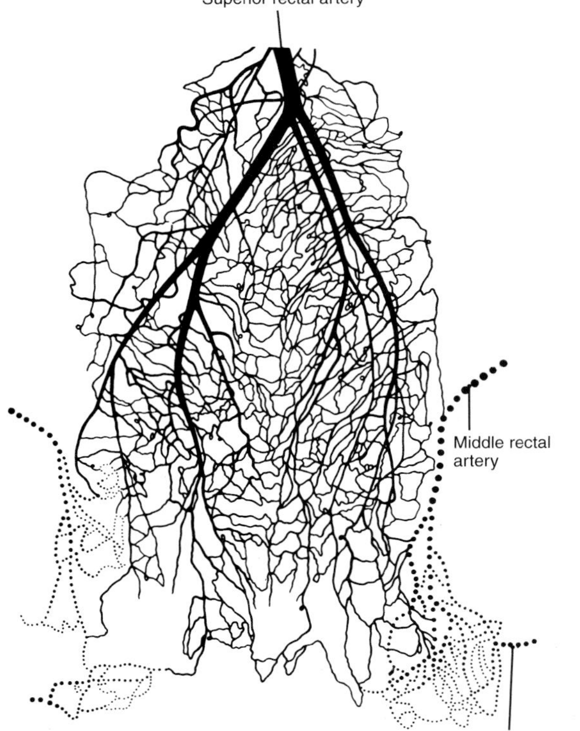
Superior rectal artery
Middle rectal artery
Inferior rectal artery

Figure 310.2 Distribution Pattern of the Rectal Arteries

NOTE: (1) This figure shows the distribution of the **superior, middle,** and **inferior rectal arteries** as they supply the rectum and the anal canal.

(2) The region of distribution of the superior rectal artery is much greater than either the middle or inferior rectal arteries.

(3) The rich anastomoses among these three vessels.

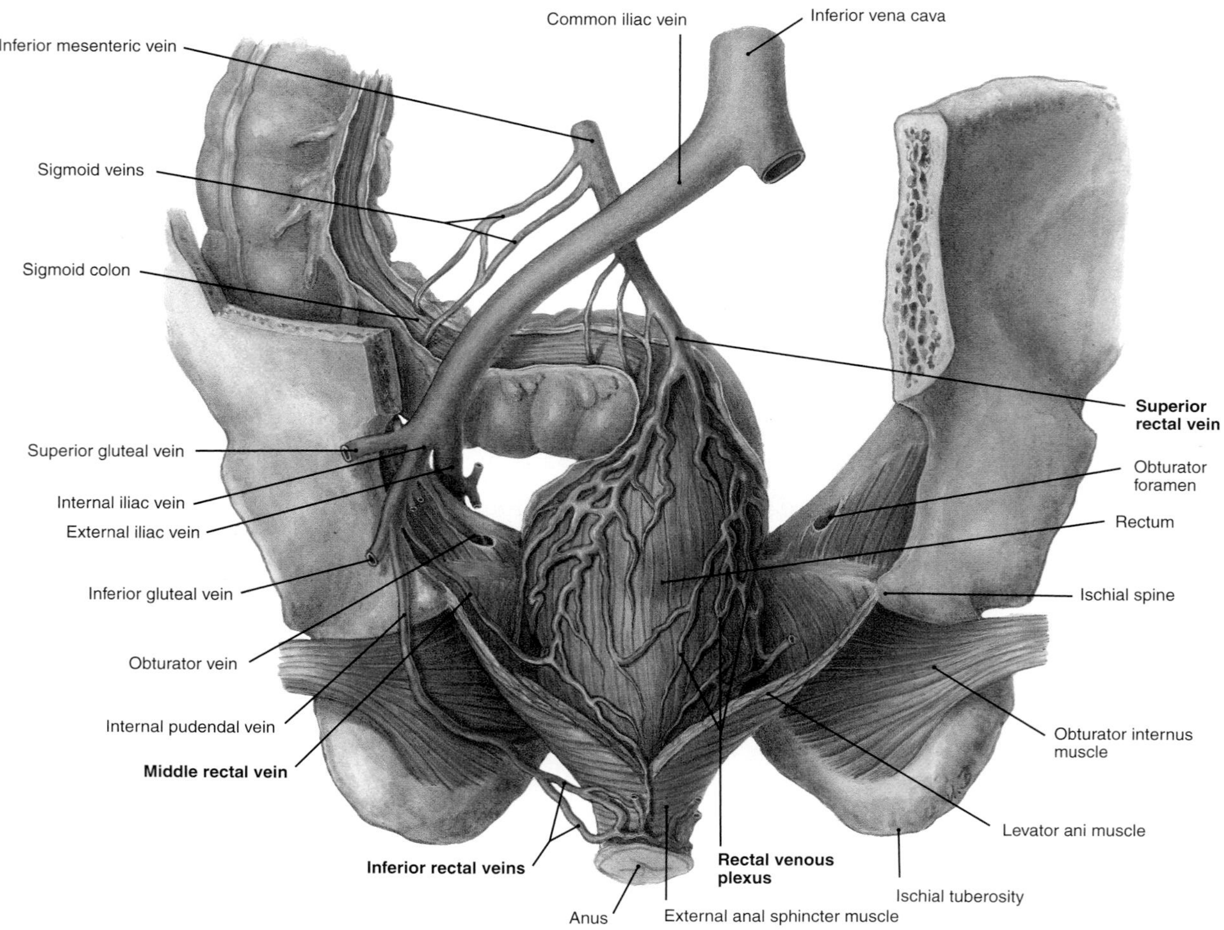
Common iliac vein
Inferior vena cava
Inferior mesenteric vein
Sigmoid veins
Sigmoid colon
Superior rectal vein
Obturator foramen
Rectum
Superior gluteal vein
Internal iliac vein
External iliac vein
Inferior gluteal vein
Ischial spine
Obturator vein
Internal pudendal vein
Obturator internus muscle
Middle rectal vein
Levator ani muscle
Inferior rectal veins
Rectal venous plexus
Ischial tuberosity
Anus
External anal sphincter muscle

Figure 311.1 Venous Drainage of the Rectum (Posterior View)

NOTE: Blood from the middle and inferior rectal veins eventually drains into the inferior vena cava, while blood returning from the superior rectal vein drains into the portal circulation by way of the inferior mesenteric vein. This allows a route of **collateral circulation** between these two venous systems.

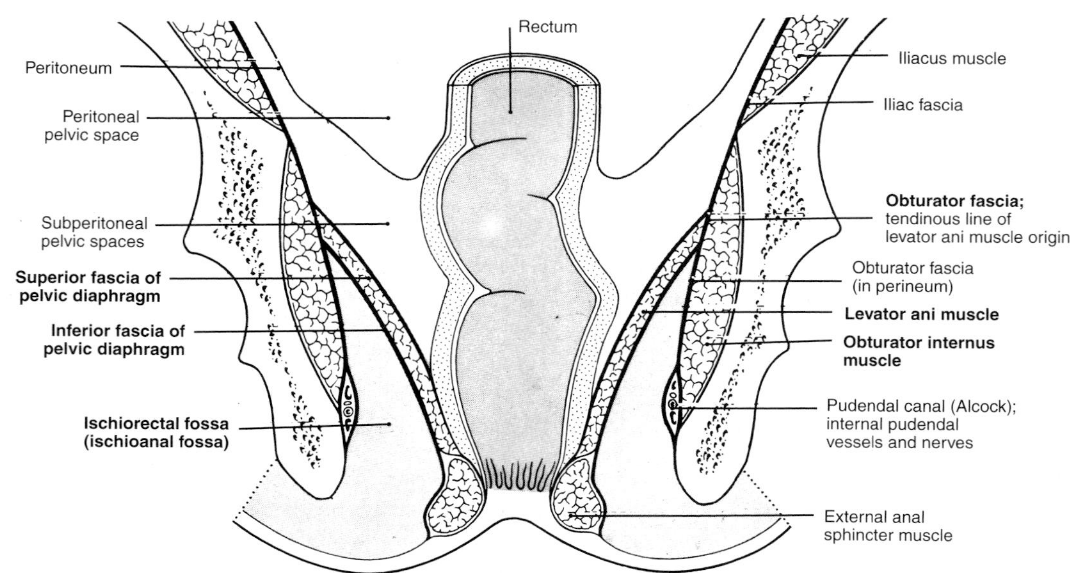
Rectum
Peritoneum
Iliacus muscle
Iliac fascia
Peritoneal pelvic space
Obturator fascia; tendinous line of levator ani muscle origin
Subperitoneal pelvic spaces
Obturator fascia (in perineum)
Superior fascia of pelvic diaphragm
Levator ani muscle
Inferior fascia of pelvic diaphragm
Obturator internus muscle
Pudendal canal (Alcock); internal pudendal vessels and nerves
Ischiorectal fossa (ischioanal fossa)
External anal sphincter muscle

Figure 311.2 Diagram of Frontal Section through Pelvis and Perineum

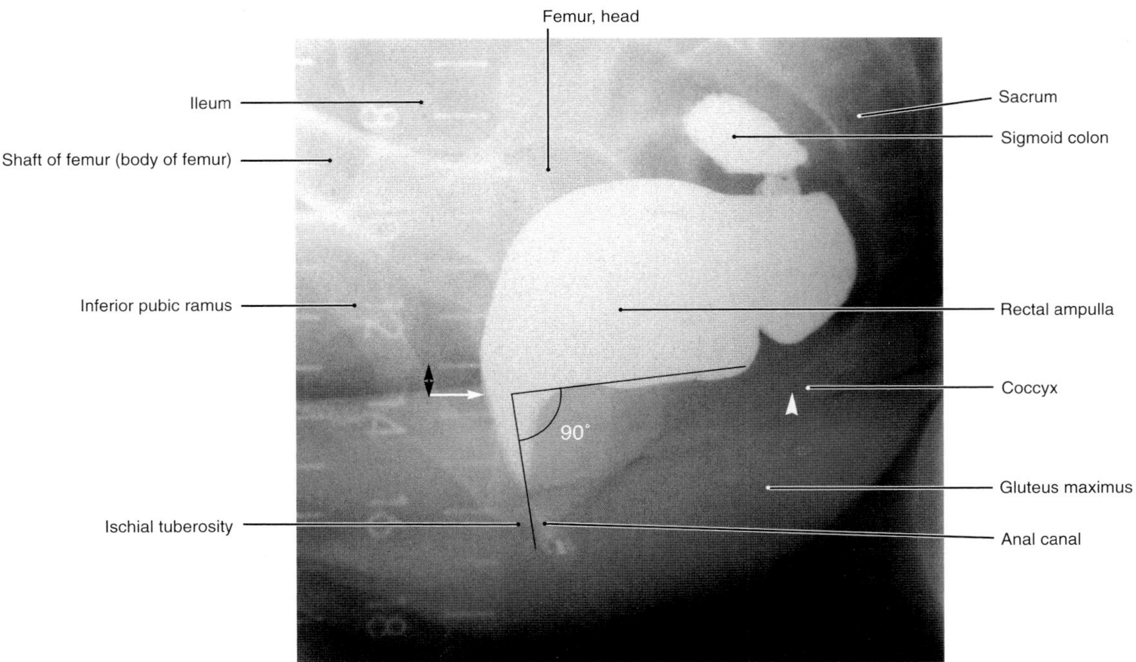
Femur, head
Ileum
Shaft of femur (body of femur)
Inferior pubic ramus
Ischial tuberosity
Sacrum
Sigmoid colon
Rectal ampulla
Coccyx
Gluteus maximus
Anal canal
90°

Figure 312.1 Rectum Filled with Contrast Medium (Lateral Radiograph)

NOTE: (1) With the anus closed voluntarily the contrast medium is retained in the rectal ampulla.

(2) The junction between the anal canal and the rectum (thin white arrow) is located approximately at the level of the tip of the coccyx (white arrowhead).

(3) The angle between the anal canal and the rectum is about 90 degrees and is due to the **puborectalis** loop of the levator ani muscle.

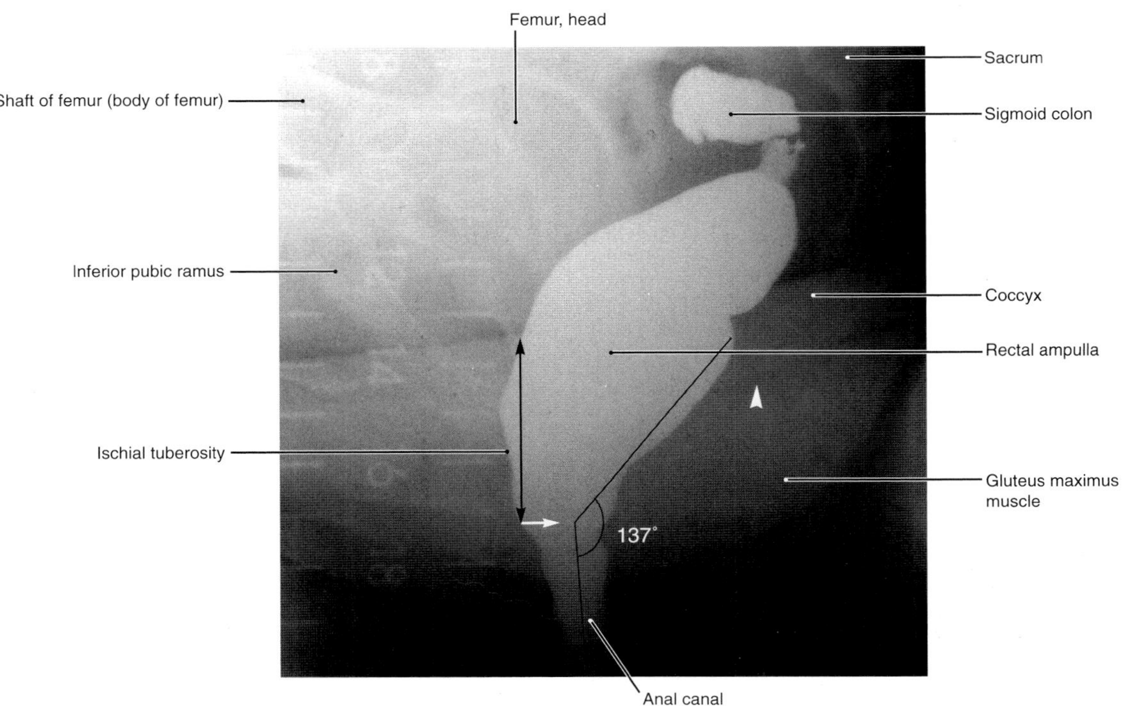
Femur, head
Shaft of femur (body of femur)
Inferior pubic ramus
Ischial tuberosity
Sacrum
Sigmoid colon
Coccyx
Rectal ampulla
Gluteus maximus muscle
137°
Anal canal

Figure 312.2 Rectum during Defecation (Lateral Radiograph)

NOTE: (1) This radiograph shows the rectum containing a contrast medium during the act of defecation (compare this radiograph with Fig. 312.1).

(2) The angle between the anal canal and the rectum has increased (in this instance to 137 degrees). At this time the puborectalis muscle and the anal sphincters have relaxed, allowing defecation to occur. Observe that increasing the anorectal angle makes this lowest region of the gastrointestinal tract more nearly vertical.

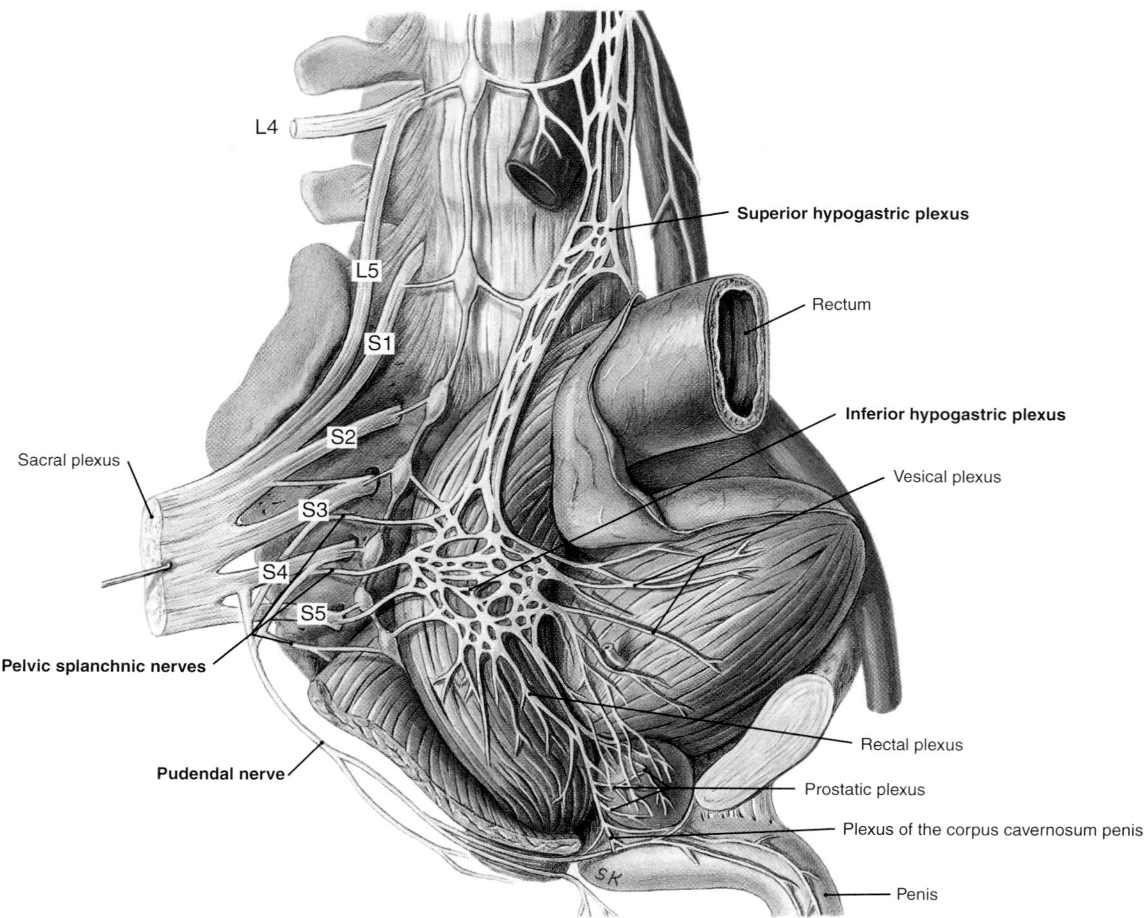
L4
L5
S1
S2
S3
S4
S5
Superior hypogastric plexus
Rectum
Inferior hypogastric plexus
Vesical plexus
Sacral plexus
Pelvic splanchnic nerves
Pudendal nerve
Rectal plexus
Prostatic plexus
Plexus of the corpus cavernosum penis
Penis

Figure 313.1 Autonomic and Visceral Afferent Innervation of the Pelvic Organs

NOTE: (1) *Post*ganglionic *sympathetic fibers* course downward in the **superior hypogastric plexus** from lower lumbar ganglia and continue in the specific visceral plexuses (i.e., rectal, vesical, etc.) to supply pelvic organs with sympathetic innervation.

(2) *Pre*ganglionic *parasympathetic fibers* to the pelvic organs emerge from the S2, S3, and S4 spinal nerves to form the **pelvic splanchnic nerves.** They also course through the specific visceral plexuses and then synapse with postganglionic parasympathetic neurons within the walls of the viscera.

(3) **Visceral afferent fibers** from the pelvic organs course centrally along with these autonomic fibers. Their cell bodies lie in their respective dorsal-root ganglia, and they enter the spinal cord by way of the dorsal roots from these ganglia.

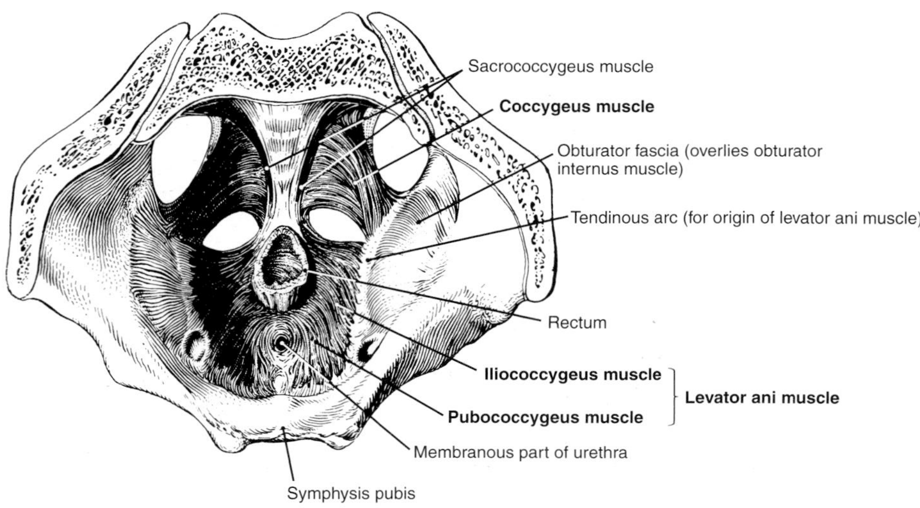
Sacrococcygeus muscle
Coccygeus muscle
Obturator fascia (overlies obturator internus muscle)
Tendinous arc (for origin of levator ani muscle)
Rectum
Iliococcygeus muscle
Pubococcygeus muscle
Levator ani muscle
Membranous part of urethra
Symphysis pubis

Figure 313.2 Muscular Floor of the Pelvis: Pelvic Diaphragm

NOTE: (1) The **pelvic diaphragm** consists of the **levator ani** (iliococcygeus and pubococcygeus parts) **muscle** and the **coccygeus muscle** along with two fascial layers, which cover the *pelvic* (supra-anal fascia) and *perineal* (infra-anal fascia) surfaces of these two muscles.

(2) The muscles composing the pelvic diaphragm stretch across the pelvic floor in a concave sling-like manner and separate the structures of the pelvis from those in the perineum below. In males, the pelvic diaphragm is perforated by the anal canal and urethra.

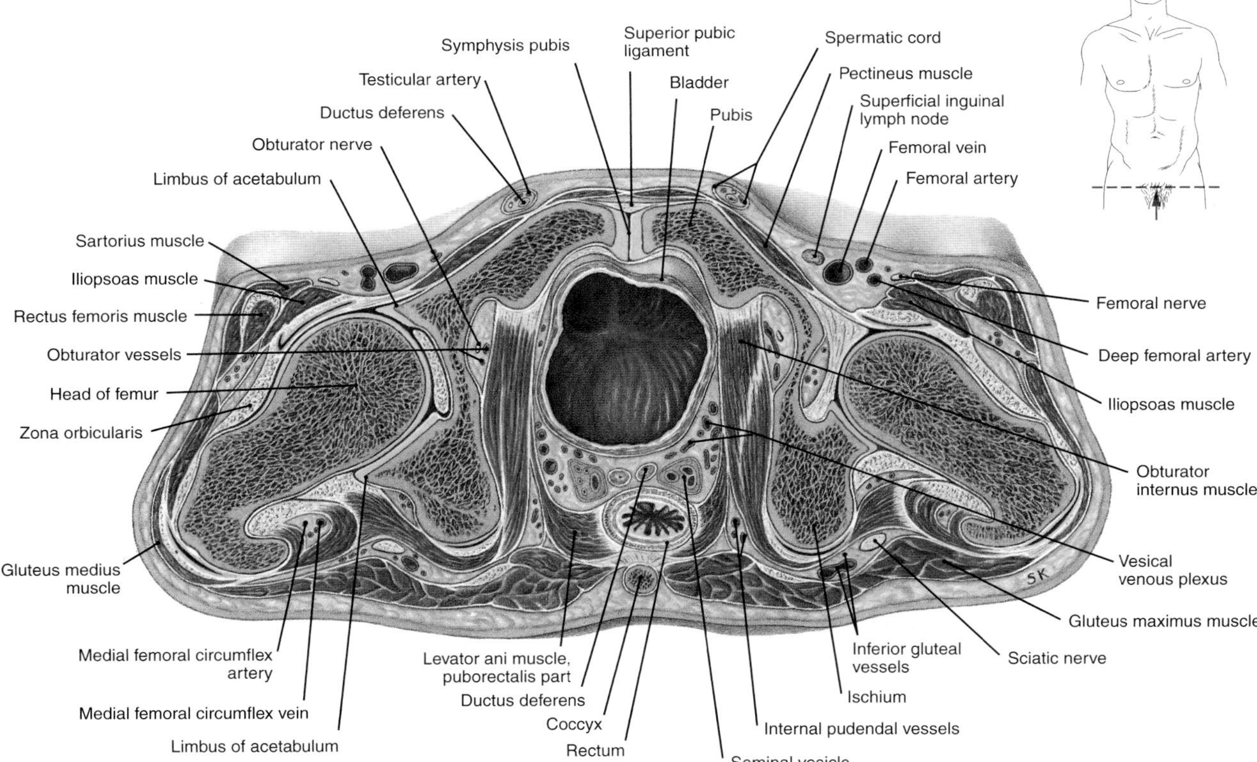
Symphysis pubis
Superior pubic ligament
Spermatic cord
Testicular artery
Bladder
Pectineus muscle
Ductus deferens
Pubis
Superficial inguinal lymph node
Obturator nerve
Femoral vein
Limbus of acetabulum
Femoral artery
Sartorius muscle
Iliopsoas muscle
Rectus femoris muscle
Obturator vessels
Head of femur
Zona orbicularis
Femoral nerve
Deep femoral artery
Iliopsoas muscle
Obturator internus muscle
Vesical venous plexus
Gluteus maximus muscle
Gluteus medius muscle
Medial femoral circumflex artery
Medial femoral circumflex vein
Limbus of acetabulum
Levator ani muscle, puborectalis part
Ductus deferens
Coccyx
Rectum
Inferior gluteal vessels
Ischium
Internal pudendal vessels
Seminal vesicle
Sciatic nerve
SK

Figure 314.1 Cross Section of the Male Pelvis at the Level of the Symphysis Pubis

NOTE: (1) The **ductus deferens** and the **seminal vesicle** are located behind the **bladder** on both sides, and behind these, observe the position of the **rectum.**

(2) The **obturator internus muscle** forms the lateral wall of the true pelvis and the levator ani (in this figure, its puborectalis part) arises from the obturator fascia that covers its medial surface.

(3) The **vesical plexus of veins** surrounding the bladder. This plexus anastomoses with the prostatic plexus below, and both drain into the internal iliac vein. Thus, venous blood from the bladder and prostate usually enters the inferior vena cava and goes to the lungs, although anastomoses also exist with the rectal system of veins and with the vertebral system of veins.

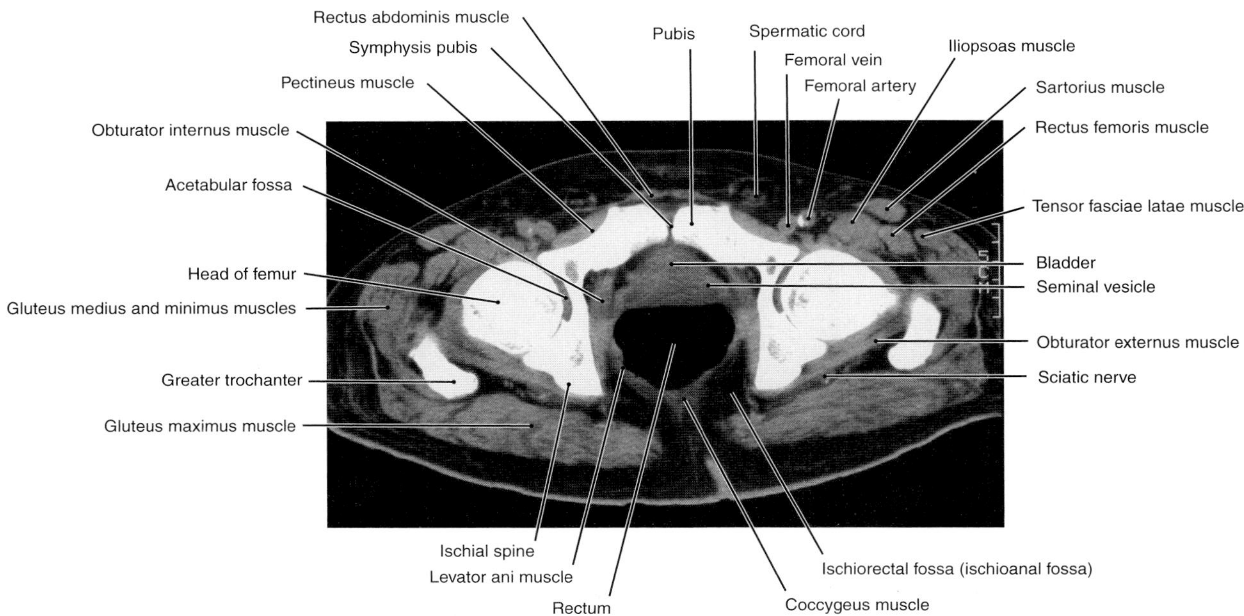
Rectus abdominis muscle
Symphysis pubis
Pubis
Spermatic cord
Femoral vein
Femoral artery
Iliopsoas muscle
Pectineus muscle
Sartorius muscle
Obturator internus muscle
Rectus femoris muscle
Acetabular fossa
Tensor fasciae latae muscle
Head of femur
Bladder
Seminal vesicle
Gluteus medius and minimus muscles
Obturator externus muscle
Greater trochanter
Sciatic nerve
Gluteus maximus muscle
Ischial spine
Levator ani muscle
Rectum
Ischiorectal fossa (ischioanal fossa)
Coccygeus muscle

Figure 314.2 CT of the Male Pelvis Taken from Below

Parietal peritoneum
Sigmoid arteries
Internal iliac vein
Omental appendices (fatty appendices of colon)
Ductus deferens (vas deferens)
Rectal ampulla
Ischioanal fossa
Anal columns
Ilium
Sigmoid colon
Ureter
Seminal gland (seminal vesicle)
Obturator internus
Levator ani
Internal pudendal artery and vein
Ischial tuberosity
Biceps femoris; semitendinosus; semimembranosus
SK
Skin
Internal anal sphincter
Lavator ani, puborectalis
External anal sphincter

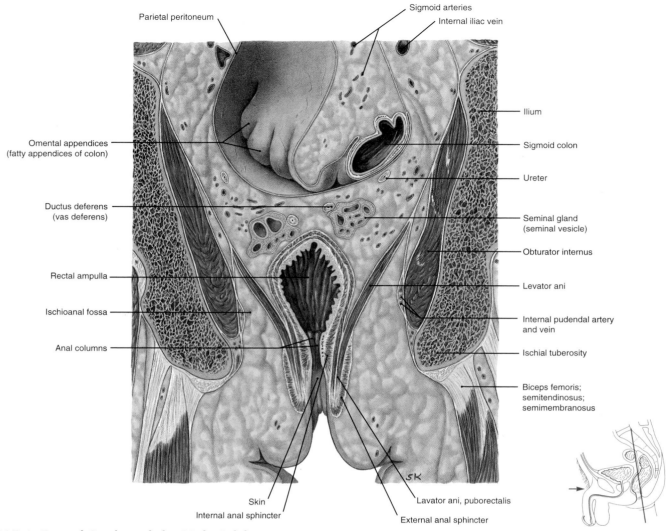

Figure 315.1 Frontal Section of the Male Pelvis

NOTE: (1) This frontal section goes through the seminal vesicles, rectal ampulla, and anal canal.

(2) The levator ani muscles arise from the obturator internus fascia and form a sling that separates the pelvis superiorly from the perineum inferiorly.

(3) The internal and external sphincters are shown. Observe also the fat-filled ischiorectal (ischioanal) fossa on both sides and that the obturator internus muscles help form the lateral walls of the pelvis and the lateral borders of the ischiorectal fossae.

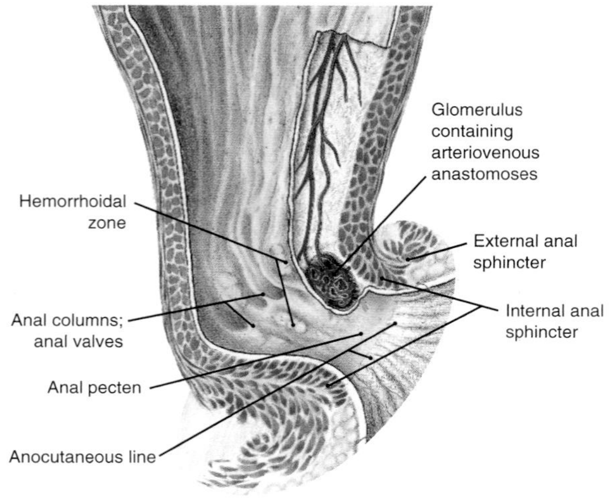
Glomerulus containing arteriovenous anastomoses
Hemorrhoidal zone
External anal sphincter
Internal anal sphincter
Anal columns; anal valves
Anal pecten
Anocutaneous line

Figure 315.2 Median Section of the Rectum and Anal Canal

NOTE: (1) The anal canal commences where the ampulla of the rectum narrows and it ends at the anus.

(2) There are 6 to 11 vertical folds called **anal columns,** each of which contains arteriovenous anastomoses. The anal columns are joined by folds of mucous membranes called **anal valves.**

(3) The anal valves are situated along a line called the **pectinate line** or **anal pecten.** Adjacent is the **anocutaneous** line, where usually there is a transition to stratified squamous epithelium from the columnar epithelium of the gastrointestinal tract.

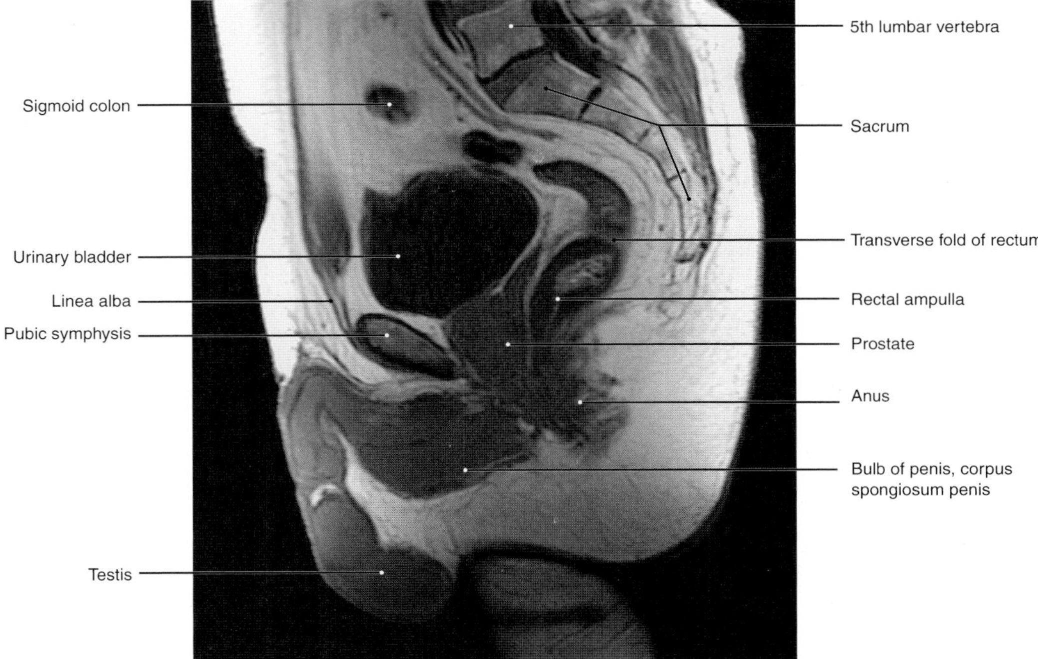
5th lumbar vertebra
Sigmoid colon
Sacrum
Transverse fold of rectum
Urinary bladder
Rectal ampulla
Linea alba
Pubic symphysis
Prostate
Anus
Bulb of penis, corpus spongiosum penis
Testis

Figure 316.1 Magnetic Resonance Tomograph of the Male Pelvis

NOTE: (1) This paramedian section (nearly a median section) goes through the linea alba and symphysis pubis anteriorly and the prostate, bladder, and rectal ampulla within the pelvis.

(2) The testis within the scrotal sac in the perineum and the anus posteriorly (in the anal triangle).

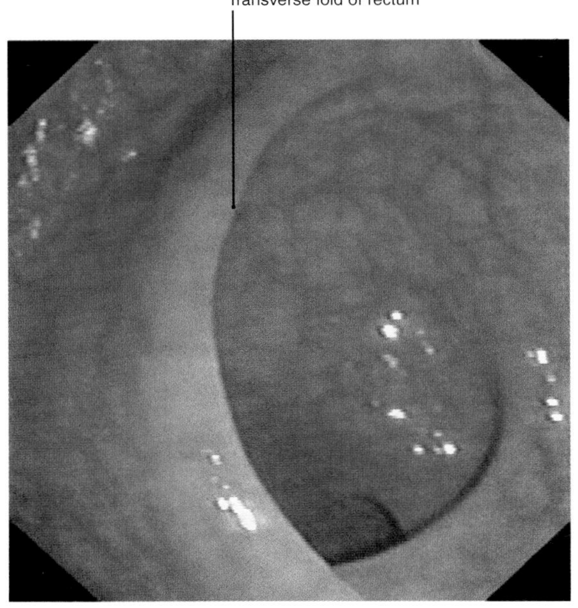
Transverse fold of rectum

Figure 316.2 Endoscopic View of the Rectal Ampulla

NOTE: (1) The relatively smooth and glistening mucous membrane on the inner surface of the rectum.

(2) The **transverse rectal fold;** compare this with Fig. 309.1.

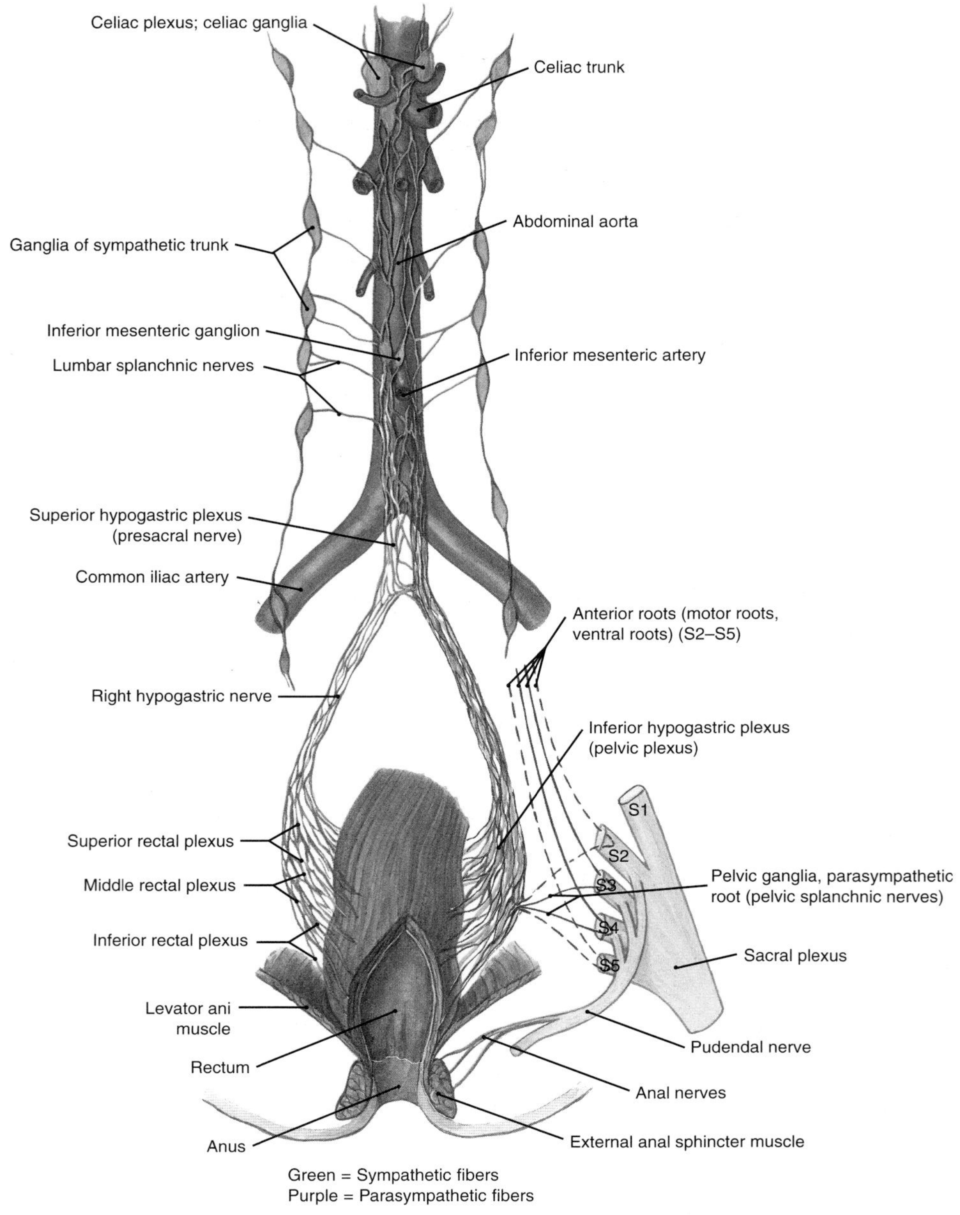
Celiac plexus; celiac ganglia
Celiac trunk
Ganglia of sympathetic trunk
Abdominal aorta
Inferior mesenteric ganglion
Lumbar splanchnic nerves
Inferior mesenteric artery
Superior hypogastric plexus
(presacral nerve)
Common iliac artery
Anterior roots (motor roots, ventral roots) (S2–S5)
Right hypogastric nerve
Inferior hypogastric plexus
(pelvic plexus)
S1
S2
S3
S4
S5
Superior rectal plexus
Middle rectal plexus
Pelvic ganglia, parasympathetic root (pelvic splanchnic nerves)
Inferior rectal plexus
Sacral plexus
Levator ani muscle
Rectum
Pudendal nerve
Anal nerves
Anus
External anal sphincter muscle
Green = Sympathetic fibers
Purple = Parasympathetic fibers

Figure 317 Autonomic (Visceral Efferent) Innervation of the Rectum

NOTE: (1) **Preganglionic** sympathetic fibers (shown in green) to pelvic organs emerge from the spinal cord in the L1 to L3 spinal segments, and they synapse in sympathetic ganglia along the lower lumbar part of the sympathetic chain and in other associated sympathetic ganglia.

(2) From these synapses, **postganglionic** sympathetic fibers course along the third and fourth lumbar splanchnic nerves and contribute to the formation of the **superior hypogastric plexus,** located anterior to the abdominal aorta. (This plexus is at times referred to as the presacral nerve, even though it lies anterior to the bodies of the third and fourth lumbar vertebrae.);

(3) The superior hypogastric plexus then divides into right and left hypogastric nerves. These divide to form **inferior hypogastric plexuses** on the two sides that also receive preganglionic parasympathetic fibers from the (S2), S3, S4, (S5) spinal segments (shown in purple).

(4) From the inferior hypogastric plexuses, autonomic fibers surround the pelvic organs and supply the seminal vesicle, prostate, bladder, and rectum in the male and the rectum, bladder, uterine cervix, and the vagina surrounding the cervix in females.

(5) This figure shows only the autonomic fibers that supply the rectum.

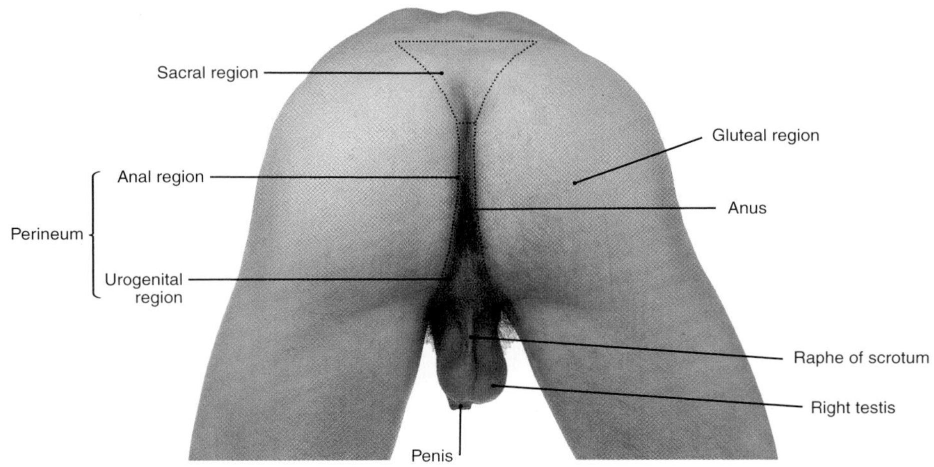
Sacral region
Gluteal region
Perineum
Anal region
Anus
Urogenital region
Raphe of scrotum
Right testis
Penis

Figure 318.1 Surface Anatomy of the Male Perineum

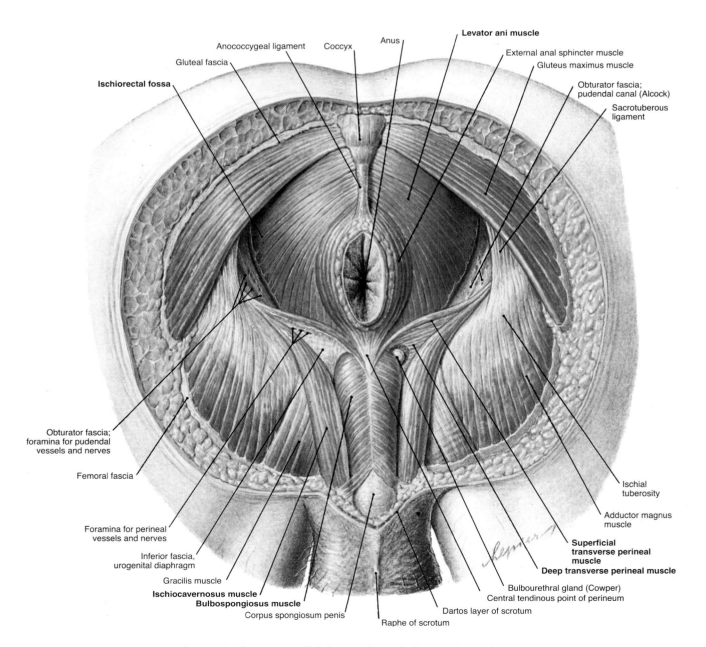

Anococcygeal ligament
Coccyx
Anus
Levator ani muscle
External anal sphincter muscle
Gluteus maximus muscle
Gluteal fascia
Ischiorectal fossa
Obturator fascia; pudendal canal (Alcock)
Sacrotuberous ligament
Obturator fascia; foramina for pudendal vessels and nerves
Femoral fascia
Foramina for perineal vessels and nerves
Inferior fascia, urogenital diaphragm
Gracilis muscle
Ischiocavernosus muscle
Bulbospongiosus muscle
Corpus spongiosum penis
Raphe of scrotum
Dartos layer of scrotum
Central tendinous point of perineum
Bulbourethral gland (Cowper)
Deep transverse perineal muscle
Superficial transverse perineal muscle
Adductor magnus muscle
Ischial tuberosity

Figure 318.2 Superficial Muscles of the Male Perineum

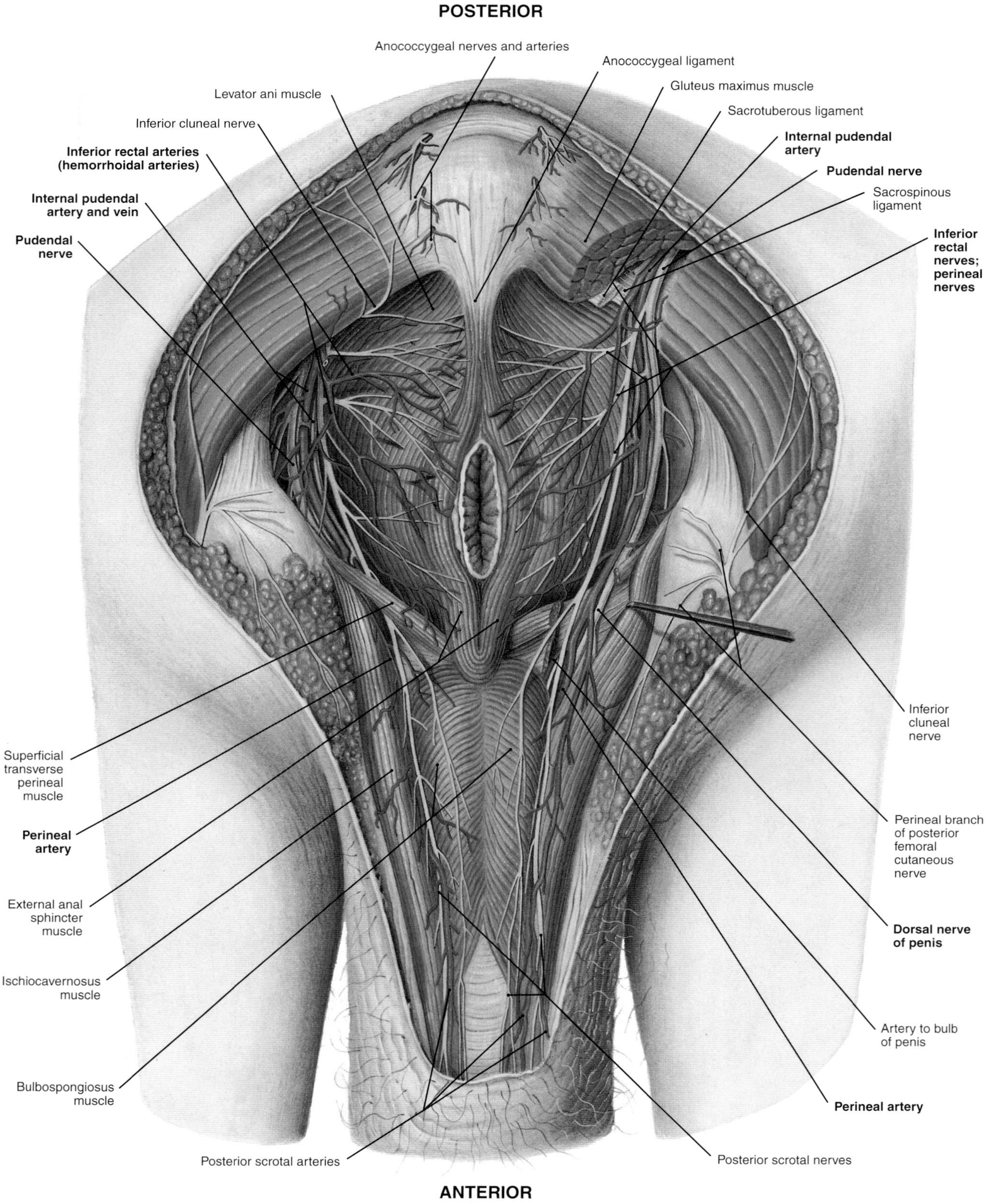

POSTERIOR

Anococcygeal nerves and arteries
Anococcygeal ligament
Levator ani muscle
Gluteus maximus muscle
Sacrotuberous ligament
Inferior cluneal nerve
Inferior rectal arteries (hemorrhoidal arteries)
Internal pudendal artery
Pudendal nerve
Internal pudendal artery and vein
Sacrospinous ligament
Pudendal nerve
Inferior rectal nerves; perineal nerves
Inferior cluneal nerve
Superficial transverse perineal muscle
Perineal branch of posterior femoral cutaneous nerve
Perineal artery
External anal sphincter muscle
Dorsal nerve of penis
Ischiocavernosus muscle
Artery to bulb of penis
Bulbospongiosus muscle
Perineal artery
Posterior scrotal arteries
Posterior scrotal nerves

ANTERIOR

Figure 319 Nerves and Blood Vessels of the Male Perineum

NOTE: (1) The skin of the perineum and the fat of the ischiorectal fossa have been removed to expose the muscles, vessels, and nerves of both the **anal** and **urogenital regions.**

(2) The **internal pudendal vessels** and **nerves** emerge from the pelvis to the gluteal region and then course to the perineum by way of the **pudendal canal** (of Alcock). At the lateral border of the **ischiorectal fossa** their branches, the **inferior rectal vessels** and **nerves**, cross the fossa transversely to supply the levator ani and external anal sphincter muscles.

(3) The main trunks of the vessels and nerve continue anteriorly, pierce the urogenital diaphragm, and become the **perineal vessels** and **nerve** and the **dorsal vessels** and **nerve of the penis**. The muscles of the urogenital triangle are innervated by the perineal nerve, while the dorsal nerve of the penis is the main sensory nerve of that organ.

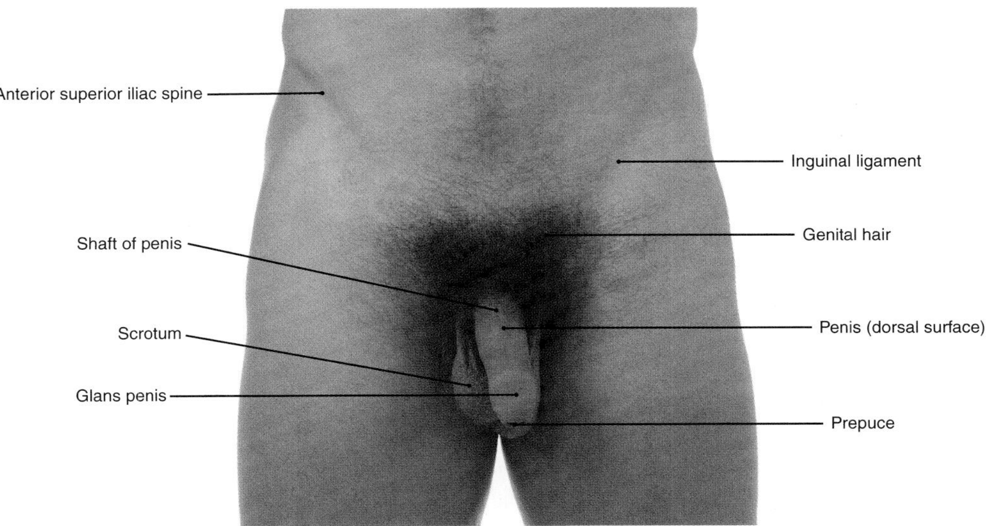
Anterior superior iliac spine
Inguinal ligament
Shaft of penis
Genital hair
Scrotum
Penis (dorsal surface)
Glans penis
Prepuce

Figure 320.1 Surface Anatomy of the Male External Genitalia

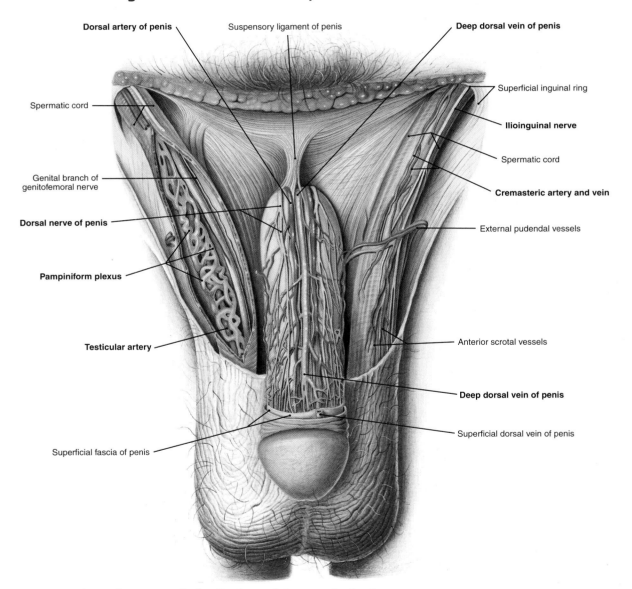

Dorsal artery of penis
Suspensory ligament of penis
Deep dorsal vein of penis
Superficial inguinal ring
Spermatic cord
Ilioinguinal nerve
Spermatic cord
Genital branch of genitofemoral nerve
Cremasteric artery and vein
Dorsal nerve of penis
External pudendal vessels
Pampiniform plexus
Testicular artery
Anterior scrotal vessels
Deep dorsal vein of penis
Superficial dorsal vein of penis
Superficial fascia of penis

Figure 320.2 Vessels and Nerves of the Penis and Spermatic Cord

NOTE: (1) The skin has been removed from the anterior pubic region and the penis, revealing the superficial vessels and nerves of the penis and left **spermatic cord.** The right spermatic cord has been slit open to show the deeper structures within (see Fig. 322.1).

(2) Along the surface of the spermatic cord course the **ilioinguinal nerve** and the **cremasteric artery** and **vein.** Within the cord are found the **ductus deferens** and **testicular artery** surrounded by the **pampiniform plexus of veins.**

(3) Beneath the fascia of the penis and in the midline courses the unpaired **deep dorsal vein of the penis.** Along the sides of the vein, observe the paired **dorsal arteries** and **nerves of the penis.**

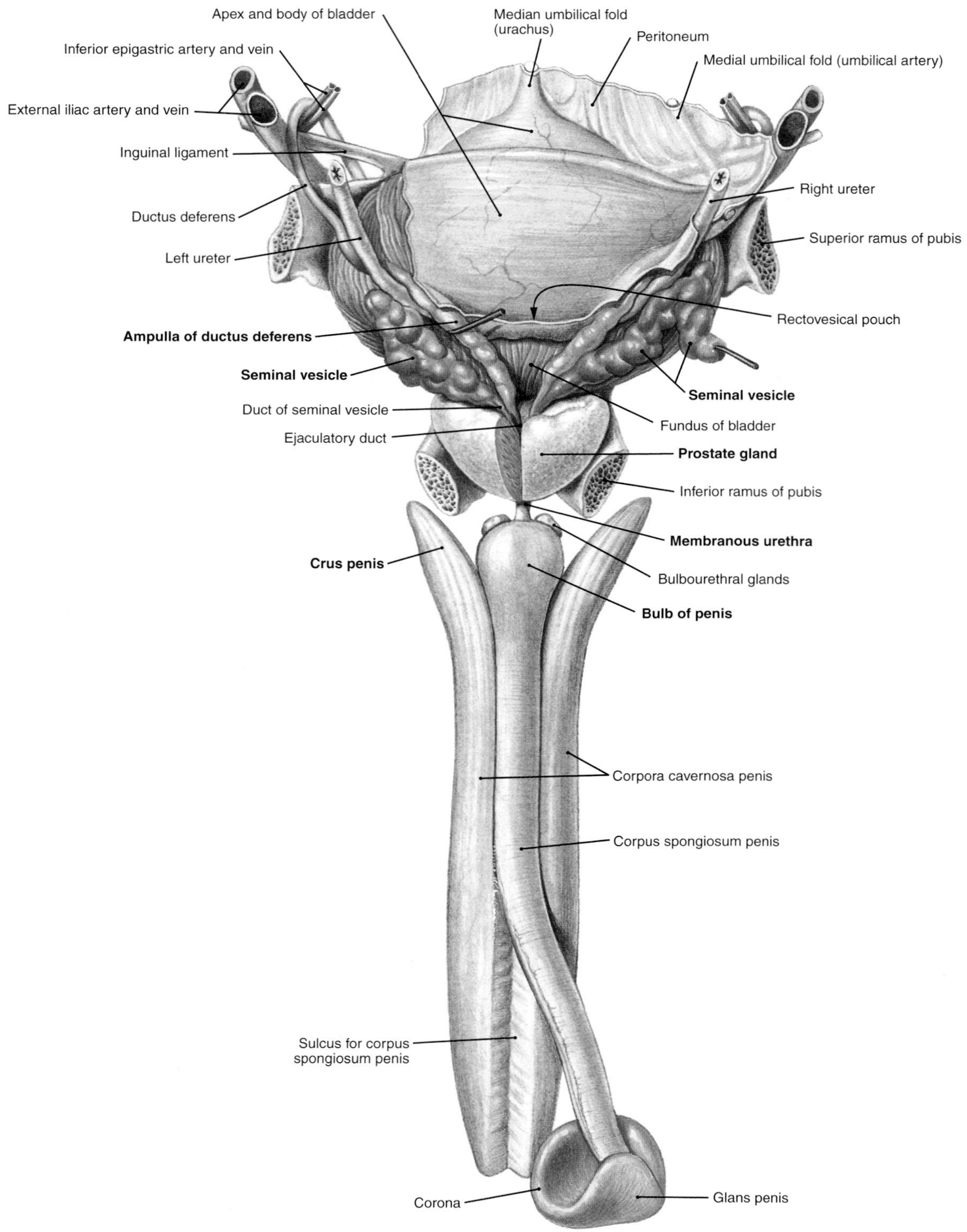
Apex and body of bladder
Median umbilical fold (urachus)
Peritoneum
Medial umbilical fold (umbilical artery)
Inferior epigastric artery and vein
External iliac artery and vein
Inguinal ligament
Ductus deferens
Left ureter
Right ureter
Superior ramus of pubis
Rectovesical pouch
Ampulla of ductus deferens
Seminal vesicle
Seminal vesicle
Duct of seminal vesicle
Ejaculatory duct
Fundus of bladder
Prostate gland
Inferior ramus of pubis
Membranous urethra
Crus penis
Bulbourethral glands
Bulb of penis
Corpora cavernosa penis
Corpus spongiosum penis
Sulcus for corpus spongiosum penis
Corona
Glans penis

Figure 321 Erectile Bodies of the Penis Attached to the Bladder and Other Organs by the Membranous Urethra

NOTE: (1) The deep fascia, which closely invests the erectile bodies of the penis, has been removed, and the distal part of the **corpus spongiosum penis** (which contains the penile urethra), has been displaced from its position between the two **corpora cavernosa penis.**

(2) The posterior surface of the **bladder** and **prostate** and the associated **seminal vesicles, ductus deferens,** and **bulbourethral glands** are also demonstrated. These structures all communicate with the **urethra,** the membranous part of which is in continuity with the **penile urethra.**

(3) The tapered **crura** of the corpora cavernosa penis, which diverge laterally to become adherent to the ischial and pubic rami. They are surrounded by fibers of the ischiocavernosus muscles (see Fig. 319). The base of the corpus spongiosum penis is also expanded, and is called the **bulb of the penis.** It is surrounded by the bulbocavernosus muscle (see Fig. 318.2).

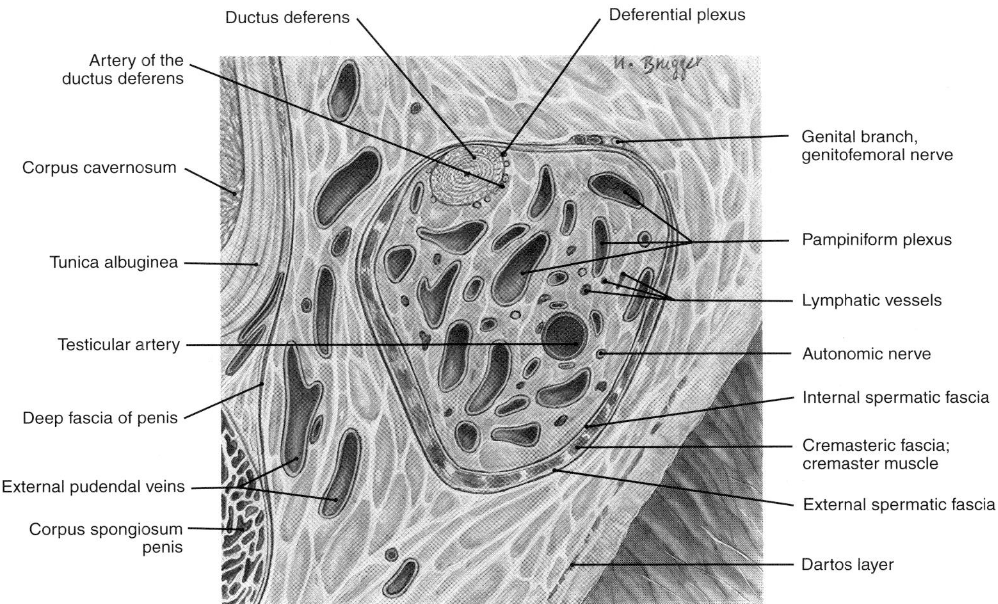
Ductus deferens
Deferential plexus
Artery of the ductus deferens
Corpus cavernosum
Tunica albuginea
Testicular artery
Deep fascia of penis
External pudendal veins
Corpus spongiosum penis
Genital branch, genitofemoral nerve
Pampiniform plexus
Lymphatic vessels
Autonomic nerve
Internal spermatic fascia
Cremasteric fascia; cremaster muscle
External spermatic fascia
Dartos layer

Figure 322.1 Transverse Section of the Spermatic Cord within the Scrotum

NOTE: (1) The spermatic cord contains the: (a) ductus deferens, (b) artery of the ductus deferens, (c) testicular artery, (d) cremasteric artery, (e) pampiniform plexus of veins, (f) lymphatic vessels, and (g) sympathetic and sensory nerve fibers and some fat. These are surrounded by the internal and external spermatic fascial layers and the cremaster muscle.

(2) The spermatic cord traverses the superficial inguinal ring, the inguinal canal, and the abdominal inguinal ring.

(3) The arteries and nerves descend to the testis from the abdomen, while the ductus deferens, the veins. and the lymphatics ascend to the abdomen from the scrotum.

(4) The spermatic cord is covered by the external spermatic fascia, the internal spermatic fascia, and the cremaster muscle.

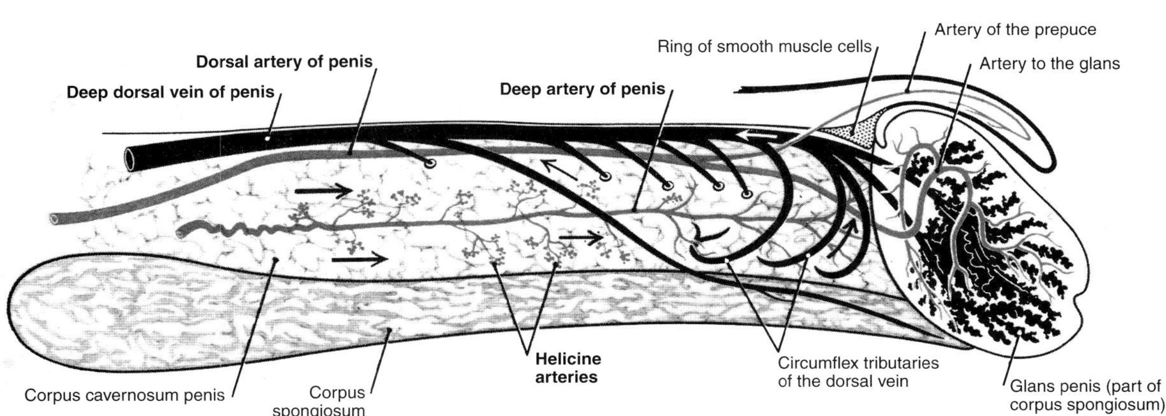
Artery of the prepuce
Ring of smooth muscle cells
Artery to the glans
Dorsal artery of penis
Deep dorsal vein of penis
Deep artery of penis
Helicine arteries
Circumflex tributaries of the dorsal vein
Corpus cavernosum penis
Corpus spongiosum
Glans penis (part of corpus spongiosum)

Figure 322.2 Longitudinal Section through the Penis, Showing Its Vascular Circulation

NOTE: (1) The dorsal and deep arteries of the penis supply blood principally to the corpora cavernosa but also to the glans penis of the corpus spongiosum.

(2) The **helicine branches** of the deep artery and the **circumflex tributaries** of the deep dorsal vein that return blood from the corpora and the glans.

(3) The venous drainage from the glans penis, the corpora cavernosa, and the corpus spongiosum is along the **deep dorsal vein of the penis,** while the superficial dorsal vein (not shown in this figure) drains the prepuce and skin of the penis.

Figure 323.1 Section through Middle of Penis (see Fig. 323.4)

NOTE: (1) The penis is composed of two corpora cavernosa penis containing erectile tissue and one corpus spongiosum penis seen ventrally and in the midline that contains the penile portion of the urethra.

(2) The three corpora are surrounded by a closely investing layer of deep fascia. In erection, blood fills the erectile tissue, causing the corpora to become rigid. The thin-walled veins are compressed between the corpora and the deep fascia. Erection is maintained by preventing venous blood from draining back into the general circulation.

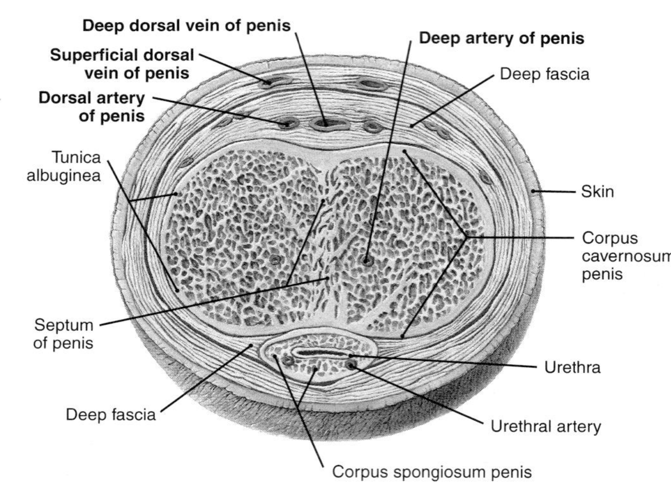
Deep dorsal vein of penis
Superficial dorsal vein of penis
Dorsal artery of penis
Tunica albuginea
Septum of penis
Deep fascia
Deep artery of penis
Deep fascia
Skin
Corpus cavernosum penis
Urethra
Urethral artery
Corpus spongiosum penis

Prepuce
Corona of glans penis
Tunica albuginea of corpus spongiosum
Tunica albuginea of corpus cavernosum
Urethra
Septum of penis

Figure 323.2 Section at Neck of the Glans Penis (see Fig. 323.4)

NOTE: This section is taken from the proximal part of the glans penis. The corpora cavernosa penis become smaller distally, while the corona of the glans penis is formed by the spongy tissue of the corpus spongiosum penis.

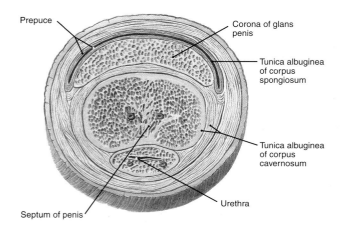

Figure 323.3 Section Midway along the Glans Penis

NOTE: This cross section at the level of the middle of the glans penis shows that the corpora cavernosa penis are diminishing in size. At this site, the glans occupies a larger portion of the cross section.

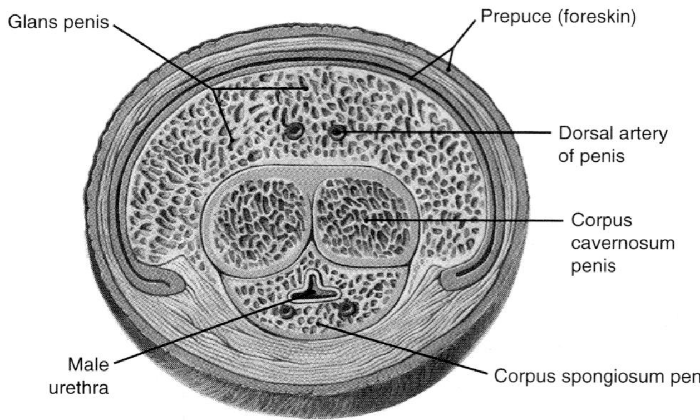
Glans penis
Prepuce (foreskin)
Dorsal artery of penis
Corpus cavernosum penis
Male urethra
Corpus spongiosum penis

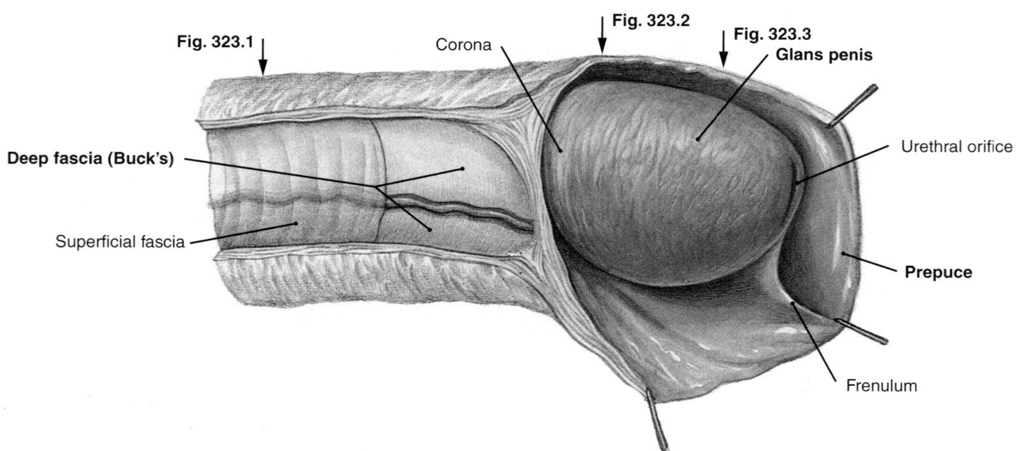
Fig. 323.1
Corona
Fig. 323.2
Fig. 323.3
Glans penis
Deep fascia (Buck's)
Superficial fascia
Urethral orifice
Prepuce
Frenulum

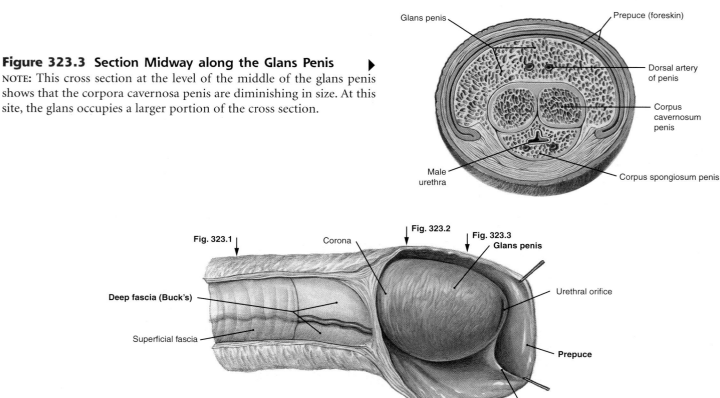

Figure 323.4 Distal End of Penis

NOTE: The distal end of the penis consists of the glans penis, which is attached by the frenulum to a duplicated fold of skin, the prepuce. Observe that the skin of the penis is thin and delicate and is loosely attached to the underlying deep fascia and corpora, accounting for its freely movable nature. (Arrows indicate cross sections seen above.)

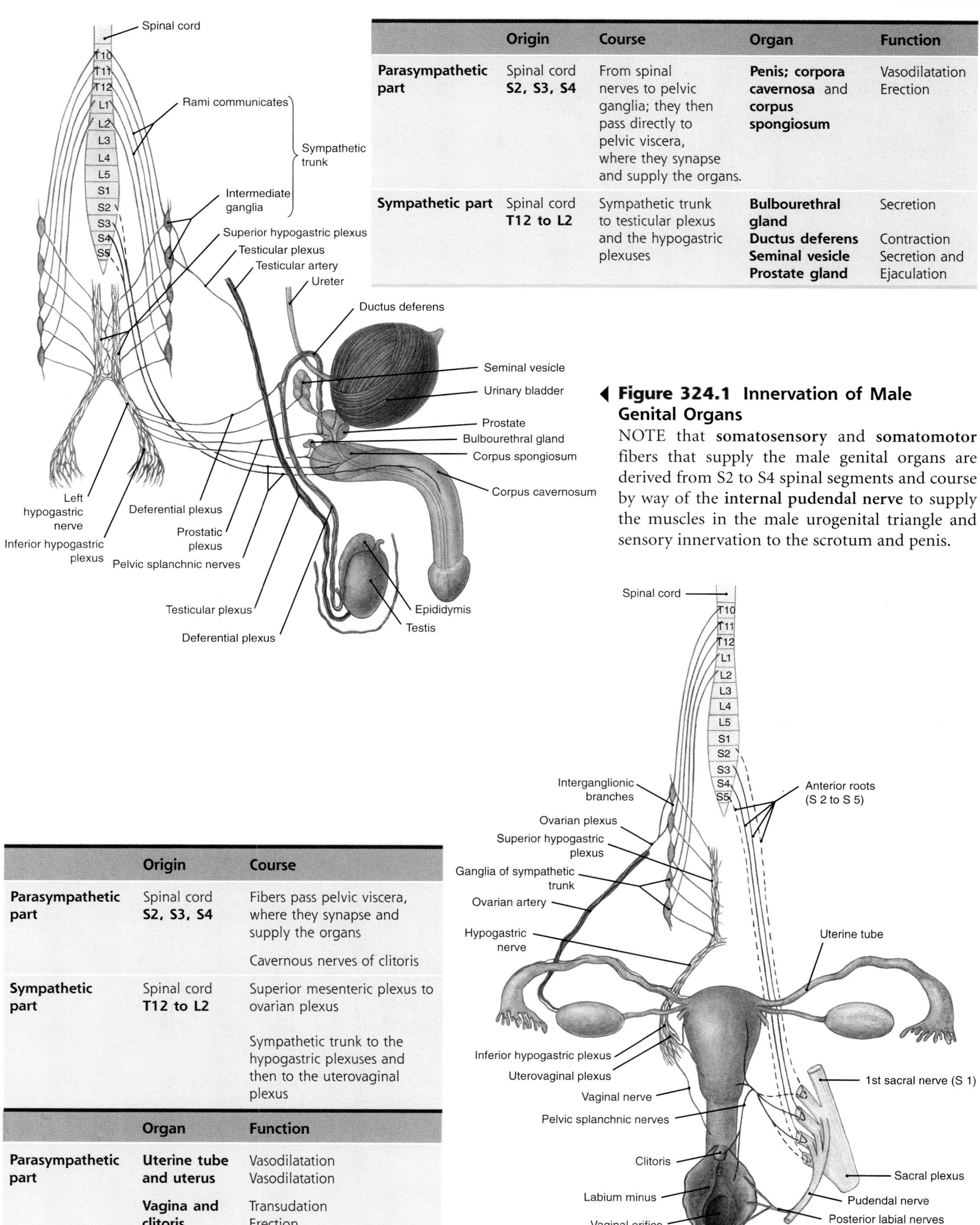

Spinal cord
T10
T11
T12
L1
L2
L3
L4
L5
S1
S2
S3
S4
S5
Rami communicates
Sympathetic trunk
Intermediate ganglia
Superior hypogastric plexus
Testicular plexus
Testicular artery
Ureter
Ductus deferens
Seminal vesicle
Urinary bladder
Prostate
Bulbourethral gland
Corpus spongiosum
Corpus cavernosum
Left hypogastric nerve
Inferior hypogastric plexus
Deferential plexus
Prostatic plexus
Pelvic splanchnic nerves
Testicular plexus
Deferential plexus
Epididymis
Testis
Spinal cord
Interganglionic branches
Ovarian plexus
Superior hypogastric plexus
Ganglia of sympathetic trunk
Ovarian artery
Hypogastric nerve
Anterior roots (S 2 to S 5)
Uterine tube
Inferior hypogastric plexus
Uterovaginal plexus
Vaginal nerve
Pelvic splanchnic nerves
1st sacral nerve (S 1)
Clitoris
Labium minus
Vaginal orifice
Sacral plexus
Pudendal nerve
Posterior labial nerves

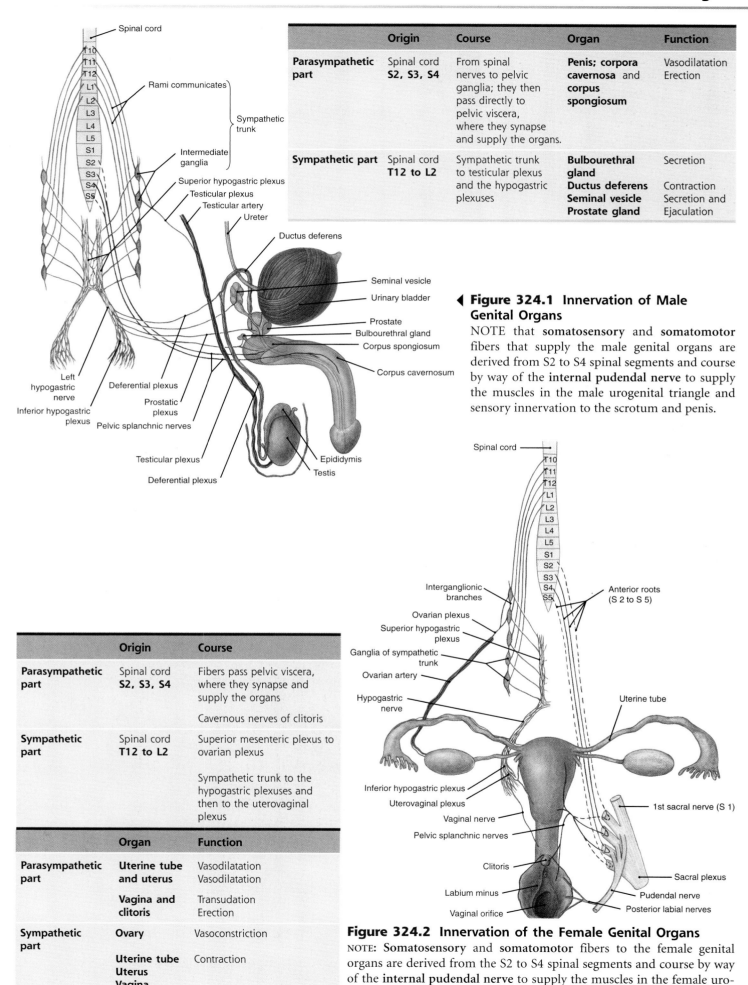

	Origin	Course	Organ	Function
Parasympathetic part	Spinal cord **S2, S3, S4**	From spinal nerves to pelvic ganglia; they then pass directly to pelvic viscera, where they synapse and supply the organs.	**Penis; corpora cavernosa** and **corpus spongiosum**	Vasodilatation Erection
Sympathetic part	Spinal cord **T12 to L2**	Sympathetic trunk to testicular plexus and the hypogastric plexuses	**Bulbourethral gland** **Ductus deferens** **Seminal vesicle** **Prostate gland**	Secretion Contraction Secretion and Ejaculation

Figure 324.1 Innervation of Male Genital Organs

NOTE that **somatosensory** and **somatomotor** fibers that supply the male genital organs are derived from S2 to S4 spinal segments and course by way of the **internal pudendal nerve** to supply the muscles in the male urogenital triangle and sensory innervation to the scrotum and penis.

	Origin	Course
Parasympathetic part	Spinal cord **S2, S3, S4**	Fibers pass pelvic viscera, where they synapse and supply the organs
		Cavernous nerves of clitoris
Sympathetic part	Spinal cord **T12 to L2**	Superior mesenteric plexus to ovarian plexus
		Sympathetic trunk to the hypogastric plexuses and then to the uterovaginal plexus

	Organ	Function
Parasympathetic part	**Uterine tube and uterus**	Vasodilatation Vasodilatation
	Vagina and clitoris	Transudation Erection
Sympathetic part	**Ovary**	Vasoconstriction
	Uterine tube Uterus Vagina	Contraction

Figure 324.2 Innervation of the Female Genital Organs

NOTE: **Somatosensory** and **somatomotor** fibers to the female genital organs are derived from the S2 to S4 spinal segments and course by way of the **internal pudendal nerve** to supply the muscles in the female urogenital triangle and sensory innervation to the clitoris and labia.

THE BACK, VERTEBRAL COLUMN, AND SPINAL CORD

5

PLATES

5 The Back, Vertebral Column, and Spinal Cord

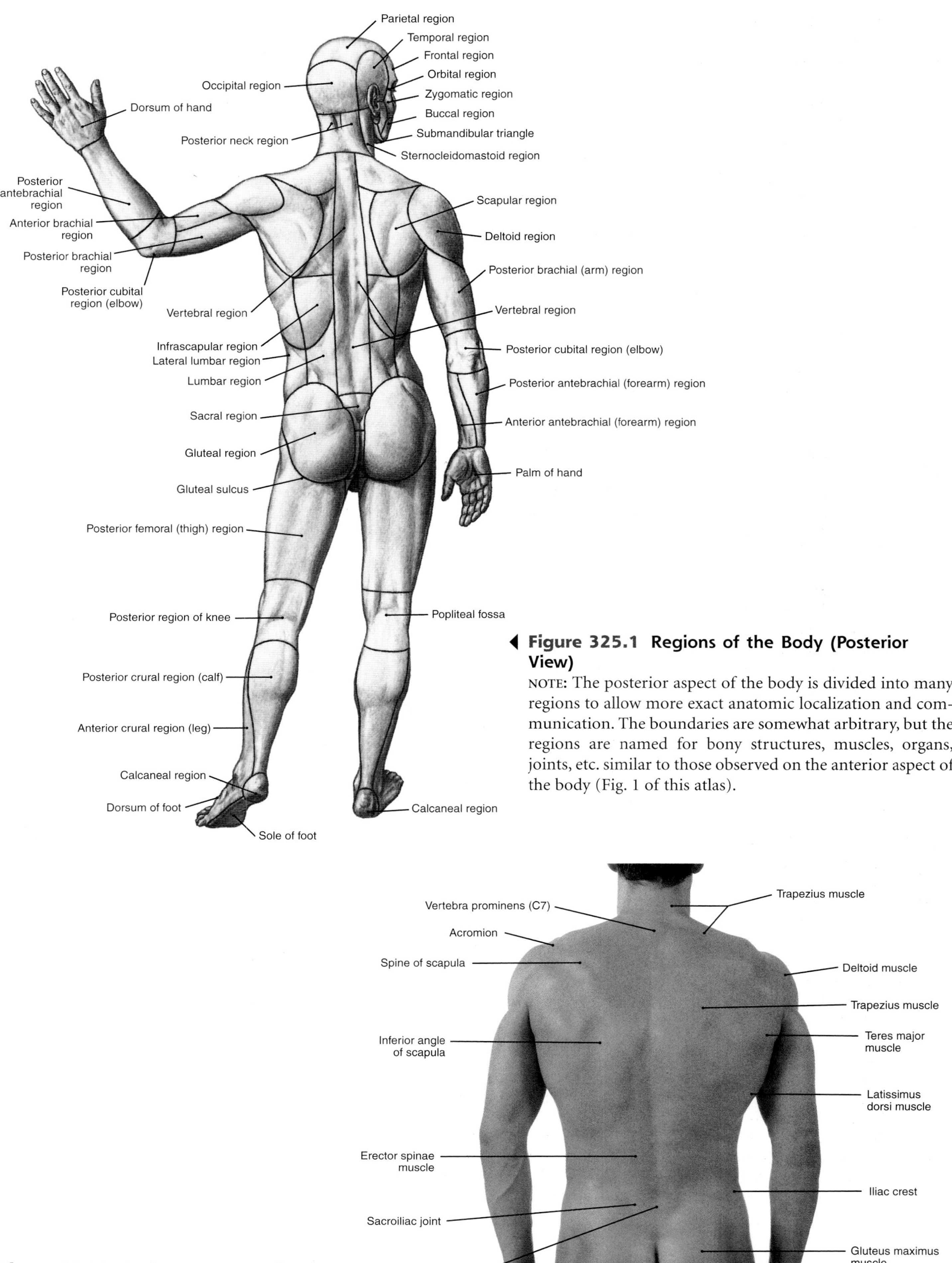
Parietal region
Temporal region
Frontal region
Orbital region
Zygomatic region
Buccal region
Submandibular triangle
Sternocleidomastoid region
Occipital region
Dorsum of hand
Posterior neck region
Posterior antebrachial region
Anterior brachial region
Posterior brachial region
Posterior cubital region (elbow)
Vertebral region
Scapular region
Deltoid region
Posterior brachial (arm) region
Vertebral region
Infrascapular region
Lateral lumbar region
Lumbar region
Posterior cubital region (elbow)
Posterior antebrachial (forearm) region
Sacral region
Anterior antebrachial (forearm) region
Gluteal region
Palm of hand
Gluteal sulcus
Posterior femoral (thigh) region
Posterior region of knee
Popliteal fossa
Posterior crural region (calf)
Anterior crural region (leg)
Calcaneal region
Dorsum of foot
Sole of foot
Calcaneal region
Vertebra prominens (C7)
Trapezius muscle
Acromion
Spine of scapula
Deltoid muscle
Trapezius muscle
Inferior angle of scapula
Teres major muscle
Latissimus dorsi muscle
Erector spinae muscle
Iliac crest
Sacroiliac joint
Gluteus maximus muscle
5th lumbar vertebra (spinous process)

Figure 325.1 Regions of the Body (Posterior View)

NOTE: The posterior aspect of the body is divided into many regions to allow more exact anatomic localization and communication. The boundaries are somewhat arbitrary, but the regions are named for bony structures, muscles, organs, joints, etc. similar to those observed on the anterior aspect of the body (Fig. 1 of this atlas).

Figure 325.2 Surface Anatomy of the Back

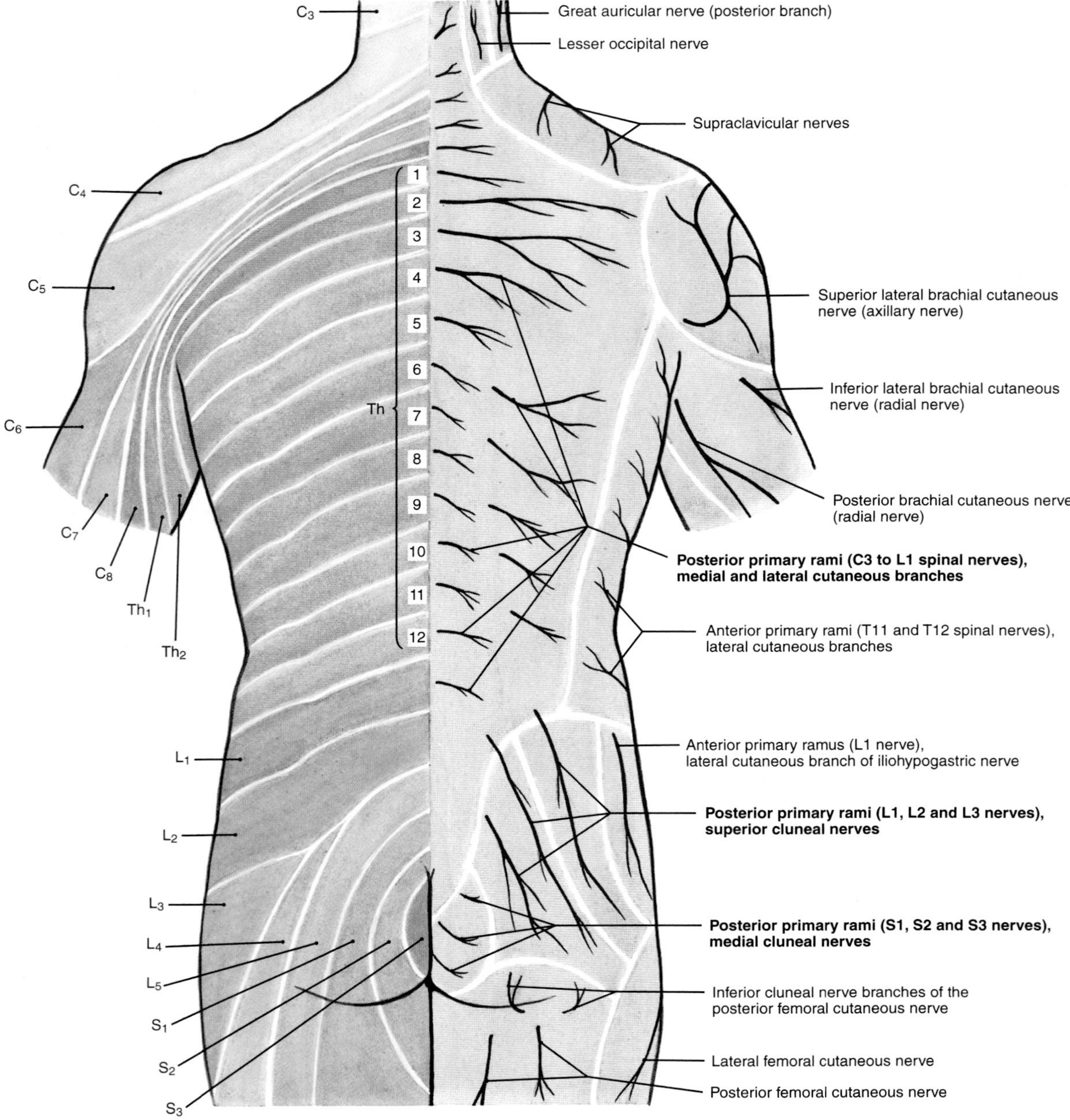
C3
Great auricular nerve (posterior branch)
Lesser occipital nerve
Supraclavicular nerves
C4
C5
Superior lateral brachial cutaneous nerve (axillary nerve)
Inferior lateral brachial cutaneous nerve (radial nerve)
C6
Th
1
2
3
4
5
6
7
8
9
10
11
12
Posterior brachial cutaneous nerve (radial nerve)
C7
C8
Th1
Th2
Posterior primary rami (C3 to L1 spinal nerves), medial and lateral cutaneous branches
Anterior primary rami (T11 and T12 spinal nerves), lateral cutaneous branches
L1
Anterior primary ramus (L1 nerve), lateral cutaneous branch of iliohypogastric nerve
L2
Posterior primary rami (L1, L2 and L3 nerves), superior cluneal nerves
L3
L4
L5
Posterior primary rami (S1, S2 and S3 nerves), medial cluneal nerves
S1
Inferior cluneal nerve branches of the posterior femoral cutaneous nerve
S2
Lateral femoral cutaneous nerve
S3
Posterior femoral cutaneous nerve

Figure 326 Dermatomes and Cutaneous Nerve Distribution (Posterior Aspect of the Body)

NOTE: (1) **Dermatomes** are shown on the left and the **cutaneous nerve** distribution and surface areas for the dorsum of the trunk are shown on the right.

(2) An area of skin supplied by the cutaneous branches of a single nerve is called a dermatome. There is considerable overlap between adjacent segmental nerves and, although the loss of a single spinal nerve produces an area of altered sensation, it does not result in total sensory loss.

(3) Destruction of at least three consecutive spinal nerves is required to produce a total sensory loss of the dermatome supplied by the middle nerve of the three.

(4) Mapping of skin areas affected by herpes zoster (shingles) has added to our knowledge of dermatome distribution. Another experimental procedure is that of "remaining sensibility." In the latter, dermatome areas are established in animals after severance of several roots above and below the intact root whose dermatome is being studied.

(5) The posterior primary rami of spinal nerves C3 through L1 (boldface) supply the posterior skin of the trunk, while the lateral neck, upper limb, and lateral trunk are supplied by anterior primary rami.

(6) The posterior primary rami (boldface) of L1, L2, and L3 (superior cluneal nerves) as well as the posterior primary rami (boldface) of S1, S2, and S3 (medial cluneal nerves) supply the gluteal and sacral regions. The remaining nerves of the posterior lower trunk and limbs are from anterior primary rami.

Figure 327.1 Branching of a Typical Spinal Nerve

NOTE: (1) Fibers from both dorsal and ventral roots join to form a spinal nerve that soon divides into a **posterior** and an **anterior primary ramus.** The posterior primary ramus courses dorsally to innervate the muscles and skin of the back. The anterior primary ramus courses laterally and anteriorly around the body to innervate the rest of the segment.

(2) The posterior primary rami of typical spinal nerves are smaller in diameter than the anterior rami, and each usually divides into medial and lateral branches, which contain both motor and sensory fibers innervating structures in the back.

(3) Unlike anterior primary rami, which join to form the cervical, brachial, and lumbosacral plexuses, the peripheral nerves derived from the posterior rami do not, as a rule, intercommunicate and form plexuses. There is, however, some segmental overlap of peripheral sensory fields, as seen with the anterior rami.

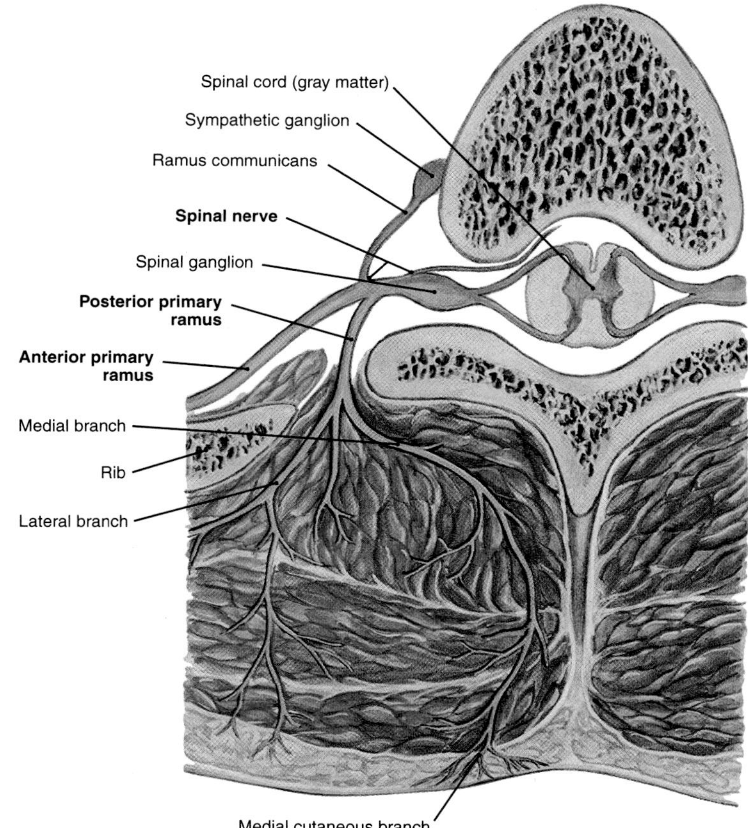
Spinal cord (gray matter)
Sympathetic ganglion
Ramus communicans
Spinal nerve
Spinal ganglion
Posterior primary ramus
Anterior primary ramus
Medial branch
Rib
Lateral branch
Medial cutaneous branch

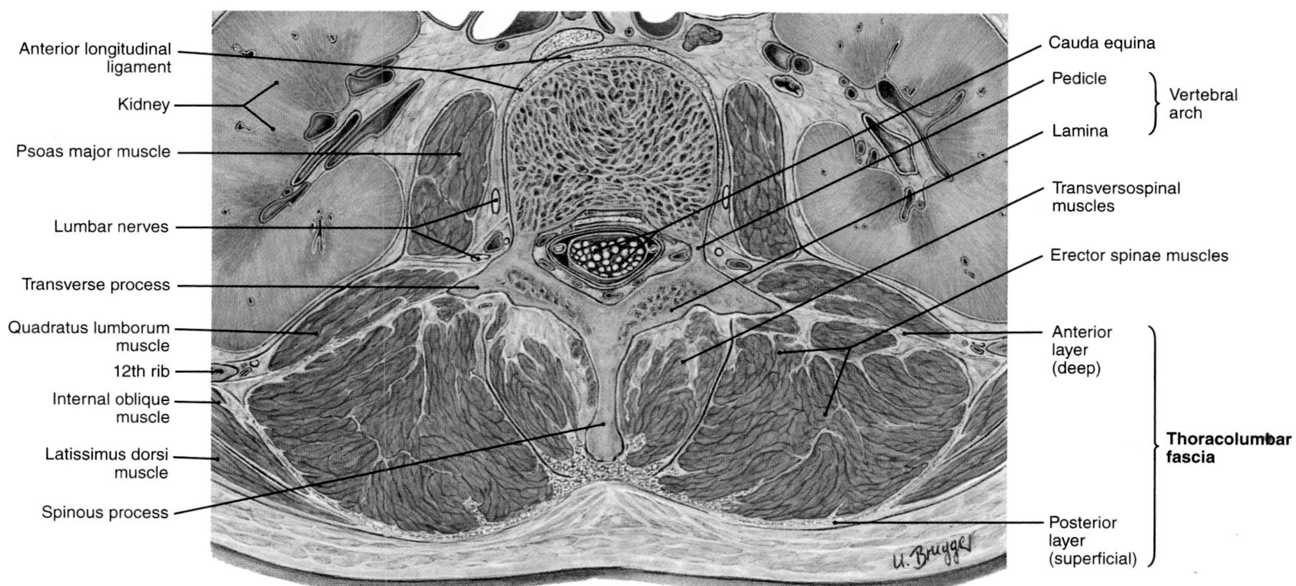
Anterior longitudinal ligament
Kidney
Psoas major muscle
Lumbar nerves
Transverse process
Quadratus lumborum muscle
12th rib
Internal oblique muscle
Latissimus dorsi muscle
Spinous process
Cauda equina
Pedicle
Lamina
Vertebral arch
Transversospinal muscles
Erector spinae muscles
Anterior layer (deep)
Posterior layer (superficial)
Thoracolumbar fascia
U. Brugger

Figure 327.2 Cross Section at the L2 Vertebral Level: Deep Back Muscles and Thoracolumbar Fascia

NOTE: (1) This cross section of the deep back shows the lumbar part of the thoracolumbar fascia as it encloses the divisions of the erector spinae and transversospinal muscles. The fascia is formed by a posterior (superficial) layer and an anterior (deep) layer.

(2) Medially, the layers of the thoracolumbar fascia attach to the spinous and transverse processes of the lumbar vertebrae and laterally they become continuous with the aponeuroses and fascias of the latissimus dorsi and anterior abdominal muscles.

(3) The quadratus lumborum and psoas major muscles located deep to the erector spinae. Observe the relationship of the kidneys anterior to the quadratus lumborum muscles.

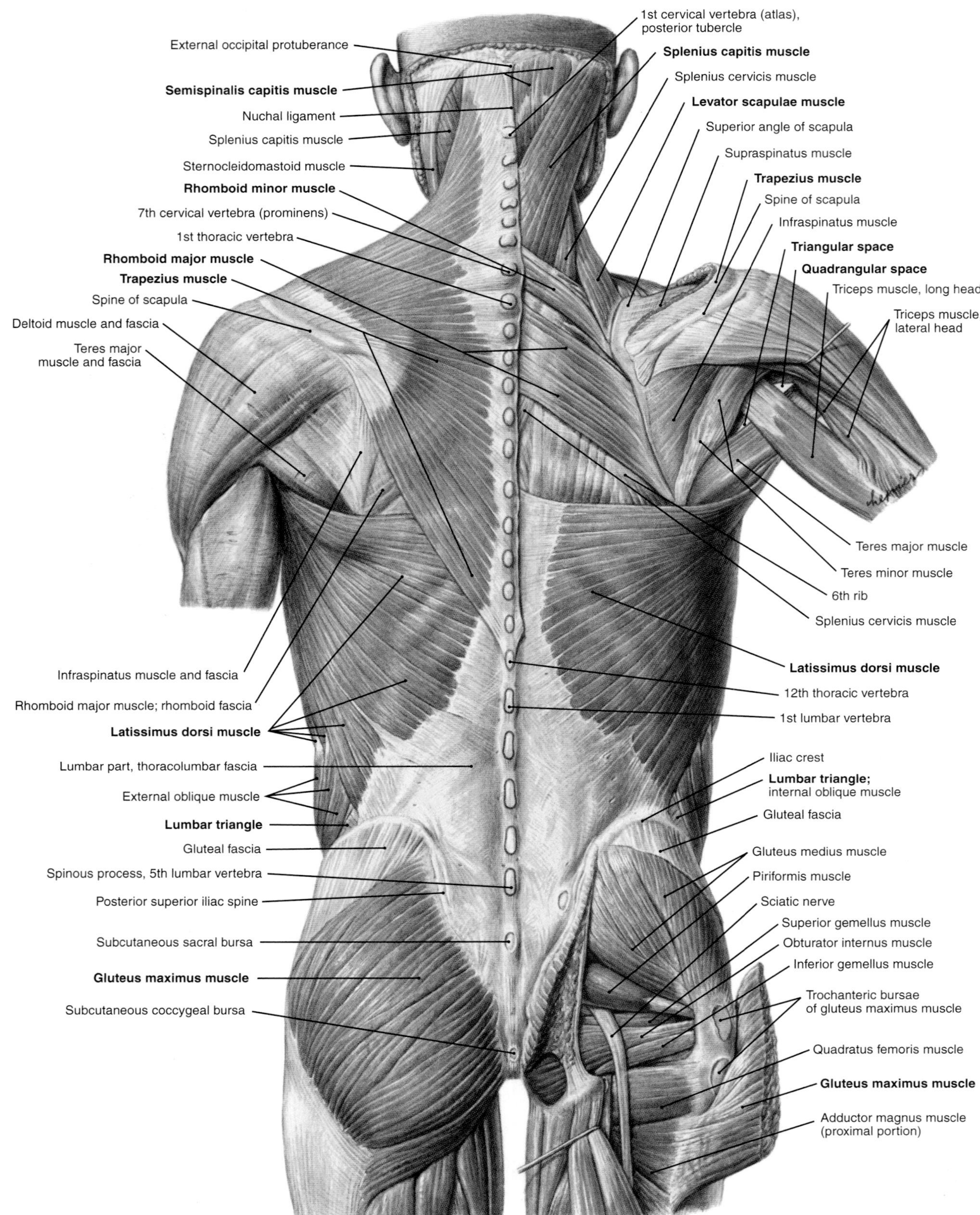

1st cervical vertebra (atlas), posterior tubercle
External occipital protuberance
Splenius capitis muscle
Semispinalis capitis muscle
Splenius cervicis muscle
Nuchal ligament
Levator scapulae muscle
Splenius capitis muscle
Superior angle of scapula
Sternocleidomastoid muscle
Supraspinatus muscle
Rhomboid minor muscle
Trapezius muscle
7th cervical vertebra (prominens)
Spine of scapula
Infraspinatus muscle
1st thoracic vertebra
Triangular space
Rhomboid major muscle
Quadrangular space
Trapezius muscle
Triceps muscle, long head
Spine of scapula
Triceps muscle, lateral head
Deltoid muscle and fascia
Teres major muscle and fascia
Teres major muscle
Teres minor muscle
6th rib
Splenius cervicis muscle
Latissimus dorsi muscle
Infraspinatus muscle and fascia
12th thoracic vertebra
Rhomboid major muscle; rhomboid fascia
1st lumbar vertebra
Latissimus dorsi muscle
Iliac crest
Lumbar part, thoracolumbar fascia
Lumbar triangle; internal oblique muscle
External oblique muscle
Gluteal fascia
Lumbar triangle
Gluteal fascia
Gluteus medius muscle
Spinous process, 5th lumbar vertebra
Piriformis muscle
Posterior superior iliac spine
Sciatic nerve
Superior gemellus muscle
Subcutaneous sacral bursa
Obturator internus muscle
Inferior gemellus muscle
Gluteus maximus muscle
Trochanteric bursae of gluteus maximus muscle
Subcutaneous coccygeal bursa
Quadratus femoris muscle
Gluteus maximus muscle
Adductor magnus muscle (proximal portion)

Figure 328 Muscles of the Posterior Neck, Shoulder, Back, and Gluteal Region

NOTE: The most superficial layer of back muscles includes the **latissimus dorsi** and the **trapezius.** Beneath the trapezius, the **levator scapulae** and **rhomboid major** and **minor muscles** attach along the vertebral border of the scapula. In the neck, the **splenius capitis** and **semispinalis capitis** lie directly under the trapezius.

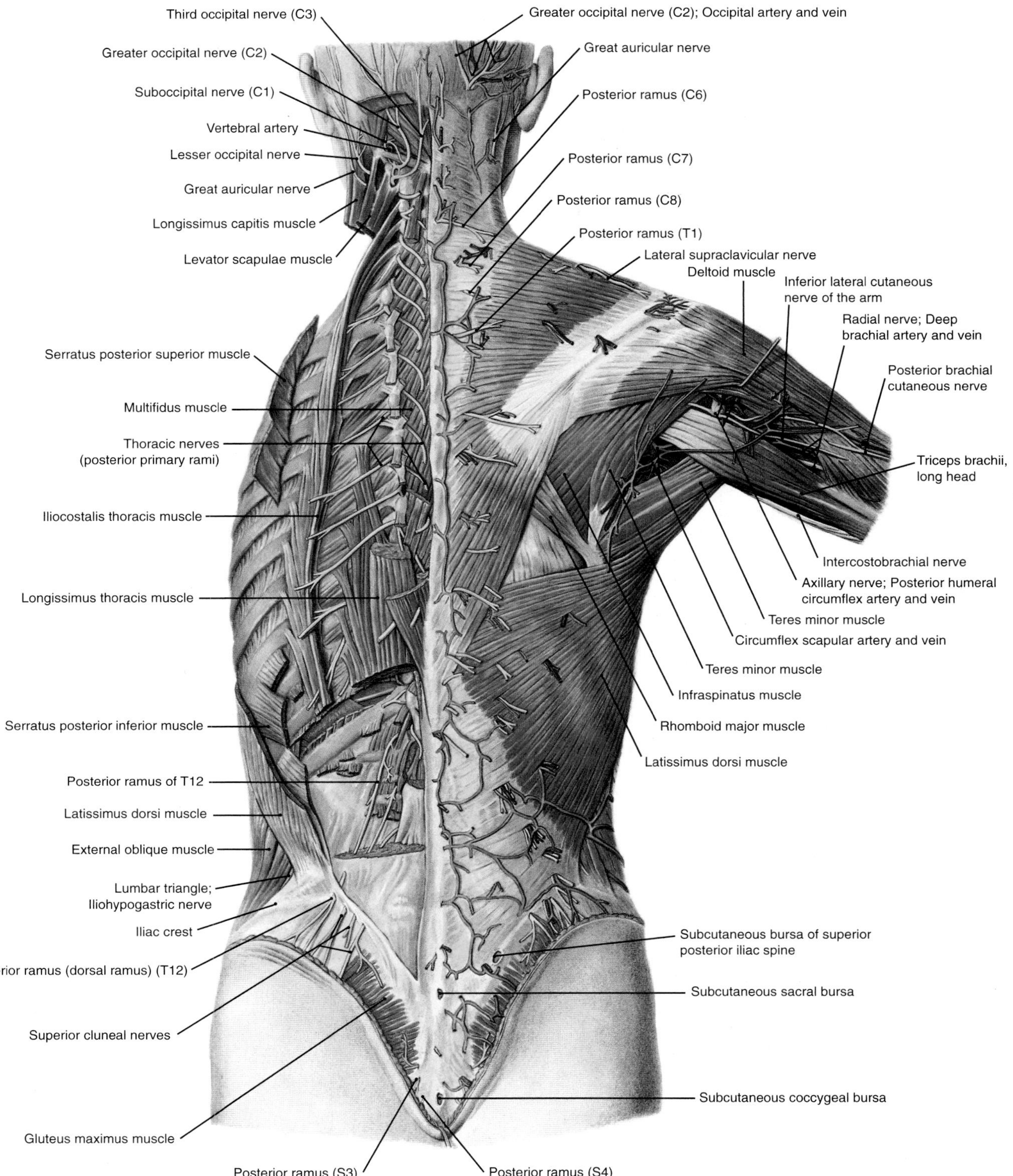
Third occipital nerve (C3)
Greater occipital nerve (C2)
Suboccipital nerve (C1)
Vertebral artery
Lesser occipital nerve
Great auricular nerve
Longissimus capitis muscle
Levator scapulae muscle
Greater occipital nerve (C2); Occipital artery and vein
Great auricular nerve
Posterior ramus (C6)
Posterior ramus (C7)
Posterior ramus (C8)
Posterior ramus (T1)
Lateral supraclavicular nerve
Deltoid muscle
Inferior lateral cutaneous nerve of the arm
Radial nerve; Deep brachial artery and vein
Posterior brachial cutaneous nerve
Triceps brachii, long head
Serratus posterior superior muscle
Multifidus muscle
Thoracic nerves (posterior primary rami)
Iliocostalis thoracis muscle
Longissimus thoracis muscle
Intercostobrachial nerve
Axillary nerve; Posterior humeral circumflex artery and vein
Teres minor muscle
Circumflex scapular artery and vein
Teres minor muscle
Infraspinatus muscle
Rhomboid major muscle
Latissimus dorsi muscle
Serratus posterior inferior muscle
Posterior ramus of T12
Latissimus dorsi muscle
External oblique muscle
Lumbar triangle; Iliohypogastric nerve
Iliac crest
Posterior ramus (dorsal ramus) (T12)
Superior cluneal nerves
Gluteus maximus muscle
Subcutaneous bursa of superior posterior iliac spine
Subcutaneous sacral bursa
Subcutaneous coccygeal bursa
Posterior ramus (S3)
Posterior ramus (S4)

Figure 329 Blood Vessels and Nerves of the Superficial and Deep Back

NOTE: (1) On the left side, the posterior primary rami of the spinal nerves are seen penetrating the soft structures to a varying level depending on how much muscle tissue has been removed.

(2) In the lower back on the left, all of the superficial and deep muscles have been removed, while in the thoracic and cervical regions the nerves are seen penetrating the deep muscles.

(3) On the right side, the nerves and vessels are seen penetrating the superficial muscle layer of the back (the trapezius and latissimus dorsi muscles) to get to the superficial muscle layer and the skin; the latissimus dorsi and trapezius muscles are *NOT supplied by these posterior primary rami*— they are supplied by the thoracodorsal and spinal accessory nerves, respectively.

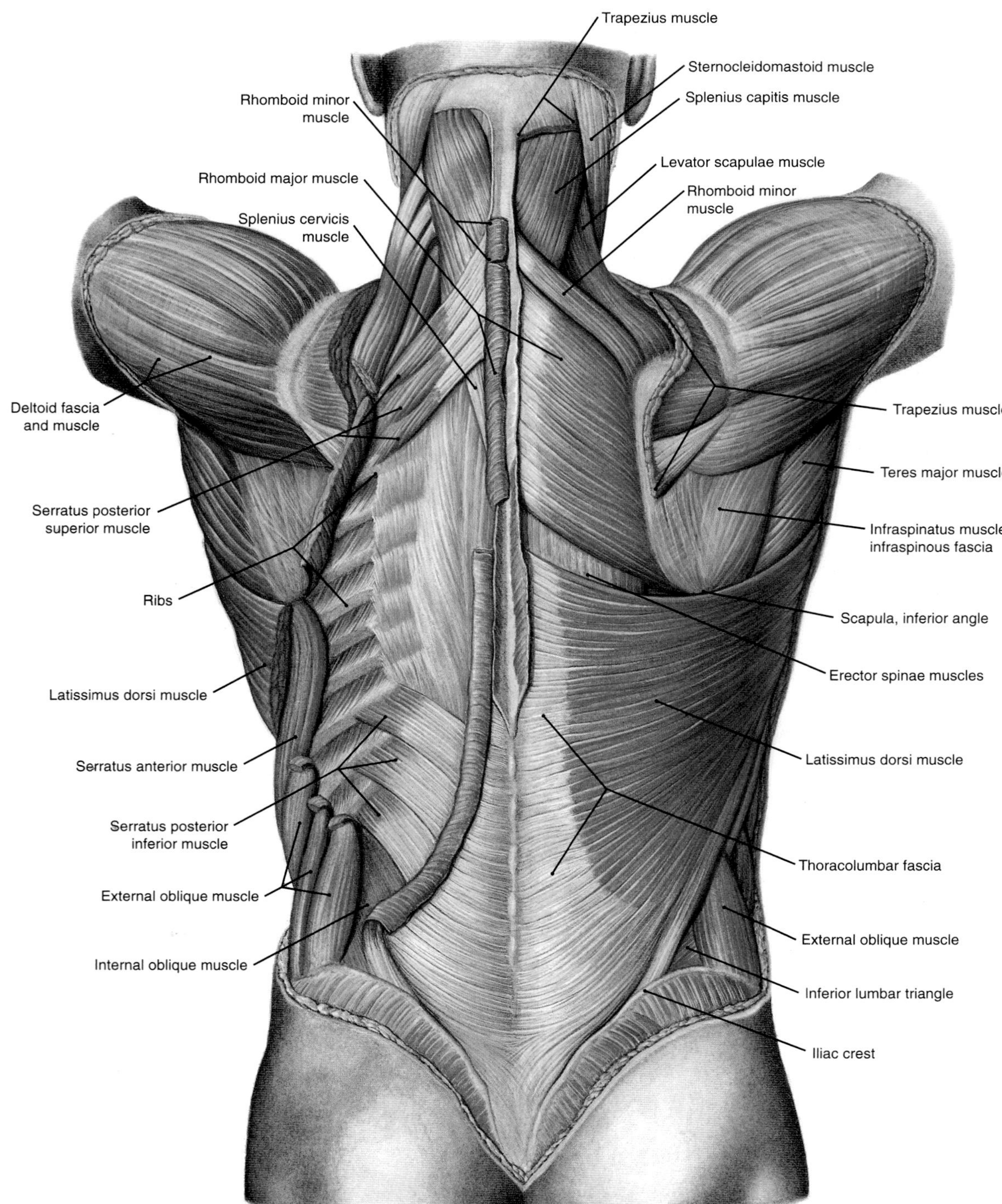
Trapezius muscle
Sternocleidomastoid muscle
Splenius capitis muscle
Rhomboid minor muscle
Rhomboid major muscle
Splenius cervicis muscle
Levator scapulae muscle
Rhomboid minor muscle
Deltoid fascia and muscle
Trapezius muscle
Teres major muscle
Serratus posterior superior muscle
Infraspinatus muscle, infraspinous fascia
Ribs
Scapula, inferior angle
Erector spinae muscles
Latissimus dorsi muscle
Latissimus dorsi muscle
Serratus anterior muscle
Serratus posterior inferior muscle
Thoracolumbar fascia
External oblique muscle
External oblique muscle
Internal oblique muscle
Inferior lumbar triangle
Iliac crest

Figure 330 Superficial and Intermediate Back Muscles (Posterior View)

NOTE: (1) On the right side, the trapezius has been removed to reveal the rhomboid muscles, the levator scapulae, and the splenius capitis. The latissimus dorsi and the thoracolumbar fascia are still intact.

(2) On the left side, the trapezius, the latissimus dorsi, and the rhomboid muscles have been removed to expose the serratus posterior superior, the serratus posterior inferior, and several ribs.

(3) The erector spinae muscles and its overlying fascia (labeled on the right and shown extensively on the left but not labeled) extends longitudinally and considered the strongest and most important deep back muscle (see Fig. 331).

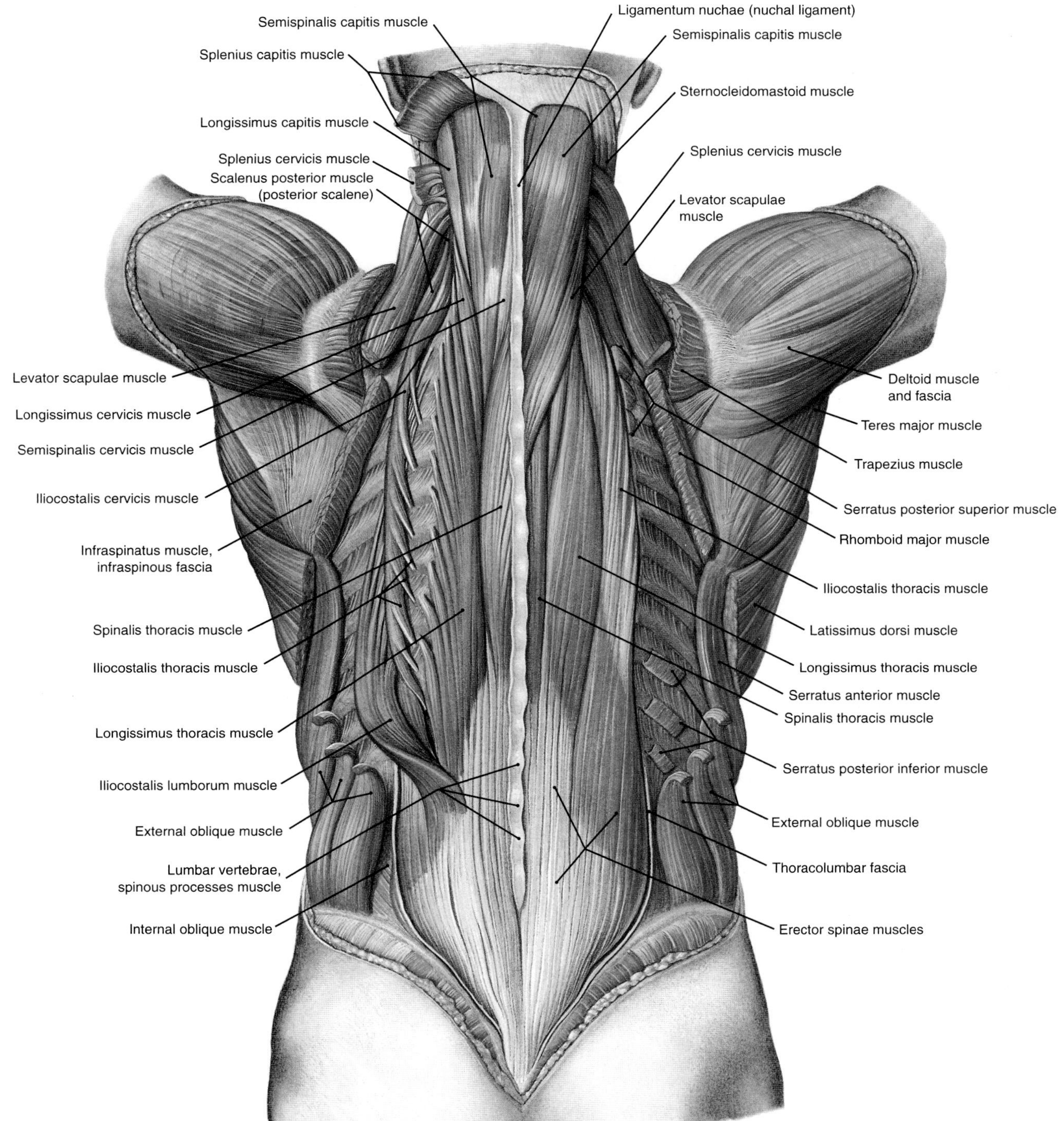
Semispinalis capitis muscle
Splenius capitis muscle
Longissimus capitis muscle
Splenius cervicis muscle
Scalenus posterior muscle (posterior scalene)
Ligamentum nuchae (nuchal ligament)
Semispinalis capitis muscle
Sternocleidomastoid muscle
Splenius cervicis muscle
Levator scapulae muscle
Levator scapulae muscle
Longissimus cervicis muscle
Semispinalis cervicis muscle
Iliocostalis cervicis muscle
Infraspinatus muscle, infraspinous fascia
Spinalis thoracis muscle
Iliocostalis thoracis muscle
Longissimus thoracis muscle
Iliocostalis lumborum muscle
External oblique muscle
Lumbar vertebrae, spinous processes muscle
Internal oblique muscle
Deltoid muscle and fascia
Teres major muscle
Trapezius muscle
Serratus posterior superior muscle
Rhomboid major muscle
Iliocostalis thoracis muscle
Latissimus dorsi muscle
Longissimus thoracis muscle
Serratus anterior muscle
Spinalis thoracis muscle
Serratus posterior inferior muscle
External oblique muscle
Thoracolumbar fascia
Erector spinae muscles

Figure 331 Erector Spinae Muscles and Semispinalis Capitis Muscles

NOTE: (1) The trapezius and latissimus dorsi muscles have been removed, as have the rhomboid muscles and the serratus posterior (superior and inferior) muscles.

(2) The erector spinae muscle is seen intact on the right side, while its iliocostalis, longissimus, and spinalis columns have been separated on the left side. This muscle is a strong extensor and lateral flexor of the vertebral column (and head).

(3) The two semispinalis capitis muscles superiorly following the removal of the splenius capitis muscles. Observe the tendinous intersections that are characteristic of this muscle.

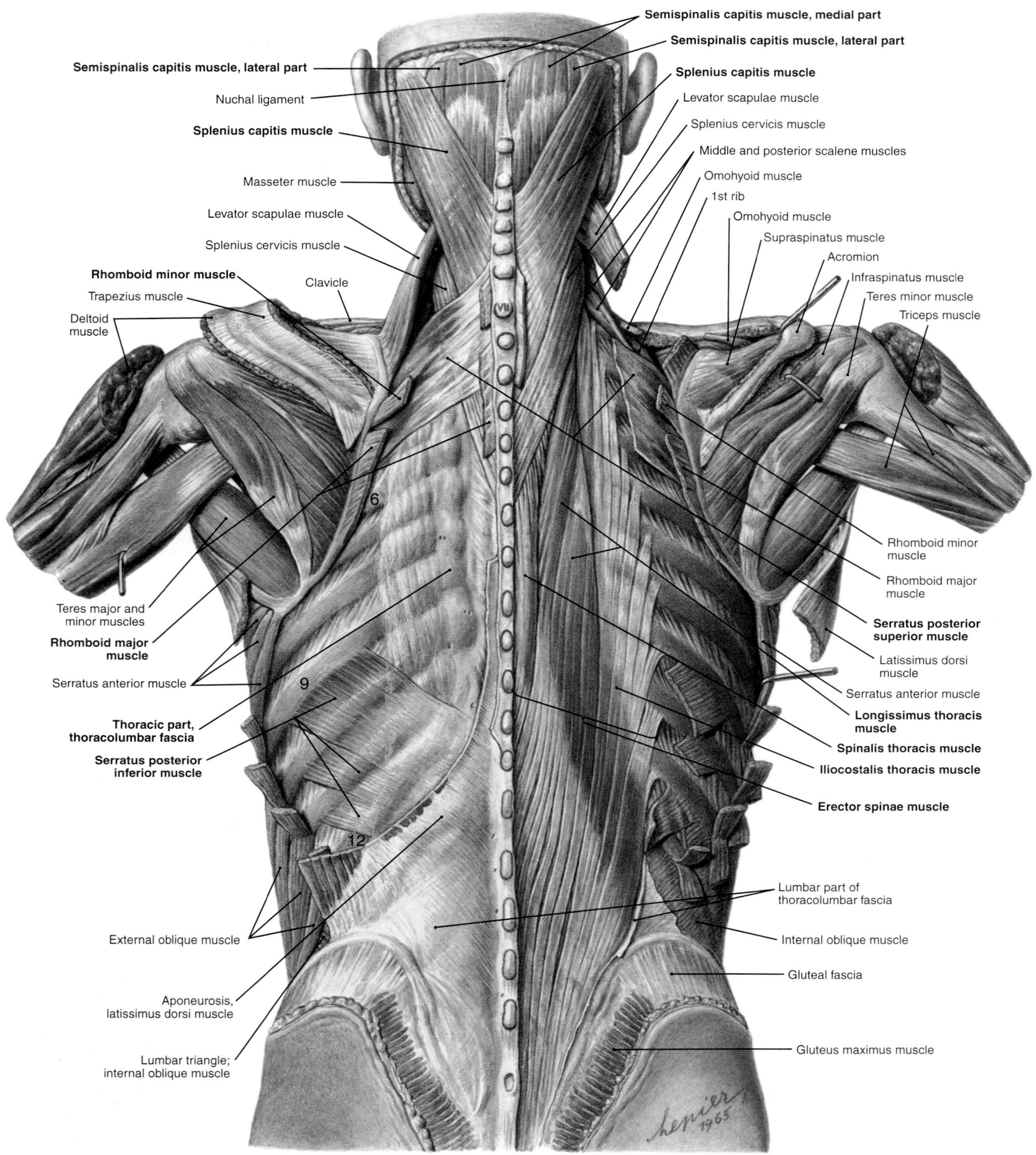
Semispinalis capitis muscle, medial part
Semispinalis capitis muscle, lateral part
Splenius capitis muscle
Levator scapulae muscle
Splenius cervicis muscle
Middle and posterior scalene muscles
Omohyoid muscle
1st rib
Omohyoid muscle
Supraspinatus muscle
Acromion
Infraspinatus muscle
Teres minor muscle
Triceps muscle
Semispinalis capitis muscle, lateral part
Nuchal ligament
Splenius capitis muscle
Masseter muscle
Levator scapulae muscle
Splenius cervicis muscle
Rhomboid minor muscle
Clavicle
Trapezius muscle
Deltoid muscle
6
VII
Teres major and minor muscles
Rhomboid major muscle
Serratus anterior muscle
9
Thoracic part, thoracolumbar fascia
Serratus posterior inferior muscle
12
Rhomboid minor muscle
Rhomboid major muscle
Serratus posterior superior muscle
Latissimus dorsi muscle
Serratus anterior muscle
Longissimus thoracis muscle
Spinalis thoracis muscle
Iliocostalis thoracis muscle
Erector spinae muscle
Lumbar part of thoracolumbar fascia
Internal oblique muscle
Gluteal fascia
Gluteus maximus muscle
External oblique muscle
Aponeurosis, latissimus dorsi muscle
Lumbar triangle; internal oblique muscle
Lenier 1965

Figure 332 Muscles of the Back: Intermediate Layer (Left), Deep Layer (Right)

NOTE: (1) On the left side, the superficial back muscles (trapezius and latissimus dorsi) have been cut, as have the rhomboids, which attach the vertebral border of the scapula to the vertebral column. Observe the underlying serratus posterior superior and inferior muscles.

(2) On the right side, the serratus posterior muscles and the thoracolumbar fascia have been removed, exposing the erector spinae muscle (formerly called sacrospinalis muscle).

(3) In the neck, the splenius cervicis, splenius capitis, and semispinalis capitis underlie the trapezius.

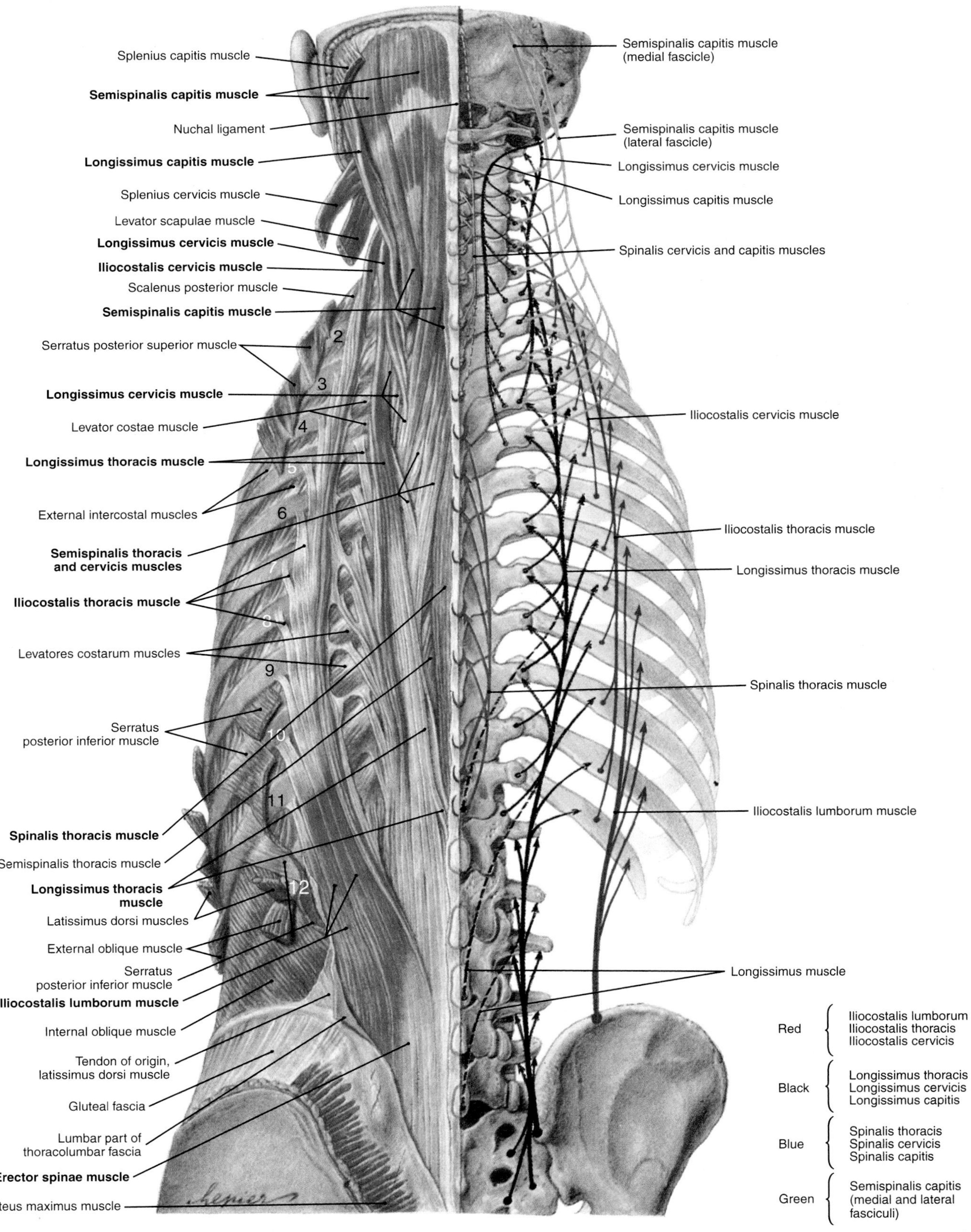
Splenius capitis muscle
Semispinalis capitis muscle
Nuchal ligament
Longissimus capitis muscle
Splenius cervicis muscle
Levator scapulae muscle
Longissimus cervicis muscle
Iliocostalis cervicis muscle
Scalenus posterior muscle
Semispinalis capitis muscle
Serratus posterior superior muscle
Longissimus cervicis muscle
Levator costae muscle
Longissimus thoracis muscle
External intercostal muscles
Semispinalis thoracis and cervicis muscles
Iliocostalis thoracis muscle
Levatores costarum muscles
Serratus posterior inferior muscle
Spinalis thoracis muscle
Semispinalis thoracis muscle
Longissimus thoracis muscle
Latissimus dorsi muscles
External oblique muscle
Serratus posterior inferior muscle
Iliocostalis lumborum muscle
Internal oblique muscle
Tendon of origin, latissimus dorsi muscle
Gluteal fascia
Lumbar part of thoracolumbar fascia
Erector spinae muscle
Gluteus maximus muscle
2
3
4
5
6
7
8
9
10
11
12
Semispinalis capitis muscle (medial fascicle)
Semispinalis capitis muscle (lateral fascicle)
Longissimus cervicis muscle
Longissimus capitis muscle
Spinalis cervicis and capitis muscles
Iliocostalis cervicis muscle
Iliocostalis thoracis muscle
Longissimus thoracis muscle
Spinalis thoracis muscle
Iliocostalis lumborum muscle
Longissimus muscle
Red: Iliocostalis lumborum, Iliocostalis thoracis, Iliocostalis cervicis
Black: Longissimus thoracis, Longissimus cervicis, Longissimus capitis
Blue: Spinalis thoracis, Spinalis cervicis, Spinalis capitis
Green: Semispinalis capitis (medial and lateral fasciculi)

Figure 333 Deep Muscles of the Back and Neck: Erector Spinae Muscle

NOTE: (1) **On the left,** the erector spinae (sacrospinalis) muscle is separated into iliocostalis, longissimus, and spinalis parts. In the neck, observe the semispinalis capitis, which has both medial and lateral fascicles. The semispinalis cervicis and thoracis extend inferiorly from above and lie deep to the sacrospinalis layer of musculature.

(2) **On the right,** all of the muscles have been removed and their attachments have been diagrammed by means of colored lines and arrows.

SUPERFICIAL MUSCLES OF THE BACK

Muscle	Origin	Insertion	Innervation	Action
Trapezius	Middle third of the superior nuchal line; external occipital protuberance; ligamentum nuchae; spinous processes of C7 and T1 to T12 vertebrae	Lateral third of the clavicle; medial margin of acromion; spine of the scapula	Motor fibers from spinal part of the accessory nerve (XI); sensory fibers from C3, C4	Assists serratus anterior in rotating the scapula during abduction of the humerus between 90 and 180 degrees; upper fibers elevate the scapula; lower fibers depress the scapula; middle fibers adduct the scapula; occipital fibers draw the head laterally
Latissimus dorsi	Thoracolumbar fascia; spinous processes of lower six thoracic vertebrae and five lumbar vertebrae and the sacrum; iliac crest; lower three or four ribs	Floor of the intertubercular sulcus of the humerus	Thoracodorsal nerve from the posterior cord of the brachial plexus (C6, C7, C8)	Extends, adducts, and medially rotates humerus; with insertion fixed, it elevates the trunk to the arms, as in climbing

INTERMEDIATE MUSCLES OF THE BACK

Muscle	Origin	Insertion	Innervation	Action
Rhomboid major	Spinous processes of T2 to T5 thoracic vertebrae	Medial border of scapula between the scapular spine and inferior angle	Dorsal scapular nerve (C5)	Adducts the scapula by pulling it medially toward the vertebral column; rotates the scapula by depressing the lateral angle; helps fix scapula to thoracic wall
Rhomboid minor	Spinous process of C7 and T1 vertebrae	Medial border of scapula at the level of the spine of the scapula	Dorsal scapular nerve (C5)	Assists the rhomboid major muscle
Levator scapulae	Transverse processes of atlas and axis and the posterior tubercles of the transverse processes of C3 and C4 vertebrae	Superior angle and upper medial border of scapula	C3 and C4 nerves and the dorsal scapular nerve (C5)	Elevates superior border of scapula; rotates scapula laterally thereby tilting the glenoid cavity downward
Serratus posterior superior	Spinous processes of C7 and T1 to T3 thoracic vertebrae	Onto the upper borders of the second, third, fourth and fifth ribs	Ventral primary rami of T1 to T4 spinal nerves	Elevates the second to fifth ribs
Serratus posterior inferior	Spinous processes of T11, T12 and upper three lumbar vertebrae	Onto the inferior border of the lower four ribs	Ventral primary rami of T9, T10, T11, and T12 spinal nerves	Draws the lower four ribs downward and backward

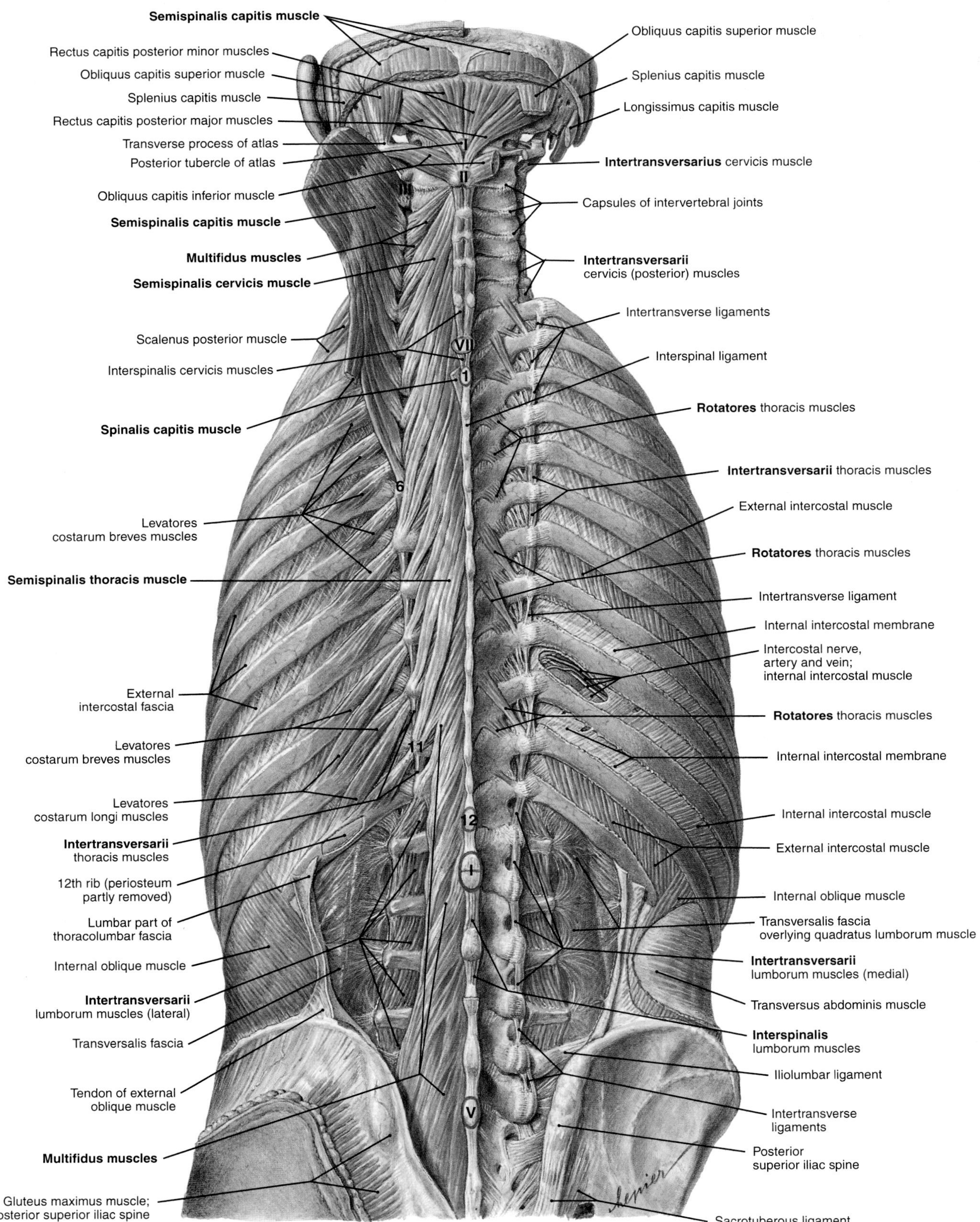
Semispinalis capitis muscle
Rectus capitis posterior minor muscles
Obliquus capitis superior muscle
Splenius capitis muscle
Rectus capitis posterior major muscles
Transverse process of atlas
Posterior tubercle of atlas
Obliquus capitis inferior muscle
Semispinalis capitis muscle
Multifidus muscles
Semispinalis cervicis muscle
Scalenus posterior muscle
Interspinalis cervicis muscles
Spinalis capitis muscle
Levatores costarum breves muscles
Semispinalis thoracis muscle
External intercostal fascia
Levatores costarum breves muscles
Levatores costarum longi muscles
Intertransversarii thoracis muscles
12th rib (periosteum partly removed)
Lumbar part of thoracolumbar fascia
Internal oblique muscle
Intertransversarii lumborum muscles (lateral)
Transversalis fascia
Tendon of external oblique muscle
Multifidus muscles
Gluteus maximus muscle; posterior superior iliac spine
Obliquus capitis superior muscle
Splenius capitis muscle
Longissimus capitis muscle
Intertransversarius cervicis muscle
Capsules of intervertebral joints
Intertransversarii cervicis (posterior) muscles
Intertransverse ligaments
Interspinal ligament
Rotatores thoracis muscles
Intertransversarii thoracis muscles
External intercostal muscle
Rotatores thoracis muscles
Intertransverse ligament
Internal intercostal membrane
Intercostal nerve, artery and vein; internal intercostal muscle
Rotatores thoracis muscles
Internal intercostal membrane
Internal intercostal muscle
External intercostal muscle
Internal oblique muscle
Transversalis fascia overlying quadratus lumborum muscle
Intertransversarii lumborum muscles (medial)
Transversus abdominis muscle
Interspinalis lumborum muscles
Iliolumbar ligament
Intertransverse ligaments
Posterior superior iliac spine
Sacrotuberous ligament
I
II
III
VII
1
6
11
12
I
V

Figure 335 Deep Muscles of the Back and Neck: Transversospinal Group

NOTE: (1) The **transversospinal** groups of muscles lie deep to the **erector spinae,** and they extend between the transverse processes of the vertebrae to the spinous processes of higher vertebrae. These muscles are extensors of the vertebral column or acting individually and on one side, they bend and rotate the vertebrae of that side.

(2) Within this group of muscles are the **semispinalis** (thoracis, cervicis, and capitis), the **multifidus,** the **rotatores** (lumborum, thoracis, cervicis), the **interspinales** (lumborum, thoracis, cervicis), and the **intertransversarii.**

DEEP MUSCLES OF THE BACK

Muscle	Origin	Insertion	Innervation	Action
ERECTOR SPINAE MUSCLES				
ILIOCOSTALIS MUSCLE (Lateral column)				
Iliocostalis lumborum	Posteromedial part of the iliac crest and from the most lateral part of the common tendon of the erector spinae muscle	By six or seven muscle fascicles onto the inferior borders of the lower six or seven ribs at their angles	Dorsal primary rami of lower thoracic and upper lumbar nerves	Extends, laterally flexes, and assists in rotation of the vertebral column; can depress the ribs
Iliocostalis thoracis	Upper borders of the lower six ribs at their angles	Upper borders of the first six ribs at their angles and on the transverse process of the seventh cervical vertebra	Dorsal primary rami of the C8 and upper six thoracic spinal nerves	Extends, laterally flexes, and assists in rotation of the thoracic vertebrae
Iliocostalis cervicis	Angles of the third, fourth, fifth, and sixth ribs	Posterior tubercles of transverse processes of fourth, fifth, and sixth cervical vertebrae	Dorsal primary rami of the lower cervical and upper thoracic spinal nerves	Extends, laterally flexes, and assists in rotation of lower cervical and upper thoracic vertebrae
LONGISSIMUS MUSCLE (Intermediate column)				
Longissimus thoracis	Intermediate continuation of the erector spinae muscle; transverse processes of the lumbar vertebrae	Onto the tips of transverse processes of all thoracic vertebrae; onto the lower 9 or 10 ribs between their tubercles and angles	Dorsal primary rami of the thoracic and lumbar spinal nerves	Extends and laterally flexes the vertebral column; also able to depress the ribs
Longissimus cervicis muscle	Tips of transverse processes of upper four or five thoracic vertebrae	Posterior tubercles of transverse processes of C2 to C6 cervical vertebrae	Dorsal primary rami of upper thoracic and lower cervical spinal nerves	Extends vertebral column and bends it to one side
Longissimus capitis	From transverse processes of upper four or five thoracic vertebrae; articular processes of lower three or four cervical vertebrae	Posterior margin of the mastoid process of the temporal bone	Dorsal primary rami of middle and lower cervical spinal nerves	Extends the head; muscle of one side bends head to the same side and turns face to that side
SPINALIS MUSCLE (Medial column)				
Spinalis thoracis	From spinous processes of T11, T12, L1, and L2 vertebrae	Spinous processes of upper four to eight thoracic vertebrae	Dorsal primary rami of thoracic spinal nerves	Extends vertebral column
Spinalis cervicis	Spinous processes of C7, T1, and T2 vertebrae and ligamentum nuchae	Spinous process of the axis and those of the C3 and C4	Dorsal primary rami of lower cervical spinal nerves	Extends the cervical vertebrae
Spinalis capitis	Spinous processes of lower cervical and upper thoracic vertebrae	Inserts with the semispinalis capitis muscle between the superior and inferior nuchal lines of the occipital bone	Dorsal primary rami of upper cervical spinal nerves	Extends the head
TRANSVERSOSPINALIS GROUP OF MUSCLES				
SEMISPINALIS MUSCLES				
Semispinalis thoracis	Transverse processes of the 6th to 10th thoracic vertebrae	Spinous processes of C7, C8 and upper four thoracic vertebrae	Dorsal primary rami of lower cervical and upper thoracic spinal nerves	Extends vertebral column and rotates it to the opposite side
Semispinalis cervicis	Transverse processes of upper five or six thoracic vertebrae	Spinous processes of the axis and third, fourth, and fifth cervical vertebrae	Dorsal primary rami of the middle cervical spinal nerves	Extends cervical spinal column; rotates vertebrae to opposite side
Semispinalis capitis	Tips of transverse processes of the C7 and upper six or seven thoracic vertebrae	Between the superior and inferior nuchal lines on the occipital bone	Dorsal primary rami of the cervical spinal nerves	Extends the head and rotates it such that the face is turned to the opposite side

DEEP MUSCLES OF THE BACK

Muscle	Origin	Insertion	Innervation	Action
MULTIFIDUS MUSCLES **Lumbrum thoracis cervicis**	From the back of the sacrum; mamillary processes of lumbar vertebrae; transverse processes of all thoracic vertebrae; articular processes of lower four cervical vertebrae	Onto the spinous processes of higher vertebrae; each multifidus muscle spans two to four vertebrae	Supplied segmentally by dorsal primary rami of the lumbar, thoracic spinal nerves	Bends or laterally flexes the vertebral column and rotates it to the opposite side; both multifidi columns acting together extend the vertebral column
ROTATORES MUSCLES **Rotatores thoracis**	From transverse processes of thoracic vertebrae deep to the multifidus muscles	On the base of the spine of thoracic vertebra above the origin or the one above that	Dorsal primary rami of the thoracic spinal nerves	Extend the vertebral column and bend it toward the opposite side
Rotatores cervicis (These are less well defined.)	From the articular processes of the cervical vertebrae	To the base of the spines of the cervical vertebra immediately above	Dorsal primary rami of cervical spinal nerves	Extend cervical vertebrae and bend them to the opposite side
Rotatores lumborum (These are less well defined.)	From the mamillary processes of the lumbar vertebrae	To the base of the spines of the lumbar vertebra immediately above	Dorsal primary rami of lumbar spinal nerves	Extend lumbar vertebrae and bend them to the opposite side

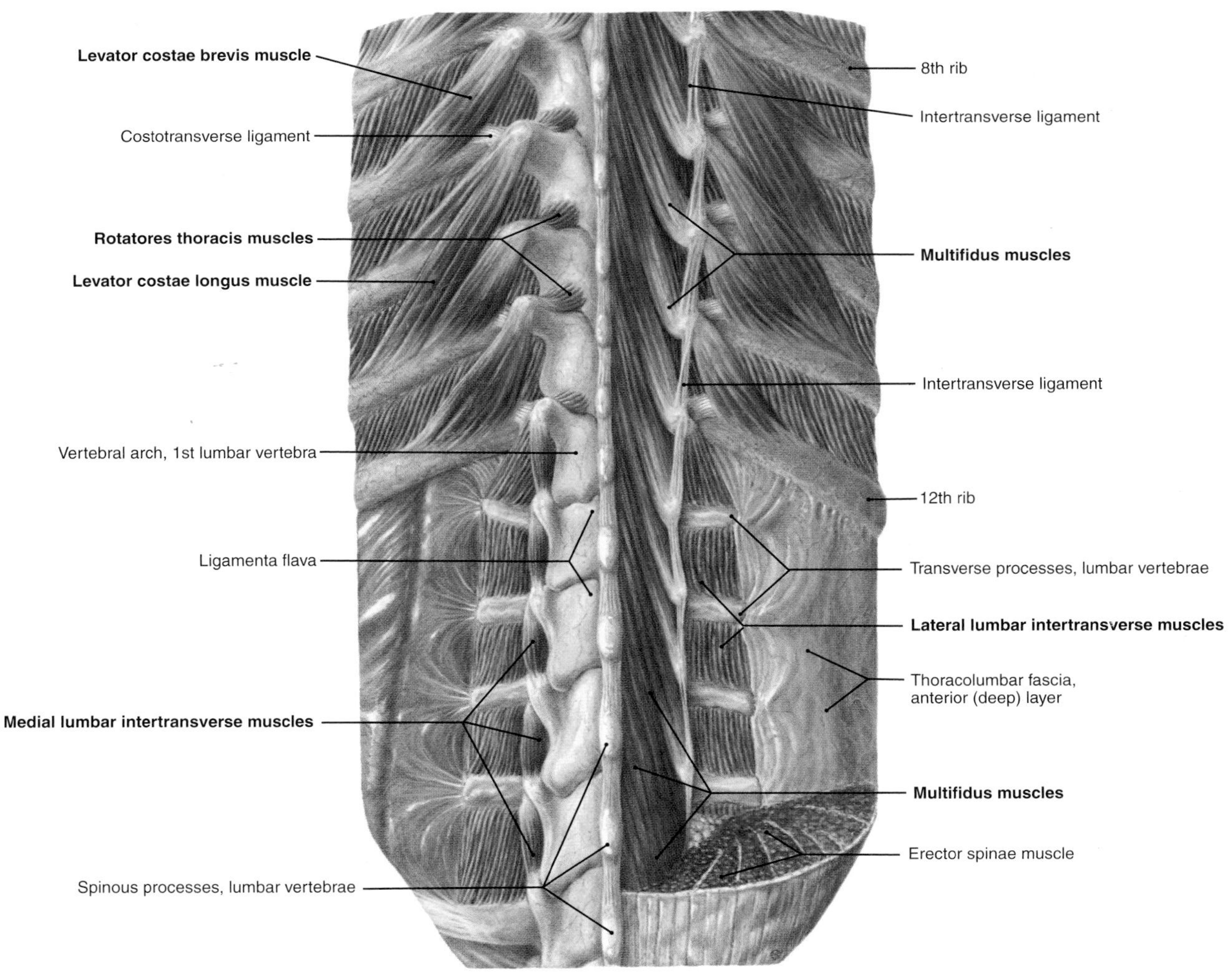
Levator costae brevis muscle
Costotransverse ligament
Rotatores thoracis muscles
Levator costae longus muscle
Vertebral arch, 1st lumbar vertebra
Ligamenta flava
Medial lumbar intertransverse muscles
Spinous processes, lumbar vertebrae
8th rib
Intertransverse ligament
Multifidus muscles
Intertransverse ligament
12th rib
Transverse processes, lumbar vertebrae
Lateral lumbar intertransverse muscles
Thoracolumbar fascia, anterior (deep) layer
Multifidus muscles
Erector spinae muscle

Figure 337 Multifidus, Rotator, Levator Costae, and Intertransverse Muscles of the Deep Back
NOTE: The erector spinae and semispinalis muscles have been removed.

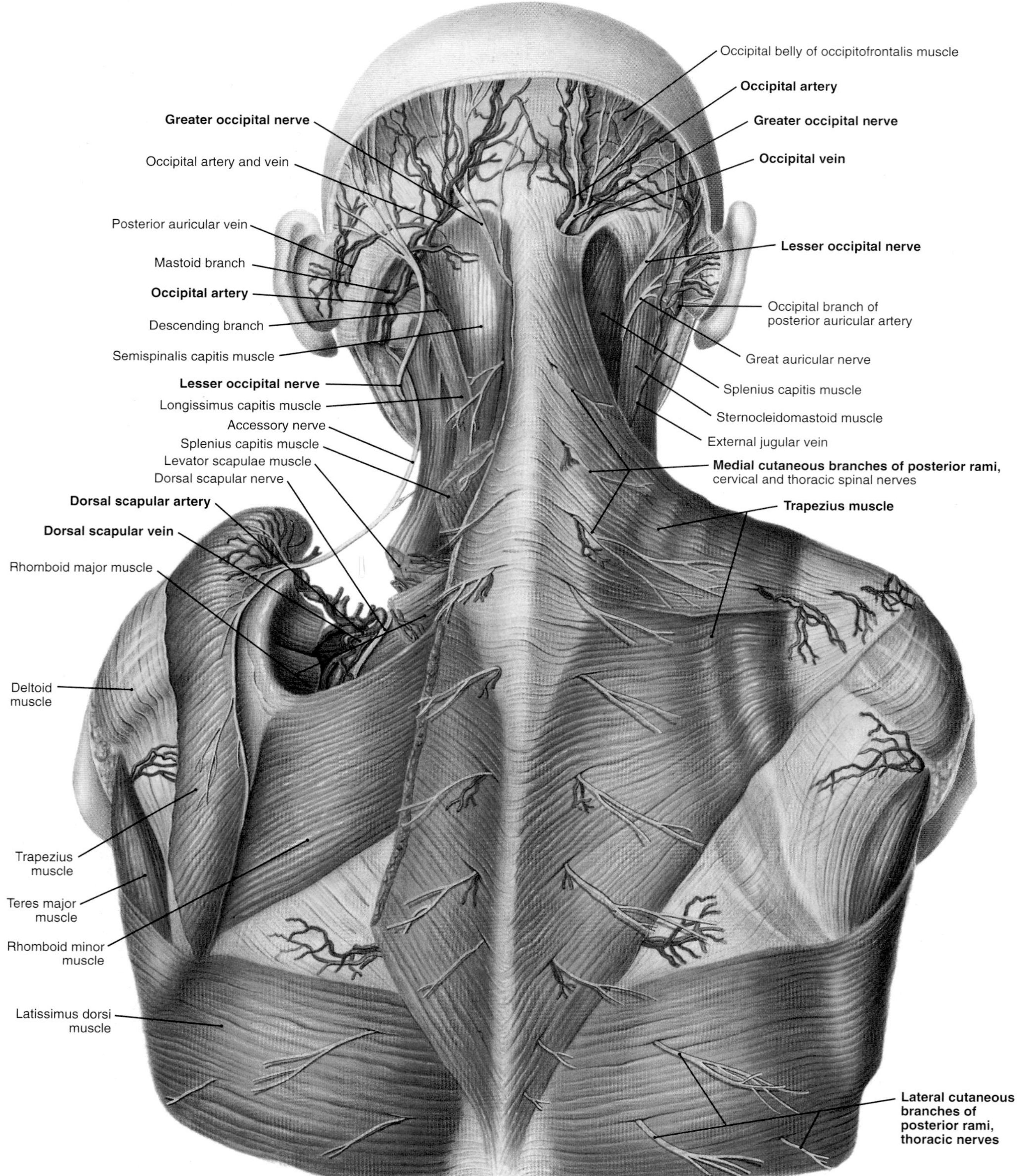
Occipital belly of occipitofrontalis muscle
Occipital artery
Greater occipital nerve
Occipital vein
Greater occipital nerve
Occipital artery and vein
Posterior auricular vein
Mastoid branch
Occipital artery
Descending branch
Semispinalis capitis muscle
Lesser occipital nerve
Longissimus capitis muscle
Accessory nerve
Splenius capitis muscle
Levator scapulae muscle
Dorsal scapular nerve
Dorsal scapular artery
Dorsal scapular vein
Rhomboid major muscle
Lesser occipital nerve
Occipital branch of posterior auricular artery
Great auricular nerve
Splenius capitis muscle
Sternocleidomastoid muscle
External jugular vein
Medial cutaneous branches of posterior rami, cervical and thoracic spinal nerves
Trapezius muscle
Deltoid muscle
Trapezius muscle
Teres major muscle
Rhomboid minor muscle
Latissimus dorsi muscle
Lateral cutaneous branches of posterior rami, thoracic nerves

Figure 338 Nerves and Vessels of the Superficial and Intermediate Muscle Layers of the Upper Back and Posterior Neck

NOTE: (1) The cutaneous branches of the **posterior primary rami** of the cervical and thoracic spinal nerves supplying the posterior neck and back segmentally. Observe the **accessory nerve (XI)** as it descends to supply the trapezius and sternocleidomastoid muscles.

(2) The **greater occipital nerve,** a sensory nerve from the posterior primary ramus of the C2 spinal nerve. It is accompanied by the occipital vessels. Observe also the **lesser occipital nerve,** which courses to the skin of the lateral posterior scalp and arises from the **anterior primary ramus** of C2.

(3) The **dorsal scapular nerve** and **vessels** that course beneath the **levator scapulae** and **rhomboid muscles.**

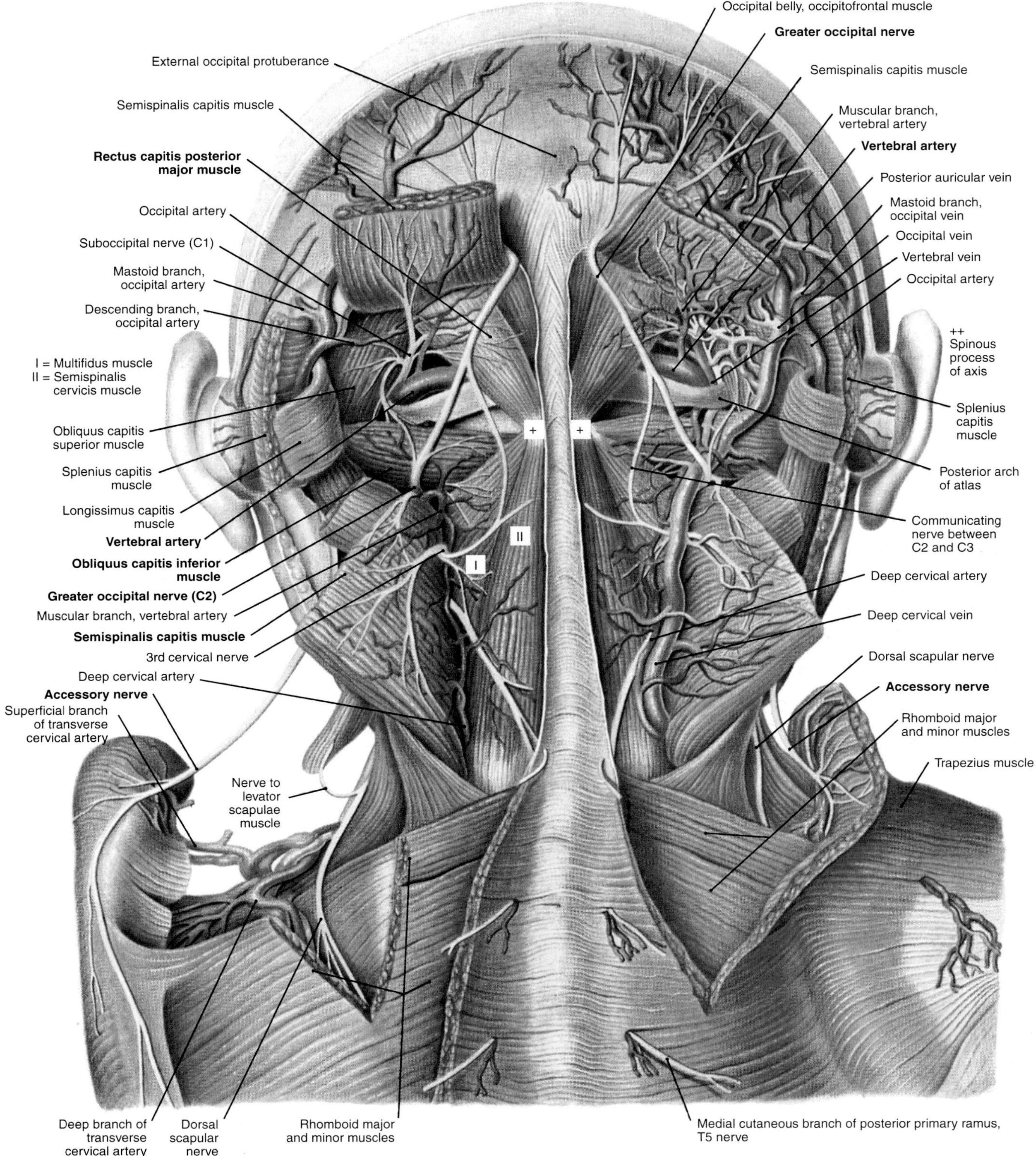
Occipital belly, occipitofrontal muscle
Greater occipital nerve
Semispinalis capitis muscle
Muscular branch, vertebral artery
Vertebral artery
Posterior auricular vein
Mastoid branch, occipital vein
Occipital vein
Vertebral vein
Occipital artery
++ Spinous process of axis
Splenius capitis muscle
Posterior arch of atlas
Communicating nerve between C2 and C3
Deep cervical artery
Deep cervical vein
Dorsal scapular nerve
Accessory nerve
Rhomboid major and minor muscles
Trapezius muscle
External occipital protuberance
Semispinalis capitis muscle
Rectus capitis posterior major muscle
Occipital artery
Suboccipital nerve (C1)
Mastoid branch, occipital artery
Descending branch, occipital artery
I = Multifidus muscle
II = Semispinalis cervicis muscle
Obliquus capitis superior muscle
Splenius capitis muscle
Longissimus capitis muscle
Vertebral artery
Obliquus capitis inferior muscle
Greater occipital nerve (C2)
Muscular branch, vertebral artery
Semispinalis capitis muscle
3rd cervical nerve
Deep cervical artery
Accessory nerve
Superficial branch of transverse cervical artery
Nerve to levator scapulae muscle
Deep branch of transverse cervical artery
Dorsal scapular nerve
Rhomboid major and minor muscles
Medial cutaneous branch of posterior primary ramus, T5 nerve

Figure 339 Deep Vessels and Nerves of the Suboccipital Region and Upper Back; Suboccipital Triangle

NOTE: (1) The **suboccipital triangle** lies deep to the semispinalis muscle and is bounded by the **rectus capitis posterior major, obliquus capitis superior,** and **obliquus capitis inferior.**

(2) The **vertebral artery** crosses the base of the suboccipital triangle, while the **suboccipital nerve** (posterior primary ramus of C1) courses *through* the triangle to supply motor innervation to the three muscles that bound the triangle as well as to the rectus capitis posterior minor and the overlying semispinalis capitis muscle.

(3) The **greater occipital nerve** (posterior primary ramus of C2), a sensory nerve, emerges below the obliquus capitis inferior and then courses medially and superiorly to become subcutaneous just lateral to and below the external occipital protuberance.

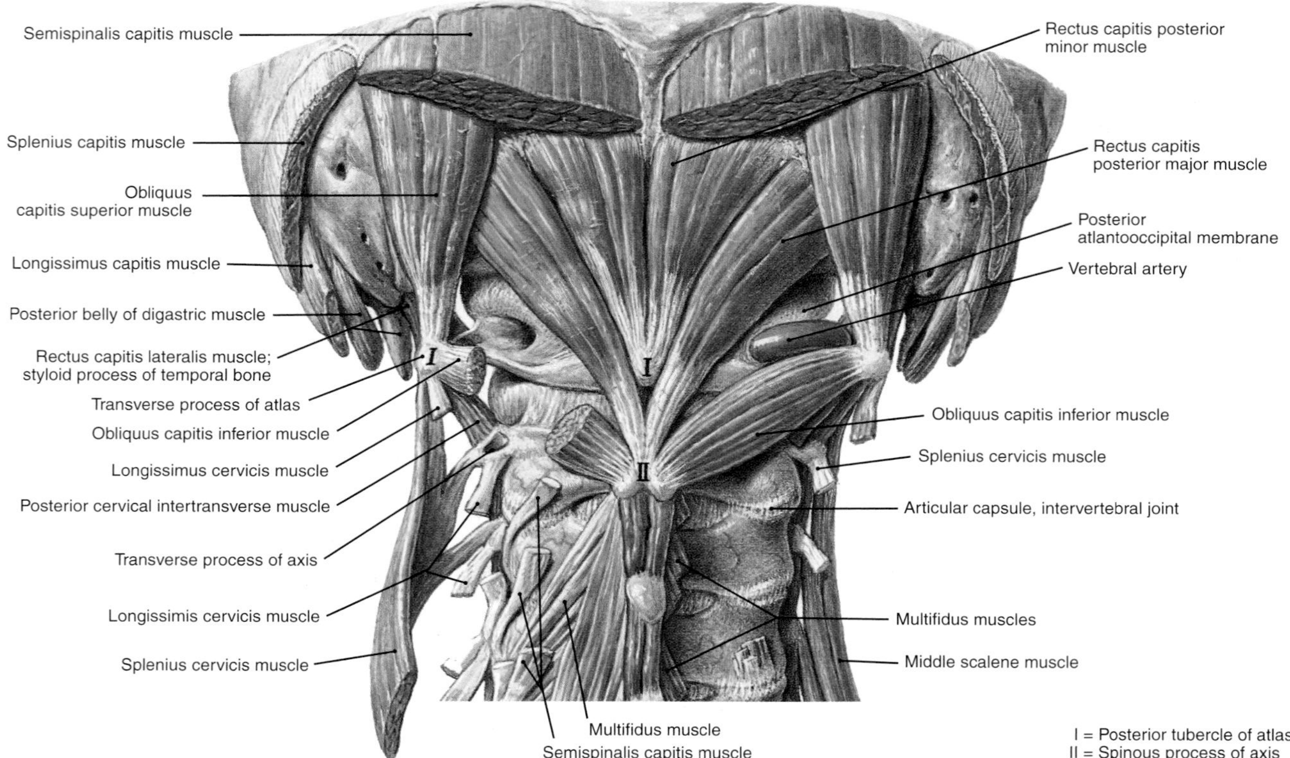
Semispinalis capitis muscle
Splenius capitis muscle
Obliquus capitis superior muscle
Longissimus capitis muscle
Posterior belly of digastric muscle
Rectus capitis lateralis muscle; styloid process of temporal bone
Transverse process of atlas
Obliquus capitis inferior muscle
Longissimus cervicis muscle
Posterior cervical intertransverse muscle
Transverse process of axis
Longissimis cervicis muscle
Splenius cervicis muscle
Multifidus muscle
Semispinalis capitis muscle
Rectus capitis posterior minor muscle
Rectus capitis posterior major muscle
Posterior atlantooccipital membrane
Vertebral artery
Obliquus capitis inferior muscle
Splenius cervicis muscle
Articular capsule, intervertebral joint
Multifidus muscles
Middle scalene muscle
I
II
I = Posterior tubercle of atlas
II = Spinous process of axis

Figure 340.1 Muscles of the Suboccipital Triangle

NOTE: (1) The **obliquus capitis inferior, obliquus capitis superior,** and **rectus capitis posterior major muscles** outline the **suboccipital triangle.**

(2) The **vertebral artery** crosses the floor of the triangle and penetrates the posterior atlantooccipital membrane to enter the foramen magnum. There the two vertebral arteries join to form the **basilar artery** on the ventral aspect of the brainstem.

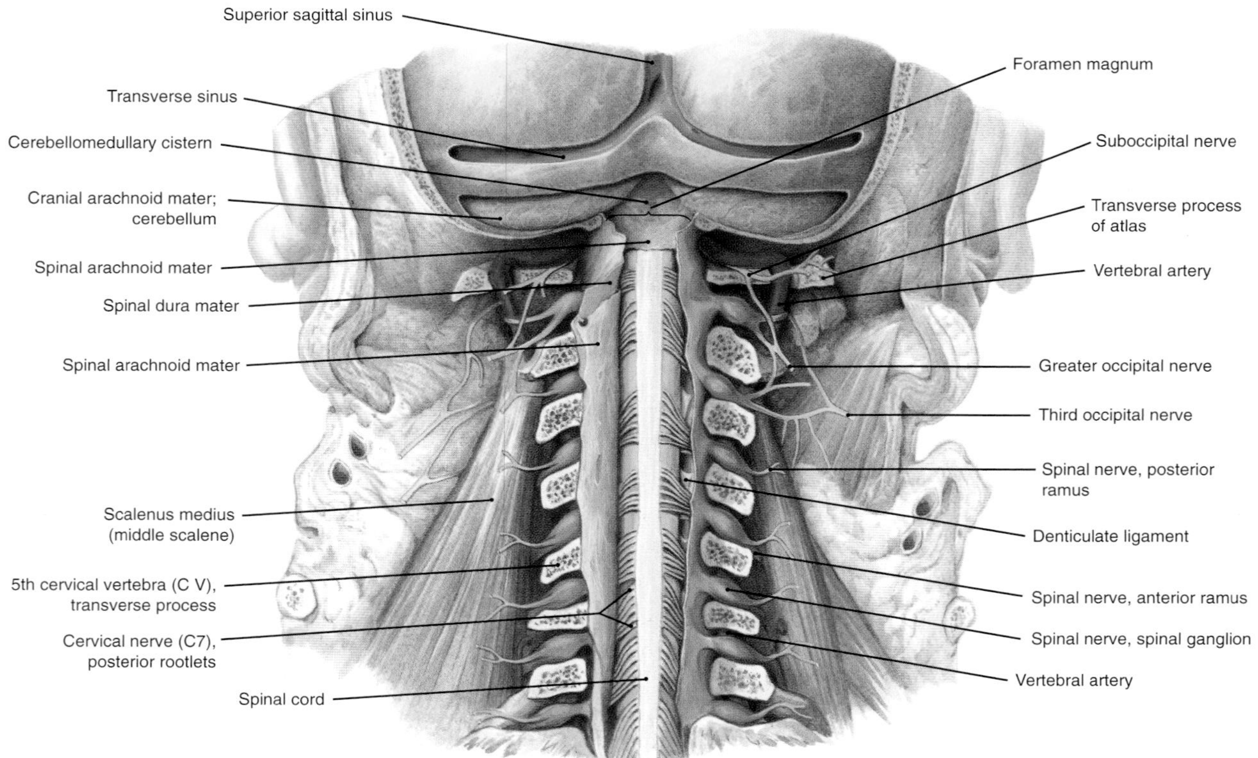
Superior sagittal sinus
Transverse sinus
Cerebellomedullary cistern
Cranial arachnoid mater; cerebellum
Spinal arachnoid mater
Spinal dura mater
Spinal arachnoid mater
Scalenus medius (middle scalene)
5th cervical vertebra (C V), transverse process
Cervical nerve (C7), posterior rootlets
Spinal cord
Foramen magnum
Suboccipital nerve
Transverse process of atlas
Vertebral artery
Greater occipital nerve
Third occipital nerve
Spinal nerve, posterior ramus
Denticulate ligament
Spinal nerve, anterior ramus
Spinal nerve, spinal ganglion
Vertebral artery

Figure 340.2 Suboccipital Region: Vertebral Artery and Occipital Nerves

NOTE: The assent and 90-degree turn medially taken by the vertebral arteries along the superior border of the atlas to achieve the ventral surface of the medulla oblongata.

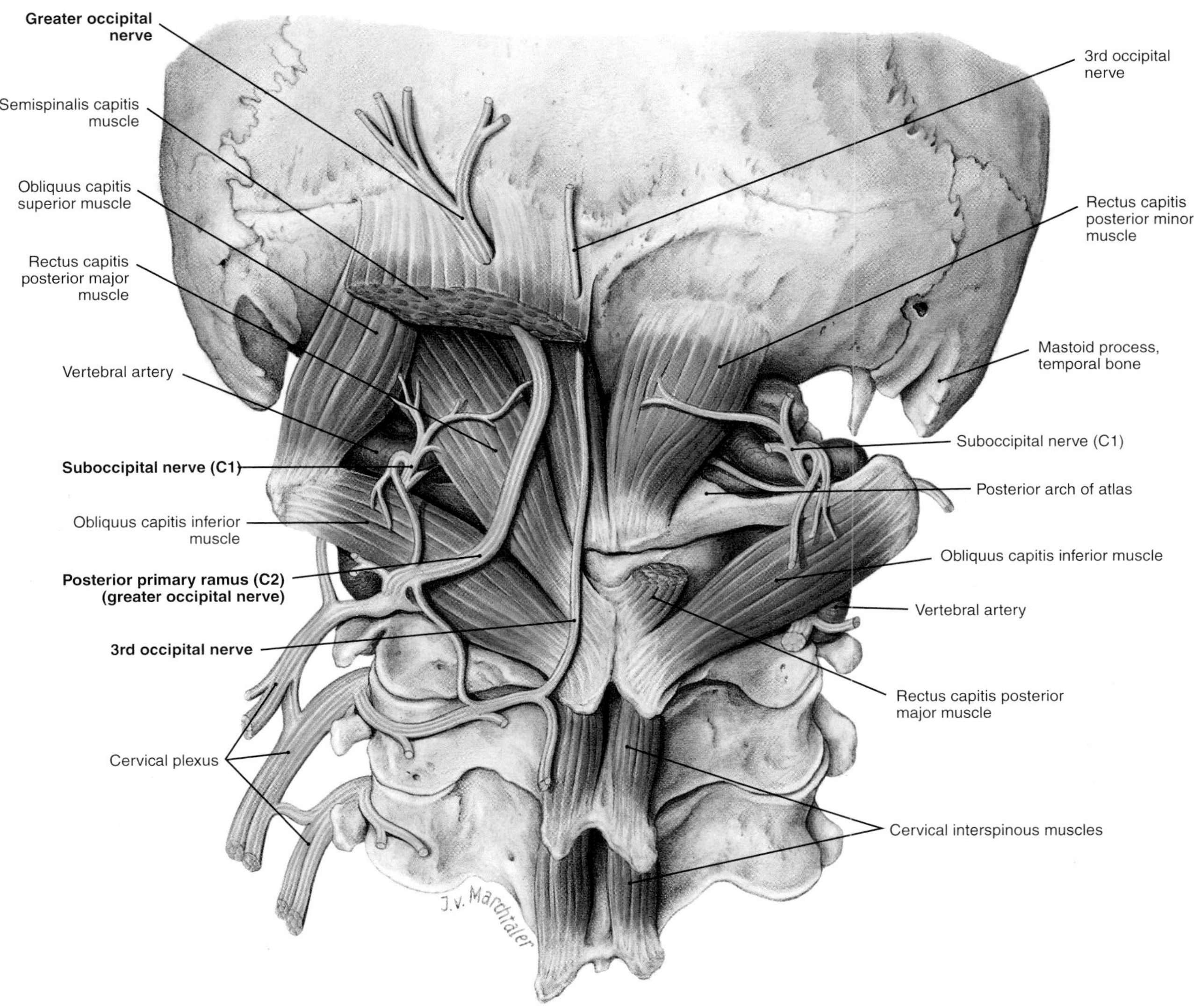
Greater occipital nerve
Semispinalis capitis muscle
Obliquus capitis superior muscle
Rectus capitis posterior major muscle
Vertebral artery
Suboccipital nerve (C1)
Obliquus capitis inferior muscle
Posterior primary ramus (C2) (greater occipital nerve)
3rd occipital nerve
Cervical plexus
3rd occipital nerve
Rectus capitis posterior minor muscle
Mastoid process, temporal bone
Suboccipital nerve (C1)
Posterior arch of atlas
Obliquus capitis inferior muscle
Vertebral artery
Rectus capitis posterior major muscle
Cervical interspinous muscles
J.v. Marchtaler

Figure 341 Nerves of the Suboccipital Region

NOTE: (1) The **suboccipital nerve (C1)**, primarily a motor nerve, emerges from the spinal cord above the atlas, courses through the suboccipital triangle and supplies motor innervation to all four suboccipital muscles.

(2) The **greater occipital** (C2) and **third occipital** (C3) **nerves** branch from the posterior primary rami of those segments. After passing through the deep muscles of the back, they become purely sensory to supply the skin on the posterior scalp and neck.

MUSCLES OF THE SUBOCCIPITAL REGION

	Origin	Insertion	Innervation	Action
Rectus capitis posterior major	Spinous process of axis	Lateral part of inferior nuchal line of occipital bone	Suboccipital nerve (dorsal ramus of C1)	Extends the head and rotates it to the same side
Rectus capitis posterior minor	Tubercle on the posterior arch of the atlas	Medial part of inferior nuchal line of occipital bone	Suboccipital nerve (dorsal ramus of C1)	Extends the head
Obliquus capitis superior	Upper surface of transverse process of the atlas	Onto occipital bone between superior and inferior nuchal lines	Suboccipital nerve (dorsal ramus of C1)	Extends the head and bends it laterally
Obliquus capitis inferior	Apex of spinous process of axis	Inferior and dorsal part of transverse process of the atlas	Suboccipital nerve (dorsal ramus of C1)	Rotates the atlas and thereby turns the face toward the same side

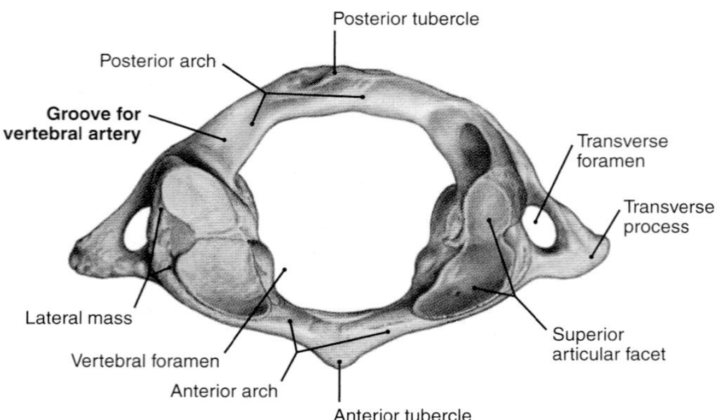
Posterior tubercle
Posterior arch
Groove for vertebral artery
Transverse foramen
Transverse process
Lateral mass
Vertebral foramen
Anterior arch
Anterior tubercle
Superior articular facet

Figure 342.1 Atlas, Viewed from Above

NOTE: The superior articular facets are the sites of the occipito-atlantal joints behind which are the grooves for the vertebral arteries.

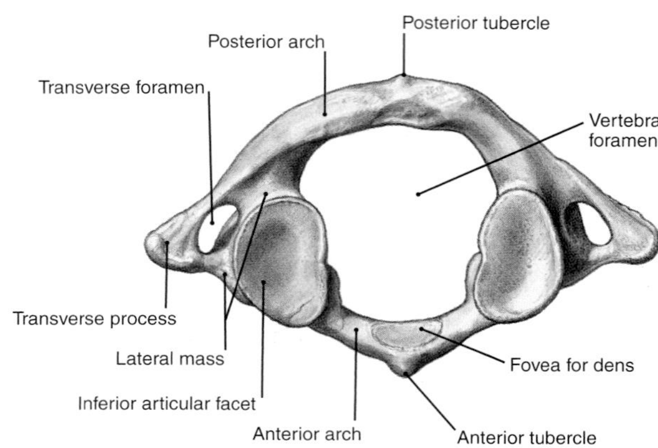
Posterior arch
Posterior tubercle
Transverse foramen
Vertebral foramen
Transverse process
Lateral mass
Inferior articular facet
Anterior arch
Fovea for dens
Anterior tubercle

Figure 342.2 Atlas (Caudal View)

NOTE: The inferior articular facets on the inferior surface of the lateral mass articulate with the axis below.

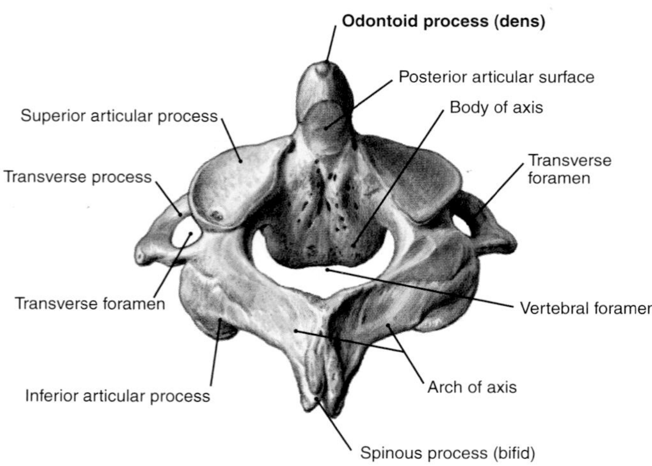
Odontoid process (dens)
Posterior articular surface
Body of axis
Superior articular process
Transverse process
Transverse foramen
Transverse foramen
Vertebral foramen
Inferior articular process
Arch of axis
Spinous process (bifid)

Figure 342.3 Posterior View of the Axis

NOTE: The large body and the odontoid process of the axis and the posterior articular facet articulates with the anterior arch of the atlas.

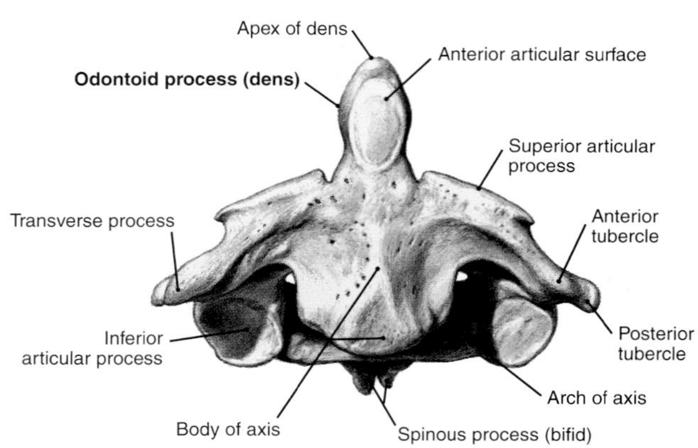
Apex of dens
Anterior articular surface
Odontoid process (dens)
Superior articular process
Transverse process
Anterior tubercle
Inferior articular process
Posterior tubercle
Arch of axis
Body of axis
Spinous process (bifid)

Figure 342.4 Anterior View of the Axis

NOTE: The articular facet on the anterior surface of the odontoid process behind (posterior) extends the transverse ligament of the atlas.

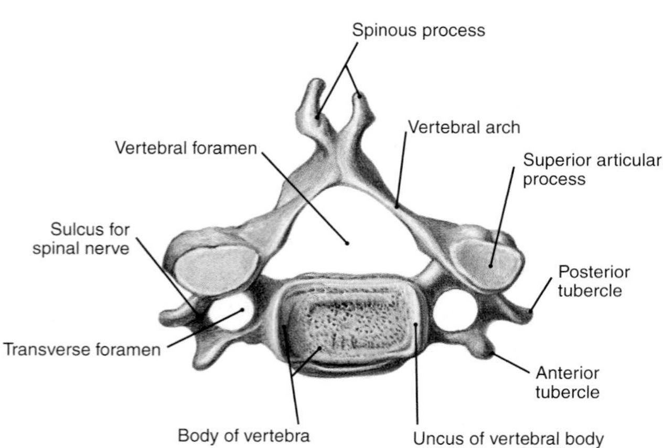
Spinous process
Vertebral arch
Vertebral foramen
Superior articular process
Sulcus for spinal nerve
Posterior tubercle
Transverse foramen
Anterior tubercle
Body of vertebra
Uncus of vertebral body

Figure 342.5 Fifth Cervical Vertebra (from Above)

NOTE: The fifth cervical vertebra is typical of third, fourth, and sixth cervical vertebrae, and different from the first (atlas), second (axis), and seventh, which present special features. Also note the delicate structure of this vertebra.

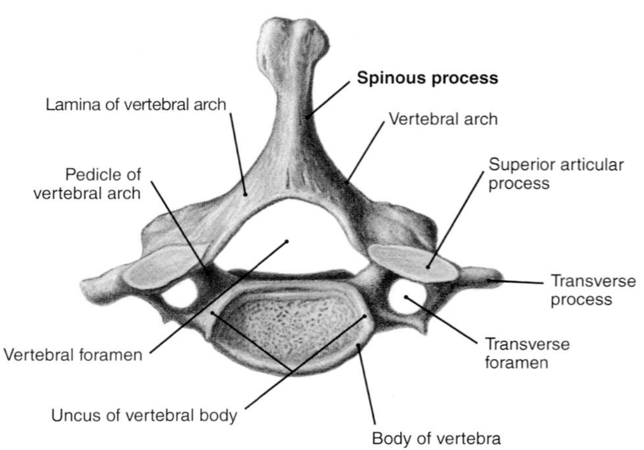
Spinous process
Lamina of vertebral arch
Vertebral arch
Pedicle of vertebral arch
Superior articular process
Transverse process
Vertebral foramen
Transverse foramen
Uncus of vertebral body
Body of vertebra

Figure 342.6 Seventh Cervical Vertebra (from Above)

NOTE: The seventh cervical vertebra, being transitional between cervical and thoracic vertebrae, has a transverse foramen similar to the cervical and a large spinous process similar to the thoracic. The latter gives it the name **vertebra prominens.**

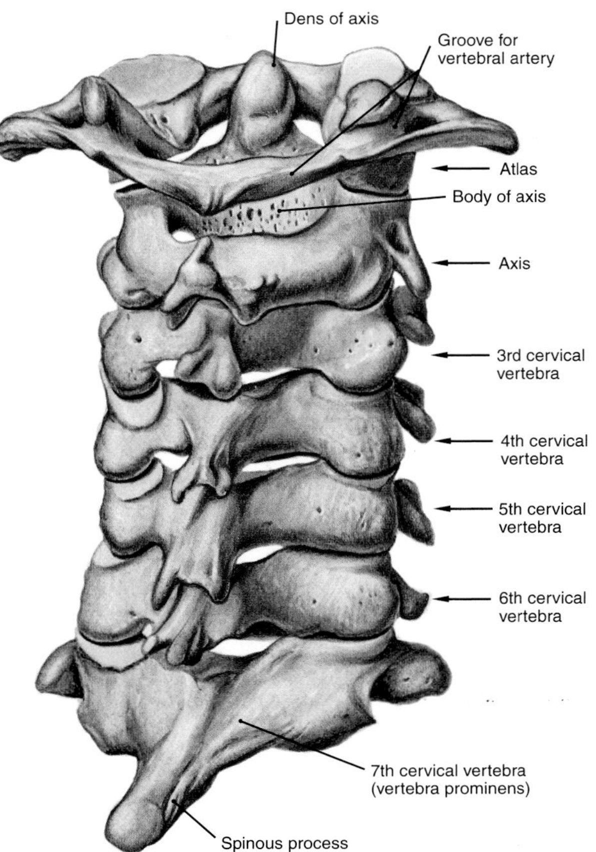
Dens of axis
Groove for vertebral artery
Atlas
Body of axis
Axis
3rd cervical vertebra
4th cervical vertebra
5th cervical vertebra
6th cervical vertebra
7th cervical vertebra (vertebra prominens)
Spinous process

Figure 343.1 Cervical Spinal Column (Dorsal)
NOTE: While flexion and extension of the head are performed at the atlantooccipital joint, turning of the head to the left or right is the result of rotation of the atlas on the axis.

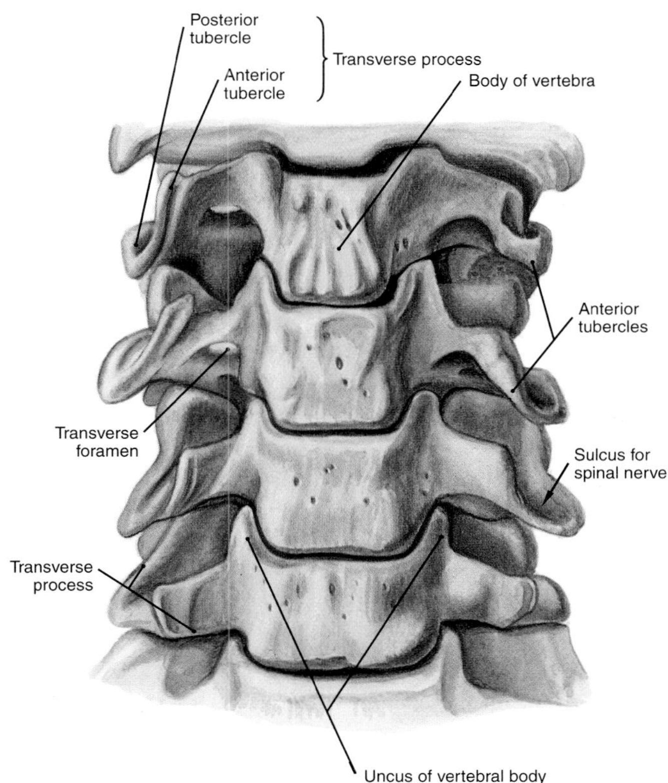
Posterior tubercle
Anterior tubercle
Transverse process
Body of vertebra
Anterior tubercles
Transverse foramen
Sulcus for spinal nerve
Transverse process
Uncus of vertebral body

Figure 343.2 Cervical Vertebrae (Ventral View)
NOTE: Only a small part of the second to seventh cervical vertebrae are shown above and below the convex anterior surfaces of the bodies of the third to sixth vertebrae.

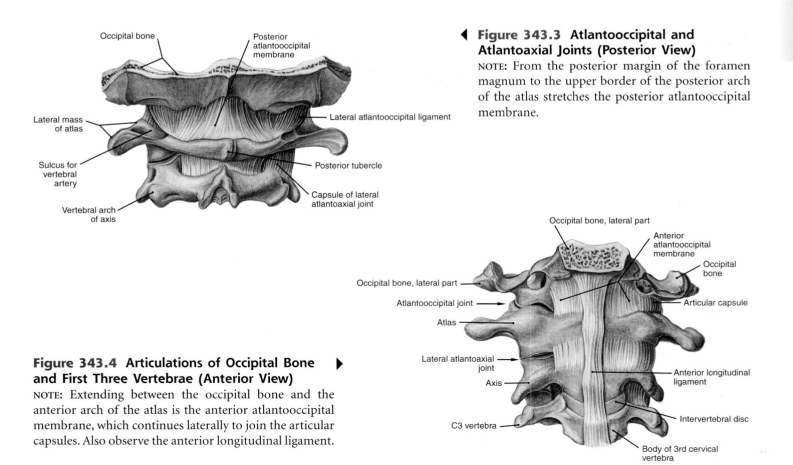

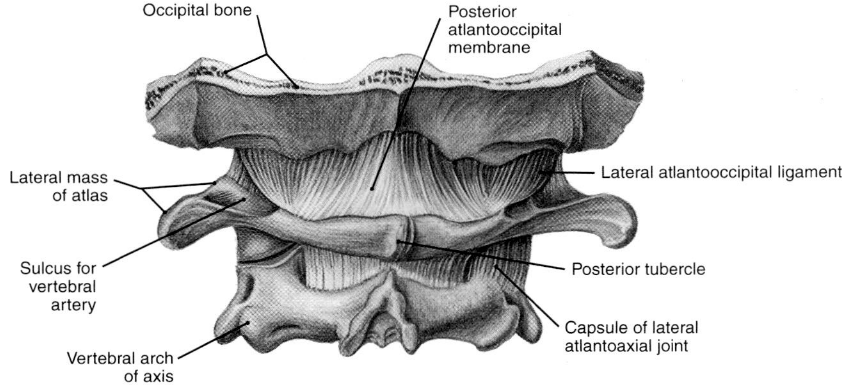
Occipital bone
Posterior atlantooccipital membrane
Lateral mass of atlas
Lateral atlantooccipital ligament
Sulcus for vertebral artery
Posterior tubercle
Capsule of lateral atlantoaxial joint
Vertebral arch of axis

Figure 343.3 Atlantooccipital and Atlantoaxial Joints (Posterior View)
NOTE: From the posterior margin of the foramen magnum to the upper border of the posterior arch of the atlas stretches the posterior atlantooccipital membrane.

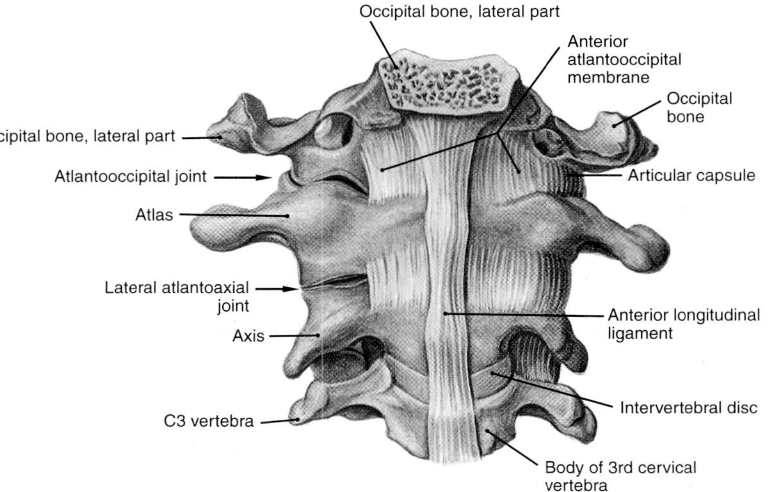
Occipital bone, lateral part
Anterior atlantooccipital membrane
Occipital bone
Occipital bone, lateral part
Atlantooccipital joint
Articular capsule
Atlas
Lateral atlantoaxial joint
Axis
Anterior longitudinal ligament
Intervertebral disc
C3 vertebra
Body of 3rd cervical vertebra

Figure 343.4 Articulations of Occipital Bone and First Three Vertebrae (Anterior View)
NOTE: Extending between the occipital bone and the anterior arch of the atlas is the anterior atlantooccipital membrane, which continues laterally to join the articular capsules. Also observe the anterior longitudinal ligament.

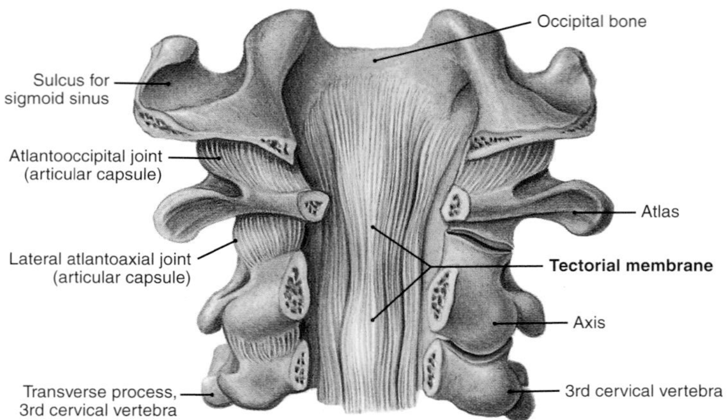
Occipital bone
Sulcus for sigmoid sinus
Atlantooccipital joint (articular capsule)
Atlas
Lateral atlantoaxial joint (articular capsule)
Tectorial membrane
Axis
Transverse process, 3rd cervical vertebra
3rd cervical vertebra

Figure 344.1 Tectorial Membrane (Dorsal View)

NOTE: The tectorial membrane is a broadened upward extension of the posterior longitudinal ligament and attaches the axis to the occipital bone (see also, Fig. 345.1). It covers the posterior surface of the odontoid process and lies dorsal to the cruciform ligament, covering it as well.

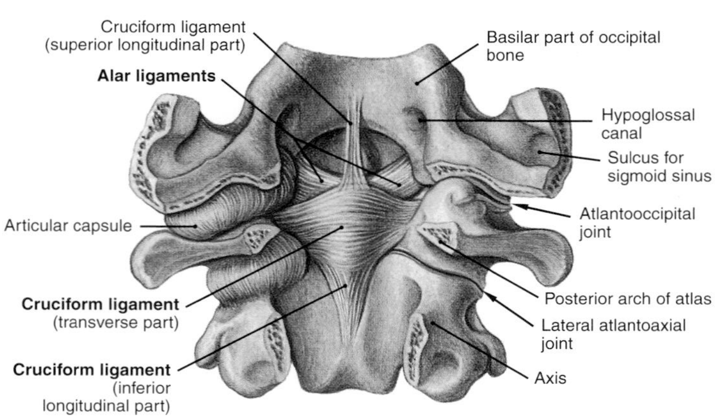
Cruciform ligament (superior longitudinal part)
Basilar part of occipital bone
Alar ligaments
Hypoglossal canal
Sulcus for sigmoid sinus
Atlantooccipital joint
Articular capsule
Posterior arch of atlas
Cruciform ligament (transverse part)
Lateral atlantoaxial joint
Cruciform ligament (inferior longitudinal part)
Axis

Figure 344.2 Atlantooccipital and Atlantoaxial Joints Showing the Cruciform Ligament (Posterior View)

NOTE: The posterior arches to the atlas and axis have been removed, and the cruciform ligament is seen from this posterior view. It consists of the transverse ligament (see Fig. 344.4) and the longitudinal fascicles that extend superiorly and inferiorly.

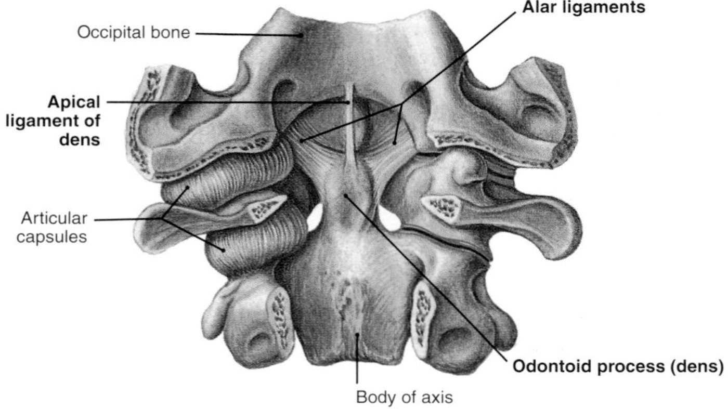
Alar ligaments
Occipital bone
Apical ligament of dens
Articular capsules
Odontoid process (dens)
Body of axis

Figure 344.3 Alar and Apical Ligaments (Posterior View)

NOTE: This figure is oriented the same as Fig. 344.2. The cruciform ligament has been removed to reveal the odontoid process of the axis. This is attached superiorly to the occipital bone by the two alar ligaments and the apical ligament of the dens. These ligaments tend to limit lateral rotation of the skull.

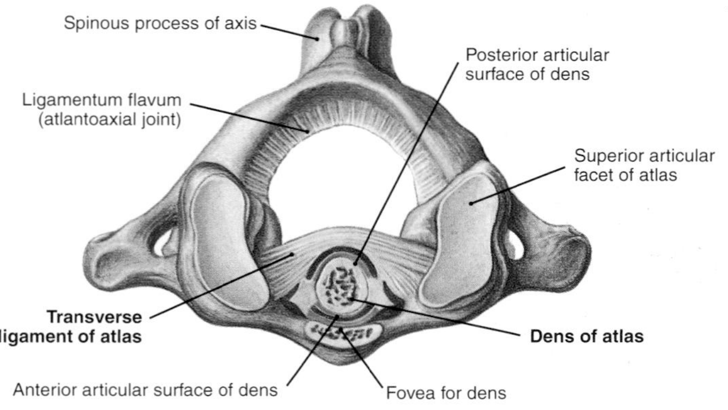
Spinous process of axis
Posterior articular surface of dens
Ligamentum flavum (atlantoaxial joint)
Superior articular facet of atlas
Transverse ligament of atlas
Dens of atlas
Anterior articular surface of dens
Fovea for dens

Figure 344.4 Median Atlantoaxial Joint (from Above)

NOTE: The odontoid process of the axis articulates with the anterior arch of the atlas, thereby forming the median atlantoaxial joint, and the thick and strong transverse ligament (part of the cruciform) of the atlas retains the dens on its posterior surface.

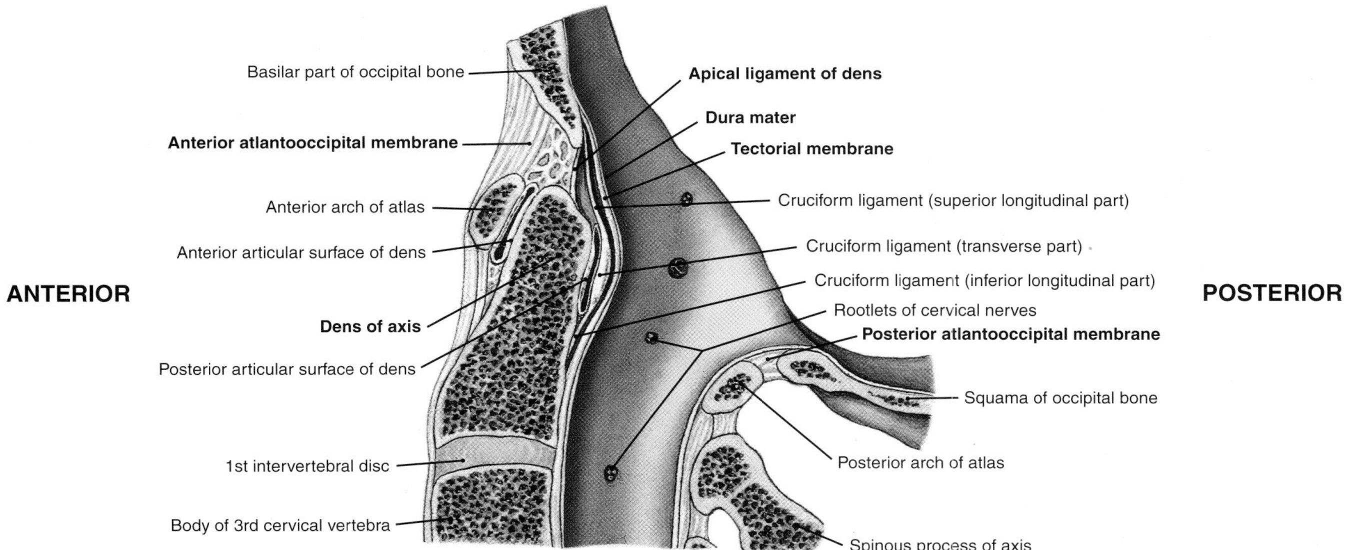
Basilar part of occipital bone
Anterior atlantooccipital membrane
Anterior arch of atlas
Anterior articular surface of dens
ANTERIOR
Dens of axis
Posterior articular surface of dens
1st intervertebral disc
Body of 3rd cervical vertebra
Apical ligament of dens
Dura mater
Tectorial membrane
Cruciform ligament (superior longitudinal part)
Cruciform ligament (transverse part)
Cruciform ligament (inferior longitudinal part)
POSTERIOR
Rootlets of cervical nerves
Posterior atlantooccipital membrane
Squama of occipital bone
Posterior arch of atlas
Spinous process of axis

Figure 345.1 Median Sagittal Section of Atlantooccipital and Atlantoaxial Regions

NOTE: The relationships from anterior to posterior of the following structures: the anterior arch of the atlas, the joint between the atlas and the odontoid process (median atlantoaxial joint), the "joint" between the odontoid process and the transverse ligament of the atlas, the tectorial membrane and finally, the dura mater covering the spinal cord.

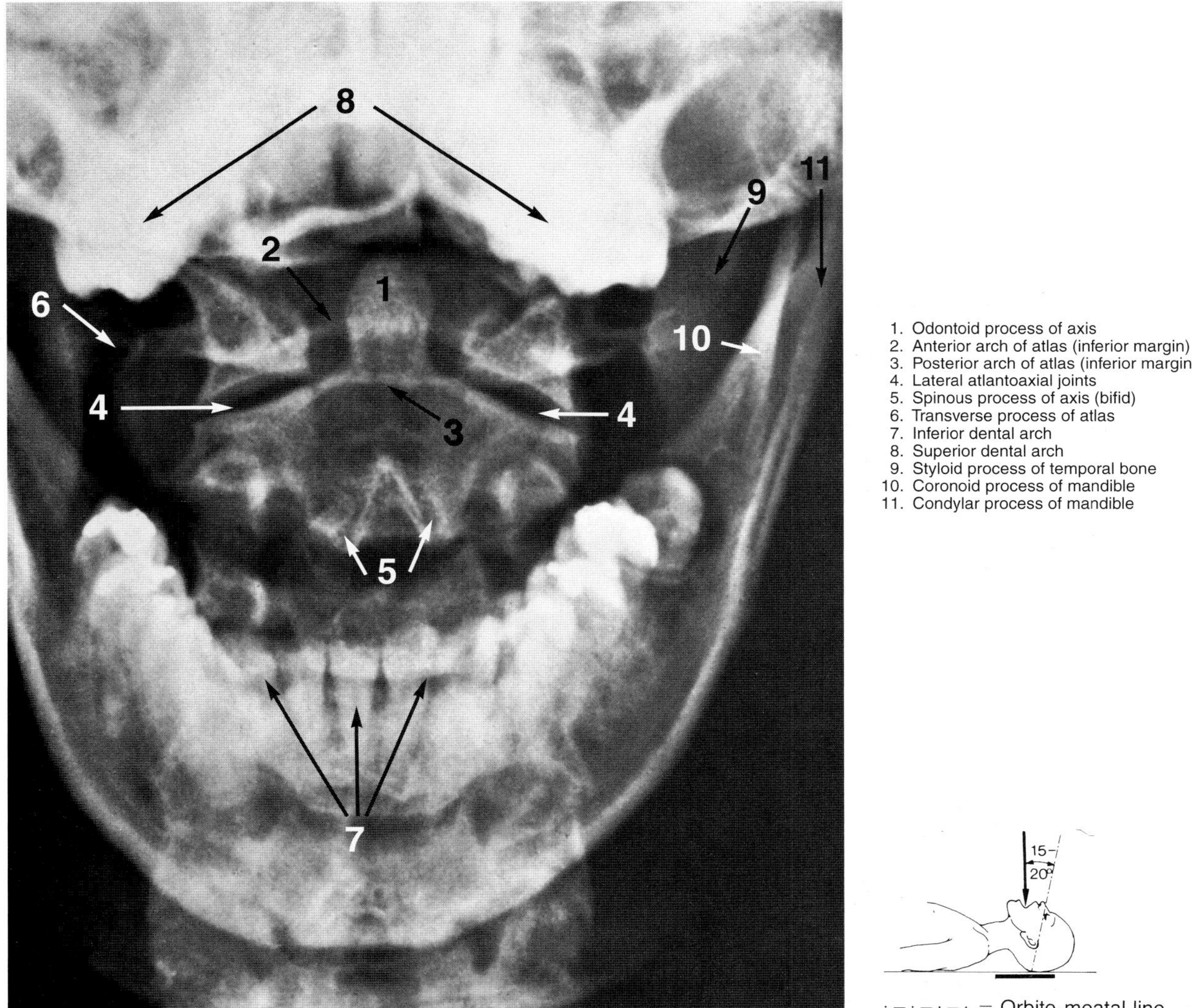
8
2
1
6
9
11
10
4
4
3
5
7
1. Odontoid process of axis
2. Anterior arch of atlas (inferior margin)
3. Posterior arch of atlas (inferior margin)
4. Lateral atlantoaxial joints
5. Spinous process of axis (bifid)
6. Transverse process of atlas
7. Inferior dental arch
8. Superior dental arch
9. Styloid process of temporal bone
10. Coronoid process of mandible
11. Condylar process of mandible
15–20°
= Orbito-meatal line

Figure 345.2 Radiograph of the Odontoid Process and the Atlantoaxial Joints

NOTE: This is an anteroposterior projection taken through the oral cavity as shown in the diagram.

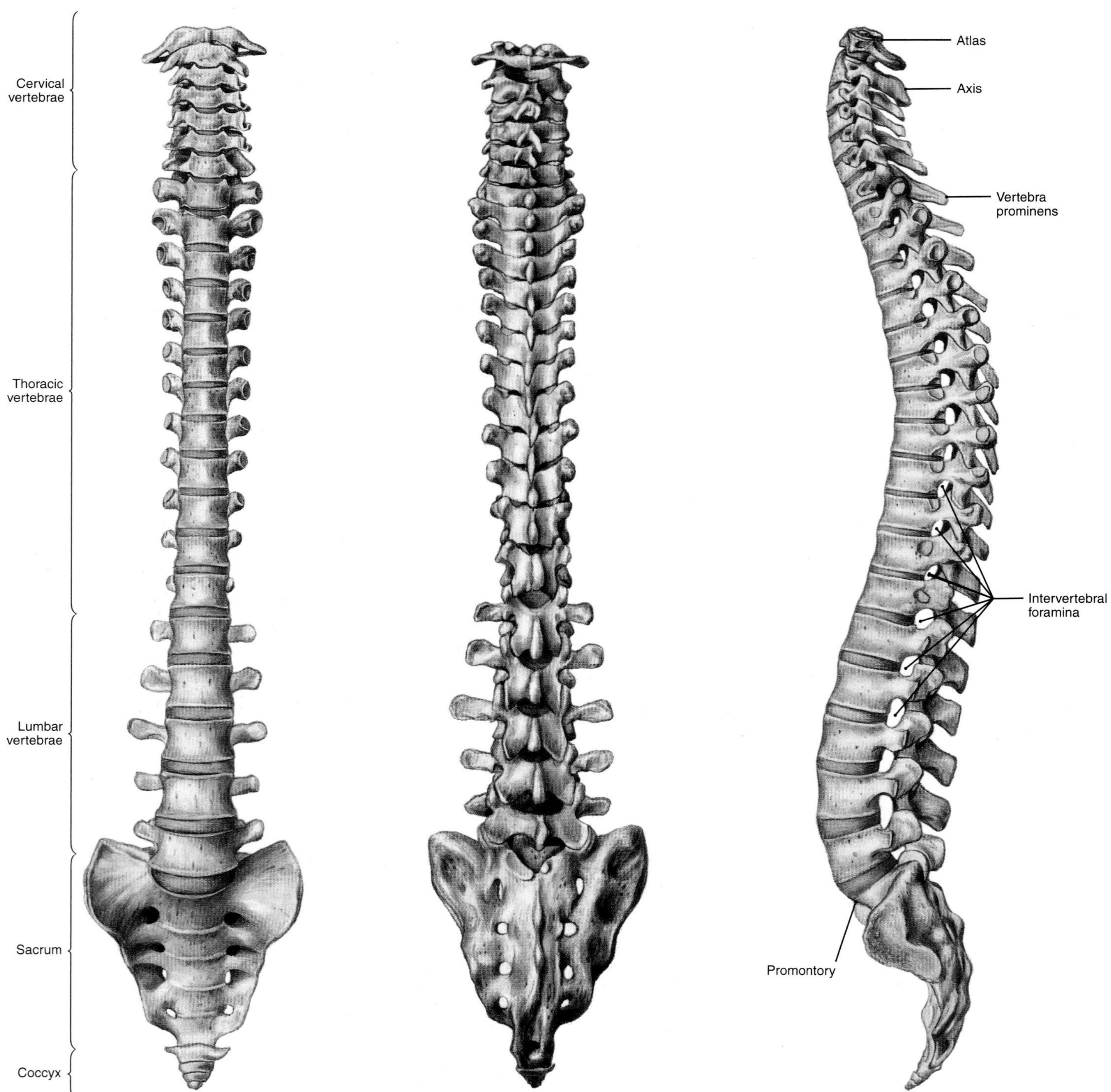
Cervical vertebrae
Thoracic vertebrae
Lumbar vertebrae
Sacrum
Coccyx
Atlas
Axis
Vertebra prominens
Intervertebral foramina
Promontory

Figure 346.1 Anterior View **Figure 346.2 Posterior View** **Figure 346.3 Left Lateral View**

Figures 346.1–346.3 Vertebral Column, Including the Sacrum and Coccyx

NOTE: (1) The vertebral column normally consists of 7 **cervical**, 12 **thoracic**, and 5 **lumbar** vertebrae and the **sacrum** and **coccyx.** Its principal functions are to assist in the maintenance of the erect posture in humans, to encase and protect the spinal cord, and to allow attachments of the musculature important for movements of the head and trunk.

(2) From a dorsal or ventral view, the normal spinal column is straight. When viewed from the side, the vertebral column presents two ventrally convex curvatures (cervical and lumbar) and two dorsally convex curvatures (thoracic and sacral).

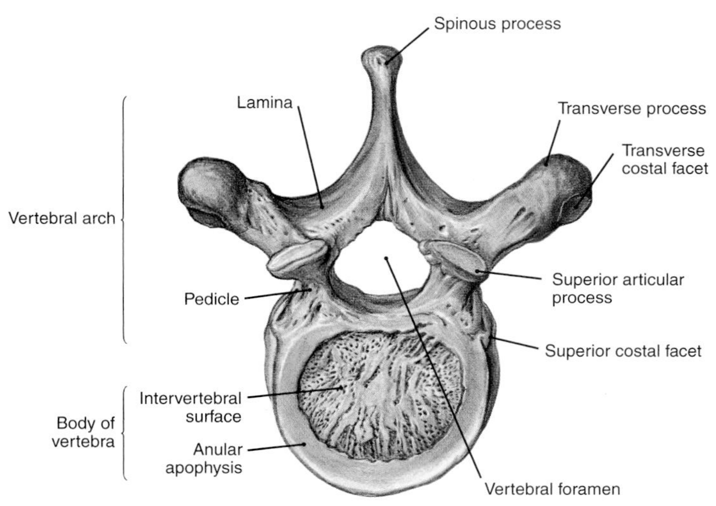
Spinous process
Lamina
Transverse process
Transverse costal facet
Vertebral arch
Superior articular process
Pedicle
Superior costal facet
Intervertebral surface
Body of vertebra
Anular apophysis
Vertebral foramen

Figure 347.1 Sixth Thoracic Vertebra (from Above)

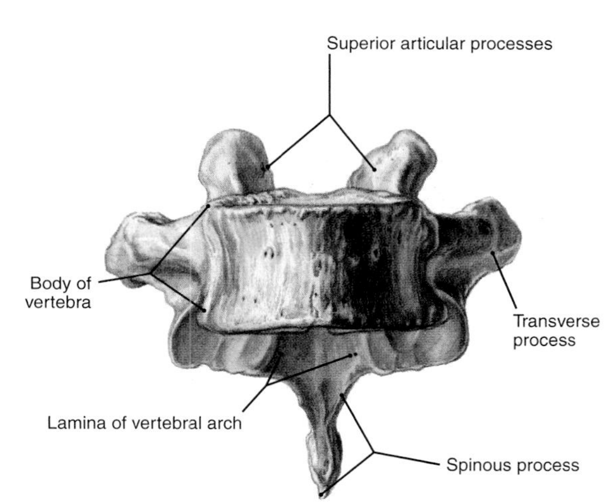
Superior articular processes
Body of vertebra
Transverse process
Lamina of vertebral arch
Spinous process

Figure 347.2 Tenth Thoracic Vertebra (Ventral View)

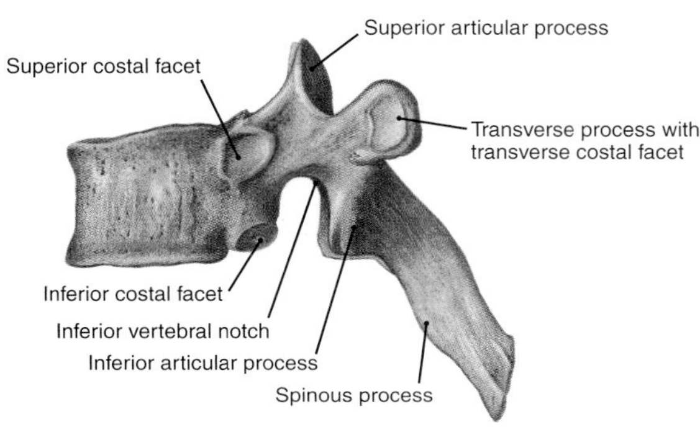
Superior articular process
Superior costal facet
Transverse process with transverse costal facet
Inferior costal facet
Inferior vertebral notch
Inferior articular process
Spinous process

Figure 347.3 Sixth Thoracic Vertebra (from Left Lateral Side)

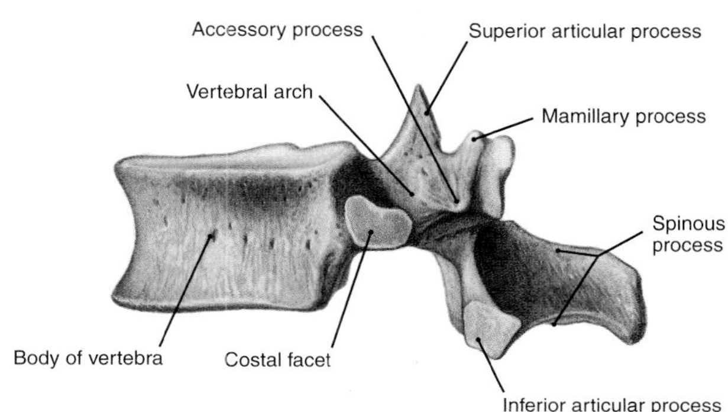
Accessory process
Superior articular process
Vertebral arch
Mamillary process
Spinous process
Body of vertebra
Costal facet
Inferior articular process

Figure 347.4 Twelfth Thoracic Vertebra (Lateral View)

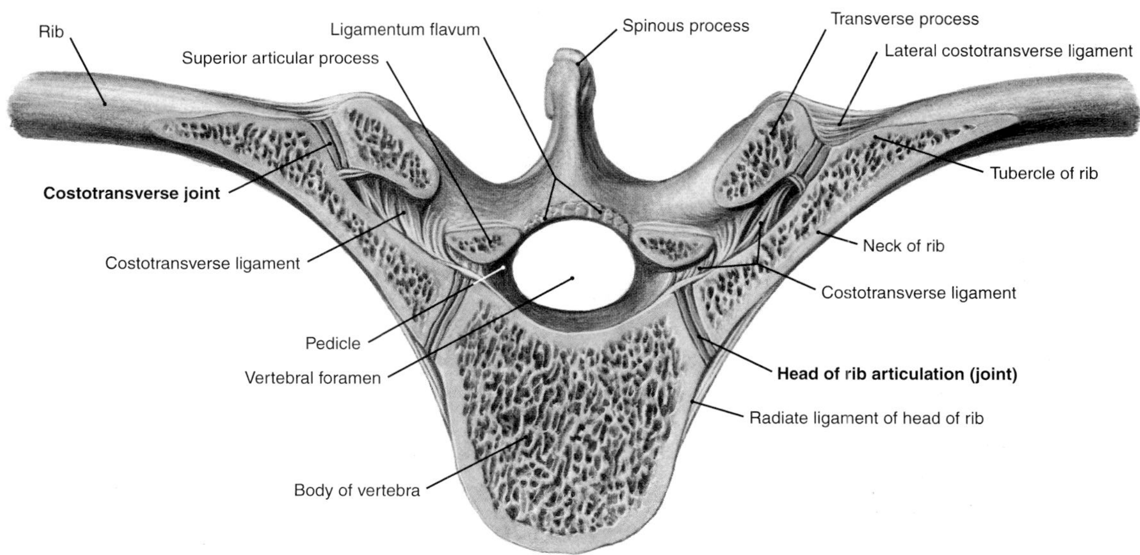
Rib
Ligamentum flavum
Superior articular process
Spinous process
Transverse process
Lateral costotransverse ligament
Tubercle of rib
Costotransverse joint
Neck of rib
Costotransverse ligament
Costotransverse ligament
Pedicle
Vertebral foramen
Head of rib articulation (joint)
Radiate ligament of head of rib
Body of vertebra

Figure 347.5 Costovertebral Joints, Transverse Section as Seen from Above

NOTE: Each rib articulates with the thoracic vertebrae at two places: (a) the **head of the rib** with the **vertebral body** and (b) the **tubercle** on the **neck of the rib** with the **transverse process** of the vertebra.

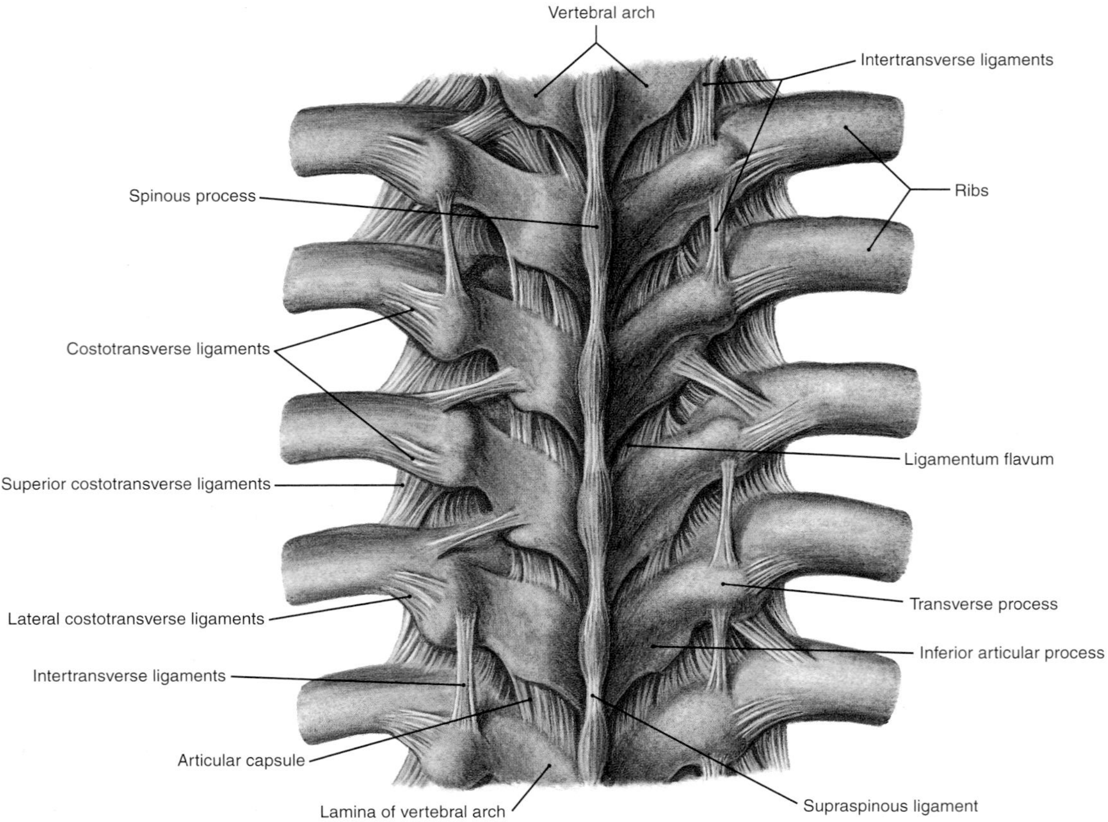
Vertebral arch
Intertransverse ligaments
Ribs
Spinous process
Costotransverse ligaments
Ligamentum flavum
Superior costotransverse ligaments
Transverse process
Lateral costotransverse ligaments
Inferior articular process
Intertransverse ligaments
Articular capsule
Lamina of vertebral arch
Supraspinous ligament

Figure 348.1 Lower Costovertebral Joints (Posterior View)

NOTE: (1) Five pairs of costovertebral joints, viewed from behind, show to advantage the articulations between the necks and tubercles of the ribs and the transverse processes of the thoracic vertebrae.

(2) The ligaments that connect these gliding joints are the **costotransverse, lateral costotransverse**, and **superior costotransverse.**

(3) The costotransverse joints (neck of rib with transverse process) are not to be confused with the joints between the heads of the ribs and the bodies of the vertebrae.

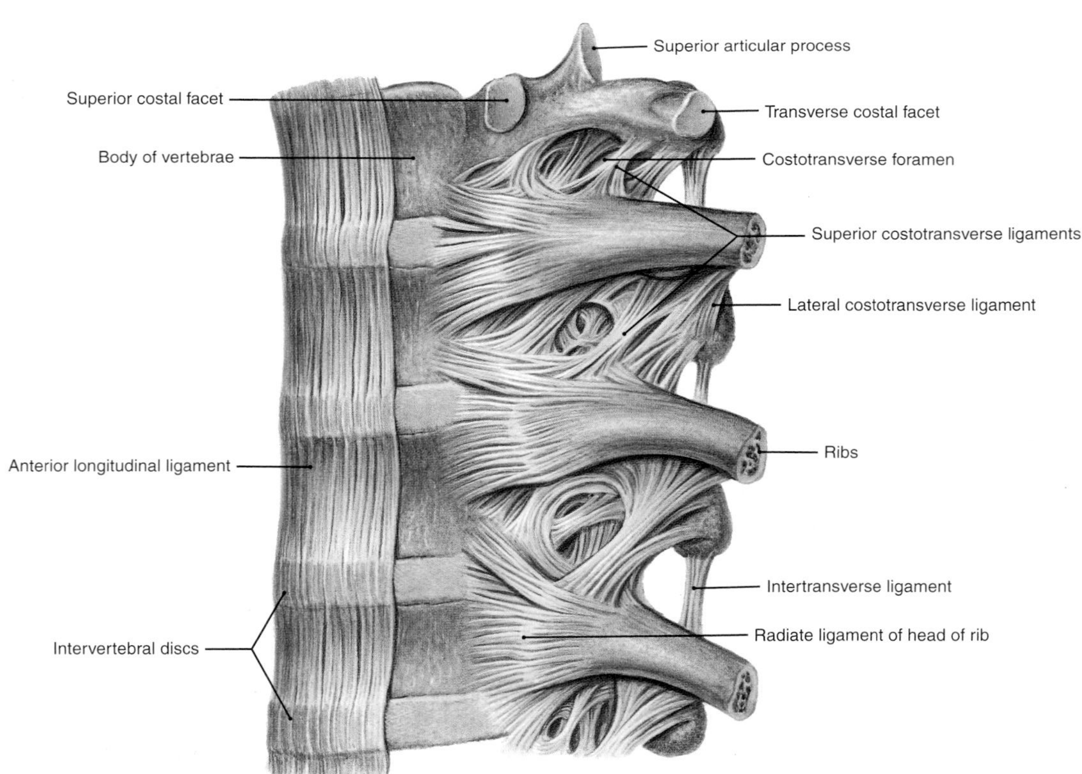
Superior articular process
Superior costal facet
Transverse costal facet
Body of vertebrae
Costotransverse foramen
Superior costotransverse ligaments
Lateral costotransverse ligament
Ribs
Anterior longitudinal ligament
Intertransverse ligament
Radiate ligament of head of rib
Intervertebral discs

Figure 348.2 Costovertebral Joints (Lateral View Showing the Radiate Ligaments of the Heads of the Ribs)

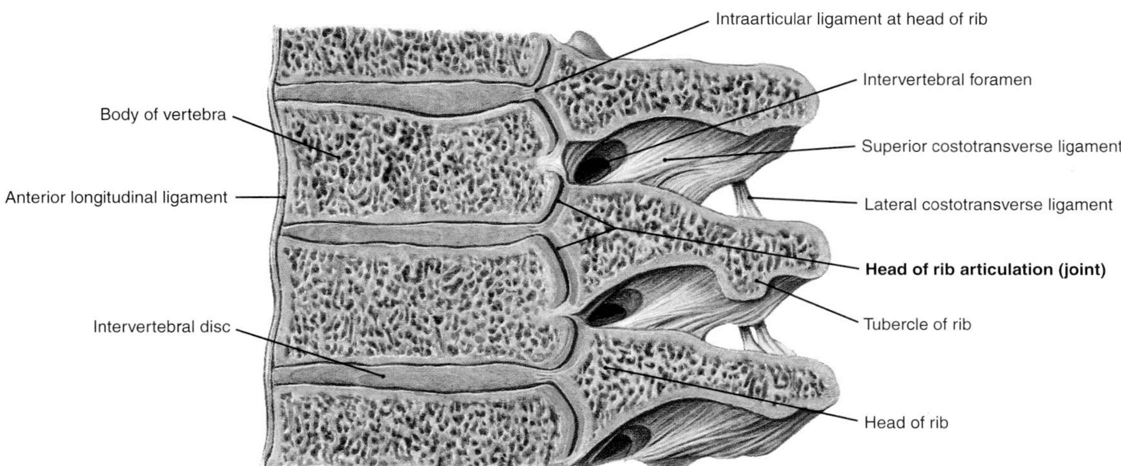
Intraarticular ligament at head of rib
Intervertebral foramen
Body of vertebra
Superior costotransverse ligament
Anterior longitudinal ligament
Lateral costotransverse ligament
Head of rib articulation (joint)
Intervertebral disc
Tubercle of rib
Head of rib

Figure 349.1 Sagittal Section through the Spinal Column Showing the Costovertebral Joints

NOTE: The following important structures are shown: the intervertebral disks, the intraarticular and costotransverse ligaments, and the intervertebral foramina, which transmit the spinal nerves and their accompanying vessels.

Figure 349.2 Anterior Longitudinal Ligament (Ventral View)

NOTE: The **anterior longitudinal ligament** extends from the axis to the sacrum along the anterior aspect of the bodies of the vertebrae and the intervertebral disks to which it is firmly attached. Its fibers are white and glistening and can readily be identified.

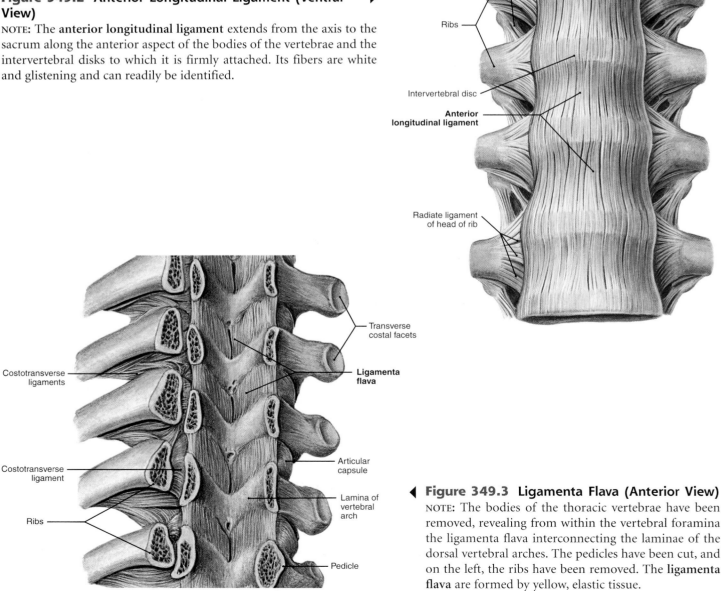

Figure 349.3 Ligamenta Flava (Anterior View)

NOTE: The bodies of the thoracic vertebrae have been removed, revealing from within the vertebral foramina the ligamenta flava interconnecting the laminae of the dorsal vertebral arches. The pedicles have been cut, and on the left, the ribs have been removed. The **ligamenta flava** are formed by yellow, elastic tissue.

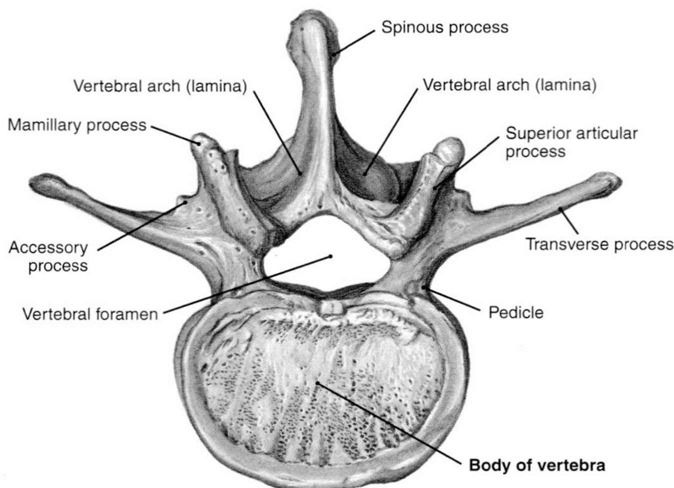
Spinous process
Vertebral arch (lamina)
Vertebral arch (lamina)
Mamillary process
Superior articular process
Accessory process
Transverse process
Vertebral foramen
Pedicle
Body of vertebra

Figure 350.1 Lumbar Vertebra (Cranial View)

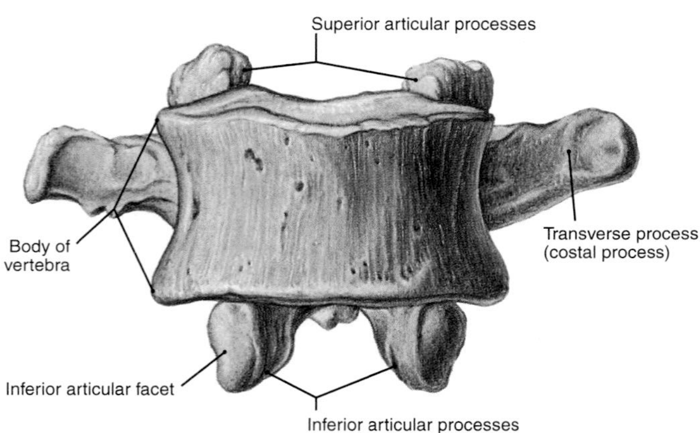
Superior articular processes
Body of vertebra
Transverse process (costal process)
Inferior articular facet
Inferior articular processes

Figure 350.2 Lumbar Vertebra (Anterior View)

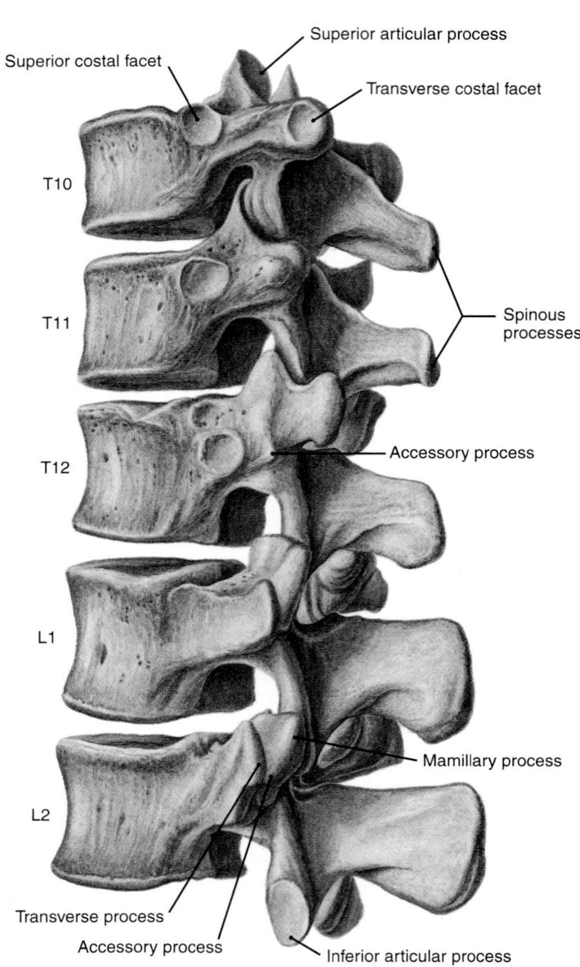
Superior articular process
Superior costal facet
Transverse costal facet
T10
T11
Spinous processes
T12
Accessory process
L1
Mamillary process
L2
Transverse process
Accessory process
Inferior articular process

Figure 350.3 Last Three Thoracic and First Two Lumbar Vertebrae (Lateral View)

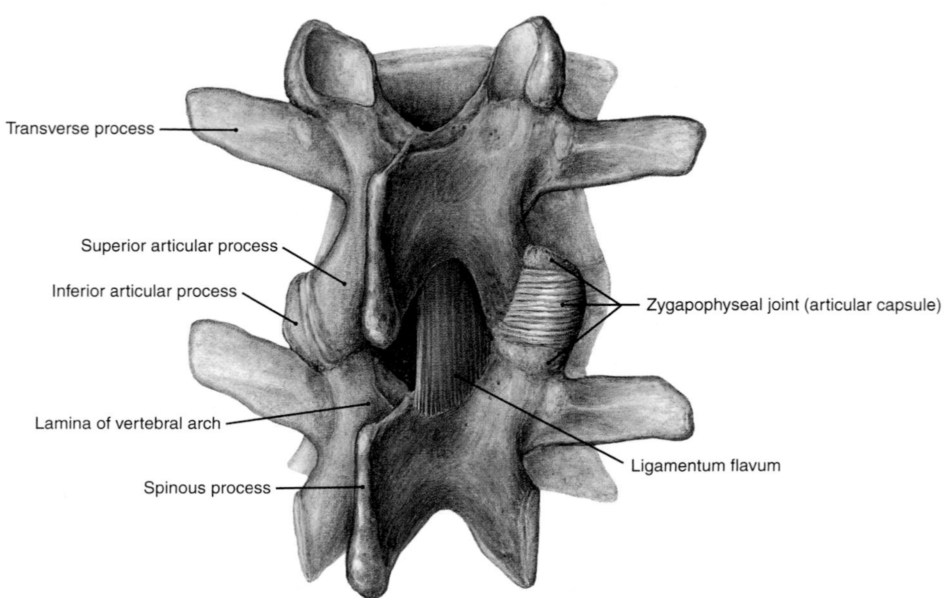
Transverse process
Superior articular process
Inferior articular process
Zygapophyseal joint (articular capsule)
Lamina of vertebral arch
Ligamentum flavum
Spinous process

Figure 350.4 Zygapophyseal Joints and Ligamenta Flava between Adjacent Lumbar Vertebrae

NOTE: (1) In this posterior view, the articular capsule of the zygapophyseal joint (between the articular processes) and the ligamentum flavum have been removed on the left side.

(2) Each ligamentum flavum is attached to the anterior surface of the lamina above and to the posterior surface of the lamina below. They are elastic and permit separation of the laminae during flexion of the spine, and they inhibit abrupt and extreme movements of the vertebral column, thus protecting the intervertebral disks (see also, Fig. 349.3).

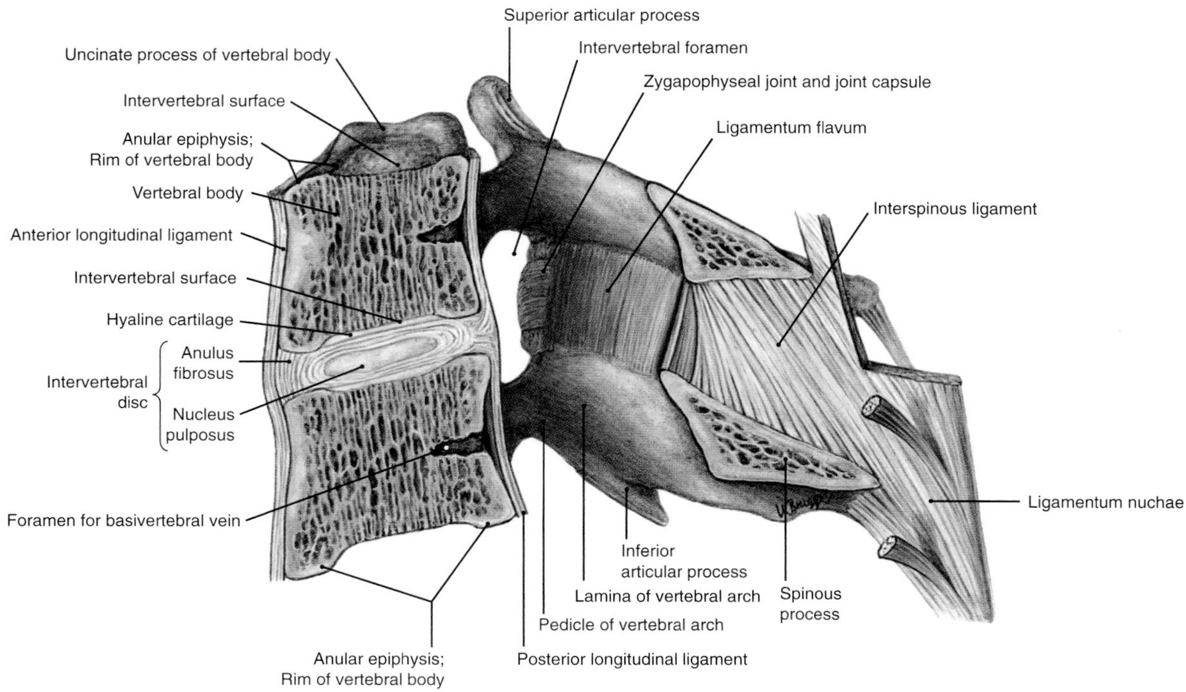
Superior articular process
Intervertebral foramen
Uncinate process of vertebral body
Zygapophyseal joint and joint capsule
Intervertebral surface
Ligamentum flavum
Anular epiphysis; Rim of vertebral body
Vertebral body
Interspinous ligament
Anterior longitudinal ligament
Intervertebral surface
Hyaline cartilage
Intervertebral disc
Anulus fibrosus
Nucleus pulposus
Ligamentum nuchae
Foramen for basivertebral vein
Inferior articular process
Lamina of vertebral arch
Spinous process
Pedicle of vertebral arch
Anular epiphysis; Rim of vertebral body
Posterior longitudinal ligament

Figure 351.1 Cervical Intervertebral Joints: Median Sagittal Section

NOTE: (1) The long spinous processes of the cervical vertebrae and the strong interspinous ligaments. Observe the blending of fibers of the interspinous ligaments with the ligamentum nuchae of the dorsal cervical region.

(2) The intervertebral disk between the bodies of the two cervical vertebrae are shown; note also the nucleus pulposus surrounded by the annulus fibrosis.

(3) The anterior and posterior longitudinal ligaments and the foramina for the basivertebral veins.

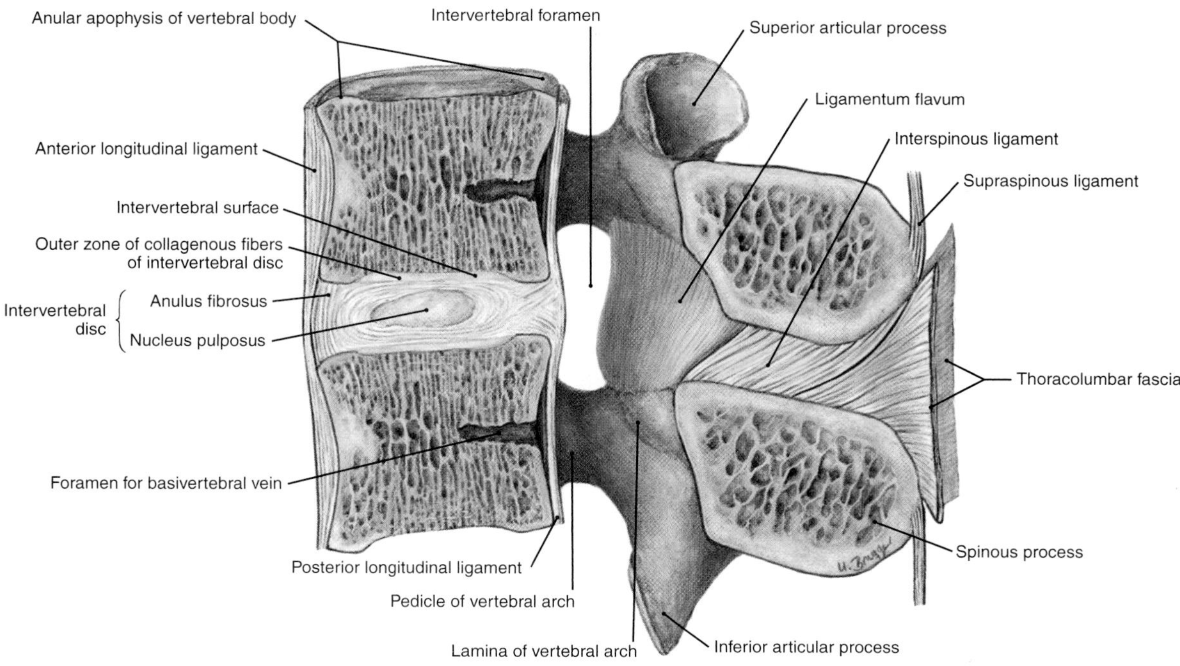
Anular apophysis of vertebral body
Intervertebral foramen
Superior articular process
Ligamentum flavum
Anterior longitudinal ligament
Interspinous ligament
Supraspinous ligament
Intervertebral surface
Outer zone of collagenous fibers of intervertebral disc
Intervertebral disc
Anulus fibrosus
Nucleus pulposus
Thoracolumbar fascia
Foramen for basivertebral vein
Spinous process
Posterior longitudinal ligament
Pedicle of vertebral arch
Lamina of vertebral arch
Inferior articular process

Figure 351.2 Median Sagittal Section through Two Lumbar Vertebrae and an Intervertebral Disk

NOTE: (1) The anterior and posterior longitudinal ligaments ventral and dorsal to the bodies of the lumbar vertebrae.

(2) The ligamentum flavum forms an important ligamentous connection between the laminae of adjacent vertebral arches on the dorsal aspect of the vertebral canal.

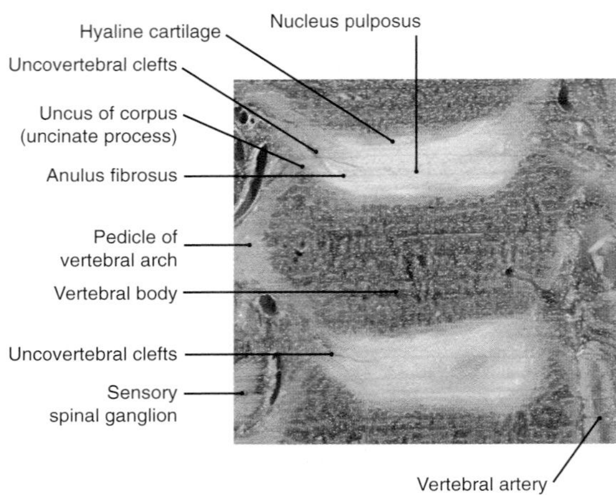
Hyaline cartilage
Nucleus pulposus
Uncovertebral clefts
Uncus of corpus
(uncinate process)
Anulus fibrosus
Pedicle of
vertebral arch
Vertebral body
Uncovertebral clefts
Sensory
spinal ganglion
Vertebral artery

Figure 352.1 Two Cervical Intervertebral Disks: Frontal Section through the Centers of the Vertebral Bodies

NOTE: (1) The intervertebral disks are located between the bodies of adjacent vertebrae (in this case cervical vertebrae).

(2) Hyaline cartilage covers the end plates of the vertebral bodies and lies adjacent to the anulus fibrosus.

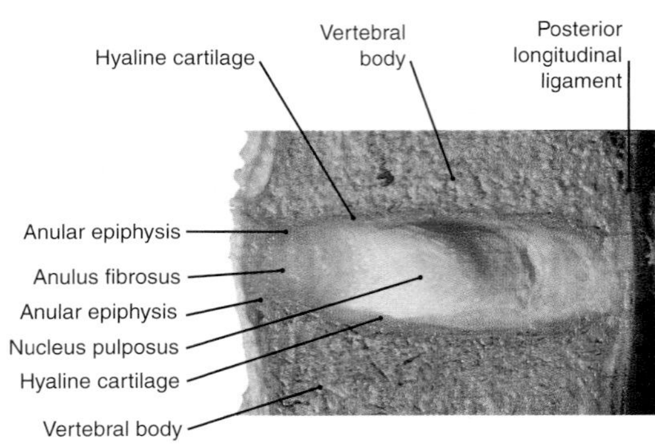
Hyaline cartilage
Vertebral
body
Posterior
longitudinal
ligament
Anular epiphysis
Anulus fibrosus
Anular epiphysis
Nucleus pulposus
Hyaline cartilage
Vertebral body

Figure 352.2 Median Sagittal Section through a Lumbar Intervertebral Disk

NOTE: (1) The **nucleus pulposus** that forms the inner core is soft and gelatinous in early years and consists of mucoid material and a few cells.

(2) After 10 or 12 years of age the mucoid material is gradually replaced by fibrocartilage, and the center of the disk becomes more like the anulus that surrounds it. (See notes for Fig. 352.3).

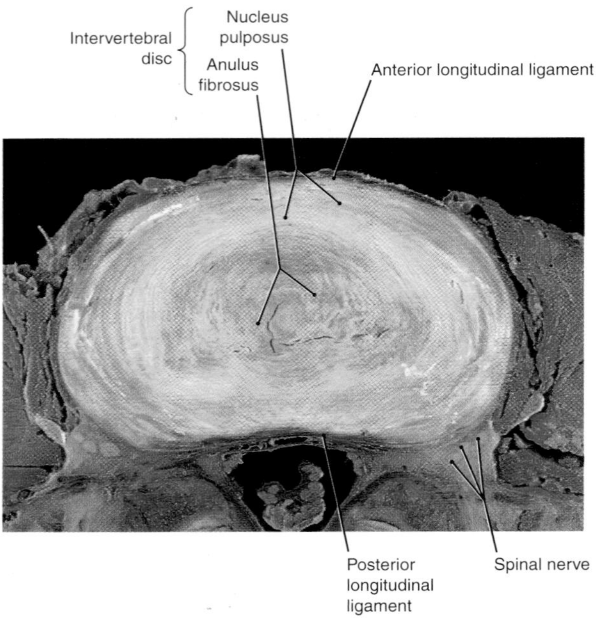
Intervertebral
disc
Nucleus
pulposus
Anulus
fibrosus
Anterior longitudinal ligament
Posterior
longitudinal
ligament
Spinal nerve

Figure 352.3 Photograph of a Lumbar Intervertebral Disk (Viewed from Above)

NOTE: (1) The anulus fibrosus consists of a thin band of collagenous fibers and a thicker band of fibrocartilage.

(2) In later adolescence and in the young adult, the intervertebral disks are strong and can withstand most vertical forces that impinge on the vertebral column, such as jumping or sitting upright.

(3) After several decades, some degeneration may occur that weakens the anulus fibrosus. These changes may account for the fact that in the elderly there may be a displacement of the nucleus pulposus (after even a mild strain) into or through the anulus, resulting in pain.

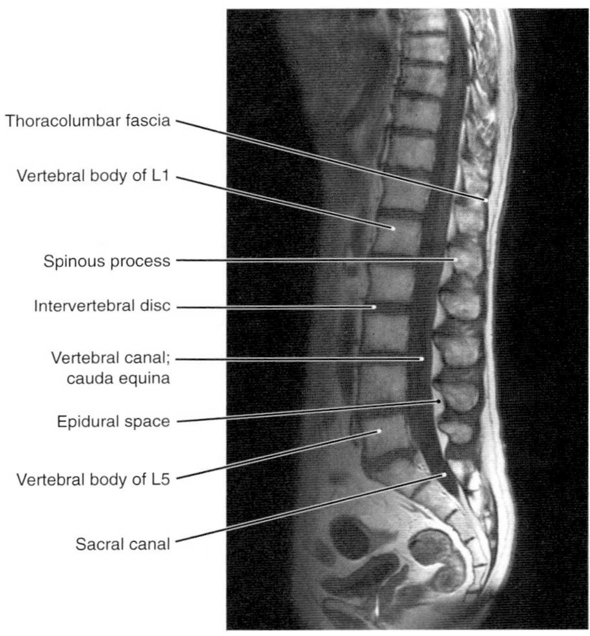
Thoracolumbar fascia
Vertebral body of L1
Spinous process
Intervertebral disc
Vertebral canal;
cauda equina
Epidural space
Vertebral body of L5
Sacral canal

Figure 352.4 Magnetic Resonance Image of the Lumbar Vertebrae (Median Sagittal Section)

NOTE: (1) The spinous processes and the bodies of the lumbar vertebrae.

(2) The intervertebral disks arranged sequentially between the vertebral bodies.

(3) The so-called disk problem that results from displacement of disk material is most likely to occur in the cervical or lumbar regions and especially between the L4-L5 vertebral body.

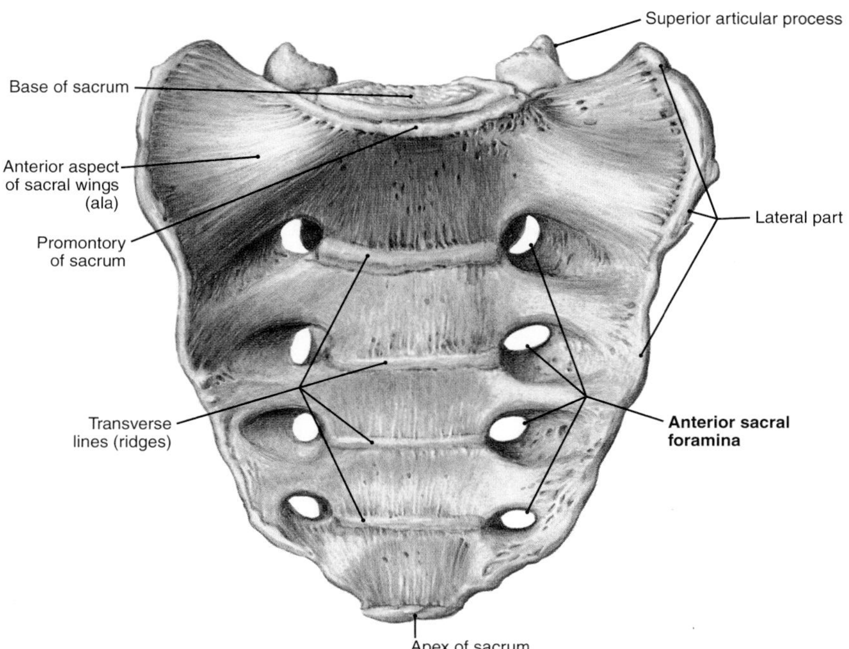
Superior articular process
Base of sacrum
Anterior aspect of sacral wings (ala)
Promontory of sacrum
Lateral part
Transverse lines (ridges)
Anterior sacral foramina
Apex of sacrum

Figure 353.1 Sacrum, Anterior or Pelvic Surface

NOTE: (1) The sacrum is a large triangular bone formed by the fusion of five sacral vertebrae, and it is wedged between the two hip bones, with which it articulates laterally.

(2) Superiorly, the sacrum articulates with the fifth lumbar vertebra, and inferiorly with the coccyx.

(3) The anterior (pelvic) surface of the sacrum is concave and shows four pelvic foramina on each side. These transmit the ventral rami of the upper four sacral nerves.

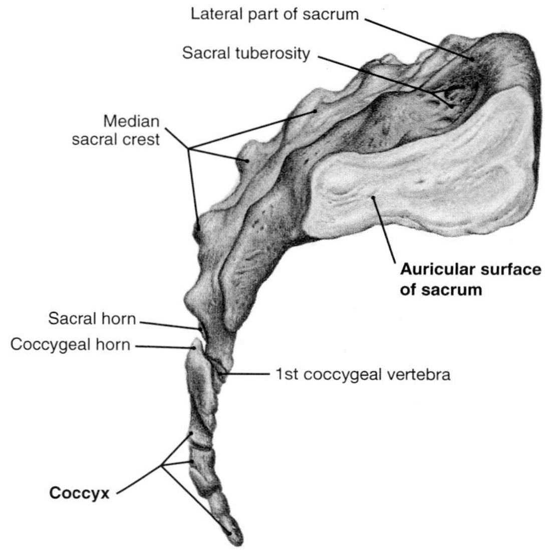
Lateral part of sacrum
Sacral tuberosity
Median sacral crest
Auricular surface of sacrum
Sacral horn
Coccygeal horn
1st coccygeal vertebra
Coccyx

Figure 353.2 Sacrum and Coccyx (Lateral View)

NOTE: The auricular (ear-shaped) surface of the sacrum articulates with the iliac portion of the pelvis. Inferiorly, the sacral apex joins the coccyx.

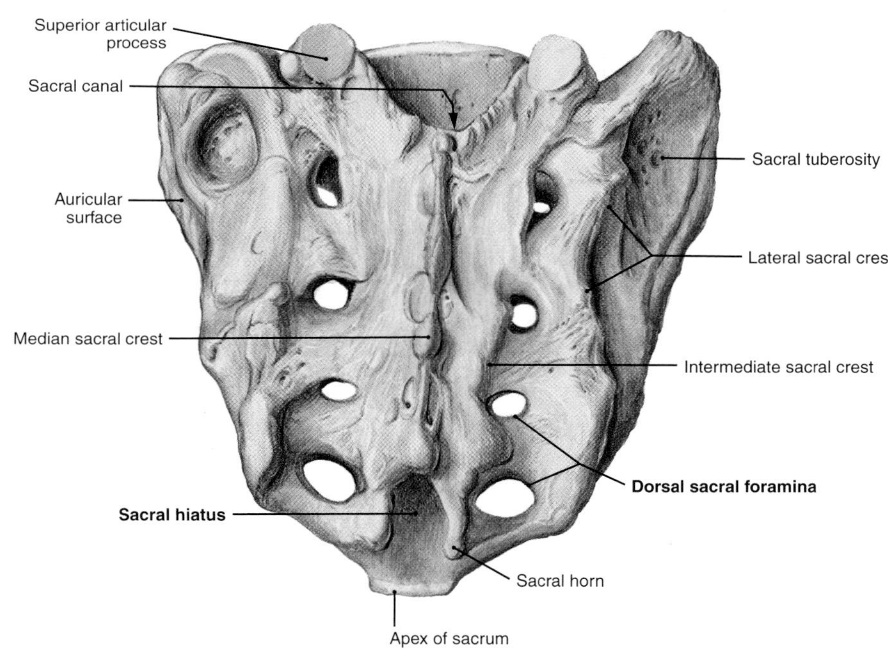
Superior articular process
Sacral canal
Sacral tuberosity
Auricular surface
Lateral sacral crest
Median sacral crest
Intermediate sacral crest
Dorsal sacral foramina
Sacral hiatus
Sacral horn
Apex of sacrum

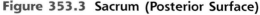

Figure 353.3 Sacrum (Posterior Surface)

NOTE: On the dorsal surface of the sacrum, the foramina transmit the dorsal rami of the sacral nerves. The dorsal laminae of the fifth sacral vertebra fails to fuse, thereby leaving a midline opening into the sacral canal called the sacral hiatus.

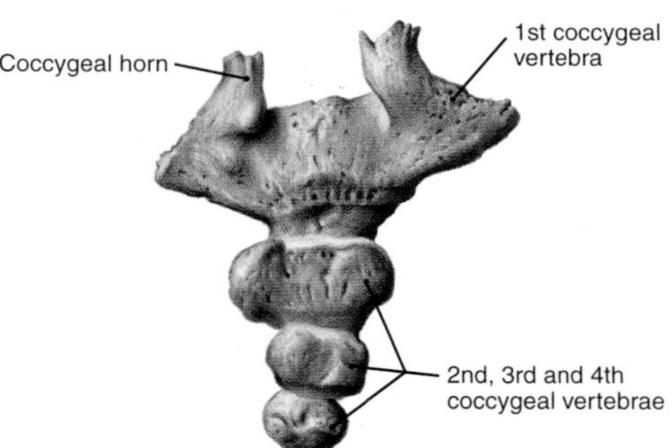
Coccygeal horn
1st coccygeal vertebra
2nd, 3rd and 4th coccygeal vertebrae

Figure 353.4 Coccyx (Dorsal View)

NOTE: This coccyx has four segments, but in many people there are three or five.

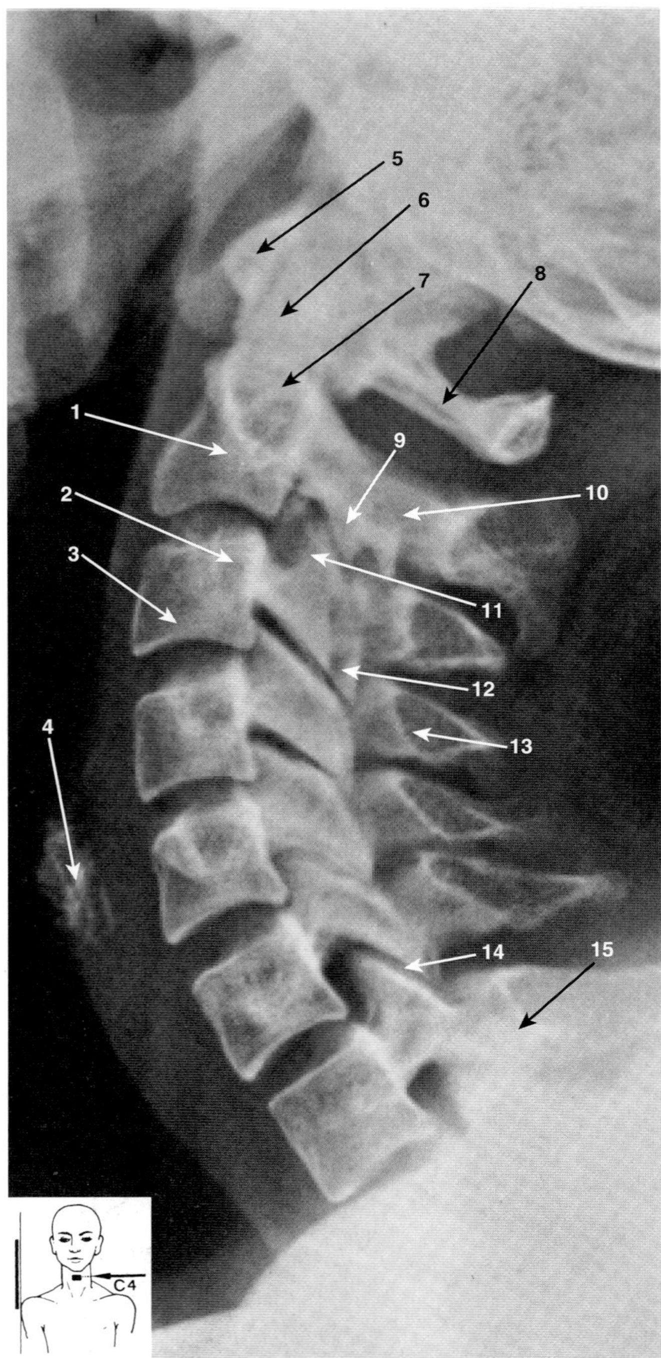
5
6
7
8
1
9
10
2
3
11
12
13
4
14
15
C4

Figure 354.1 Cervical Spinal Column (Lateral View)

1. Body of axis
2. Transverse process of C3 vertebra
3. Body of C3 vertebra
4. Lamina of cricoid cartilage
5. Anterior arch of atlas
6. Odontoid process of axis
7. Transverse process of axis
8. Posterior arch of atlas
9. Inferior articular process
10. Spinous process
11. Superior articular process
12. Inferior articular process
13. Spinous process
14. Intervertebral articulation
15. Spinous process, vertebra prominens (C7)

(From Wicke, 6th ed.)

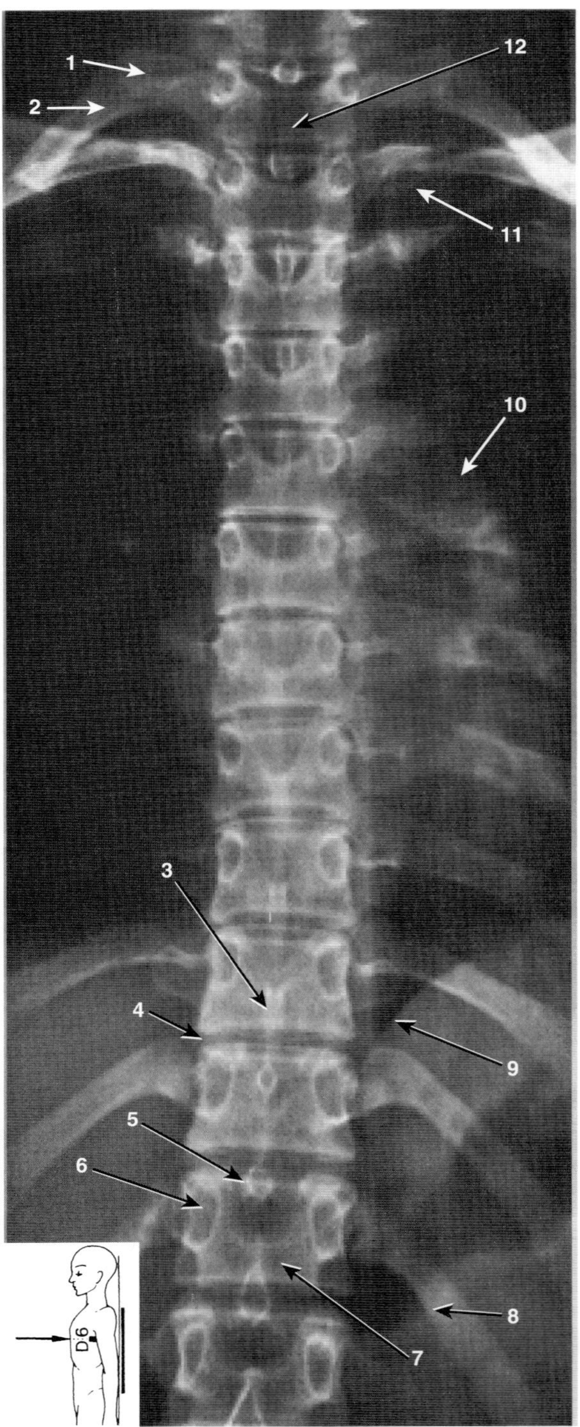
1
12
2
11
10
3
4
9
5
6
8
7
D6

Figure 354.2 Spinal Column, Thoracic Region (Anteroposterior Projection)

1. Neck of first rib
2. First rib
3. Spinous process
4. Inferior articular process
5. Superior articular process
6. Pedicle of vertebral arch
7. Twelfth thoracic vertebra
8. Twelfth rib
9. Diaphragm
10. Left contour of the heart
11. Clavicle
12. T1 vertebra

(From Wicke, 6th ed.)

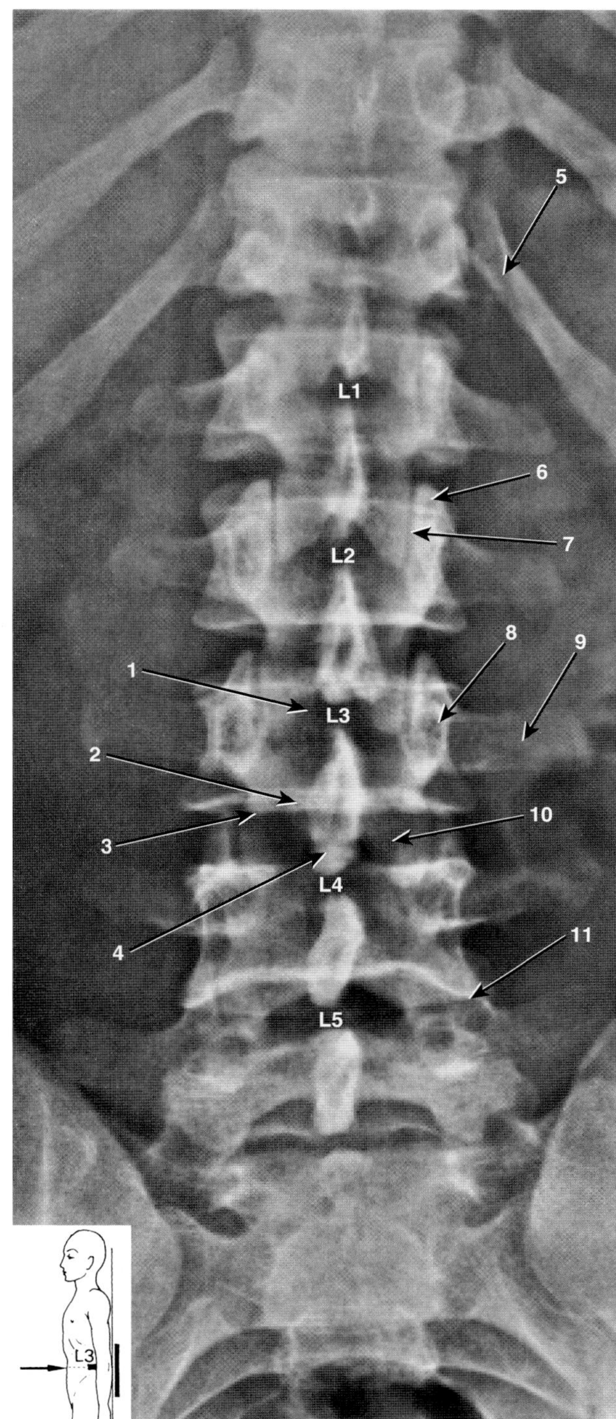
5
L1
6
7
L2
8
9
1
L3
2
10
3
L4
4
11
L5
L3

Figure 355.1 Spinal Column, Lumbar Region (Anteroposterior Projection)

1. Body of L3 vertebra
2. Posterior margin of L3 vertebra
3. Anterior margin of L4 vertebra
4. Spinous process of L3
5. Twelfth rib
6. Superior articular process
7. Intervertebral articulation (zygapophyseal joint)
8. Pedicle of vertebral arch
9. Costal process
10. Lamina of vertebral arch
11. Inferior articular process

(From Wicke, 6th ed.)

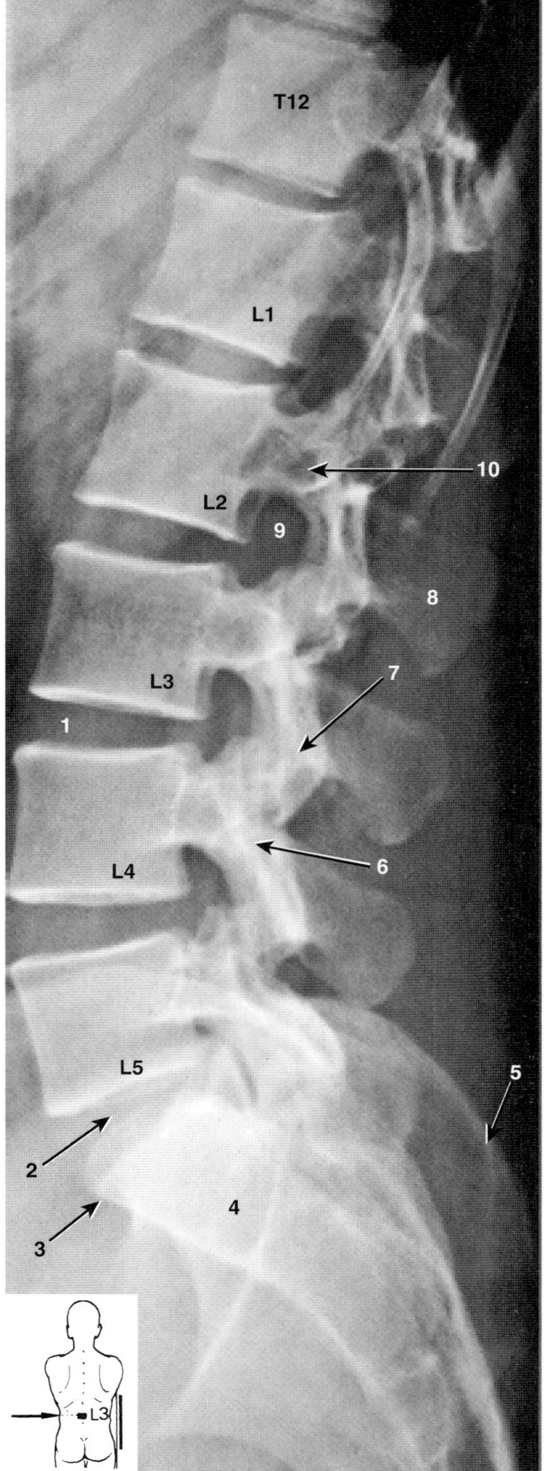
T12
L1
10
L2
9
8
L3
7
1
L4
6
L5
5
2
4
3
L3

Figure 355.2 Spinal Column, Lumbar Region (Lateral Projection)

1. Intervertebral disk space
2. Lumbosacral joint
3. Promontory
4. Sacrum
5. Iliac crest
6. Superior articular process of L4 vertebra
7. Inferior articular process of L3 vertebra
8. Spinous process of L2 vertebra
9. Intervertebral foramen
10. Costal process

(From Wicke, 6th ed.)

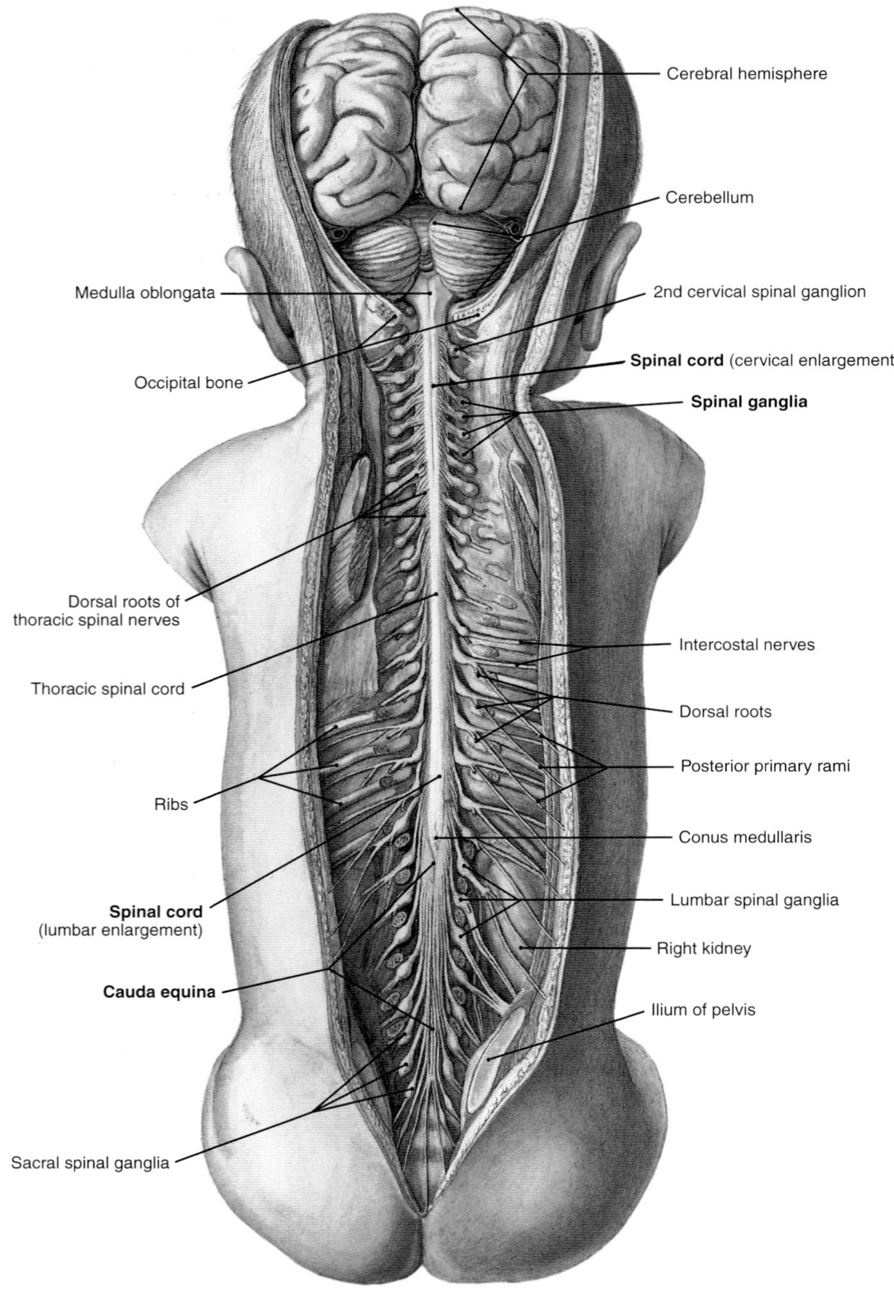
Cerebral hemisphere
Cerebellum
Medulla oblongata
2nd cervical spinal ganglion
Occipital bone
Spinal cord (cervical enlargement)
Spinal ganglia
Dorsal roots of thoracic spinal nerves
Thoracic spinal cord
Intercostal nerves
Dorsal roots
Posterior primary rami
Ribs
Conus medullaris
Spinal cord (lumbar enlargement)
Lumbar spinal ganglia
Right kidney
Cauda equina
Ilium of pelvis
Sacral spinal ganglia

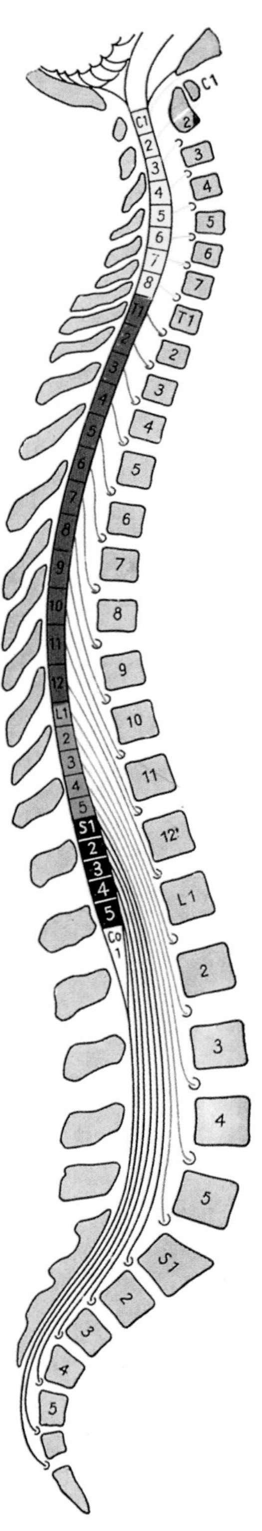

Figure 356.1 Spinal Cord and Brain of a Newborn Child (Posterior View)

NOTE: (1) The central nervous system has been exposed by the removal of the dorsal part of the spinal column and of the dorsal cranium. The spinal ganglia have been dissected, as have their corresponding spinal nerves.

(2) Although in this dissection it appears as though the substance of the spinal cord terminates at about L1, it is more usual in the newborn for the cord to end at about L3 or L4, thereby filling the spinal canal more completely than in the adult.

(3) The dorsal root ganglion of the first cervical nerve may be very small and often absent (see small ganglion above that of C2). Both anterior and posterior primary rami of C1 are principally motor, although from time to time C1 will have a small cutaneous branch.

Figure 356.2 Emerging Spinal Nerves and Segments in the Adult

Yellow: Cervical segments (C1–C8)
Red: Thoracic segments (T1–T12)
Blue: Lumbar segments (L1–L5)
Black: Sacral segments (S1–S5)
White: Coccygeal segments (C0)

NOTE: Many spinal nerves travel long distances before they leave the vertebral canal in the adult.

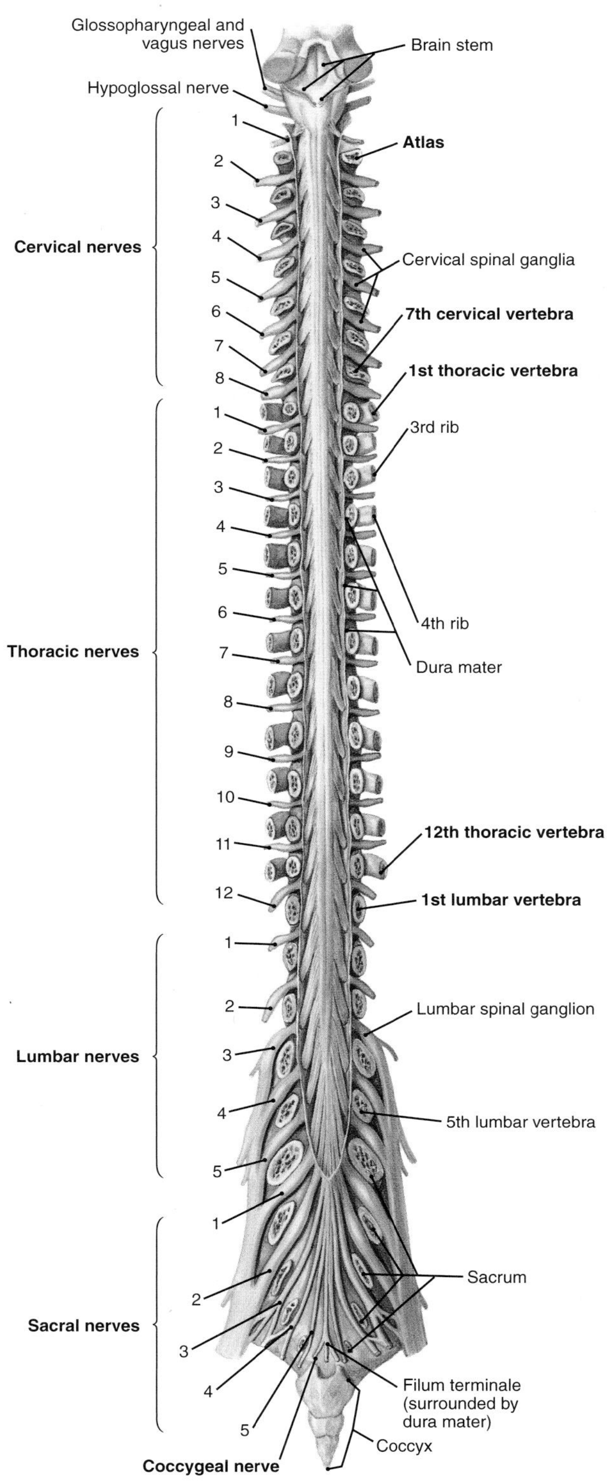
Glossopharyngeal and vagus nerves
Brain stem
Hypoglossal nerve
Atlas
Cervical nerves
1
2
3
4
5
6
7
8
Cervical spinal ganglia
7th cervical vertebra
1st thoracic vertebra
3rd rib
Thoracic nerves
1
2
3
4
5
6
7
8
9
10
11
12
4th rib
Dura mater
12th thoracic vertebra
1st lumbar vertebra
Lumbar nerves
1
2
3
4
5
Lumbar spinal ganglion
5th lumbar vertebra
Sacral nerves
1
2
3
4
5
Sacrum
Filum terminale (surrounded by dura mater)
Coccyx
Coccygeal nerve

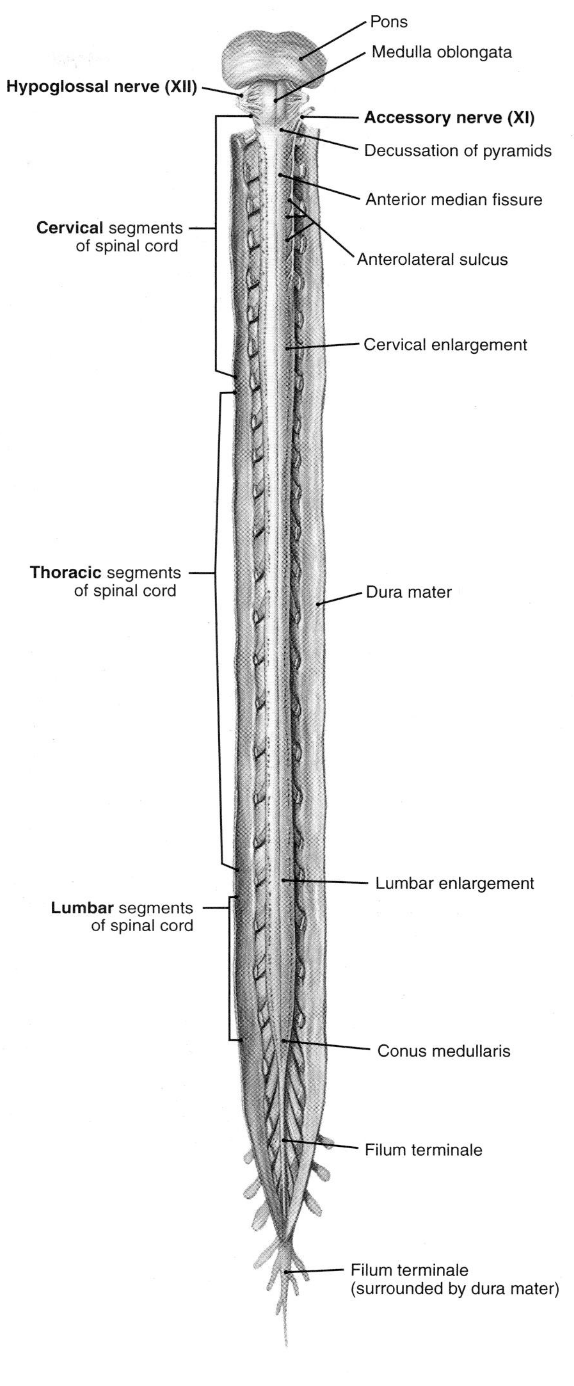
Pons
Medulla oblongata
Hypoglossal nerve (XII)
Accessory nerve (XI)
Decussation of pyramids
Anterior median fissure
Cervical segments of spinal cord
Anterolateral sulcus
Cervical enlargement
Thoracic segments of spinal cord
Dura mater
Lumbar enlargement
Lumbar segments of spinal cord
Conus medullaris
Filum terminale
Filum terminale (surrounded by dura mater)

Figure 357.1 Spinal Cord within the Vertebral Canal (Dorsal View)

NOTE: (1) The first cervical nerve emerges above the first vertebra and the eighth cervical nerve emerges below the seventh vertebra.

(2) The cervical spinal cord is continuous above with the medulla oblongata of the brainstem.

(3) Each spinal nerve is formed by the union of the dorsal and ventral roots of that segment, and it emerges between the two adjacent vertebrae through the intervertebral foramen.

Figure 357.2 Spinal Cord (Ventral View)

NOTE: (1) The origin of the spinal portion of the accessory nerve (XI) arising from the cervical spinal cord and ascending to join the bulbar portion of that nerve.

(2) The alignment of the rootlets of the hypoglossal nerve (XII) with the ventral roots of the spinal cord.

(3) The anterior median fissure is located in the longitudinal midline of the spinal cord. Within this fissure courses the anterior spinal artery (see Fig. 358.1)

(4) The cervical and lumbar enlargements caused by the large numbers of sensory and motor neurons located in these regions that are required to supply innervation to the upper and lower limbs.

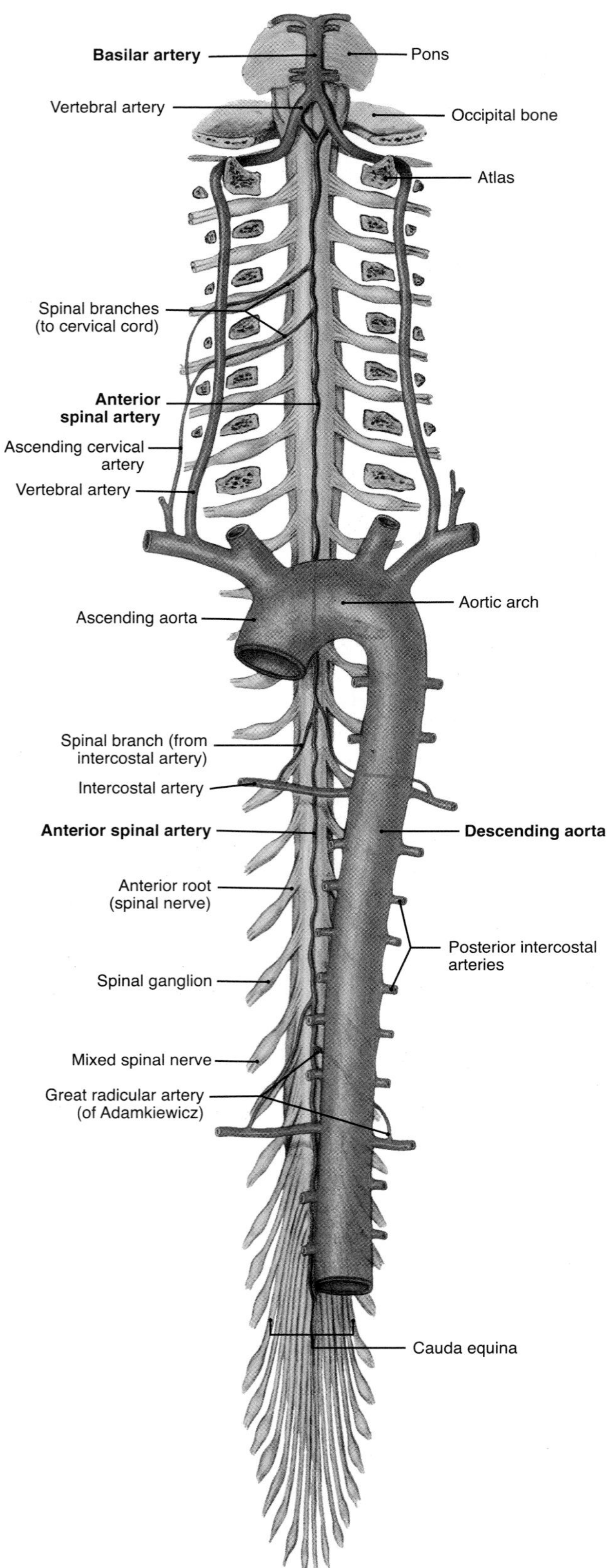
Basilar artery
Pons
Vertebral artery
Occipital bone
Atlas
Spinal branches (to cervical cord)
Anterior spinal artery
Ascending cervical artery
Vertebral artery
Ascending aorta
Aortic arch
Spinal branch (from intercostal artery)
Intercostal artery
Anterior spinal artery
Descending aorta
Anterior root (spinal nerve)
Posterior intercostal arteries
Spinal ganglion
Mixed spinal nerve
Great radicular artery (of Adamkiewicz)
Cauda equina

Figure 358.1 Anterior Spinal Artery

NOTE: The anterior spinal artery is formed by vessels from the vertebral arteries. It receives anastomotic branches from certain cervical, thoracic, and lumbar segmental arteries along the spinal roots. An especially large branch (artery of Adamkiewicz) arises in the lower thoracic or upper lumbar region.

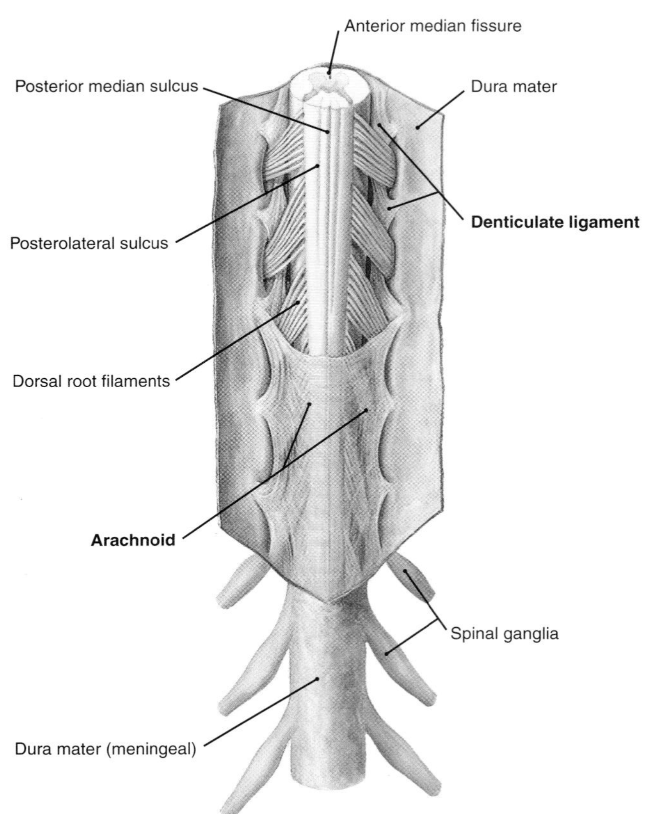
Anterior median fissure
Posterior median sulcus
Dura mater
Denticulate ligament
Posterolateral sulcus
Dorsal root filaments
Arachnoid
Spinal ganglia
Dura mater (meningeal)

Figure 358.2 Spinal Cord with Dura Mater Dissected Open (Dorsal View)

NOTE: Extensions of the pia mater to the meningeal dura mater between the roots of the spinal nerves are called **denticulate ligaments.** The arachnoid sends fine attachments to both the pia and dura.

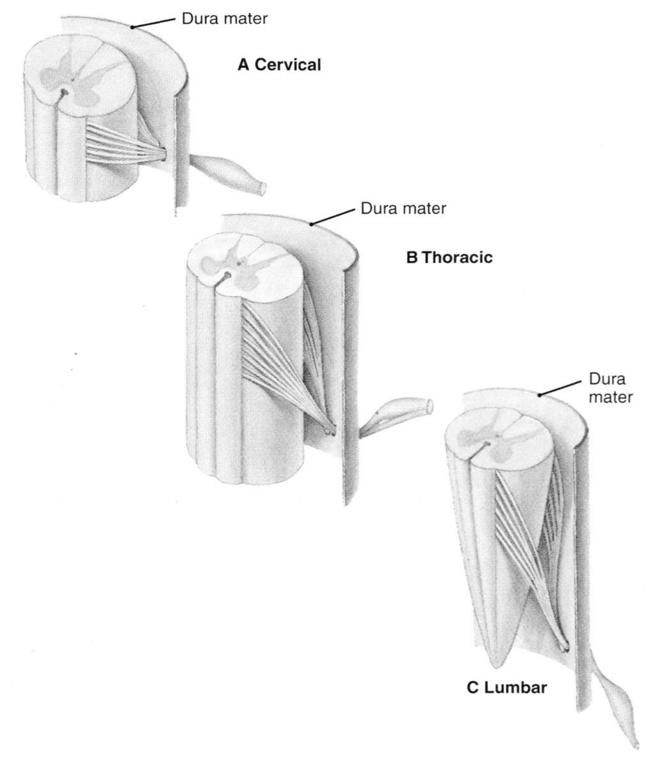
Dura mater
A Cervical
Dura mater
B Thoracic
Dura mater
C Lumbar

Figure 358.3A–C Relationship of the Dorsal and Ventral Roots to the Dura Mater (Various Spinal Levels)

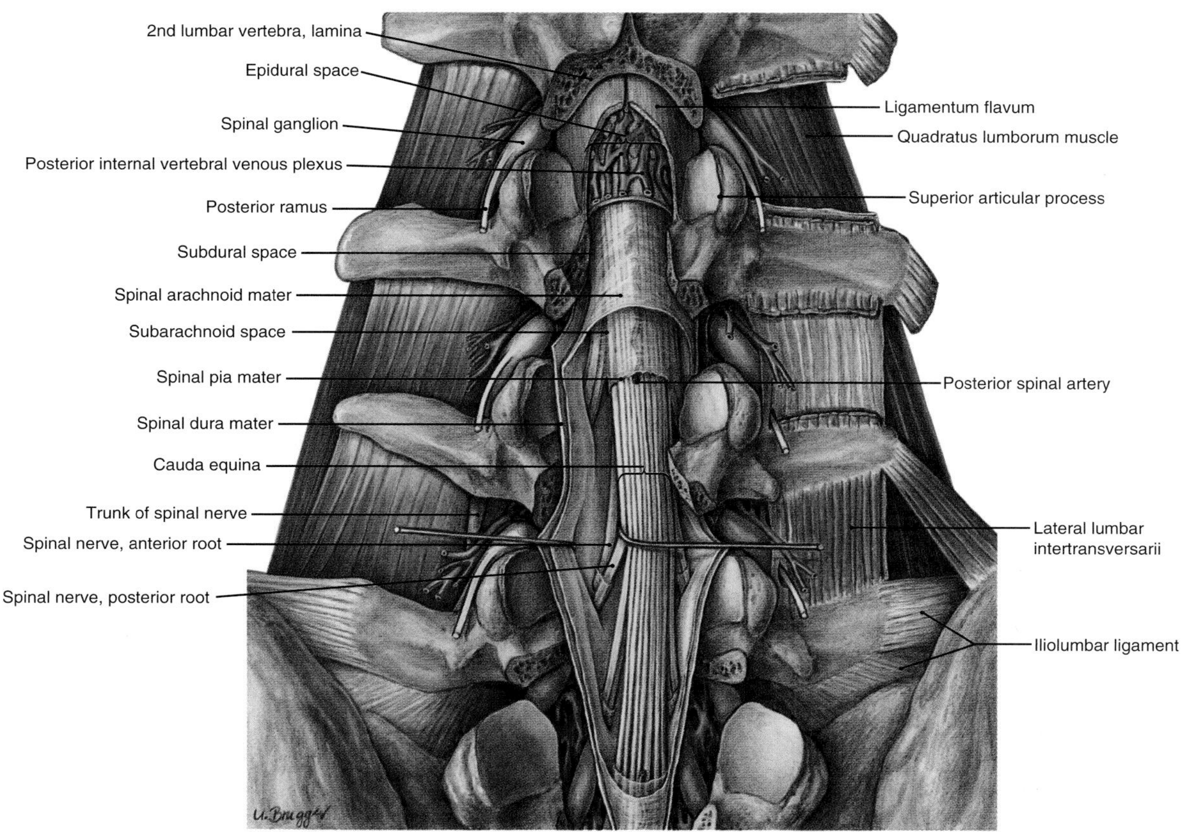
2nd lumbar vertebra, lamina
Epidural space
Spinal ganglion
Posterior internal vertebral venous plexus
Posterior ramus
Subdural space
Spinal arachnoid mater
Subarachnoid space
Spinal pia mater
Spinal dura mater
Cauda equina
Trunk of spinal nerve
Spinal nerve, anterior root
Spinal nerve, posterior root
Ligamentum flavum
Quadratus lumborum muscle
Superior articular process
Posterior spinal artery
Lateral lumbar intertransversarii
Iliolumbar ligament

Figure 359.1 Dorsal View of the Vertebral Canal from the Second to the Fifth Lumbar Vertebral Level

NOTE: (1) The vertebral arches have been removed to show the vertebral canal below the conus medullaris.

(2) The anterior (ventral) and posterior (dorsal) roots coursing together through the intervertebral foramina in the lumbar region.

(3) The dorsal root ganglia at each segmental lumbar level.

(4) The formation of spinal roots below the conus medullaris (L2 level of the spinal cord) is often called the **cauda equina** (horse's tail).

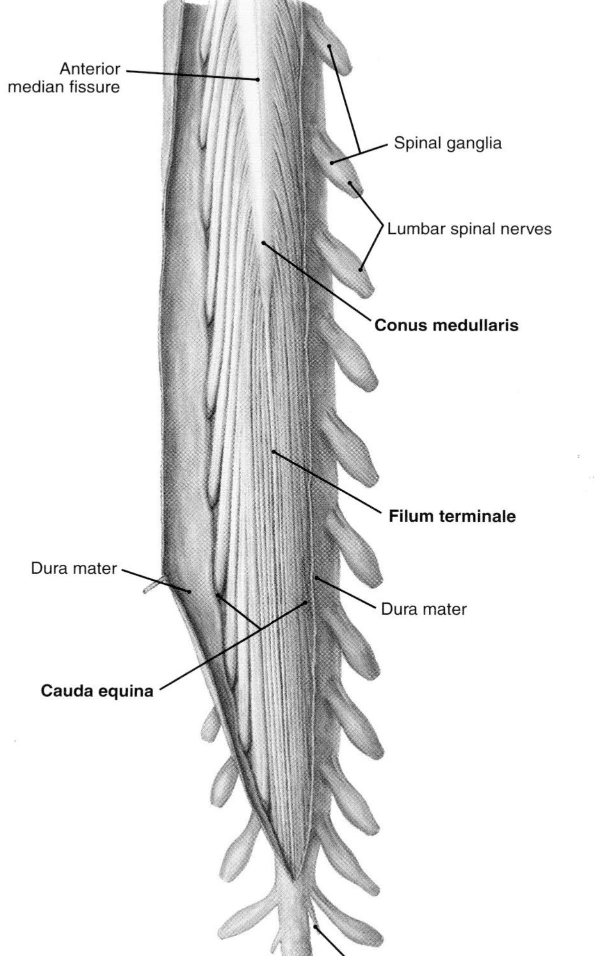
Anterior median fissure
Spinal ganglia
Lumbar spinal nerves
Conus medullaris
Filum terminale
Dura mater
Dura mater
Cauda equina
Coccygeal nerve

Figure 359.2 Conus Medullaris and Cauda Equina (Ventral)

NOTE: (1) The termination of the neural part of the spinal cord at the conus medullaris. Its membranous continuation as the filum terminale measures about 20 cm and extends as far as the coccyx.

(2) The cauda equina refers to the roots of the spinal nerves below the conus, and these are seen to surround the filum.

(3) Prolongations of the dura continue to cover the spinal nerves for some distance as they enter the intervertebral foramen.

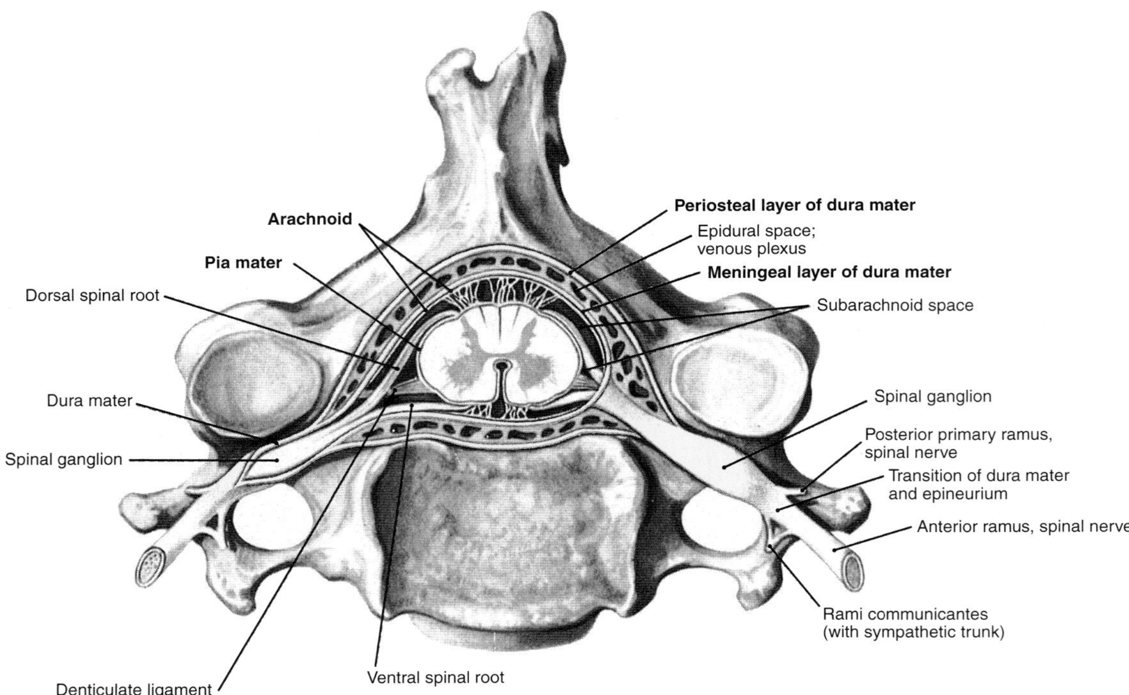
Arachnoid
Pia mater
Dorsal spinal root
Dura mater
Spinal ganglion
Periosteal layer of dura mater
Epidural space;
venous plexus
Meningeal layer of dura mater
Subarachnoid space
Spinal ganglion
Posterior primary ramus,
spinal nerve
Transition of dura mater
and epineurium
Anterior ramus, spinal nerve
Rami communicantes
(with sympathetic trunk)
Ventral spinal root
Denticulate ligament

Figure 360.1 Meninges of the Spinal Cord Shown at Cervical Level (Transverse Section)

NOTE: (1) The meningeal dura mater (inner layer of yellow) surrounds the spinal cord and continues along the spinal nerve through the intervertebral foramen. Its outer periosteal layer is formed of connective tissue that closely adheres to the bone of the vertebrae forming the vertebral canal.

(2) The delicate film-like arachnoid, which lies between the meningeal layer of the dura mater and the vascularized pia mater, which is closely applied to the cord.

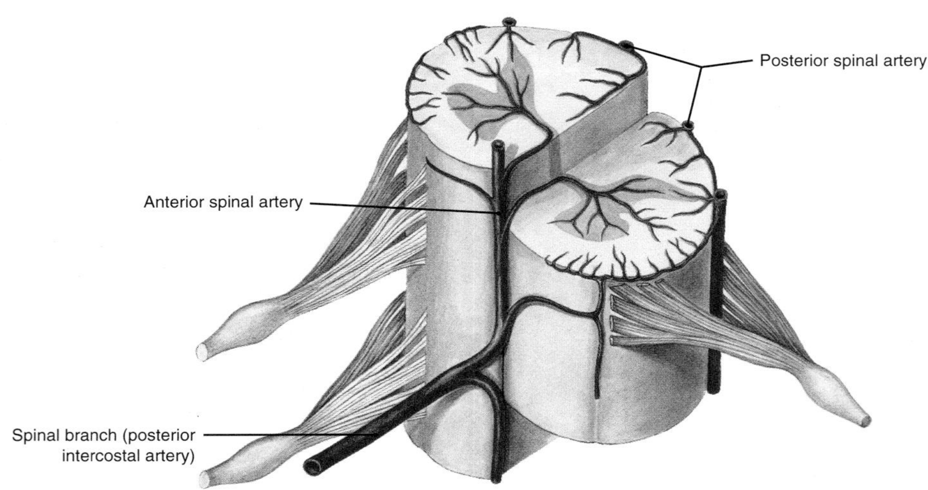
Posterior spinal artery
Anterior spinal artery
Spinal branch (posterior
intercostal artery)

Figure 360.2 Spinal Arteries and Their Sulcal Branches

NOTE: (1) As the **anterior spinal artery** descends in the anterior median sulcus, it gives off **sulcal branches** that penetrate the spinal cord.

(2) These sulcal branches usually arise singly, and each turns to the right or left to supply that half of the spinal cord. When each branch is given off it *does not bifurcate* to supply both sides.

(3) Each sulcal branch turns to one side of the cord, and the next branch turns to the other. This alternating pattern (as shown in this figure) occurs along the length of the spinal cord.

(4) Each of the two **posterior spinal arteries** supply their respective sides of the cord.

(5) The spinal arteries anastomose with the spinal branches of the segmental arteries (especially those from the intercostal and lumbar arteries).

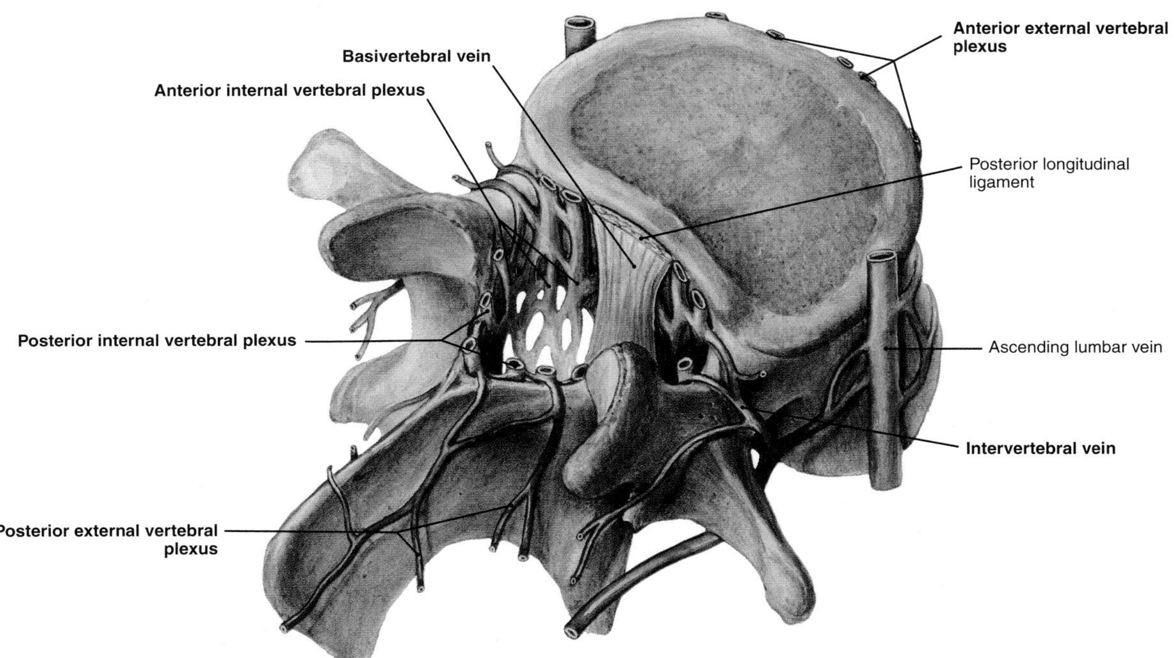
Basivertebral vein
Anterior internal vertebral plexus
Anterior external vertebral plexus
Posterior longitudinal ligament
Posterior internal vertebral plexus
Ascending lumbar vein
Intervertebral vein
Posterior external vertebral plexus

Figure 361.1 Veins of the Vertebral Column

NOTE: (1) The veins drain blood from the vertebrae, and the contents of the spinal canal form plexuses that extend the entire length of the spinal column (Batson's veins).

(2) The plexuses are grouped according to whether they lie external to or within the vertebral canal. Thus, they include **external vertebral, internal vertebral, basivertebral, intervertebral** and **veins of the spinal cord.**

(3) The basivertebral veins drain the bodies of the vertebrae and may flow into anterior external or anterior internal vertebral plexuses.

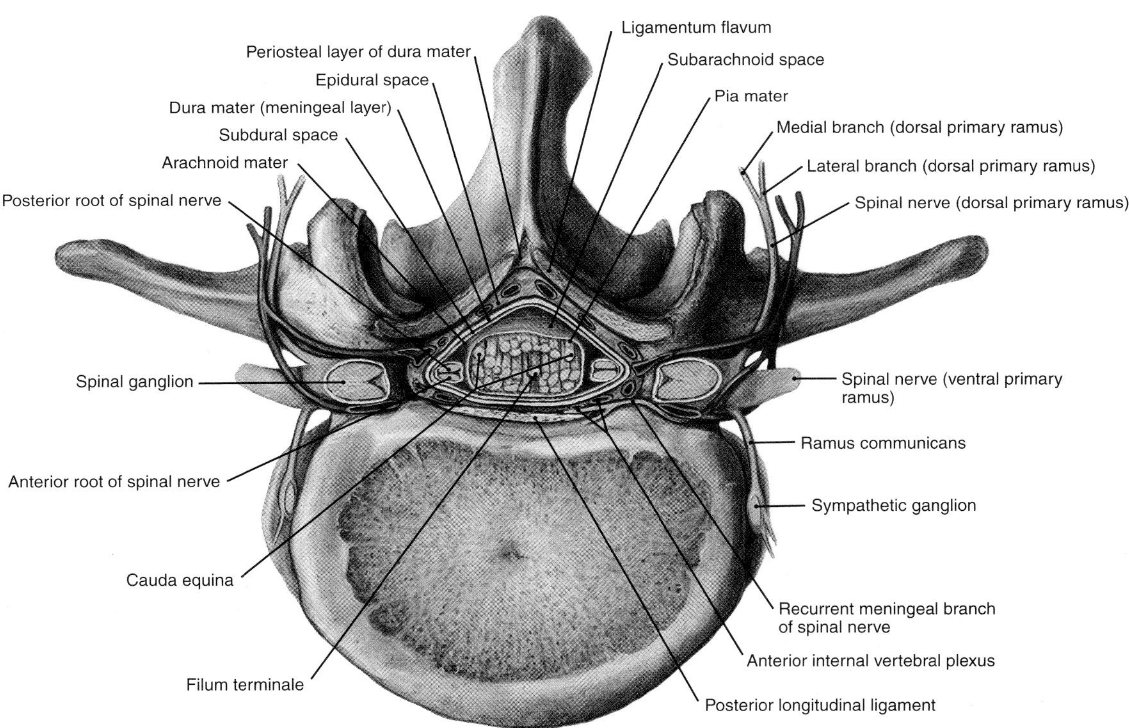
Ligamentum flavum
Periosteal layer of dura mater
Subarachnoid space
Epidural space
Pia mater
Dura mater (meningeal layer)
Medial branch (dorsal primary ramus)
Subdural space
Lateral branch (dorsal primary ramus)
Arachnoid mater
Spinal nerve (dorsal primary ramus)
Posterior root of spinal nerve
Spinal ganglion
Spinal nerve (ventral primary ramus)
Ramus communicans
Anterior root of spinal nerve
Sympathetic ganglion
Cauda equina
Recurrent meningeal branch of spinal nerve
Anterior internal vertebral plexus
Filum terminale
Posterior longitudinal ligament

Figure 361.2 Cross Section of the Cauda Equina within the Vertebral Canal

NOTE: (1) This cross section is at the level of the third lumbar vertebra, one segment or more below the site where the spinal cord ends.

(2) Specimens of cerebrospinal fluid may be obtained by performing lumbar punctures between the laminae or spines of the third and fourth or fourth and fifth lumbar vertebrae.

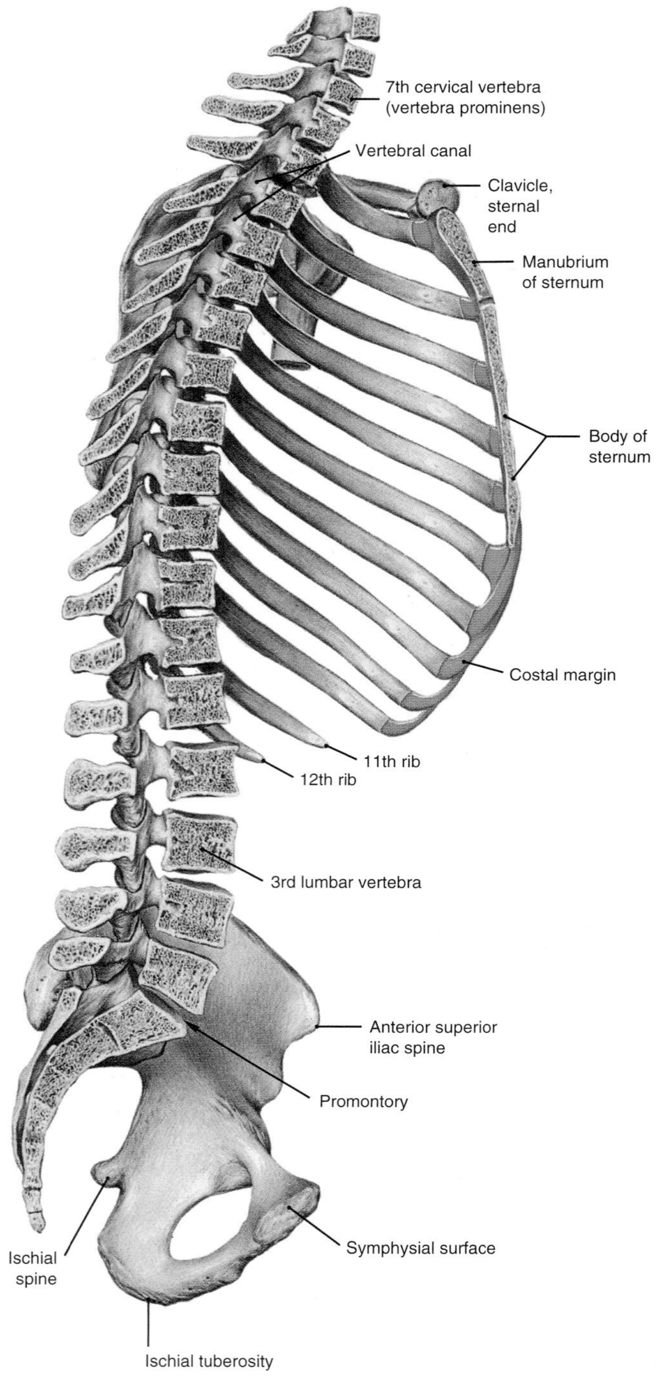
7th cervical vertebra (vertebra prominens)
Vertebral canal
Clavicle, sternal end
Manubrium of sternum
Body of sternum
Costal margin
11th rib
12th rib
3rd lumbar vertebra
Anterior superior iliac spine
Promontory
Symphysial surface
Ischial spine
Ischial tuberosity

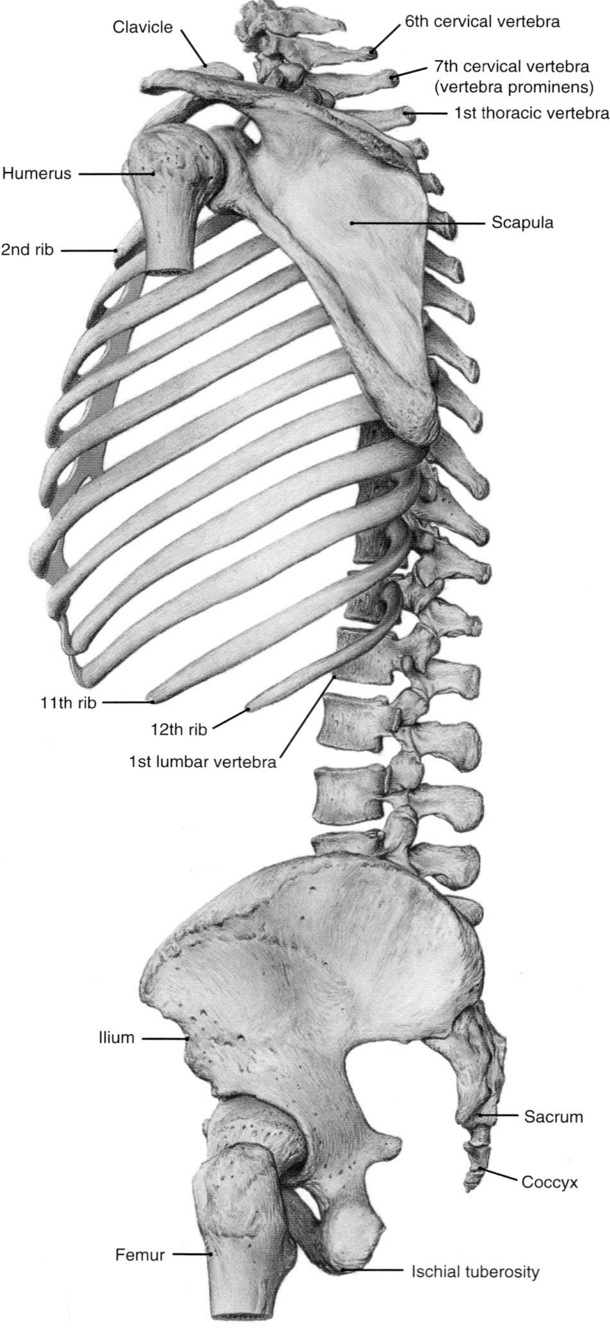
Clavicle
6th cervical vertebra
7th cervical vertebra (vertebra prominens)
1st thoracic vertebra
Humerus
Scapula
2nd rib
11th rib
12th rib
1st lumbar vertebra
Ilium
Sacrum
Coccyx
Femur
Ischial tuberosity

Figure 362.1 Left Medial Surface of the Vertebral Column Sectioned in the Median Plane

NOTE: (1) The sectioned vertebral column is shown from vertebra C5 inferiorly to the tip of the coccyx.

(2) The **vertebral canal** within which descends the spinal cord from the medulla oblongata of the brain.

(3) The C7 vertebra has a spinous process that is usually longer than the other cervical vertebrae and, therefore, is often called the **vertebra prominens.**

Figure 362.2 Left Lateral Surface of the Vertebral Column Sectioned in the Median Plane

NOTE: The scapula does not articulate with the vertebral column, whereas the pelvis articulates with the sacrum to form the **sacroiliac joint.**

THE LOWER LIMB

6

PLATES

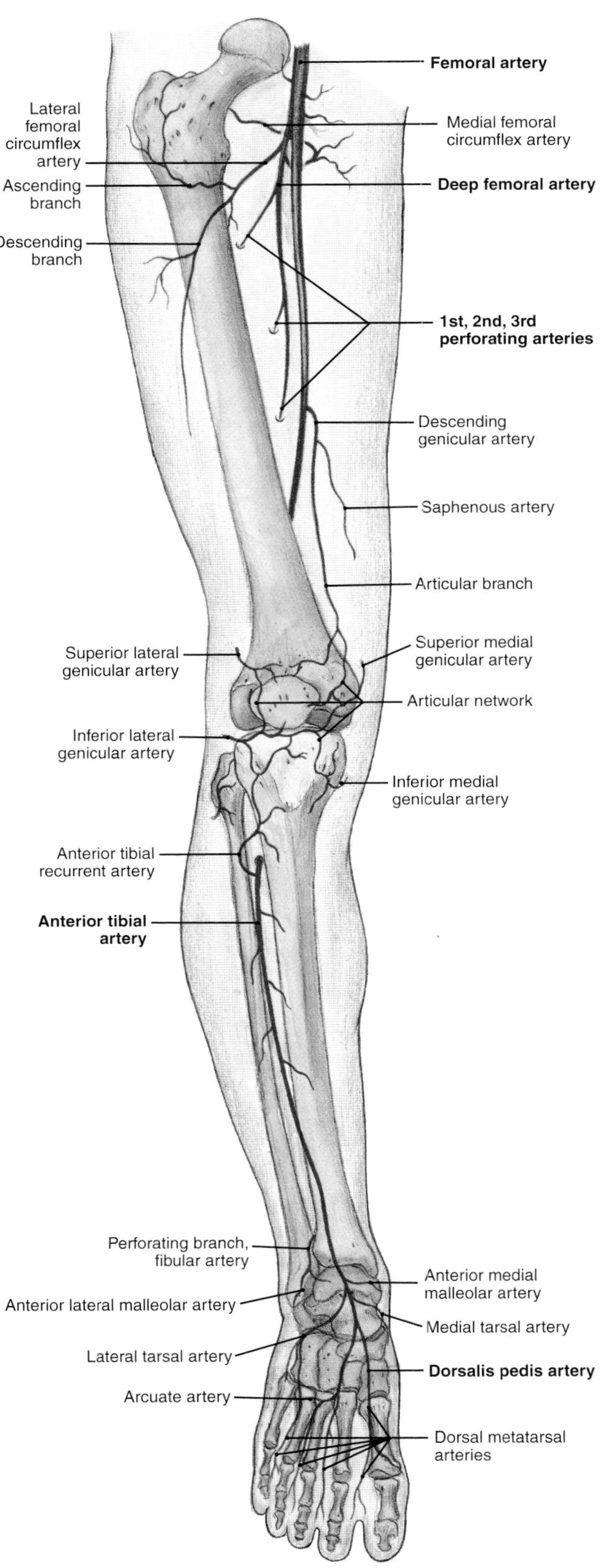

Femoral artery
Lateral femoral circumflex artery
Medial femoral circumflex artery
Ascending branch
Deep femoral artery
Descending branch
1st, 2nd, 3rd perforating arteries
Descending genicular artery
Saphenous artery
Articular branch
Superior lateral genicular artery
Superior medial genicular artery
Articular network
Inferior lateral genicular artery
Inferior medial genicular artery
Anterior tibial recurrent artery
Anterior tibial artery
Perforating branch, fibular artery
Anterior medial malleolar artery
Anterior lateral malleolar artery
Medial tarsal artery
Lateral tarsal artery
Dorsalis pedis artery
Arcuate artery
Dorsal metatarsal arteries

Figure 363.1 Arteries and Bones of the Lower Limb (Anterior View)

NOTE: The anastomoses in the hip and knee regions, and the **perforating branches** of the **deep femoral artery.** In the anterior leg, the **anterior tibial artery** descends between the tibia and fibula to achieve the malleolar region and the foot dorsum.

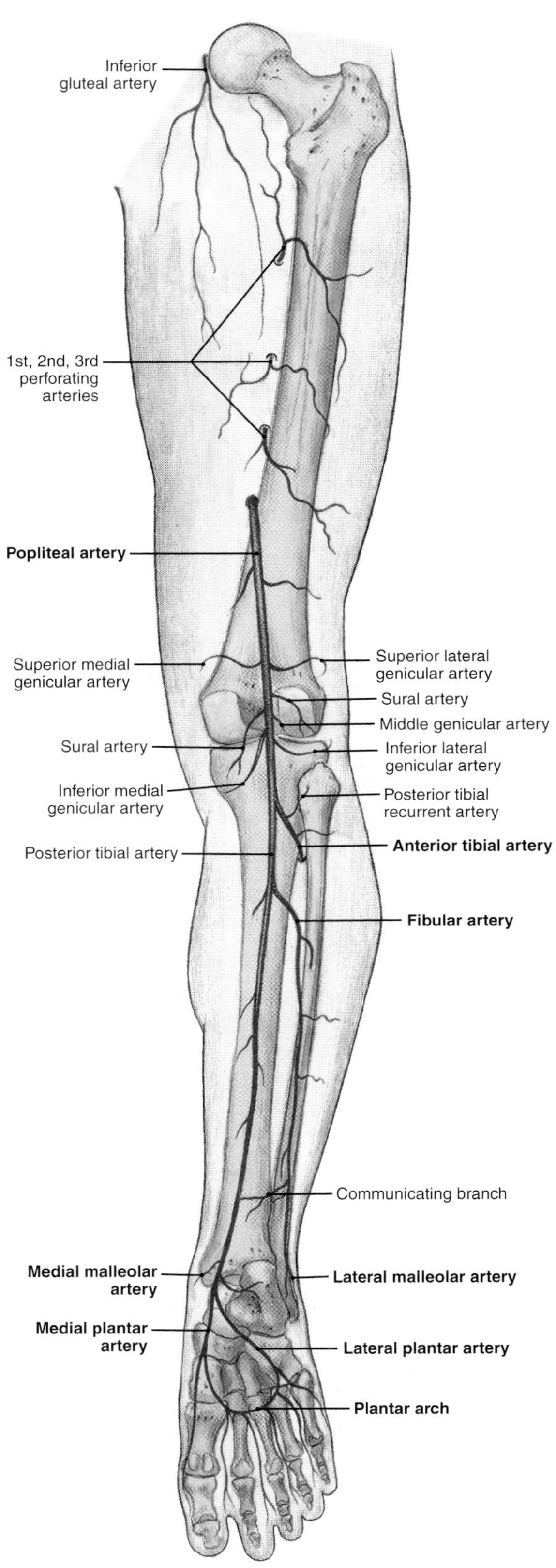

Inferior gluteal artery
1st, 2nd, 3rd perforating arteries
Popliteal artery
Superior medial genicular artery
Superior lateral genicular artery
Sural artery
Middle genicular artery
Sural artery
Inferior lateral genicular artery
Inferior medial genicular artery
Posterior tibial recurrent artery
Anterior tibial artery
Posterior tibial artery
Fibular artery
Communicating branch
Medial malleolar artery
Lateral malleolar artery
Medial plantar artery
Lateral plantar artery
Plantar arch

Figure 363.2 Arteries and Bones of the Lower Limb (Posterior View)

NOTE: The branches of the **popliteal artery** at the knee and its continuation as the **posterior tibial artery.** In the foot this vessel divides to form the **medial** and **lateral plantar arteries,** which then anastomose to form the **plantar arch.**

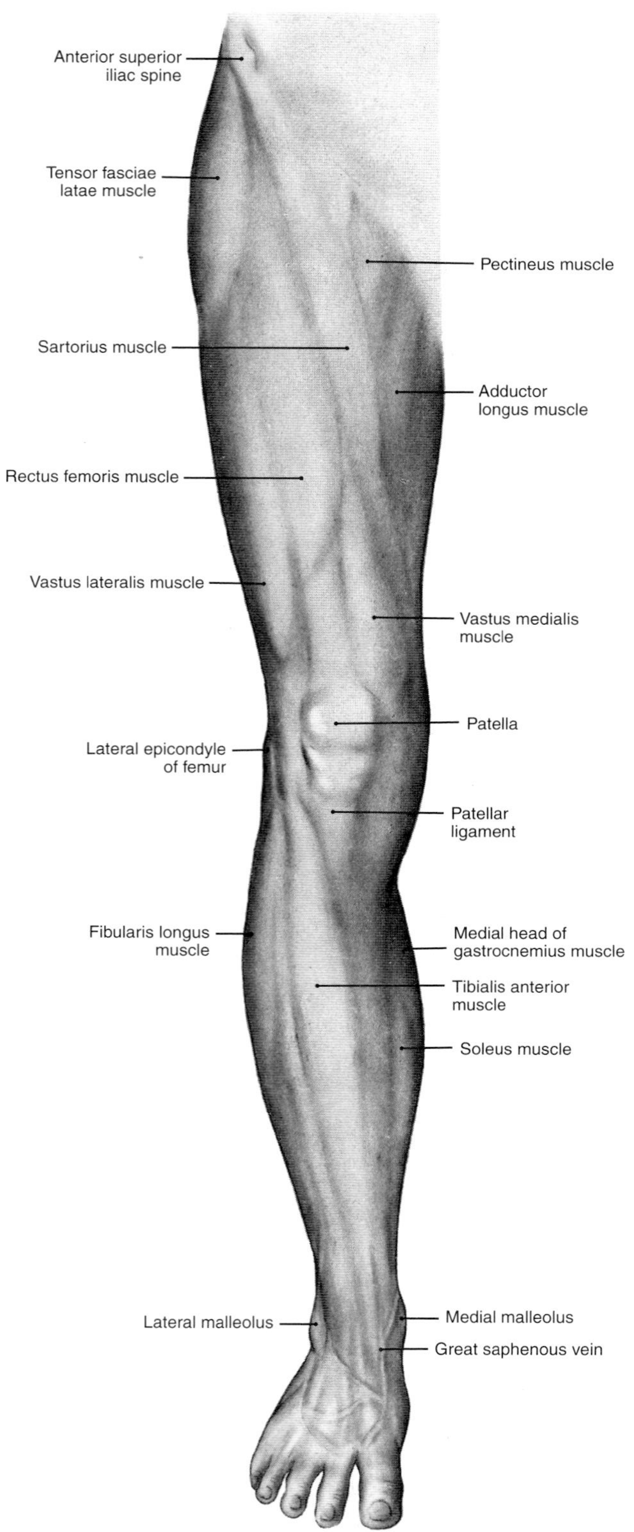
Anterior superior iliac spine
Tensor fasciae latae muscle
Pectineus muscle
Sartorius muscle
Adductor longus muscle
Rectus femoris muscle
Vastus lateralis muscle
Vastus medialis muscle
Patella
Lateral epicondyle of femur
Patellar ligament
Fibularis longus muscle
Medial head of gastrocnemius muscle
Tibialis anterior muscle
Soleus muscle
Lateral malleolus
Medial malleolus
Great saphenous vein

Figure 364.1 Surface Anatomy of the Right Lower Limb (Anterior View)

NOTE: (1) The pectineus and adductor longus muscles forming the floor of the femoral triangle. Observe also the sartorius muscle coursing inferomedially and the tensor fasciae latae that shapes the rounded upper lateral contour of the thigh.

(2) The leg is shaped laterally by the fibularis muscles, anteriorly by the tibialis anterior, and medially by the gastrocnemius and soleus muscles.

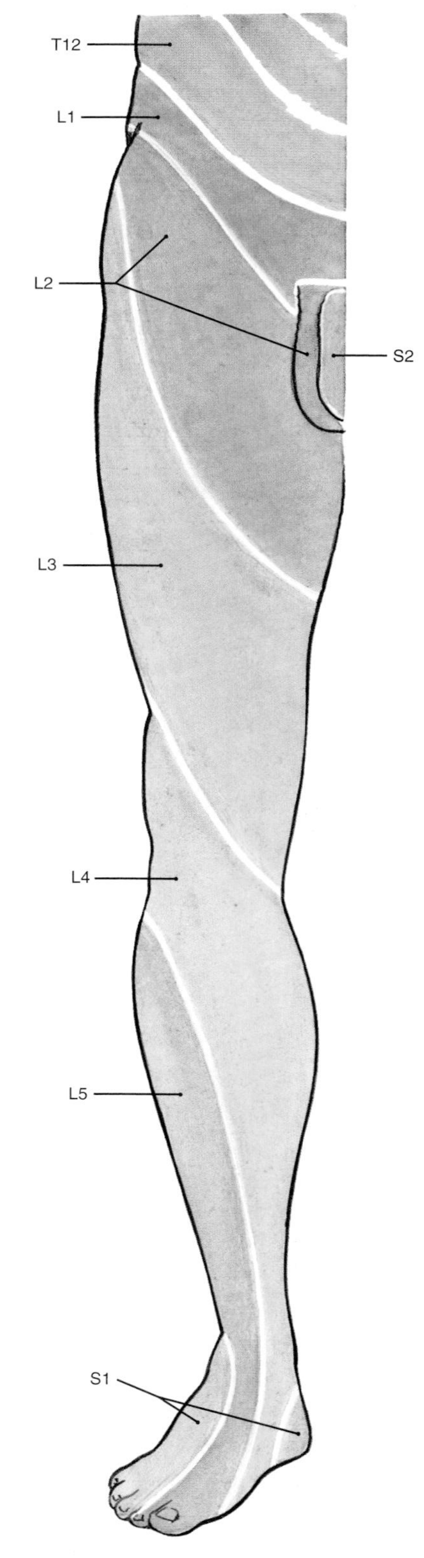
T12
L1
L2
S2
L3
L4
L5
S1

Figure 364.2 Segmental Cutaneous Innervation of the Right Lower Extremity (Dermatomes: Anterior View)

NOTE: (1) As a rule, the lumbar segments of the spinal cord supply cutaneous innervation to the anterior aspect of the lower limb, and the dermatomes are segmentally arranged in order from L1 to L5.

(2) The first sacral segment supplies the skin over the medial malleolus and the dorsolateral aspect of the foot.

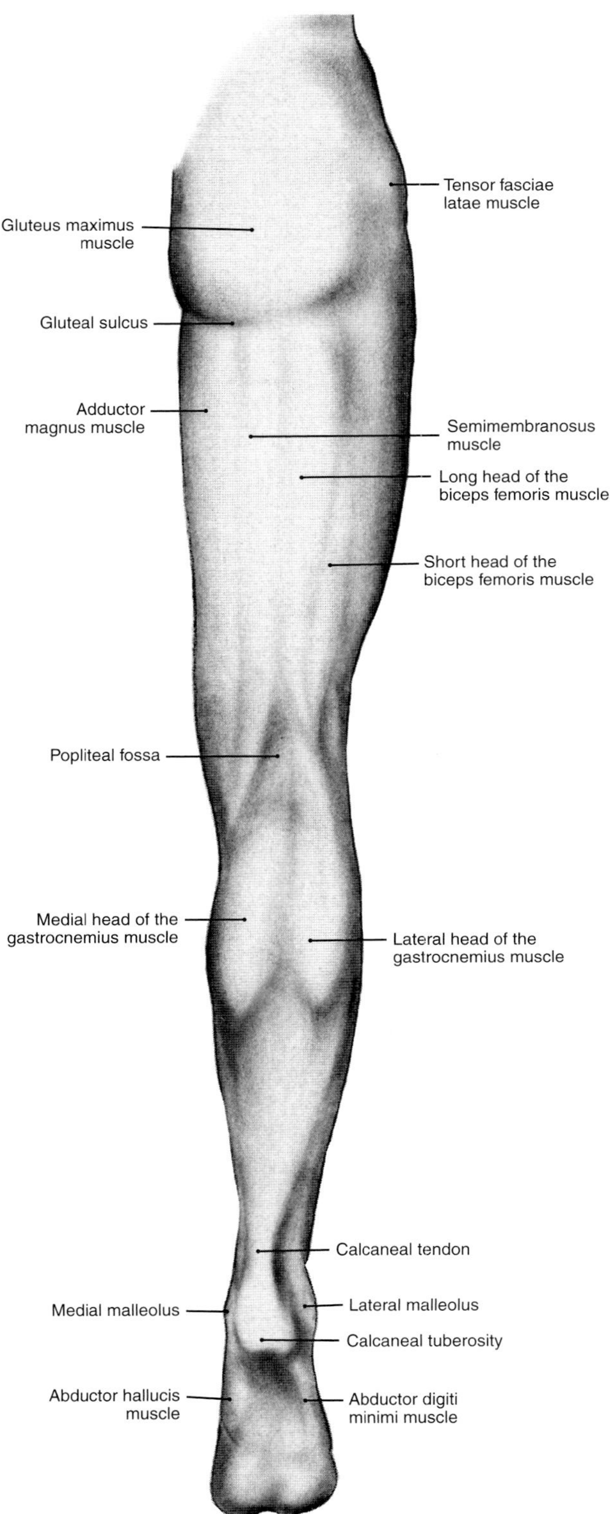
Tensor fasciae latae muscle
Gluteus maximus muscle
Gluteal sulcus
Adductor magnus muscle
Semimembranosus muscle
Long head of the biceps femoris muscle
Short head of the biceps femoris muscle
Popliteal fossa
Medial head of the gastrocnemius muscle
Lateral head of the gastrocnemius muscle
Calcaneal tendon
Medial malleolus
Lateral malleolus
Calcaneal tuberosity
Abductor hallucis muscle
Abductor digiti minimi muscle

Figure 365.1 Surface Anatomy of the Right Lower Limb (Posterior View)

NOTE: (1) The rounded contour of the buttock formed by the gluteus maximus muscle.

(2) The outline of the hamstring muscles (semitendinosus, semimembranosus, and biceps femoris) in the posterior thigh.

(3) The popliteal fossa, below which are the heads of the gastrocnemius muscle. Note also the calcaneal tendon, which inserts between the two malleoli onto the calcaneus. On the plantar surface of the foot see the abductor hallucis medially and the abductor digiti minimi laterally.

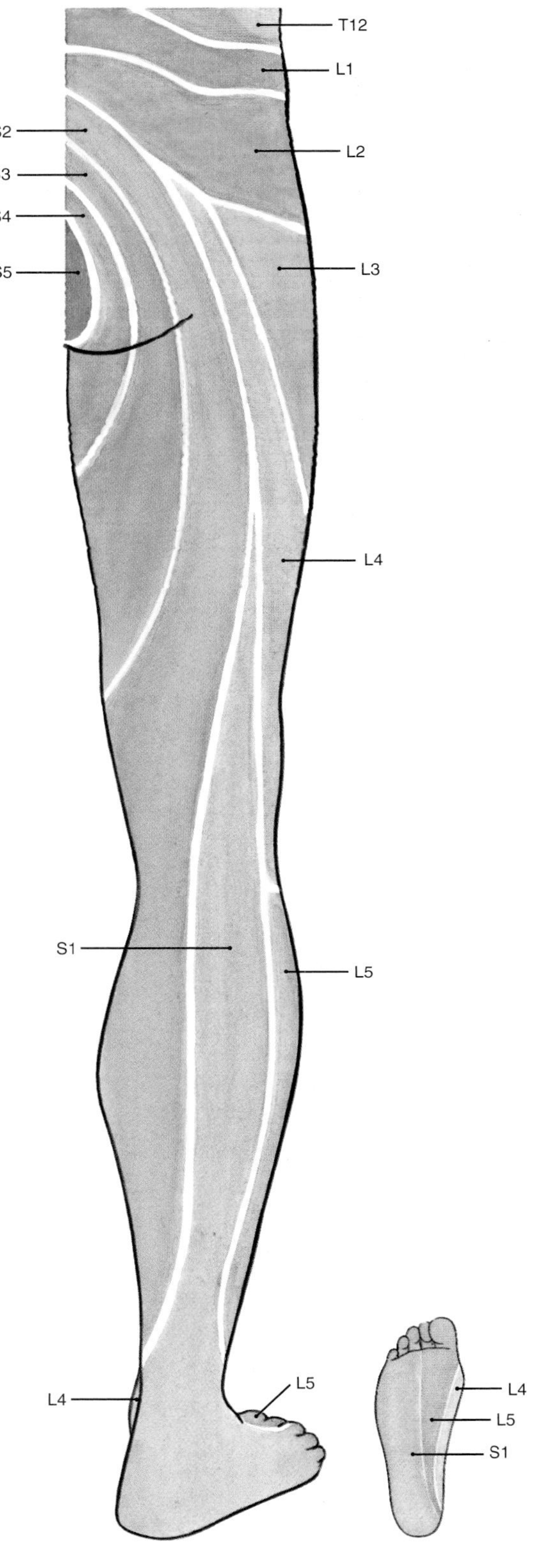
T12
L1
S2
L2
S3
S4
S5
L3
L4
S1
L5
L4
L5
L4
L5
S1

Figure 365.2 Segmental Cutaneous Innervation of the Right Lower Extremity (Dermatomes: Posterior View)

NOTE: (1) Sensory innervation to: (a) the **posterior thigh** is by the posterior femoral cutaneous nerve (S1, S2, S3), (b) the **medial calf** by the saphenous nerve (femoral: L2, L3, L4), and (c) the **lateral calf** by the sural nerve (S1, S2).

(2) The **heel** is supplied by the tibial nerve (S1, S2), and the **plantar foot** by the medial plantar nerve (L4, L5) and the lateral plantar nerve (S1, S2).

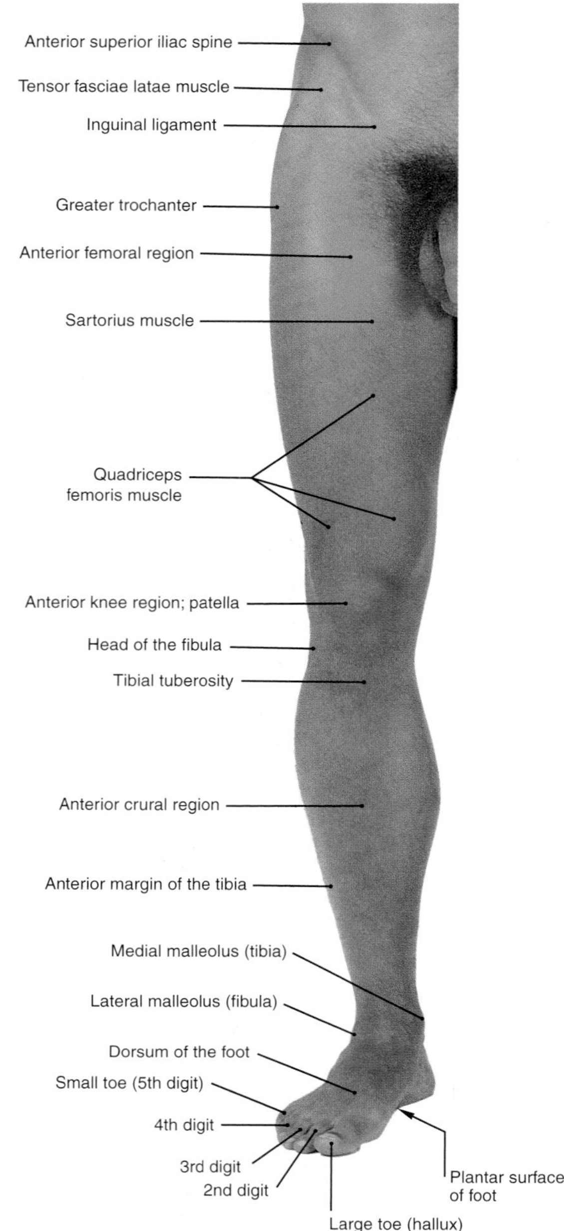
Anterior superior iliac spine
Tensor fasciae latae muscle
Inguinal ligament
Greater trochanter
Anterior femoral region
Sartorius muscle
Quadriceps femoris muscle
Anterior knee region; patella
Head of the fibula
Tibial tuberosity
Anterior crural region
Anterior margin of the tibia
Medial malleolus (tibia)
Lateral malleolus (fibula)
Dorsum of the foot
Small toe (5th digit)
4th digit
3rd digit
2nd digit
Large toe (hallux)
Plantar surface of foot

Figure 366.1 Photograph of the Anterior Surface of the Lower Limb

NOTE: (1) The following bony landmarks are shown:

(a) Anterior superior iliac spine
(b) Greater trochanter
(c) Patella
(d) Head of the fibula
(e) Tibial tuberosity
(f) Anterior margin of the tibia
(g) Medial and lateral malleoli

(2) The inguinal ligament, which forms the lower anterior boundary of the abdominal wall, separating it from the anterior thigh inferiorly.

(3) Deep to the surface areas shown in this figure course branches of the cutaneous nerves that supply the anterior and lateral aspects of the thigh and leg and the dorsum of the foot. These branches are shown in Figure 367.1.

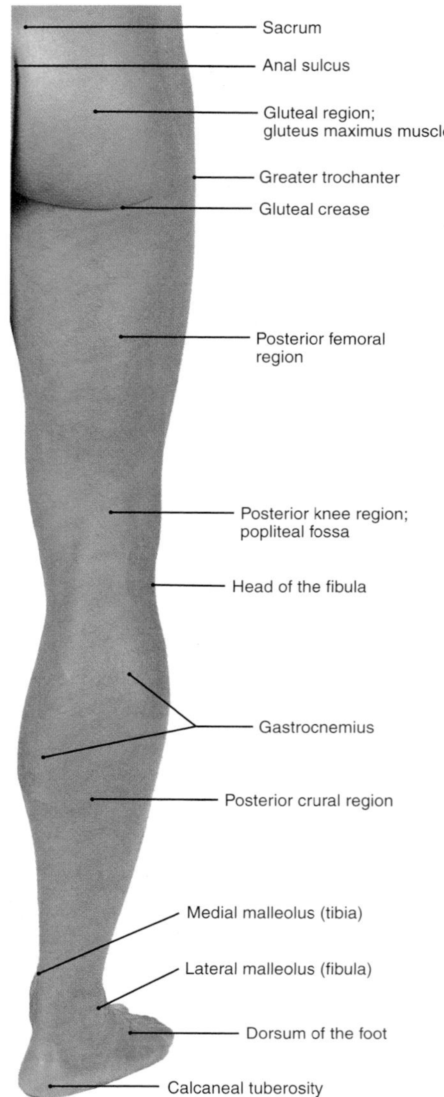
Sacrum
Anal sulcus
Gluteal region; gluteus maximus muscle
Greater trochanter
Gluteal crease
Posterior femoral region
Posterior knee region; popliteal fossa
Head of the fibula
Gastrocnemius
Posterior crural region
Medial malleolus (tibia)
Lateral malleolus (fibula)
Dorsum of the foot
Calcaneal tuberosity

Figure 366.2 Photograph of the Posterior Surface of the Lower Limb

NOTE: (1) The following bony landmarks are shown:

(a) Sacrum
(b) Greater trochanter
(c) Head of the fibula
(d) Medial and lateral malleoli
(e) Calcaneal tuberosity

(2) The **gluteal crease.** Midway between the greater trochanter laterally and the ischial tuberosity medially and deep to this crease is found the large **sciatic nerve** descending in the posterior thigh. **The nerve is vulnerable at this site because only skin and superficial fascia overlie it.**

(3) The **popliteal fossa** located behind the knee joint. Deep to the skin at this site are found the tibial and fibular divisions of the sciatic nerve and the popliteal artery and vein.

(4) The **calcaneal tuberosity** into which inserts the calcaneus tendon formed as the common tendon of the gastrocnemius, soleus, and plantaris muscles.

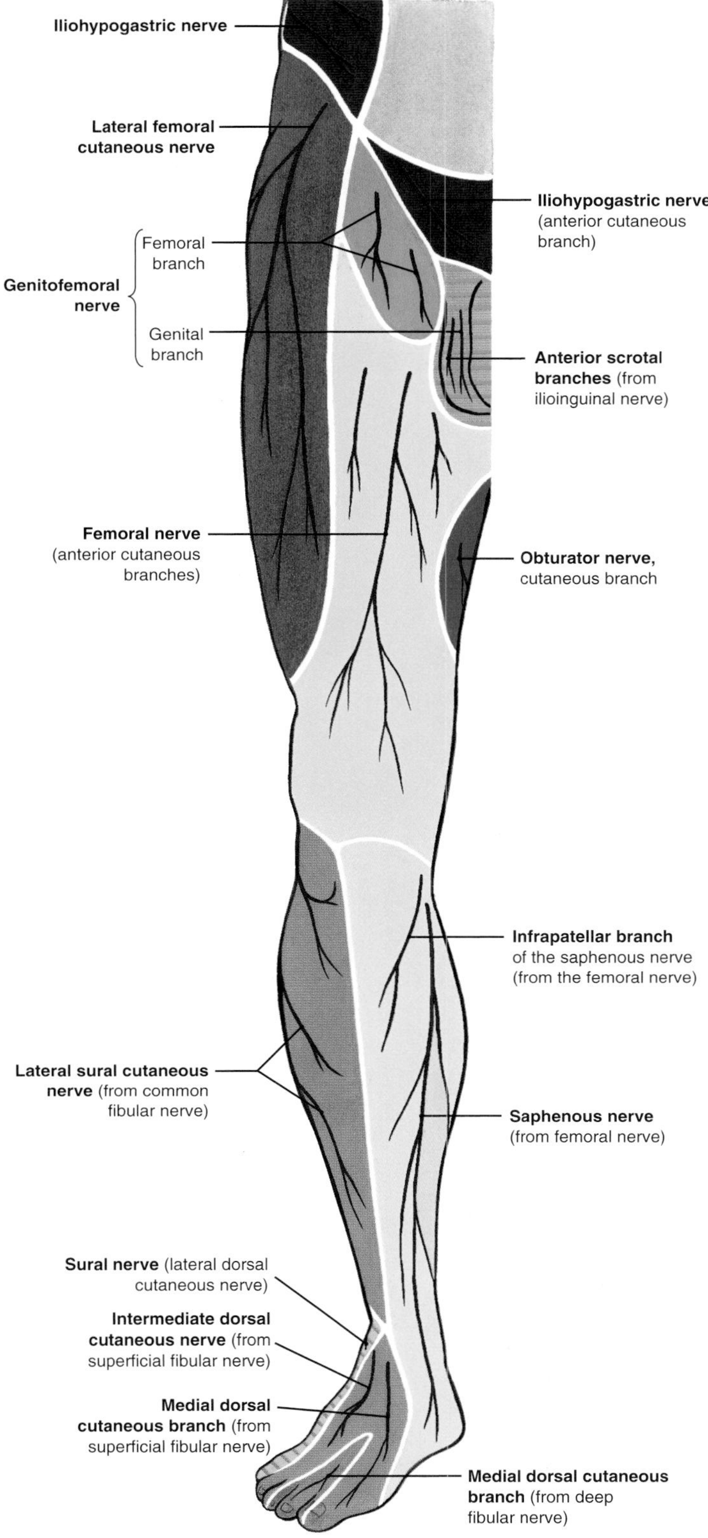
Iliohypogastric nerve
Lateral femoral cutaneous nerve
Genitofemoral nerve
Femoral branch
Genital branch
Iliohypogastric nerve (anterior cutaneous branch)
Anterior scrotal branches (from ilioinguinal nerve)
Femoral nerve (anterior cutaneous branches)
Obturator nerve, cutaneous branch
Infrapatellar branch of the saphenous nerve (from the femoral nerve)
Lateral sural cutaneous nerve (from common fibular nerve)
Saphenous nerve (from femoral nerve)
Sural nerve (lateral dorsal cutaneous nerve)
Intermediate dorsal cutaneous nerve (from superficial fibular nerve)
Medial dorsal cutaneous branch (from superficial fibular nerve)
Medial dorsal cutaneous branch (from deep fibular nerve)

Figure 367.1 Cutaneous Nerve Branches (Anterior Surface)

NOTE: (1) Cutaneous branches of the femoral nerve supply the skin of the anteromedial thigh, and the **saphenous nerve** supplies the anteromedial and posteromedial leg.

(2) The **lateral sural branch** of the **common fibular nerve** supplies the anterolateral and posterolateral leg skin.

(3) The fields supplied by the **superficial and deep fibular nerves** on the anterior leg and foot dorsum.

(4) The knowledge of the course of these nerves is important in administering local anesthesia.

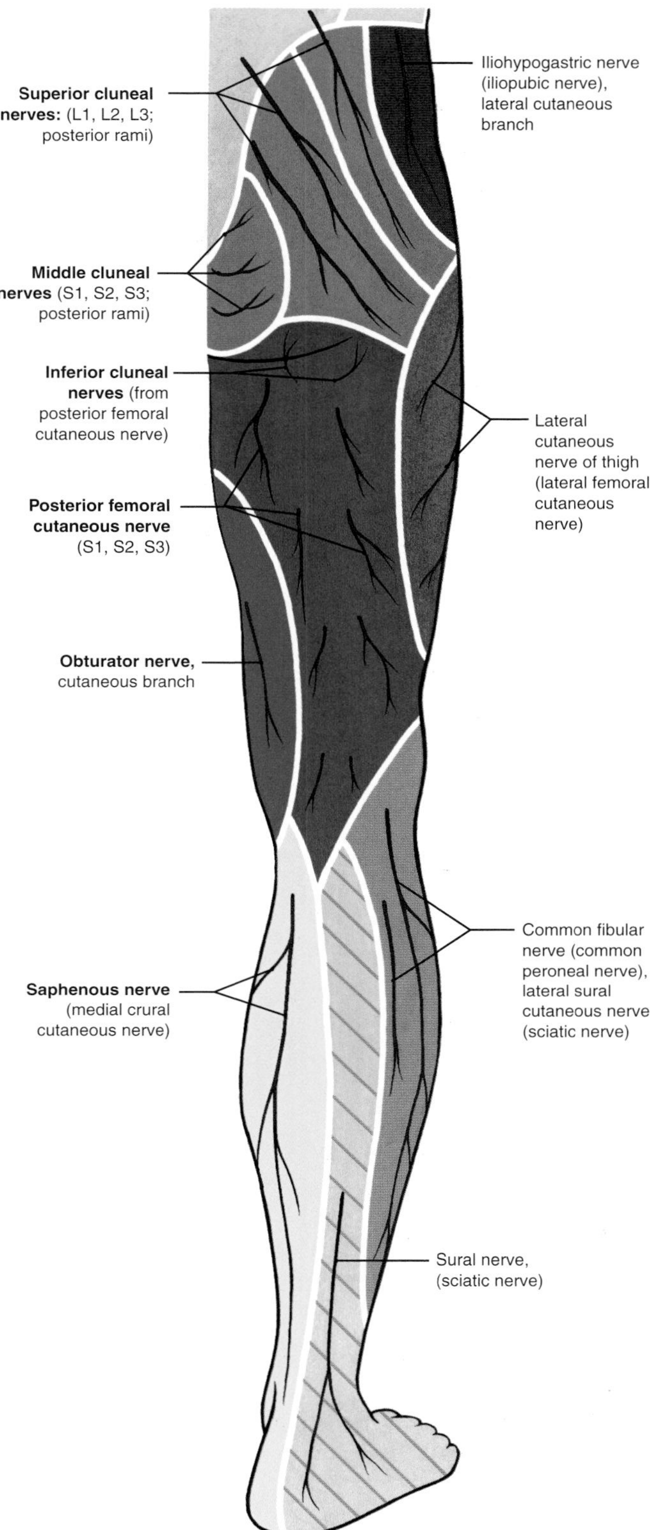
Superior cluneal nerves: (L1, L2, L3; posterior rami)
Iliohypogastric nerve (iliopubic nerve), lateral cutaneous branch
Middle cluneal nerves (S1, S2, S3; posterior rami)
Inferior cluneal nerves (from posterior femoral cutaneous nerve)
Lateral cutaneous nerve of thigh (lateral femoral cutaneous nerve)
Posterior femoral cutaneous nerve (S1, S2, S3)
Obturator nerve, cutaneous branch
Common fibular nerve (common peroneal nerve), lateral sural cutaneous nerve (sciatic nerve)
Saphenous nerve (medial crural cutaneous nerve)
Sural nerve, (sciatic nerve)

Figure 367.2 Cutaneous Nerve Branches (Posterior Surface)

NOTE: (1) Cutaneous innervation of the gluteal region:

(a) Lateral branch of **iliohypogastric nerve** (anterior ramus: L1)

(b) **Superior cluneal nerves** (posterior rami: L1–L3)

(c) Middle cluneal nerves (posterior rami: S1–S3)

(d)Inferior cluneal nerves (S1–S3)

(2) Skin of posterior thigh supplied by the **posterior and lateral femoral cutaneous nerves** and **obturator nerve.**

(3) Skin of posterior leg supplied the **saphenous, sural,** and **lateral sural nerves.**

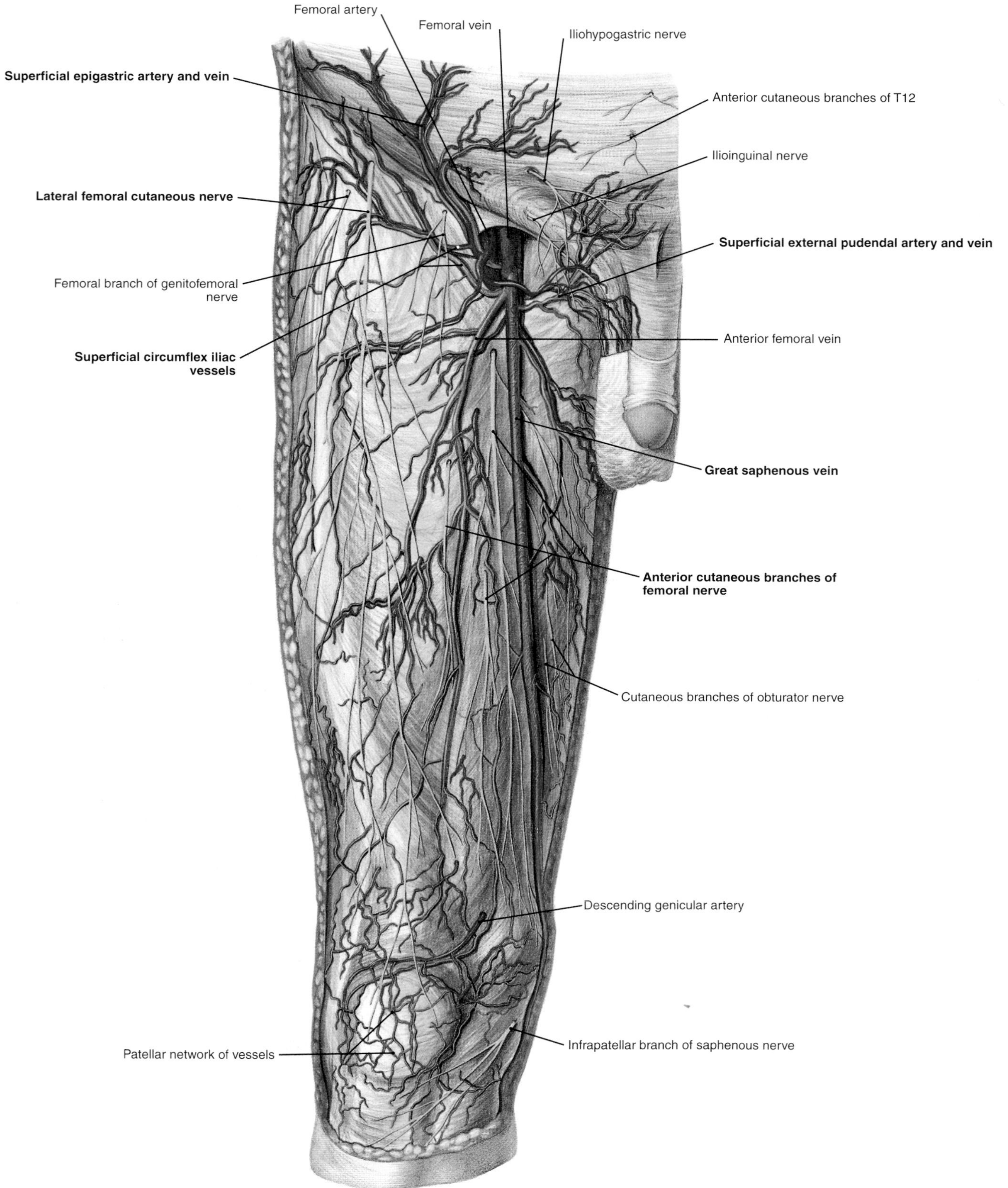
Femoral artery
Femoral vein
Iliohypogastric nerve
Superficial epigastric artery and vein
Anterior cutaneous branches of T12
Ilioinguinal nerve
Lateral femoral cutaneous nerve
Superficial external pudendal artery and vein
Femoral branch of genitofemoral nerve
Superficial circumflex iliac vessels
Anterior femoral vein
Great saphenous vein
Anterior cutaneous branches of femoral nerve
Cutaneous branches of obturator nerve
Descending genicular artery
Patellar network of vessels
Infrapatellar branch of saphenous nerve

Figure 368 Superficial Nerves and Blood Vessels of the Anterior Thigh

NOTE: (1) The **great saphenous vein** as it ascends the anterior and medial aspect of the thigh. Just below ($1\frac{1}{2}$ inches) the inguinal ligament, it penetrates the deep fascia through the **saphenous opening** to enter the **femoral vein.**

(2) The superficial branches of the **femoral artery** and the superficial vessels drain into the **great saphenous vein.** These include the: (1) **superficial epigastric,** (2) **external pudendal,** and (3) **superficial circumflex iliac** arteries and veins.

(3) The principal cutaneous nerves of the anterior thigh. Compare these with those shown in Figure 367.1.

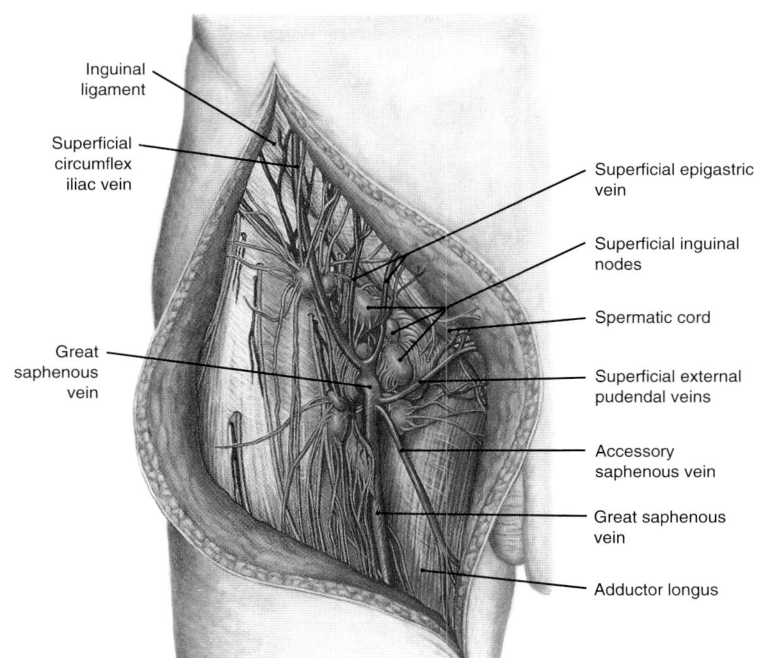
Inguinal ligament
Superficial circumflex iliac vein
Great saphenous vein
Superficial epigastric vein
Superficial inguinal nodes
Spermatic cord
Superficial external pudendal veins
Accessory saphenous vein
Great saphenous vein
Adductor longus

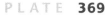

Figure 369.1 Superficial Inguinal Lymph Nodes

NOTE: (1) The superficial tissues of the genitalia, lower anterior abdominal wall, inguinal region, and anterior thigh drain into the **superficial inguinal lymphatic nodes.**

(2) These nodes are located around the femoral vessels just inferior to the inguinal ligament and usually number between 10 and 15. In turn, these nodes drain into the external iliac nodes within the pelvis.

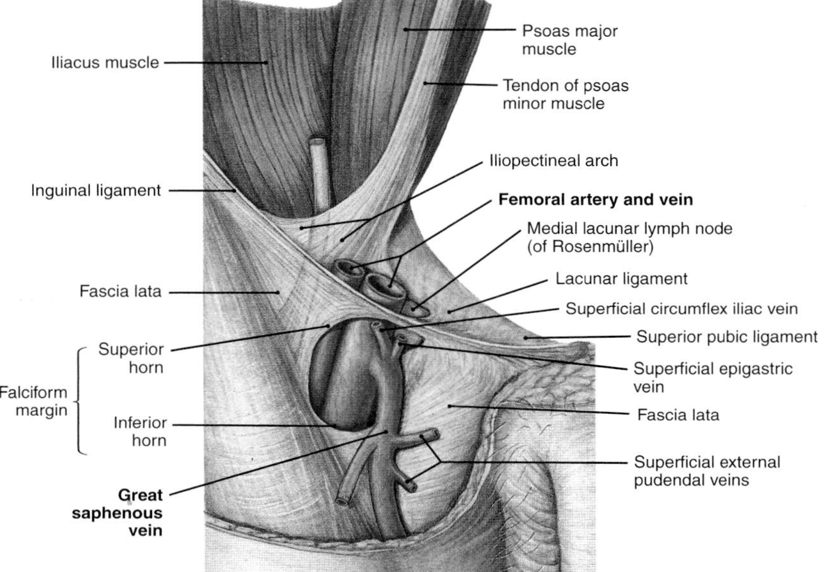
Iliacus muscle
Psoas major muscle
Tendon of psoas minor muscle
Inguinal ligament
Iliopectineal arch
Femoral artery and vein
Medial lacunar lymph node (of Rosenmüller)
Lacunar ligament
Fascia lata
Superficial circumflex iliac vein
Superior pubic ligament
Falciform margin
Superior horn
Inferior horn
Superficial epigastric vein
Fascia lata
Superficial external pudendal veins
Great saphenous vein

Figure 369.2 Saphenous Opening in the Fascia Lata

NOTE: (1) The *femoral sheath* (dense connective tissue that surrounds the femoral artery and vein) has been removed in this dissection, revealing the sharply defined **falciform margin** of the **saphenous opening.**

(2) The great saphenous vein receives its superficial tributaries before it enters the saphenous opening.

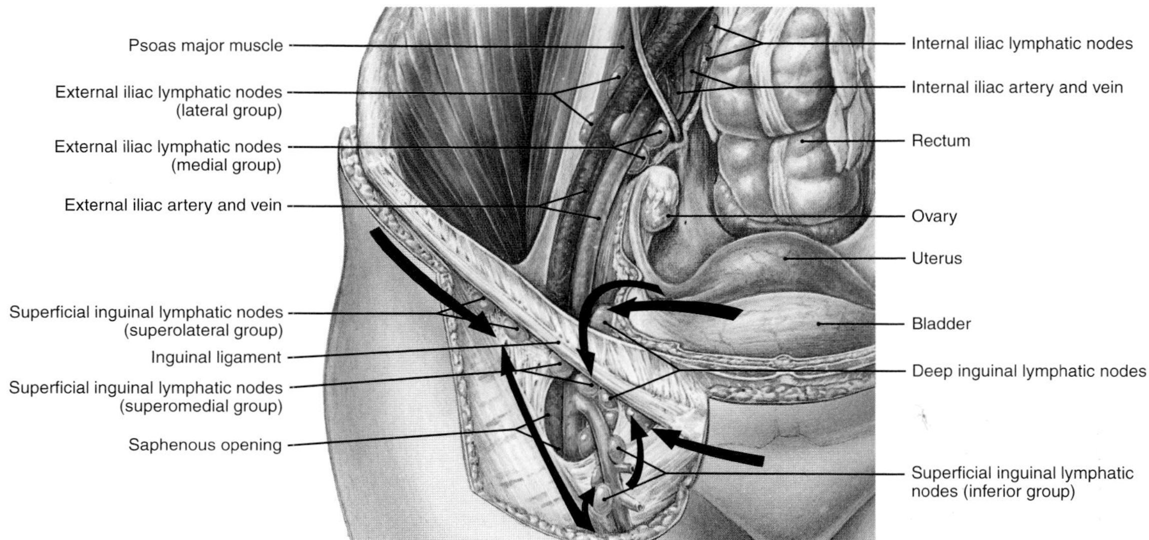
Psoas major muscle
External iliac lymphatic nodes (lateral group)
External iliac lymphatic nodes (medial group)
External iliac artery and vein
Superficial inguinal lymphatic nodes (superolateral group)
Inguinal ligament
Superficial inguinal lymphatic nodes (superomedial group)
Saphenous opening
Internal iliac lymphatic nodes
Internal iliac artery and vein
Rectum
Ovary
Uterus
Bladder
Deep inguinal lymphatic nodes
Superficial inguinal lymphatic nodes (inferior group)

Figure 369.3 Superficial and Deep Inguinal Lymphatic Nodes

NOTE: The directions of flow (arrows) of lymph from adjacent tissues into the superficial and deep inguinal nodes. The superficial nodes are divided into superolateral, superomedial, and inferomedial groups, while the deep nodes are closest to the femoral vessels.

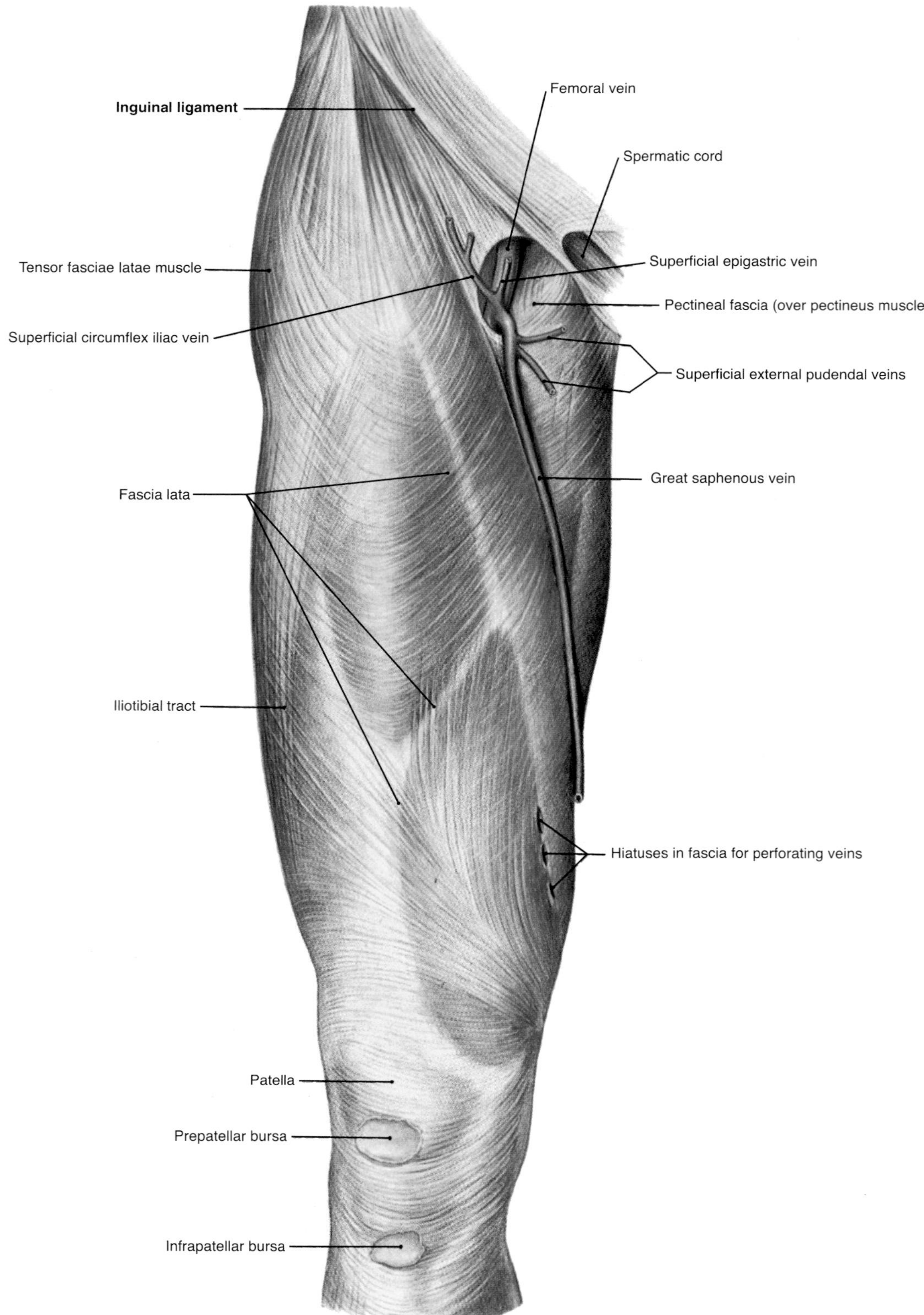
Femoral vein
Inguinal ligament
Spermatic cord
Tensor fasciae latae muscle
Superficial epigastric vein
Pectineal fascia (over pectineus muscle)
Superficial circumflex iliac vein
Superficial external pudendal veins
Great saphenous vein
Fascia lata
Iliotibial tract
Hiatuses in fascia for perforating veins
Patella
Prepatellar bursa
Infrapatellar bursa

Figure 370 Fascia of the Anterior Thigh, Fascia Lata (Right)

NOTE: (1) The dense fascia, which closely invests the muscles of the hip and thigh, is called the **fascia lata.** It is attached above to the ischial and pubic rami and inguinal ligament anteriorly, the crest of the ilium laterally, and the ischial tuberosity, sacrotuberous ligament, sacrum, and coccyx posteriorly.

(2) The fascia lata is most strong laterally, where it forms the **iliotibial tract.** This thickened band descends to the lateral condyle of the tibia. Above, the fascia lata surrounds a muscle called the **tensor fascia latae,** which, by pulling on the iliotibial tract, can extend and laterally rotate the leg at the knee joint.

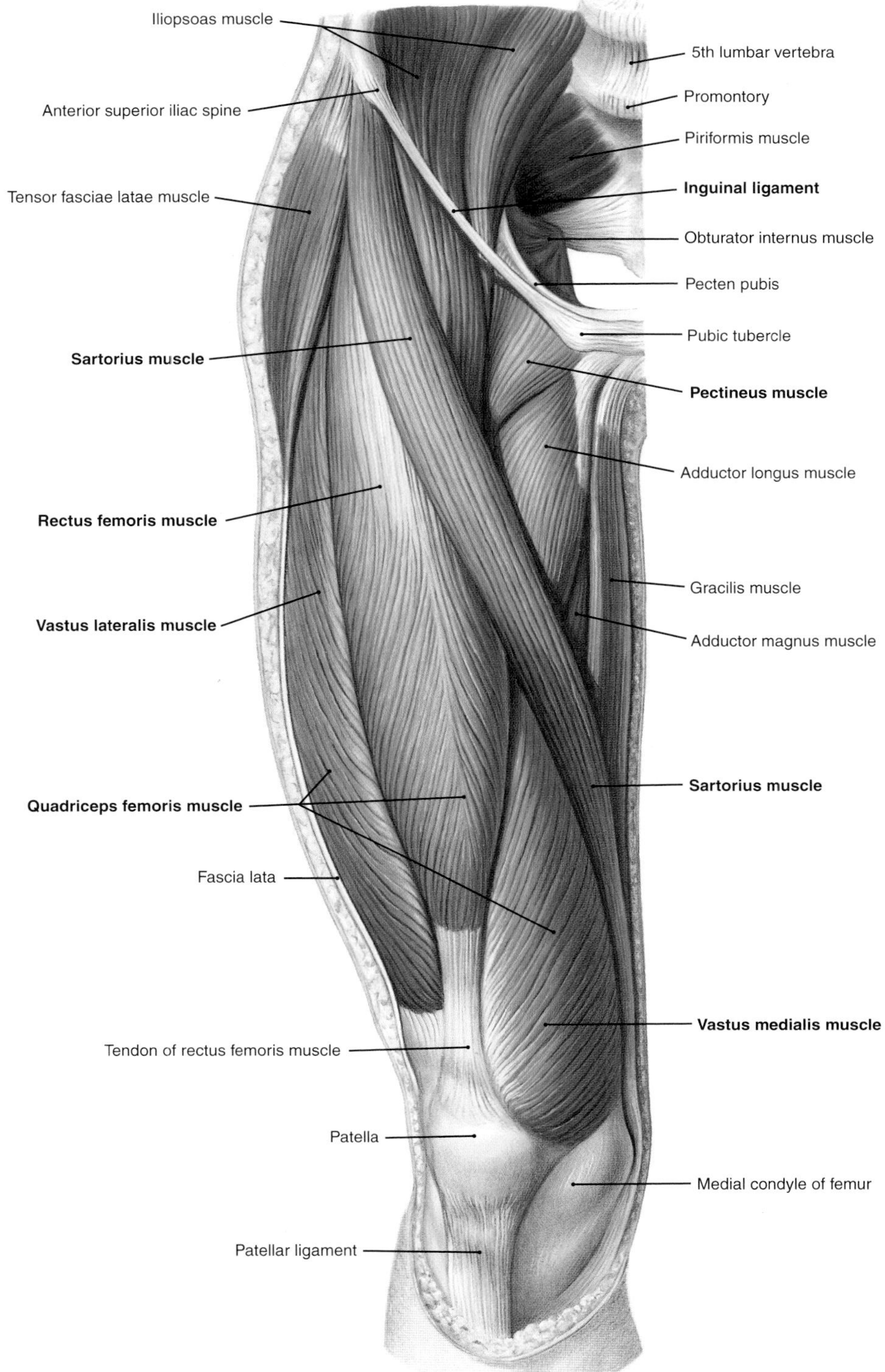
Iliopsoas muscle
Anterior superior iliac spine
Tensor fasciae latae muscle
Sartorius muscle
Rectus femoris muscle
Vastus lateralis muscle
Quadriceps femoris muscle
Fascia lata
Tendon of rectus femoris muscle
Patella
Patellar ligament
5th lumbar vertebra
Promontory
Piriformis muscle
Inguinal ligament
Obturator internus muscle
Pecten pubis
Pubic tubercle
Pectineus muscle
Adductor longus muscle
Gracilis muscle
Adductor magnus muscle
Sartorius muscle
Vastus medialis muscle
Medial condyle of femur

Figure 371 Anterior Muscles of the Thigh: Superficial View (Right)

NOTE: (1) The long narrow **sartorius muscle,** which arises on the anterior superior iliac spine and passes obliquely across the anterior femoral muscles to insert on the medial aspect of the body of the tibia. The sartorius flexes, abducts, and rotates the thigh laterally at the hip joint, and it flexes and rotates the leg medially at the knee joint.

(2) The **quadriceps femoris muscle** forms the bulk of the anterior femoral muscles, and both the sartorius and quadriceps muscles are innervated by the femoral nerve.

(3) Above and medial to the sartorius muscle are visible, in order, the iliopsoas, pectineus, adductor longus, adductor magnus, and gracilis muscles.

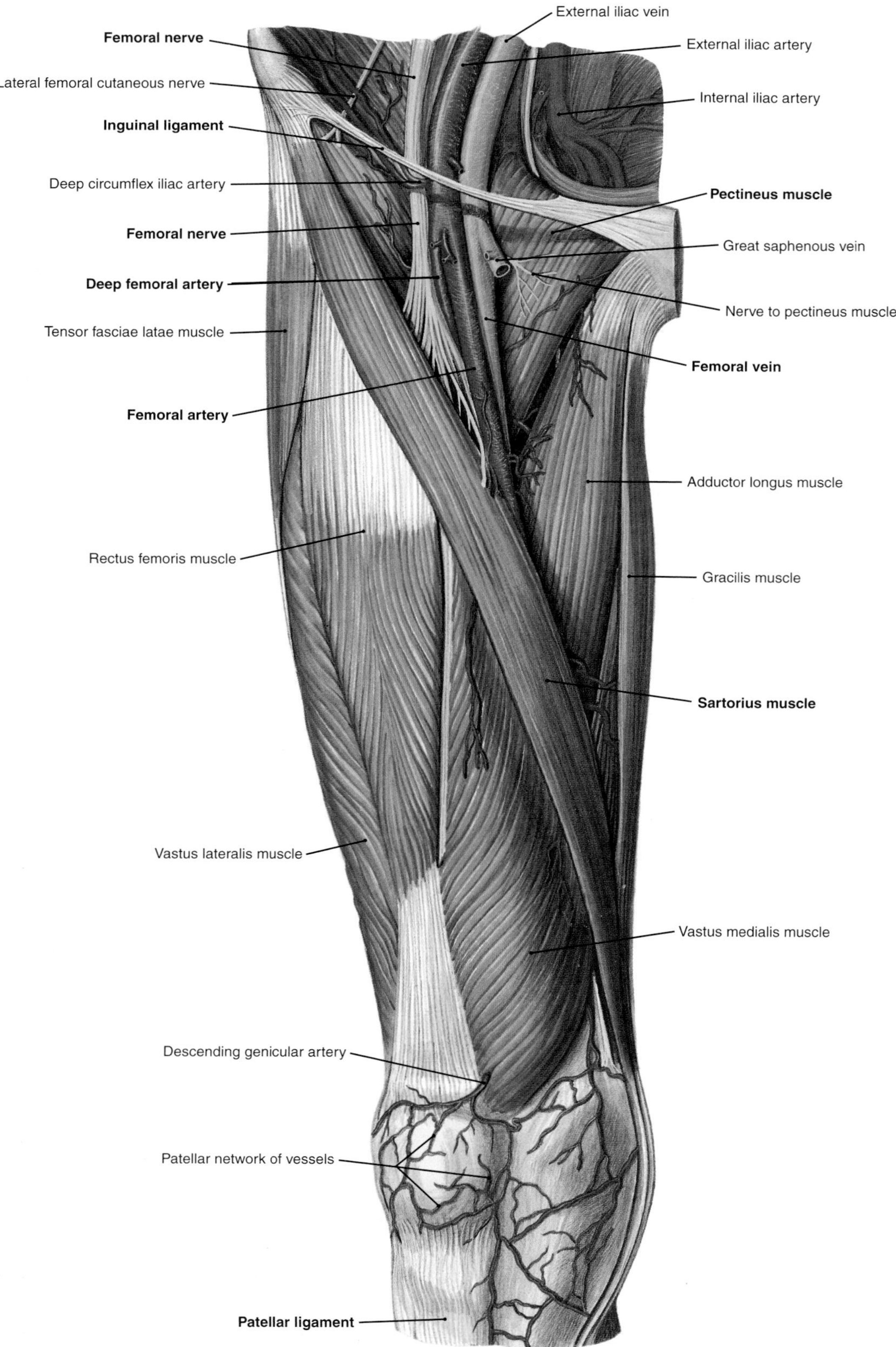
External iliac vein
Femoral nerve
External iliac artery
Lateral femoral cutaneous nerve
Internal iliac artery
Inguinal ligament
Deep circumflex iliac artery
Pectineus muscle
Femoral nerve
Great saphenous vein
Deep femoral artery
Nerve to pectineus muscle
Tensor fasciae latae muscle
Femoral vein
Femoral artery
Adductor longus muscle
Rectus femoris muscle
Gracilis muscle
Sartorius muscle
Vastus lateralis muscle
Vastus medialis muscle
Descending genicular artery
Patellar network of vessels
Patellar ligament

Figure 372 Femoral Triangle

NOTE: (1) The boundaries of the **femoral triangle** are the inguinal ligament above, the medial border of the sartorius muscle laterally, and the medial border of the adductor longus muscle medially. The floor is formed by the iliopsoas and pectineus muscles. The **femoral nerve, artery**, and **vein** traverse the triangle beneath the inguinal ligament.

(2) Of the neurovascular structures, the nerve is the most lateral within the triangle, then descend the artery and vein. The femoral artery can easily be located because it courses downward *midway* between the anterior superior iliac spine and the public tubercle, just below the inguinal ligament.

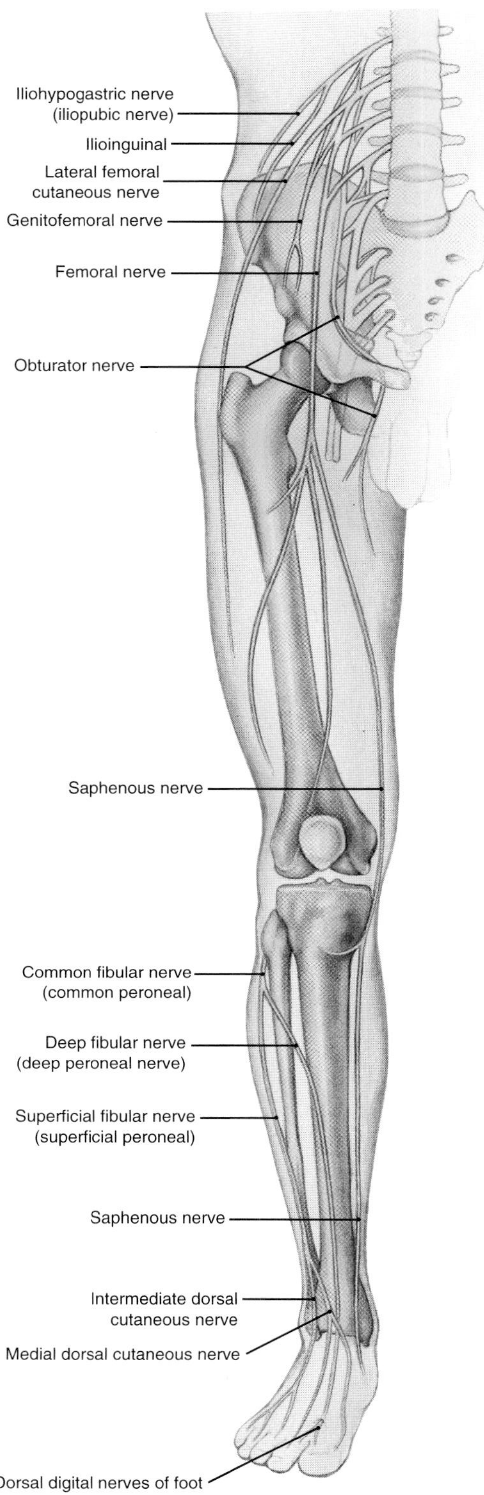
Iliohypogastric nerve
(iliopubic nerve)
Ilioinguinal
Lateral femoral
cutaneous nerve
Genitofemoral nerve
Femoral nerve
Obturator nerve
Saphenous nerve
Common fibular nerve
(common peroneal)
Deep fibular nerve
(deep peroneal nerve)
Superficial fibular nerve
(superficial peroneal)
Saphenous nerve
Intermediate dorsal
cutaneous nerve
Medial dorsal cutaneous nerve
Dorsal digital nerves of foot

Figure 373.1 Nerves of the Lower Limb (Anterior Aspect)

NOTE: (1) The **femoral nerve** is the principal nerve of the anterior thigh, but the **obturator nerve** supplies muscles of the medial thigh.

(2) The **lateral femoral cutaneous nerve** (L2, L3) supplies the skin of the lateral thigh.

(3) The **saphenous nerve** (a sensory branch of the femoral nerve) supplies the skin of the medial leg.

(4) All **other branches** below the knee are derived from the **sciatic nerve.**

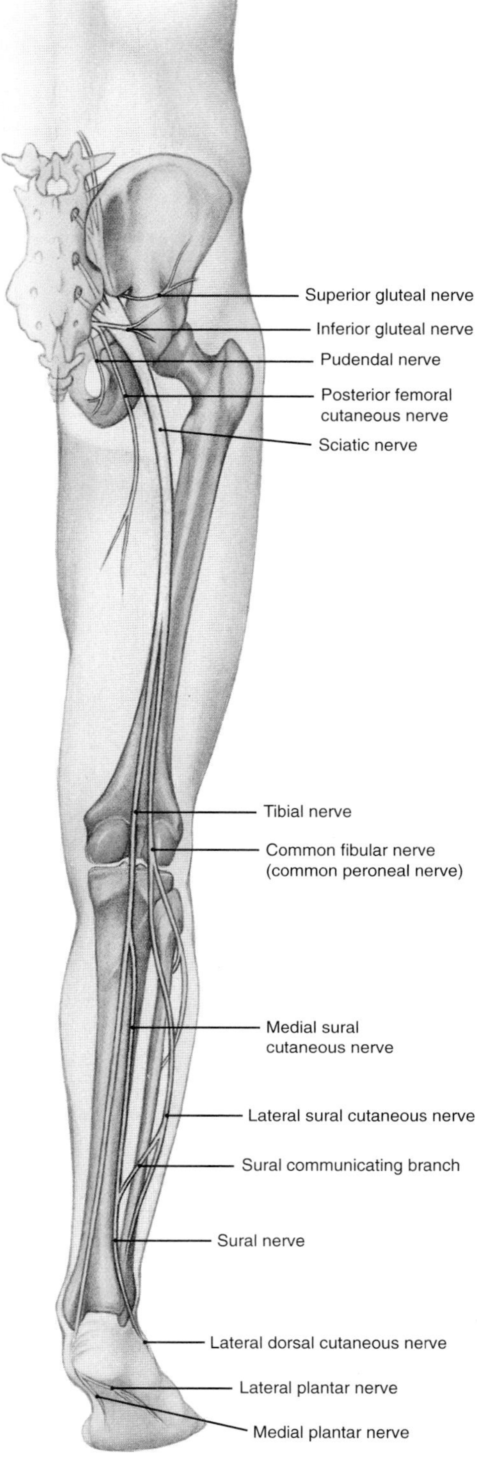
Superior gluteal nerve
Inferior gluteal nerve
Pudendal nerve
Posterior femoral
cutaneous nerve
Sciatic nerve
Tibial nerve
Common fibular nerve
(common peroneal nerve)
Medial sural
cutaneous nerve
Lateral sural cutaneous nerve
Sural communicating branch
Sural nerve
Lateral dorsal cutaneous nerve
Lateral plantar nerve
Medial plantar nerve

Figure 373.2 Nerves of the Lower Limb (Posterior Aspect)

NOTE: (1) The **sciatic nerve** supplies the posterior thigh and all other structures below the knee *EXCEPT* the skin of the medial leg, which is supplied by the **saphenous nerve,** a branch of the **femoral nerve.**

(2) The **fibular nerves** (**superficial** and **deep**) supply all of the muscles of the leg and foot and the skin of the dorsal and plantar surfaces of the foot.

(3) The **common fibular nerve** divides into superficial and deep fibular branches as it courses around the head of the fibula (see Fig. 373.1).

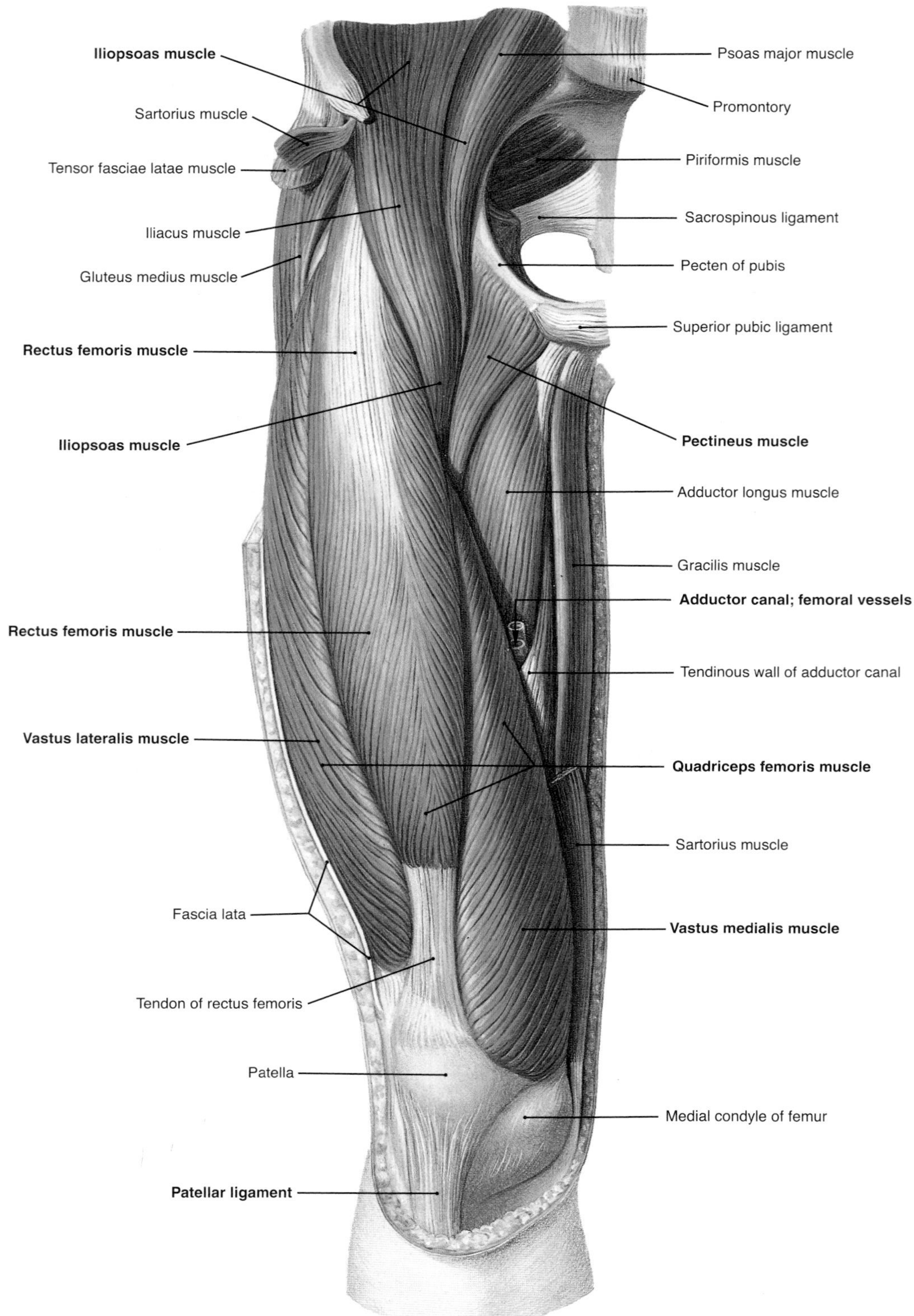
Iliopsoas muscle
Sartorius muscle
Tensor fasciae latae muscle
Iliacus muscle
Gluteus medius muscle
Rectus femoris muscle
Iliopsoas muscle
Rectus femoris muscle
Vastus lateralis muscle
Fascia lata
Tendon of rectus femoris
Patella
Patellar ligament
Psoas major muscle
Promontory
Piriformis muscle
Sacrospinous ligament
Pecten of pubis
Superior pubic ligament
Pectineus muscle
Adductor longus muscle
Gracilis muscle
Adductor canal; femoral vessels
Tendinous wall of adductor canal
Quadriceps femoris muscle
Sartorius muscle
Vastus medialis muscle
Medial condyle of femur

Figure 374 Quadriceps Femoris, Iliopsoas, and Pectineus Muscles

NOTE: (1) The **quadriceps femoris muscle** consists of the rectus femoris and the three vastus muscles (lateralis, intermedius, and medialis) as it converges inferiorly to form a powerful tendon that encases the patella and inserts onto the **tuberosity of the tibia.** The entire quadriceps extends the leg at the knee, while the rectus femoris also flexes the thigh at the hip.

(2) The **iliopsoas muscle** is the most powerful flexor of the thigh at the hip joint, and it inserts on the **lesser trochanter.**

(3) The quadrangular and flat **pectineus muscle** medial to the iliopsoas. Sometimes called the key to the femoral triangle, this muscle is normally supplied by the femoral nerve, but in slightly over 10% of cases it also receives a branch from one of the obturator nerves.

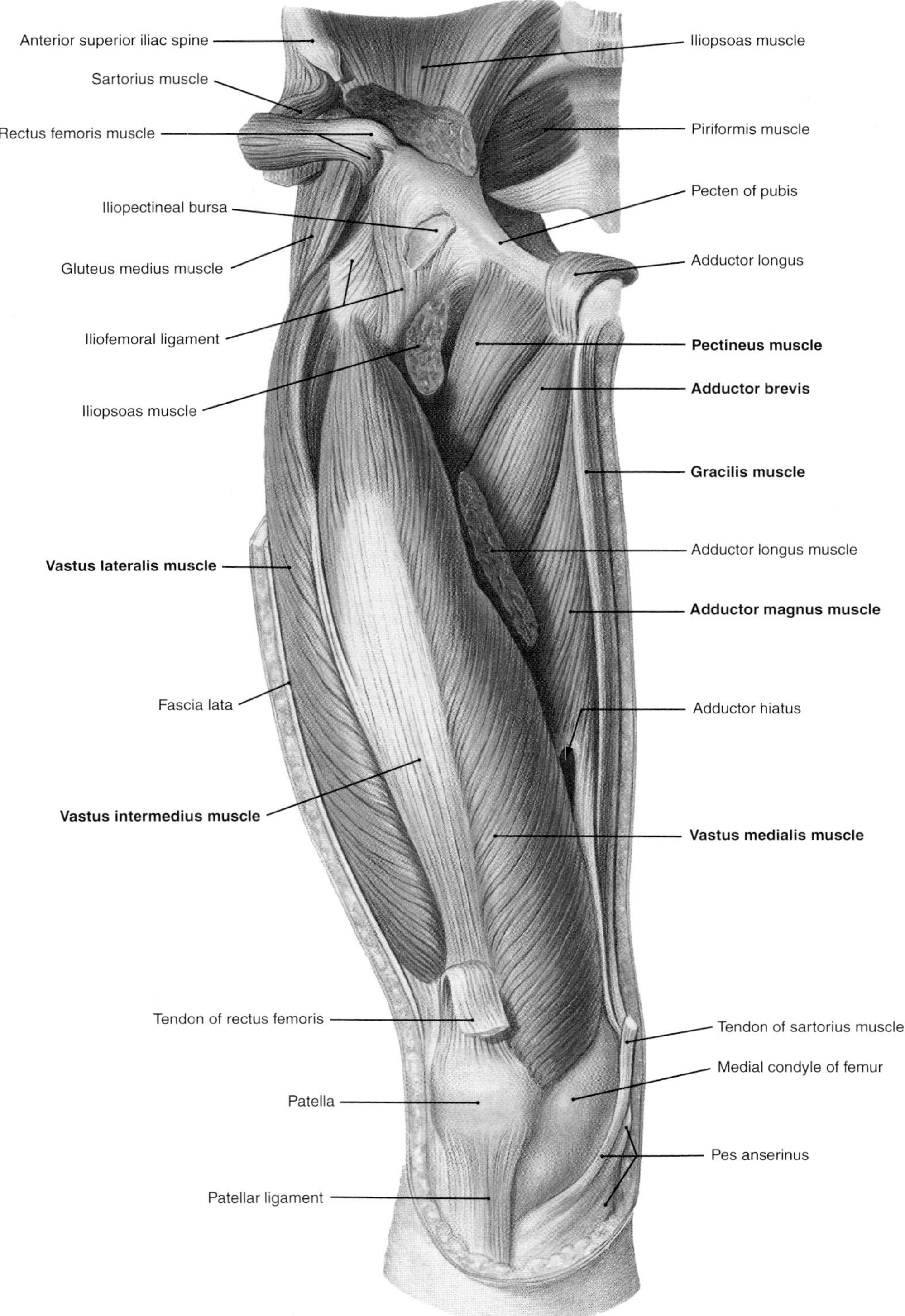
Anterior superior iliac spine
Sartorius muscle
Rectus femoris muscle
Iliopectineal bursa
Gluteus medius muscle
Iliofemoral ligament
Iliopsoas muscle
Vastus lateralis muscle
Fascia lata
Vastus intermedius muscle
Tendon of rectus femoris
Patella
Patellar ligament
Iliopsoas muscle
Piriformis muscle
Pecten of pubis
Adductor longus
Pectineus muscle
Adductor brevis
Gracilis muscle
Adductor longus muscle
Adductor magnus muscle
Adductor hiatus
Vastus medialis muscle
Tendon of sartorius muscle
Medial condyle of femur
Pes anserinus

Figure 375 Intermediate Layer of Anterior and Medial Thigh Muscles

NOTE: (1) The **rectus femoris** and **iliopsoas muscles** are cut to expose the underlying **vastus intermedius,** situated between the **vastus lateralis** and **vastus medialis.**

(2) The **adductor longus** has also been reflected. This displays the **pectineus, adductor brevis,** and **magnus muscles** and the long **gracilis muscle.**

(3) The quadriceps femoris is the most powerful extensor of the leg. During extension, however, there is a natural tendency to displace the patella laterally out of its groove on the patellar surface of the femur because of the natural angulation of the femur with respect to the bones of the leg.

(4) The muscle fibers of the **vastus medialis** descend further inferiorly than those of the vastus lateralis, and the lowest fibers insert directly along the medial border of the patella. The medial pull of these fibers is thought to be essential in maintaining the stability of the patella on the femur.

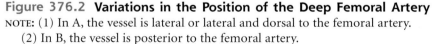

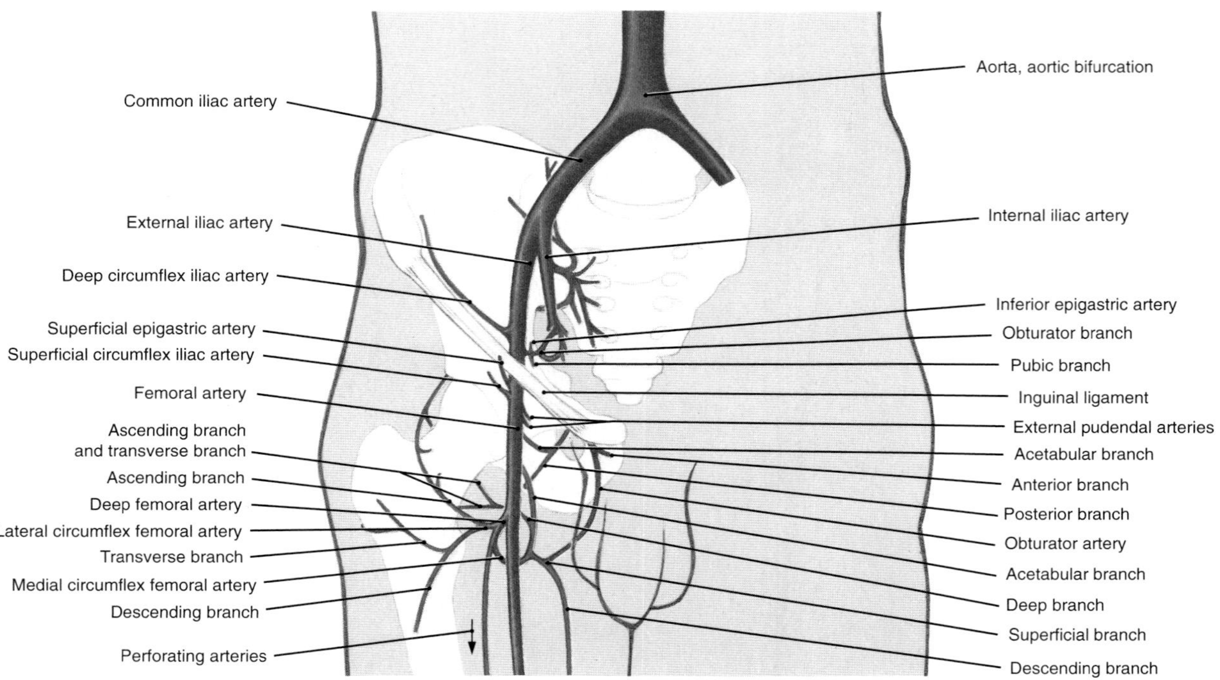
Aorta, aortic bifurcation
Common iliac artery
Internal iliac artery
External iliac artery
Deep circumflex iliac artery
Inferior epigastric artery
Obturator branch
Superficial epigastric artery
Superficial circumflex iliac artery
Pubic branch
Inguinal ligament
Femoral artery
External pudendal arteries
Ascending branch
and transverse branch
Acetabular branch
Ascending branch
Anterior branch
Deep femoral artery
Posterior branch
Lateral circumflex femoral artery
Obturator artery
Transverse branch
Acetabular branch
Medial circumflex femoral artery
Deep branch
Descending branch
Superficial branch
Perforating arteries
Descending branch

Figure 376.1 Arteries of the Right Hip Region and the Thigh

NOTE: (1) The branching pattern of the deep femoral artery (profundus femoris) shown in this drawing is observed in 55% to 60% of cases studied.

(2) A number of the branches of the internal iliac artery are not labeled in this figure, but these can be seen in Figures 282 to 284.

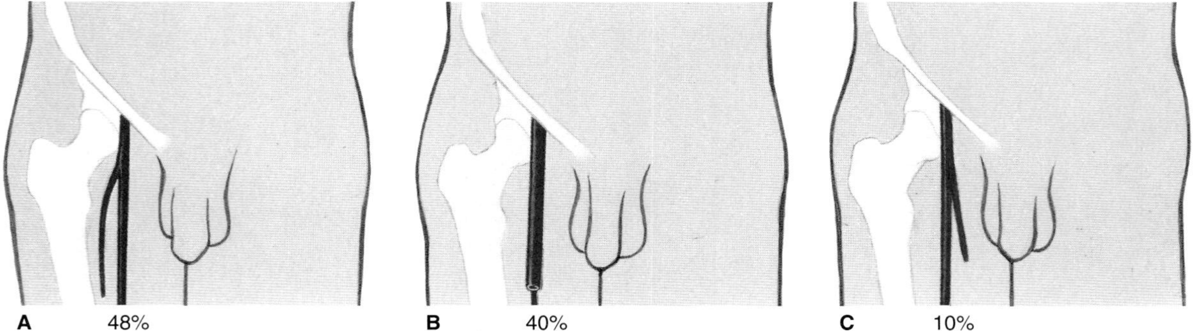
A 48%
B 40%
C 10%

Figure 376.2 Variations in the Position of the Deep Femoral Artery

NOTE: (1) In A, the vessel is lateral or lateral and dorsal to the femoral artery.

(2) In B, the vessel is posterior to the femoral artery.

(3) In C, the vessel is medial to the femoral artery.

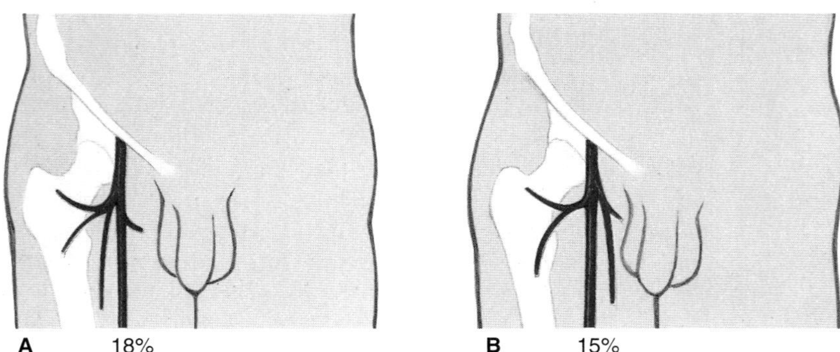
A 18%
B 15%

Figure 376.3 Variations in the Origins of the Femoral Circumflex Arteries

NOTE: (1) In A, the separate origin of the medial femoral circumflex artery is shown.

(2) In B, the separate origin of the lateral femoral circumflex artery is shown.

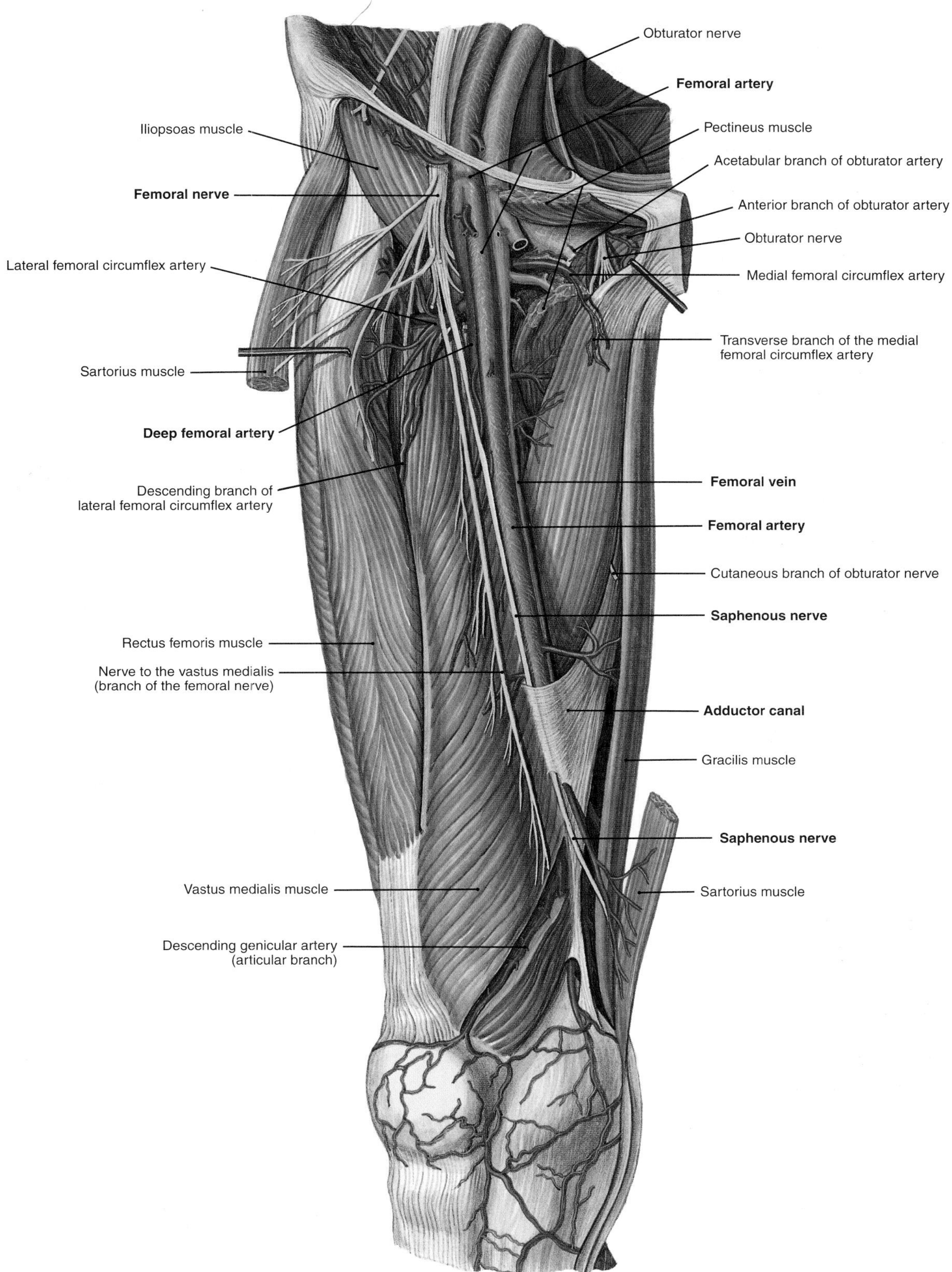
Obturator nerve
Femoral artery
Pectineus muscle
Acetabular branch of obturator artery
Anterior branch of obturator artery
Obturator nerve
Medial femoral circumflex artery
Transverse branch of the medial femoral circumflex artery
Iliopsoas muscle
Femoral nerve
Lateral femoral circumflex artery
Sartorius muscle
Deep femoral artery
Descending branch of lateral femoral circumflex artery
Femoral vein
Femoral artery
Cutaneous branch of obturator nerve
Saphenous nerve
Rectus femoris muscle
Nerve to the vastus medialis (branch of the femoral nerve)
Adductor canal
Gracilis muscle
Saphenous nerve
Vastus medialis muscle
Sartorius muscle
Descending genicular artery (articular branch)

Figure 377 **Femoral Vessels and Nerves**

NOTE: (1) The femoral vessels, the saphenous branch of the femoral nerve, and the nerve to the vastus medialis all enter the **adductor canal** (**of Hunter**).

(2) The **saphenous nerve,** after coursing some distance in the canal, penetrates the overlying fascia to reach the superficial leg region; the **nerve to the vastus medialis** traverses the more proximal part of the canal and then divides into muscular branches to supply the vastus medialis muscle.

(3) The **femoral artery and vein** course through the entire canal and then leave it by way of an opening in the adductor magnus muscle called the **adductor hiatus.** The vessels course to the back of the lower limb to become the **popliteal artery and vein.**

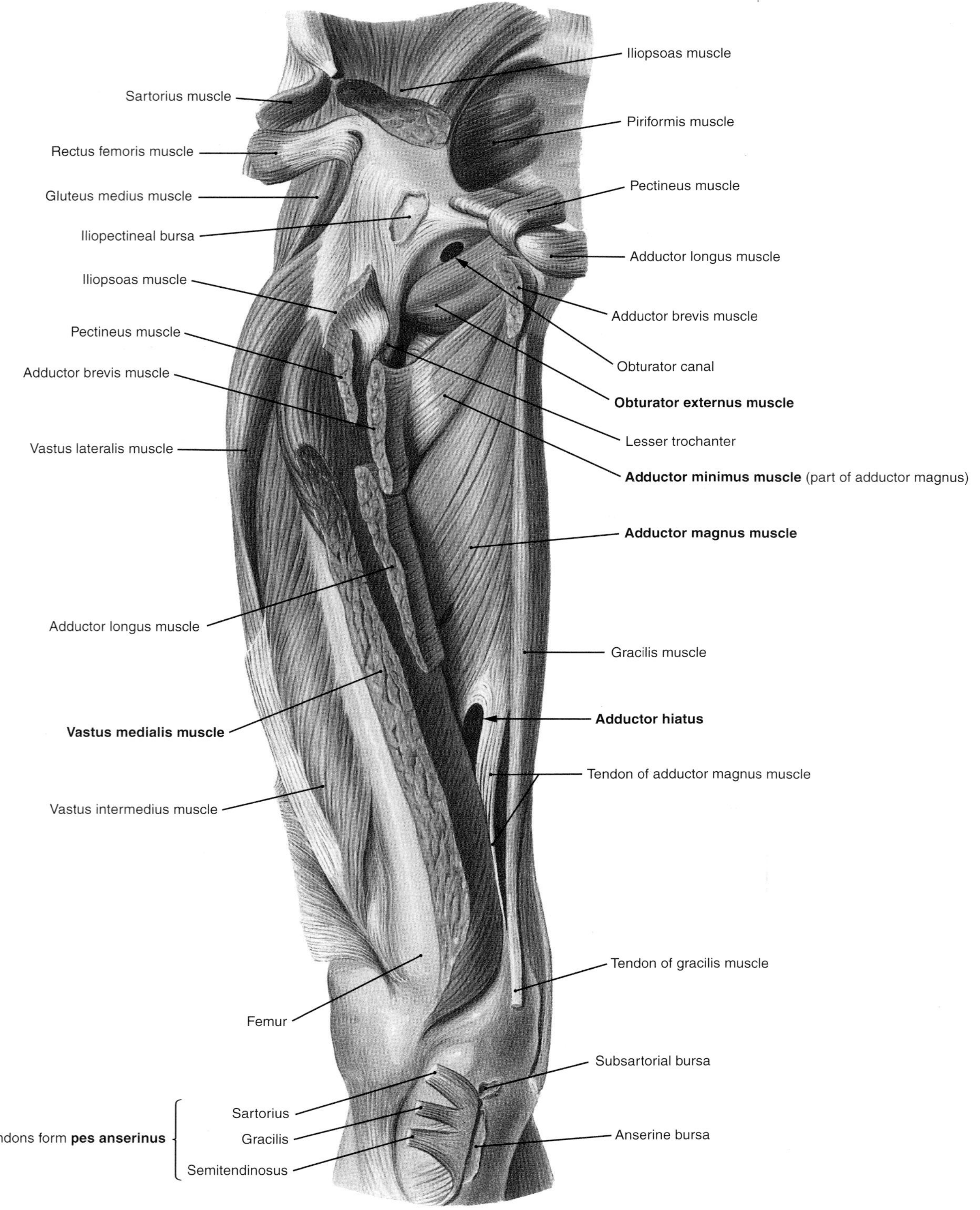
Iliopsoas muscle
Sartorius muscle
Piriformis muscle
Rectus femoris muscle
Pectineus muscle
Gluteus medius muscle
Iliopectineal bursa
Adductor longus muscle
Iliopsoas muscle
Adductor brevis muscle
Pectineus muscle
Obturator canal
Adductor brevis muscle
Obturator externus muscle
Lesser trochanter
Vastus lateralis muscle
Adductor minimus muscle (part of adductor magnus)
Adductor magnus muscle
Adductor longus muscle
Gracilis muscle
Adductor hiatus
Vastus medialis muscle
Tendon of adductor magnus muscle
Vastus intermedius muscle
Tendon of gracilis muscle
Femur
Subsartorial bursa
Sartorius
Tendons form pes anserinus
Gracilis
Anserine bursa
Semitendinosus

Figure 378 Deep Layer of Anterior and Medial Thigh Muscles (Right)

NOTE: (1) The rectus femoris and vastus medialis have been removed, thereby exposing the shaft of the femur. Likewise, the adductor longus and brevis and the pectineus muscles have been reflected, exposing the **obturator externus**, the **adductor magnus** and the **adductor minimus** (which usually is just the upper portion of the adductor magnus).

(2) The common insertion of the tendons of the **sartorius, gracilis,** and **semitendinosus muscles** on the medial aspect of the medial condyle of the tibia. The divergent nature of this insertion resembles a goose's foot (pes anserinus). This tendinous formation can be used by surgeons to strengthen the medial aspect of the capsule of the knee joint.

(3) The tendinous opening on the adductor magnus, called the **adductor hiatus,** through which the femoral vessels course to (or from) the popliteal fossa.

(4) The **obturator externus muscle** stretching across the inferior surface of the obturator membrane to insert laterally on the neck of the femur. This muscle rotates the femur laterally, and it is not part of the adductor group of muscles.

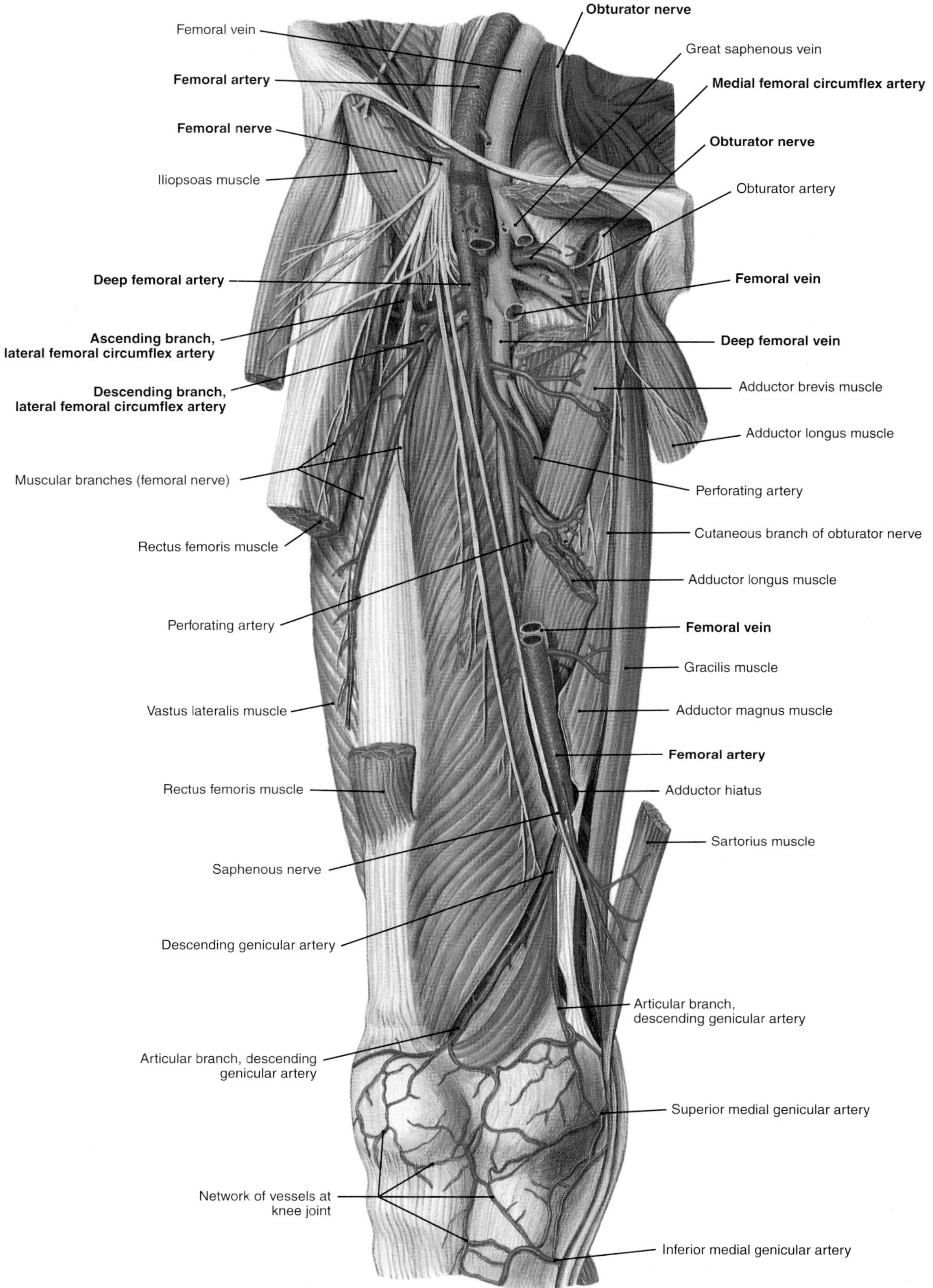
Femoral vein
Femoral artery
Femoral nerve
Iliopsoas muscle
Deep femoral artery
Ascending branch, lateral femoral circumflex artery
Descending branch, lateral femoral circumflex artery
Muscular branches (femoral nerve)
Rectus femoris muscle
Perforating artery
Vastus lateralis muscle
Rectus femoris muscle
Saphenous nerve
Descending genicular artery
Articular branch, descending genicular artery
Network of vessels at knee joint
Obturator nerve
Great saphenous vein
Medial femoral circumflex artery
Obturator nerve
Obturator artery
Femoral vein
Deep femoral vein
Adductor brevis muscle
Adductor longus muscle
Perforating artery
Cutaneous branch of obturator nerve
Adductor longus muscle
Femoral vein
Gracilis muscle
Adductor magnus muscle
Femoral artery
Adductor hiatus
Sartorius muscle
Articular branch, descending genicular artery
Superior medial genicular artery
Inferior medial genicular artery

Figure 379 Femoral and Obturator Nerves and Deep Femoral Artery

NOTE: (1) The **obturator nerve** supplies the adductor muscles, the gracilis, and the obturator externus (not shown, see Fig. 378), while the femoral nerve innervates all the other anterior thigh muscles.

(2) The **deep femoral artery** is the largest branch of the femoral artery, and it gives off both the **medial** and **lateral femoral circumflex arteries.** Observe the femoral vessels traversing the femoral canal.

(3) In about 50% of cases, the deep femoral artery branches from the lateral side of the femoral artery; in 40%, it branches from the posterior aspect of the femoral and courses behind it; in 10%, the deep femoral arises from the medial side of the femoral.

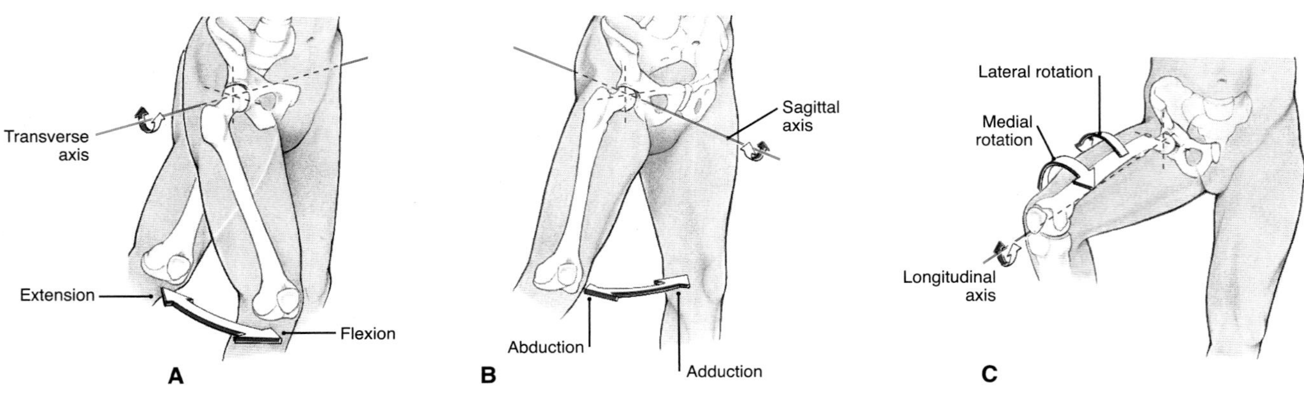
Transverse axis
Extension
Flexion
A
Sagittal axis
Abduction
Adduction
B
Lateral rotation
Medial rotation
Longitudinal axis
C

Figure 380 Movements of the Thigh at the Hip Joint
In A, **flexion** and **extension** occur through the transverse axis of the hip joint.
In B, **abduction** and **adduction** occur through the sagittal axis of the hip joint.
In C, **medial rotation** and **lateral rotation** occur around the longitudinal axis of the hip joint.

ANTERIOR MUSCLES OF THE HIP

Muscle	Origin	Insertion	Innervation	Action
Rectus femoris head of the quadriceps femoris	Straight head: Anterior inferior iliac spine. Reflected head: The groove above the acetabulum.	With the other three parts of the quadriceps femoris, the rectus form a common tendon that encases the patella and inserts onto the tibial tuberosity.	Femoral nerve (L2, L3, L4)	All four parts extend the leg at the knee joint; the rectus femoris also helps to flex the thigh at the hip joint
Psoas major	Transverse process and body of T12 and upper four lumbar vertebrae; intervertebral disks between T12 and L5	Lesser trochanter of femur (receives also the fibers of iliacus muscle)	Branches from upper four lumbar nerves	Powerful flexor of thigh at hip; when femurs are fixed, they flex the trunk, as in sitting up from a supine position
Psoas minor (muscle present in about 40% of cadavers)	Lateral surface of bodies of T12 and L1 vertebrae	Pectineal line and iliopectineal eminence and the iliac fascia (often merges with psoas major tendon)	Branch from L1 nerve	Weak flexor of the trunk
Iliacus	Iliac fossa; anterior inferior iliac spine	Lesser trochanter of femur in common with tendon of psoas major muscle	Femoral nerve (L2, L3)	Powerful flexor of thigh at the hip joint

ANTERIOR THIGH MUSCLES

Muscle	Origin	Insertion	Innervation	Action
Sartorius	Anterior superior iliac spine	Superior part of the medial surface of the tibia	Femoral nerve (L2, L3)	Flexes, abducts, and laterally rotates the thigh at the hip joint; flexes and medially rotates the leg at the knee joint
Quadriceps femoris muscle Rectus femoris	Straight head: Anterior inferior iliac spine. Reflected head: the groove above the acetabulum.	All four parts of the quadriceps femoris form a common tendon that encases the patella and finally inserts onto the tibial tuberosity	Femoral nerve (L2, L3, L4)	All four parts extend the leg at the knee joint; the rectus femoris also helps to flex the thigh at the hip joint.
Vastus medialis	Intertrochanteric line and the medial lip of the linea aspera on the femur			
Vastus lateralis	Greater trochanter and the lateral lip of the linea aspera			
Vastus intermedius	Anterior and lateral surface of the body of the femur			
Articularis genu	Anterior surface of the lower part of the femur	Upper part of the synovial membrane of the knee joint	Femoral nerve (L2, L3, L4)	Draws the synovial membrane upward during extension of the leg to prevent its compression

MEDIAL THIGH MUSCLES

Muscle	Origin	Insertion	Innervation	Action
Pectineus	Pectineal line of the pubis	Along the pectineal line of the femur, between the lesser trochanter and the linea aspera	Femoral nerve (L2, L3); may also receive a branch from the obturator or the accessory obturator nerve when present	Flexes, adducts, and medially rotates the femur
Adductor longus	From the anterior pubis, where the pubic crest joins the symphysis pubis	Middle third of the femur along the linea aspera	Obturator nerve (L2, L3, L4)	Adducts, flexes, and medially rotates the femur
Adductor brevis	Outer surface of the inferior pubic ramus between the gracilis and the obturator externus	Along the pectineal line of the femur and the upper part of the linea aspera behind the pectineus	Obturator nerve (L2, L3, L4)	Adducts, flexes, and medially rotates the femur
Adductor magnus	Inferior ramus of pubis; ramus of the ischium and the ischial tuberosity	Medial lip of the upper two-thirds of the linea aspera; the medial supracondylar line and the adductor tubercle	Obturator nerve (L2, L3, L4): sciatic nerve (tibial division) for the hamstring part of the muscle	Powerful adductor of the thigh; upper part flexes and medially rotates the thigh; lower part extends and laterally rotates the thigh
Adductor minimus	The upper more horizontal part of the adductor magnus, which receives the name adductor minimus when it forms a distinct muscle			
Gracilis	From the body of the pubis and the adjacent inferior pubic ramus	Upper part of the medial surface of the tibia below the medial condyle	Obturator nerve (L2, L3)	Adducts the thigh; also flexes the leg at the knee and medially rotates the leg
Obturator externus	Medial part of the outer surface of obturator membrane and medial margin of obturator foramen	Trochanteric fossa of the femur	Obturator nerve (L3, L4)	Laterally rotates the thigh

LATERAL THIGH MUSCLE

Muscle	Origin	Insertion	Innervation	Action
Tensor fasciae latae	Outer lip of the iliac crest; also from the anterior superior iliac spine	Iliotibial tract, which then descends to attach to the lateral condyle of the tibia	Superior gluteal nerve (L4, L5)	Abducts, flexes, and medially rotates the thigh; tenses the iliotibial tract, thereby helping to extend the leg at the knee

POSTERIOR THIGH MUSCLES

Muscle	Origin	Insertion	Innervation	Action
Biceps femoris	Long head: Ischial tuberosity in common with other hamstring muscles, Short head: Lateral lip of the linea aspera of the femur.	Lateral surface of the head of the fibula and a small slip to lateral condyle of the tibia	Long head: Tibial part of sciatic nerve (S1, S2, S3). Short head: Commom fibular part sciatic nerve (L5, S1, S2).	Flexes the leg and rotates the tibia laterally; long head also extends the thigh at the hip joint
Semitendinosus	Ischial tuberosity in common with other hamstring muscles	Medial surface of the upper part of the body of the tibia	Tibial part of the sciatic nerve (L5, S1, S2)	Flexes the leg and rotates the tibia medially; extends the thigh
Semimembranosus	Ischial tuberosity in common with other hamstring muscles	Posterior aspect of the medial condyle of the tibia	Tibial part of the sciatic nerve (L5, S1, S2)	Flexes the leg and rotates it medially; extends the thigh

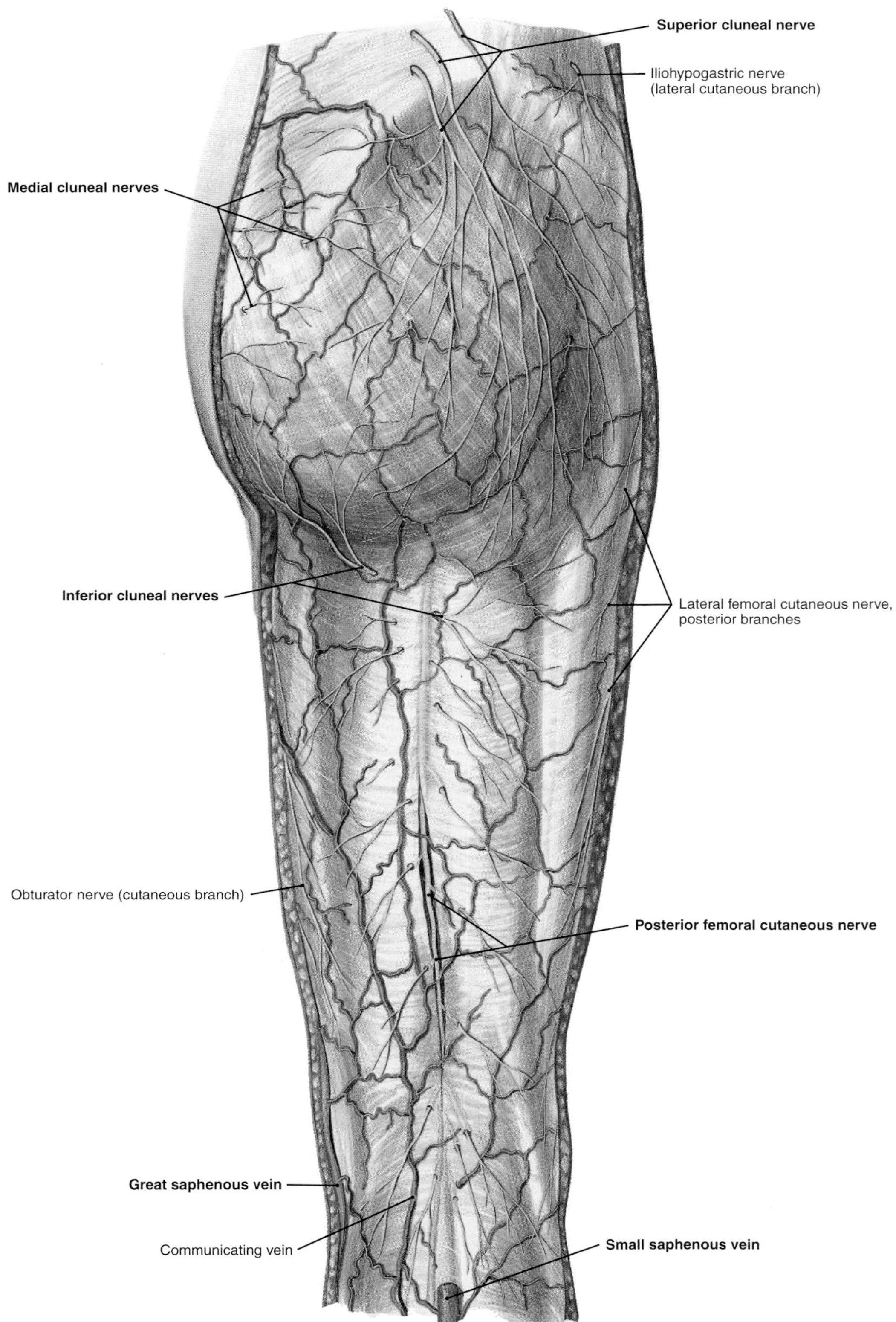
Superior cluneal nerve
Iliohypogastric nerve
(lateral cutaneous branch)
Medial cluneal nerves
Inferior cluneal nerves
Lateral femoral cutaneous nerve,
posterior branches
Obturator nerve (cutaneous branch)
Posterior femoral cutaneous nerve
Great saphenous vein
Communicating vein
Small saphenous vein

Figure 382 Superficial Veins and Nerves of the Gluteal Region and Posterior Thigh

NOTE: (1) The principal cutaneous nerves supplying the **gluteal region** are the:

(a) **Superior cluneal nerves** (from the posterior primary rami of L1, L2, L3),

(b) **Medial cluneal nerves** (from the posterior primary rami of S1, S2, S3), and

(c) **Inferior cluneal nerves** (from the posterior femoral cutaneous nerve: anterior primary rami of S1, S2, S3).

(2) The skin of the **posterior thigh** is supplied primarily by the **posterior femoral cutaneous nerve (S1, S2, S3)**, but posterolaterally it also receives branches from the lateral femoral cutaneous nerve, and posteromedially, cutaneous branches from the obturator nerve.

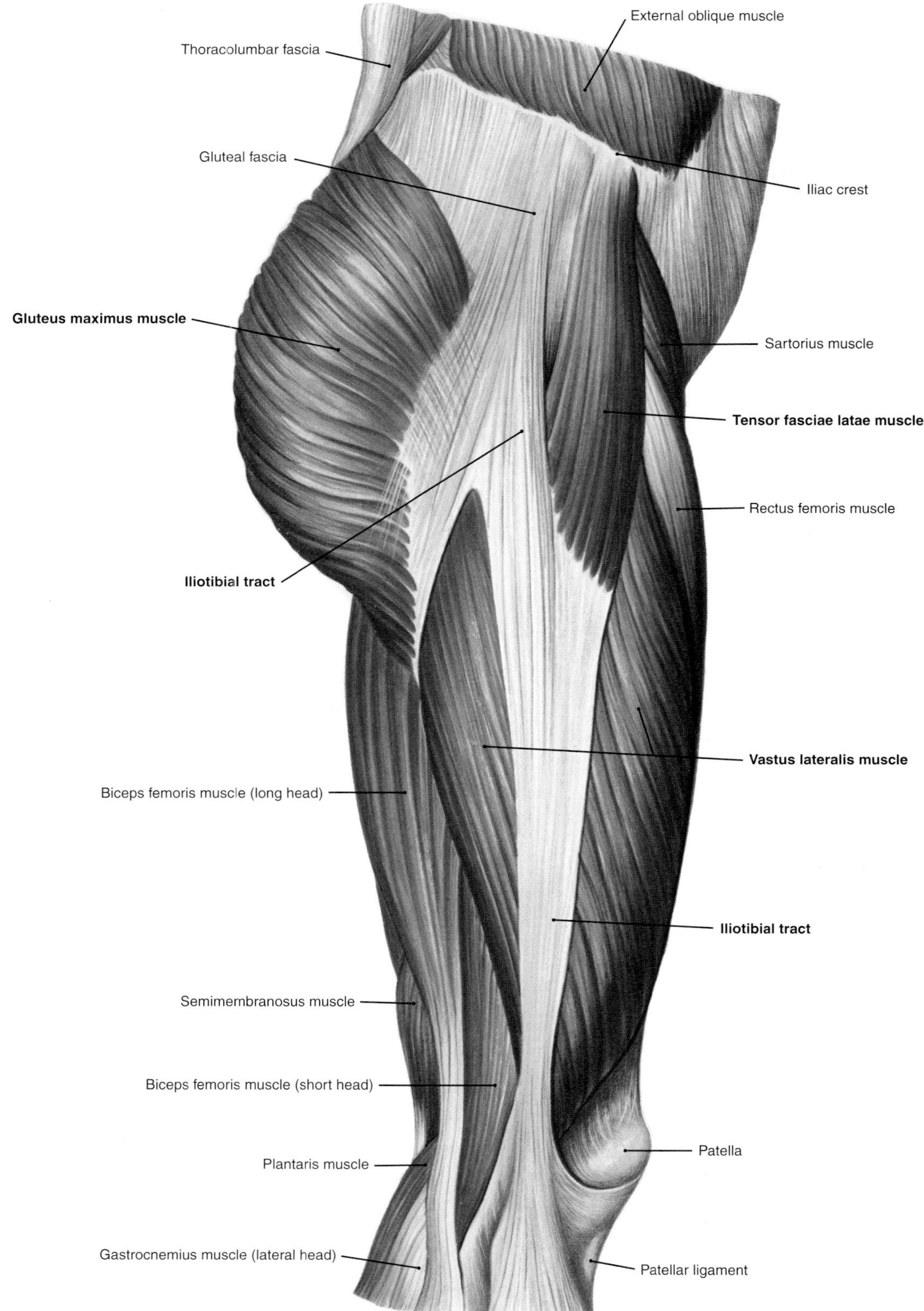
External oblique muscle
Thoracolumbar fascia
Gluteal fascia
Iliac crest
Gluteus maximus muscle
Sartorius muscle
Tensor fasciae latae muscle
Rectus femoris muscle
Iliotibial tract
Vastus lateralis muscle
Biceps femoris muscle (long head)
Iliotibial tract
Semimembranosus muscle
Biceps femoris muscle (short head)
Patella
Plantaris muscle
Gastrocnemius muscle (lateral head)
Patellar ligament

Figure 383 Superficial Thigh and Gluteal Muscles (Lateral View)

NOTE: (1) The massive size of the **vastus lateralis, biceps femoris,** and **gluteus maximus muscles** is seen from this lateral side.

(2) The **iliotibial tract** (or band) stretches, superficially, the length of the thigh. Its muscle, the **tensor fasciae latae,** helps to keep the dense fascia lata taut.

(3) The fascia lata is a very tight layer of deep fascia that surrounds the thigh muscles (see Fig. 370). Because of this, the tensor fasciae latae assists in extension of the leg at the knee joint and in helping to maintain an erect posture.

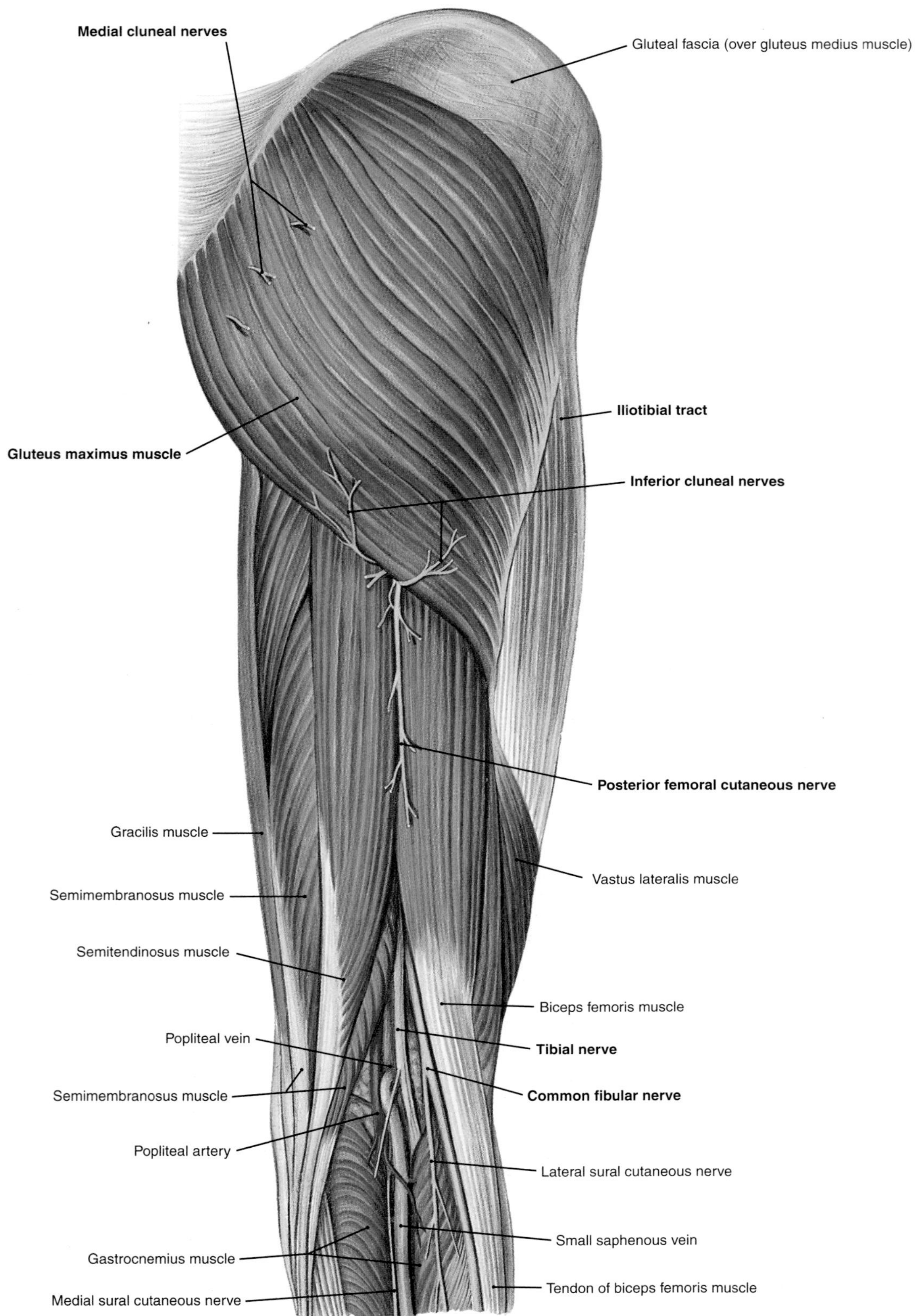
Medial cluneal nerves
Gluteal fascia (over gluteus medius muscle)
Iliotibial tract
Gluteus maximus muscle
Inferior cluneal nerves
Posterior femoral cutaneous nerve
Gracilis muscle
Vastus lateralis muscle
Semimembranosus muscle
Semitendinosus muscle
Biceps femoris muscle
Popliteal vein
Tibial nerve
Semimembranosus muscle
Common fibular nerve
Popliteal artery
Lateral sural cutaneous nerve
Small saphenous vein
Gastrocnemius muscle
Tendon of biceps femoris muscle
Medial sural cutaneous nerve

Figure 384 Hamstring Muscles of Posterior Thigh and Gluteus Maximus (Superficial Dissection)

NOTE: (1) The emergence of the posterior femoral cutaneous nerve below the inferior border of the gluteus maximus muscle, and its descent down the middle of the thigh.

(2) The appearance of the major vessels (popliteal artery and vein) and the sciatic nerve (tibial and common fibular nerves) in the popliteal fossa.

(3) The posterior thigh contains the **hamstring muscles.** These include four muscles, the **long head of the biceps femoris,** the **semitendinosus muscle,** the **semimembranosus muscle,** and the ischiocondylar part of the **adductor magnus muscle.**

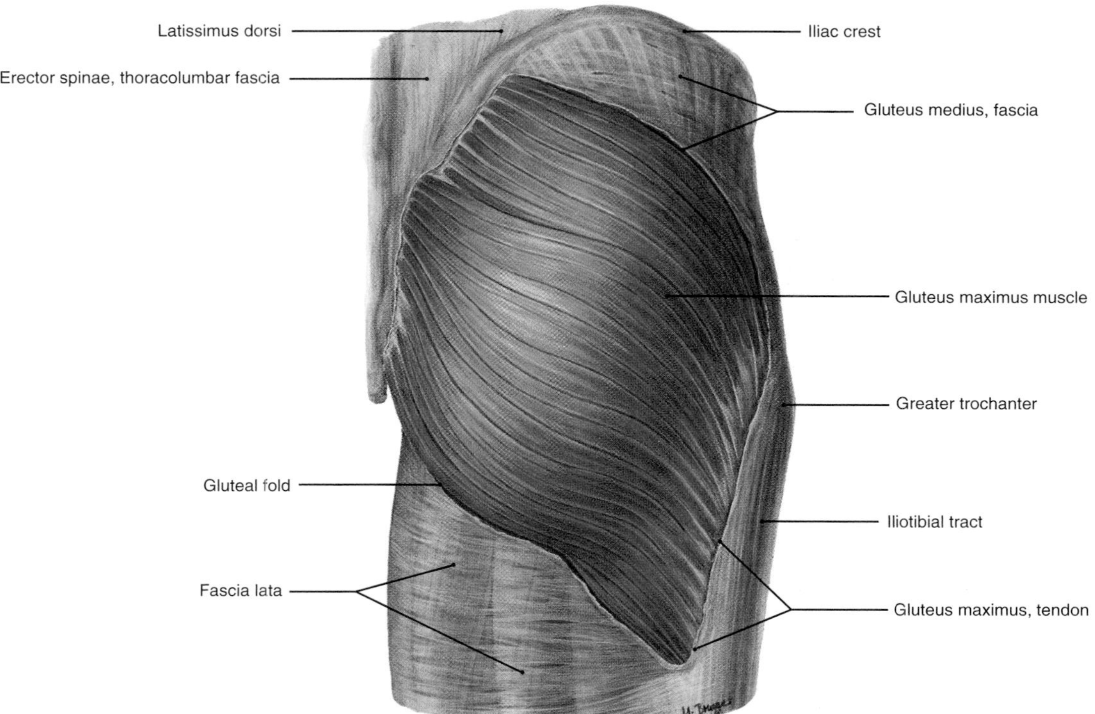
Latissimus dorsi
Erector spinae, thoracolumbar fascia
Iliac crest
Gluteus medius, fascia
Gluteus maximus muscle
Greater trochanter
Gluteal fold
Iliotibial tract
Fascia lata
Gluteus maximus, tendon

Figure 385.1 Right Gluteus Maximus Muscle (Posterior View)

NOTE: (1) The gluteus maximus muscle forms the contour of the buttocks. It arises from the posterior gluteal line of the ilium and the posterior surfaces of the sacrum, coccyx, and sacrotuberous ligament.

(2) The muscle fibers extend inferolaterally and end in a broad tendon that crosses the greater trochanter to insert on the iliotibial band of the fascia lata and the gluteal tuberosity of the femur.

(3) While the gluteus maximus is a powerful extensor and lateral rotator of the thigh, its upper fibers abduct the thigh and its lower fibers adduct the thigh.

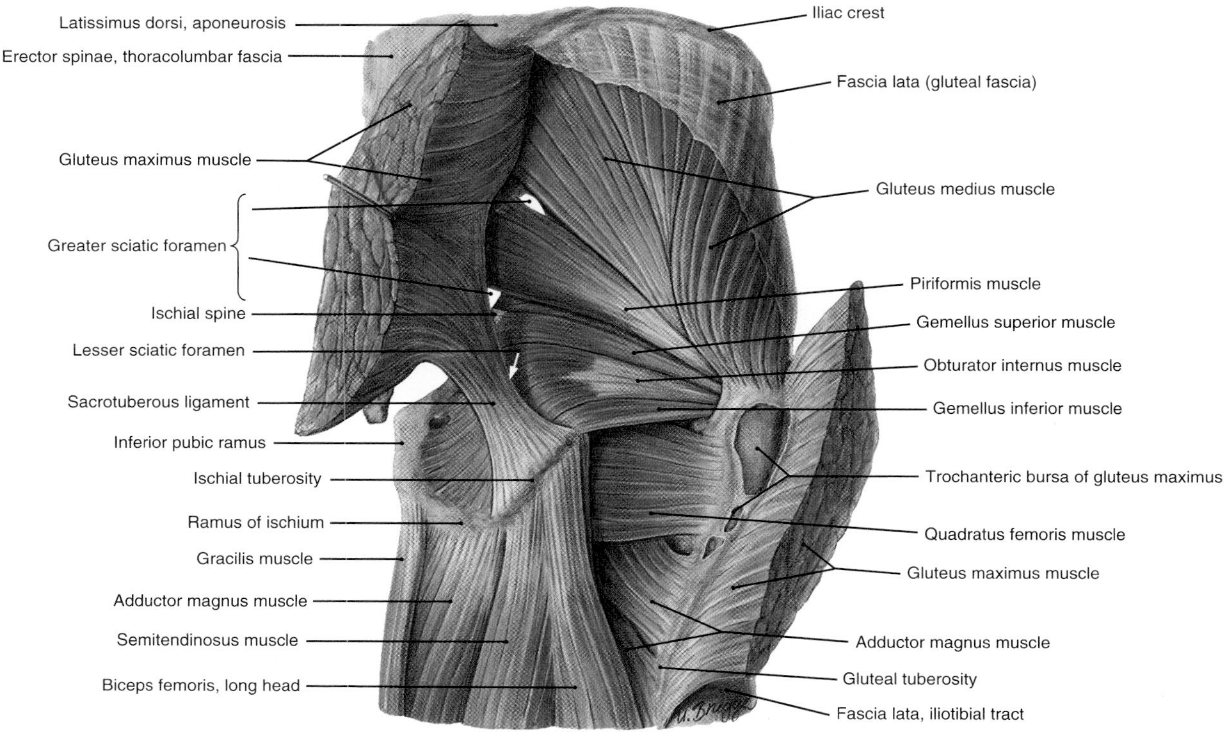
Latissimus dorsi, aponeurosis
Erector spinae, thoracolumbar fascia
Iliac crest
Fascia lata (gluteal fascia)
Gluteus maximus muscle
Gluteus medius muscle
Greater sciatic foramen
Piriformis muscle
Ischial spine
Gemellus superior muscle
Lesser sciatic foramen
Obturator internus muscle
Sacrotuberous ligament
Gemellus inferior muscle
Inferior pubic ramus
Ischial tuberosity
Trochanteric bursa of gluteus maximus
Ramus of ischium
Quadratus femoris muscle
Gracilis muscle
Gluteus maximus muscle
Adductor magnus muscle
Semitendinosus muscle
Adductor magnus muscle
Gluteal tuberosity
Biceps femoris, long head
Fascia lata, iliotibial tract

Figure 385.2 Deep Muscles of the Gluteal and Hip Regions (Posterior View)

NOTE: (1) Deep to the gluteus maximus are found the gluteus medius, gluteus minimus, piriformis, the two gemellus muscles (superior and inferior), the obturator internus, and the quadratus femoris.

(2) The gluteus medius (and the gluteus minimus deep to the medius) are abductors and **medial** rotators, while the other gluteal muscles are also abductors, but they are **lateral** rotators of the thigh. The piriformis also helps to abduct the flexed thigh.

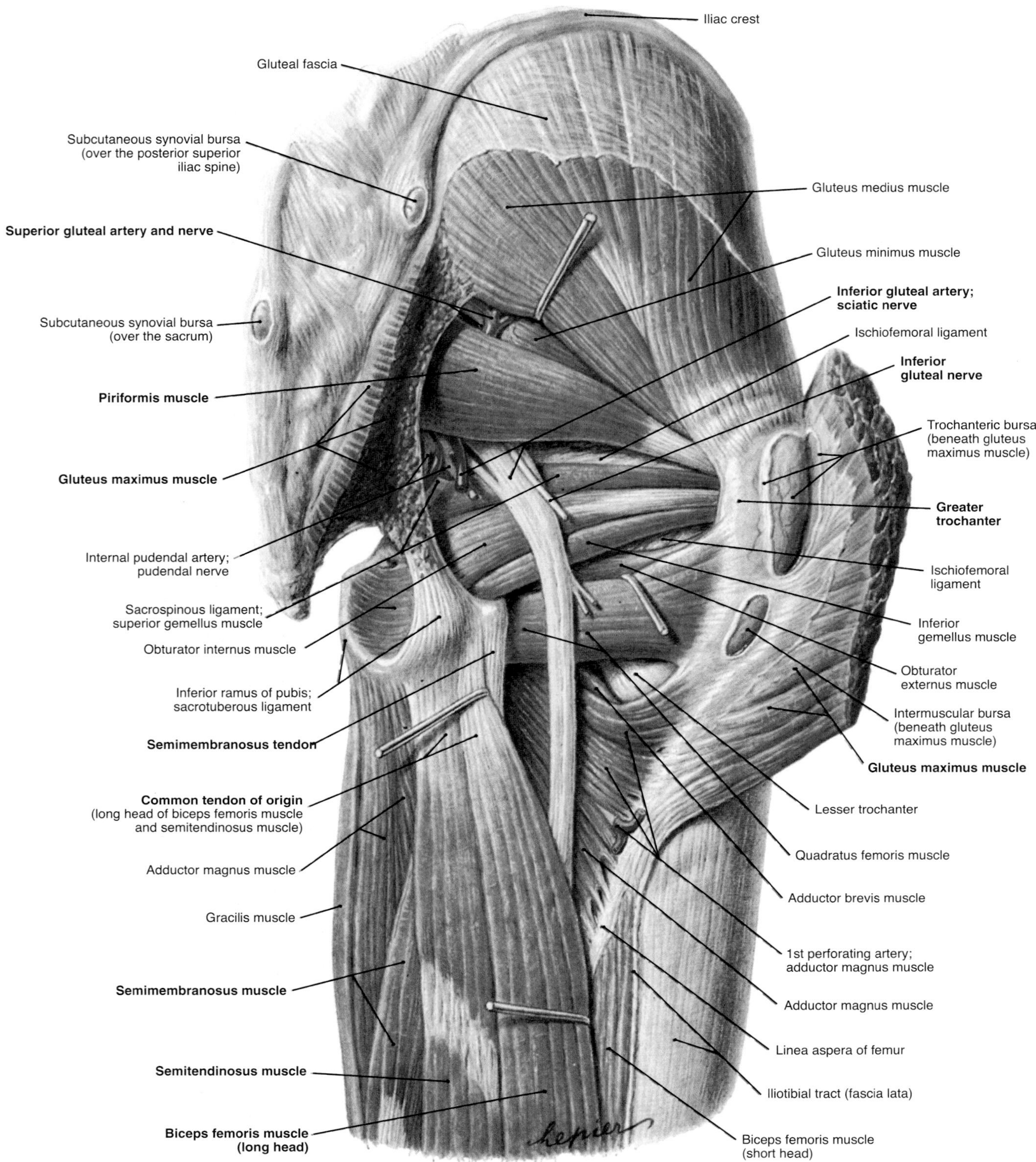
Iliac crest
Gluteal fascia
Subcutaneous synovial bursa (over the posterior superior iliac spine)
Superior gluteal artery and nerve
Subcutaneous synovial bursa (over the sacrum)
Piriformis muscle
Gluteus maximus muscle
Internal pudendal artery; pudendal nerve
Sacrospinous ligament; superior gemellus muscle
Obturator internus muscle
Inferior ramus of pubis; sacrotuberous ligament
Semimembranosus tendon
Common tendon of origin (long head of biceps femoris muscle and semitendinosus muscle)
Adductor magnus muscle
Gracilis muscle
Semimembranosus muscle
Semitendinosus muscle
Biceps femoris muscle (long head)
Gluteus medius muscle
Gluteus minimus muscle
Inferior gluteal artery; sciatic nerve
Ischiofemoral ligament
Inferior gluteal nerve
Trochanteric bursa (beneath gluteus maximus muscle)
Greater trochanter
Ischiofemoral ligament
Inferior gemellus muscle
Obturator externus muscle
Intermuscular bursa (beneath gluteus maximus muscle)
Gluteus maximus muscle
Lesser trochanter
Quadratus femoris muscle
Adductor brevis muscle
1st perforating artery; adductor magnus muscle
Adductor magnus muscle
Linea aspera of femur
Iliotibial tract (fascia lata)
Biceps femoris muscle (short head)

Figure 386 Middle and Deep Gluteal Muscles and the Sciatic Nerve

NOTE: (1) The gluteus maximus has been reflected to show the centrally located **piriformis muscle,** which is the key structure in understanding the anatomy of this region.

(2) The piriformis muscle, as do most other structures that leave the pelvis to enter the gluteal region, passes through the **greater sciatic foramen.** The nerves and vessels enter the gluteal region from the pelvis either above or below the piriformis muscle. The important **sciatic nerve** enters the gluteal region **below** the piriformis.

(3) In addition to the piriformis, observe the **gluteus medius, the obturator internus**, with two **gemelli** above and below it, and the **quadratus femoris** muscles. The gluteus medius and minimus muscles are abductors and medial rotators of the thigh and all the other muscles are lateral rotators.

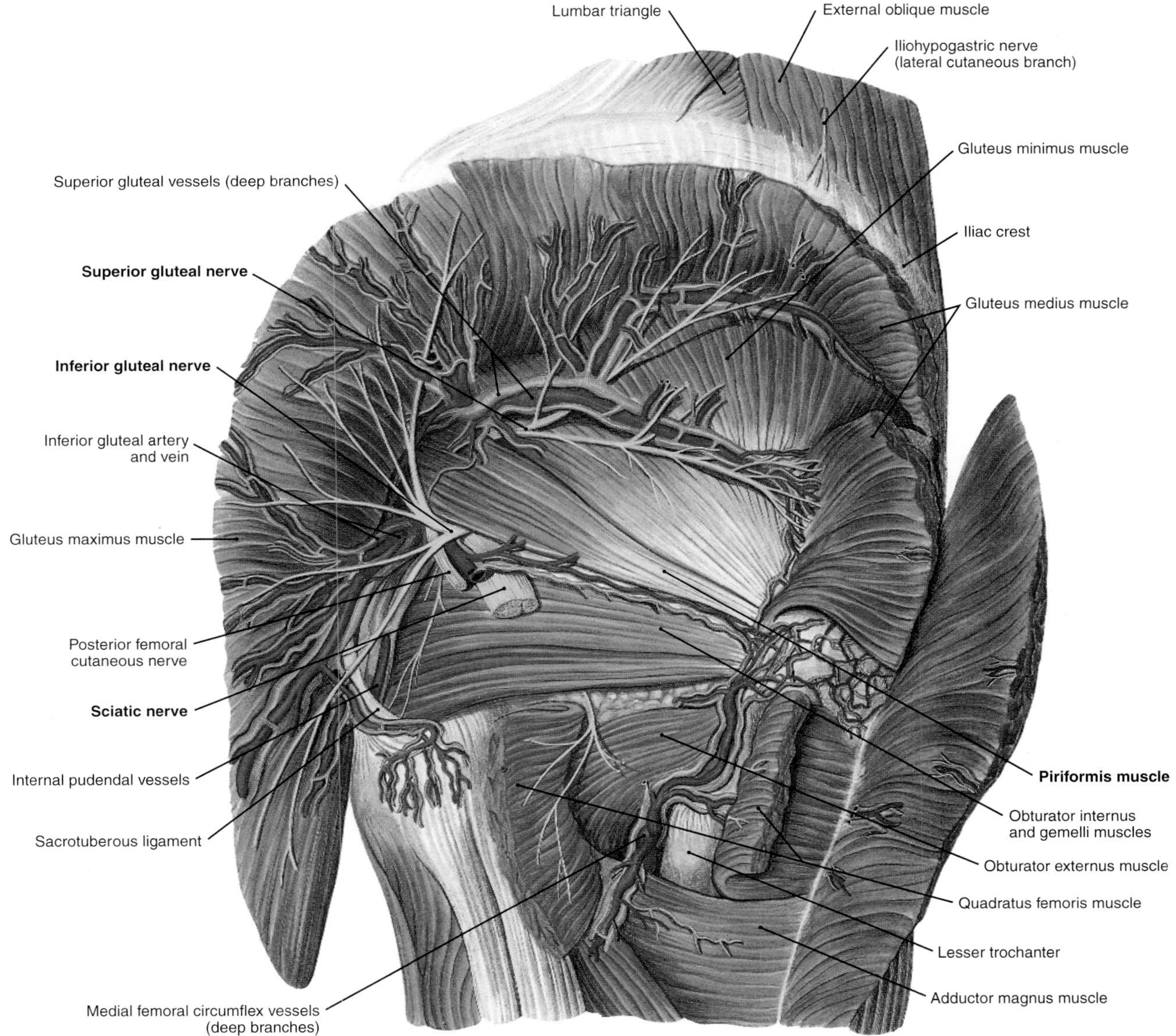
Lumbar triangle
External oblique muscle
Iliohypogastric nerve
(lateral cutaneous branch)
Gluteus minimus muscle
Superior gluteal vessels (deep branches)
Iliac crest
Superior gluteal nerve
Gluteus medius muscle
Inferior gluteal nerve
Inferior gluteal artery
and vein
Gluteus maximus muscle
Posterior femoral
cutaneous nerve
Sciatic nerve
Internal pudendal vessels
Piriformis muscle
Obturator internus
and gemelli muscles
Sacrotuberous ligament
Obturator externus muscle
Quadratus femoris muscle
Lesser trochanter
Adductor magnus muscle
Medial femoral circumflex vessels
(deep branches)

Figure 387 Deep Vessels and Nerves of the Gluteal Region

NOTE: (1) The gluteus maximus and gluteus medius muscles and the sciatic nerve have been cut to expose the short lateral rotators and the **gluteus minimus muscle.**

(2) **Above the piriformis** the **superior gluteal artery, vein,** and **nerve** enter the gluteal region through the greater sciatic foramen; **below the piriformis** the following structures enter the gluteal region by way of the greater sciatic foramen: the **inferior gluteal vessels** and **nerve,** the **sciatic nerve,** the **nerve to the obturator internus muscle,** the **posterior femoral cutaneous nerve,** the **nerve to the quadratus femoris muscle,** and the **internal pudendal vessels** and **pudendal nerve.**

(3) The internal pudendal artery and vein and the pudendal nerve, after entering the gluteal region through the greater sciatic foramen, cross the sacrospinous ligament and reenter the pelvis through the **lesser sciatic foramen** and course in the pudendal canal to get to the perineum. The other structure that passes through the lesser sciatic foramen is the **tendon of the obturator internus muscle.**

(4) To separate the gluteus medius muscle from the gluteus minimus muscle as shown in this figure, dissect along the course of the superior gluteal vessels and nerve, since these structures lie in the plane between the medius and minimus.

MUSCLES OF THE GLUTEAL REGION

Muscle	Origin	Insertion	Innervation	Action
Gluteus maximus	Outer surface of the ilium and iliac crest; dorsal surface of the sacrum; lateral side of coccyx and the sacrotuberous ligament	Into the iliotibial band, which then descends to attach to the lateral condyle of tibia; also onto the gluteal tuberosity of the femur	Inferior gluteal nerve (L5, S1, S2)	Powerful extensor of the thigh; lateral rotator of the thigh; helps steady the extended leg; extends the trunk when distal end is fixed
Gluteus medius	External surface of the ilium between the anterior and posterior gluteal lines	Lateral surface of greater trochanter of the femur	Superior gluteal nerve (L4, L5, S1)	Abducts and medially rotates the thigh; helps steady the pelvis
Gluteus minimus	Outer surface of ilium between the anterior and inferior gluteal lines	Anterior border of greater trochanter and on the fibrous capsule of the hip joint	Superior gluteal nerve (L4, L5, S1)	Abducts and medially rotates the thigh; helps steady the pelvis
Piriformis	Anterior (pelvic) surface of the sacrum and the inner surface of sacrotuberous ligament	Upper border of the greater trochanter of the femur	Muscular branches from the S1 and S2 nerves	Laterally rotates the extended thigh; when the thigh is flexed, it abducts the femur
Obturator internus	Pelvic surface of obturator membrane and from the bone surrounding the obturator foramen	Medial surface of greater trochanter proximal to the trochanteric fossa	Nerve to the obturator internus (L5, S1)	Laterally rotates the extended thigh and abducts the flexed thigh
Superior gemellus	Outer surface of the ischial spine	Medial surface of greater trochanter with tendon of the obturator interius	Nerve to the obturator internus (L5, S1)	Laterally rotates the extended thigh and abducts the flexed thigh
Inferior gemellus	From the ischial tuberosity	Medial surface of greater trochanter with tendon of the obturator internus	Nerve to the quadratus femoris (L5, S1)	Laterally rotates the extended thigh and abducts the flexed thigh
Quadratus femoris	Lateral border of the ischial tuberosity	Quadrate tubercle on the posterior surface of the femur; also onto the intertrochanteric crest of the femur	Nerve to the quadratus femoris (L5, S1)	Laterally rotates the thigh

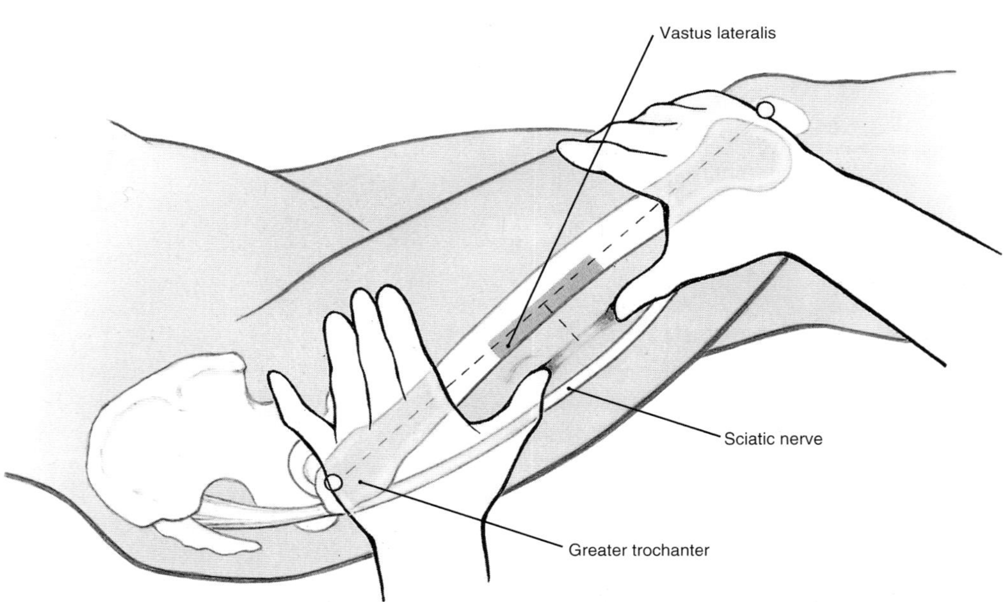
Vastus lateralis
Sciatic nerve
Greater trochanter

Figure 388 Intramuscular Injection into the Middle of the Lateral Thigh

NOTE: (1) The lateral thigh is a relatively safe site for intramuscular injections, since there exist only small branches of the lateral femoral cutaneous nerve and femoral artery in this region of the vastus lateralis muscle.

(2) Become oriented as to the position of the femur. Insert the needle toward the bone within the belly of the vastus lateralis muscle.

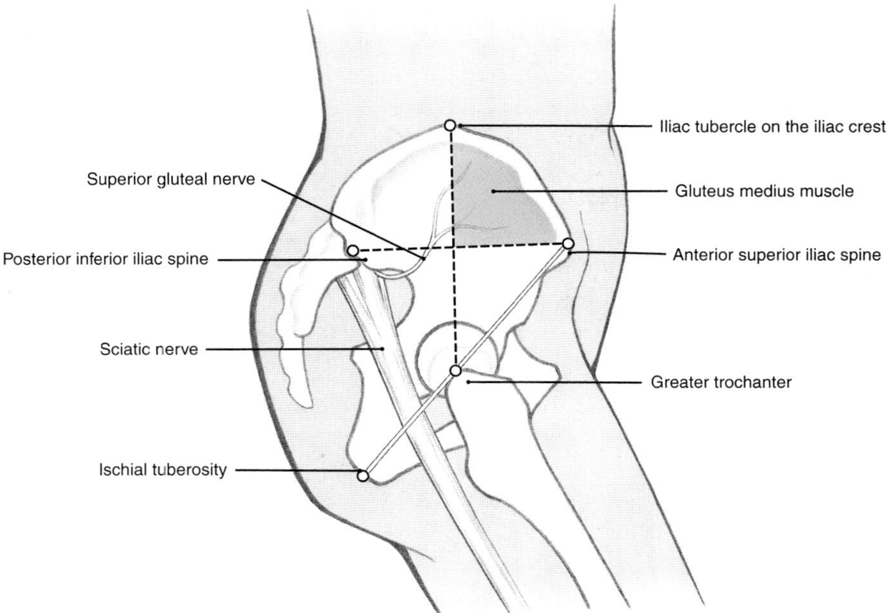
Iliac tubercle on the iliac crest
Superior gluteal nerve
Gluteus medius muscle
Posterior inferior iliac spine
Anterior superior iliac spine
Sciatic nerve
Greater trochanter
Ischial tuberosity

Figure 389.1 Safe Quadrant for Injections into the Gluteal Region

NOTE: In this figure the four quadrants of the gluteal region are determined by a **transverse line** between the **anterior superior iliac spine** anteriorly and the **posterior inferior iliac spine** posteriorly that intersects a **vertical line** between the **greater trochanter** inferiorly and the **iliac crest** superiorly. The colored upper lateral quadrant is the safe zone for intramuscular injection.

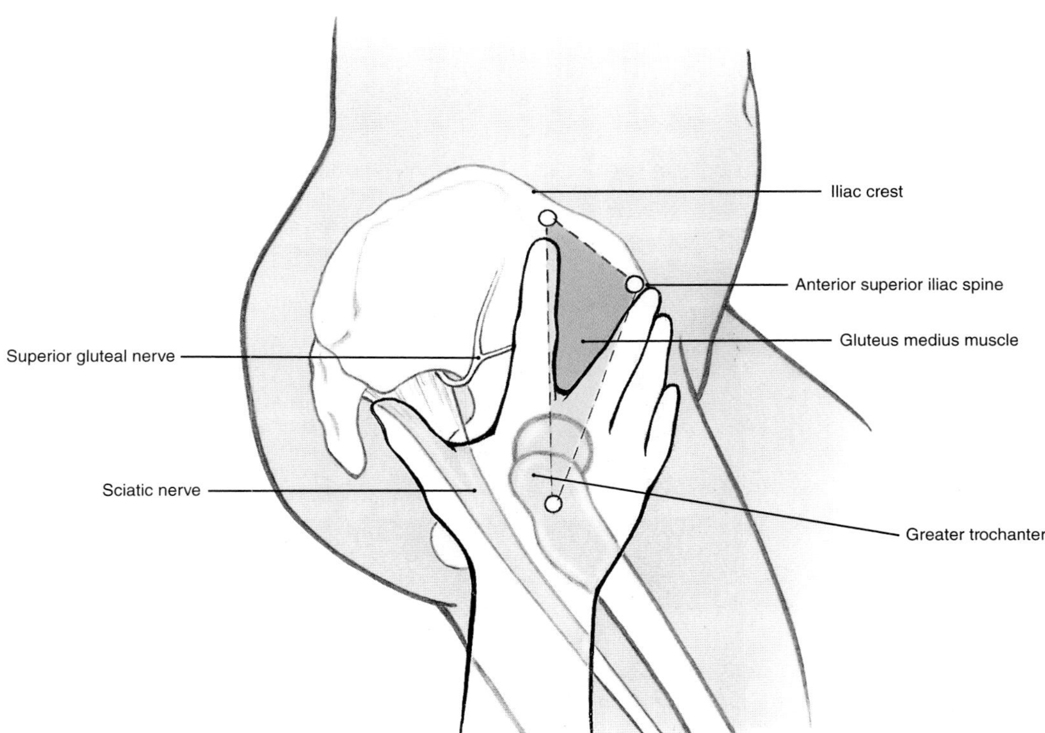
Iliac crest
Anterior superior iliac spine
Gluteus medius muscle
Superior gluteal nerve
Sciatic nerve
Greater trochanter

Figure 389.2 Quick Method of Determining the Safe Zone for Intramuscular Gluteal Injection

NOTE: The safe zone can be visualized quickly by:

(1) Placing the palm of the right hand over the right greater trochanter (or left hand over the left greater trochanter),

(2) Directing the index finger vertically to the iliac crest and spreading the middle finger to the anterior superior iliac spine,

(3) The colored region shown in this diagram between the index and middle fingers is the safe zone and avoids the superior gluteal vessels and nerve as well as the sciatic nerve and other important gluteal structures.

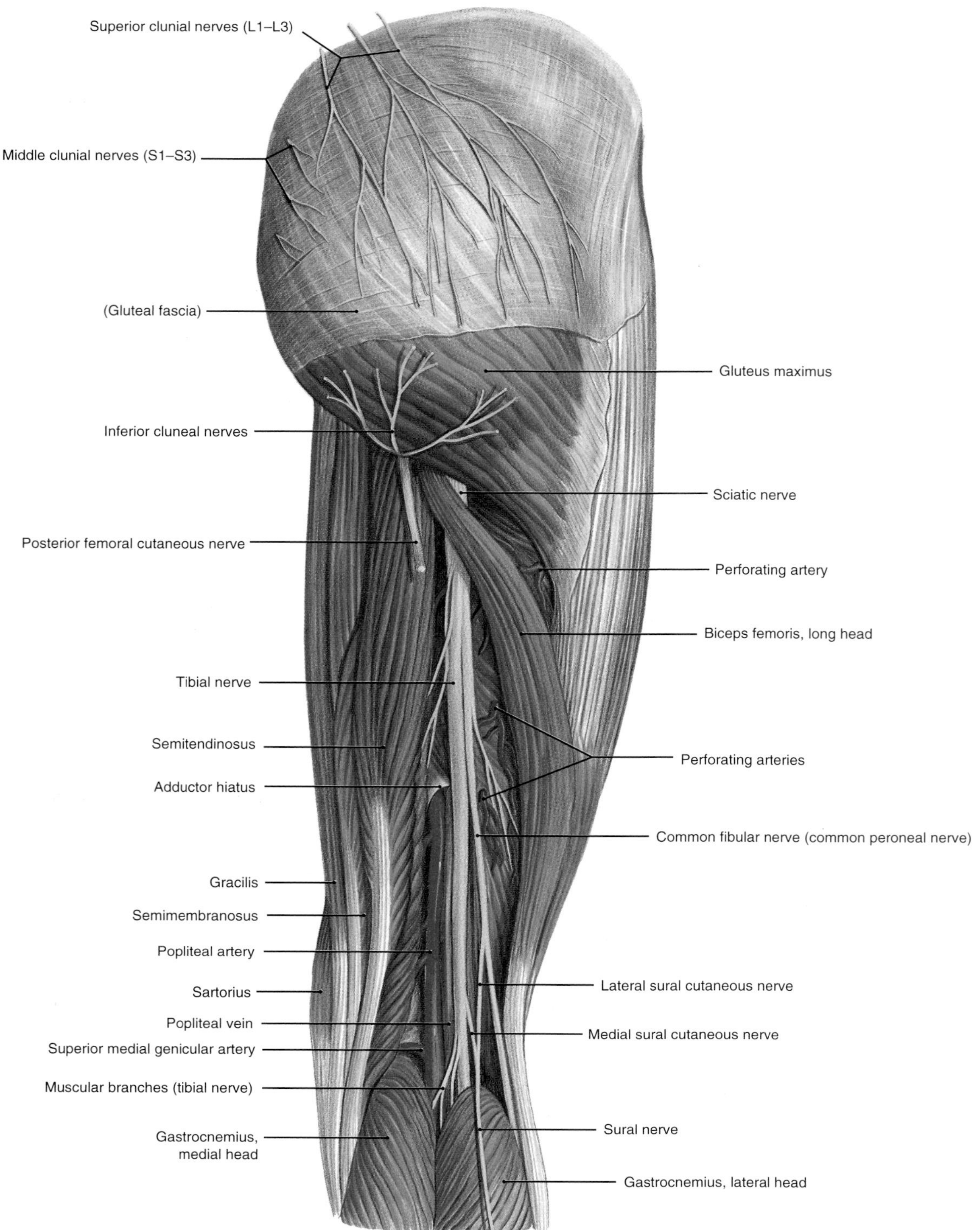
Superior clunial nerves (L1–L3)
Middle clunial nerves (S1–S3)
(Gluteal fascia)
Gluteus maximus
Inferior cluneal nerves
Sciatic nerve
Posterior femoral cutaneous nerve
Perforating artery
Biceps femoris, long head
Tibial nerve
Semitendinosus
Perforating arteries
Adductor hiatus
Common fibular nerve (common peroneal nerve)
Gracilis
Semimembranosus
Popliteal artery
Lateral sural cutaneous nerve
Sartorius
Popliteal vein
Medial sural cutaneous nerve
Superior medial genicular artery
Muscular branches (tibial nerve)
Sural nerve
Gastrocnemius, medial head
Gastrocnemius, lateral head

Figure 390 **Descent of the Sciatic Nerve from the Gluteus Maximus to the Popliteal Fossa; the Popliteal Vessels**

POSTERIOR THIGH MUSCLES

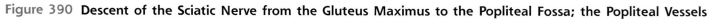

Muscle	Origin	Insertion	Innervation	Function
Biceps femoris	Long head: Ischial tuberosity in common with other hamstring muscles. Short head: Lateral lip of the linea aspera of the femur.	Lateral surface of the head of the fibula and a small slip to lateral condyle of tibia	Long head: Tibial part of sciatic nerve (S1, S2, S3). Short head: Peroneal part of the sciatic nerve (L5, S1, S2).	Flexes the leg and rotates the tibia laterally; long head also extends the thigh at the hip joint
Semitendinosus	Ischial tuberosity in common with other hamstring muscles	Medial surface of the upper part of the body of the tibia	Tibial part of the sciatic nerve (L5, S1, S2)	Flexes the leg and rotates the tibia medially; extends the thigh
Semimembranosus	Ischial tuberosity in common with other hamstring muscles	Posterior aspect of the medial condyle of the tibia	Tibial part of the sciatic nerve (L5, S1, S2)	Flexes the leg and rotates it medially; extends the thigh

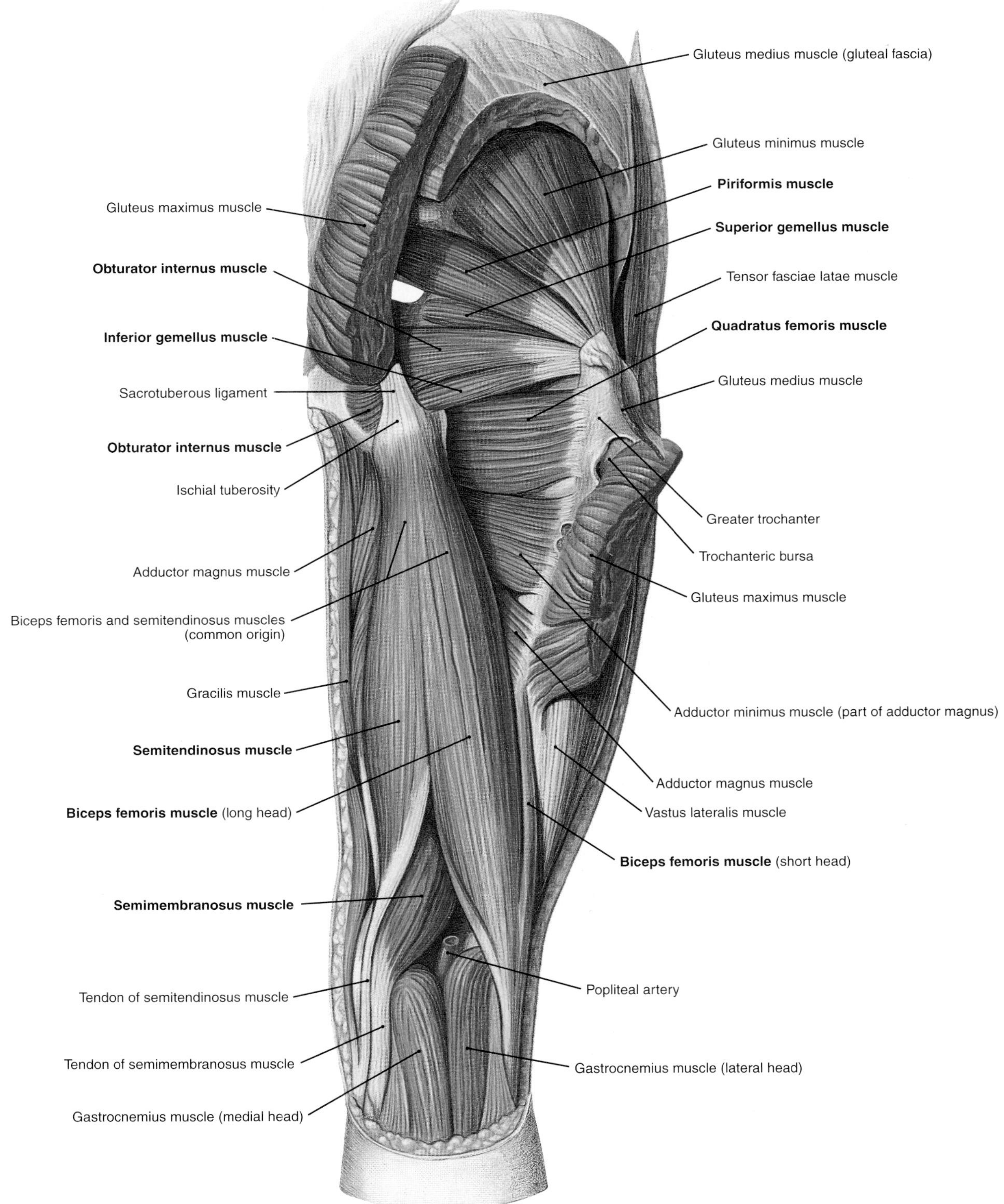
Gluteus medius muscle (gluteal fascia)
Gluteus minimus muscle
Piriformis muscle
Superior gemellus muscle
Tensor fasciae latae muscle
Quadratus femoris muscle
Gluteus medius muscle
Gluteus maximus muscle
Obturator internus muscle
Inferior gemellus muscle
Sacrotuberous ligament
Obturator internus muscle
Ischial tuberosity
Greater trochanter
Trochanteric bursa
Gluteus maximus muscle
Adductor magnus muscle
Biceps femoris and semitendinosus muscles (common origin)
Gracilis muscle
Adductor minimus muscle (part of adductor magnus)
Semitendinosus muscle
Biceps femoris muscle (long head)
Adductor magnus muscle
Vastus lateralis muscle
Biceps femoris muscle (short head)
Semimembranosus muscle
Popliteal artery
Tendon of semitendinosus muscle
Tendon of semimembranosus muscle
Gastrocnemius muscle (lateral head)
Gastrocnemius muscle (medial head)

Figure 391 Hamstring Muscles of Posterior Thigh and Deep Muscles of Gluteal Region

NOTE: (1) For a muscle to be considered a **hamstring muscle**, it must:

(a) arise from the **ischial tuberosity**,

(b) receive innervation from the **tibial division of the sciatic nerve**, and

(c) cross **both** the hip and knee joints.

(2) The long head of the biceps is a hamstring, but the short head is not, because it arises from the femur and is supplied by the common fibular division of the sciatic nerve.

(3) The **ischiocondylar part** of the adductor magnus meets two criteria as a hamstring, but only crosses the hip joint. Its insertion, however, on the adductor tubercle is embryologically continuous with the tibial collateral ligament, which does attach below on the tibia.

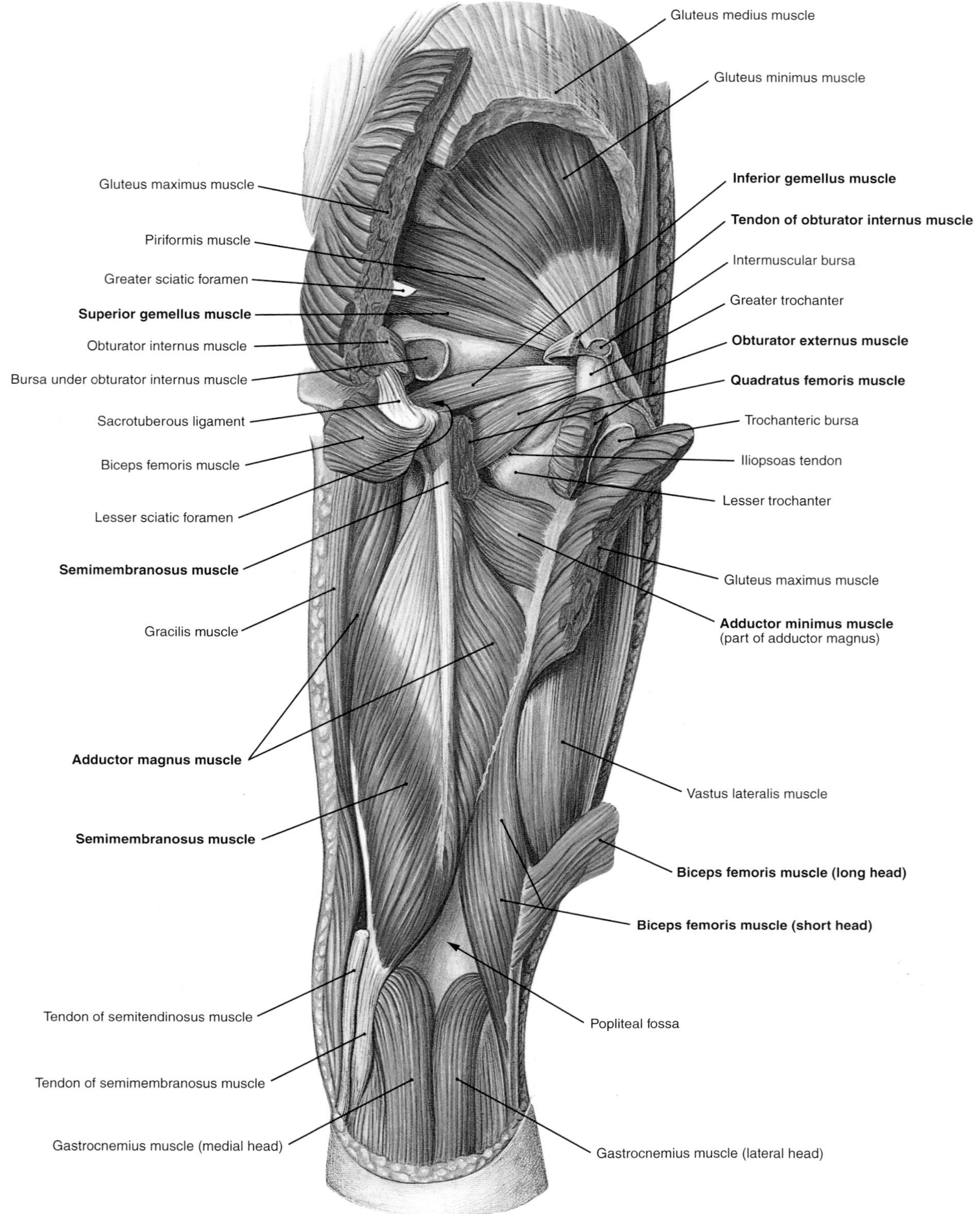
Gluteus medius muscle
Gluteus minimus muscle
Gluteus maximus muscle
Inferior gemellus muscle
Tendon of obturator internus muscle
Piriformis muscle
Intermuscular bursa
Greater sciatic foramen
Greater trochanter
Superior gemellus muscle
Obturator externus muscle
Obturator internus muscle
Bursa under obturator internus muscle
Quadratus femoris muscle
Sacrotuberous ligament
Trochanteric bursa
Biceps femoris muscle
Iliopsoas tendon
Lesser trochanter
Lesser sciatic foramen
Semimembranosus muscle
Gluteus maximus muscle
Adductor minimus muscle
(part of adductor magnus)
Gracilis muscle
Adductor magnus muscle
Vastus lateralis muscle
Semimembranosus muscle
Biceps femoris muscle (long head)
Biceps femoris muscle (short head)
Tendon of semitendinosus muscle
Popliteal fossa
Tendon of semimembranosus muscle
Gastrocnemius muscle (medial head)
Gastrocnemius muscle (lateral head)

Figure 392 Hamstring Muscles of Posterior Thigh (Deep Dissection) and Deep Gluteal Muscles

NOTE: (1) The common tendon of the long head of the biceps femoris and semitendinosus muscles has been cut in the thigh close to the ischial tuberosity. This exposes the origin of the **semimembranosus muscle,** the breadth of the **adductor magnus muscle,** and the **short head of the biceps femoris muscle.**

(2) The **short head of the biceps femoris muscle** arising from the lateral lip of the linea aspera of the femur, between the attachments of the vastus lateralis and the adductor magnus muscles. It descends to join the tendon of the long head before insertion.

(3) In the gluteal region, the quadratus femoris muscle has been severed and reflected, thereby revealing the **obturator externus muscle** beneath. Also, the tendon of the obturator internus muscle has been cut (between the gemelli) exposing the bursa deep to that tendon.

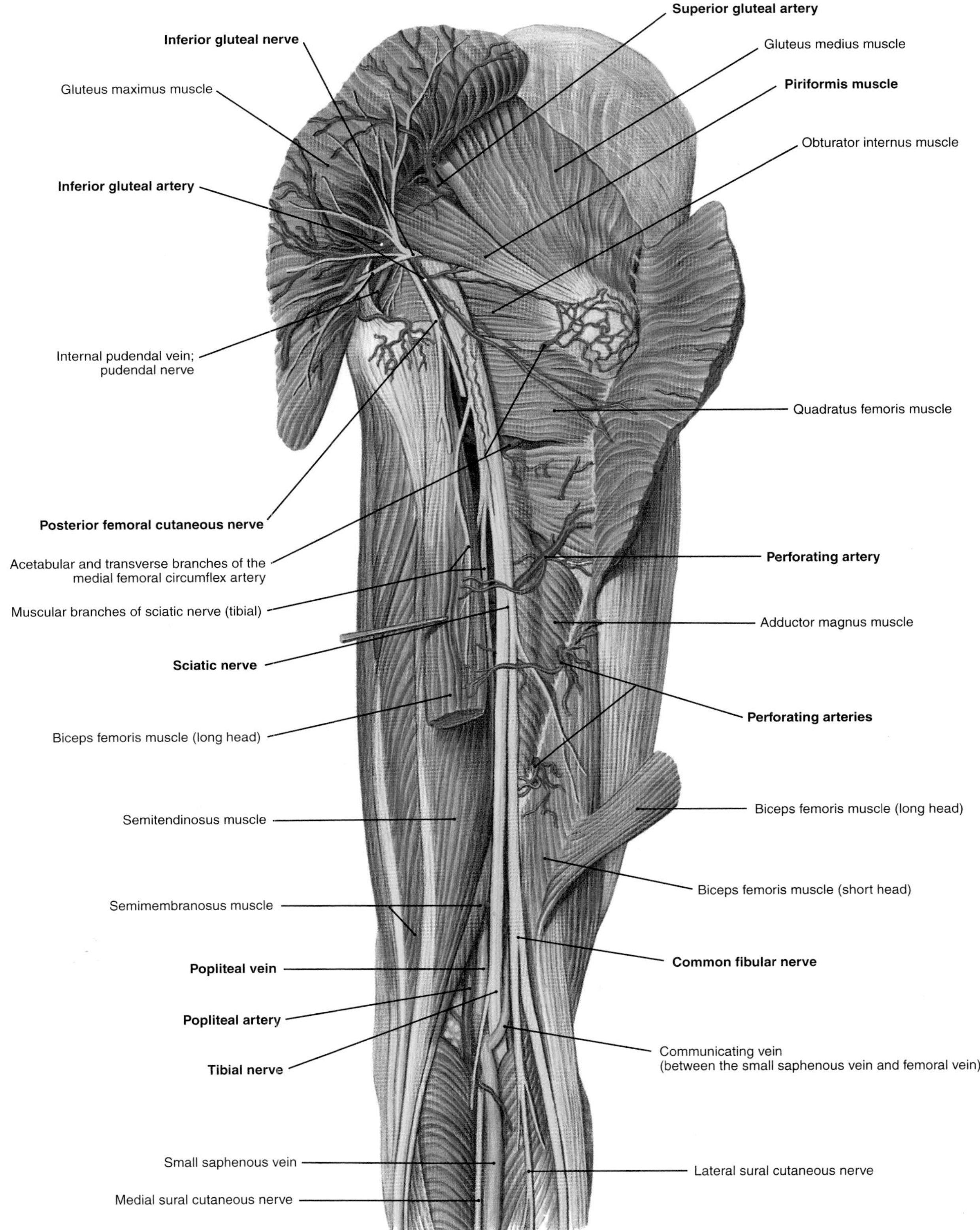
Superior gluteal artery
Inferior gluteal nerve
Gluteus medius muscle
Gluteus maximus muscle
Piriformis muscle
Obturator internus muscle
Inferior gluteal artery
Internal pudendal vein; pudendal nerve
Quadratus femoris muscle
Posterior femoral cutaneous nerve
Perforating artery
Acetabular and transverse branches of the medial femoral circumflex artery
Muscular branches of sciatic nerve (tibial)
Adductor magnus muscle
Sciatic nerve
Perforating arteries
Biceps femoris muscle (long head)
Biceps femoris muscle (long head)
Semitendinosus muscle
Biceps femoris muscle (short head)
Semimembranosus muscle
Common fibular nerve
Popliteal vein
Popliteal artery
Communicating vein
(between the small saphenous vein and femoral vein)
Tibial nerve
Small saphenous vein
Lateral sural cutaneous nerve
Medial sural cutaneous nerve

Figure 393 Vessels and Nerves of the Posterior Thigh and Gluteal Region (Deep Dissection)

NOTE: (1) The course of the **sciatic nerve** as it passes through the greater sciatic foramen in the gluteal region, inferior to the piriformis muscle, lateral to the ischial tuberosity and under cover of the gluteus maximus muscle. It enters the thigh nearly midway between the ischial tuberosity and the greater trochanter.

(2) The **superior and inferior gluteal arteries** and the **posterior femoral cutaneous nerve** in the gluteal region. In the thigh, observe the **perforating arteries**, branches of the **deep femoral artery**, and the fact that the sciatic nerve splits to become the **tibial and common fibular nerves.**

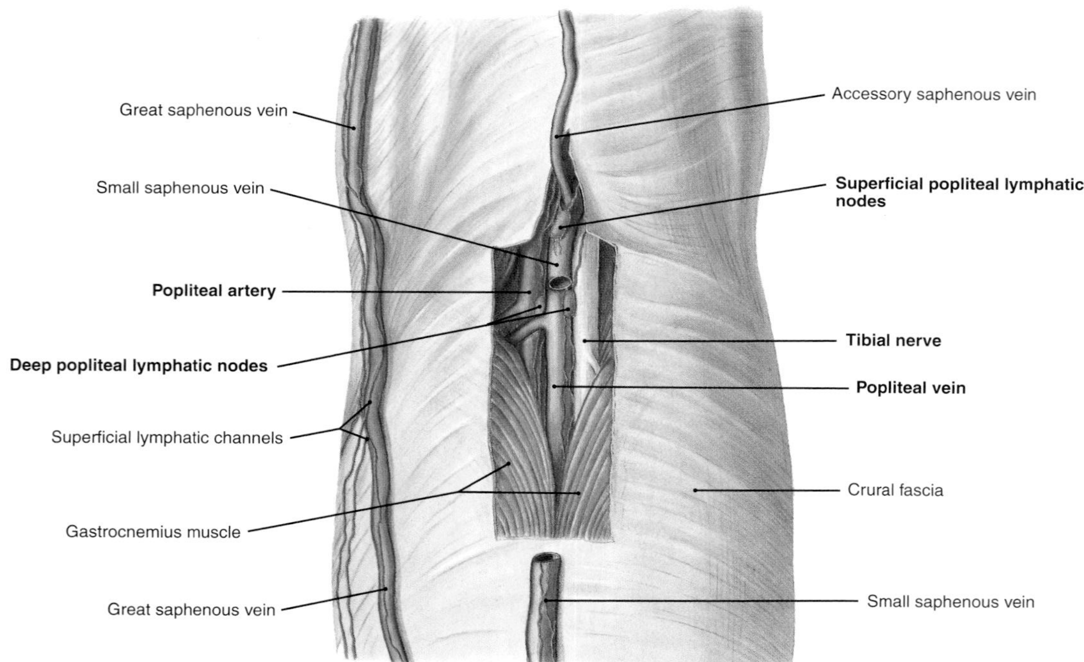
Great saphenous vein
Small saphenous vein
Popliteal artery
Deep popliteal lymphatic nodes
Superficial lymphatic channels
Gastrocnemius muscle
Great saphenous vein
Accessory saphenous vein
Superficial popliteal lymphatic nodes
Tibial nerve
Popliteal vein
Crural fascia
Small saphenous vein

Figure 394.1 Subcutaneous Dissection of the Popliteal Fossa

NOTE: The skin and crural fascia have been removed over the popliteal fossa and a part of the small saphenous vein has been resected. Observe the popliteal vessels and nerves and the **popliteal lymphatic nodes** and **channels** deeper in the fossa.

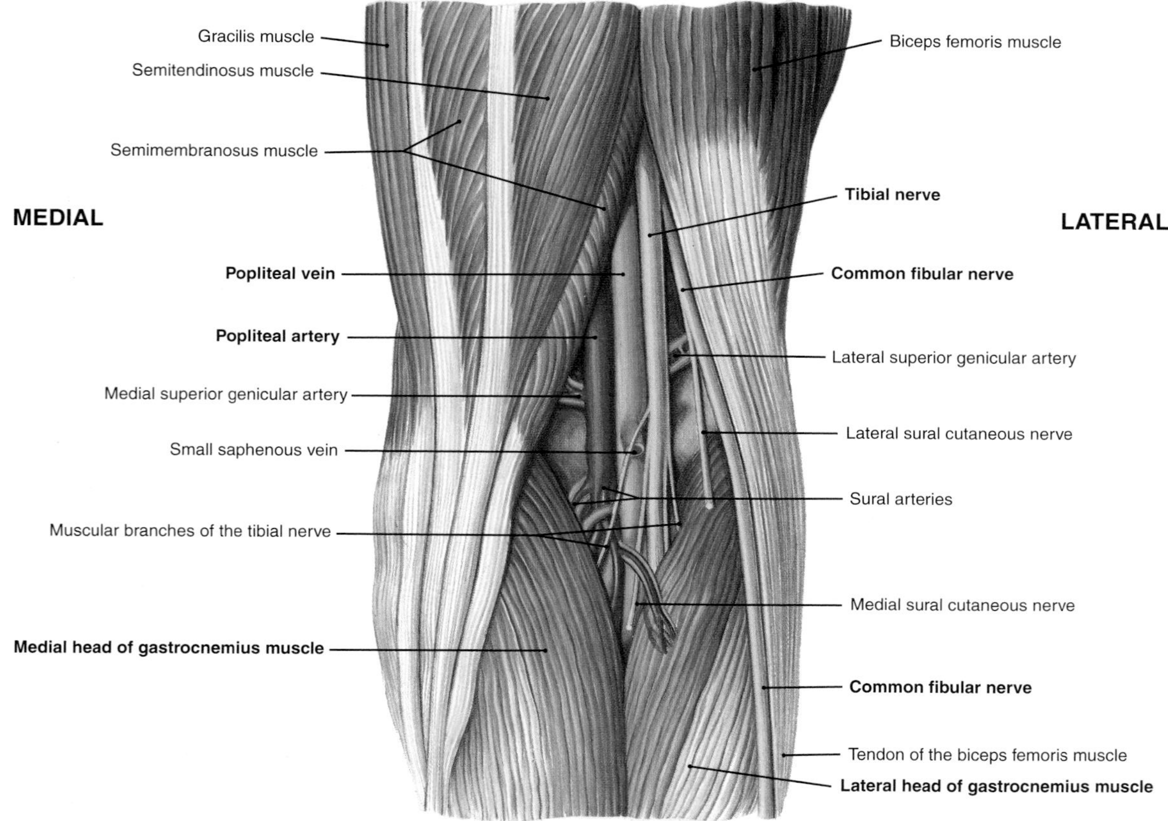
Gracilis muscle
Semitendinosus muscle
Semimembranosus muscle
MEDIAL
Popliteal vein
Popliteal artery
Medial superior genicular artery
Small saphenous vein
Muscular branches of the tibial nerve
Medial head of gastrocnemius muscle
Biceps femoris muscle
Tibial nerve
LATERAL
Common fibular nerve
Lateral superior genicular artery
Lateral sural cutaneous nerve
Sural arteries
Medial sural cutaneous nerve
Common fibular nerve
Tendon of the biceps femoris muscle
Lateral head of gastrocnemius muscle

Figure 394.2 Nerves and Vessels of the Popliteal Fossa (Superficial View)

NOTE: (1) The relationships of the **popliteal vessels** and **nerve** within the popliteal fossa. The **sciatic nerve** has already divided into the laterally directed **common fibular nerve** and the **tibial nerve,** which continues directly into the calf. Both the common fibular and the tibial nerves lie superficial to the vessels in the popliteal fossa.

(2) The popliteal vein is located between the tibial nerve and popliteal artery, while the artery is the deepest (most anterior) and most medial of three structures.

(3) The two muscular branches of the tibial nerve innervating the two heads of the gastrocnemius muscle, and a descending sensory branch, the **medial sural cutaneous nerve,** to the calf. Also note the **lateral sural cutaneous nerve** from the common fibular nerve.

(4) The popliteal fossa is about 2.5 cm (1 in.) wide at its maximum, and in the undissected specimen, the fossa is filled with fat, and the vessels and nerves are initially difficult to see.

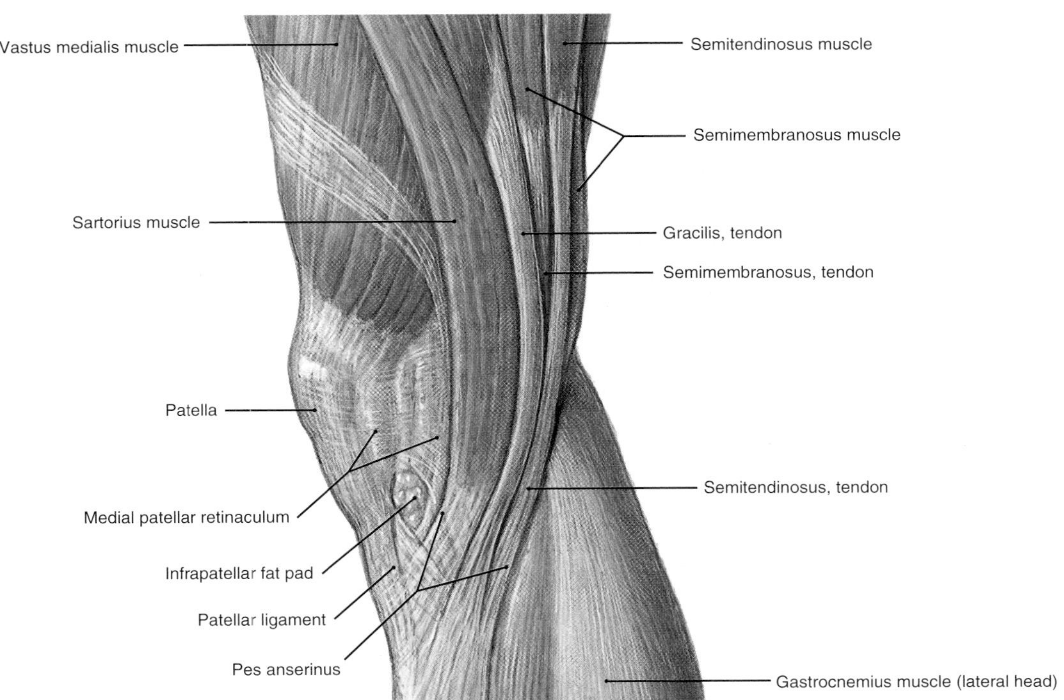
Vastus medialis muscle
Semitendinosus muscle
Semimembranosus muscle
Sartorius muscle
Gracilis, tendon
Semimembranosus, tendon
Patella
Semitendinosus, tendon
Medial patellar retinaculum
Infrapatellar fat pad
Patellar ligament
Pes anserinus
Gastrocnemius muscle (lateral head)

Figure 395.1 Medial Surface of the Knee Region

NOTE: The tendons of the sartorius, gracilis, and semitendinosus form the so-called pes anserinus (goose's foot). This formation of tendons strengthens the medial aspect of the knee joint.

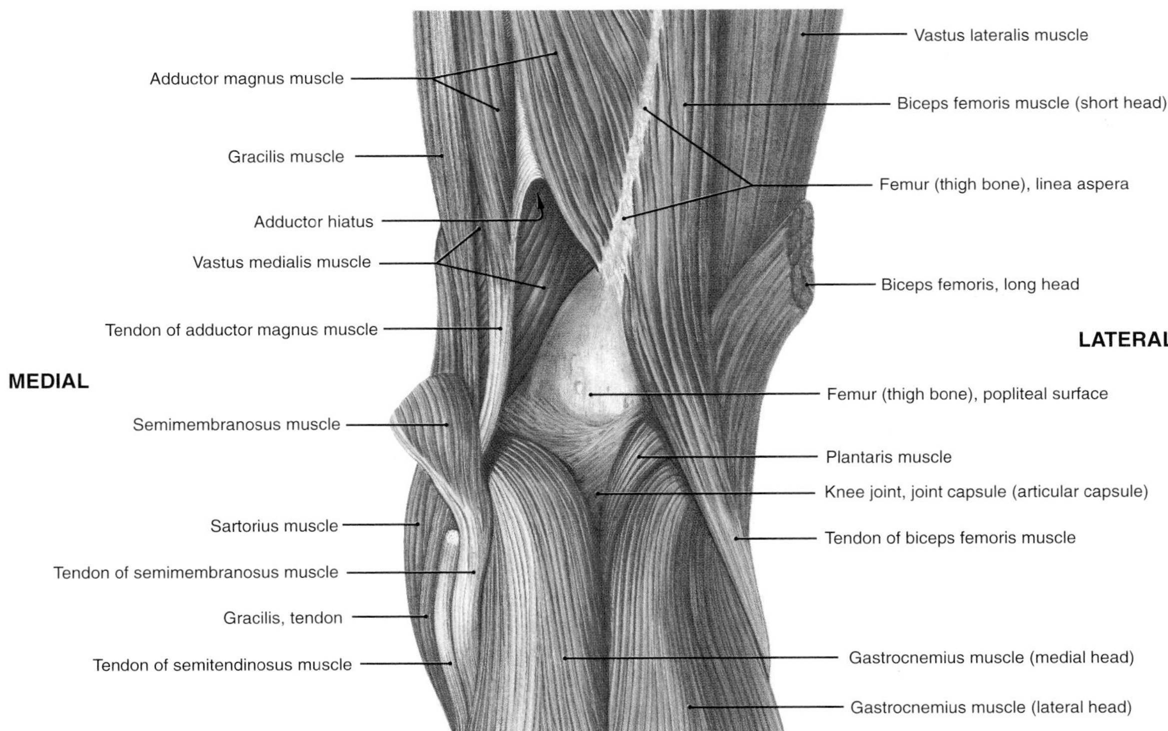
Vastus lateralis muscle
Adductor magnus muscle
Biceps femoris muscle (short head)
Gracilis muscle
Femur (thigh bone), linea aspera
Adductor hiatus
Vastus medialis muscle
Biceps femoris, long head
Tendon of adductor magnus muscle
LATERAL
MEDIAL
Femur (thigh bone), popliteal surface
Semimembranosus muscle
Plantaris muscle
Knee joint, joint capsule (articular capsule)
Sartorius muscle
Tendon of biceps femoris muscle
Tendon of semimembranosus muscle
Gracilis, tendon
Tendon of semitendinosus muscle
Gastrocnemius muscle (medial head)
Gastrocnemius muscle (lateral head)

Figure 395.2 Deep Muscles That Bound the Popliteal Fossa

NOTE: (1) The **popliteal fossa** is a diamond-shaped space behind the knee joint. Its *superior boundaries* are the **long head of the biceps femoris muscle** laterally and the **semimembranosus** and **semitendinosus muscles** medially (see Fig. 394.2). All three of these muscles have been cut in this dissection, exposing the more deeply located **adductor magnus** and **vastus medialis** medially and the **short head of the biceps femoris** laterally.

(2) The *inferior boundaries* of the fossa are the **medial** and **lateral heads of the gastrocnemius muscle,** which arise from the medial and lateral condyles of the femur.

(3) The inferior opening of the **adductor canal** (the adductor hiatus), which transmits the **femoral artery** and **vein** from and to the anterior aspect of the thigh.

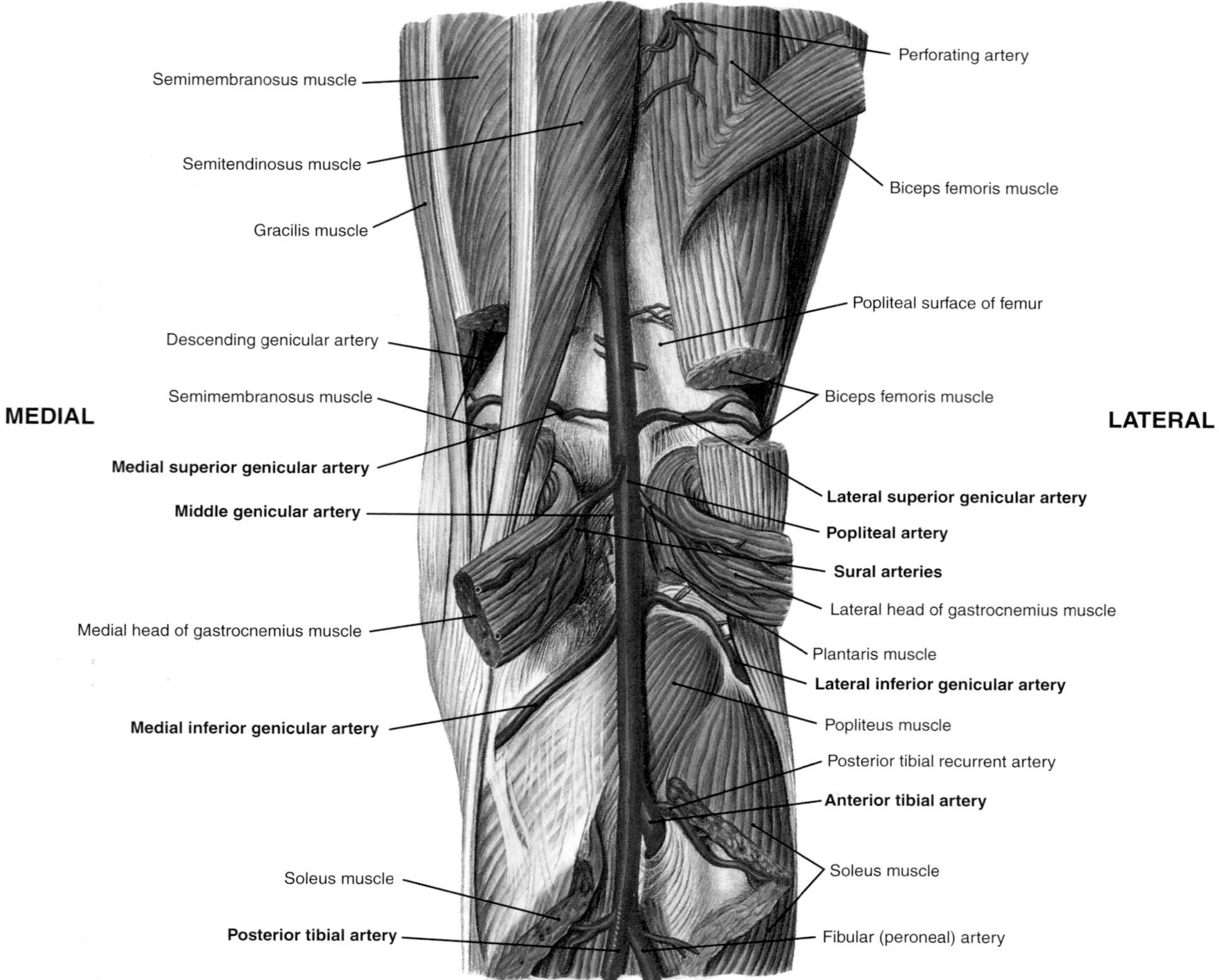

Semimembranosus muscle
Semitendinosus muscle
Gracilis muscle
Descending genicular artery
Semimembranosus muscle
MEDIAL
Medial superior genicular artery
Middle genicular artery
Medial head of gastrocnemius muscle
Medial inferior genicular artery
Soleus muscle
Posterior tibial artery
Perforating artery
Biceps femoris muscle
Popliteal surface of femur
Biceps femoris muscle
LATERAL
Lateral superior genicular artery
Popliteal artery
Sural arteries
Lateral head of gastrocnemius muscle
Plantaris muscle
Lateral inferior genicular artery
Popliteus muscle
Posterior tibial recurrent artery
Anterior tibial artery
Soleus muscle
Fibular (peroneal) artery

Figure 396.1 Branches of the Popliteal Artery

NOTE: (1) Within the popliteal fossa, the popliteal artery most frequently gives rise to two **superior (lateral and medial) genicular,** one **middle genicular,** and two **inferior (lateral and medial) genicular arteries.**

(2) The **popliteal artery** bifurcates into the **posterior tibial** and the **anterior tibial.** The latter penetrates an aperture above the interosseous membrane to reach the anterior compartment. Somewhat lower, the **fibular artery** branches from the posterior tibial. The pattern shown here occurs in about **90% of cases.** Variations in this pattern are shown in Figure 396.2.

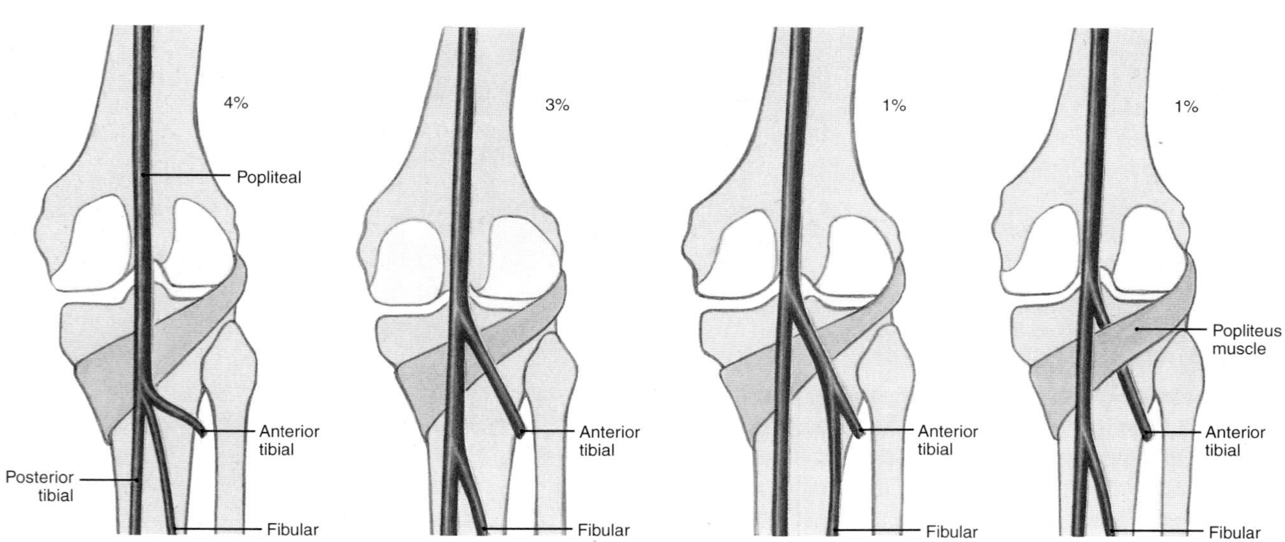

4%
Popliteal
Anterior tibial
Posterior tibial
Fibular
3%
Anterior tibial
Fibular
1%
Anterior tibial
Fibular
1%
Popliteus muscle
Anterior tibial
Fibular

Figure 396.2 Variations in the Branching Pattern of the Anterior Tibial and Fibular Arteries

See NOTE 2 under Figure 396.1

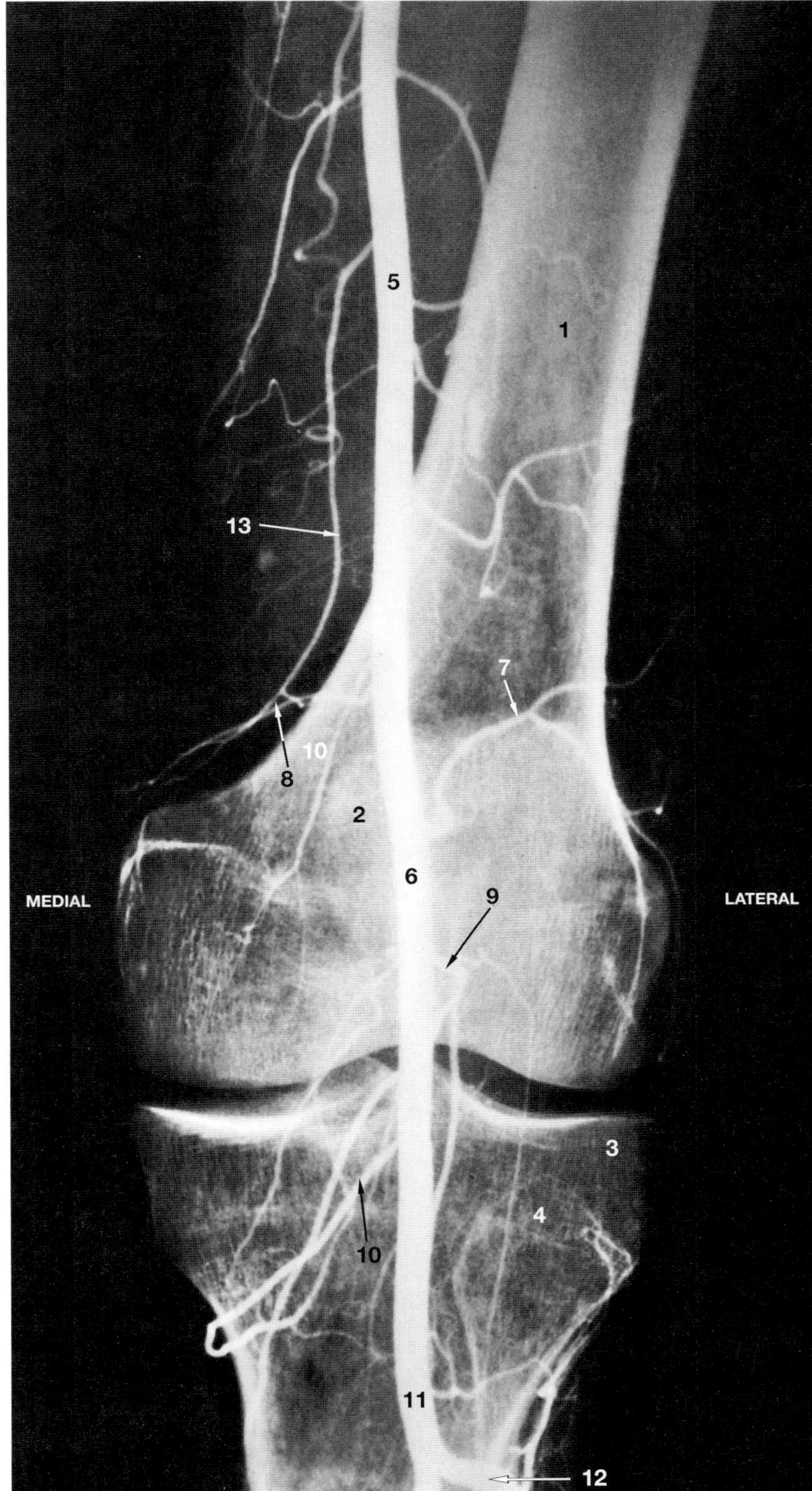
5
1
13
7
10
8
2
6
MEDIAL
9
LATERAL
3
4
10
11
12

1. Femur
2. Patella
3. Tibia
4. Head of fibula
5. Femoral artery
6. Popliteal artery
7. Lateral superior genicular artery
8. Medial superior genicular artery
9. Middle genicular artery
10. Inferior genicular artery
11. Popliteal artery
12. Anterior tibial artery
13. Descending genicular artery

Figure 397 Arteriogram of the Left Femoral–Popliteal–Tibial Arterial Tree (Anteroposterior Projection)

NOTE: (1) This arteriogram shows the branches from the femoral, popliteal, and tibial arteries in the lower third of the thigh and the upper part of the calf. Observe the following bony structures: **femur** (1), **patella** (2), **tibia** (3), and **fibula** (4).

(2) The course of the **femoral artery** (5) as it becomes the **popliteal artery** (6) just above the popliteal fossa. Observe the following branches from the popliteal artery: **superior genicular** (7, 8), **middle genicular** (9), and single **inferior genicular** (10) in this patient.

(3) Below the popliteal fossa the **popliteal artery** (11) can be seen giving off the **anterior and posterior tibial arteries** just above the lower edge of the angiogram.

(4) The **descending genicular artery** (13), a branch of the femoral above the popliteal fossa, as it courses downward to participate in the anastomosis around the knee joint.

(From Wicke, 6th ed.)

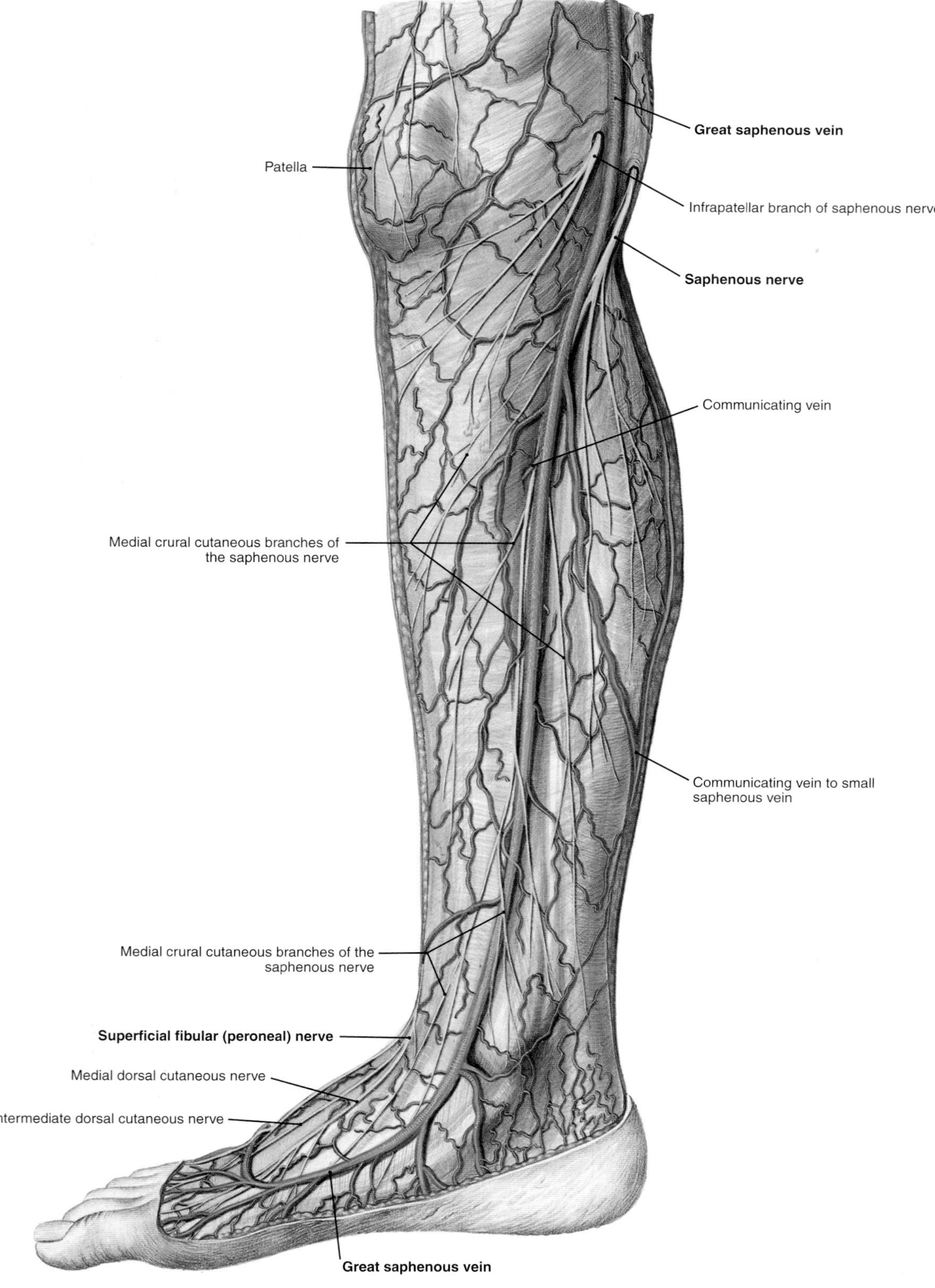
Great saphenous vein
Patella
Infrapatellar branch of saphenous nerve
Saphenous nerve
Communicating vein
Medial crural cutaneous branches of the saphenous nerve
Communicating vein to small saphenous vein
Medial crural cutaneous branches of the saphenous nerve
Superficial fibular (peroneal) nerve
Medial dorsal cutaneous nerve
Intermediate dorsal cutaneous nerve
Great saphenous vein

Figure 398 Superficial Veins and Nerves on the Anterior and Medial Aspects of the Leg and Foot

NOTE: (1) The **great saphenous vein** is formed on the medial aspect of the foot, courses anterior to the medial malleolus, and ascends along the medial side of the leg.

(2) Branches of the **saphenous nerve** accompany the great saphenous vein below the knee. This nerve becomes superficial medially just below the knee and is the largest branch of the femoral nerve. It functions as the sensory nerve that supplies the skin over most of the medial half of the leg region (i.e., between the knee and ankle).

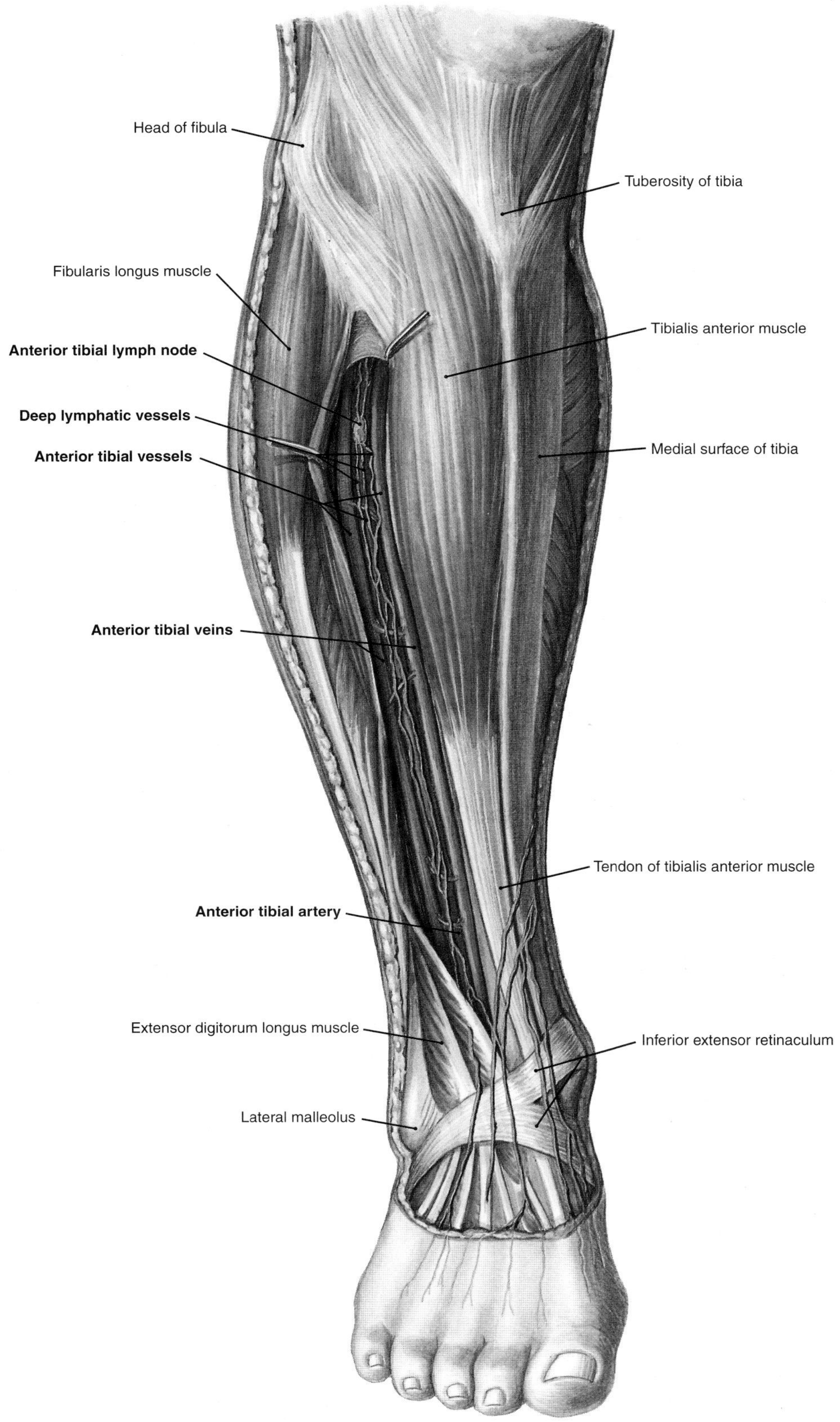
Head of fibula
Tuberosity of tibia
Fibularis longus muscle
Tibialis anterior muscle
Anterior tibial lymph node
Deep lymphatic vessels
Medial surface of tibia
Anterior tibial vessels
Anterior tibial veins
Tendon of tibialis anterior muscle
Anterior tibial artery
Extensor digitorum longus muscle
Inferior extensor retinaculum
Lateral malleolus

Figure 401 Anterior Tibial Vessels and Lymphatic Channels in the Anterior Compartment

NOTE: (1) By separating the **tibialis anterior muscle** from the other muscles in the anterior compartment, the **anterior tibial artery** is exposed descending in the anterior compartment to the dorsum of the foot.

(2) The artery is accompanied by a pair of **anterior tibial veins (venae comitantes)**, which ascend to join the posterior tibial vein posteriorly to help form the popliteal vein.

(3) Lymphatic channels from the dorsum of the foot course superiorly along the path of these vessels, and at times a lymph node can be found just below the knee.

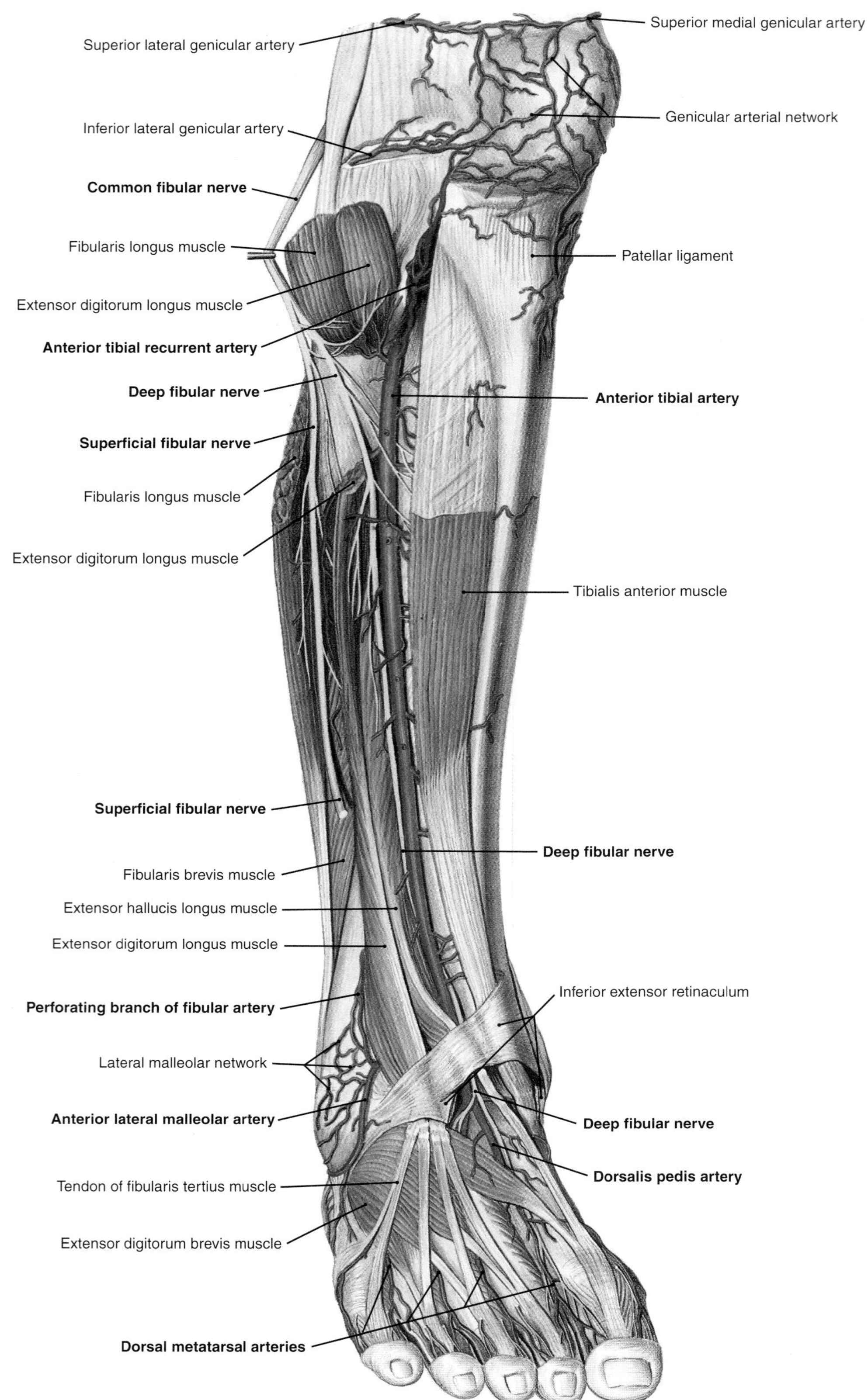
Superior lateral genicular artery
Superior medial genicular artery
Genicular arterial network
Inferior lateral genicular artery
Common fibular nerve
Fibularis longus muscle
Patellar ligament
Extensor digitorum longus muscle
Anterior tibial recurrent artery
Deep fibular nerve
Anterior tibial artery
Superficial fibular nerve
Fibularis longus muscle
Extensor digitorum longus muscle
Tibialis anterior muscle
Superficial fibular nerve
Deep fibular nerve
Fibularis brevis muscle
Extensor hallucis longus muscle
Extensor digitorum longus muscle
Inferior extensor retinaculum
Perforating branch of fibular artery
Lateral malleolar network
Anterior lateral malleolar artery
Deep fibular nerve
Dorsalis pedis artery
Tendon of fibularis tertius muscle
Extensor digitorum brevis muscle
Dorsal metatarsal arteries

Figure 402 Deep Dissection of the Anterior and Lateral Compartments: Nerves and Arteries

NOTE: (1) As the **common fibular nerve** courses laterally around the head of the fibula, it divides into the **superficial** and **deep fibular nerves,** which innervate the muscles of the lateral and anterior compartments.

(2) The deep fibular nerve is joined by the **anterior tibial artery**, which descends toward the foot, where it becomes the **dorsalis pedis artery.**

(3) The superficial fibular nerve becomes cutaneous about 7 inches above the lateral malleolus, while the deep fibular nerve becomes cutaneous between the large and second toes.

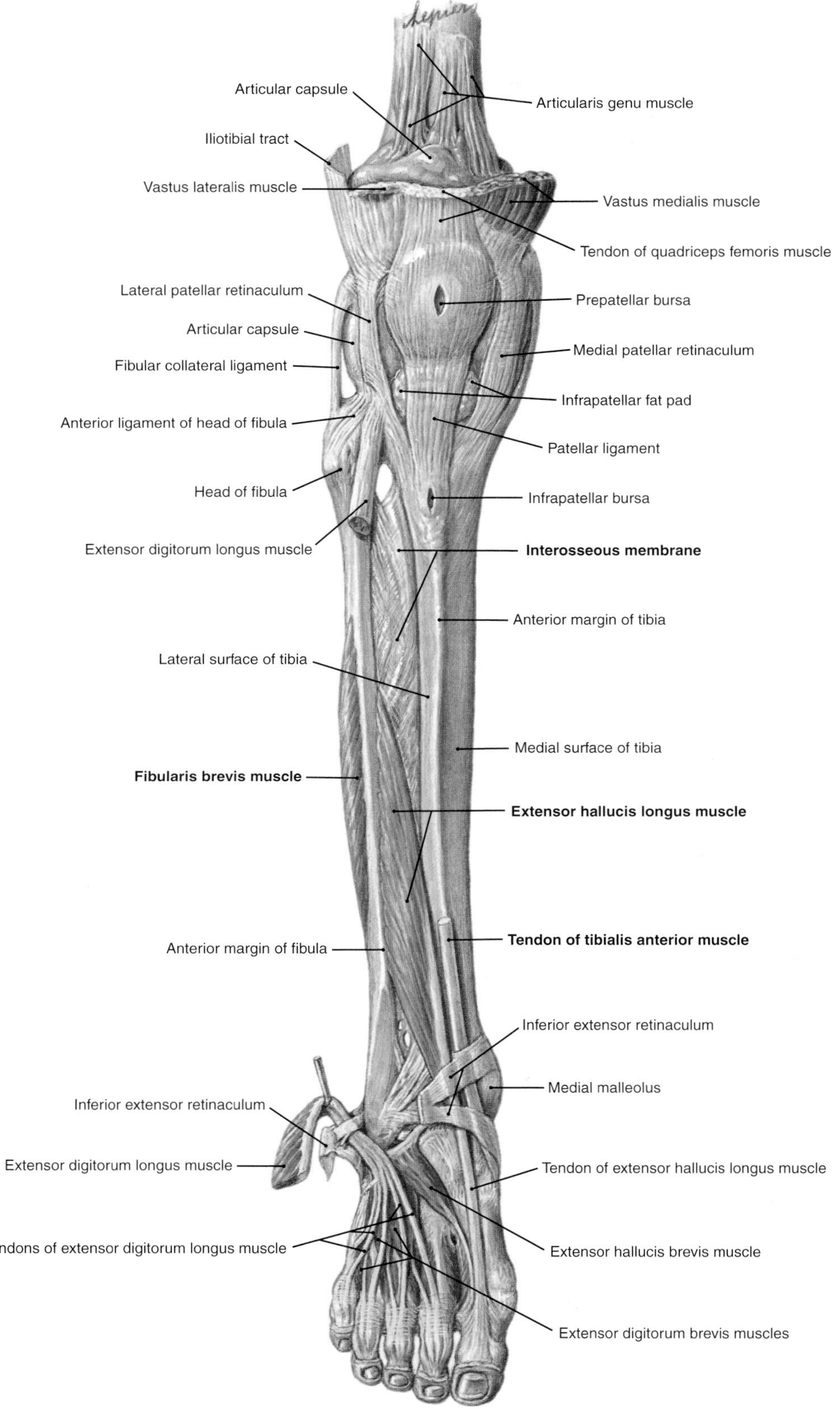
Articular capsule
Iliotibial tract
Vastus lateralis muscle
Lateral patellar retinaculum
Articular capsule
Fibular collateral ligament
Anterior ligament of head of fibula
Head of fibula
Extensor digitorum longus muscle
Lateral surface of tibia
Fibularis brevis muscle
Anterior margin of fibula
Inferior extensor retinaculum
Extensor digitorum longus muscle
Tendons of extensor digitorum longus muscle
Articularis genu muscle
Vastus medialis muscle
Tendon of quadriceps femoris muscle
Prepatellar bursa
Medial patellar retinaculum
Infrapatellar fat pad
Patellar ligament
Infrapatellar bursa
Interosseous membrane
Anterior margin of tibia
Medial surface of tibia
Extensor hallucis longus muscle
Tendon of tibialis anterior muscle
Inferior extensor retinaculum
Medial malleolus
Tendon of extensor hallucis longus muscle
Extensor hallucis brevis muscle
Extensor digitorum brevis muscles

Figure 403 Deep Dissection of the Anterior and Lateral Compartments: Muscles

NOTE: (1) The bellies of the tibialis anterior and fibularis longus muscles have been removed and the extensor digitorum longus muscle has been reflected. Observe the full extent of the **extensor hallucis longus** and the belly of the **fibularis brevis muscle.**

(2) The interosseous membrane between the tibia and the fibula and the opening above its upper border through which course the anterior tibial vessels.

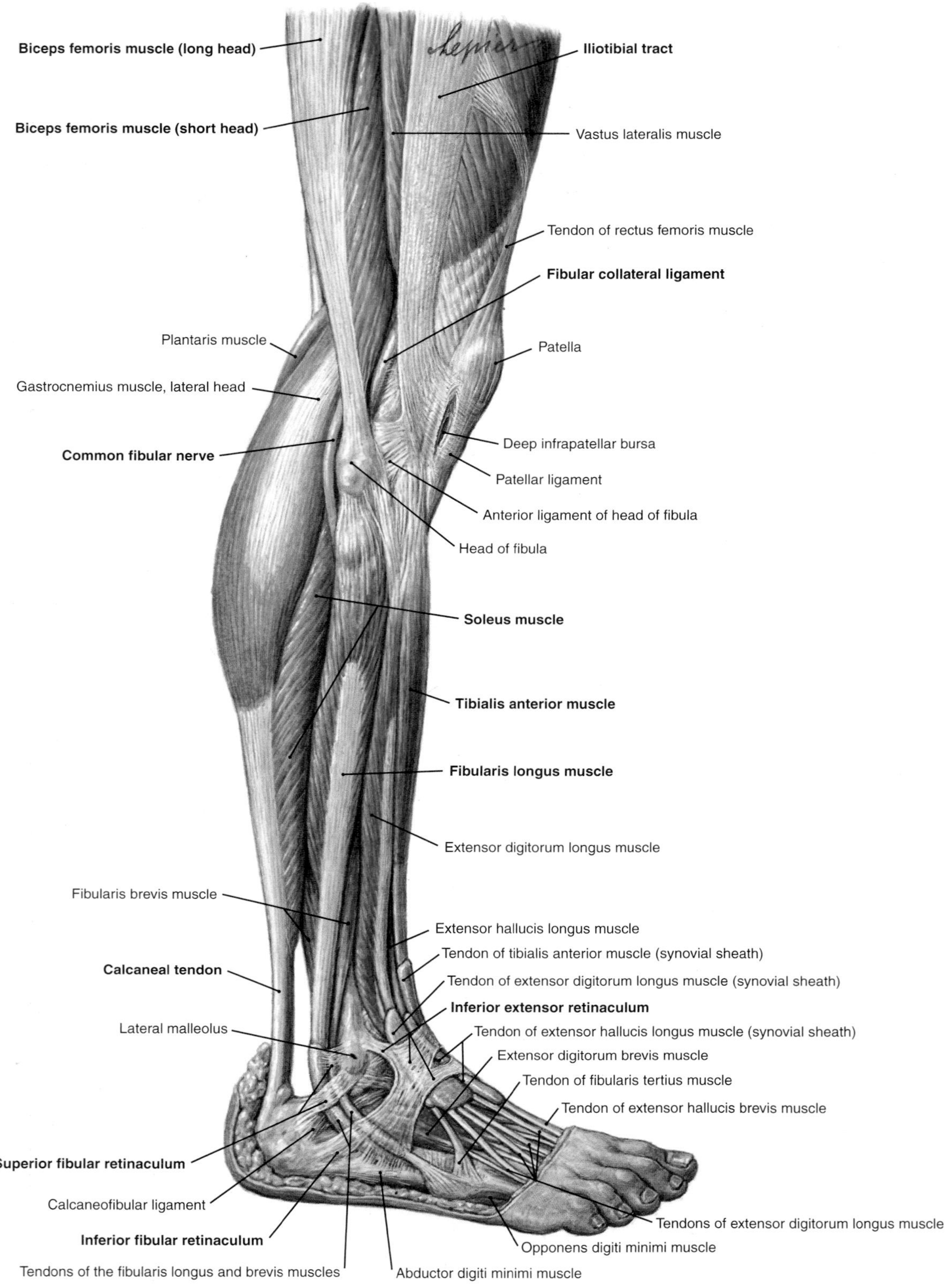
Biceps femoris muscle (long head)
Biceps femoris muscle (short head)
Iliotibial tract
Vastus lateralis muscle
Tendon of rectus femoris muscle
Fibular collateral ligament
Plantaris muscle
Patella
Gastrocnemius muscle, lateral head
Common fibular nerve
Deep infrapatellar bursa
Patellar ligament
Anterior ligament of head of fibula
Head of fibula
Soleus muscle
Tibialis anterior muscle
Fibularis longus muscle
Extensor digitorum longus muscle
Fibularis brevis muscle
Extensor hallucis longus muscle
Tendon of tibialis anterior muscle (synovial sheath)
Calcaneal tendon
Tendon of extensor digitorum longus muscle (synovial sheath)
Inferior extensor retinaculum
Lateral malleolus
Tendon of extensor hallucis longus muscle (synovial sheath)
Extensor digitorum brevis muscle
Tendon of fibularis tertius muscle
Tendon of extensor hallucis brevis muscle
Superior fibular retinaculum
Calcaneofibular ligament
Tendons of extensor digitorum longus muscle
Inferior fibular retinaculum
Opponens digiti minimi muscle
Tendons of the fibularis longus and brevis muscles
Abductor digiti minimi muscle

Figure 404 Lateral Compartment Muscles and Tendons of the Right Leg (Lateral View)

NOTE: (1) The **fibularis longus** and **brevis** occupy the lateral compartment of the leg, and their tendons descend into the foot behind the lateral malleolus. The fibularis longus tendon crosses the sole of the foot to insert on the base of the first metatarsal bone, while the fibularis brevis inserts directly onto fifth metatarsal bone.

(2) The superficial location of the **head of the fibula** and its relationship to the **common fibular nerve.** Trauma to the lateral side of the leg could cause injury to this nerve, resulting in a condition called foot drop, because the dorsiflexors would be denervated and the action of the plantar flexors in the posterior compartment would no longer be opposed.

(3) The tendons of the anterior and lateral compartment muscles enter the foot beneath the extensor and fibular retinacula and are surrounded by tendon sheaths (in blue).

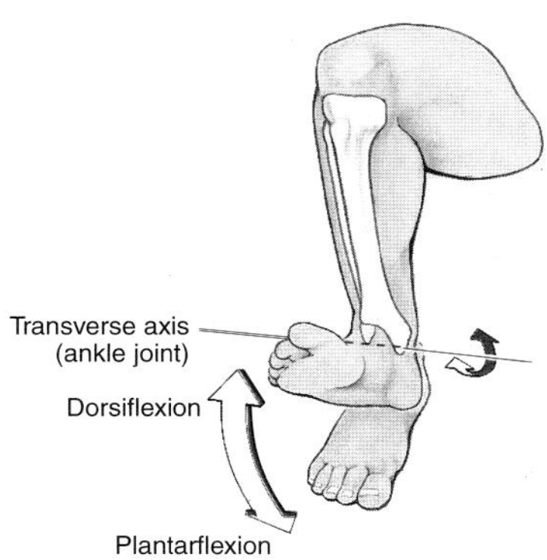
Transverse axis
(ankle joint)
Dorsiflexion
Plantarflexion

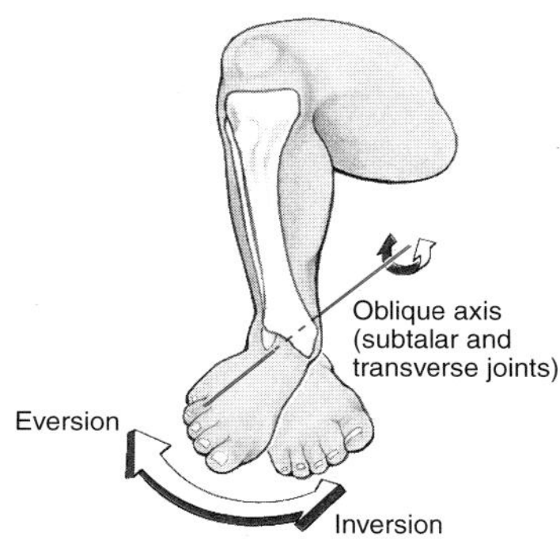
Oblique axis
(subtalar and
transverse joints)
Eversion
Inversion

Figure 405.1 Dorsiflexion and Plantar Flexion of the Foot (at Ankle Joint)

Dorsiflexion:

1. Attempts to approximate the dorsum of the foot to the anterior leg surface.
2. Is considered as extension at ankle joint.
3. Is performed by muscles in the anterior compartment of the leg.

Plantar flexion:

1. Reverses dorsiflexion and also occurs when one stands on one's toes.
2. Is considered as flexion at ankle joint.
3. Is performed by muscles in the posterior compartment of the leg.

Figure 405.2 Inversion and Eversion of the Foot (at Subtalar and Transverse Joint)

Inversion:

1. Attempts to supinate the foot, i.e., to turn the sole medially or inward.
2. Is performed by muscles in the leg that attach medially on the foot (tibialis anterior *and* posterior; extensor *and* flexor hallucis longus).

Eversion:

1. Attempts to pronate the foot, i.e., to turn the sole laterally or outward.
2. Is performed by muscles in the leg that attach laterally on the foot such as fibularis longus, brevis, and tertius.

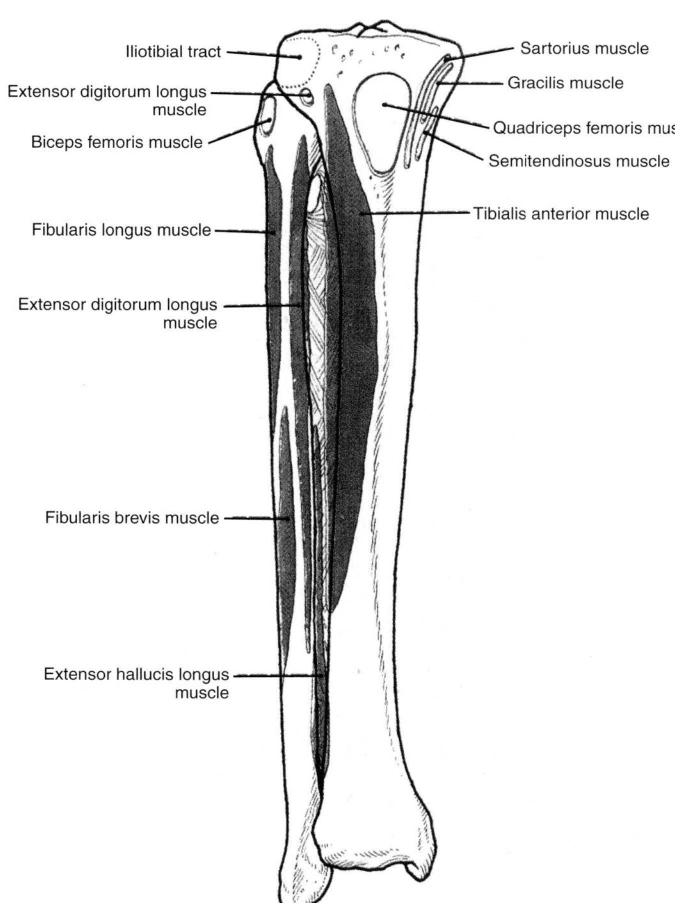
Iliotibial tract
Extensor digitorum longus muscle
Biceps femoris muscle
Fibularis longus muscle
Extensor digitorum longus muscle
Fibularis brevis muscle
Extensor hallucis longus muscle
Sartorius muscle
Gracilis muscle
Quadriceps femoris muscle
Semitendinosus muscle
Tibialis anterior muscle

Figure 405.3 Muscle Attachments on the Right Tibia and Fibula (Anterior Surface)

NOTE: (1) Most of the upper three-fourths of the anterior surface of the fibula gives attachment to muscles, while much of the anterior tibia is free of muscles, attachments.

(2) The only muscle of the anterior and lateral compartments that does *not* arise from the fibula is the tibialis anterior. The only muscle of the thigh that attaches to the fibula is the biceps femoris.

(3) Portions of the anterior surface of the interosseous membrane are used by all three muscles of the anterior compartment for their origin, whereas neither of the lateral compartment muscles extends that far medially.

(4) The sartorius, gracilis, and semitendinosus muscles insert on the medial condyle of the tibia forming a tendinous expansion sometimes called the pes anserinus (goose's foot), while onto the tibial tuberosity inserts the large quadriceps femoris muscle.

(5) Onto the lateral condyle of the tibia inserts the biceps femoris muscle.

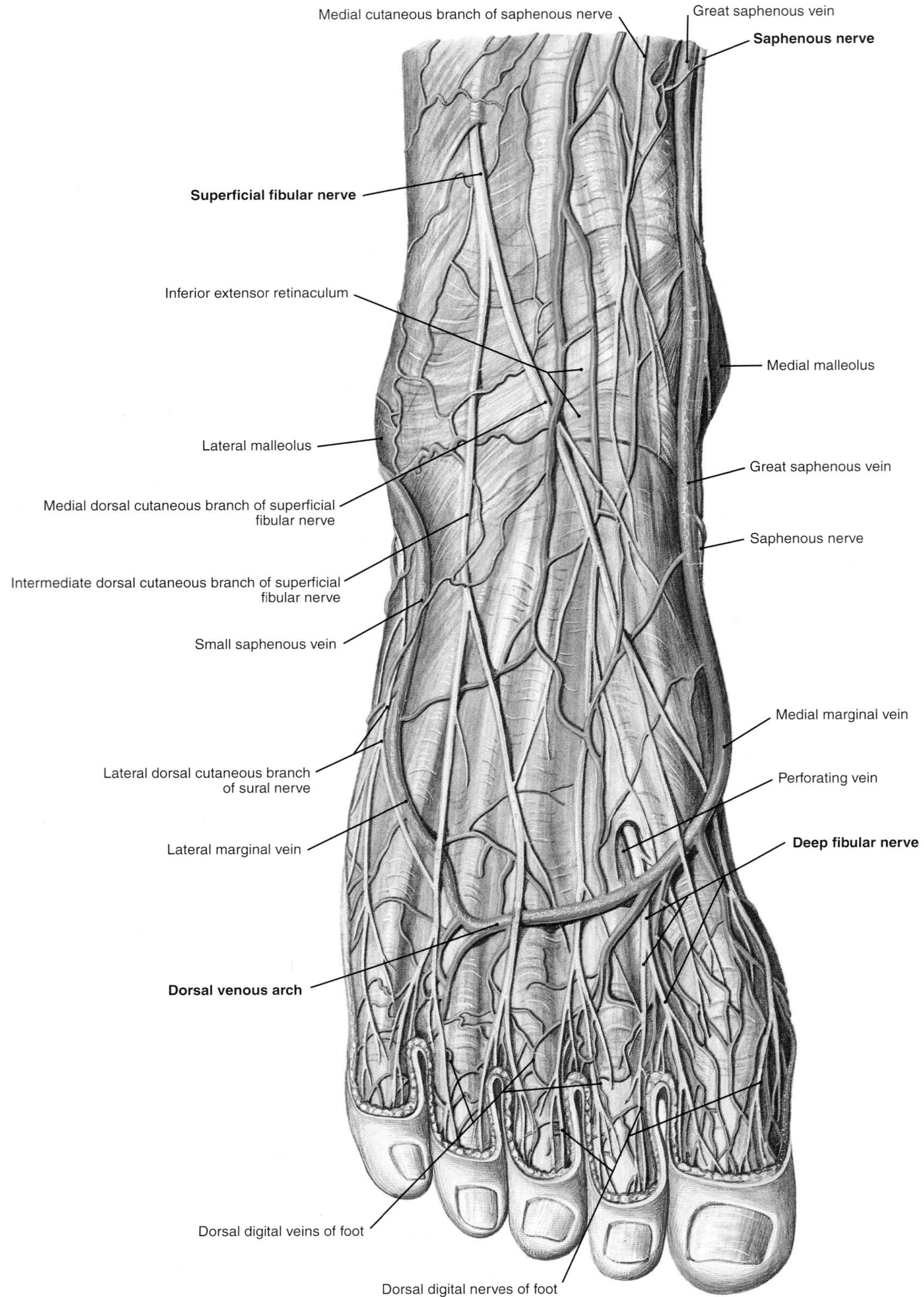
Medial cutaneous branch of saphenous nerve
Great saphenous vein
Saphenous nerve
Superficial fibular nerve
Inferior extensor retinaculum
Medial malleolus
Lateral malleolus
Great saphenous vein
Medial dorsal cutaneous branch of superficial fibular nerve
Saphenous nerve
Intermediate dorsal cutaneous branch of superficial fibular nerve
Small saphenous vein
Medial marginal vein
Lateral dorsal cutaneous branch of sural nerve
Perforating vein
Lateral marginal vein
Deep fibular nerve
Dorsal venous arch
Dorsal digital veins of foot
Dorsal digital nerves of foot

Figure 406 Superficial Nerves and Veins of the Dorsal Right Foot

NOTE: (1) Cutaneous innervation of the dorsal foot is supplied principally by the **superficial fibular nerve** (L4, L5, S1). In addition, the **deep fibular nerve** (L4, L5) supplies the adjacent sides of the first and second toes, while the **lateral dorsal cutaneous nerve** (S1, S2; terminal branch of the sural nerve in the foot) supplies the lateral and dorsal aspects of the fifth digit.

(2) The digital and metatarsal veins drain back from the toes to form the dorsal venous arch of the foot. From this arch, the **great saphenous vein** ascends medially and the **small saphenous vein** laterally on the foot dorsum.

(3) The cutaneous branch of the **saphenous nerve** extends downward as far as the ankle joint anteriorly. Medially, the main trunk of the saphenous nerve can extend inferiorly as far as the metatarsophalangeal joint of the large toe.

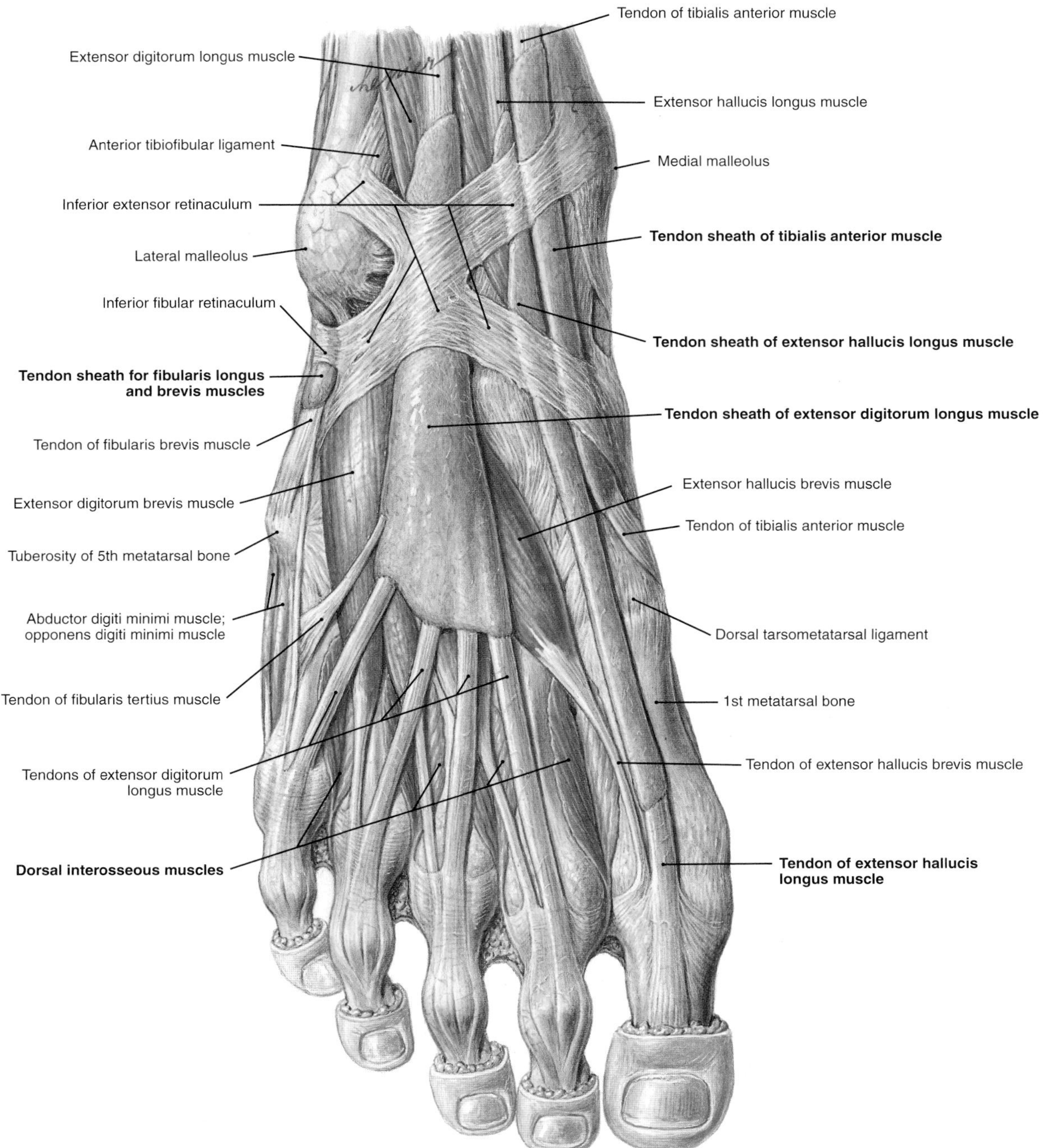

Tendon of tibialis anterior muscle
Extensor digitorum longus muscle
Extensor hallucis longus muscle
Anterior tibiofibular ligament
Medial malleolus
Inferior extensor retinaculum
Tendon sheath of tibialis anterior muscle
Lateral malleolus
Inferior fibular retinaculum
Tendon sheath of extensor hallucis longus muscle
Tendon sheath for fibularis longus and brevis muscles
Tendon sheath of extensor digitorum longus muscle
Tendon of fibularis brevis muscle
Extensor hallucis brevis muscle
Extensor digitorum brevis muscle
Tendon of tibialis anterior muscle
Tuberosity of 5th metatarsal bone
Abductor digiti minimi muscle; opponens digiti minimi muscle
Dorsal tarsometatarsal ligament
Tendon of fibularis tertius muscle
1st metatarsal bone
Tendon of extensor hallucis brevis muscle
Tendons of extensor digitorum longus muscle
Dorsal interosseous muscles
Tendon of extensor hallucis longus muscle

Figure 407 Muscles, Tendons, and Tendon Sheaths of the Dorsal Right Foot (Superficial View)

NOTE: (1) The tendons of the tibialis anterior, extensor hallucis longus, and extensor digitorum longus are bound by the Y-shaped (or X-shaped) inferior extensor retinaculum as they enter the dorsum of the foot at the level of the ankle joint.

(2) The extensor tendons insert onto the dorsal aspect of the distal phalanx of each toe. In addition, the tendons of the extensor digitorum longus also insert onto the dorsum of the middle phalanx of the four lateral toes.

(3) The tendon of the fibularis tertius inserts on the base of the fifth metatarsal bone (and at times the fourth also).

(4) Separate synovial sheaths (shown in blue) surround the tendons of the tibialis anterior and extensor hallucis longus. Also note the common synovial sheath for the main tendon and the individual digital tendons of the extensor digitorum longus.

(5) The tendon sheaths laterally and medially under the two malleoli are shown in Figures 408.1 and 408.2.

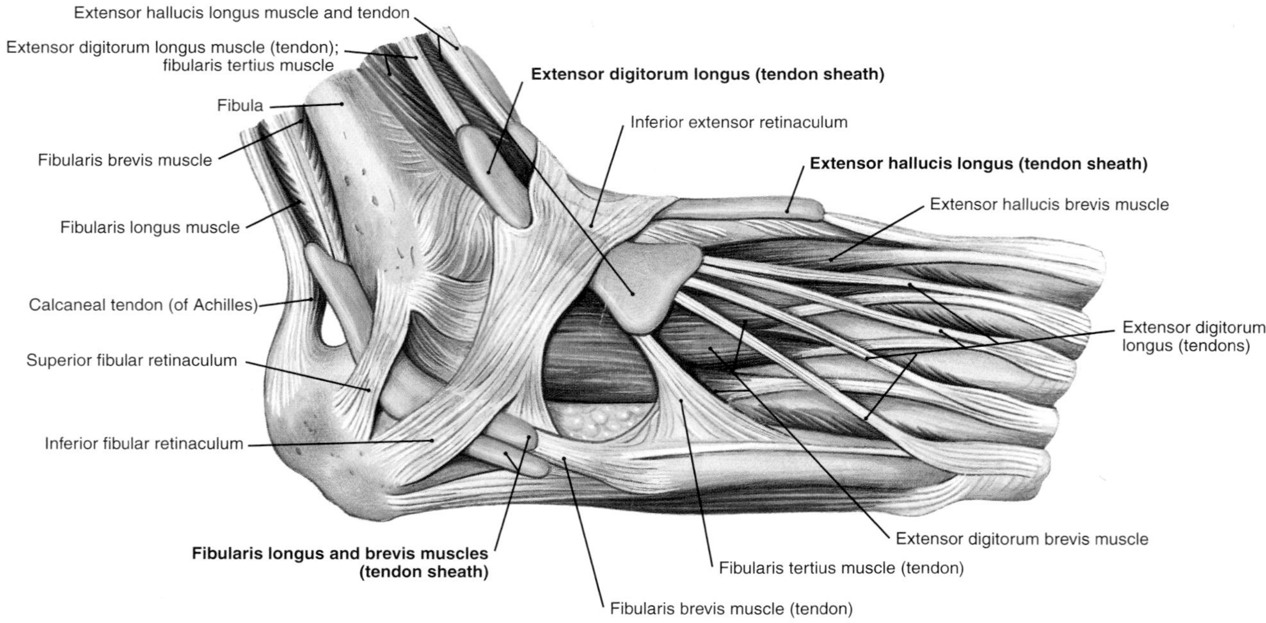
Extensor hallucis longus muscle and tendon
Extensor digitorum longus muscle (tendon); fibularis tertius muscle
Fibula
Fibularis brevis muscle
Fibularis longus muscle
Calcaneal tendon (of Achilles)
Superior fibular retinaculum
Inferior fibular retinaculum
Fibularis longus and brevis muscles (tendon sheath)
Extensor digitorum longus (tendon sheath)
Inferior extensor retinaculum
Extensor hallucis longus (tendon sheath)
Extensor hallucis brevis muscle
Extensor digitorum longus (tendons)
Extensor digitorum brevis muscle
Fibularis tertius muscle (tendon)
Fibularis brevis muscle (tendon)

Figure 408.1 Tendons and Synovial Sheaths: Right Dorsum of Foot and Ankle Region (Lateral View)

NOTE: (1) Similar to the wrist, tendons at the ankle region passing from the leg into the foot are bound by closely investing **retinacula** and are surrounded by **synovial sheaths**, which are indicated in blue in this figure and in Fig. 408.2.

(2) Anterior to the ankle joint and on the dorsum of the foot are three separate synovial sheaths, one that includes the extensor digitorum longus and the fibularis tertius, a second for the extensor hallucis longus and a third for the tibialis anterior (see Figs. 404 and 407).

(3) Behind the lateral malleolus is a single tendon sheath for the fibularis longus and brevis muscles, which then splits distally to continue along each individual tendon for some distance.

(4) The inferior extensor retinaculum and the superior and inferior fibular retinacula, which bind the tendons and their sheaths close to the bone.

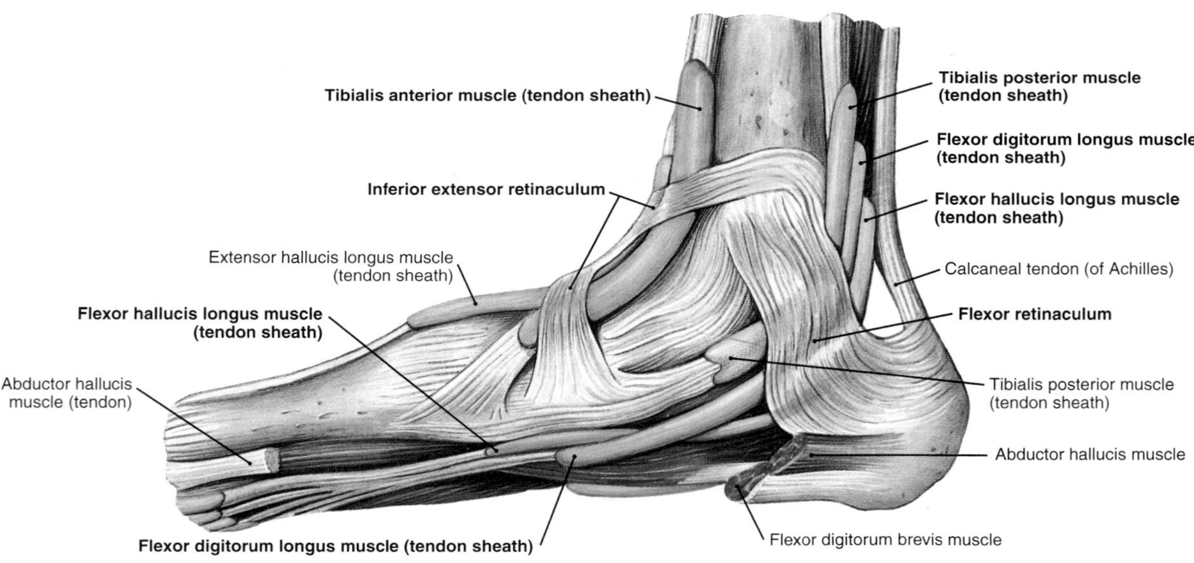
Tibialis anterior muscle (tendon sheath)
Inferior extensor retinaculum
Extensor hallucis longus muscle (tendon sheath)
Flexor hallucis longus muscle (tendon sheath)
Abductor hallucis muscle (tendon)
Flexor digitorum longus muscle (tendon sheath)
Tibialis posterior muscle (tendon sheath)
Flexor digitorum longus muscle (tendon sheath)
Flexor hallucis longus muscle (tendon sheath)
Calcaneal tendon (of Achilles)
Flexor retinaculum
Tibialis posterior muscle (tendon sheath)
Abductor hallucis muscle
Flexor digitorum brevis muscle

Figure 408.2 Tendons and Synovial Sheaths: Right Dorsum of Foot and Ankle Region (Medial View)

NOTE: (1) From this medial view can be seen the synovial sheaths and tendons of the tibialis anterior and extensor hallucis longus on the dorsum of the foot, as well as the three tendons that course beneath the medial malleolus into the plantar aspect of the foot from the posterior compartment: tibialis posterior, the flexor digitorum longus, and the flexor hallucis longus.

(2) The bifurcating nature of the inferior extensor retinaculum, and the manner in which the flexor retinaculum secures the structures beneath the medial malleolus.

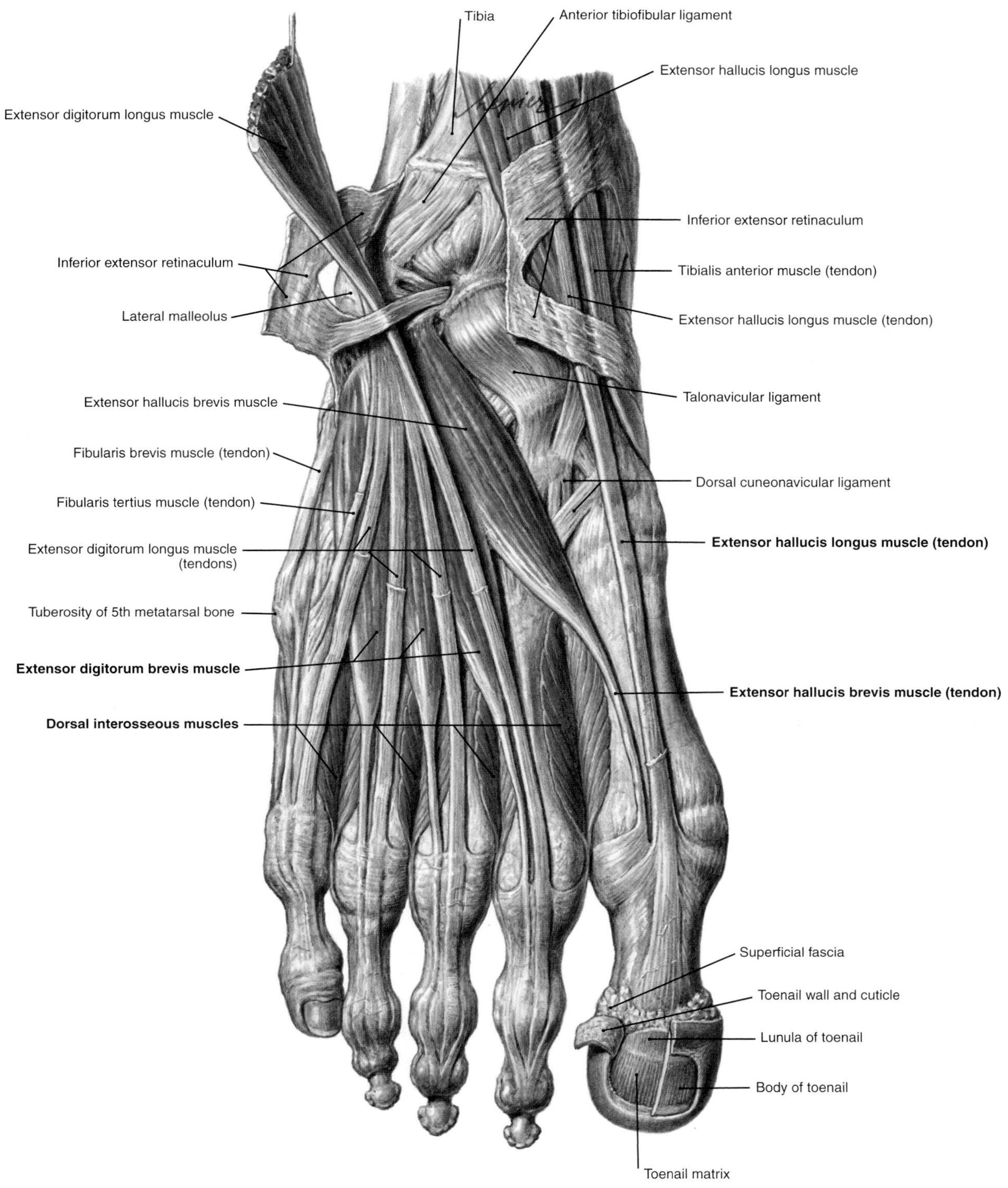
Tibia
Anterior tibiofibular ligament
Extensor hallucis longus muscle
Extensor digitorum longus muscle
Inferior extensor retinaculum
Tibialis anterior muscle (tendon)
Inferior extensor retinaculum
Extensor hallucis longus muscle (tendon)
Lateral malleolus
Talonavicular ligament
Extensor hallucis brevis muscle
Fibularis brevis muscle (tendon)
Dorsal cuneonavicular ligament
Fibularis tertius muscle (tendon)
Extensor hallucis longus muscle (tendon)
Extensor digitorum longus muscle (tendons)
Tuberosity of 5th metatarsal bone
Extensor digitorum brevis muscle
Extensor hallucis brevis muscle (tendon)
Dorsal interosseous muscles
Superficial fascia
Toenail wall and cuticle
Lunula of toenail
Body of toenail
Toenail matrix

Figure 409 **Muscles and Tendons on the Dorsal Aspect of the Right Foot**

MUSCLES ON THE DORSUM OF THE FOOT

Muscle	Origin	Insertion	Innervation	Function
Extensor hallucis brevis	Dorsal aspect of the calcaneus bone	Lateral side of the base of the proximal phalanx of the great toe	Deep fibular nerve (L5, S1)	Helps to extend the proximal phalanx of the great toe
Extensor digitorum brevis	Dorsal and lateral aspect of the calcaneus bone	Lateral side of the tendons of the extensor digitorum longus muscle for the second, third, and fourth toes	Deep fibular nerve (L5, S1)	Helps to extend the proximal phalanges of the second, third, and fourth toes

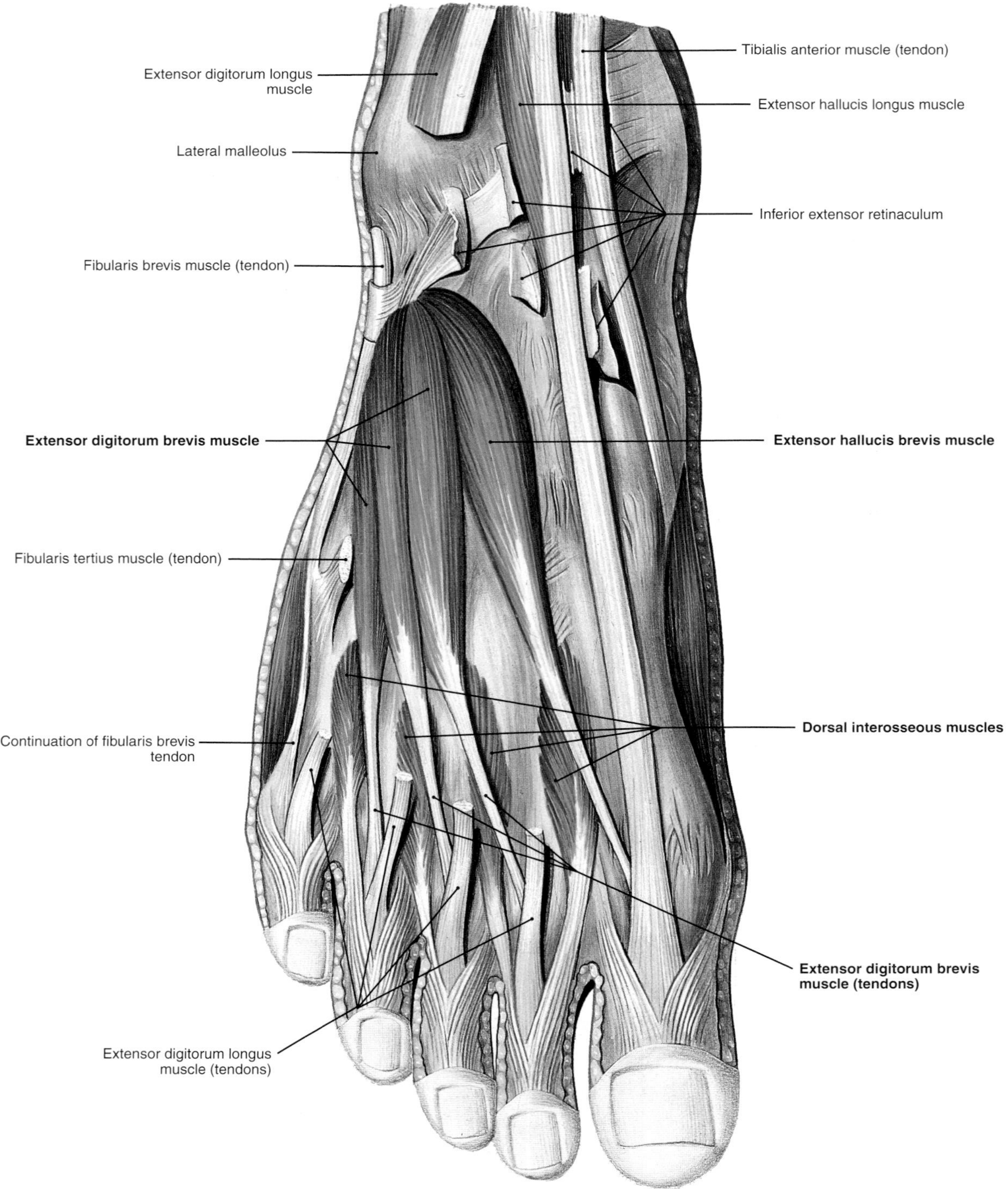
Extensor digitorum longus muscle
Lateral malleolus
Fibularis brevis muscle (tendon)
Extensor digitorum brevis muscle
Fibularis tertius muscle (tendon)
Continuation of fibularis brevis tendon
Extensor digitorum longus muscle (tendons)
Tibialis anterior muscle (tendon)
Extensor hallucis longus muscle
Inferior extensor retinaculum
Extensor hallucis brevis muscle
Dorsal interosseous muscles
Extensor digitorum brevis muscle (tendons)

Figure 410 Intrinsic Muscles of the Dorsal Foot (Right)

NOTE: (1) The inferior extensor retinaculum has been opened and the tendons of the extensor digitorum longus and fibularis tertius muscles have been severed.

(2) The **extensor hallucis brevis muscle** and the three small bellies of the **extensor digitorum brevis.** The delicate tendons of these muscles insert on the proximal phalanx of the medial four toes.

(3) The four **dorsal interosseous muscles.** These muscles abduct the toes from the longitudinal axis of the foot (down the middle of the second toe). The first dorsal interosseous muscle inserts on the medial side of the second toe, while the remaining three insert on the lateral side of the second, third, and fourth toes.

(4) Although the dorsal interosseous muscles are usually designated as the deepest layer of muscles on the **plantar** aspect of the foot, they can best be seen on the dorsal surface following reflection of the tendons of the extensor digitorum longus and brevis muscles.

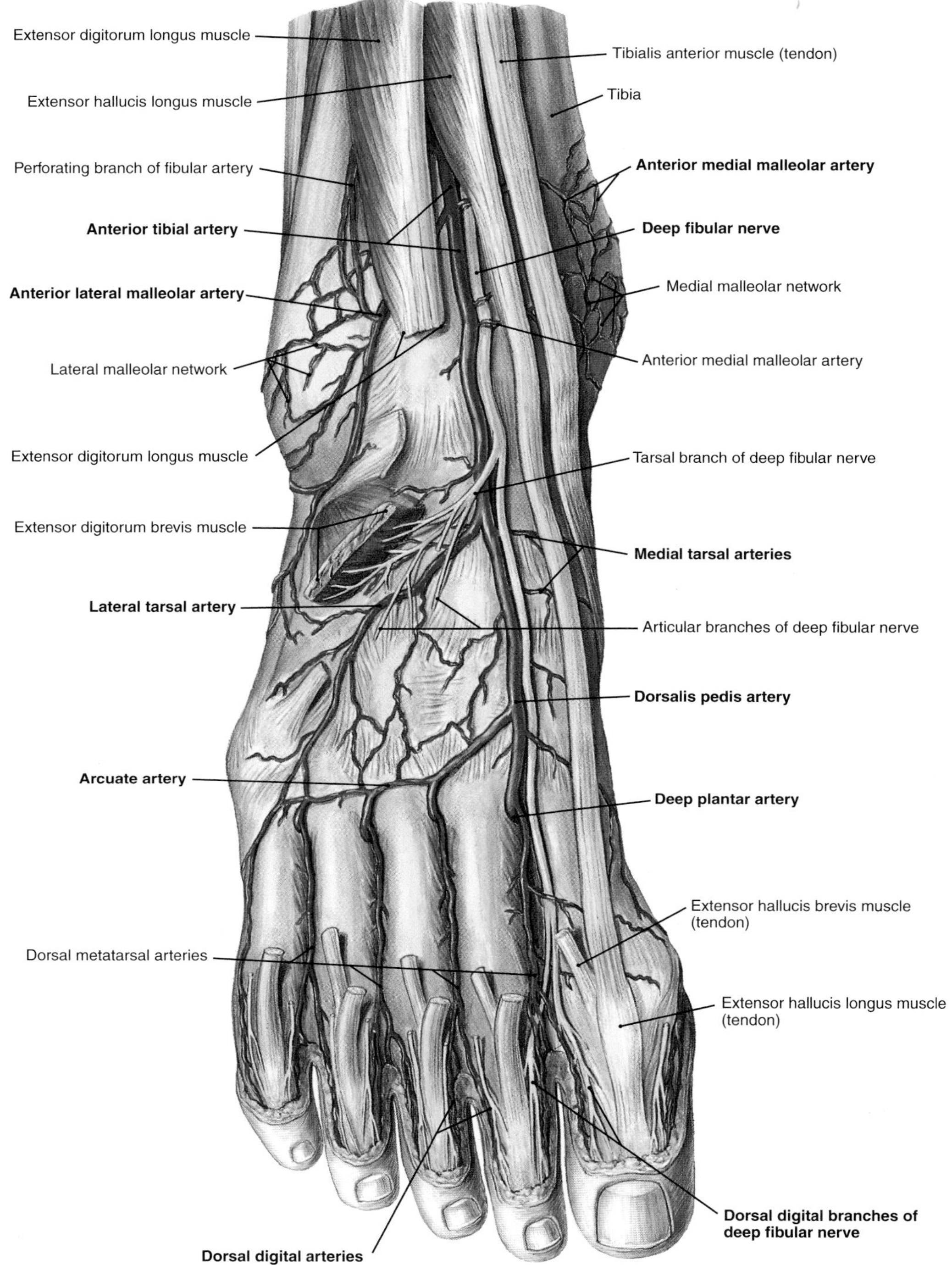
Extensor digitorum longus muscle
Extensor hallucis longus muscle
Perforating branch of fibular artery
Anterior tibial artery
Anterior lateral malleolar artery
Lateral malleolar network
Extensor digitorum longus muscle
Extensor digitorum brevis muscle
Lateral tarsal artery
Arcuate artery
Dorsal metatarsal arteries
Dorsal digital arteries
Tibialis anterior muscle (tendon)
Tibia
Anterior medial malleolar artery
Deep fibular nerve
Medial malleolar network
Anterior medial malleolar artery
Tarsal branch of deep fibular nerve
Medial tarsal arteries
Articular branches of deep fibular nerve
Dorsalis pedis artery
Deep plantar artery
Extensor hallucis brevis muscle (tendon)
Extensor hallucis longus muscle (tendon)
Dorsal digital branches of deep fibular nerve

Figure 411 Deep Nerves and Arteries of the Dorsal Foot

NOTE: (1) The deeply coursing **anterior tibial artery** and **deep fibular nerve** and their branches have been exposed. They enter the foot between tendons of the extensor hallucis longus and extensor digitorum longus muscles.

(2) The anterior tibial artery becomes the **dorsalis pedis artery** below the ankle joint. The **deep plantar artery** branches from the dorsalis pedis and perforates the tissue between the first two metatarsal bones to enter the plantar foot. Note also the **malleolar, tarsal, arcuate, dorsal metatarsal,** and **digital arteries.**

(3) The **deep fibular nerve** supplies the extensor hallucis and extensor digitorum brevis muscles in the foot and continues distally to terminate as two dorsal digital nerves, which supply sensory innervation to the adjacent sides of the great toe and the second toe. Sensory innervation on the dorsal aspect of the other toes is derived from the **superficial fibular nerve.**

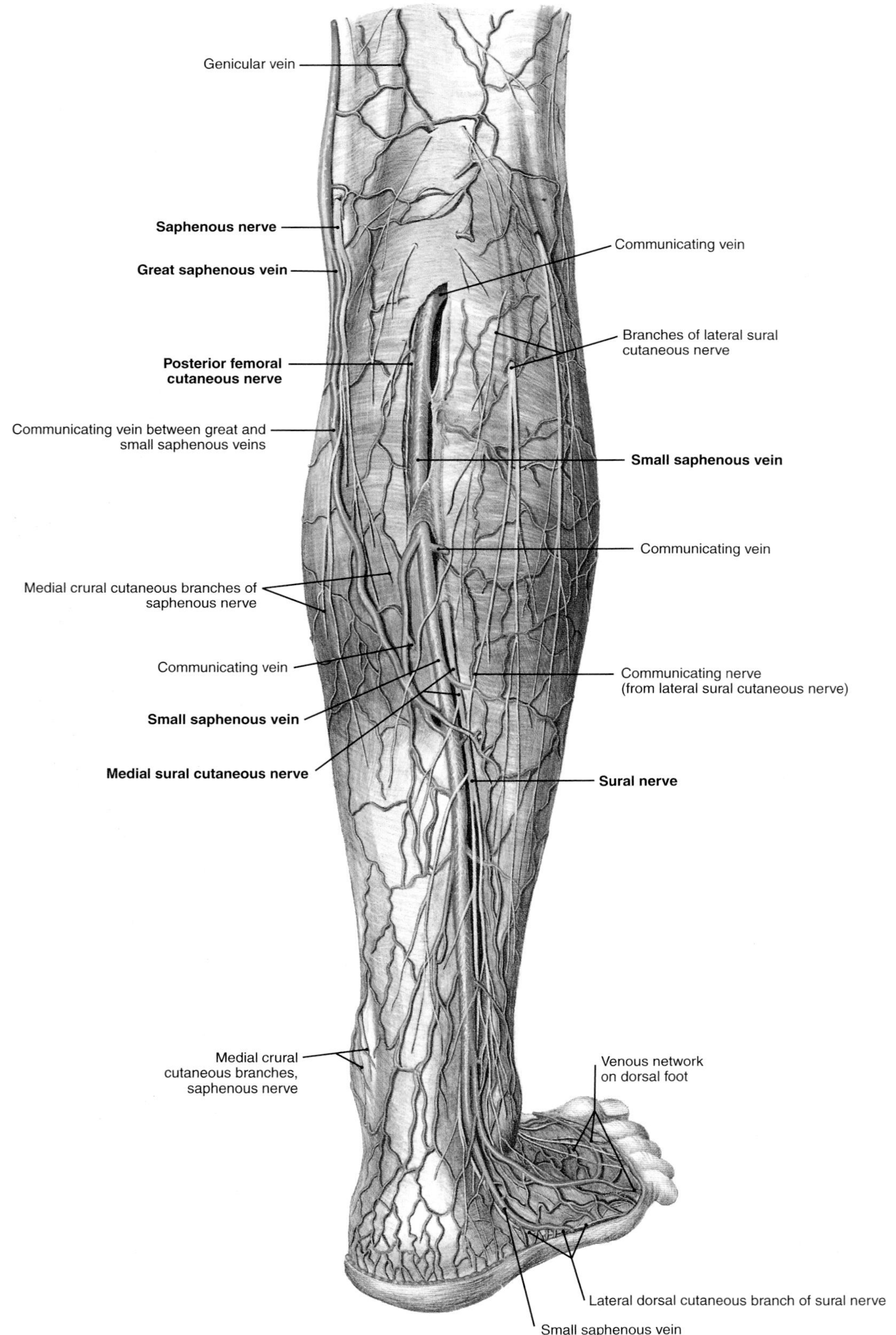
Genicular vein
Saphenous nerve
Great saphenous vein
Posterior femoral cutaneous nerve
Communicating vein between great and small saphenous veins
Medial crural cutaneous branches of saphenous nerve
Communicating vein
Small saphenous vein
Medial sural cutaneous nerve
Medial crural cutaneous branches, saphenous nerve
Communicating vein
Branches of lateral sural cutaneous nerve
Small saphenous vein
Communicating vein
Communicating nerve (from lateral sural cutaneous nerve)
Sural nerve
Venous network on dorsal foot
Lateral dorsal cutaneous branch of sural nerve
Small saphenous vein

Figure 412 Superficial Veins and Cutaneous Nerves of the Posterior Leg and Dorsal Foot

NOTE: (1) The **small saphenous vein** forms on the dorsolateral aspect of the foot and ascends to the popliteal fossa, and superficial communicating branches interconnect it to the great saphenous vein.

(2) The **sural nerve** is formed by the junction of a large branch, the medial sural cutaneous nerve (from the tibial nerve), and the lateral sural cutaneous branches from the common fibular nerve. This nerve supplies most of the posterolateral part of the leg, and medial crural cutaneous branches of the **saphenous nerve** supply the posteromedial leg.

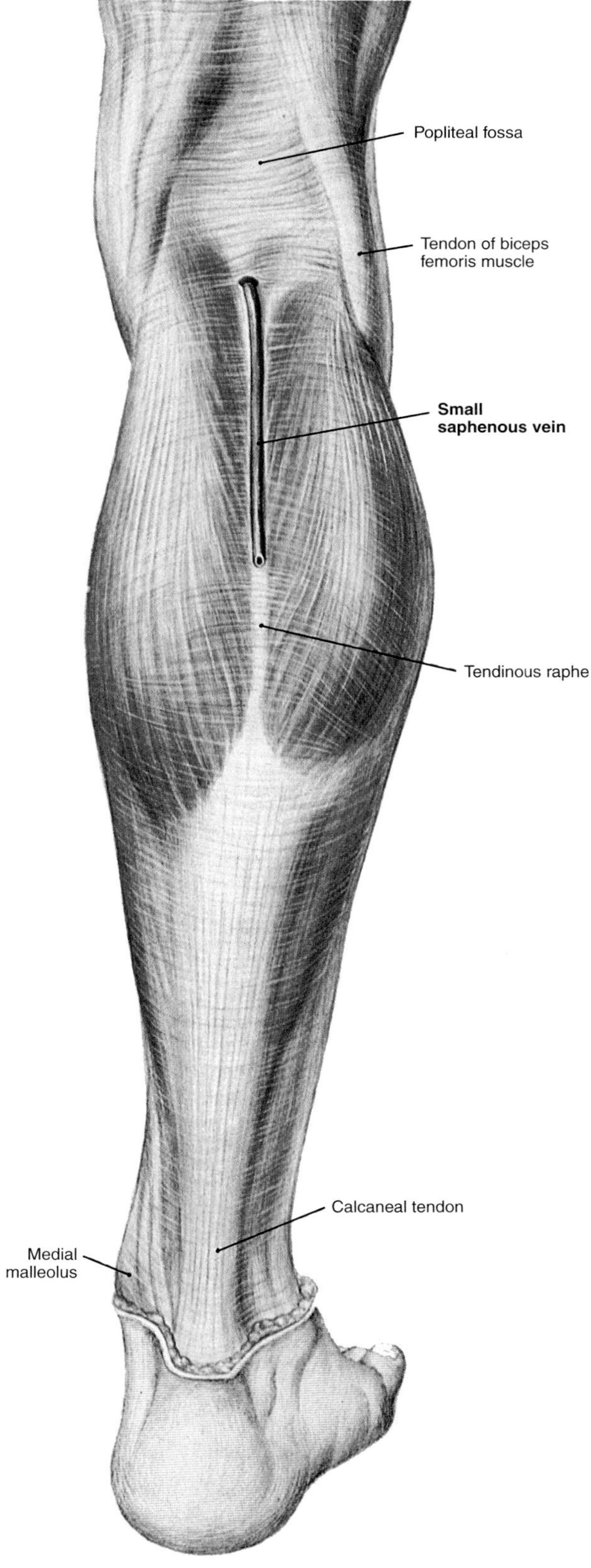
Popliteal fossa
Tendon of biceps femoris muscle
Small saphenous vein
Tendinous raphe
Calcaneal tendon
Medial malleolus

Figure 413.1 Deep Fascia of the Leg (the Crural Fascia) (Posterior View)

NOTE: The deep fascia of the leg closely invests all the muscles between the knee and ankle and forms the fascial covering over the popliteal fossa. It is continuous above with the fascia lata of the thigh and below with the retinacula that bind the tendons close to the bones in the ankle region.

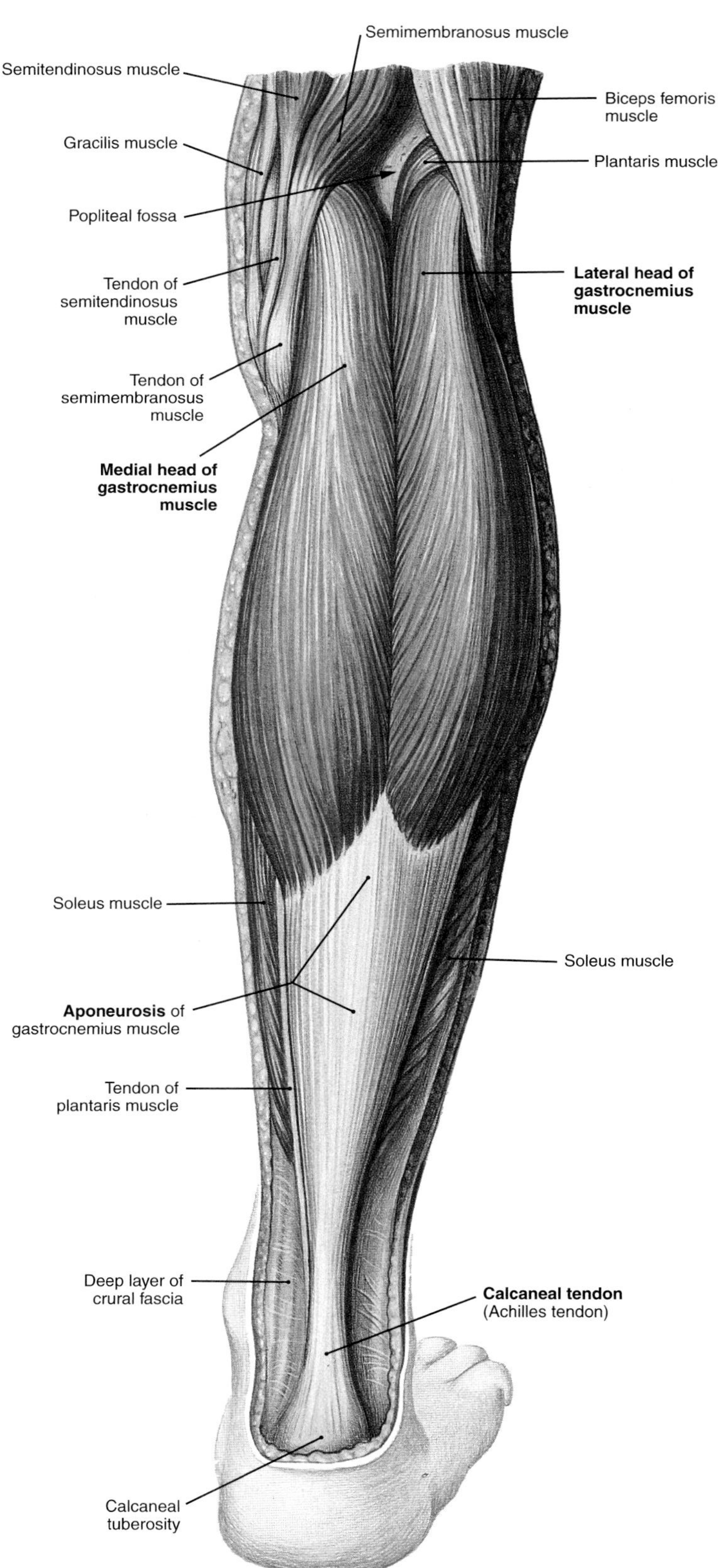
Semimembranosus muscle
Semitendinosus muscle
Biceps femoris muscle
Gracilis muscle
Plantaris muscle
Popliteal fossa
Tendon of semitendinosus muscle
Lateral head of gastrocnemius muscle
Tendon of semimembranosus muscle
Medial head of gastrocnemius muscle
Soleus muscle
Soleus muscle
Aponeurosis of gastrocnemius muscle
Tendon of plantaris muscle
Deep layer of crural fascia
Calcaneal tendon (Achilles tendon)
Calcaneal tuberosity

Figure 413.2 Muscles of the Posterior Leg: Superficial Calf Muscles

NOTE: (1) The **gastrocnemius muscle** arises by two heads from the condyles and posterior surface of the femur. It inserts by means of the strong **calcaneal tendon** onto the tuberosity of the calcaneus.

(2) The gastrocnemius is a strong plantar flexor of the foot, and its continued action also flexes the leg at the knee.

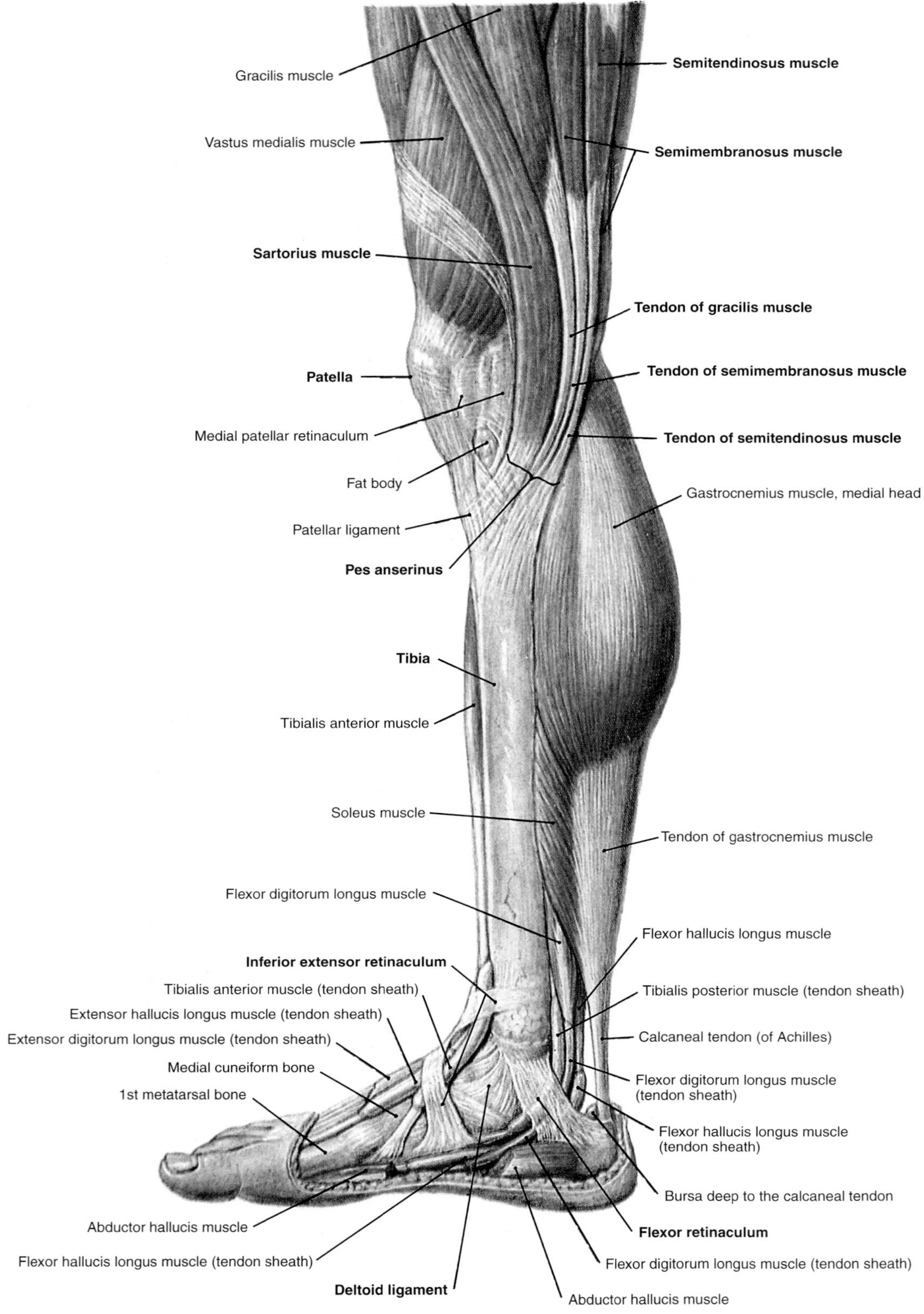
Gracilis muscle
Semitendinosus muscle
Vastus medialis muscle
Semimembranosus muscle
Sartorius muscle
Tendon of gracilis muscle
Patella
Tendon of semimembranosus muscle
Medial patellar retinaculum
Tendon of semitendinosus muscle
Fat body
Gastrocnemius muscle, medial head
Patellar ligament
Pes anserinus
Tibia
Tibialis anterior muscle
Soleus muscle
Tendon of gastrocnemius muscle
Flexor digitorum longus muscle
Flexor hallucis longus muscle
Inferior extensor retinaculum
Tibialis anterior muscle (tendon sheath)
Tibialis posterior muscle (tendon sheath)
Extensor hallucis longus muscle (tendon sheath)
Extensor digitorum longus muscle (tendon sheath)
Calcaneal tendon (of Achilles)
Medial cuneiform bone
Flexor digitorum longus muscle (tendon sheath)
1st metatarsal bone
Flexor hallucis longus muscle (tendon sheath)
Bursa deep to the calcaneal tendon
Abductor hallucis muscle
Flexor retinaculum
Flexor hallucis longus muscle (tendon sheath)
Flexor digitorum longus muscle (tendon sheath)
Deltoid ligament
Abductor hallucis muscle

Figure 414 Medial View of the Leg: Knee, Posterior Compartment, Ankle and Foot Regions

NOTE: (1) The medial head of the gastrocnemius muscle. Observe how its tendon inserts onto the tuberosity of the calcaneus, while the tendons of the tibialis posterior, flexor digitorum longus and flexor hallucis longus enter the plantar surface of the foot.

(2) The flexor retinaculum holds these deep posterior compartment muscles close to the bone, thereby increasing their efficiency when they contract. Without these retinacula, muscular contraction would result in a bowing of the tendons and a loss of power.

(3) The tendons of the sartorius, gracilis, and semitendinosus form the so-called pes anserinus (goose's foot). This tendinous formation helps protect the medial aspect of the knee, while the tendon of the semimembranosus helps reinforce the capsule of the knee joint posteriorly.

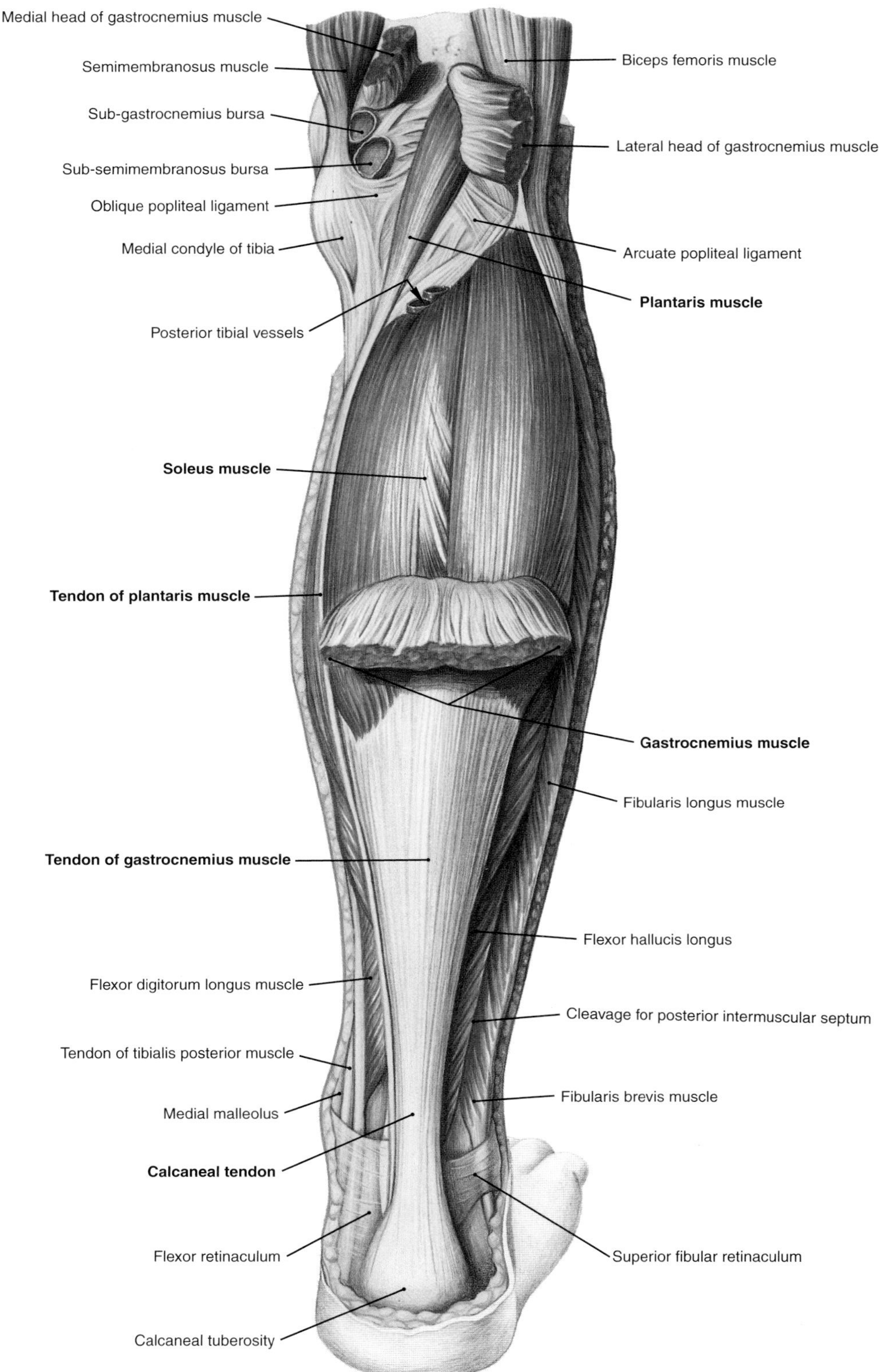
Medial head of gastrocnemius muscle
Semimembranosus muscle
Sub-gastrocnemius bursa
Sub-semimembranosus bursa
Oblique popliteal ligament
Medial condyle of tibia
Posterior tibial vessels
Soleus muscle
Tendon of plantaris muscle
Tendon of gastrocnemius muscle
Flexor digitorum longus muscle
Tendon of tibialis posterior muscle
Medial malleolus
Calcaneal tendon
Flexor retinaculum
Calcaneal tuberosity
Biceps femoris muscle
Lateral head of gastrocnemius muscle
Arcuate popliteal ligament
Plantaris muscle
Gastrocnemius muscle
Fibularis longus muscle
Flexor hallucis longus
Cleavage for posterior intermuscular septum
Fibularis brevis muscle
Superior fibular retinaculum

Figure 415 Muscles of the Posterior Leg: Soleus and Plantaris Muscles

NOTE: (1) Both heads of the gastrocnemius muscle have been severed. Observe the stumps of their origins from the femur above and the lower flap reflected downward to uncover the **soleus** and **plantaris muscles.**

(2) The soleus muscle is broad and thick and arises from the posterior surface of the fibula, the intermuscular septum, and the dorsal aspect of the tibia. Its fibers join the calcaneal tendon and insert in common with the gastrocnemius muscle.

(3) The small plantaris muscle has a long thin tendon that also joins the calcaneal tendon. Although the function of the plantaris is of little significance, its long tendon can be used by surgeons when that type of tissue is required.

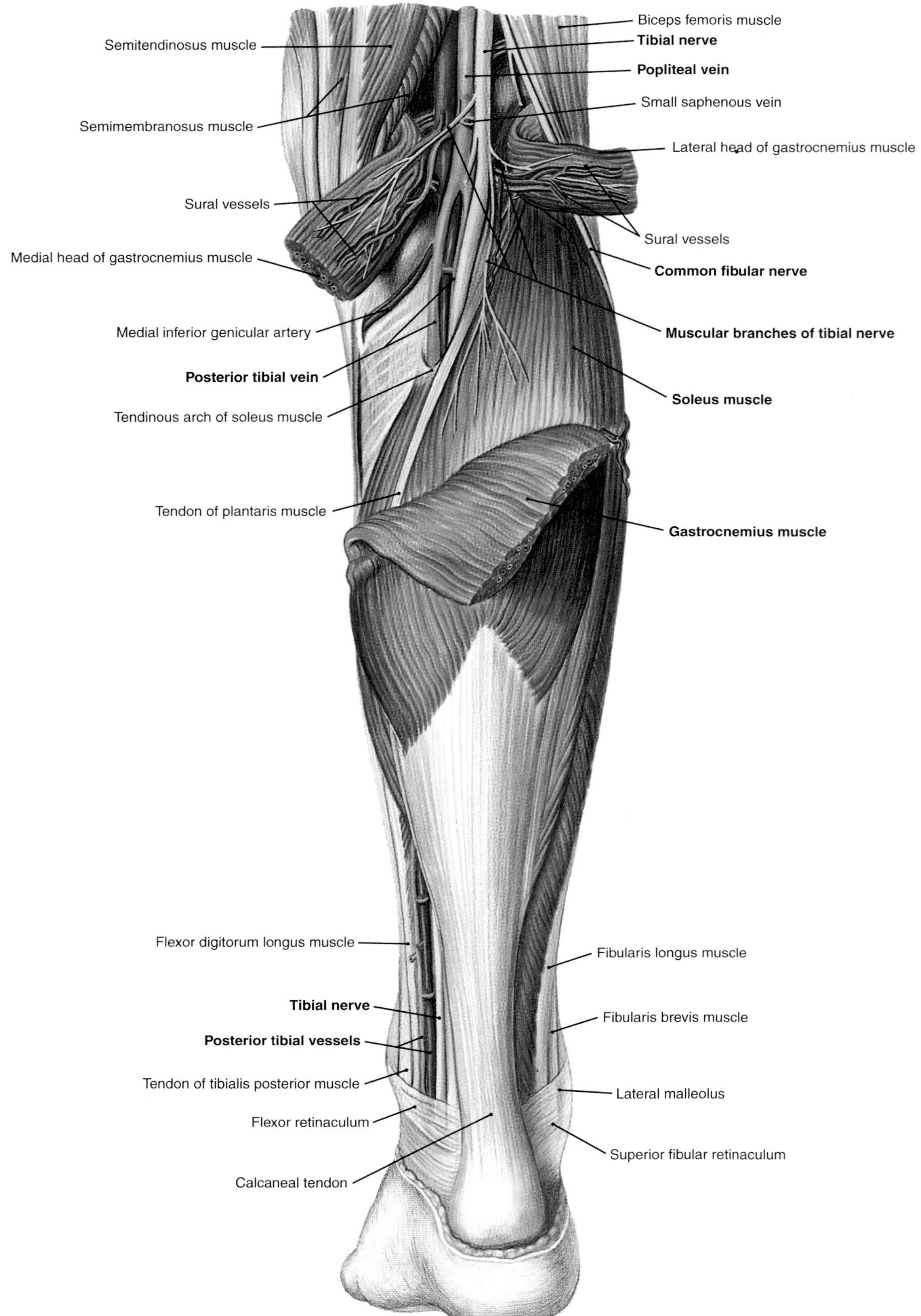
Semitendinosus muscle
Semimembranosus muscle
Sural vessels
Medial head of gastrocnemius muscle
Medial inferior genicular artery
Posterior tibial vein
Tendinous arch of soleus muscle
Tendon of plantaris muscle
Biceps femoris muscle
Tibial nerve
Popliteal vein
Small saphenous vein
Lateral head of gastrocnemius muscle
Sural vessels
Common fibular nerve
Muscular branches of tibial nerve
Soleus muscle
Gastrocnemius muscle
Flexor digitorum longus muscle
Tibial nerve
Posterior tibial vessels
Tendon of tibialis posterior muscle
Flexor retinaculum
Calcaneal tendon
Fibularis longus muscle
Fibularis brevis muscle
Lateral malleolus
Superior fibular retinaculum

Figure 416 Nerves and Vessels of the Posterior Leg above and below the Soleus Muscle

NOTE: (1) The popliteal vessels and tibial nerve, descending from the popliteal fossa into the posterior compartment and the leg, commence to course medially in a gradual manner so that at the ankle they lie behind the medial malleolus.

(2) From the popliteal fossa, sural branches of the popliteal artery and muscular branches of the tibial nerve descend to supply the gastrocnemius and soleus muscles. These neurovascular structures course through a tendinous arch in the soleus muscle and descend deep to the soleus and become superficial again several inches above the medial malleolus.

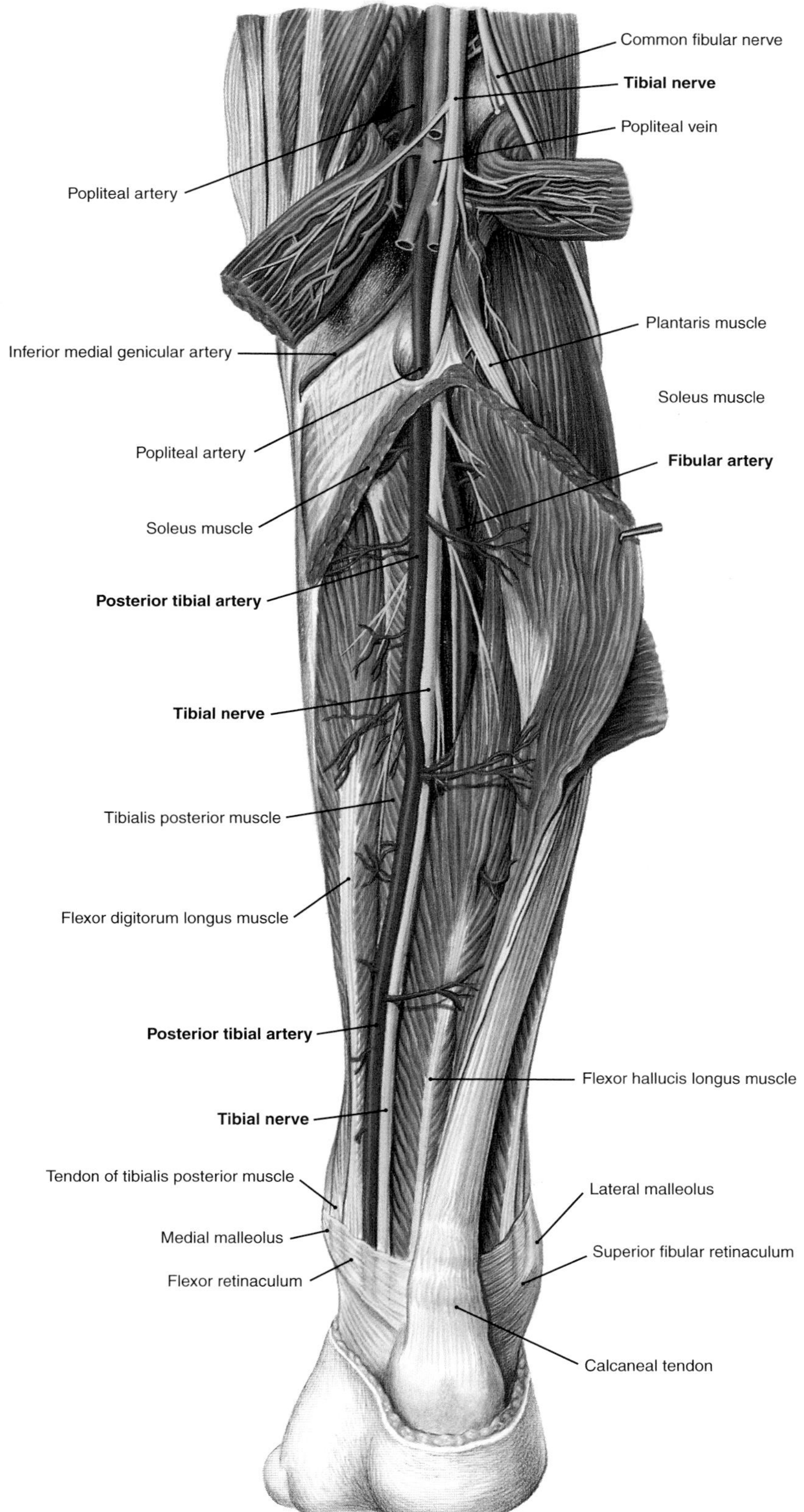
Common fibular nerve
Tibial nerve
Popliteal vein
Popliteal artery
Plantaris muscle
Inferior medial genicular artery
Soleus muscle
Popliteal artery
Fibular artery
Soleus muscle
Posterior tibial artery
Tibial nerve
Tibialis posterior muscle
Flexor digitorum longus muscle
Posterior tibial artery
Flexor hallucis longus muscle
Tibial nerve
Tendon of tibialis posterior muscle
Lateral malleolus
Medial malleolus
Superior fibular retinaculum
Flexor retinaculum
Calcaneal tendon

Figure 417 Nerves and Vessels of the Right Posterior Leg, Intermediate Dissection

NOTE: (1) The soleus muscle has been severed and reflected laterally, exposing the course of the tibial nerve and posterior tibial artery as far as the medial malleolus.

(2) This vessel and nerve descend in the leg between the superficial and deep muscles of the posterior compartment, and they lie between the flexor hallucis longus and the flexor digitorum longus and dorsal to the tibialis posterior muscle.

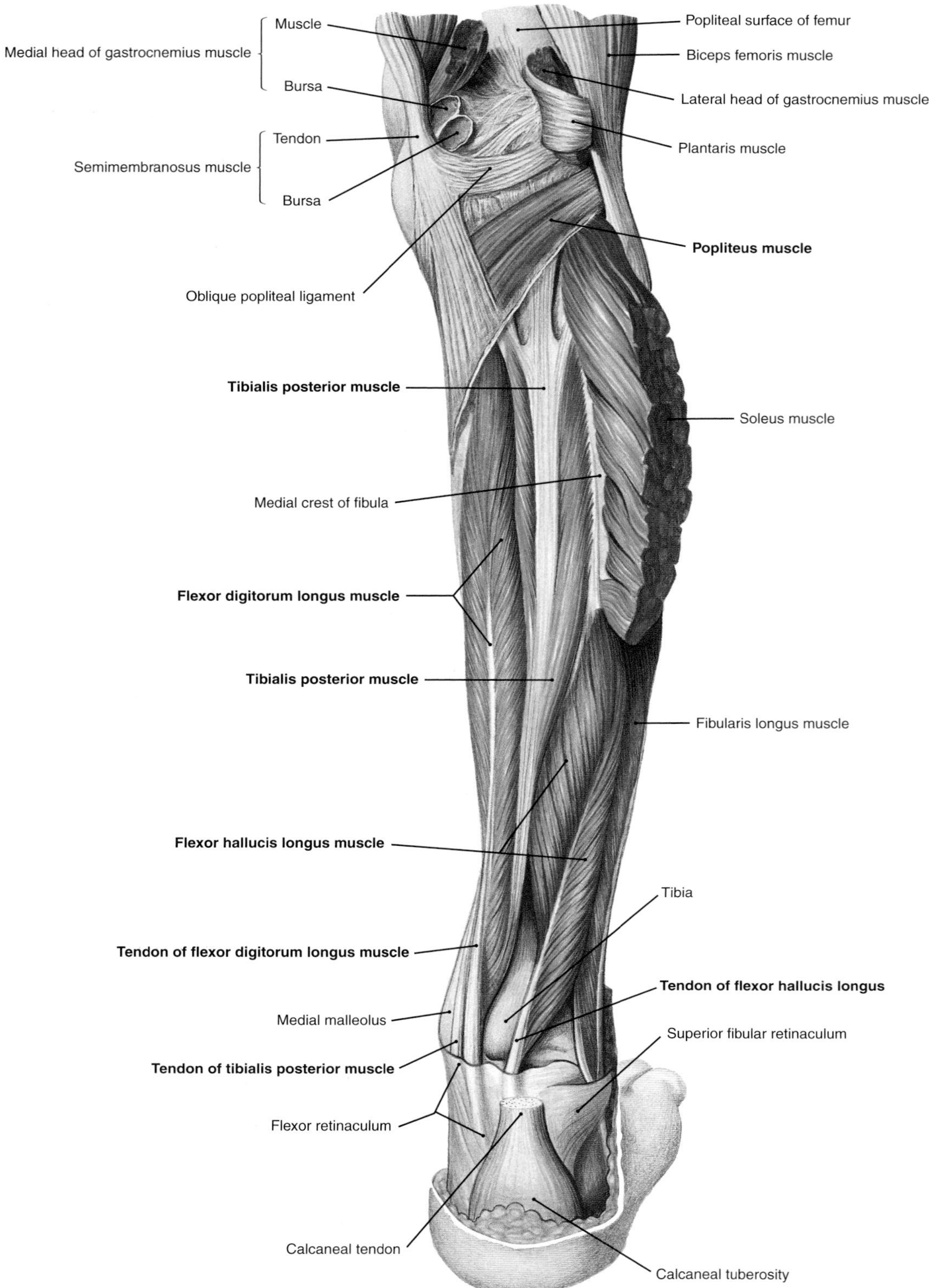
Medial head of gastrocnemius muscle
Muscle
Bursa
Semimembranosus muscle
Tendon
Bursa
Oblique popliteal ligament
Tibialis posterior muscle
Medial crest of fibula
Flexor digitorum longus muscle
Tibialis posterior muscle
Flexor hallucis longus muscle
Tendon of flexor digitorum longus muscle
Medial malleolus
Tendon of tibialis posterior muscle
Flexor retinaculum
Calcaneal tendon
Popliteal surface of femur
Biceps femoris muscle
Lateral head of gastrocnemius muscle
Plantaris muscle
Popliteus muscle
Soleus muscle
Fibularis longus muscle
Tibia
Tendon of flexor hallucis longus
Superior fibular retinaculum
Calcaneal tuberosity

Figure 418 Deep Muscles of the Posterior Compartment of the Leg

NOTE: (1) The four deep posterior compartment muscles are: (a) the **popliteus,** (b) the **flexor digitorum longus**, (c) the **tibialis posterior,** and (d) the **flexor hallucis longus.**

(2) The **popliteus** is a femorotibial muscle and it tends to rotate the leg medially; however, when the tibia is fixed and the knee joint is locked, this muscle rotates the femur laterally on the tibia and thereby it "unlocks" the knee joint.

(3) The other three muscles are cruropedal muscles, and as a group, they invert the foot, flex the toes, and assist in plantar flexion at the ankle joint.

(4) At the ankle region, the tendon of the tibialis posterior is closest to the bone behind the medial malleolus. Most lateral is the tendon of the flexor hallucis longus, with the tendon of the flexor digitorum longus in between the other two.

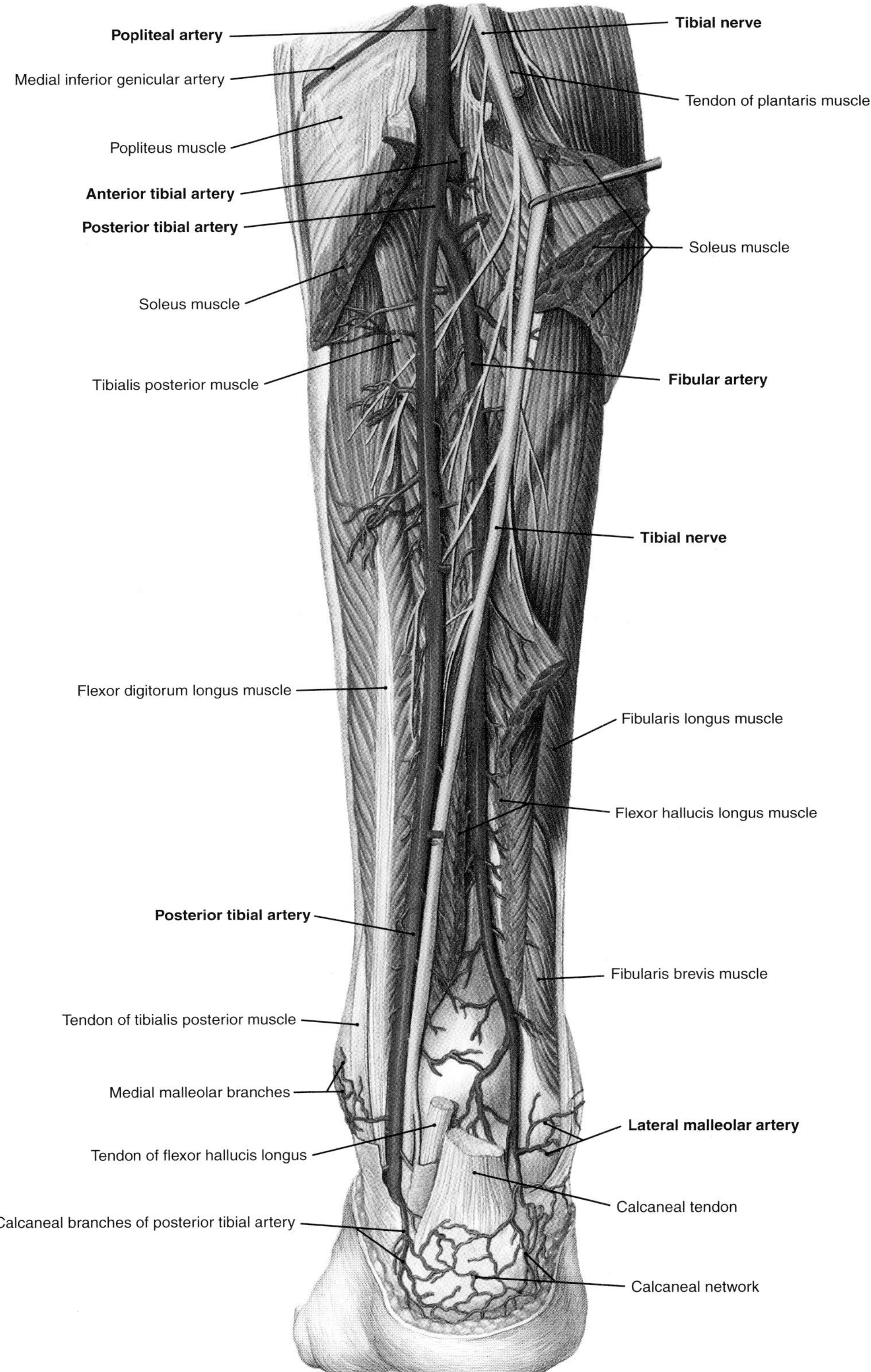
Popliteal artery
Medial inferior genicular artery
Popliteus muscle
Anterior tibial artery
Posterior tibial artery
Soleus muscle
Tibialis posterior muscle
Flexor digitorum longus muscle
Posterior tibial artery
Tendon of tibialis posterior muscle
Medial malleolar branches
Tendon of flexor hallucis longus
Calcaneal branches of posterior tibial artery
Tibial nerve
Tendon of plantaris muscle
Soleus muscle
Fibular artery
Tibial nerve
Fibularis longus muscle
Flexor hallucis longus muscle
Fibularis brevis muscle
Lateral malleolar artery
Calcaneal tendon
Calcaneal network

Figure 419 Deep Nerves and Arteries of the Posterior Compartment of the Leg

NOTE: (1) The soleus muscle was resected and the tibial nerve pulled laterally. Observe the branching of the **fibular artery** from the posterior tibial and its descending course toward the lateral malleolus.

(2) In the popliteal fossa, the tibial nerve courses superficial to the popliteal artery, whereas at the ankle, the posterior tibial artery is superficial to the tibial nerve.

(3) Behind the medial malleolus, the neurovascular structures are located between the tendons of the flexor digitorum longus and flexor hallucis longus.

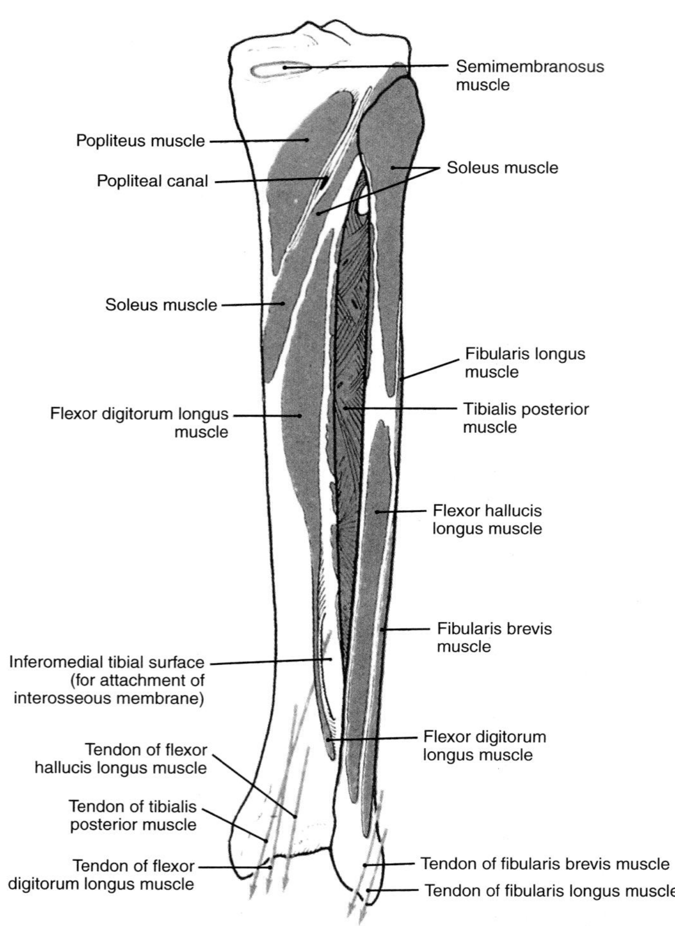

Semimembranosus muscle
Popliteus muscle
Popliteal canal
Soleus muscle
Soleus muscle
Fibularis longus muscle
Flexor digitorum longus muscle
Tibialis posterior muscle
Flexor hallucis longus muscle
Fibularis brevis muscle
Inferomedial tibial surface (for attachment of interosseous membrane)
Flexor digitorum longus muscle
Tendon of flexor hallucis longus muscle
Tendon of tibialis posterior muscle
Tendon of flexor digitorum longus muscle
Tendon of fibularis brevis muscle
Tendon of fibularis longus muscle

Figure 420 Muscle Attachments on the Right Tibia and Fibula (Posterior Surface)

NOTE: (1) Of the posterior compartment muscles, only the gastrocnemius and plantaris do not attach to the posterior surface of the tibia, fibula or interosseous membrane.

(2) Nearly the entire posterior surface of the fibula serves for the origin of muscles. The **soleus** arises from the upper third of the fibula and along the soleal line of the tibia. Inferior to the soleus, the **flexor hallucis longus** arises principally from the fibula, while the **flexor digitorum longus** arises primarily from the tibia.

(3) The **tibialis posterior** is interposed between the flexors hallucis longus and digitorum longus and arises, for the most part, from the interosseous membrane.

(4) The arrows indicate the course of the tendons into the foot from the posterior surface. The tendon of the tibialis posterior crosses from lateral to medial beneath the tendon of the flexor digitorum longus and enters the foot immediately behind the medial malleolus.

MUSCLES OF THE POSTERIOR COMPARTMENT OF THE LEG

Muscle	Origin	Insertion	Innervation	Action
		Superficial Group		
Gastrocnemius	Medial head: Medial epicondyle of the femur. Lateral head: Lateral epicondyle of the femur.	Posterior surface of the calcaneus by means of the calcaneal tendon	Tibial nerve (S1, S2)	Plantar flexes the foot; flexes the leg at knee joint, tends to supinate the foot
Soleus	Posterior surface of head and upper third or body of fibula; soleal line and medial border of tibia	Joins the tendon of the gastrocnemius to insert on the calcaneus by means of the calcaneal tendon	Tibial nerve (S1, S2)	Plantar flexes the foot; important as a postural muscle during ordinary standing
Plantaris	Posterior aspect of lateral epicondyle of femur and from the oblique popliteal ligament	Into the calcaneal tendon with the gastrocnemius and soleus muscles	Tibial nerve (S1, S2)	Assists the gastrocnemius in plantar flexion of the foot and flexing the leg (weak action)
		Deep Group		
Popliteus	Lateral epicondyle of the femur; the lateral meniscus of the knee joint	Posterior surface of the body of the tibia proximal to the soleal line	Tibial nerve (L4, L5, S1)	Flexes and medially rotates the tibia when femur is fixed; laterally rotates the femur to unlock the knee joint when the tibia is fixed
Tibialis posterior	Posterior surface of interosseous membrane; posterior surface of tibia and medial surface of the fibula	Tuberosity of the navicular bone; slips to calcaneus, the three cuneiforms, the cuboid and the second, third, and fourth metatarsal bones	Tibial nerve (L5, S1)	Plantar flexes the foot; inverts and adducts the foot (tends to supinate the foot)

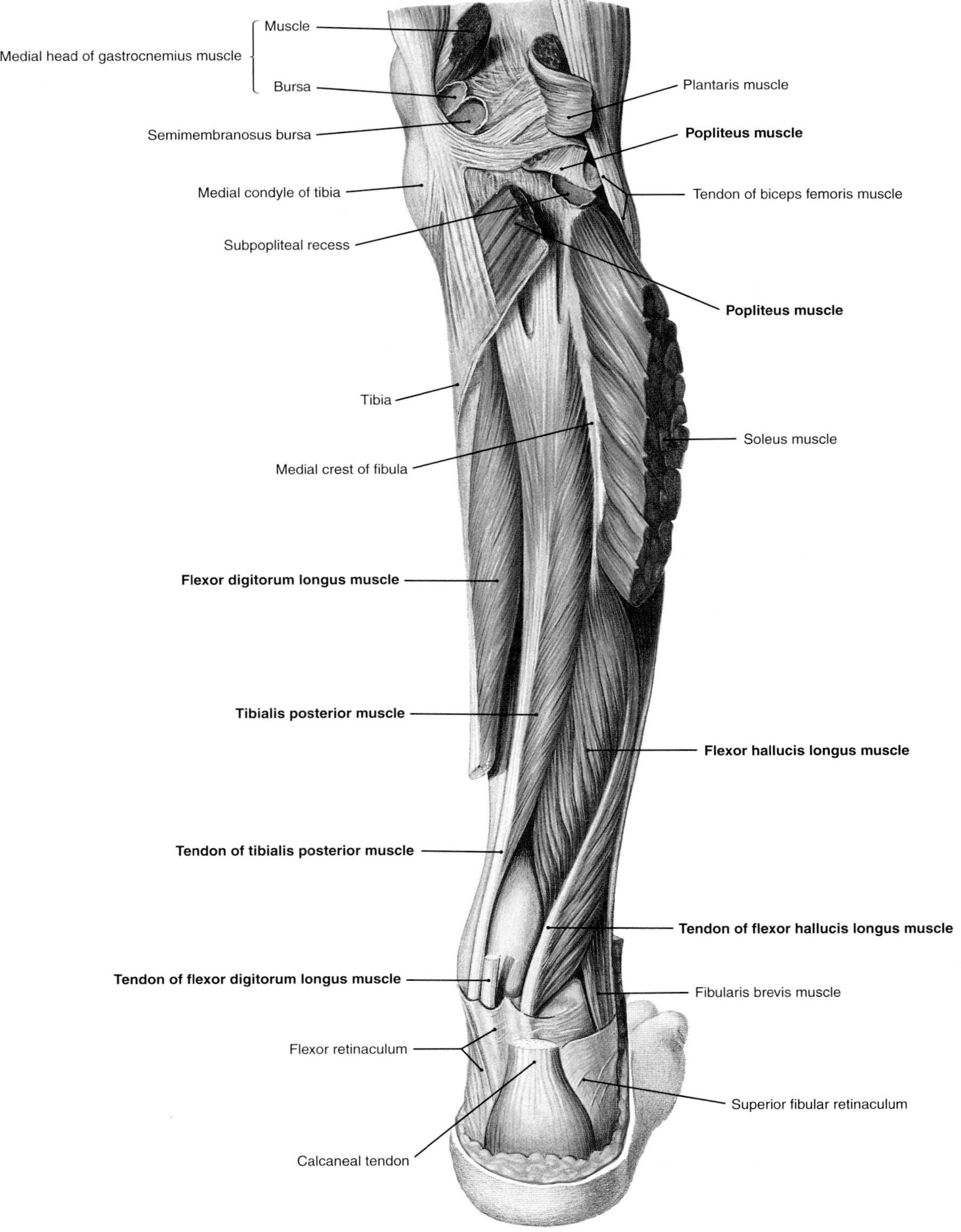
Muscle
Medial head of gastrocnemius muscle
Bursa
Semimembranosus bursa
Medial condyle of tibia
Subpopliteal recess
Tibia
Medial crest of fibula
Flexor digitorum longus muscle
Tibialis posterior muscle
Tendon of tibialis posterior muscle
Tendon of flexor digitorum longus muscle
Flexor retinaculum
Calcaneal tendon
Plantaris muscle
Popliteus muscle
Tendon of biceps femoris muscle
Popliteus muscle
Soleus muscle
Flexor hallucis longus muscle
Tendon of flexor hallucis longus muscle
Fibularis brevis muscle
Superior fibular retinaculum

Figure 421 **Tibialis Posterior and Flexor Hallucis Longus Muscles**

MUSCLES OF THE POSTERIOR COMPARTMENT OF THE LEG (CONT.)

Muscle	Origin	Insertion	Innervation	Action
Flexor digitorum longus	Posterior surface of tibia and fascia over tibialis posterior	Bases of the distal phalanx of the four lateral toes	Tibial nerve (S1, S2)	Flexes distal phalanx of lateral four toes; plantar flexes and supinates the foot
Flexor hallucis longus	Lower two-thirds of the posterior fibula and lower part of the interosseous membrane	Base of the distal phalanx of the large toe (hallux)	Tibial nerve (S1, S2)	Flexes distal phalanx of large toe; plantar flexes and supinates the foot

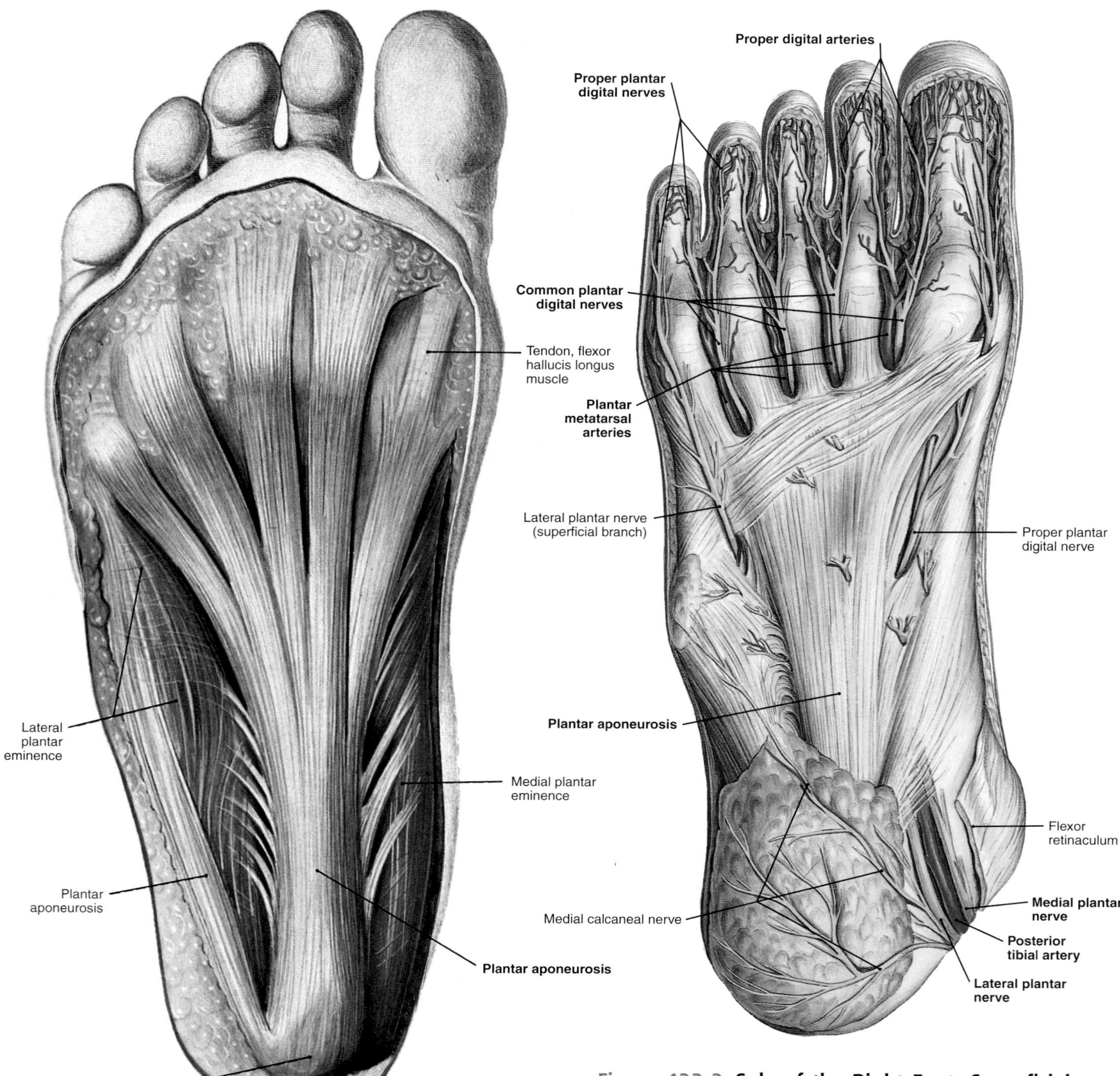
Lateral plantar eminence
Plantar aponeurosis
Calcaneal tuberosity
Tendon, flexor hallucis longus muscle
Medial plantar eminence
Plantar aponeurosis
Proper digital arteries
Proper plantar digital nerves
Common plantar digital nerves
Plantar metatarsal arteries
Lateral plantar nerve (superficial branch)
Proper plantar digital nerve
Plantar aponeurosis
Flexor retinaculum
Medial calcaneal nerve
Medial plantar nerve
Posterior tibial artery
Lateral plantar nerve

Figure 422.1 Sole of the Right Foot: Plantar Aponeurosis

NOTE: (1) The **plantar aponeurosis** stretching along the sole of the foot. Similar to the palmar aponeurosis in the hand, the plantar aponeurosis is a thickened layer of deep fascia serving a protective function to underlying muscles, vessels, and nerves.

(2) The longitudinal orientation of the plantar aponeurosis and its attachment behind to the calcaneal tuberosity. The aponeurosis divides distally into digital slips, one to each toe. At the margins, fibers partially cover the medial and lateral plantar eminences.

Figure 422.2 Sole of the Right Foot: Superficial Nerves and Arteries

NOTE: (1) The **medial** and **lateral plantar nerves** and **posterior tibial artery** as they enter the foot behind the medial malleolus and then immediately course beneath the plantar aponeurosis toward the digits. Cutaneous branches of the nerves penetrate the aponeurosis to supply the overlying skin and fascia.

(2) Between digital slips of the plantar aponeurosis, the vessels and nerves course superficially toward the toes. **Metatarsal arteries** and **common plantar digital nerves** divide to supply adjacent portions of the toes as **proper plantar digital arteries** and **nerves.**

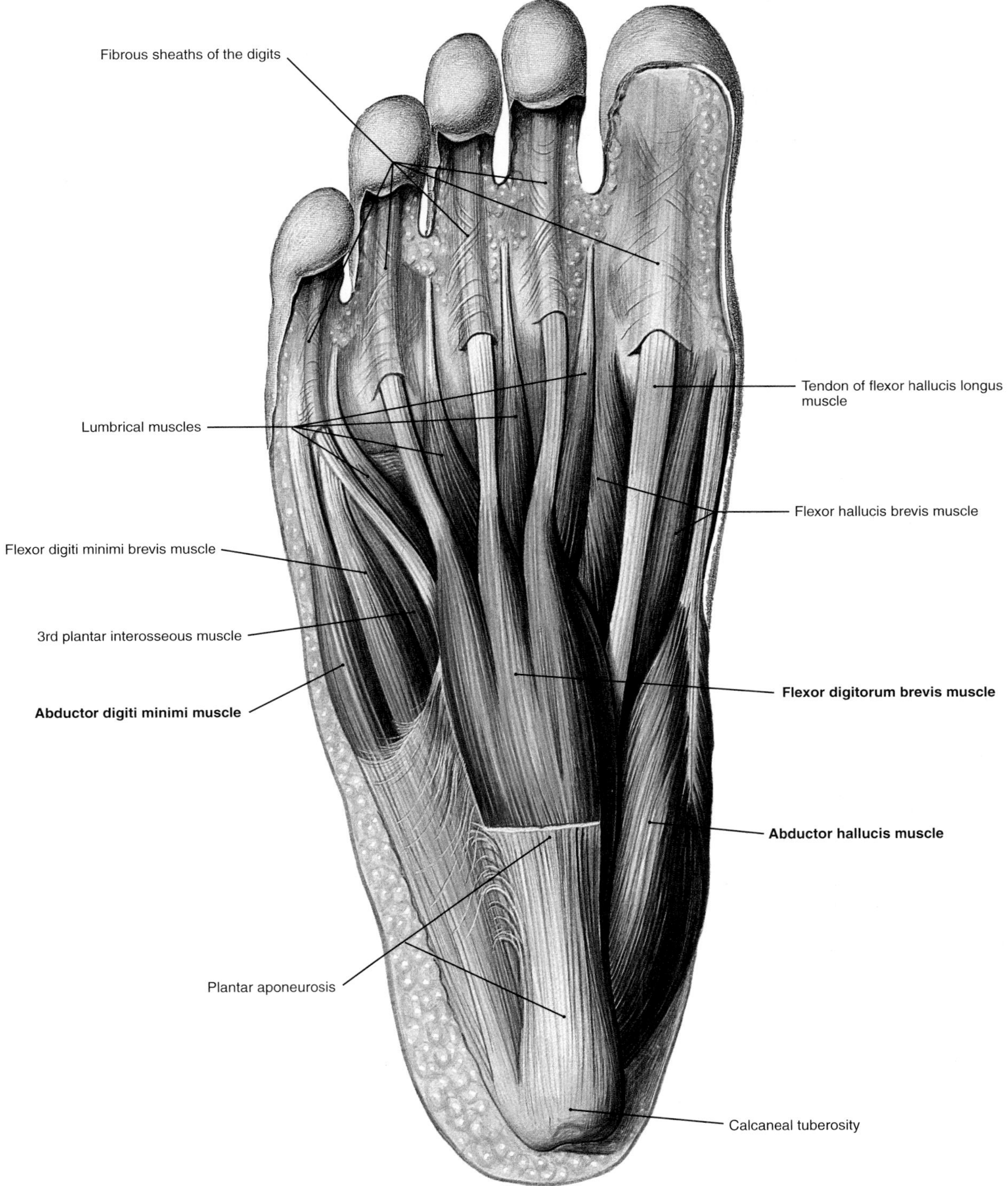
Fibrous sheaths of the digits
Lumbrical muscles
Flexor digiti minimi brevis muscle
3rd plantar interosseous muscle
Abductor digiti minimi muscle
Plantar aponeurosis
Tendon of flexor hallucis longus muscle
Flexor hallucis brevis muscle
Flexor digitorum brevis muscle
Abductor hallucis muscle
Calcaneal tuberosity

Figure 423 **Sole of the Foot: First Layer of Plantar Muscles**

NOTE: (1) With most of the plantar aponeurosis removed, three muscles comprising the first layer of plantar muscles are exposed. These are the **abductor hallucis,** the **flexor digitorum brevis,** and the **abductor digiti minimi.**

(2) All three muscles of the first layer arise from the tuberosity of the calcaneus. The abductor hallucis inserts on the proximal phalanx of the large toe. The flexor digitorum brevis separates into four tendons that insert onto the middle phalanges of the four lateral toes. The abductor digiti minimi inserts on the proximal phalanx of the small toe.

(3) The terminal parts of the tendons of the short and long flexors of the toes course within osseous–aponeurotic canals to their insertions on bone.

(4) These canals are covered inferiorly by **digital fibrous sheaths** that arch over the tendons and attach to the sides of the phalanges. Within the canals, **synovial sheaths** are closely reflected around the tendons, allowing for their movement upon muscular contraction.

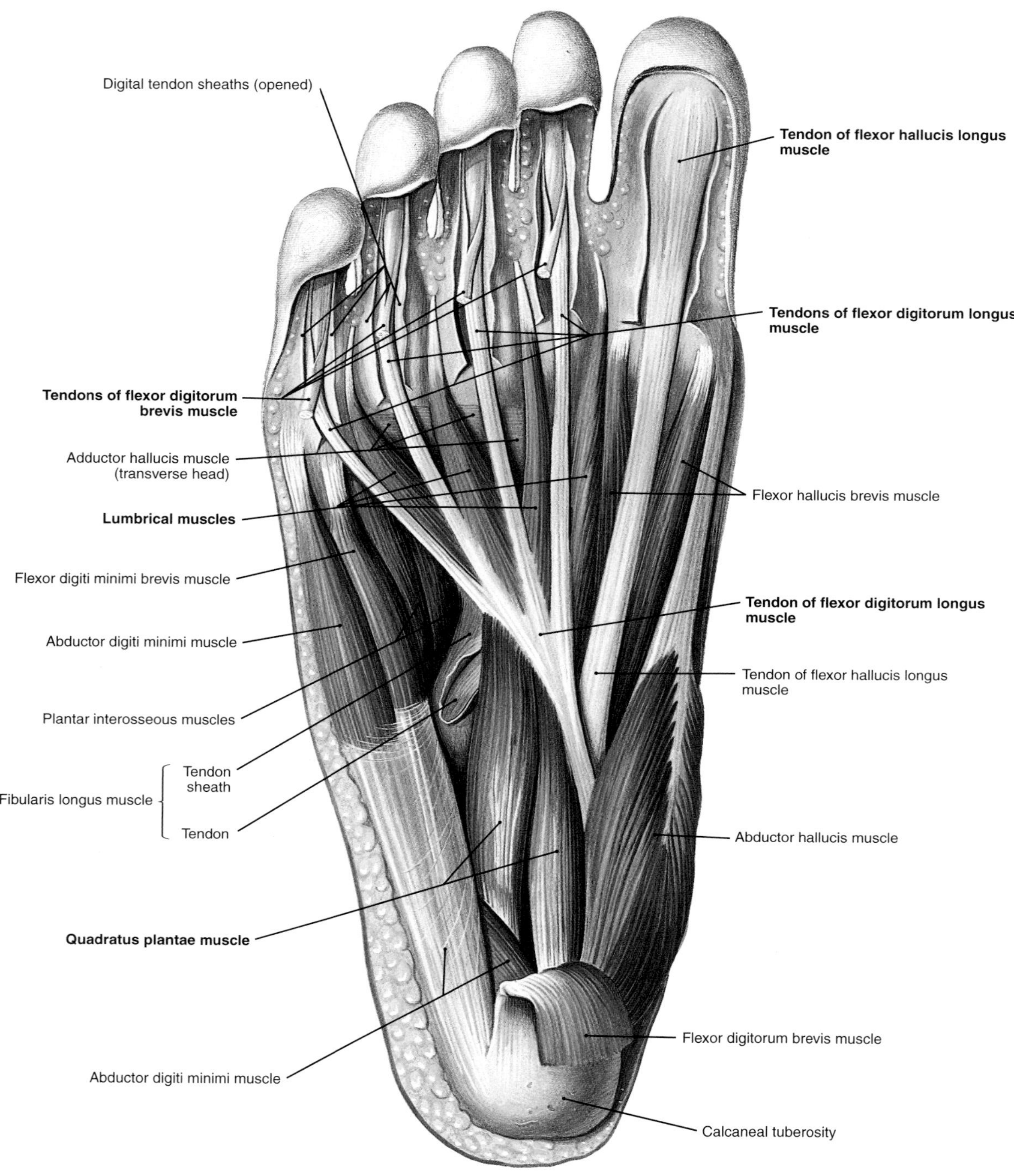

Digital tendon sheaths (opened)
Tendon of flexor hallucis longus muscle
Tendons of flexor digitorum longus muscle
Tendons of flexor digitorum brevis muscle
Adductor hallucis muscle (transverse head)
Lumbrical muscles
Flexor hallucis brevis muscle
Flexor digiti minimi brevis muscle
Tendon of flexor digitorum longus muscle
Abductor digiti minimi muscle
Tendon of flexor hallucis longus muscle
Plantar interosseous muscles
Fibularis longus muscle
Tendon sheath
Tendon
Abductor hallucis muscle
Quadratus plantae muscle
Flexor digitorum brevis muscle
Abductor digiti minimi muscle
Calcaneal tuberosity

Figure 424 Sole of the Right Foot: Second Layer of Plantar Muscles

NOTE: (1) The tendons of the flexor digitorum brevis muscle were severed and removed, thereby exposing the underlying tendons of the **flexor digitorum longus muscle.**

(2) The muscles of the **second layer** in the plantar foot include the **quadratus plantae muscle** and the four **lumbrical muscles.** The quadratus plantae arises by two heads from the calcaneus and inserts into the tendon of the flexor digitorum longus muscle.

(3) The four lumbrical muscles arise from the tendons of the flexor digitorum longus muscle. They insert on the medial aspect of the first phalanx of the lateral four toes as well as on the dorsal extensor hoods of the toes.

(4) The quadratus plantae muscle helps align the pull of the tendons of the flexor digitorum longus by straightening the diagonal vector of the long tendon.

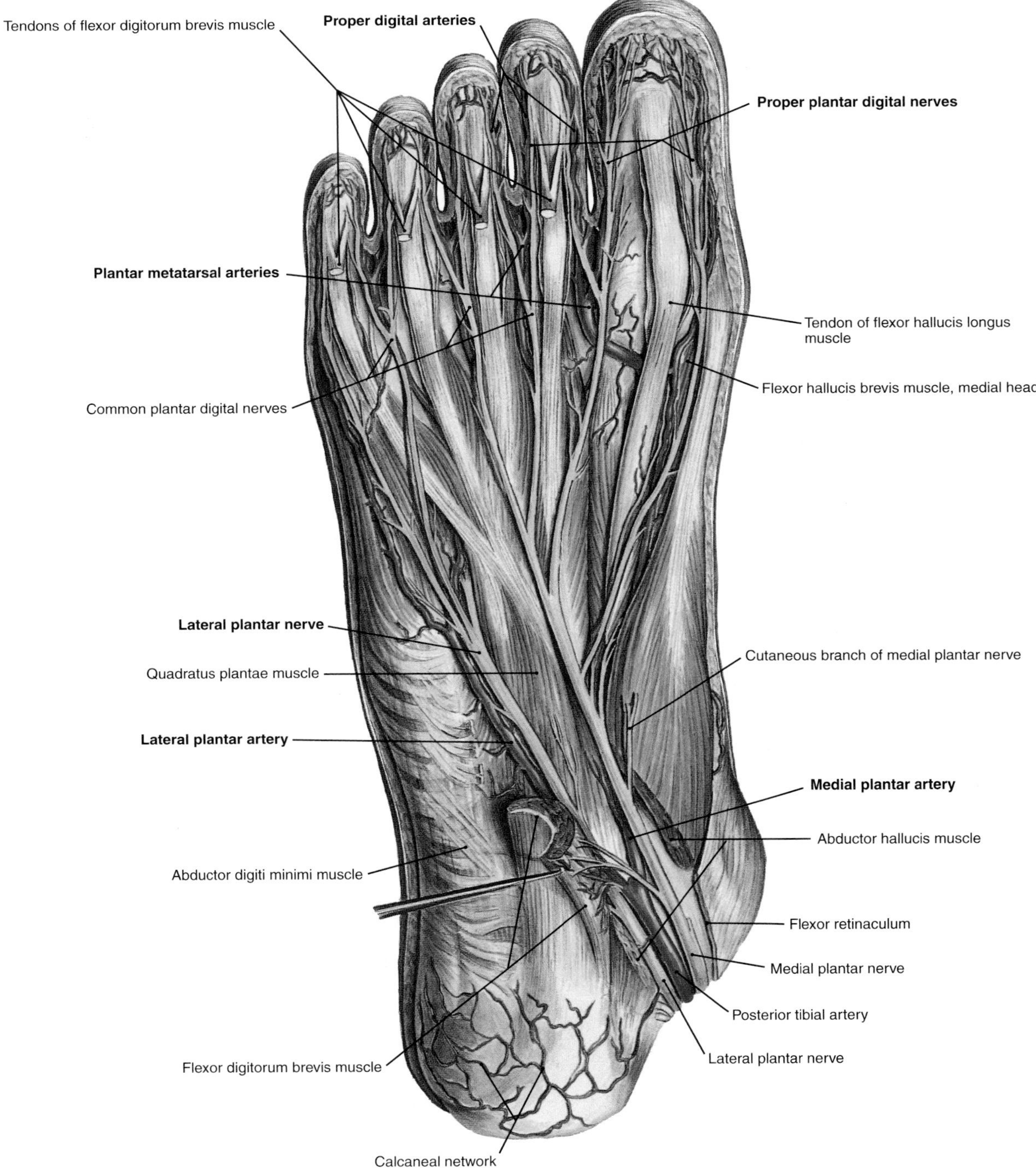
Tendons of flexor digitorum brevis muscle
Proper digital arteries
Proper plantar digital nerves
Plantar metatarsal arteries
Tendon of flexor hallucis longus muscle
Flexor hallucis brevis muscle, medial head
Common plantar digital nerves
Lateral plantar nerve
Cutaneous branch of medial plantar nerve
Quadratus plantae muscle
Lateral plantar artery
Medial plantar artery
Abductor hallucis muscle
Abductor digiti minimi muscle
Flexor retinaculum
Medial plantar nerve
Posterior tibial artery
Lateral plantar nerve
Flexor digitorum brevis muscle
Calcaneal network

Figure 425 **Sole of the Right Foot: the Plantar Nerves and Arteries**

NOTE: (1) While the tibial nerve divides into **medial** and **lateral plantar nerves** just below the medial malleolus, the posterior tibial artery enters the plantar surface of the foot as a single vessel and then divides into **medial** and **lateral plantar arteries** beneath or at the medial border of the abductor hallucis muscle.

(2) The lateral plantar nerve supplies the lateral 1½ digits with cutaneous innervation, while the medial plantar nerve supplies the medial 3 ½ digits. Observe the formation of the **common plantar digital nerves,** which then divide into the **proper plantar digital nerves.**

(3) The main trunks of the plantar vessels and nerves cross the sole of the foot from medial to lateral deep to the flexor digitorum brevis and abductor hallucis muscles (first layer), but superficial to the quadratus plantae and lumbrical muscles (second layer).

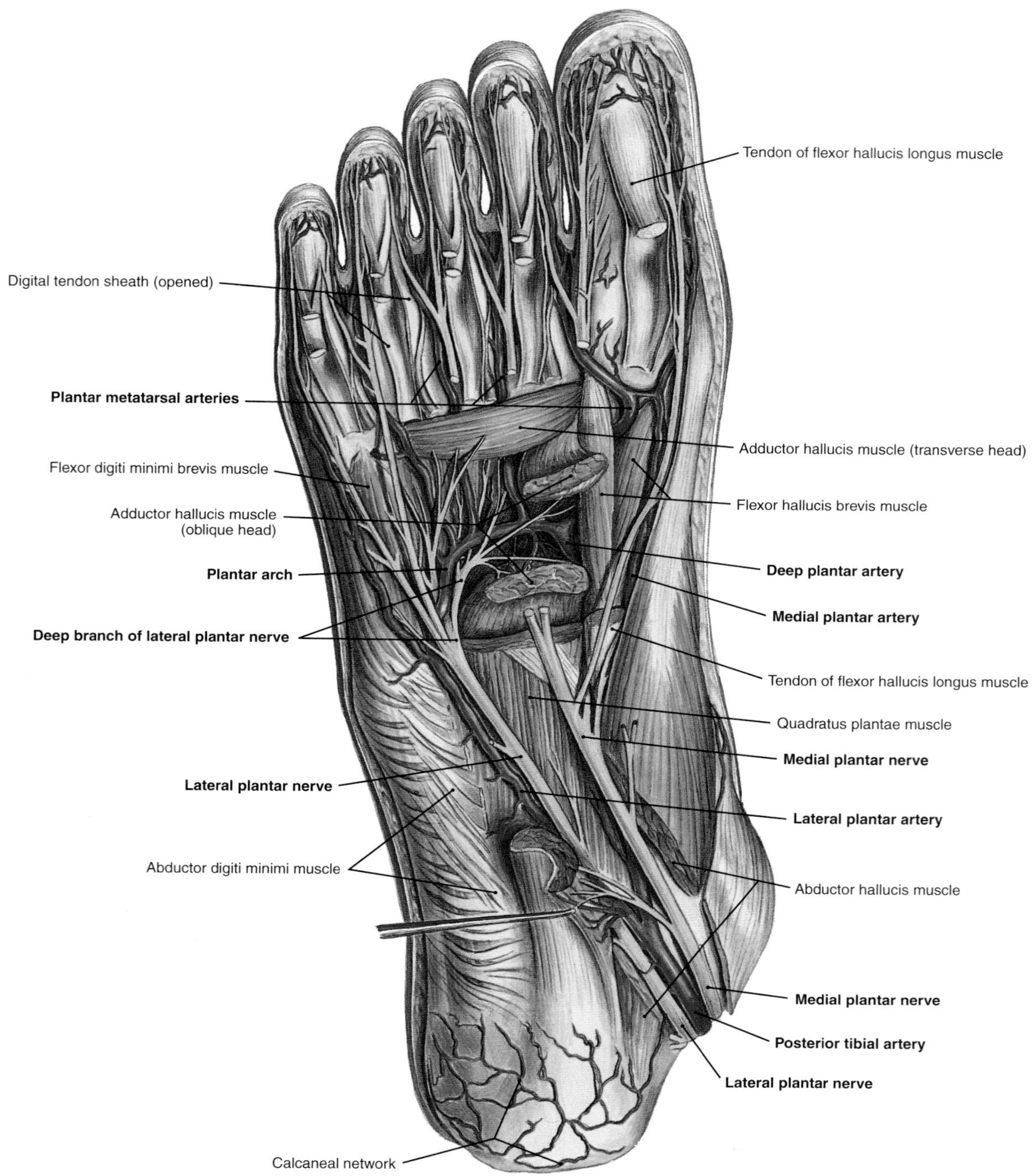
Tendon of flexor hallucis longus muscle
Digital tendon sheath (opened)
Plantar metatarsal arteries
Adductor hallucis muscle (transverse head)
Flexor digiti minimi brevis muscle
Flexor hallucis brevis muscle
Adductor hallucis muscle (oblique head)
Plantar arch
Deep plantar artery
Medial plantar artery
Deep branch of lateral plantar nerve
Tendon of flexor hallucis longus muscle
Quadratus plantae muscle
Medial plantar nerve
Lateral plantar nerve
Lateral plantar artery
Abductor digiti minimi muscle
Abductor hallucis muscle
Medial plantar nerve
Posterior tibial artery
Lateral plantar nerve
Calcaneal network

Figure 426 Sole of the Right Foot: Plantar Arch and Deep Vessels and Nerves

NOTE: (1) The formation of the **deep plantar arch** principally from the lateral plantar artery and the junction of the deep plantar arch with the deep plantar artery from the foot dorsum (see Fig. 411). From the plantar arch branch **plantar metatarsal arteries,** which divide into **proper original arteries.**

(2) The muscles of the foot are innervated in the following manner:

	Medial plantar nerve	Lateral plantar nerve
First layer	Abductor hallucis; flexor digitorum brevis	Abductor digiti minimi
Second layer	First lumbrical	Quadratus plantae; second, third, and fourth lumbrical
Third layer	Flexor hallucis brevis	Adductor hallucis; flexor digiti minimi brevis
Fourth layer		Plantar interossei; dorsal interossei

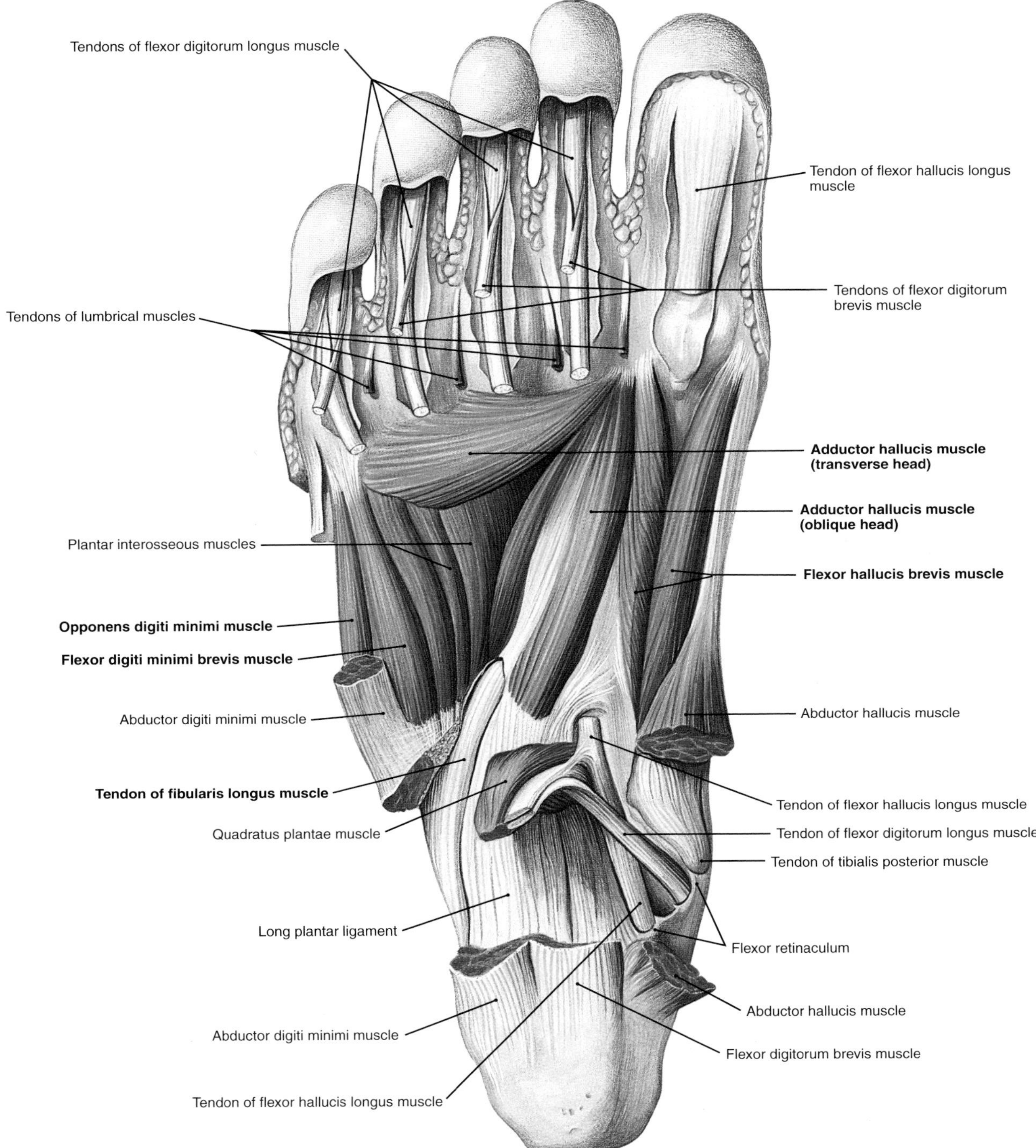
Tendons of flexor digitorum longus muscle
Tendon of flexor hallucis longus muscle
Tendons of flexor digitorum brevis muscle
Tendons of lumbrical muscles
Adductor hallucis muscle (transverse head)
Adductor hallucis muscle (oblique head)
Plantar interosseous muscles
Flexor hallucis brevis muscle
Opponens digiti minimi muscle
Flexor digiti minimi brevis muscle
Abductor digiti minimi muscle
Abductor hallucis muscle
Tendon of fibularis longus muscle
Tendon of flexor hallucis longus muscle
Quadratus plantae muscle
Tendon of flexor digitorum longus muscle
Tendon of tibialis posterior muscle
Long plantar ligament
Flexor retinaculum
Abductor hallucis muscle
Abductor digiti minimi muscle
Flexor digitorum brevis muscle
Tendon of flexor hallucis longus muscle

Figure 427 **Sole of the Right Foot: Third Layer of Plantar Muscles**

NOTE: (1) The third layer of plantar muscles consists of two flexors and an *ad*ductor (with two heads), in contrast to the first layer, which contains one flexor and two *ab*ductors. Thus, the **flexor hallucis brevis, flexor digiti minimi brevis,** and the **oblique** and **transverse heads** of the **adductor hallucis** form the third layer of plantar muscles.

(2) At times, the fibers of the flexor digiti minimi brevis that insert on the lateral side of the first phalanx of the fifth toe are referred to as a separate muscle: the **opponens digiti minimi.**

(3) The tendon of the **fibularis longus muscles,** which crosses the plantar aspect of the foot obliquely to insert on the lateral side of the base of the first metatarsal and the first (medial) cuneiform bone.

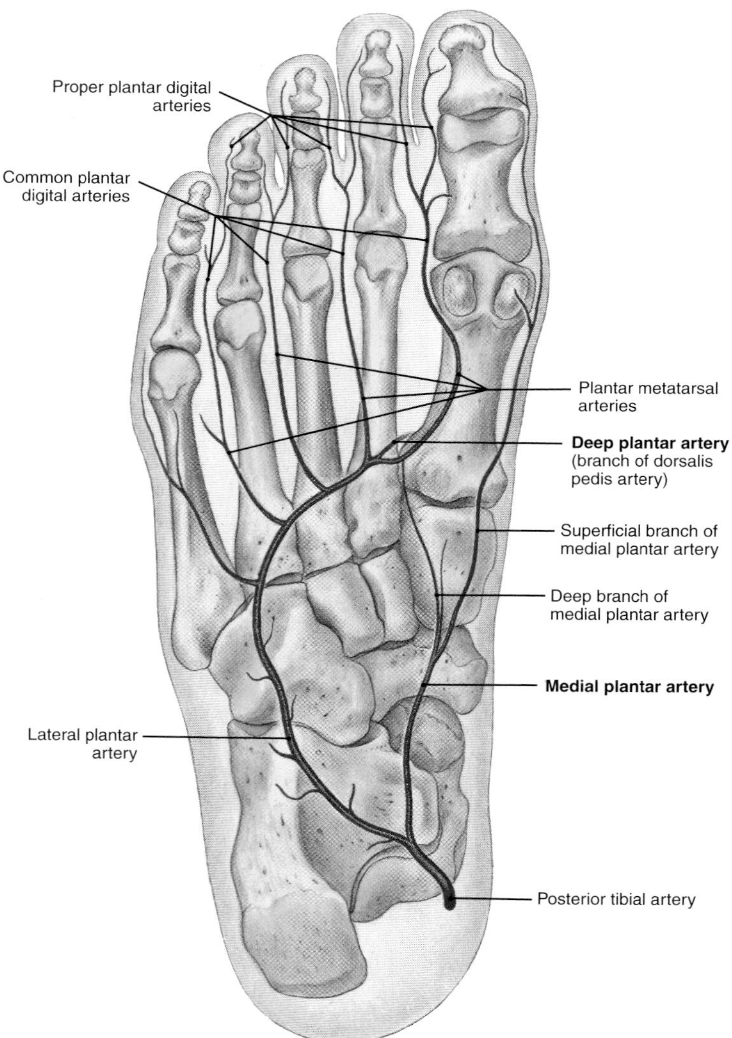
Proper plantar digital arteries
Common plantar digital arteries
Plantar metatarsal arteries
Deep plantar artery (branch of dorsalis pedis artery)
Superficial branch of medial plantar artery
Deep branch of medial plantar artery
Medial plantar artery
Lateral plantar artery
Posterior tibial artery

Figure 428.1 Plantar Aspect of the Foot: Diagram of Arteries and Bones

NOTE: The **posterior tibial artery** enters the foot medially behind the medial malleolus, divides into **medial** and **lateral plantar arteries,** and anastomoses with the deep plantar branch of the **dorsalis pedis artery** between the first and second digits.

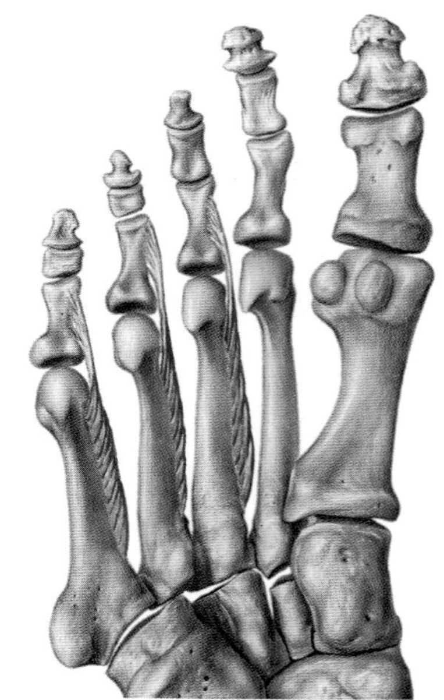

Figure 428.2 Plantar Interossei

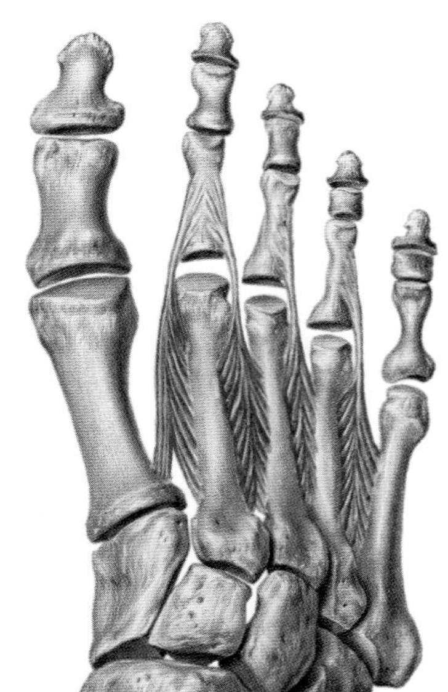

Figure 428.3 Dorsal Interossei

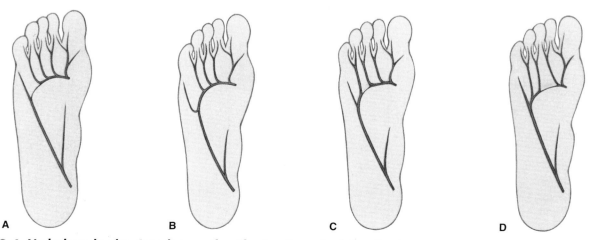

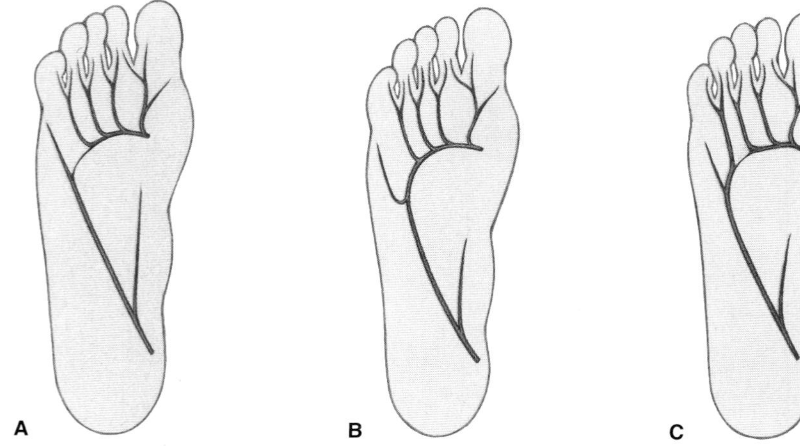
A
B
C
D

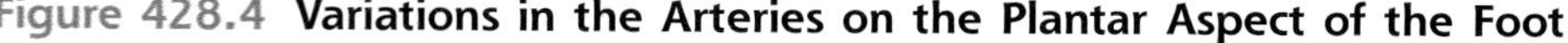

Figure 428.4 Variations in the Arteries on the Plantar Aspect of the Foot

NOTE: A. Deep plantar arch principally from the dorsalis pedis artery (from the foot dorsum).

B. Deep plantar arch supplied mainly from the lateral plantar branch of the posterior fibial artery.

C. Fifth and part of fourth toes by lateral plantar artery, medial toes by dorsalis pedis artery.

D. Fifth, fourth, and lateral part of third toe by lateral plantar artery, medial toes by dorsalis pedis artery.

MUSCLES OF THE SOLE OF THE FOOT

Muscle	Origin	Insertion	Innervation	Action
		First Layer of Muscles		
Abductor hallucis	Flexor retinaculum; medial process of calcaneal tuberosity; plantar aponeurosis	Medial side of the base of the proximal phalanx of the large toe	Medial plantar nerve (L5, S1)	Abducts and flexes the large toe; helps maintain the medial longitudinal arch
Flexor digitorum brevis	Medial process of calcaneal tuberosity; plantar aponeurosis	By four tendons onto the middle phalanx of the lateral four toes	Medial plantar nerve (L5, S1)	Flexes the lateral four toes
Abductor digiti minimi	Medial and lateral processes of the calcaneal tuberosity; plantar aponeurosis	Lateral side of the base of the proximal phalanx of the small toe	Lateral planter nerve (S2, S3)	Abducts and flexes the little toe
		Second Layer of Muscles		
Quadratus plantae	By two heads from the plantar surface of the calcaneus; long plantar ligament	Lateral and deep surfaces of the tendons of the flexor digitorum longus muscle	Lateral plantar nerve (S2, S3)	Assists the flexor digitorum longus; straightens the pull of the flexor digitorum longus along longitudinal axis of foot
First lumbrical	Medial side of the first tendon (to second toe) of the flexor digitorum longus	Passes along the medial side of second toe and inserts on its dorsal digital expansion	Medial plantar nerve (L5, S1)	Flex the proximal phalanx at the metatarsophalangeal joint; extend the interphalangeal joints
Second, third, and fourth lumbrical	Each muscle by two heads from the adjacent surfaces of the second, third and fourth tendons (to the third, fourth, and fifth toes) of the flexor digitorum longus muscle	Course along the medial sides of the third, fourth, and fifth toes and insert on their respective dorsal digital expansions	Lateral plantar nerve (S2, S3)	Action same as the first lumbrical
		Third Layer of Muscles		
Flexor hallucis brevis	Plantar surface of cuboid and lateral (third) cuneiform bones; tendon of the tibialis posterior	By two tendons onto the sides of the base of the proximal phalanx of the large toe	Medial plantar nerve (L5, S1)	Flexes the proximal phalanx of the large toe at the metatarsophalangeal joint
Flexor digiti minimi	Base of the fifth metatarsal bone; the sheath of the tendon of the fibularis longus	Lateral side of the base of the proximal phalanx of the small toe	Lateral plantar nerve (S2, S3)	Flexes the proximal phalanx of the small toe at the metatarsophalangeal joint
Adductor hallucis Transverse head	Plantar metatarsophalangeal ligaments of third, fourth, and fifth toes; deep transverse metatarsal ligaments between the toes	By a common tendon to lateral aspect of the base of the proximal phalanx of the large toe	Lateral plantar nerve (S2, S3)	Adducts large toe; flexes large toe at metatarsophalangeal joint
Oblique head	Bases of the second, third, and fourth metatarsal bones; sheath of the tendon of fibularis longus muscle			
		Fourth Layer of Muscles		
Plantar interossei (three muscles)	Bases and medial sides of third, fourth, and fifth metatarsal bones	Bases of proximal phalanx of third, fourth, and fifth toes (medial side); onto the dorsal digital expansions	Lateral plantar nerve (S2, S3)	Adduct third, fourth, and fifth toes; flex metatarsophalangeal joints; extend interphalangeal joints
Dorsal interossei (four muscles)	Each by two heads from adjacent sides of metatarsal bones	Proximal phalanx and dorsal digital expansions of second, third, and fourth toes	Lateral plantar nerve (S2, S3)	Abduct second, third, and fourth toes; flex metatarsophalangeal joints and extend interphalangeal joints

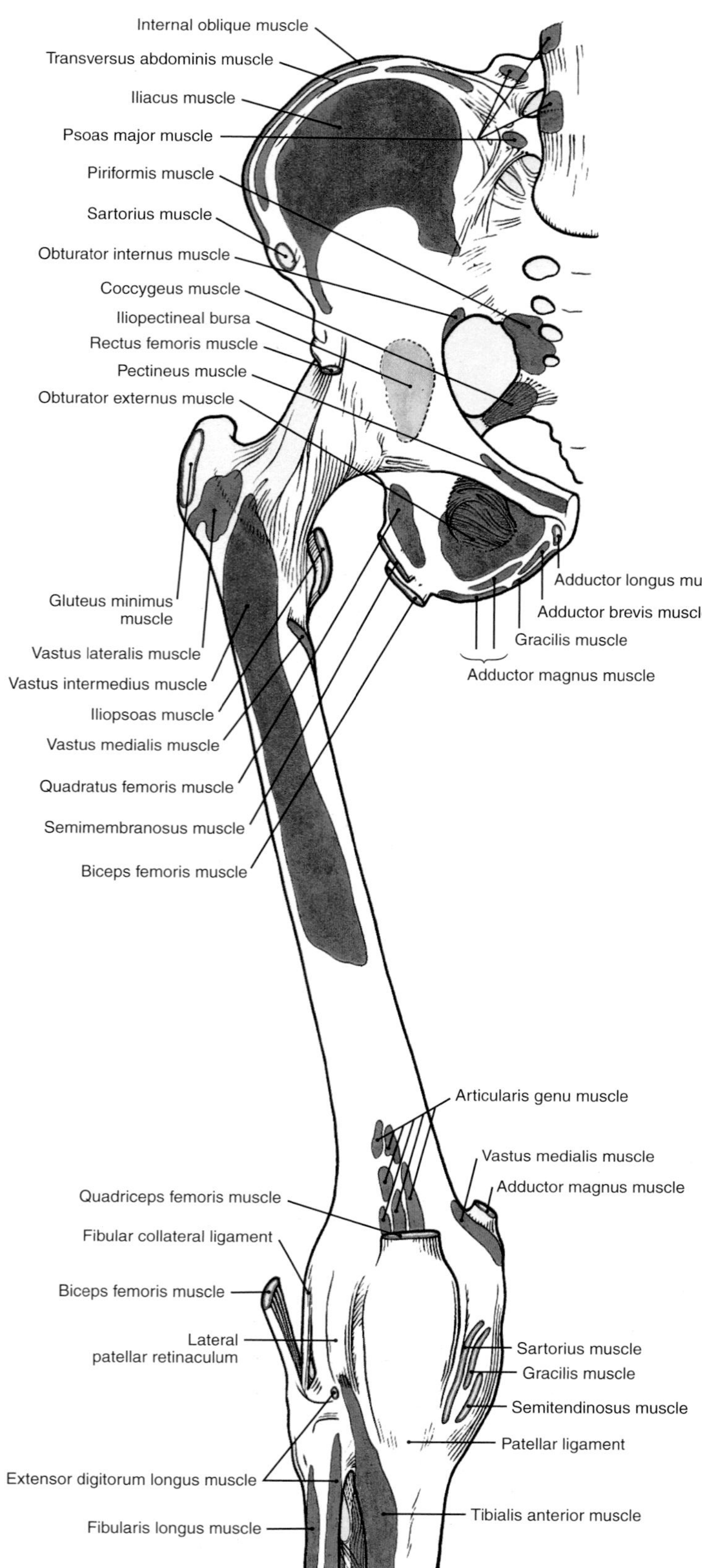
Internal oblique muscle
Transversus abdominis muscle
Iliacus muscle
Psoas major muscle
Piriformis muscle
Sartorius muscle
Obturator internus muscle
Coccygeus muscle
Iliopectineal bursa
Rectus femoris muscle
Pectineus muscle
Obturator externus muscle
Gluteus minimus muscle
Vastus lateralis muscle
Vastus intermedius muscle
Iliopsoas muscle
Vastus medialis muscle
Quadratus femoris muscle
Semimembranosus muscle
Biceps femoris muscle
Adductor longus muscle
Adductor brevis muscle
Gracilis muscle
Adductor magnus muscle
Articularis genu muscle
Vastus medialis muscle
Adductor magnus muscle
Quadriceps femoris muscle
Fibular collateral ligament
Biceps femoris muscle
Lateral patellar retinaculum
Sartorius muscle
Gracilis muscle
Semitendinosus muscle
Patellar ligament
Extensor digitorum longus muscle
Fibularis longus muscle
Tibialis anterior muscle

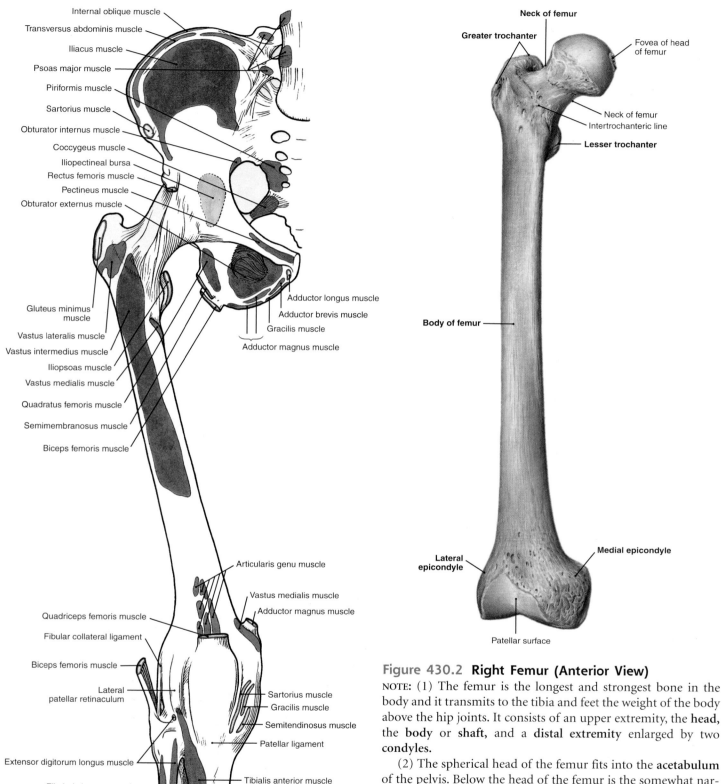

Figure 430.1 Anterior View of Right Pelvis and Femur Showing Muscle Attachments

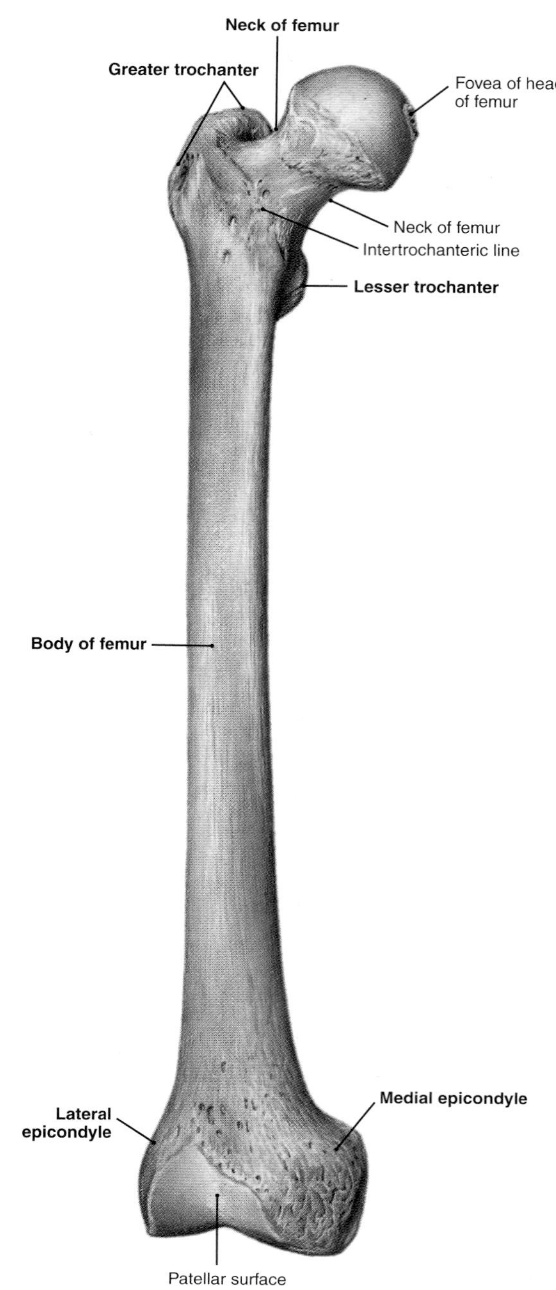
Neck of femur
Greater trochanter
Fovea of head of femur
Neck of femur
Intertrochanteric line
Lesser trochanter
Body of femur
Lateral epicondyle
Medial epicondyle
Patellar surface

Figure 430.2 Right Femur (Anterior View)

NOTE: (1) The femur is the longest and strongest bone in the body and it transmits to the tibia and feet the weight of the body above the hip joints. It consists of an upper extremity, the **head,** the **body** or **shaft,** and a **distal extremity** enlarged by two **condyles.**

(2) The spherical head of the femur fits into the **acetabulum** of the pelvis. Below the head of the femur is the somewhat narrowed femoral **neck** and two prominent tubercles, the **greater** and **lesser trochanters.**

(3) The anterior surface of the body of the femur is smooth and its proximal two-thirds gives origin to the vastus intermedius muscle.

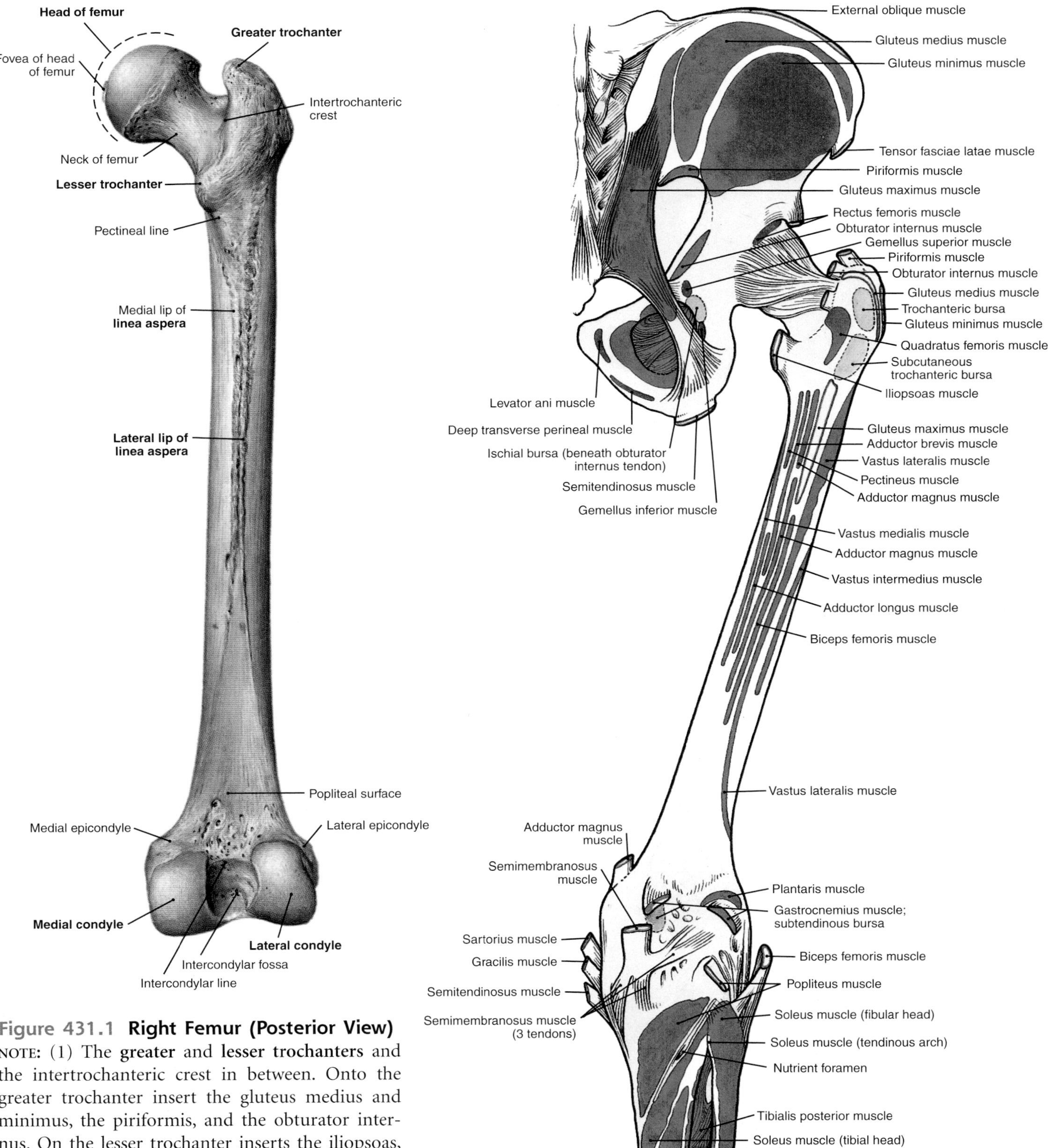
Head of femur
Fovea of head of femur
Greater trochanter
Intertrochanteric crest
Neck of femur
Lesser trochanter
Pectineal line
Medial lip of linea aspera
Lateral lip of linea aspera
Popliteal surface
Medial epicondyle
Lateral epicondyle
Medial condyle
Lateral condyle
Intercondylar fossa
Intercondylar line
External oblique muscle
Gluteus medius muscle
Gluteus minimus muscle
Tensor fasciae latae muscle
Piriformis muscle
Gluteus maximus muscle
Rectus femoris muscle
Obturator internus muscle
Gemellus superior muscle
Piriformis muscle
Obturator internus muscle
Gluteus medius muscle
Trochanteric bursa
Gluteus minimus muscle
Quadratus femoris muscle
Subcutaneous trochanteric bursa
Iliopsoas muscle
Levator ani muscle
Deep transverse perineal muscle
Ischial bursa (beneath obturator internus tendon)
Semitendinosus muscle
Gemellus inferior muscle
Gluteus maximus muscle
Adductor brevis muscle
Vastus lateralis muscle
Pectineus muscle
Adductor magnus muscle
Vastus medialis muscle
Adductor magnus muscle
Vastus intermedius muscle
Adductor longus muscle
Biceps femoris muscle
Vastus lateralis muscle
Adductor magnus muscle
Semimembranosus muscle
Plantaris muscle
Gastrocnemius muscle; subtendinous bursa
Sartorius muscle
Gracilis muscle
Biceps femoris muscle
Semitendinosus muscle
Popliteus muscle
Semimembranosus muscle (3 tendons)
Soleus muscle (fibular head)
Soleus muscle (tendinous arch)
Nutrient foramen
Tibialis posterior muscle
Soleus muscle (tibial head)
Soleus muscle (fibular head)
Flexor digitorum longus muscle

Figure 431.1 Right Femur (Posterior View)

NOTE: (1) The **greater** and **lesser trochanters** and the intertrochanteric crest in between. Onto the greater trochanter insert the gluteus medius and minimus, the piriformis, and the obturator internus. On the lesser trochanter inserts the iliopsoas, while the quadratus femoris attaches along the intertrochanteric crest.

(2) The thick, longitudinally oriented ridge, the **linea aspera,** along the posterior surface of the body of the femur. It also serves for muscle attachments.

(3) The **medial** and **lateral condyles** and **epicondyles** inferiorly. The condyles articulate with the tibia and the intercondyloid fossa affords attachment for the cruciate ligaments.

Figure 431.2 Posterior View of Right Pelvis and Femur Showing Muscle Attachments

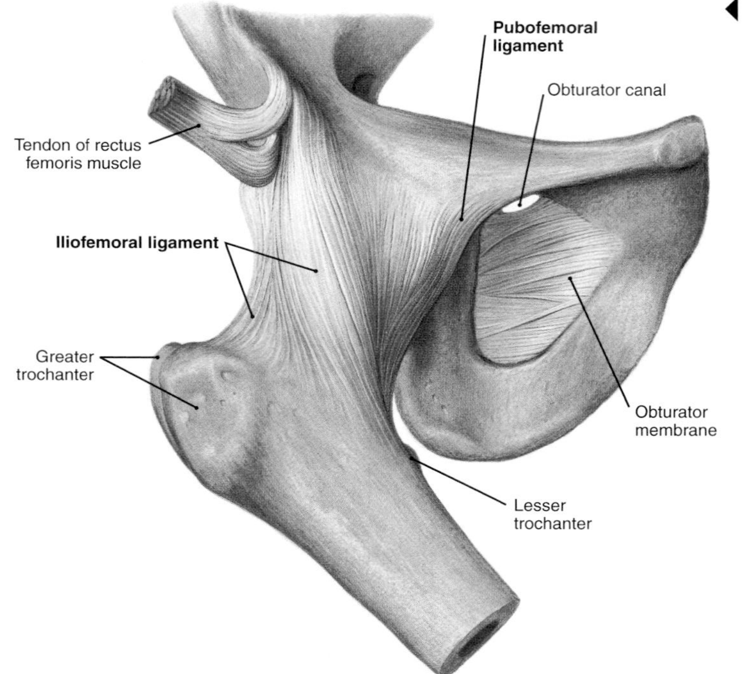
Pubofemoral ligament
Obturator canal
Tendon of rectus femoris muscle
Iliofemoral ligament
Greater trochanter
Obturator membrane
Lesser trochanter

Figure 432.1 Right Hip Joint (Anterior View)

NOTE: (1) The hip joint is a typical ball-and-socket joint and consists of the **head of the femur,** which fits snugly in a deepened cavity, the **acetabular fossa.** The bones are held in position by a series of extremely strong ligaments.

(2) The **articular capsule** of the hip joints is reinforced by the **iliofemoral, pubofemoral,** and **ischiofemoral ligaments,** the **acetabular labrum,** the **transverse acetabular ligament,** and the **ligament of the head of the femur.**

(3) The longitudinally oriented fibers of the iliofemoral and pubofemoral ligaments seen anteriorly on the capsule.

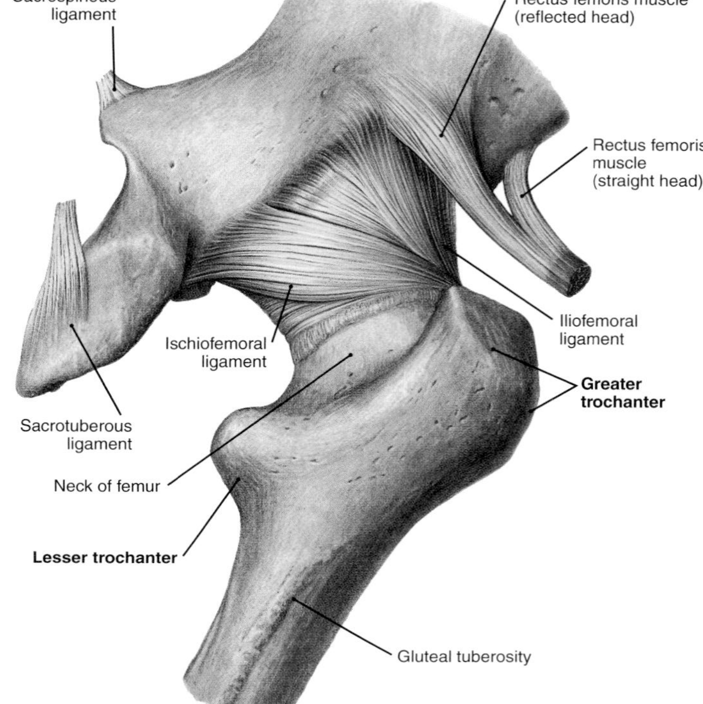
Sacrospinous ligament
Rectus femoris muscle (reflected head)
Rectus femoris muscle (straight head)
Iliofemoral ligament
Ischiofemoral ligament
Greater trochanter
Sacrotuberous ligament
Neck of femur
Lesser trochanter
Gluteal tuberosity

Figure 432.2 Right Hip Joint (Posterior View)

NOTE: Fibers of the **ischiofemoral ligament** are directed almost horizontally across the capsule of the hip joint. Whereas anteriorly (Fig. 430.2) the capsule attaches along the intertrochanteric line of the femur, posteriorly it encircles the femoral neck. The capsule is thinnest and weaker posteriorly.

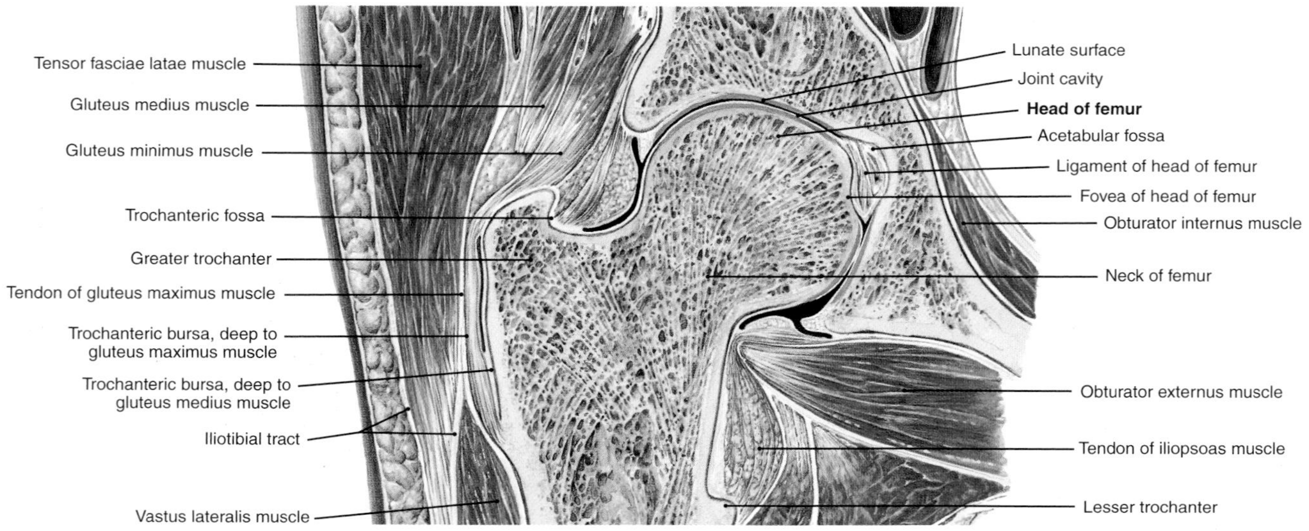
Tensor fasciae latae muscle
Gluteus medius muscle
Gluteus minimus muscle
Trochanteric fossa
Greater trochanter
Tendon of gluteus maximus muscle
Trochanteric bursa, deep to gluteus maximus muscle
Trochanteric bursa, deep to gluteus medius muscle
Iliotibial tract
Vastus lateralis muscle
Lunate surface
Joint cavity
Head of femur
Acetabular fossa
Ligament of head of femur
Fovea of head of femur
Obturator internus muscle
Neck of femur
Obturator externus muscle
Tendon of iliopsoas muscle
Lesser trochanter

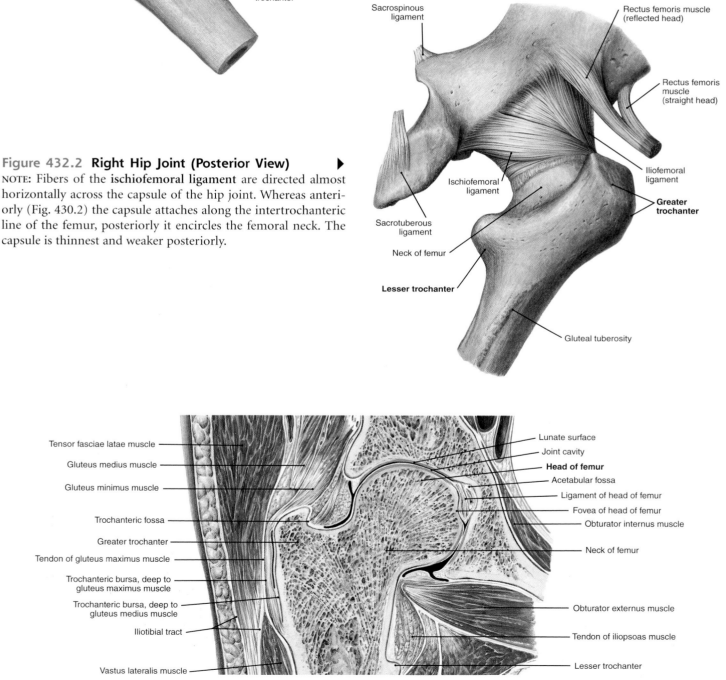

Figure 432.3 Frontal Section through the Right Hip Joint and Some Surrounding Soft Tissues

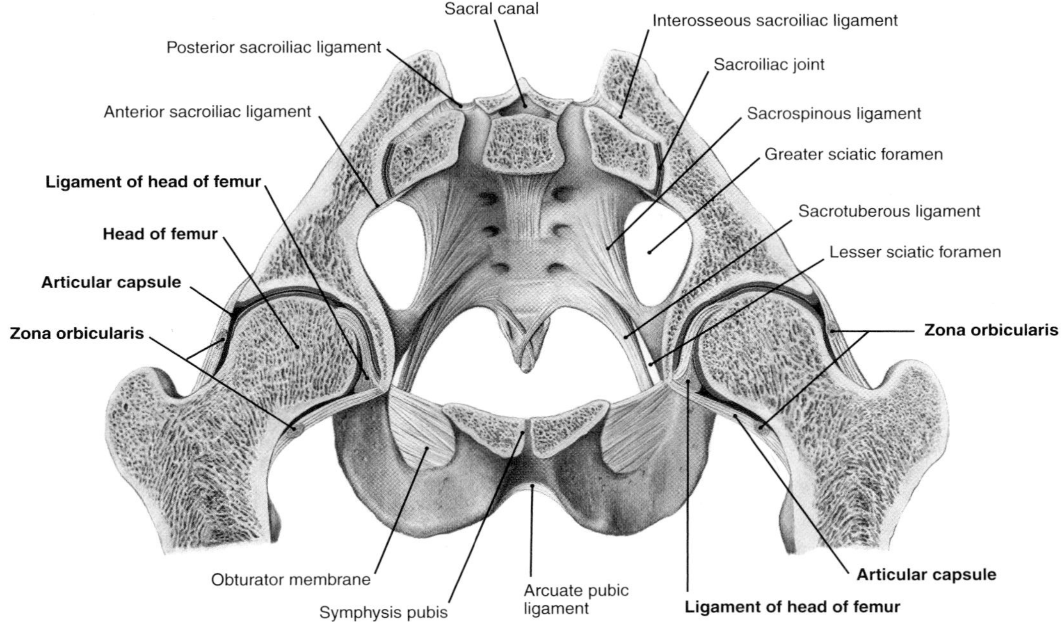
Sacral canal
Interosseous sacroiliac ligament
Posterior sacroiliac ligament
Sacroiliac joint
Anterior sacroiliac ligament
Sacrospinous ligament
Greater sciatic foramen
Ligament of head of femur
Sacrotuberous ligament
Head of femur
Lesser sciatic foramen
Articular capsule
Zona orbicularis
Zona orbicularis
Obturator membrane
Articular capsule
Symphysis pubis
Arcuate pubic ligament
Ligament of head of femur

Figure 433.1 Frontal Section of the Pelvis Showing Both Hip Joints

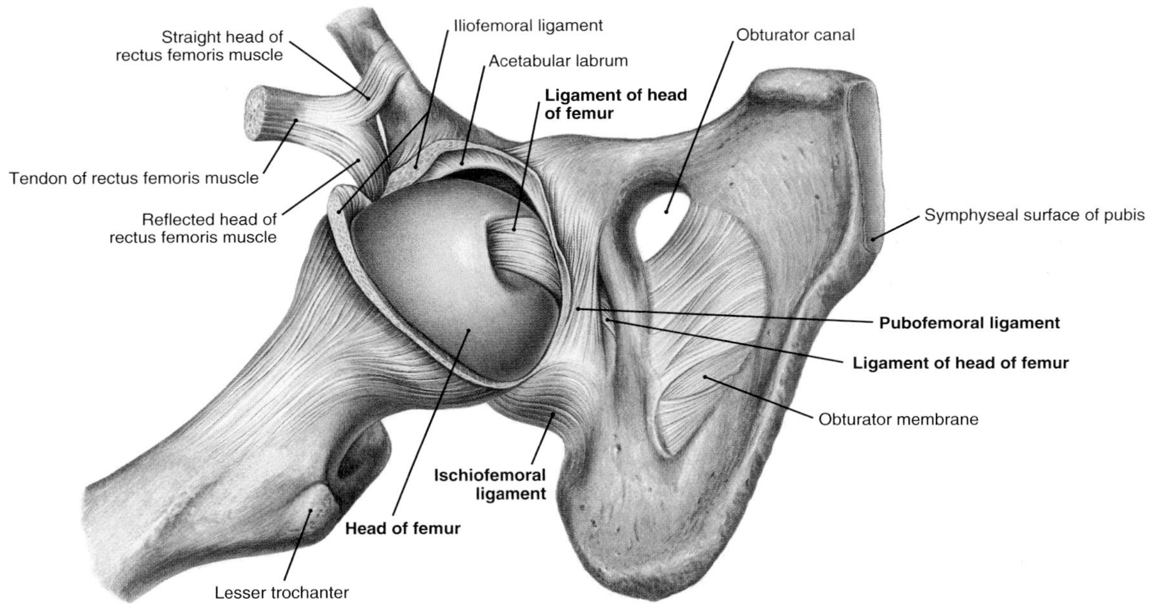
Straight head of rectus femoris muscle
Iliofemoral ligament
Obturator canal
Acetabular labrum
Ligament of head of femur
Tendon of rectus femoris muscle
Reflected head of rectus femoris muscle
Symphyseal surface of pubis
Pubofemoral ligament
Ligament of head of femur
Obturator membrane
Ischiofemoral ligament
Head of femur
Lesser trochanter

Figure 433.2 Anterior Exposure of the Right Hip Joint

NOTE: The articular capsule of the hip joint has been opened near the acetabular labrum. This exposes the cartilage-covered head of the femur within the joint cavity. Observe the ligament of the femoral head attached to the femur where cartilage is lacking.

Figure 433.3 Socket of the Right Hip Joint ▶

NOTE: (1) The acetabulum is surrounded by a fibrocartilaginous rim, the **acetabular labrum.** This deepens the joint cavity and accommodates enough of the distal head of the femur so that it cannot be pulled from its socket without injuring the acetabular labrum.

(2) The bony acetabulum is incomplete below. Here the acetabular notch is partially covered by the **transverse acetabular ligament.** Through the free portion of the acetabular notch course vessels and nerves that supply the head of the **femur.**

(3) The **ligament of the head of the femur** attaches the femoral head by two bands to either side of the acetabular notch.

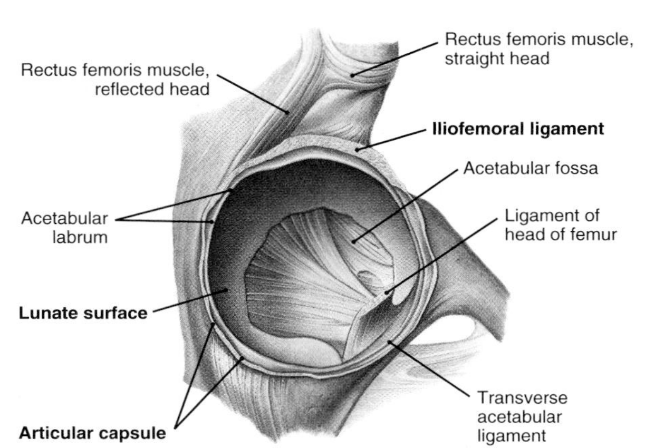
Rectus femoris muscle, straight head
Rectus femoris muscle, reflected head
Iliofemoral ligament
Acetabular fossa
Acetabular labrum
Ligament of head of femur
Lunate surface
Transverse acetabular ligament
Articular capsule

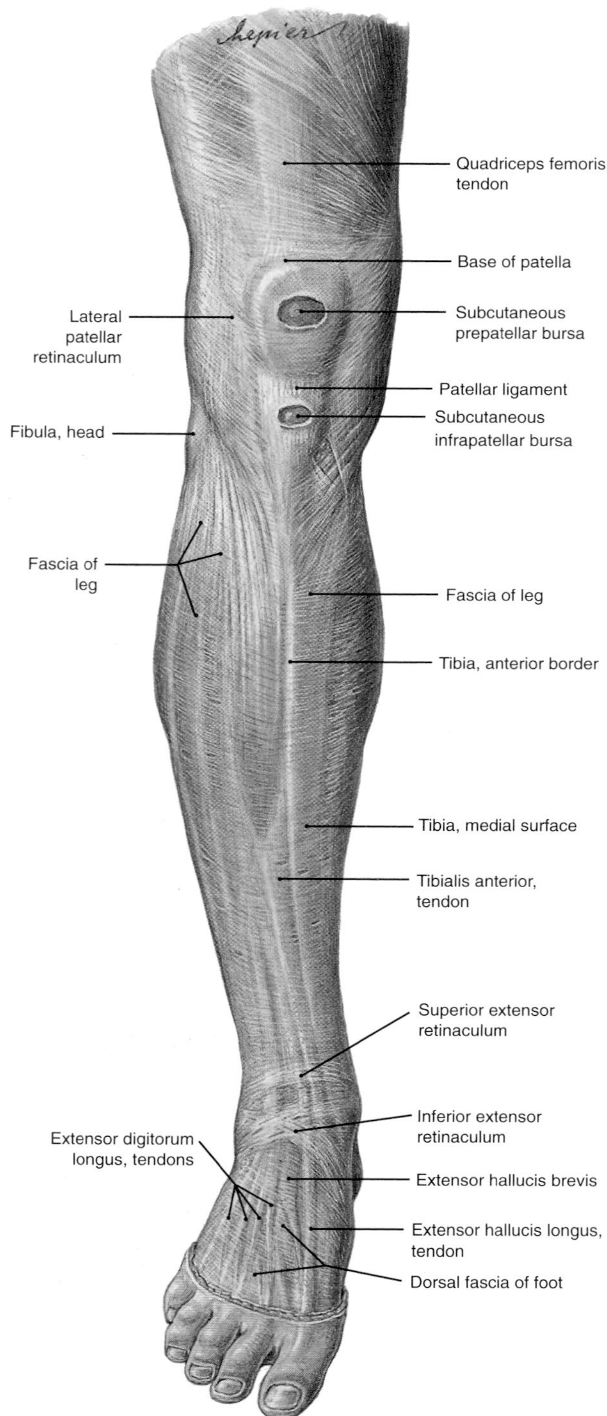
Quadriceps femoris, tendon
Base of patella
Lateral patellar retinaculum
Subcutaneous prepatellar bursa
Patellar ligament
Subcutaneous infrapatellar bursa
Fibula, head
Fascia of leg
Fascia of leg
Tibia, anterior border
Tibia, medial surface
Tibialis anterior, tendon
Superior extensor retinaculum
Inferior extensor retinaculum
Extensor digitorum longus, tendons
Extensor hallucis brevis
Extensor hallucis longus, tendon
Dorsal fascia of foot

Figure 434.1 Fascia of the Right Knee and Leg (Anterior Aspect)

NOTE: (1) The subcutaneous **infrapatellar bursa** and the **prepatellar bursa;** these bursae may become inflamed, resulting in a bursitis (sometimes called housemaid's knee, and often seen in persons who kneel a lot).

(2) The thick and dense deep fascia of the leg is continuous with the fascia lata; it is frequently called the **crural fascia.**

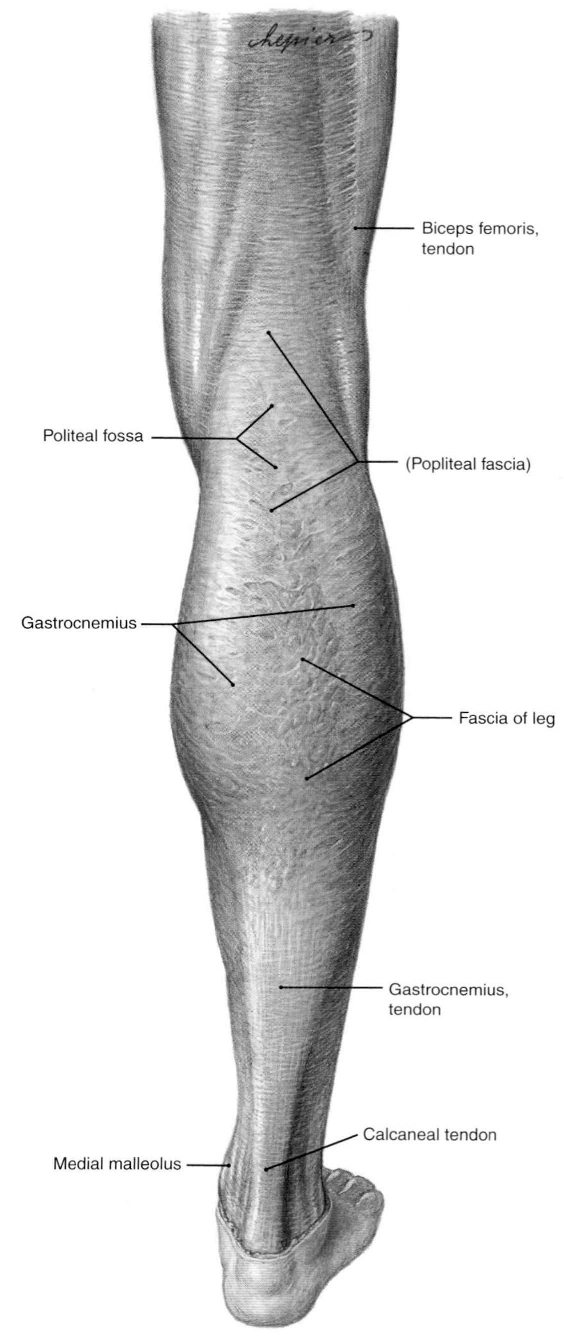
Biceps femoris, tendon
Politeal fossa
(Popliteal fascia)
Gastrocnemius
Fascia of leg
Gastrocnemius, tendon
Calcaneal tendon
Medial malleolus

Figure 434.2 Fascia of the Right Knee and Leg (Posterior Aspect)

NOTE: (1) The popliteal fascia covering the posterior aspect of the popliteal fossa.

(2) Extensions from the deep fascia of the leg, called **intermuscular septa** (medial and lateral), penetrate the crural muscles and separate them as functional groups (anterior, lateral, superficial posterior, and deep posterior).

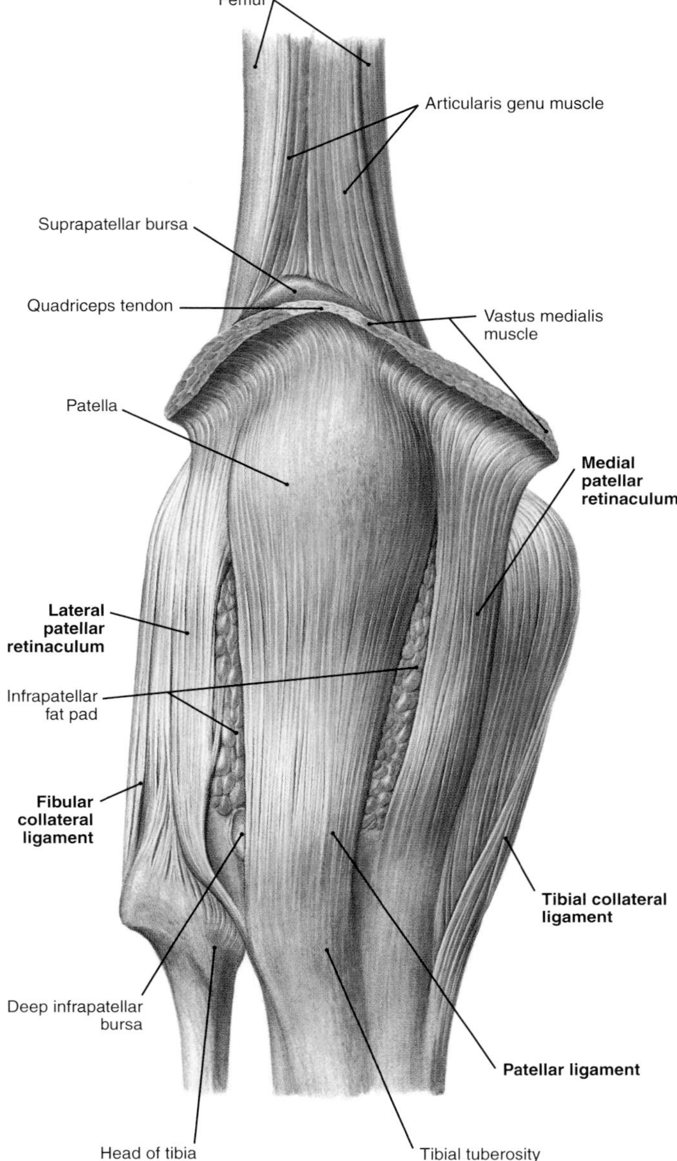
Femur
Articularis genu muscle
Suprapatellar bursa
Quadriceps tendon
Vastus medialis muscle
Patella
Medial patellar retinaculum
Lateral patellar retinaculum
Infrapatellar fat pad
Fibular collateral ligament
Tibial collateral ligament
Deep infrapatellar bursa
Patellar ligament
Head of tibia
Tibial tuberosity

Figure 435.1 Right Knee Joint (Anterior View)

NOTE: (1) The deep fascia has been removed, and the bellies of the four heads of the quadriceps femoris muscle have been cut to expose the quadriceps tendon, the patella, and the patellar ligament.

(2) The **patellar ligament** inserts onto the tibial tuberosity located on the proximal aspect of the anterior tibial surface.

(3) The **medial** and **lateral patellar retinacula.** These structures reinforce the anteromedial and anterolateral parts of the fibrous capsule of the knee joint and often (but not shown in this figure) they are attached to the borders of the patellar ligament and patella.

(4) The **tibial** and **fibular collateral ligaments** and the location of the **deep infrapatellar bursa.**

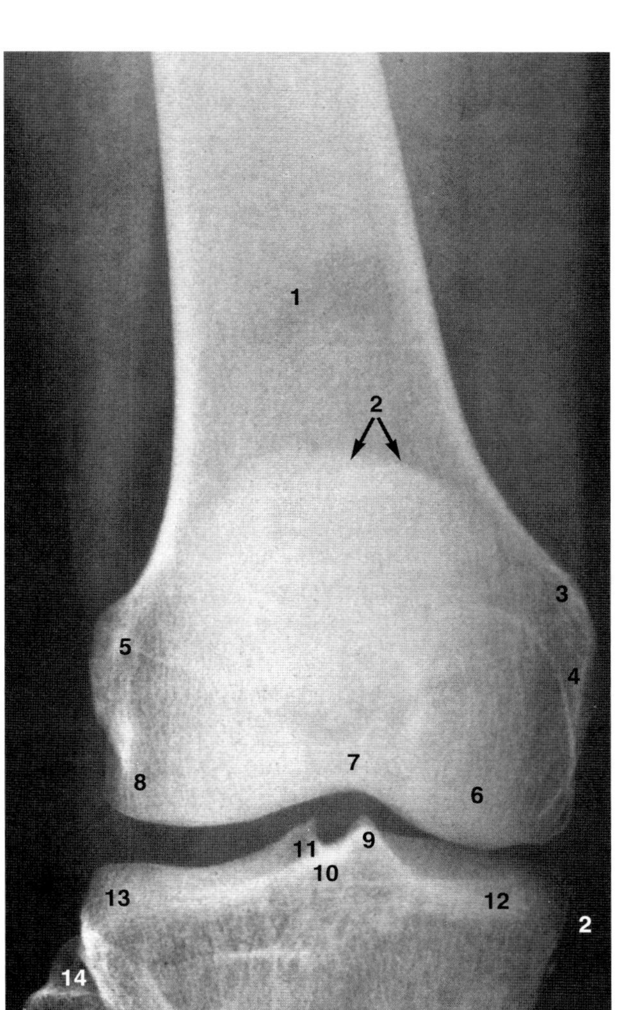
1
2
3
4
5
6
7
8
9
10
11
12
13
2
14
15
16
17

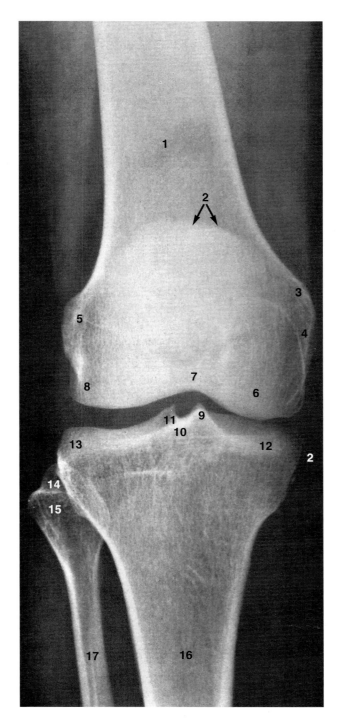

Figure 435.2 Radiograph of the Right Knee (Anteroposterior Projection)

NOTE: The following bony structures on the femur, tibia, and fibula in the region of the knee.

1. Body of femur
2. Margin of patella
3. Adductor tubercle
4. Medial epicondyle
5. Lateral epicondyle
6. Medial condyle of femur
7. Intercondylar fossa
8. Lateral condyle of femur
9. Medial intercondylar tubercle
10. Anterior intercondylar area
11. Lateral intercondylar tubercle
12. Medial condyle of tibia
13. Lateral condyle of tibia
14. Apex of head of fibula
15. Head of fibula
16. Body of tibia
17. Body of fibula

(From Wicke, 6th ed.)

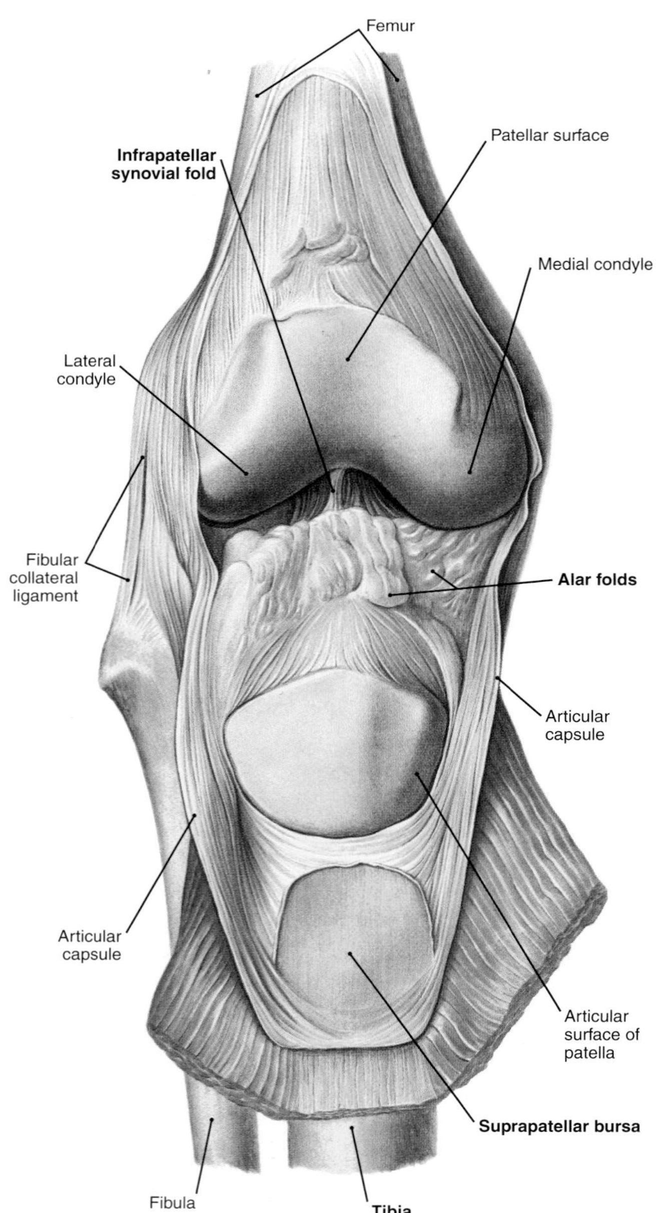
Femur
Patellar surface
Infrapatellar synovial fold
Medial condyle
Lateral condyle
Fibular collateral ligament
Alar folds
Articular capsule
Articular capsule
Articular surface of patella
Suprapatellar bursa
Fibula
Tibia

Figure 436.1 Knee Joint Opened Anteriorly

NOTE: (1) In this dissection, the anterior part of the articular capsule and the quadriceps tendon have been cut and reflected downward along with the **suprapatellar bursa.** The articular surface of the **patella** has also been pulled inferiorly away from its normal position on the femur.

(2) From the medial and lateral borders of the patella, the synovial membrane projects as fringe-like **alar folds** on each side. These converge in the midline to form the **infrapatellar synovial fold,** which attaches above to the intercondylar fossa of the femur.

(3) Upon removal of the infrapatellar synovial fold and any fat in the region, the anterior cruciate ligament and the menisci become exposed, as seen in Figure 436.2.

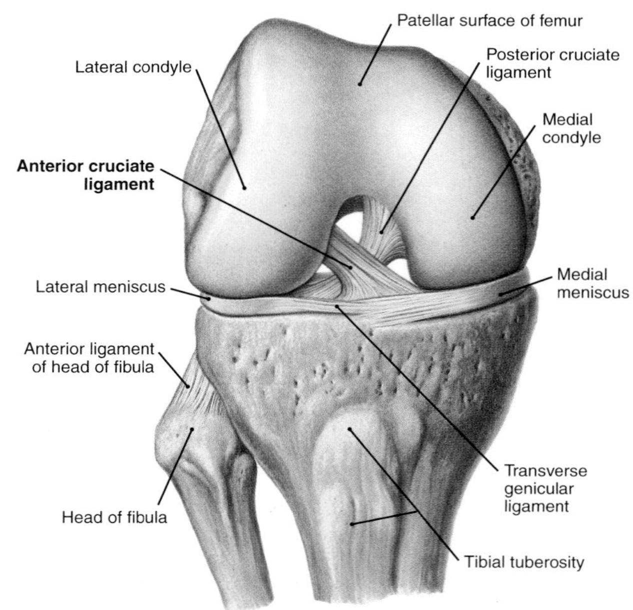
Patellar surface of femur
Lateral condyle
Posterior cruciate ligament
Medial condyle
Anterior cruciate ligament
Lateral meniscus
Medial meniscus
Anterior ligament of head of fibula
Transverse genicular ligament
Head of fibula
Tibial tuberosity

Figure 436.2 Flexed Right Knee Joint (Anterior View) Showing the Cruciate Ligaments

NOTE: (1) The **anterior cruciate ligament** is best exposed from this frontal approach. It extends from the posterior part of the medial surface of the lateral femoral condyle to the anterior surface of the tibial plateau.

(2) The anterior cruciate ligament helps prevent the posterior, or backward, displacement of the femur on the upper tibial plateau.

(3) More importantly, however, the anterior cruciate ligament limits extension of the lateral condyle to which it is attached. When it becomes taut, it causes medial rotation of the femur. This allows the medial condyle, which has a longer and more curved articular surface than the lateral condyle, to reach its full extension, placing the knee joint in a "locked position."

(4) Thus, the "locked" knee joint is achieved because:

(a) The medial condyle has a longer articular surface and a greater curvature than that of the lateral condyle.

(b) After the anterior cruciate ligament becomes taut, the lateral condyle can rotate around the "radius of the ligament" and forces the medial condyle to glide backward into its full extension.

(c) Medial rotation of the femur at the same time causes the oblique popliteal ligament and the medial and lateral collateral ligaments to tighten as well. (From Last RJ. Anatomy, Regional and Applied. Edinburgh: Churchill Livingstone, 1978.)

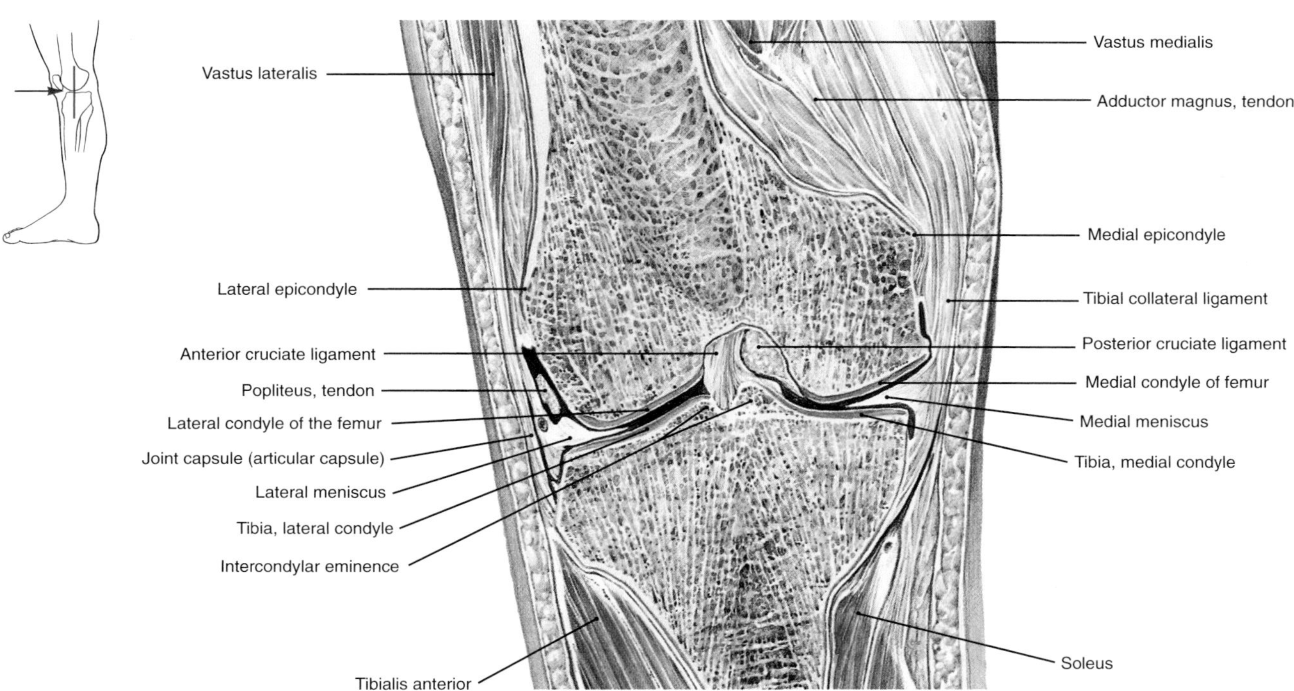

Vastus lateralis
Lateral epicondyle
Anterior cruciate ligament
Popliteus, tendon
Lateral condyle of the femur
Joint capsule (articular capsule)
Lateral meniscus
Tibia, lateral condyle
Intercondylar eminence
Tibialis anterior
Vastus medialis
Adductor magnus, tendon
Medial epicondyle
Tibial collateral ligament
Posterior cruciate ligament
Medial condyle of femur
Medial meniscus
Tibia, medial condyle
Soleus

Figure 437.1 Frontal Section through the Right Knee Joint

NOTE: (1) The anterior and posterior cruciate ligaments and the medial and lateral menisci.

(2) The tendon of the popliteus muscle adjacent to the lateral meniscus and lateral condyle. It attaches to both of these structures, and during the first phase of flexion of the knee in taking a step, this muscle retracts the meniscus in order not to have it crushed between the lateral condyles of the tibia and femur (see Fig. 418).

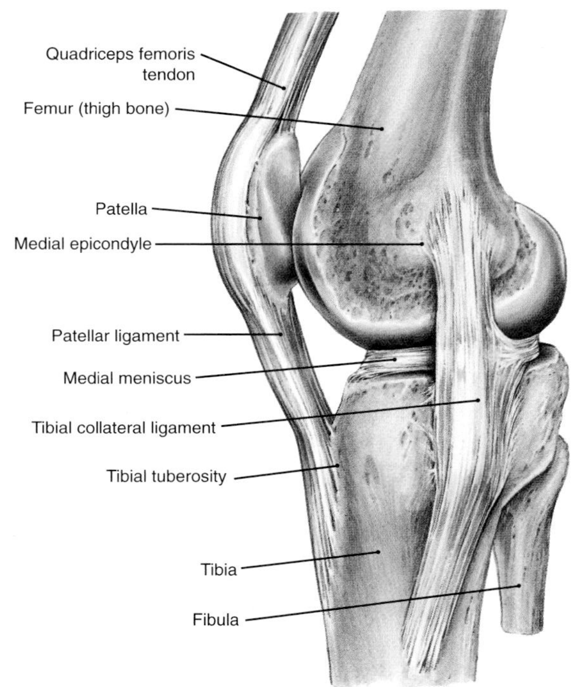

Quadriceps femoris tendon
Femur (thigh bone)
Patella
Medial epicondyle
Patellar ligament
Medial meniscus
Tibial collateral ligament
Tibial tuberosity
Tibia
Fibula

Figure 437.2 Right Knee Joint and the Tibial Collateral Ligament in Full Extension

NOTE: Only the posterior fibers of the tibial collateral ligament attach to the medial meniscus, while all the other fibers attach to the medial condyles of both the femur and tibia.

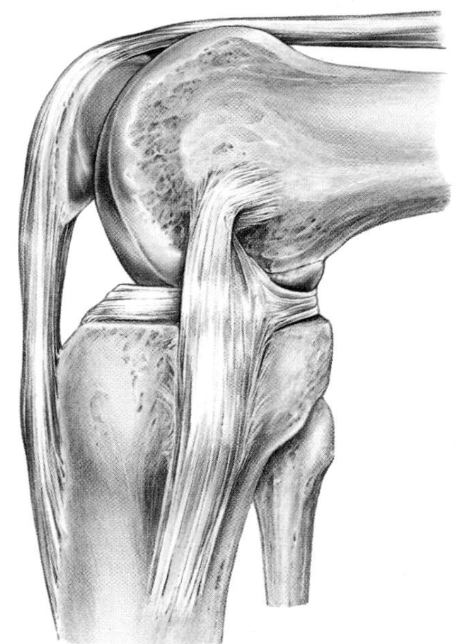

Figure 437.3 Right Knee Joint and the Tibial Collateral Ligament in Flexion

NOTE: During flexion, the posterior fibers of the tibial collateral ligament and those attaching to the femur become twisted and, thus, help to stabilize the medial meniscus to which the ligament is attached.

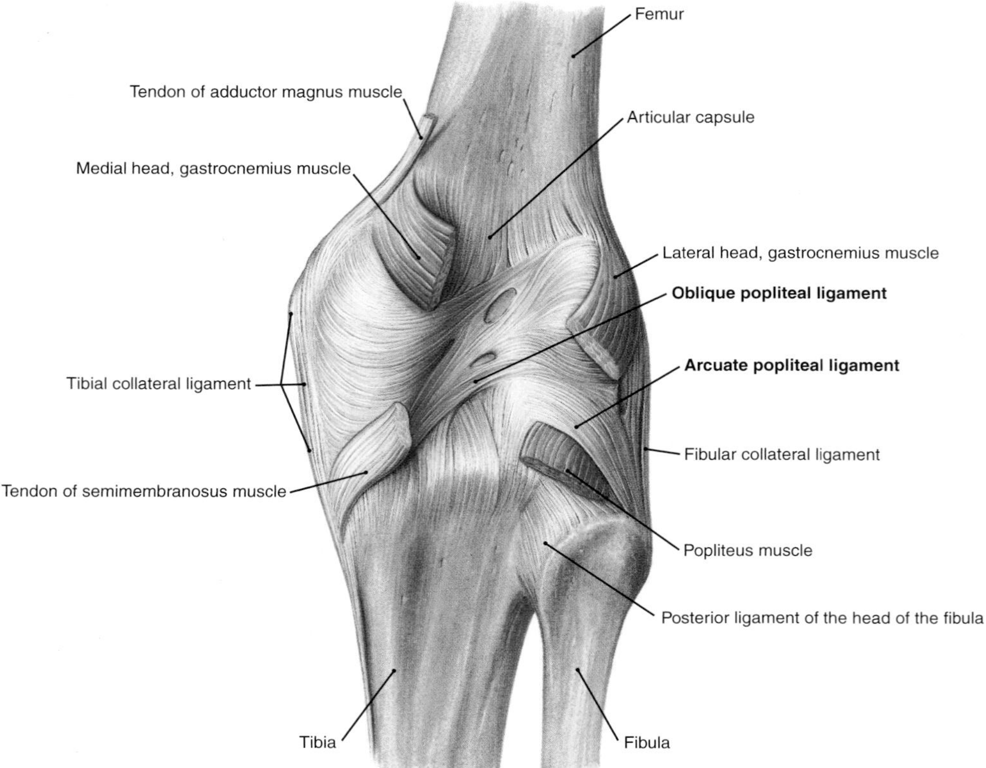
Femur
Tendon of adductor magnus muscle
Articular capsule
Medial head, gastrocnemius muscle
Lateral head, gastrocnemius muscle
Oblique popliteal ligament
Arcuate popliteal ligament
Tibial collateral ligament
Fibular collateral ligament
Tendon of semimembranosus muscle
Popliteus muscle
Posterior ligament of the head of the fibula
Tibia
Fibula

Figure 438.1 Knee Joint (Posterior View, Superficial Dissection)

NOTE: (1) The posterior aspect of the articular capsule is reinforced by the oblique and arcuate popliteal ligaments, and, to some extent, by the tendons of origin and insertion of muscles.

(2) From its insertion, the tendon of the semimembranosus muscle expands upward and laterally across the posterior surface of the articular capsule of the knee joint as the **oblique popliteal ligament.**

(3) The **arcuate popliteal ligament** is a band of fibers attached to the head of the fibula and courses superficial to the popliteal muscle to blend with the oblique popliteal ligament and the fibular collateral ligament.

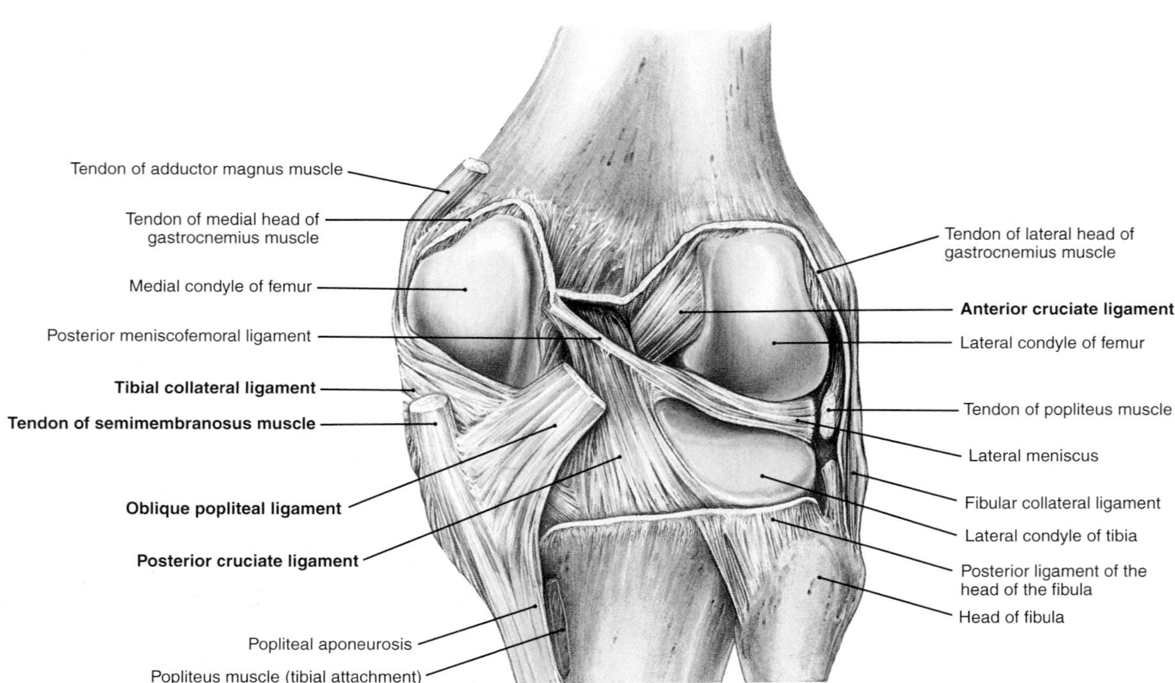
Tendon of adductor magnus muscle
Tendon of medial head of gastrocnemius muscle
Medial condyle of femur
Posterior meniscofemoral ligament
Tibial collateral ligament
Tendon of semimembranosus muscle
Oblique popliteal ligament
Posterior cruciate ligament
Popliteal aponeurosis
Popliteus muscle (tibial attachment)
Tendon of lateral head of gastrocnemius muscle
Anterior cruciate ligament
Lateral condyle of femur
Tendon of popliteus muscle
Lateral meniscus
Fibular collateral ligament
Lateral condyle of tibia
Posterior ligament of the head of the fibula
Head of fibula

Figure 438.2 Posterior View of the Knee Joint with the Articular Capsule Opened

NOTE: This more diagrammatic figure should be compared with the dissection in Figure 438.1.

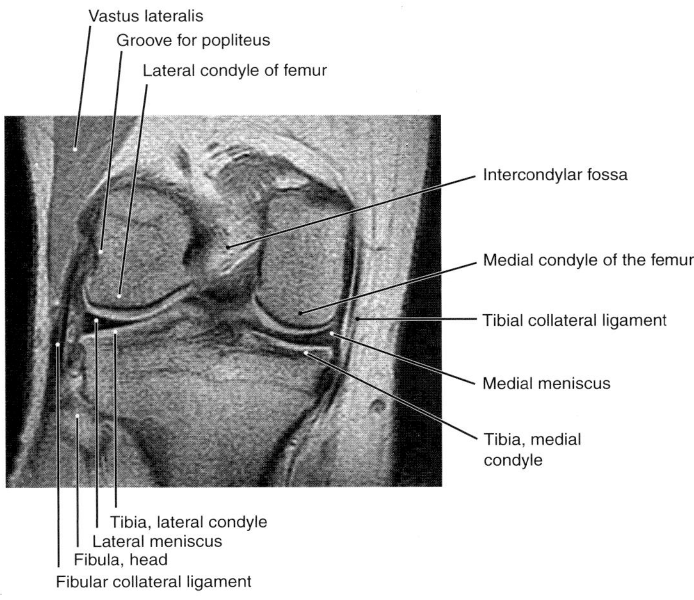
Vastus lateralis
Groove for popliteus
Lateral condyle of femur
Intercondylar fossa
Medial condyle of the femur
Tibial collateral ligament
Medial meniscus
Tibia, medial condyle
Tibia, lateral condyle
Lateral meniscus
Fibula, head
Fibular collateral ligament

Figure 439.1 MRI of the Knee Joint (Frontal Section)
NOTE: This MRI frontal section cuts through the intercondylar eminence of the tibia (not labeled) and the intercondylar fossa of the femur. Observe the menisci, which in this frontal section, have a triangular shape.

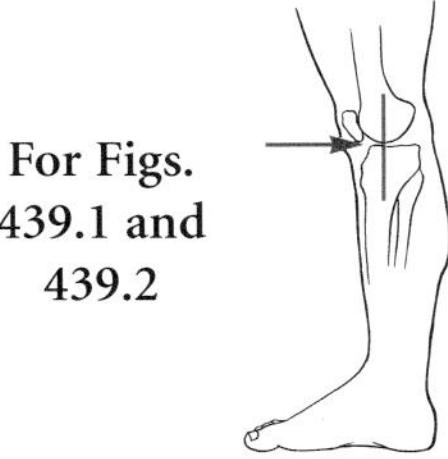

For Figs. 439.1 and 439.2

Figure 439.2 MRI of the Knee Joint (Sagittal Section)
NOTE: This sagittal section cuts through the lateral part of the knee joint and shows the **horns of the lateral meniscus,** the **tendon of the popliteus muscle,** and the **superior tibiofibular joint.** Compare this image with Figure 441.2.

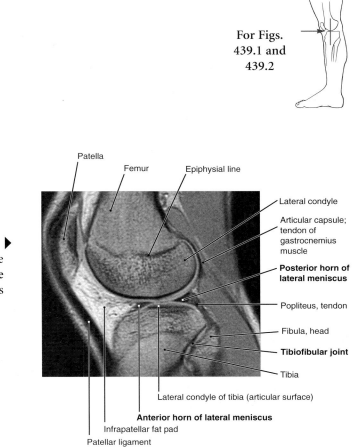

Patella
Femur
Epiphysial line
Lateral condyle
Articular capsule; tendon of gastrocnemius muscle
Posterior horn of lateral meniscus
Popliteus, tendon
Fibula, head
Tibiofibular joint
Tibia
Lateral condyle of tibia (articular surface)
Anterior horn of lateral meniscus
Infrapatellar fat pad
Patellar ligament

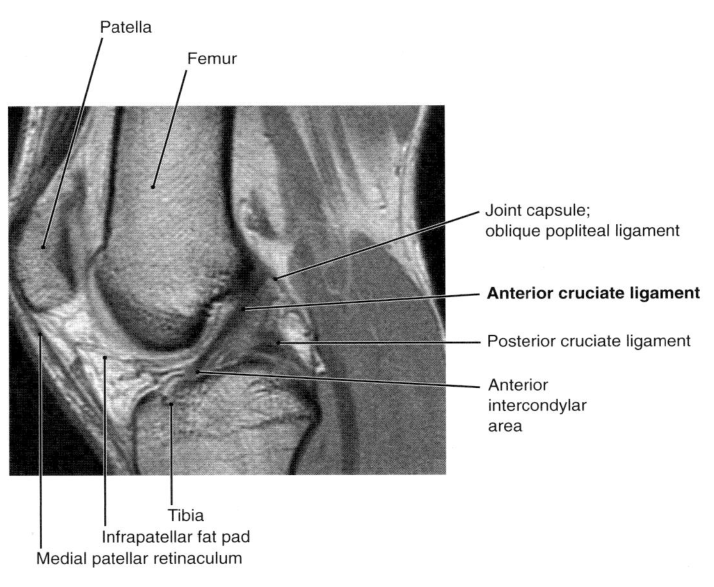
Patella
Femur
Joint capsule; oblique popliteal ligament
Anterior cruciate ligament
Posterior cruciate ligament
Anterior intercondylar area
Tibia
Infrapatellar fat pad
Medial patellar retinaculum

Figure 439.3 MRI of the Knee Joint in Extension
NOTE: This sagittal section shows both the anterior and posterior cruciate ligaments.

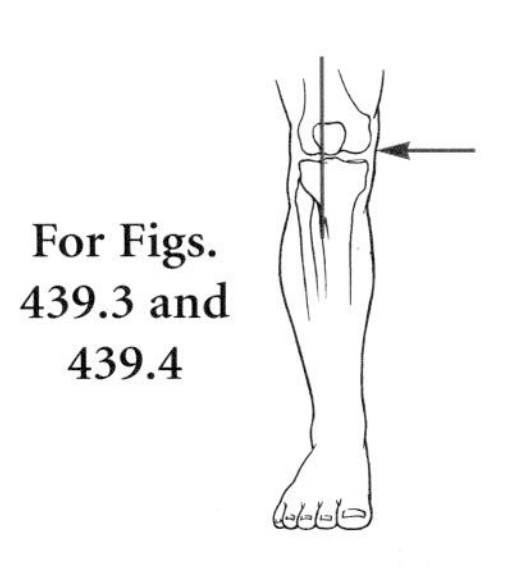

For Figs. 439.3 and 439.4

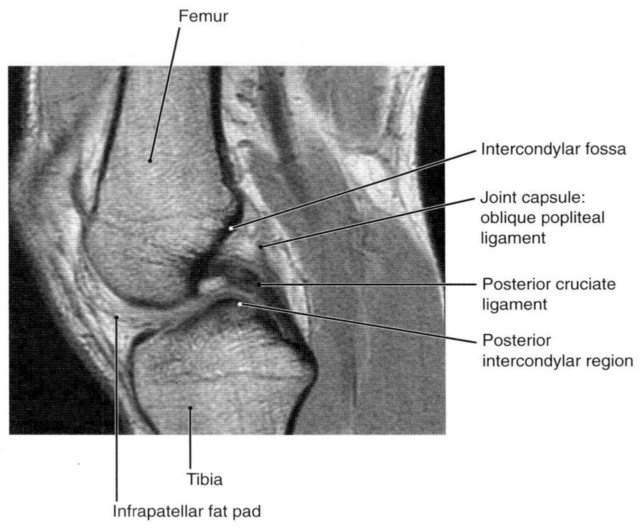
Femur
Intercondylar fossa
Joint capsule: oblique popliteal ligament
Posterior cruciate ligament
Posterior intercondylar region
Tibia
Infrapatellar fat pad

Figure 439.4 MRI of the Knee Joint in Extension
NOTE: This sagittal section shows the posterior cruciate ligament to good advantage.

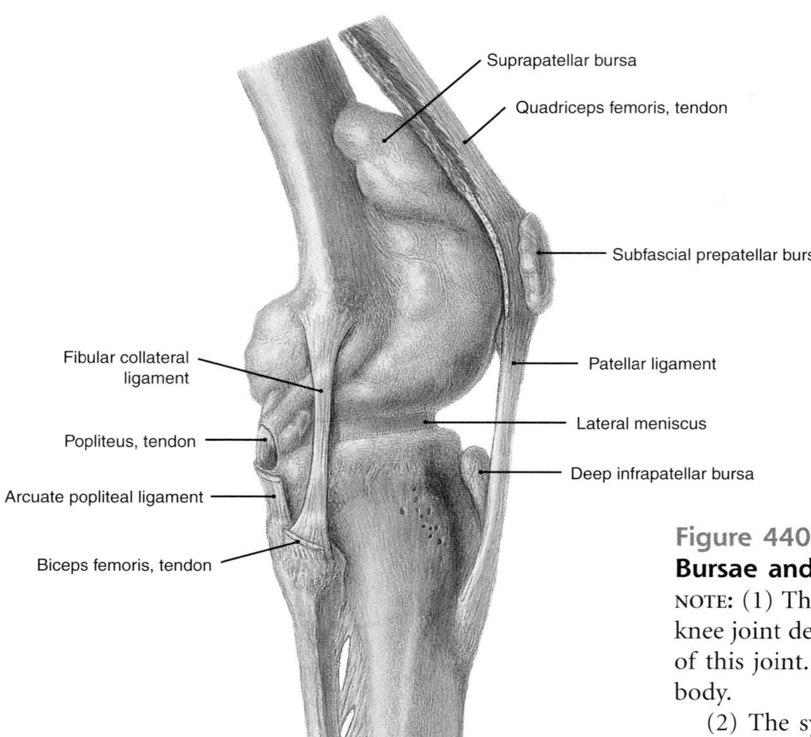
Suprapatellar bursa
Quadriceps femoris, tendon
Subfascial prepatellar bursa
Fibular collateral ligament
Patellar ligament
Lateral meniscus
Popliteus, tendon
Deep infrapatellar bursa
Arcuate popliteal ligament
Biceps femoris, tendon
SK

Figure 440.1 Cast of Knee Joint (Distended) Showing Bursae and Joint Cavity (Lateral View)

NOTE: (1) This lateral view of the distended synovial cavity of the right knee joint demonstrates the extensive nature of the synovial membrane of this joint. It is more extensive in this joint than in any other in the body.

(2) The synovial membrane reaches *superiorly* above the patella to form a large pouch called the **suprapatellar bursa. Laterally**, it courses deep to the popliteal tendon and fibular collateral ligament. **Posteriorly**, it extends above the menisci as high as the origins of the gastrocnemius muscle. **Inferiorly**, the joint cavity descends below both the lateral and medial menisci.

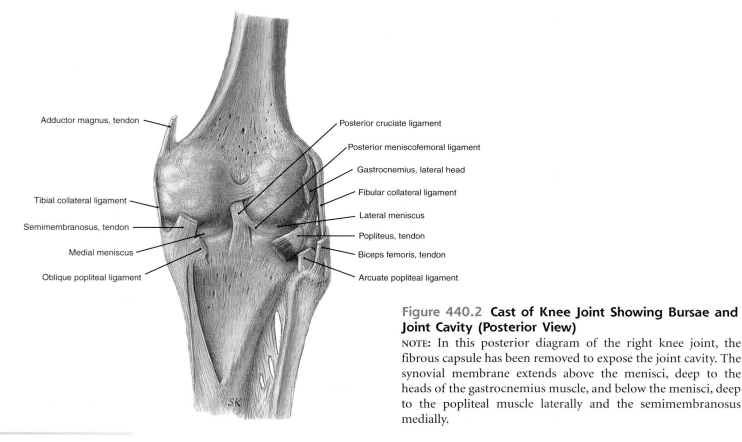

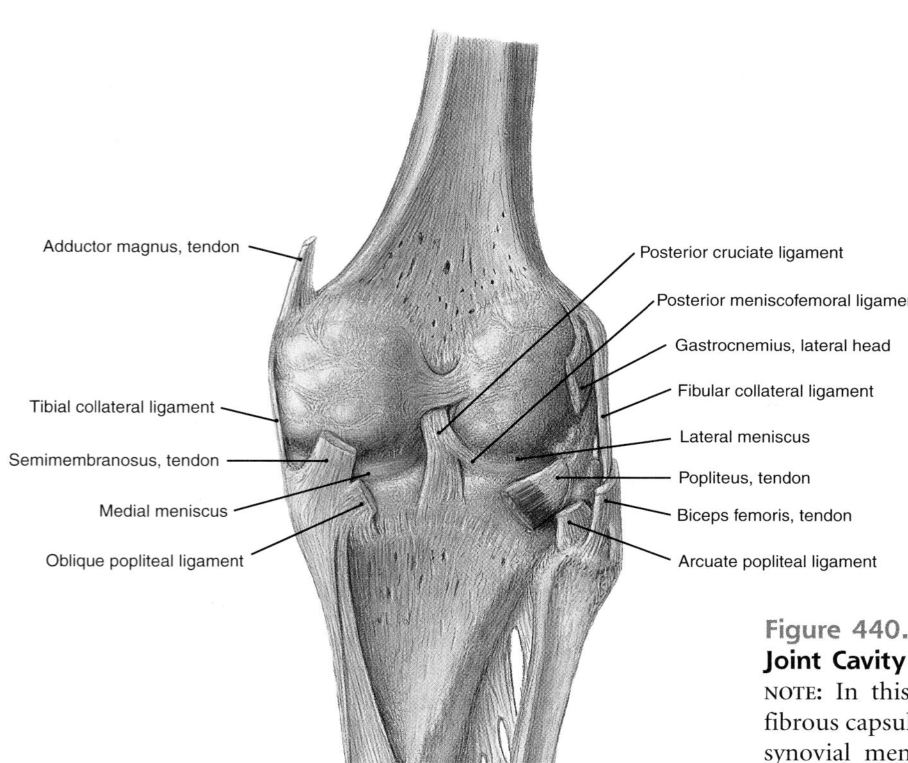
Adductor magnus, tendon
Posterior cruciate ligament
Posterior meniscofemoral ligament
Gastrocnemius, lateral head
Tibial collateral ligament
Fibular collateral ligament
Lateral meniscus
Semimembranosus, tendon
Popliteus, tendon
Medial meniscus
Biceps femoris, tendon
Oblique popliteal ligament
Arcuate popliteal ligament
SK

Figure 440.2 Cast of Knee Joint Showing Bursae and Joint Cavity (Posterior View)

NOTE: In this posterior diagram of the right knee joint, the fibrous capsule has been removed to expose the joint cavity. The synovial membrane extends above the menisci, deep to the heads of the gastrocnemius muscle, and below the menisci, deep to the popliteal muscle laterally and the semimembranosus medially.

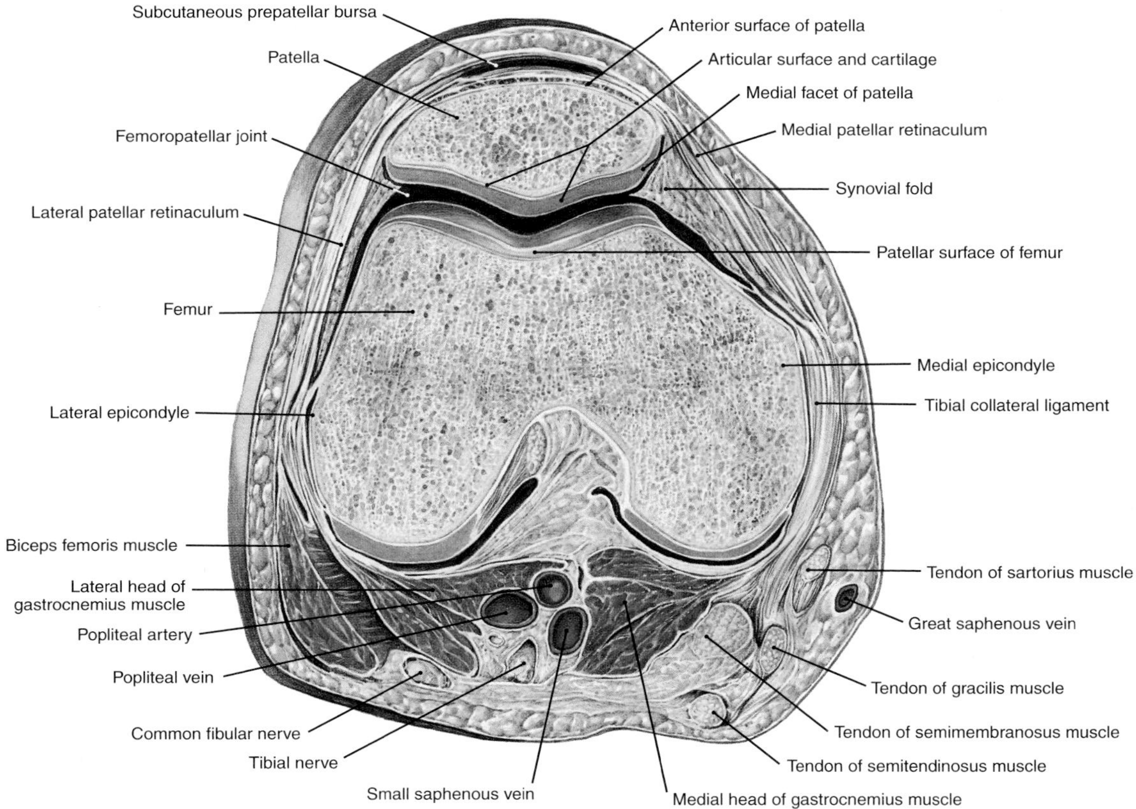
Subcutaneous prepatellar bursa
Patella
Femoropatellar joint
Lateral patellar retinaculum
Femur
Lateral epicondyle
Biceps femoris muscle
Lateral head of gastrocnemius muscle
Popliteal artery
Popliteal vein
Common fibular nerve
Tibial nerve
Small saphenous vein
Anterior surface of patella
Articular surface and cartilage
Medial facet of patella
Medial patellar retinaculum
Synovial fold
Patellar surface of femur
Medial epicondyle
Tibial collateral ligament
Tendon of sartorius muscle
Great saphenous vein
Tendon of gracilis muscle
Tendon of semimembranosus muscle
Tendon of semitendinosus muscle
Medial head of gastrocnemius muscle

Figure 441.1 Transverse Section through the Knee Joint and the Popliteal Fossa

NOTE: The relationship of the muscles, vessels, and nerves in the popliteal fossa to the bony structures of the knee joint.

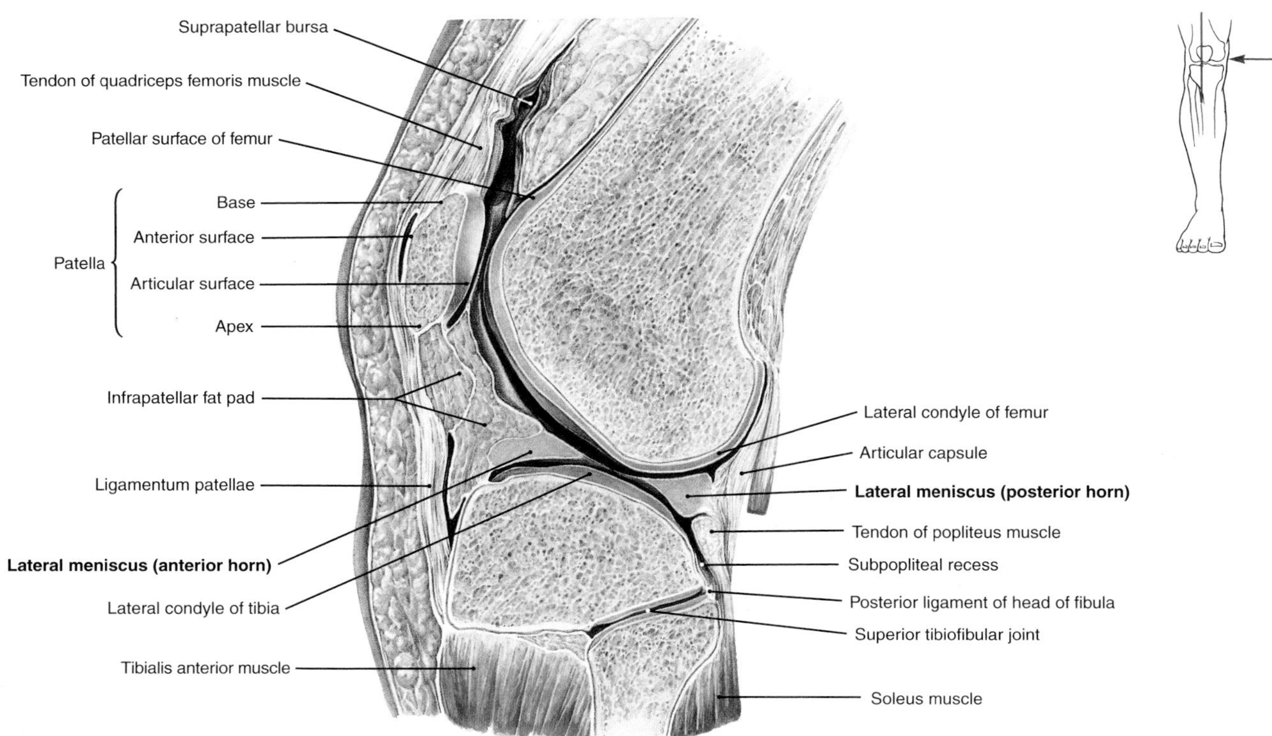
Suprapatellar bursa
Tendon of quadriceps femoris muscle
Patellar surface of femur
Patella
Base
Anterior surface
Articular surface
Apex
Infrapatellar fat pad
Ligamentum patellae
Lateral meniscus (anterior horn)
Lateral condyle of tibia
Tibialis anterior muscle
Lateral condyle of femur
Articular capsule
Lateral meniscus (posterior horn)
Tendon of popliteus muscle
Subpopliteal recess
Posterior ligament of head of fibula
Superior tibiofibular joint
Soleus muscle

Figure 441.2 Sagittal Section through the Lateral Part of the Knee Joint

NOTE: The horns of the lateral meniscus, the tendon of the popliteal muscle, and the superior tibiofibular joint. Compare these structures in this drawing with those in the MRI section seen in Figure 439.2.

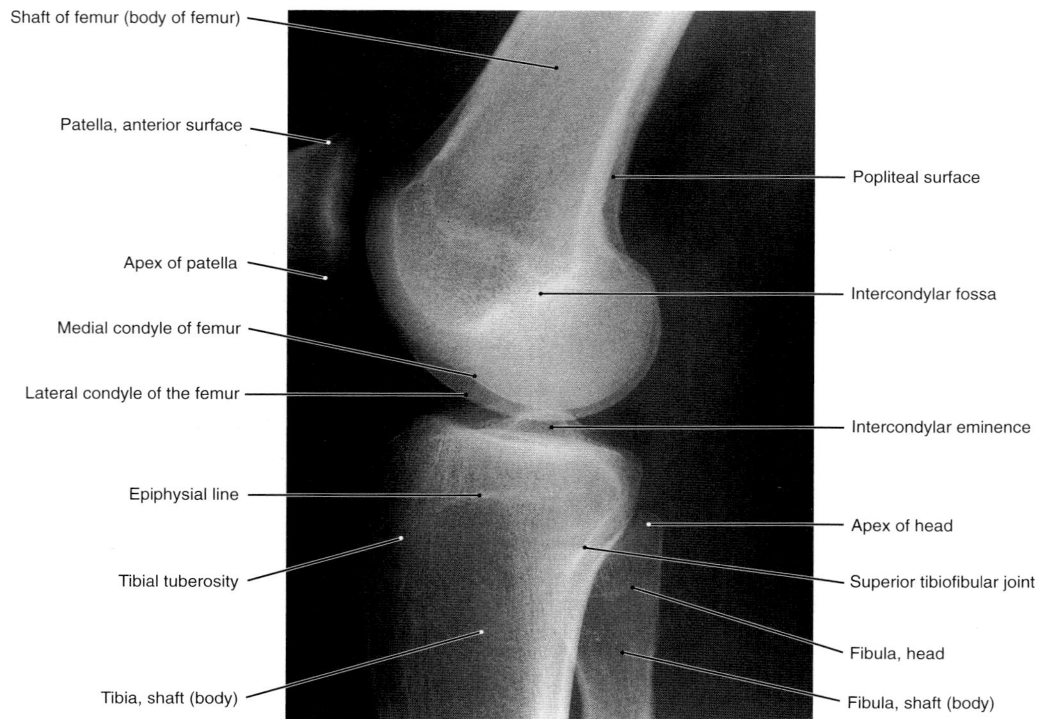
Shaft of femur (body of femur)
Patella, anterior surface
Apex of patella
Medial condyle of femur
Lateral condyle of the femur
Epiphysial line
Tibial tuberosity
Tibia, shaft (body)
Popliteal surface
Intercondylar fossa
Intercondylar eminence
Apex of head
Superior tibiofibular joint
Fibula, head
Fibula, shaft (body)

Figure 442.1 Lateral Radiograph of the Knee Joint: Subject Lying in the Supine Position

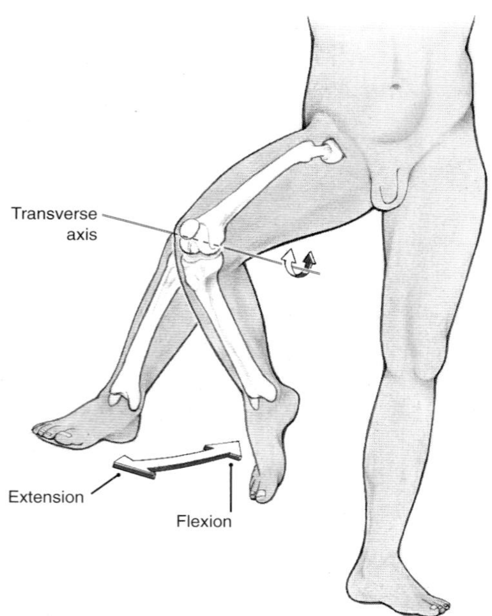
Transverse axis
Extension
Flexion

Figure 442.2 Knee Joint Movement (Sagittal Plane)

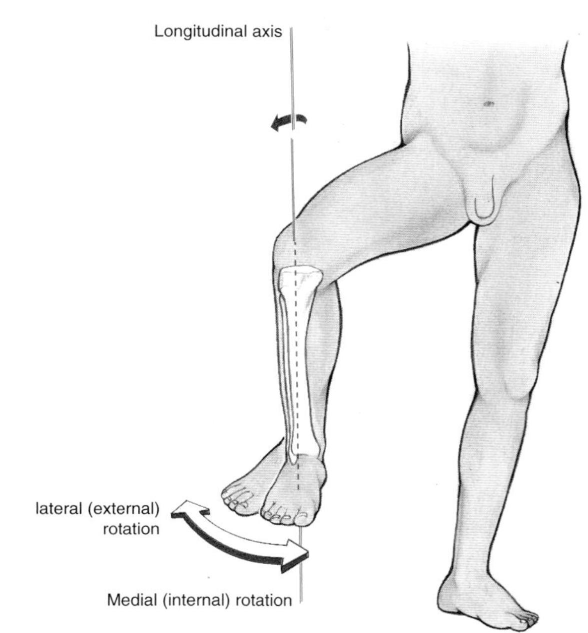
Longitudinal axis
lateral (external) rotation
Medial (internal) rotation

Figure 442.3 Knee Joint Movement (Transverse Plane)

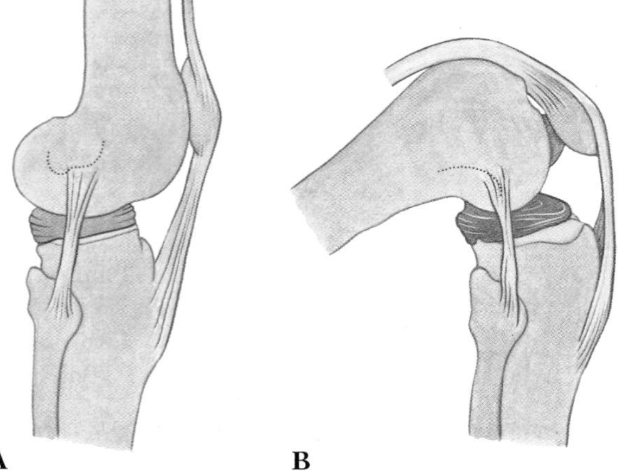
A
B

Figure 442.4 Lateral Views of the Right Knee Joint

NOTE: In A, the knee joint is extended, while in B it is flexed. When greater flexion at the knee joint occurs, the menisci (especially the lateral meniscus) are pulled posteriorly on the tibial plateau (see Figs. 443.1 and 443.2).

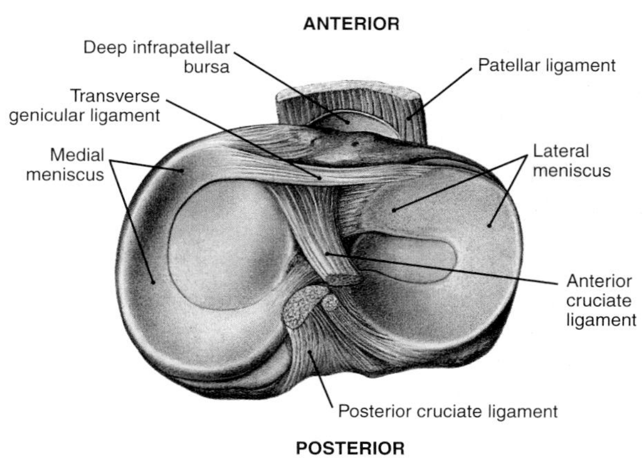
ANTERIOR
Deep infrapatellar bursa
Patellar ligament
Transverse genicular ligament
Medial meniscus
Lateral meniscus
Anterior cruciate ligament
Posterior cruciate ligament
POSTERIOR

Figure 443.1 **Condyles of the Right Tibia, Viewed from Above: Showing the Menisci and the Attachments on the Tibia of the Cruciate Ligaments**

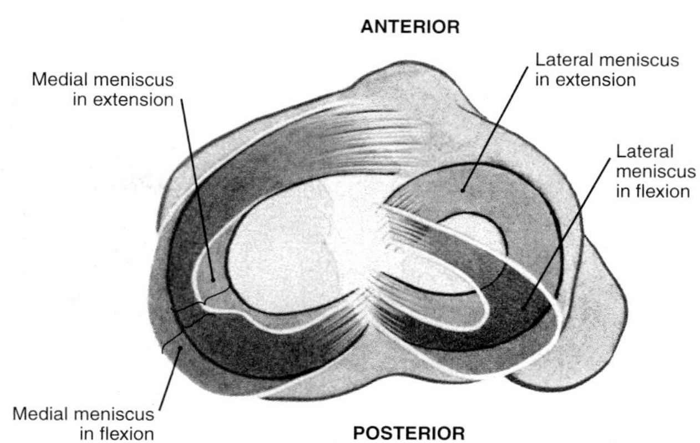
ANTERIOR
Medial meniscus in extension
Lateral meniscus in extension
Lateral meniscus in flexion
Medial meniscus in flexion
POSTERIOR

Figure 443.2 **Superior Surface of the Right Tibial Surface Showing the Locations of the Menisci during Extension (Light Blue) and Their Changes in Position during Flexion (Purple).**

NOTE: (1) The C-shaped menisci lie above the condyles of the tibia; they are triangular in cross section and composed of fibrous connective tissue and NOT of cartilage.

(2) The **medial meniscus** is larger and has a more open curve than that of the **lateral meniscus.** Both menisci are attached at their anterior and posterior horns to the tibial surface.

(3) The **lateral meniscus** receives a flat tendon of insertion from the upper fibers of the **popliteus muscle,** and this muscle comes into action during "unlocking" of the knee joint by slightly rotating the femur laterally in preparation to take a step. In addition, these fibers draw the posterior convexity of the lateral meniscus backward "out of harm's way" during flexion of the tibia at the knee joint.

(4) In addition to its attachment on the tibia, the **medial meniscus** is securely attached to the tibial collateral ligament and is frequently injured in athletes when:

(a) The foot of the victim is planted firmly on the ground and the knee is semiflexed, and

(b) The victim is hit from behind ("clipping in football"), causing the weight of the body to severely rotate the femur medially. Thus, the leg is abducted and the tibial collateral ligament and the medial meniscus can be torn.

Figure 443.3 **Arterial Supply of the Menisci, Right Knee▸**
NOTE: The **medial** and **lateral genicular arteries** encircle the tibia and supply the menisci. The **middle genicular artery** supplies the cruciate ligaments.
(From Sick and Korike.)

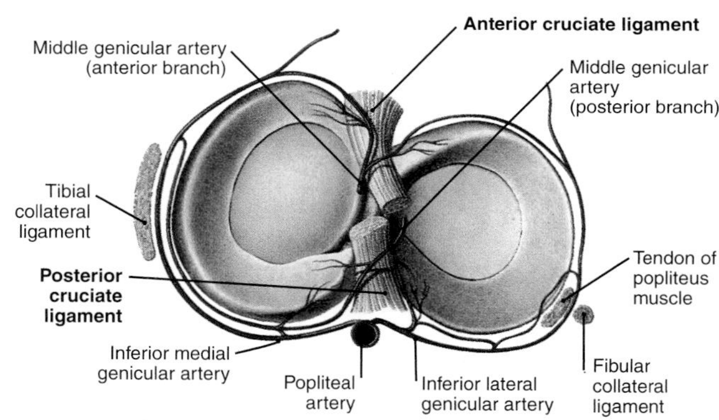
Middle genicular artery (anterior branch)
Anterior cruciate ligament
Middle genicular artery (posterior branch)
Tibial collateral ligament
Posterior cruciate ligament
Tendon of popliteus muscle
Inferior medial genicular artery
Popliteal artery
Inferior lateral genicular artery
Fibular collateral ligament

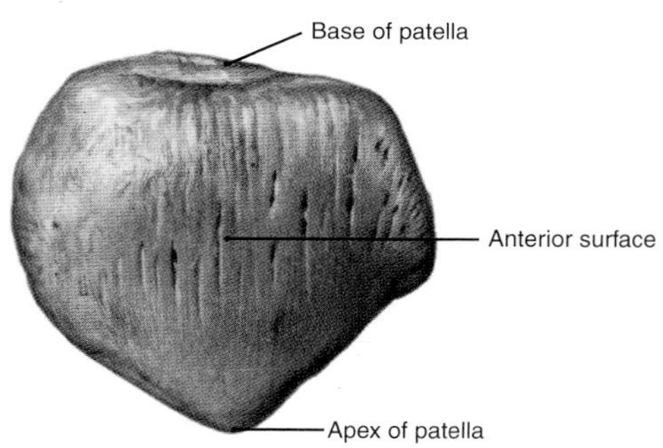
Base of patella
Anterior surface
Apex of patella

Figure 443.4 **Anterior Aspect of the Right Patella**

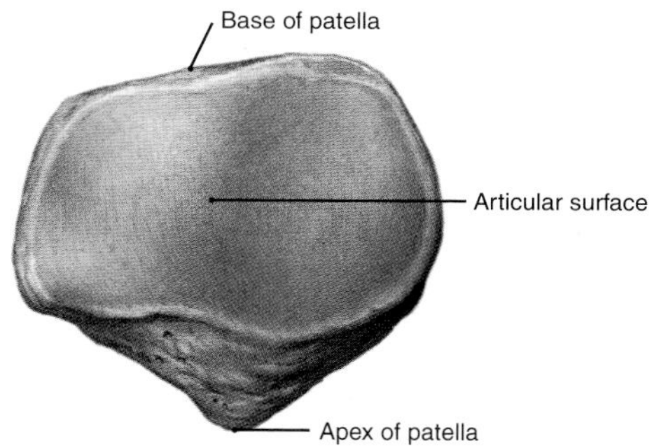
Base of patella
Articular surface
Apex of patella

Figure 443.5 **Posterior Aspect of the Right Patella**

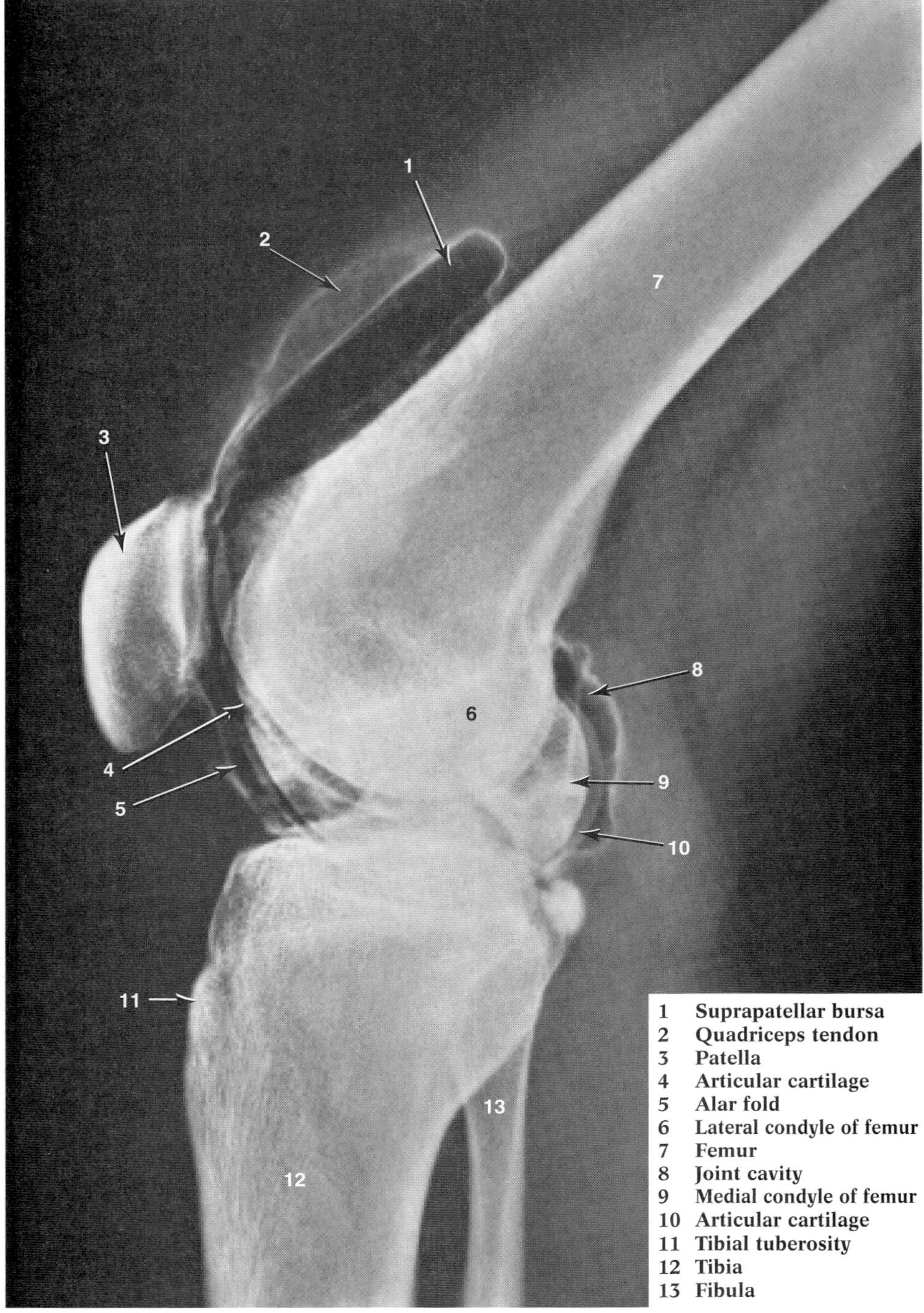
1
2
7
3
8
6
4
9
5
10
11
13
12
1 Suprapatellar bursa
2 Quadriceps tendon
3 Patella
4 Articular cartilage
5 Alar fold
6 Lateral condyle of femur
7 Femur
8 Joint cavity
9 Medial condyle of femur
10 Articular cartilage
11 Tibial tuberosity
12 Tibia
13 Fibula

Figure 444 Arthrogram of the Knee Joint

NOTE: (1) An arthrogram is a radiograph of a joint taken during arthrography, which is an examination of a joint following the injection into the joint of a radiopaque agent (or gas).

(2) An arthroscope is an instrument that uses fiber optics and permits visualization of the inside of a joint. This is a achieved by puncturing the joint through a small incision in the joint capsule (see Plate 445).

(3) The large **suprapatellar bursa.** The **patella** is a bony structure within the tendon of the quadriceps femoris muscle. The tendon then continues inferiorly to the knee and inserts onto the **tibial tuberosity** as the patellar ligament.

(4) During development, the fibers of the quadriceps tendon and the patellar ligament that attaches to the **tibial tuberosity** were continuous, but upon further development the central part of the tendon becomes ossified to form the **patella.**

(5) People that kneel a lot may have inflammation of the bursae anterior to the patella and superior to the **patella.** This is sometimes called housemaid's knee.

(From Wicke, 6th ed.)

Figure 445.1 Arthroscopic Approaches to the Knee

1. Arthroscope
2. Inlet and outlet for rinsing solution
3. Cold light source
4. Ocular or connector for visual system
5. Anterolateral approach
6. Anteromedial approach
7. Supplementary instrument

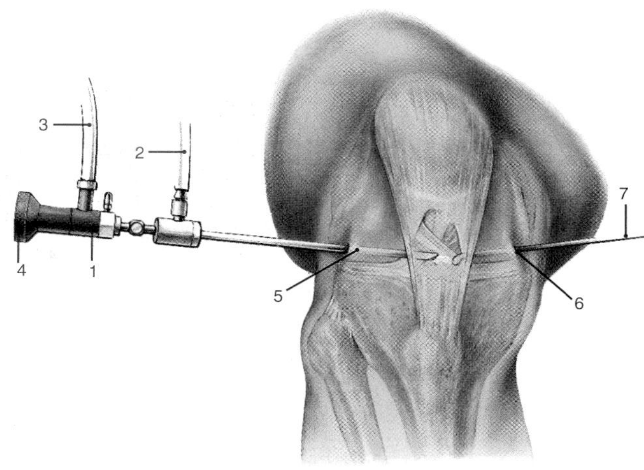
3
2
7
4
1
5
6

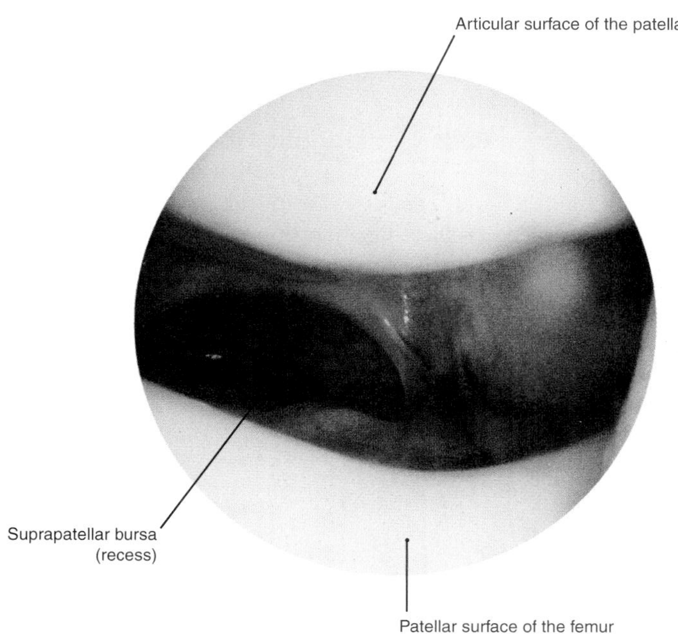
Articular surface of the patella
Suprapatellar bursa (recess)
Patellar surface of the femur

Figure 445.2 Knee Joint Arthroscopy

NOTE: This is an inferior view of the femoropatellar joint.

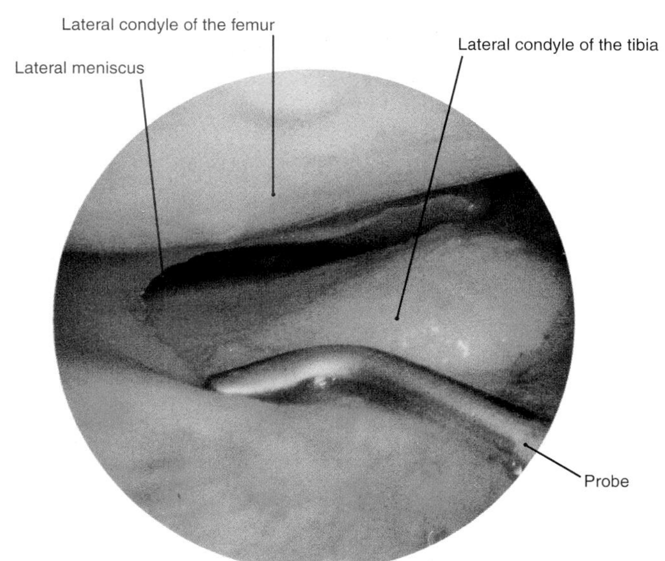
Lateral condyle of the femur
Lateral meniscus
Lateral condyle of the tibia
Probe

Figure 445.3 Knee Joint Arthroscopy

NOTE: This image shows the medial free border of the lateral meniscus; the anterior part of the meniscus is being depressed by a probe.

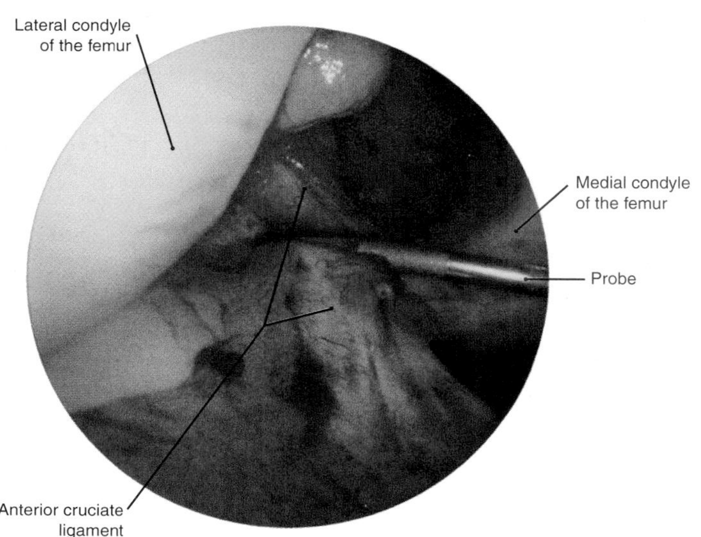
Lateral condyle of the femur
Medial condyle of the femur
Probe
Anterior cruciate ligament

Figure 445.4 Knee Joint Arthroscopy

NOTE: The distal part of the right anterior cruciate ligament is visible, and the highly vascular synovial membrane is being retracted by a probe.

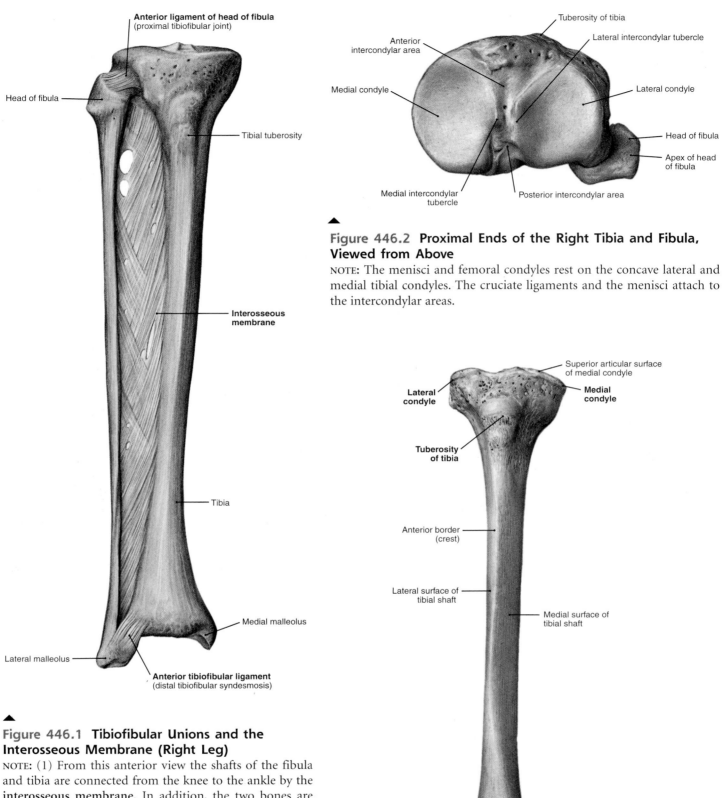

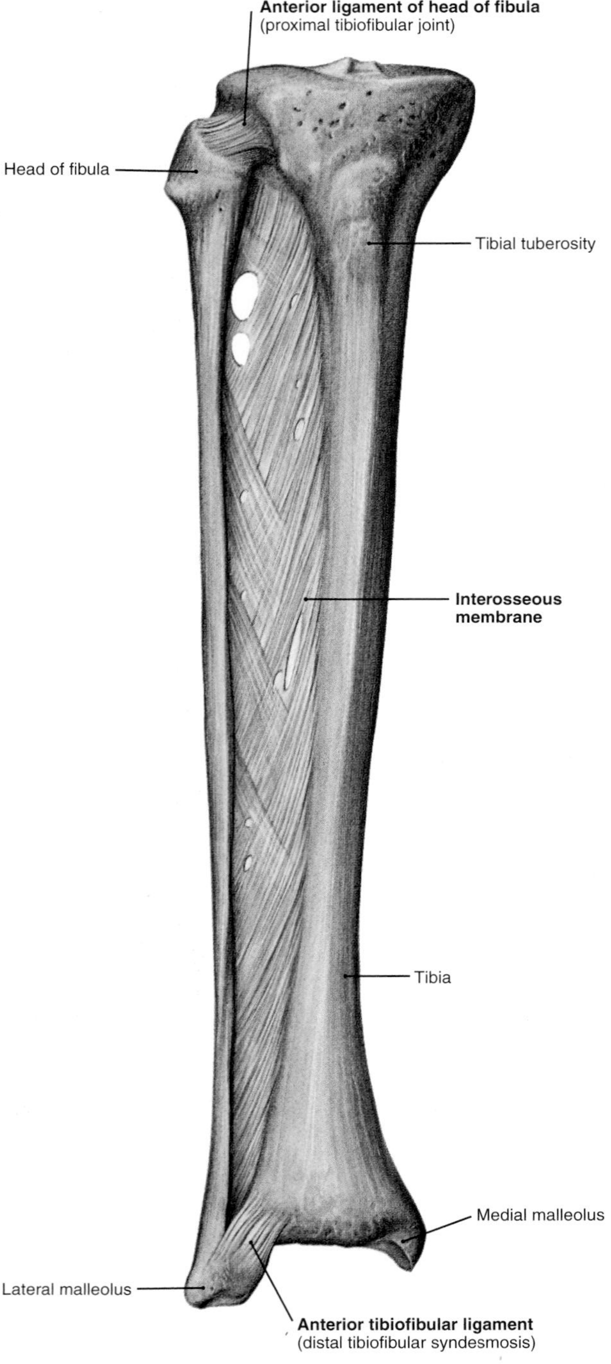

Anterior ligament of head of fibula
(proximal tibiofibular joint)
Head of fibula
Tibial tuberosity
Interosseous membrane
Tibia
Medial malleolus
Lateral malleolus
Anterior tibiofibular ligament
(distal tibiofibular syndesmosis)

Figure 446.1 **Tibiofibular Unions and the Interosseous Membrane (Right Leg)**

NOTE: (1) From this anterior view the shafts of the fibula and tibia are connected from the knee to the ankle by the **interosseous membrane.** In addition, the two bones are joined proximally (the tibiofibular joint) and distally (the tibiofibular syndesmosis).

(2) The head of the fibula articulates with the inferolateral aspect of the lateral condyle of the tibia. This is a gliding joint whose fibrous capsule is strengthened by **anterior** and **posterior ligaments of the head of the fibula.**

(3) The syndesmosis between the distal ends of the fibula and the tibia is bound by anterior and posterior tibiofibular ligaments.

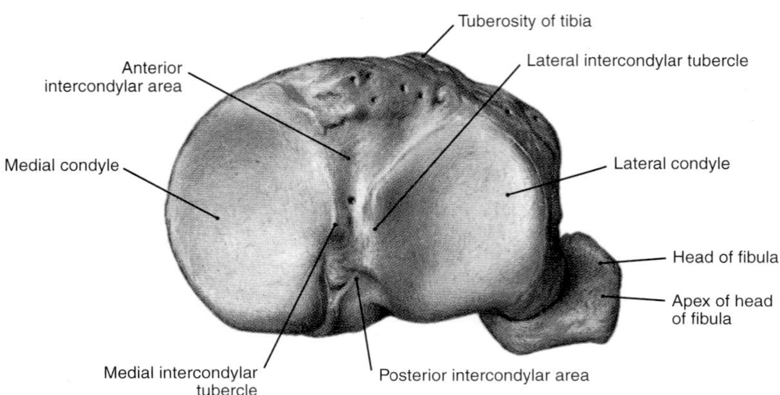

Tuberosity of tibia
Anterior intercondylar area
Lateral intercondylar tubercle
Medial condyle
Lateral condyle
Head of fibula
Apex of head of fibula
Medial intercondylar tubercle
Posterior intercondylar area

Figure 446.2 **Proximal Ends of the Right Tibia and Fibula, Viewed from Above**

NOTE: The menisci and femoral condyles rest on the concave lateral and medial tibial condyles. The cruciate ligaments and the menisci attach to the intercondylar areas.

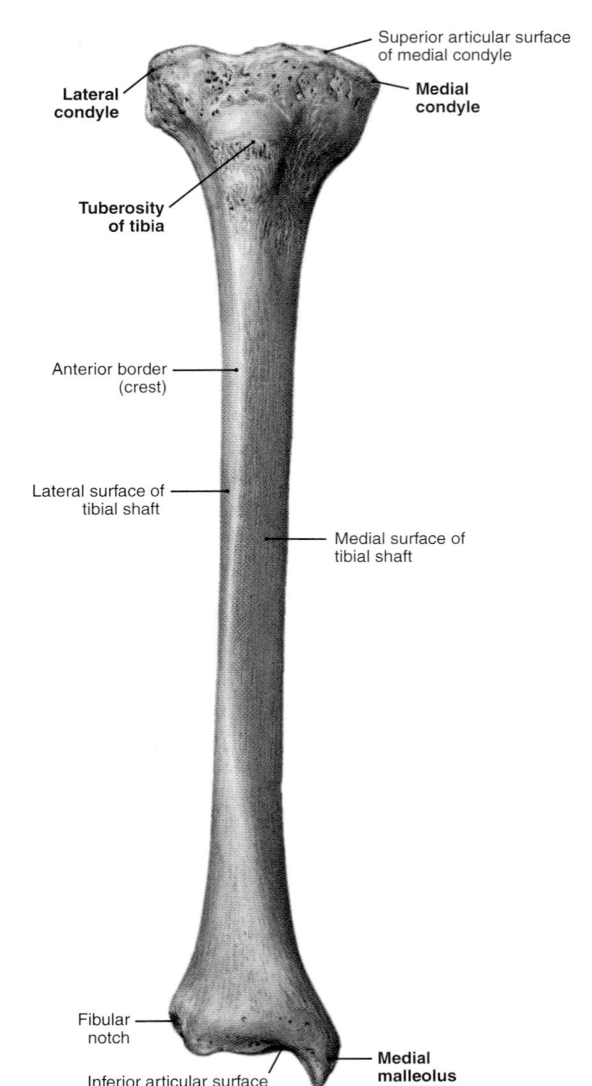

Superior articular surface of medial condyle
Lateral condyle
Medial condyle
Tuberosity of tibia
Anterior border (crest)
Lateral surface of tibial shaft
Medial surface of tibial shaft
Fibular notch
Inferior articular surface
Medial malleolus

Figure 446.3 **Right Tibia (Anterior View)**

NOTE: The proximal extremity is marked by the tibial condyles and the tibial tuberosity. The medial aspect of the distal extremity forms the medial malleolus.

Figures 447.1 and 447.2 Right Fibula (Medial and Lateral Views)

NOTE: (1) The fibula is a long slender bone situated lateral to the tibia, to which it articulates proximally and distally. The fibula expands inferiorly to form the **lateral malleolus.** The medial aspect of its inferior articular surface articulates with the tibia to form the **talocrural joint (ankle joint).**

(2) Although the fibula does not bear any weight of the trunk (not participating in the knee joint), it is important, since numerous muscles attach to its surface (see Figs. 405.3 and 420). and because it helps form the ankle joint.

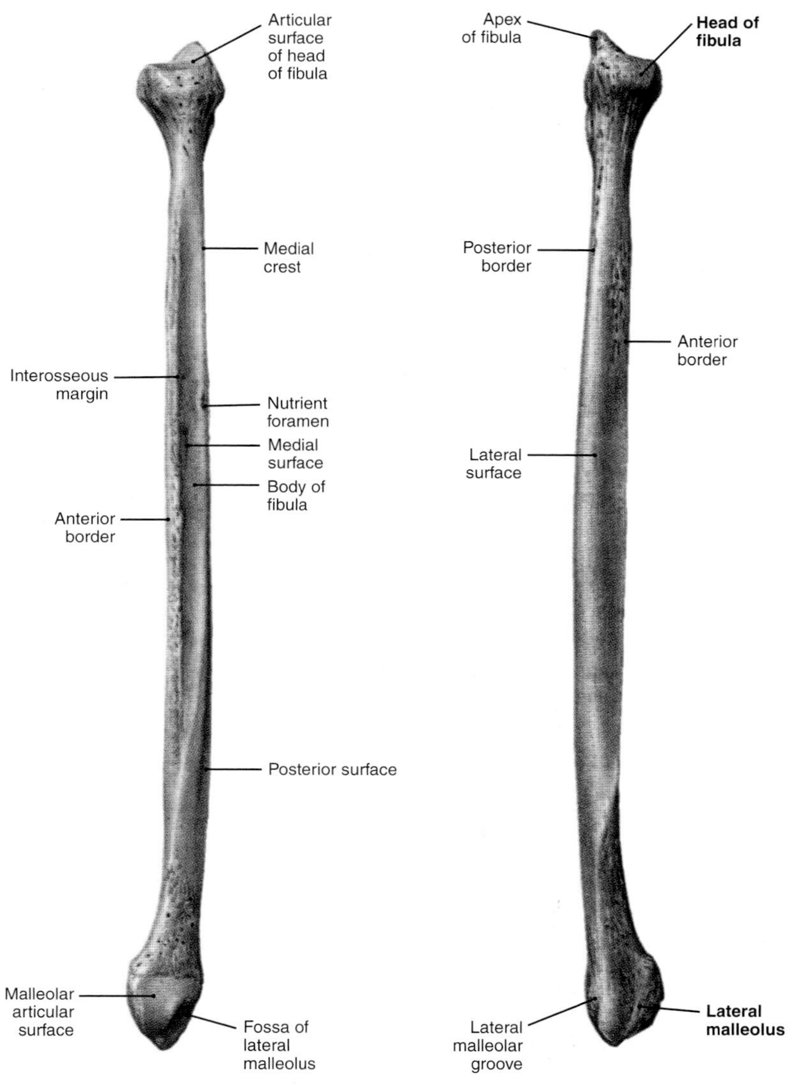
Articular surface of head of fibula
Medial crest
Interosseous margin
Nutrient foramen
Medial surface
Body of fibula
Anterior border
Posterior surface
Malleolar articular surface
Fossa of lateral malleolus
Apex of fibula
Head of fibula
Posterior border
Anterior border
Lateral surface
Lateral malleolar groove
Lateral malleolus

Figure 447.1: Medial View

Figure 447.2: Lateral View

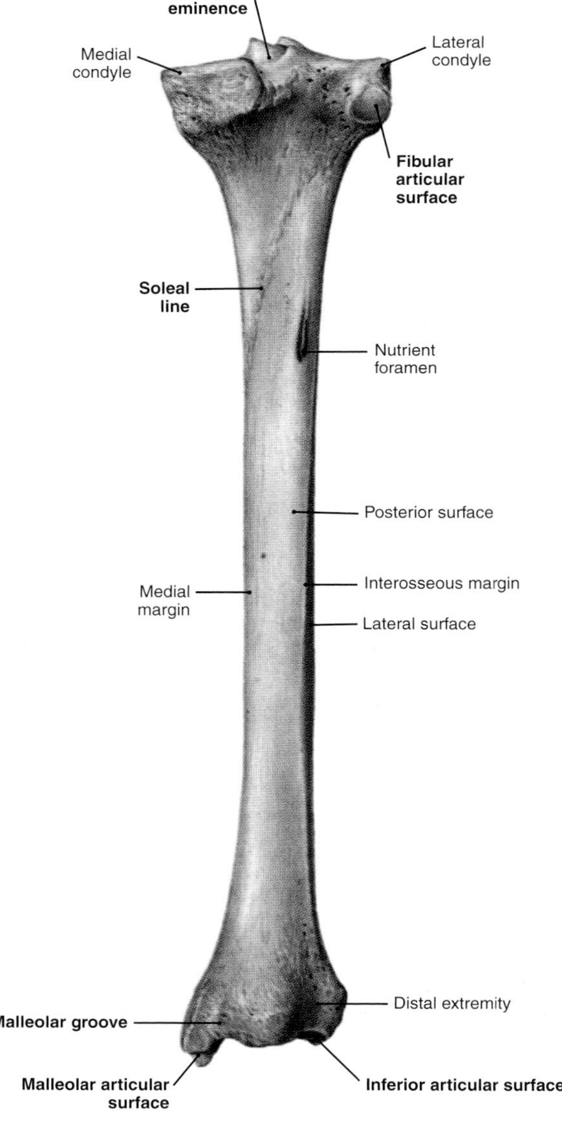
Intercondylar eminence
Medial condyle
Lateral condyle
Fibular articular surface
Soleal line
Nutrient foramen
Posterior surface
Medial margin
Interosseous margin
Lateral surface
Distal extremity
Malleolar groove
Malleolar articular surface
Inferior articular surface

Figure 447.3 Right Tibia (Posterior View)

NOTE: (1) The smooth posterior surface of the shaft of the tibia is marked by a prominent ridge, the **soleal line,** and a large oblong **nutrient foramen.** The tibial shaft tapers toward a larger proximal extremity and a somewhat less pronounced distal extremity.

(2) Proximally, the medial and lateral condyles are separated by the intercondylar eminence, anterior and posterior to which attach the cruciate ligaments. Distally, the tibia articulates with the **talus,** and on this posterior surface, presents grooves for the passage of the tendons of the tibialis posterior, flexor digitorum longus, and flexor hallucis longus.

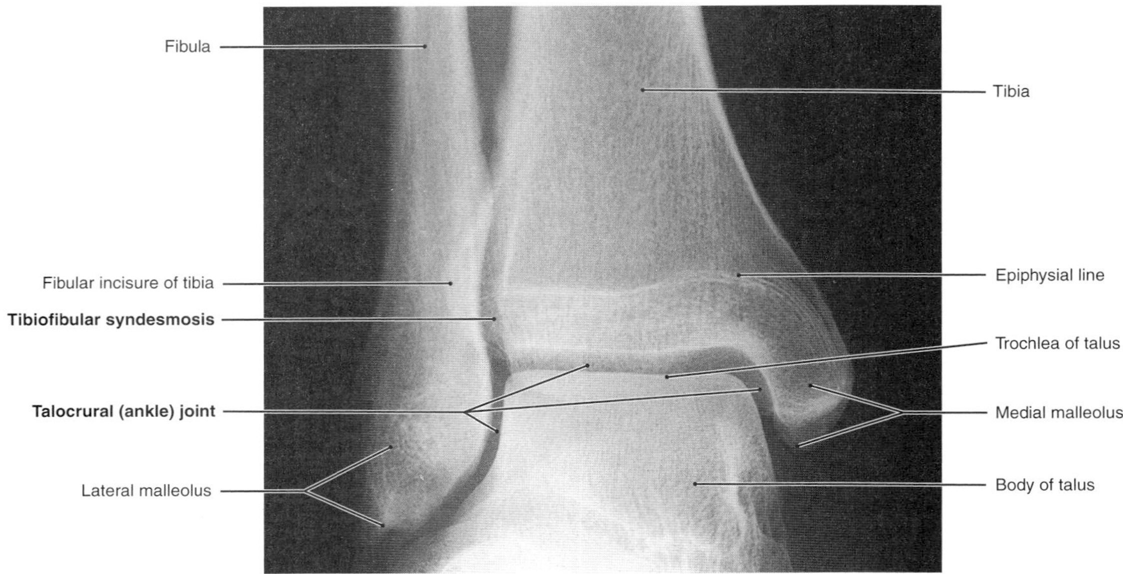
Fibula
Tibia
Fibular incisure of tibia
Tibiofibular syndesmosis
Epiphysial line
Trochlea of talus
Talocrural (ankle) joint
Medial malleolus
Lateral malleolus
Body of talus

Figure 448.1 X-Ray of the Talocrural (Ankle) Joint and the Inferior Tibiofibular Syndesmosis

NOTE: (1) This is an anteroposterior radiograph showing both the ankle joint and the tibiofibular syndesmosis.

(2) The ankle joint is a ginglymus, or hinge, joint. The bony structures participating in this joint superiorly are the distal end of the **tibia** and its **medial malleolus,** and the distal **fibula** and its **lateral malleolus.** Together these structures form a concave receptacle for the convex proximal surface of the **talus.**

(3) The inferior tibiofibular joint connects the convex or medial side of the lower part of the fibular with the concavity of the fibular notch of the tibia. These surfaces are separated by the upward prolongation (4 to 5 mm) of the synovial membrane of the talocrural joint. The part of the articulation that is fibrous is called **tibiofibular syndesmosis.**

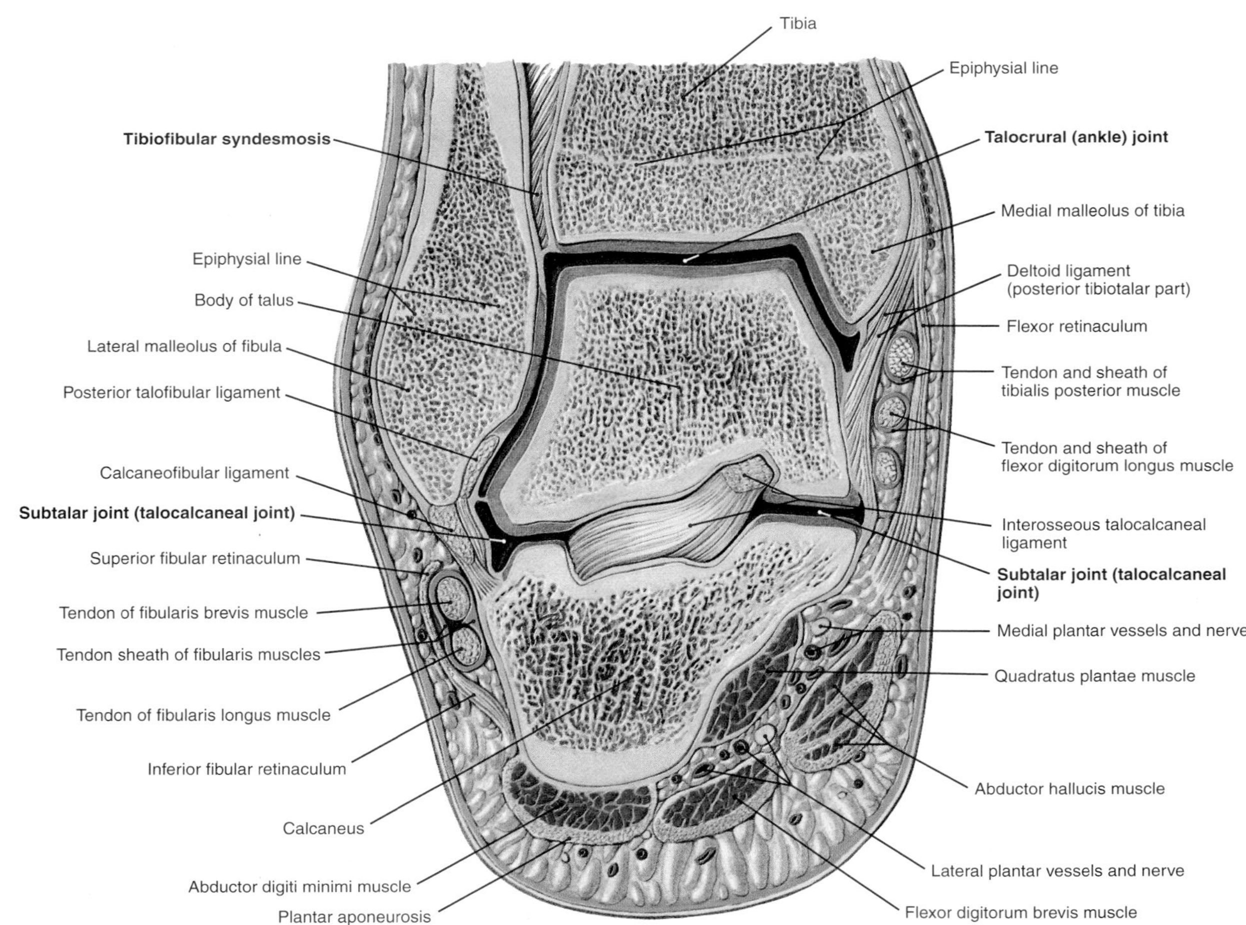
Tibia
Epiphysial line
Tibiofibular syndesmosis
Talocrural (ankle) joint
Medial malleolus of tibia
Epiphysial line
Deltoid ligament
(posterior tibiotalar part)
Body of talus
Flexor retinaculum
Lateral malleolus of fibula
Tendon and sheath of
tibialis posterior muscle
Posterior talofibular ligament
Tendon and sheath of
flexor digitorum longus muscle
Calcaneofibular ligament
Subtalar joint (talocalcaneal joint)
Interosseous talocalcaneal
ligament
Superior fibular retinaculum
Subtalar joint (talocalcaneal
joint)
Tendon of fibularis brevis muscle
Medial plantar vessels and nerve
Tendon sheath of fibularis muscles
Quadratus plantae muscle
Tendon of fibularis longus muscle
Inferior fibular retinaculum
Abductor hallucis muscle
Calcaneus
Lateral plantar vessels and nerve
Abductor digiti minimi muscle
Plantar aponeurosis
Flexor digitorum brevis muscle

Figure 448.2 Coronal Section through the Talocrural (Ankle) and Subtalar Joints and the Tibiofibular Syndesmosis

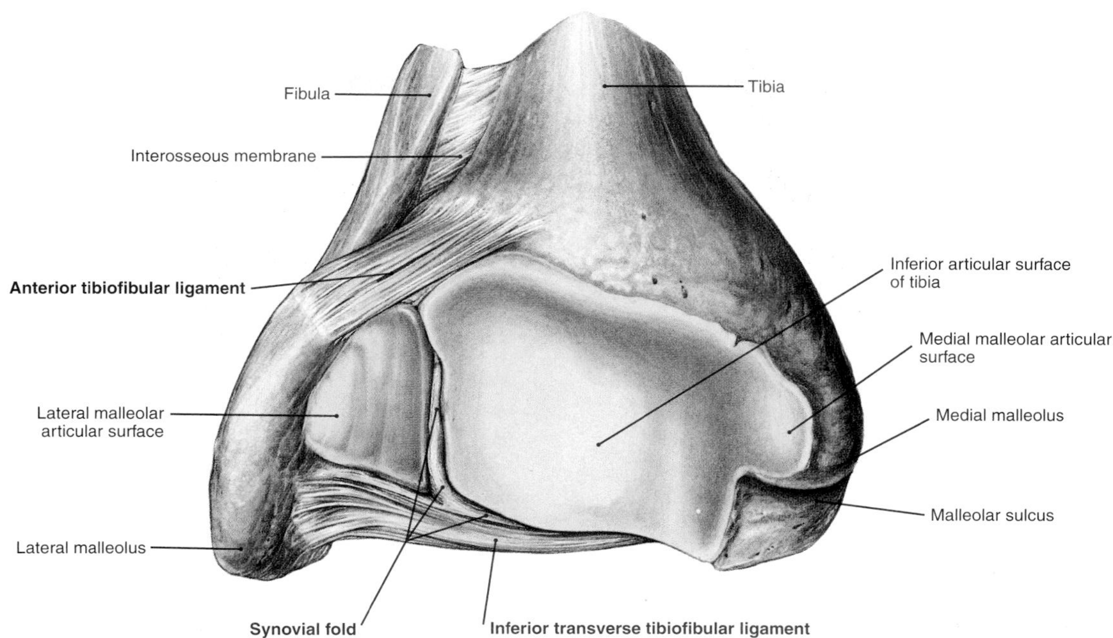
Fibula
Tibia
Interosseous membrane
Anterior tibiofibular ligament
Inferior articular surface of tibia
Medial malleolar articular surface
Lateral malleolar articular surface
Medial malleolus
Malleolar sulcus
Lateral malleolus
Synovial fold
Inferior transverse tibiofibular ligament

Figure 449.1 Inferior Articular Surface of the Tibia and Fibula at the Talocrural (Ankle) Joint

NOTE: (1) The medial and lateral sides of the upper part of the talocrural (ankle) joint are formed by the articular surfaces of the medial malleolus (tibia) and lateral malleolus (fibula). These grasp the sides of the talus.

(2) The inferior articular surface of the tibia is wider anteriorly than posteriorly to accommodate the broader anterior surface of the talus. In full dorsiflexion, the ankle joint is very stable and does not allow any side-to-side movement, but in full plantar flexion, a degree of side-to-side movement can occur.

(3) The synovial fold of the ankle joint that extends upward between the inferior surfaces of the fibula and tibia.

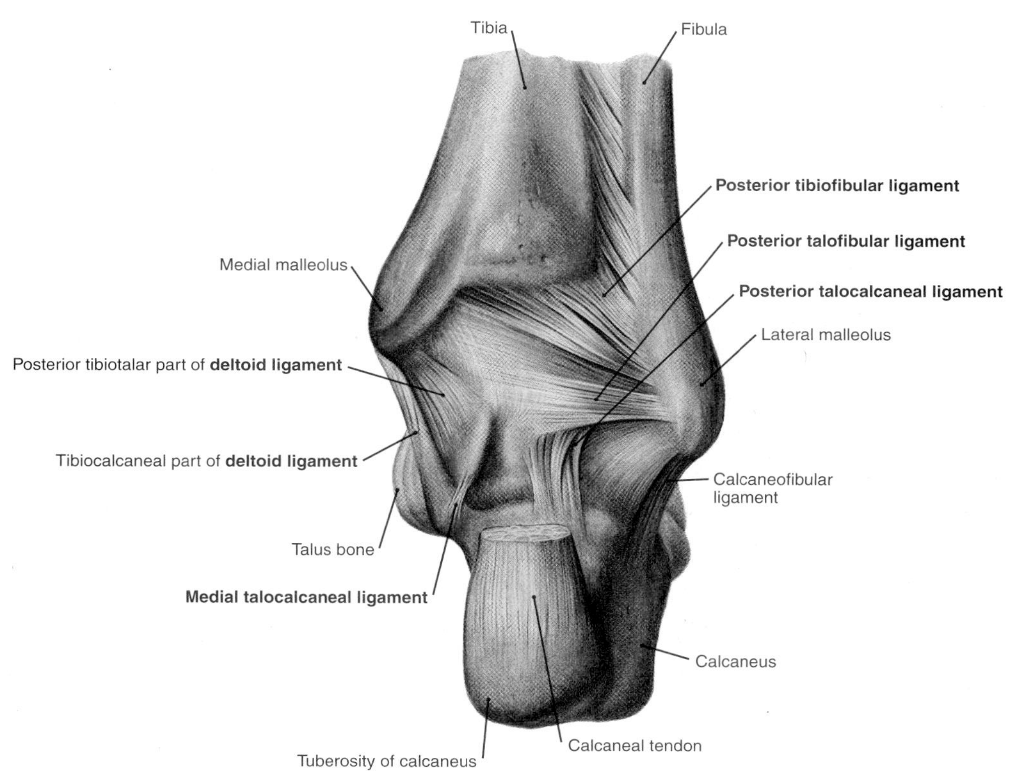
Tibia
Fibula
Posterior tibiofibular ligament
Posterior talofibular ligament
Medial malleolus
Posterior talocalcaneal ligament
Lateral malleolus
Posterior tibiotalar part of deltoid ligament
Tibiocalcaneal part of deltoid ligament
Calcaneofibular ligament
Talus bone
Medial talocalcaneal ligament
Calcaneus
Calcaneal tendon
Tuberosity of calcaneus

Figure 449.2 Ankle Joint (Talocrural) Viewed from Behind (Right Foot)

NOTE: (1) The posterior aspect of the articular capsule is somewhat strengthened by the posterior talofibular and posterior tibiofibular ligaments. The calcaneofibular ligament laterally and the strong deltoid ligament medially assist in protecting this joint.

(2) The ligamentous bands that help stabilize the talocalcaneal articulation posteriorly: the posterior and medial talocalcaneal ligaments.

Figure 450.1 Dorsal Aspect of the Bones of the Right Foot Showing the Attachments of Muscles

Red = origin; Blue = insertion

NOTE: (1) The insertion of the **calcaneal tendon** (of Achilles) on the posterior surface of the calcaneus. This tendon is the strongest in the body, and a bursa is interposed between the bone and the tendon.

(2) The only other muscle that attaches to the tarsal bones on this dorsal aspect is the **extensor digitorum brevis,** which arises from the dorsolateral surface of the calcaneus, distal to its articulation with the talus. Its medial part inserts on the proximal phalanx of the large toe, while its other three tendons insert on the middle phalanx of the second, third, and fourth toes.

(3) The insertions of the **fibularis brevis** and **tertius** onto the base of the fifth metatarsal.

(4) The four dorsal interosseous muscles, two of which insert on the second toe and the third and fourth insert on the dorsolateral aspect of the third and fourth toes.

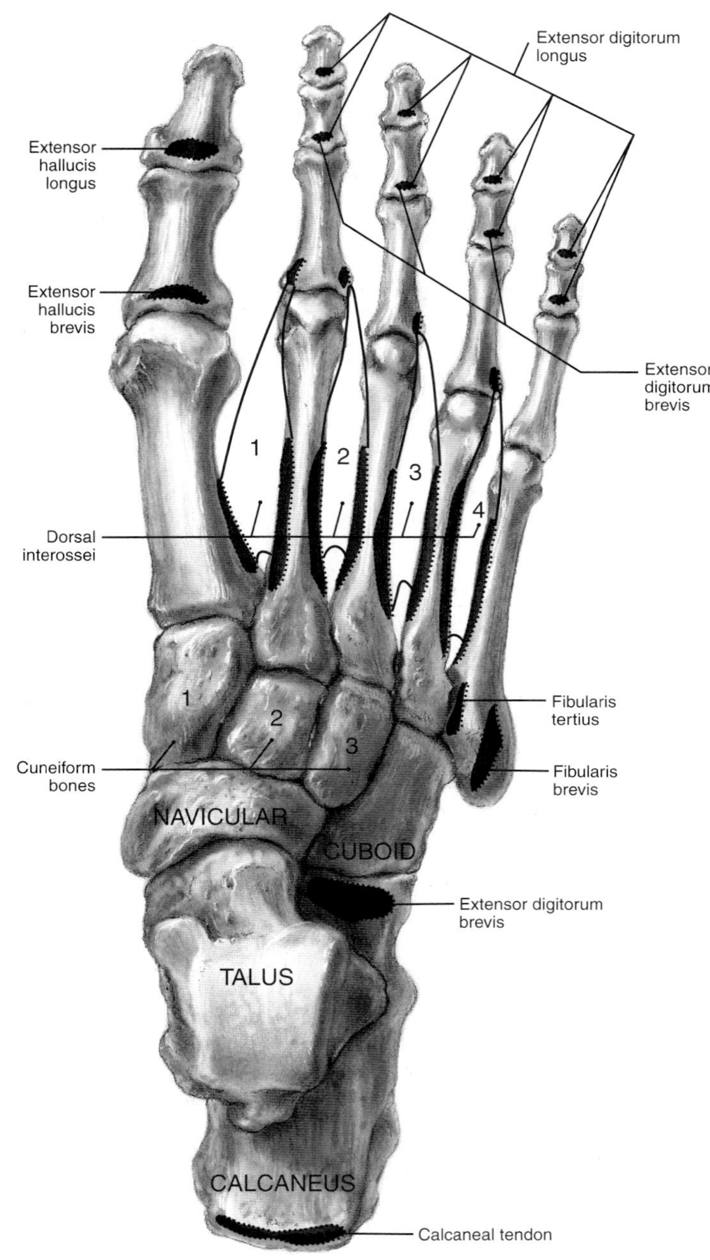
Extensor digitorum longus
Extensor hallucis longus
Extensor hallucis brevis
Extensor digitorum brevis
1
2
3
4
Dorsal interossei
1
2
3
Fibularis tertius
Cuneiform bones
Fibularis brevis
NAVICULAR
CUBOID
Extensor digitorum brevis
TALUS
CALCANEUS
Calcaneal tendon

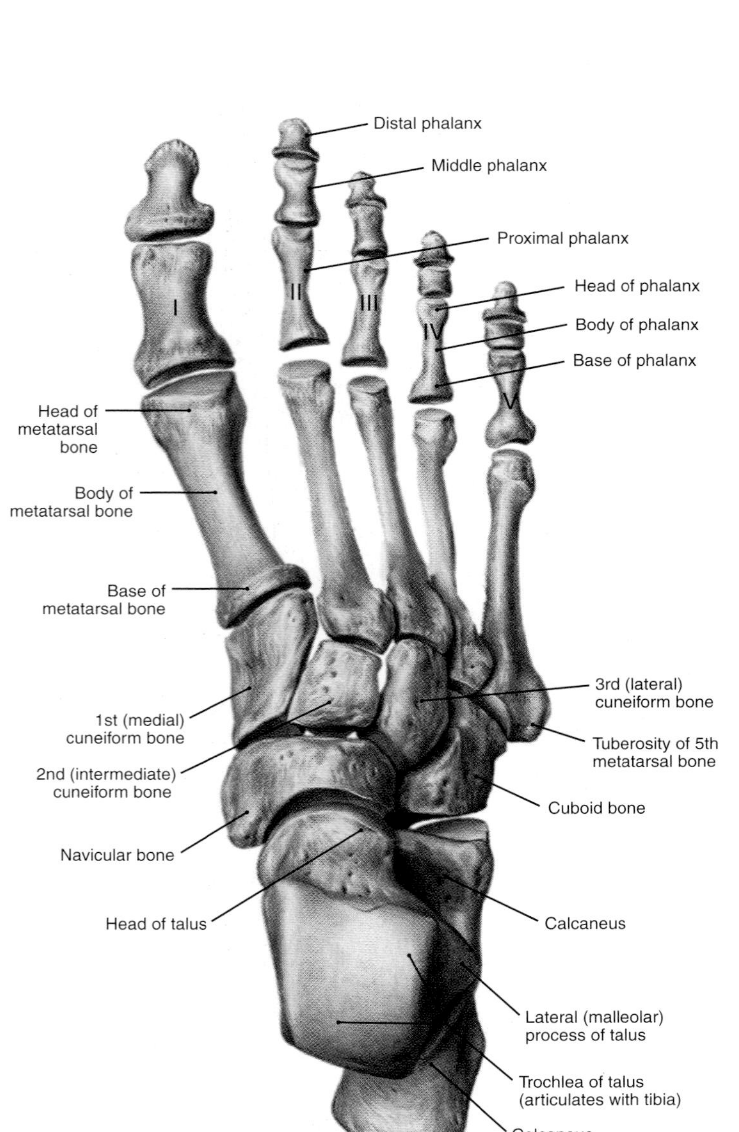
Distal phalanx
Middle phalanx
Proximal phalanx
Head of phalanx
Body of phalanx
Base of phalanx
I
II
III
IV
V
Head of metatarsal bone
Body of metatarsal bone
Base of metatarsal bone
3rd (lateral) cuneiform bone
1st (medial) cuneiform bone
Tuberosity of 5th metatarsal bone
2nd (intermediate) cuneiform bone
Cuboid bone
Navicular bone
Head of talus
Calcaneus
Lateral (malleolar) process of talus
Trochlea of talus (articulates with tibia)
Calcaneus

Figure 450.2 Bones of the Right Foot (Dorsal View)

NOTE: (1) The skeleton of the foot consists of 7 **tarsal bones,** 5 **metatarsal bones,** and 14 **phalanges.** The toes are numbered in order from medial to lateral: the large toe is the first digit, while the small toe is the fifth digit.

(2) The weight of the body is transmitted by the tibia to the **talus,** which then redistributes this weight to the **calcaneus** inferiorly (the heel of the foot) and the **navicular bone** distally (toward the heads of the metatarsals and the "ball" of the foot).

(3) Distal to the navicular and calcaneus are the three **cuneiform bones** and the **cuboid;** these articulate with the individual metatarsal bones of the digits.

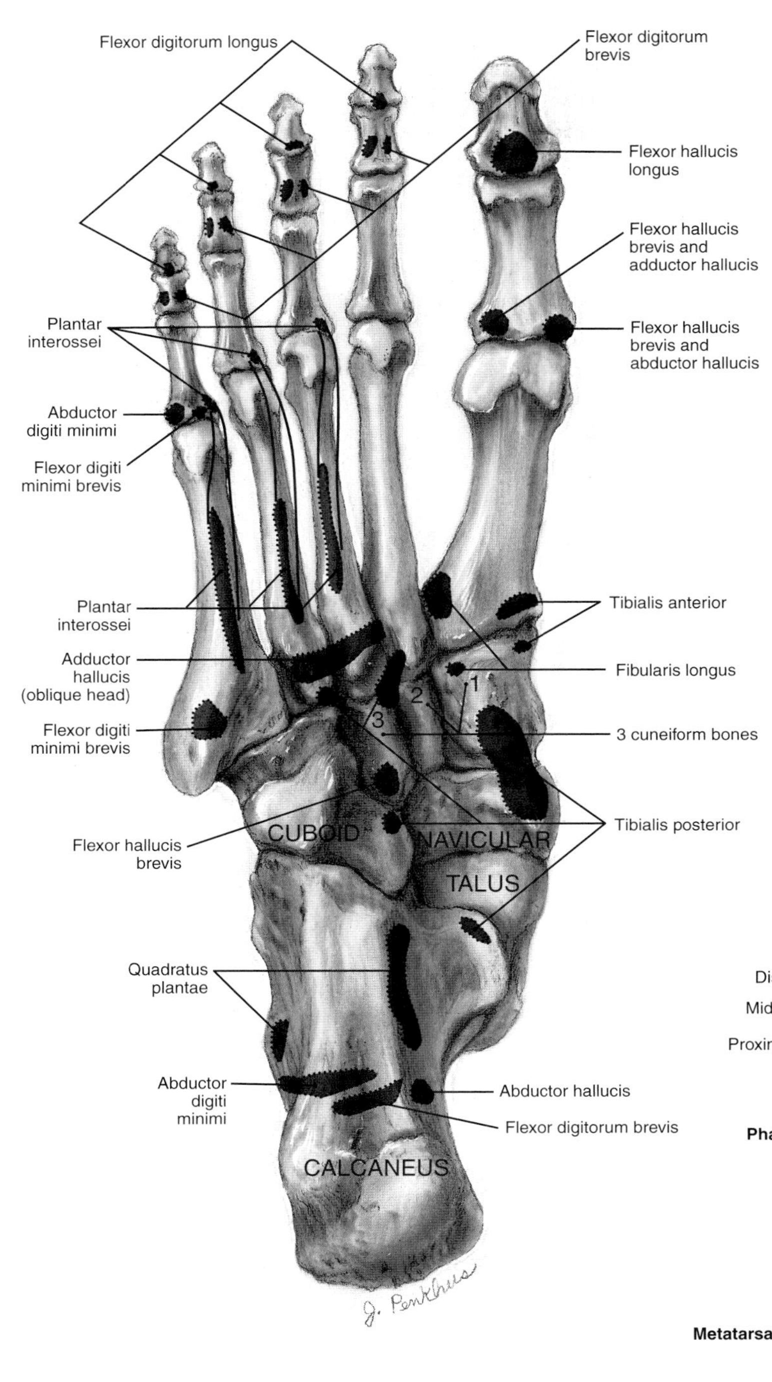
Flexor digitorum longus
Flexor digitorum brevis
Flexor hallucis longus
Flexor hallucis brevis and adductor hallucis
Flexor hallucis brevis and abductor hallucis
Plantar interossei
Abductor digiti minimi
Flexor digiti minimi brevis
Plantar interossei
Adductor hallucis (oblique head)
Flexor digiti minimi brevis
Tibialis anterior
Fibularis longus
3 cuneiform bones
1
2
3
Tibialis posterior
Flexor hallucis brevis
CUBOID
NAVICULAR
TALUS
Quadratus plantae
Abductor digiti minimi
Abductor hallucis
Flexor digitorum brevis
CALCANEUS

Figure 451.1 Plantar Aspect of the Bones of the Right Foot Showing the Attachments of Muscles

Red = origin; Blue = insertion

NOTE: (1) The muscles comprising the first and second layers (except the lumbricals) all arise from the plantar surface of the calcaneal bone. These are the **abductors hallucis** and **digiti minimi**, the **flexor digitorum brevis,** and the **quadratus plantae.**

(2) The tendons of five extrinsic muscles of the foot (arising in the leg) insert on the plantar surface. These are the **fibularis longus**, the **tibialis anterior** and **posterior,** and the **flexors hallucis longus** and **digitorum longus.** The tibialis posterior inserts on six of the seven tarsal bones (only the talus is omitted).

(3) The three **plantar interossei** act as adductors of the third, fourth, and fifth toes, moving them toward the second toe, the center of which serves as the longitudinal axis of the foot.

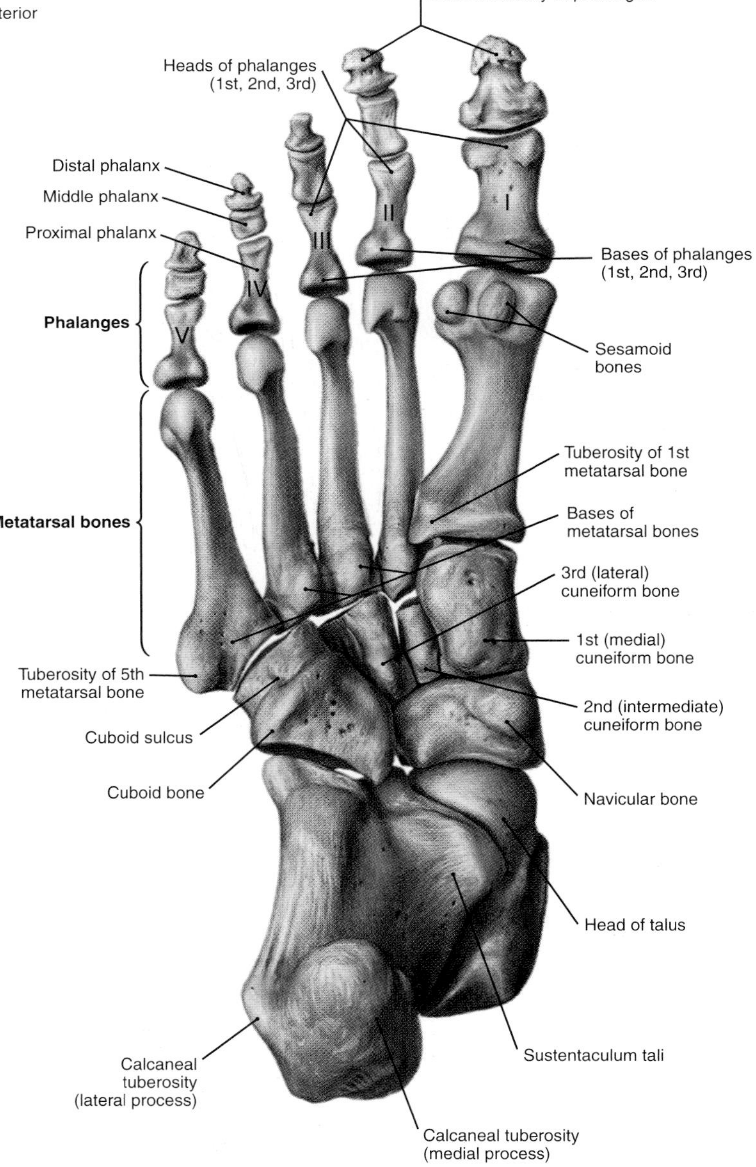
Distal tuberosity of phalanges
Heads of phalanges (1st, 2nd, 3rd)
Distal phalanx
Middle phalanx
Proximal phalanx
Bases of phalanges (1st, 2nd, 3rd)
Phalanges
I
II
III
IV
V
Sesamoid bones
Tuberosity of 1st metatarsal bone
Metatarsal bones
Bases of metatarsal bones
3rd (lateral) cuneiform bone
1st (medial) cuneiform bone
Tuberosity of 5th metatarsal bone
2nd (intermediate) cuneiform bone
Cuboid sulcus
Cuboid bone
Navicular bone
Head of talus
Sustentaculum tali
Calcaneal tuberosity (lateral process)
Calcaneal tuberosity (medial process)

Figure 451.2 Bones of the Right Foot (Plantar View)

NOTE: (1) The largest bone in the foot is the **calcaneus.** On its plantar surface can be seen the **calcaneal tuberosity,** which projects posteriorly and inferiorly (forming the heel). Observe the **sustentaculum tali,** the dorsal surface of which contains the articular facets for the talus.

(2) The **cuboid bone** and the sulcus on its plantar surface for the passage of the fibularis longus tendon that stretches across the sole of the foot.

(3) The long slender metatarsal bones, which are curved so as to be concave on their plantar surface and convex dorsally. Observe the large tuberosity on the lateral side of the base of the fifth metatarsal bone.

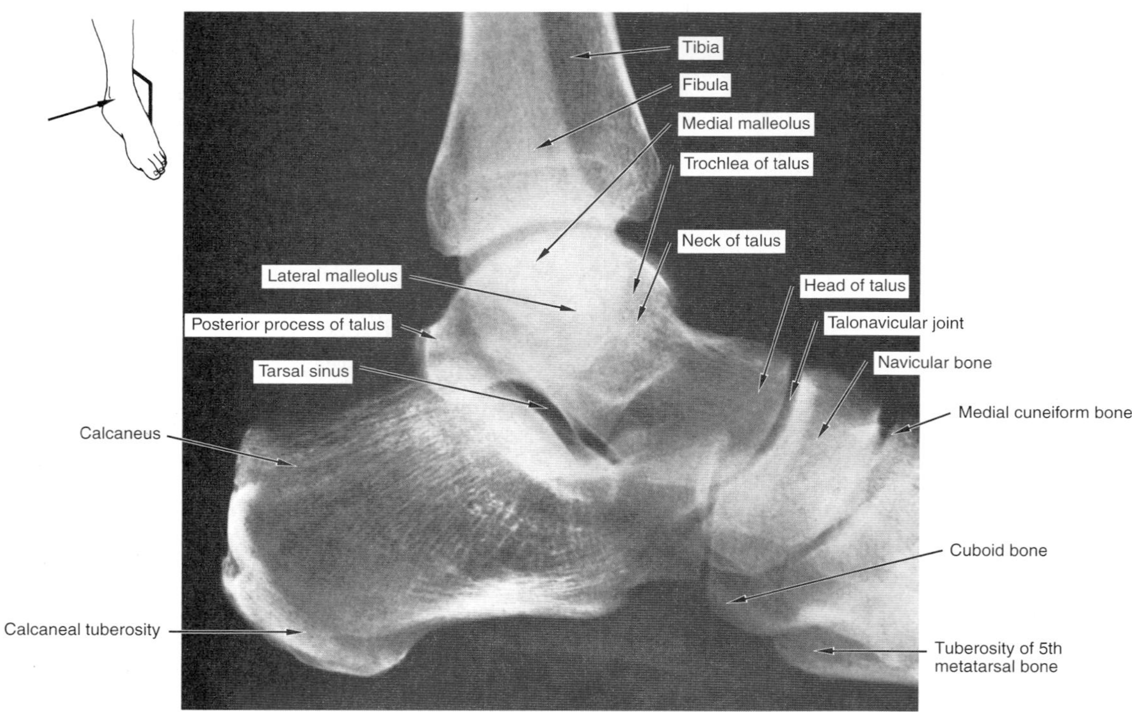
Tibia
Fibula
Medial malleolus
Trochlea of talus
Neck of talus
Lateral malleolus
Head of talus
Posterior process of talus
Talonavicular joint
Tarsal sinus
Navicular bone
Medial cuneiform bone
Calcaneus
Cuboid bone
Calcaneal tuberosity
Tuberosity of 5th metatarsal bone

Figure 452.1 Radiograph of the Talocrural (Ankle) Joint (Lateral View)

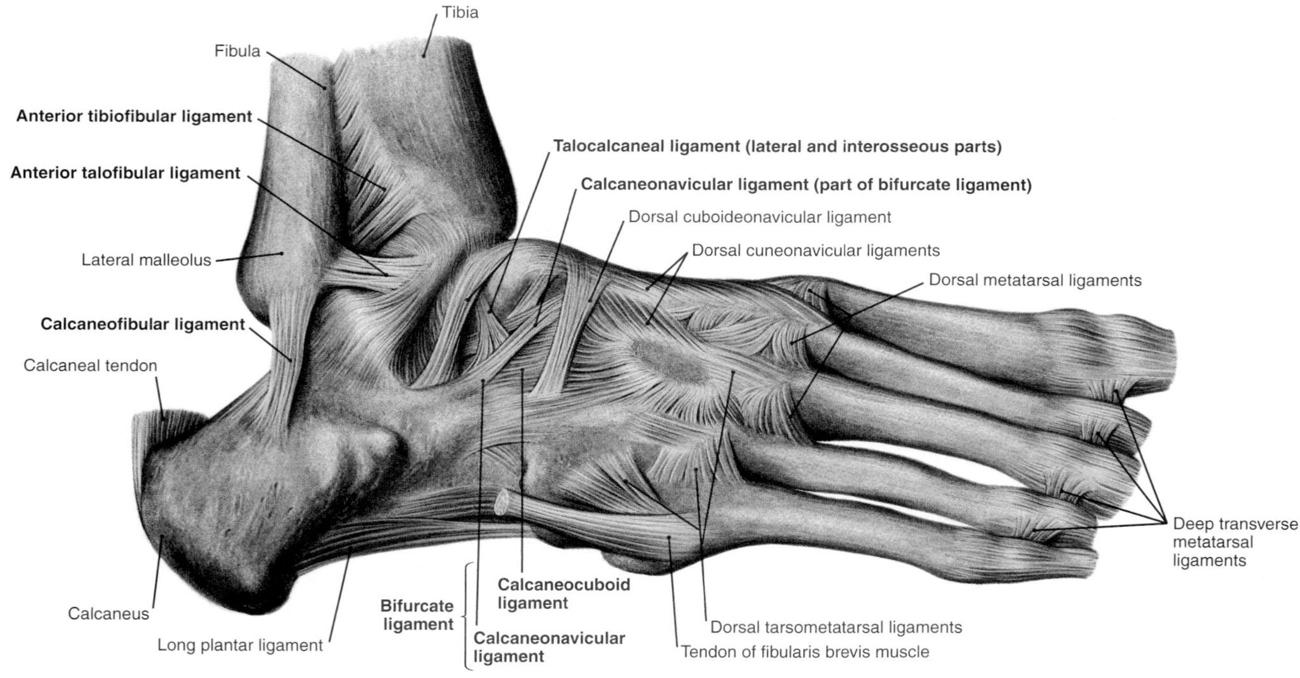
Tibia
Fibula
Anterior tibiofibular ligament
Anterior talofibular ligament
Talocalcaneal ligament (lateral and interosseous parts)
Calcaneonavicular ligament (part of bifurcate ligament)
Dorsal cuboideonavicular ligament
Dorsal cuneonavicular ligaments
Lateral malleolus
Dorsal metatarsal ligaments
Calcaneofibular ligament
Calcaneal tendon
Deep transverse metatarsal ligaments
Calcaneus
Bifurcate ligament
Calcaneocuboid ligament
Calcaneonavicular ligament
Long plantar ligament
Dorsal tarsometatarsal ligaments
Tendon of fibularis brevis muscle

Figure 452.2 Lateral Ligaments of the Ankle Joint and of the Dorsolateral Foot (Right)

NOTE: (1) The fibula is attached to the tibia distally by the **anterior (inferior) tibiofibular ligament.** In addition, the lateral malleolus of the fibula is attached to the talus by the relatively weak **anterior talofibular ligament** and the much stronger **posterior talofibular ligament** (Fig. 449.2). The fibula is attached to the calcaneus by the **calcaneofibular ligament.** Together these latter three bands constitute the lateral ligament of the ankle.

(2) The **interosseous talocalcaneal ligament** is the principal ligament that strengthens the **subtalar joint** (between talus and calcaneus); the **lateral talocalcaneal ligament** also helps strengthen this joint as does the **medial talocalcaneal ligament,** which blends with the deltoid ligament (not shown).

(3) The (dorsal) **calcaneonavicular ligament,** part of the **bifurcate ligament,** attaches the dorsolateral aspect of the navicular bone with the calcaneus. Along with this (dorsal) calcaneonavicular ligament, the (dorsal) calcaneocuboid ligament constitutes the "**bifurcate**" **ligament.**

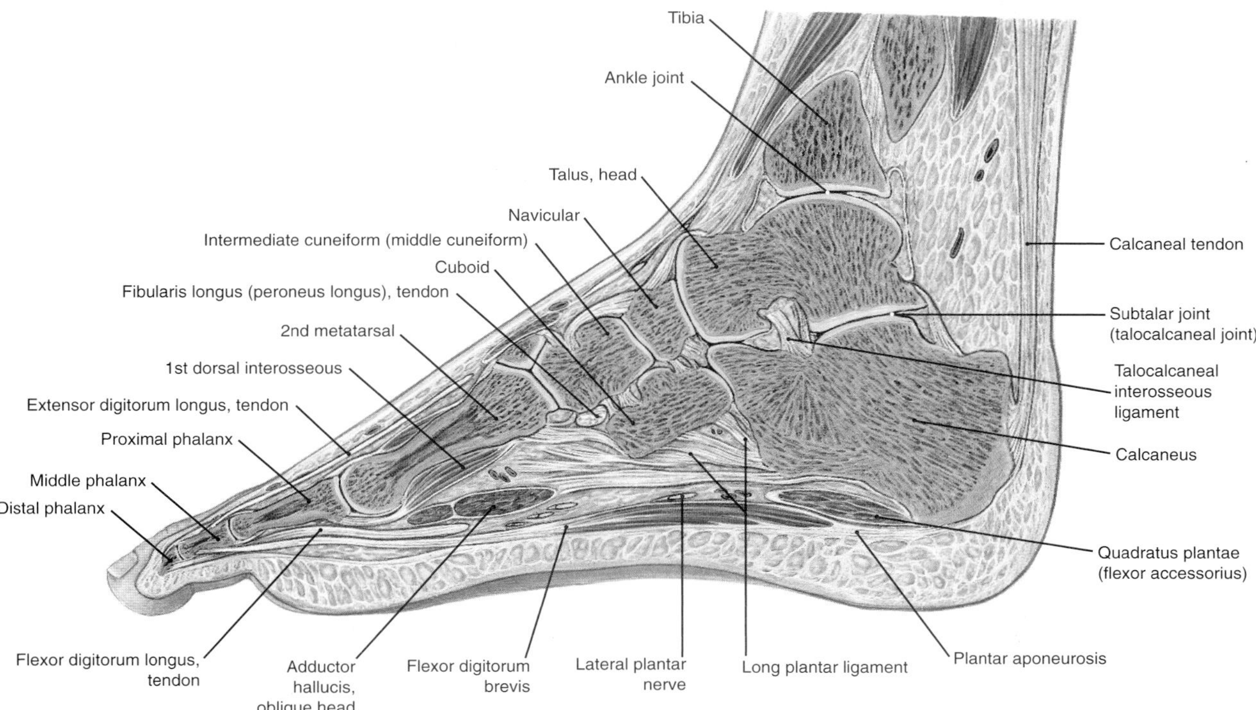
Tibia
Ankle joint
Talus, head
Navicular
Intermediate cuneiform (middle cuneiform)
Cuboid
Fibularis longus (peroneus longus), tendon
2nd metatarsal
1st dorsal interosseous
Extensor digitorum longus, tendon
Proximal phalanx
Middle phalanx
Distal phalanx
Calcaneal tendon
Subtalar joint (talocalcaneal joint)
Talocalcaneal interosseous ligament
Calcaneus
Quadratus plantae (flexor accessorius)
Flexor digitorum longus, tendon
Adductor hallucis, oblique head
Flexor digitorum brevis
Lateral plantar nerve
Long plantar ligament
Plantar aponeurosis

Figure 453.1 Sagittal Section through the Foot, Viewed from the Medial Aspect

NOTE: (1) This longitudinal section goes through the second toe.

(2) The relationship between the head of the talus proximally and the **navicular bone** distally, and the subtalar joint between the talus superiorly and the calcaneus inferiorly.

(3) The long plantar ligament. Observe this ligament also in Figure 455.1

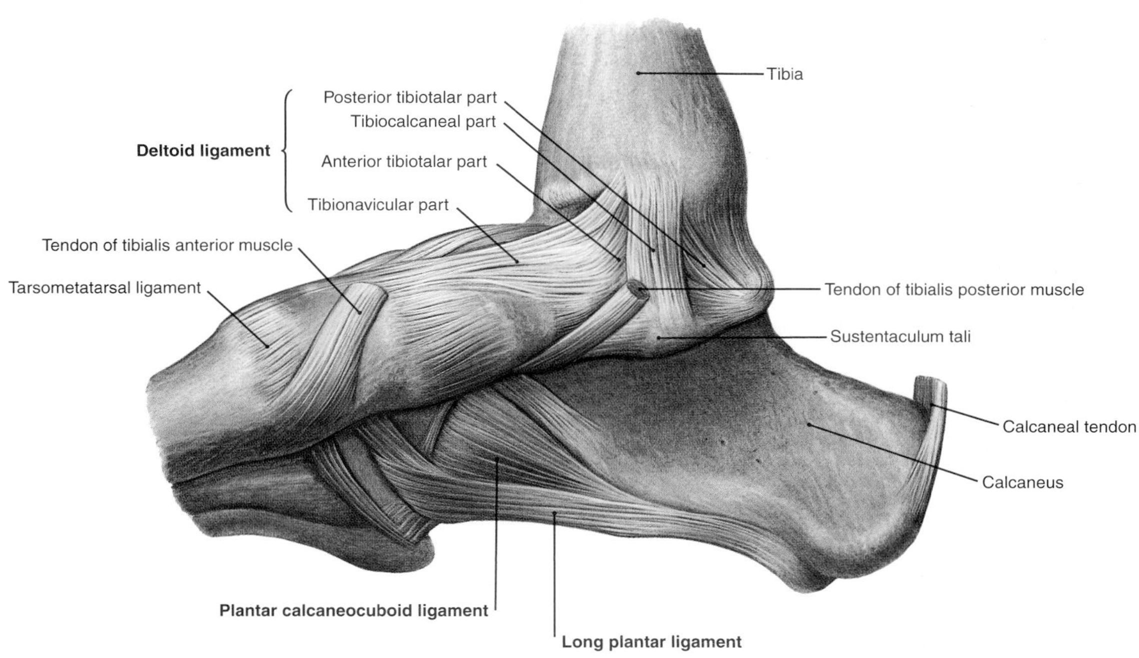
Tibia
Deltoid ligament
Posterior tibiotalar part
Tibiocalcaneal part
Anterior tibiotalar part
Tibionavicular part
Tendon of tibialis anterior muscle
Tarsometatarsal ligament
Tendon of tibialis posterior muscle
Sustentaculum tali
Calcaneal tendon
Calcaneus
Plantar calcaneocuboid ligament
Long plantar ligament

Figure 453.2 Ligaments of the Ankle and Foot: Medial View (Right Foot)

NOTE: (1) The medial aspect of the ankle joint is protected by the triangular **deltoid ligament,** which connects the tibia to the navicular, calcaneus, and talus. The deltoid ligament has four parts: (a) an anterior **tibionavicular part** that attaches the medial malleolus to the navicular, (b) a superficial **tibiocalcaneal part** attaching the malleolus to the sustentaculum tali of the calcaneus, and (c and d) the **anterior** and **posterior tibiotalar parts** that lie more deeply and attach the malleolus to the adjacent talus.

(2) The insertions of the tendons of the tibialis anterior and posterior muscles attach on this medial aspect of the foot. Also observe the **long plantar** and **plantar calcaneocuboid ligaments** on the plantar surface.

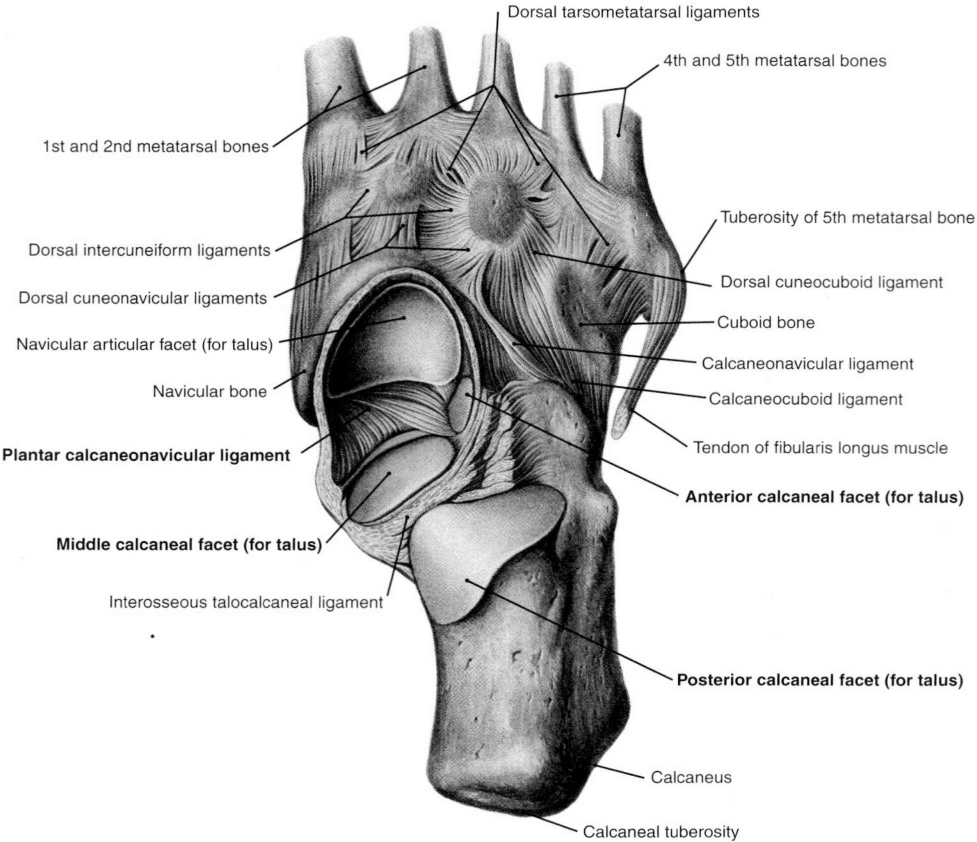
Dorsal tarsometatarsal ligaments
4th and 5th metatarsal bones
1st and 2nd metatarsal bones
Tuberosity of 5th metatarsal bone
Dorsal intercuneiform ligaments
Dorsal cuneocuboid ligament
Dorsal cuneonavicular ligaments
Cuboid bone
Navicular articular facet (for talus)
Calcaneonavicular ligament
Navicular bone
Calcaneocuboid ligament
Tendon of fibularis longus muscle
Plantar calcaneonavicular ligament
Anterior calcaneal facet (for talus)
Middle calcaneal facet (for talus)
Interosseous talocalcaneal ligament
Posterior calcaneal facet (for talus)
Calcaneus
Calcaneal tuberosity

Figure 454.1 Right Talocalcaneonavicular Joint (Viewed from Above)

NOTE: (1) The talus has been removed, which exposes the three articulations it makes inferiorly with the **calcaneus** and the one articulation it makes anteriorly with the **navicular bone.**

(2) The plantar **calcaneonavicular (spring) ligament** stretches across the plantar aspect of the talocalcaneonavicular joint.

(3) The stability of this joint is assisted dorsally by the calcaneonavicular part of the **bifurcate ligament;** however, the plantar calcaneonavicular (or spring) ligament is the principal support of the longitudinal arch of the foot.

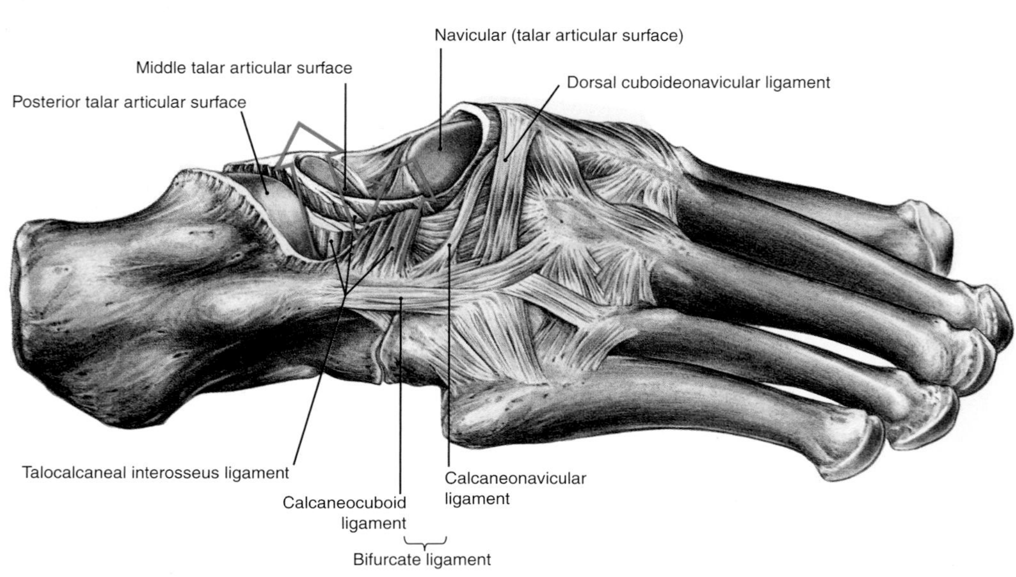
Navicular (talar articular surface)
Middle talar articular surface
Dorsal cuboideonavicular ligament
Posterior talar articular surface
Talocalcaneal interosseus ligament
Calcaneonavicular ligament
Calcaneocuboid ligament
Bifurcate ligament

Figure 454.2 Articular Surfaces of the Right Talocalcaneonavicular Joint

NOTE: (1) The posterior and middle articular surfaces of the talus articulate with the underlying calcaneus, while the anterior articular surface articulates with the navicular bone anteriorly.

(2) The **bifurcate ligament** is a strong band that attaches posteriorly to the superior surface of the calcaneus. Anteriorly, it bifurcates into the calcaneocuboid and calcaneonavicular ligaments and forms a lateral ligament of the talocalcaneonavicular joint.

(3) The two green arrows indicate the torsion of the talocalcaneal ligament.

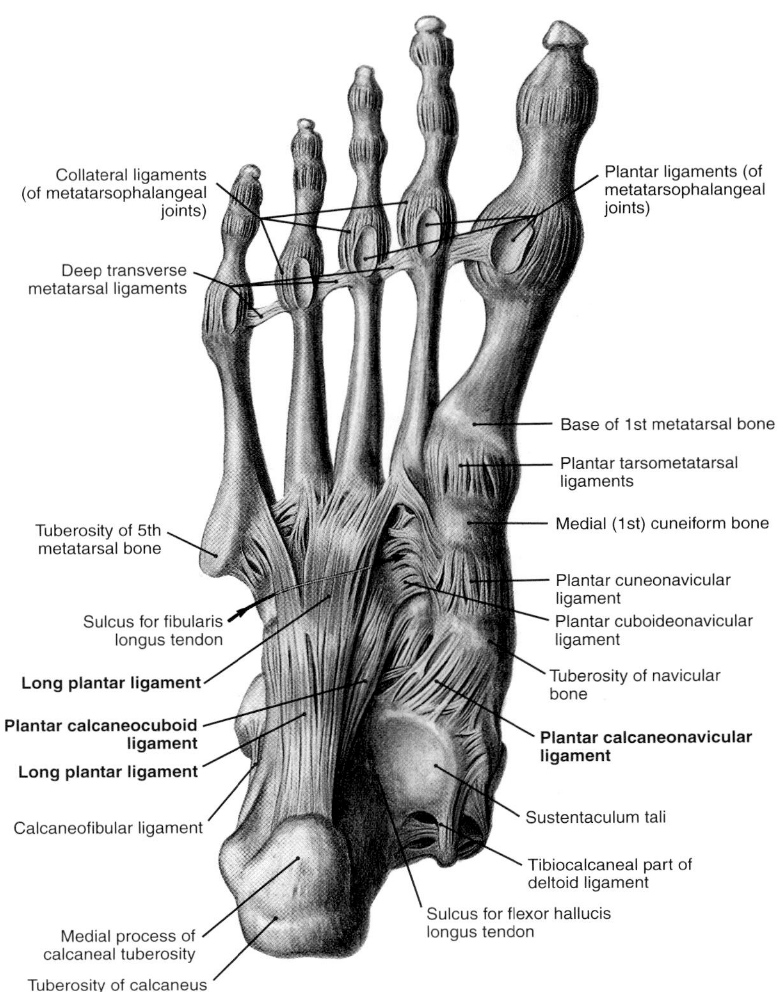
Collateral ligaments (of metatarsophalangeal joints)
Plantar ligaments (of metatarsophalangeal joints)
Deep transverse metatarsal ligaments
Base of 1st metatarsal bone
Plantar tarsometatarsal ligaments
Medial (1st) cuneiform bone
Tuberosity of 5th metatarsal bone
Plantar cuneonavicular ligament
Plantar cuboideonavicular ligament
Sulcus for fibularis longus tendon
Tuberosity of navicular bone
Long plantar ligament
Plantar calcaneocuboid ligament
Plantar calcaneonavicular ligament
Long plantar ligament
Calcaneofibular ligament
Sustentaculum tali
Tibiocalcaneal part of deltoid ligament
Sulcus for flexor hallucis longus tendon
Medial process of calcaneal tuberosity
Tuberosity of calcaneus

Figure 455.1 Ligaments on the Plantar Surface of the Right Foot (Superficial)

NOTE: (1) The **long plantar ligament** is the longest and most superficial of the plantar tarsal ligaments. It stretches from the calcaneus posteriorly to an oblique ridge on the plantar surface of the cuboid, where most of its fibers terminate.

(2) The superficial fibers of the long plantar ligament pass over the cuboid to insert on the bases of the lateral three metatarsal bones, thereby forming a tunnel for the **fibularis longus tendon.**

(3) The **plantar calcaneocuboid** or **short plantar ligament** is very strong and lies deep to the long plantar ligament and closer to the bones.

(4) Identify the **plantar calcaneonavicular (spring) ligament** medially. It is attached to the sustentaculum tali of the calcaneus and extends along the entire inferior surface of the navicular bone. It is important for the support of the medial arch of the foot.

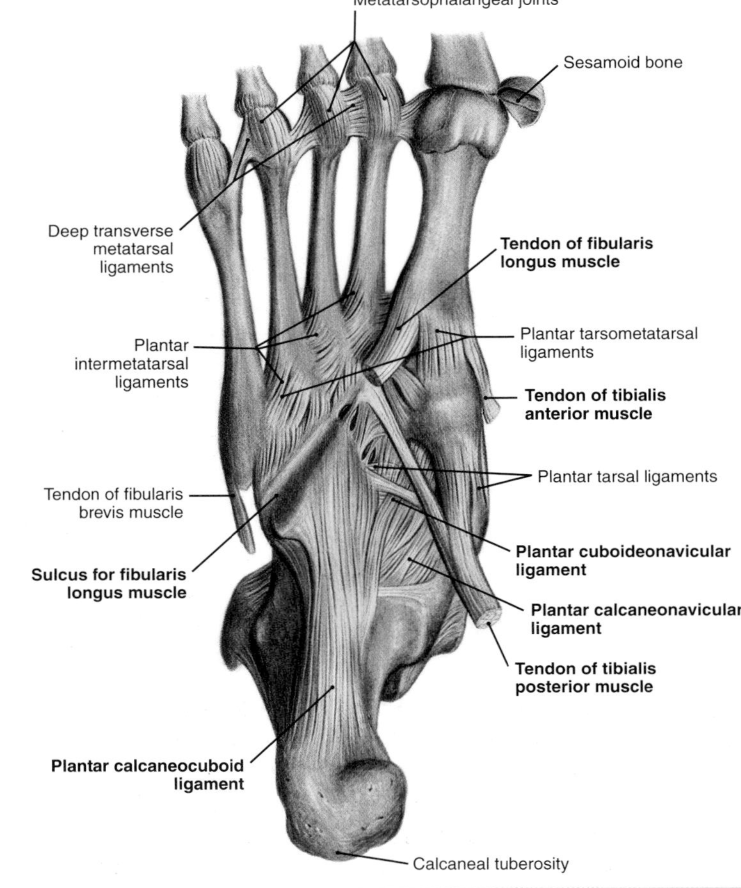
Metatarsophalangeal joints
Sesamoid bone
Deep transverse metatarsal ligaments
Tendon of fibularis longus muscle
Plantar intermetatarsal ligaments
Plantar tarsometatarsal ligaments
Tendon of tibialis anterior muscle
Plantar tarsal ligaments
Tendon of fibularis brevis muscle
Sulcus for fibularis longus muscle
Plantar cuboideonavicular ligament
Plantar calcaneonavicular ligament
Tendon of tibialis posterior muscle
Plantar calcaneocuboid ligament
Calcaneal tuberosity

Figure 455.2 Plantar Calcaneonavicular Ligament and the Insertions of Three Tendons (Right Foot)

NOTE: (1) The metatarsal extensions of the long plantar ligament have been cut away to reveal the groove for the tendon of the fibularis longus muscle. This tendon inserts onto the base of the first metatarsal bone and the first (medial) cuneiform bone.

(2) Two other tendons insert on the medial side of the plantar surface: the tibialis anterior and posterior tendons.

(3) The fibers of the calcaneocuboid (short plantar) and calcaneonavicular (spring) ligaments all stem from the calcaneus and then diverge in a radial manner toward the medial side of the foot.

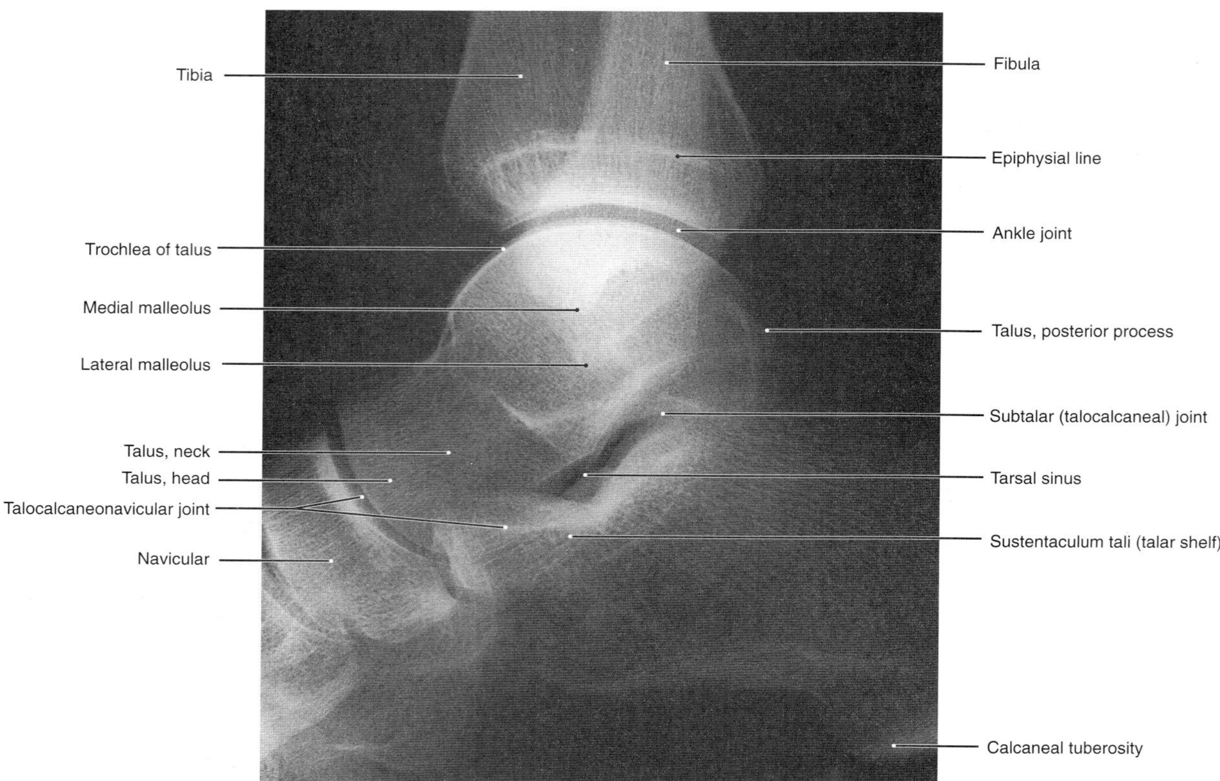
Tibia
Fibula
Epiphysial line
Ankle joint
Trochlea of talus
Medial malleolus
Talus, posterior process
Lateral malleolus
Subtalar (talocalcaneal) joint
Talus, neck
Talus, head
Tarsal sinus
Talocalcaneonavicular joint
Sustentaculum tali (talar shelf)
Navicular
Calcaneal tuberosity

Figure 456.1 Lateral Radiograph of the Subtalar and Talocalcaneonavicular Joints
NOTE: The convex head of the talus articulates with the oval, concave posterior surface of the navicular bone.

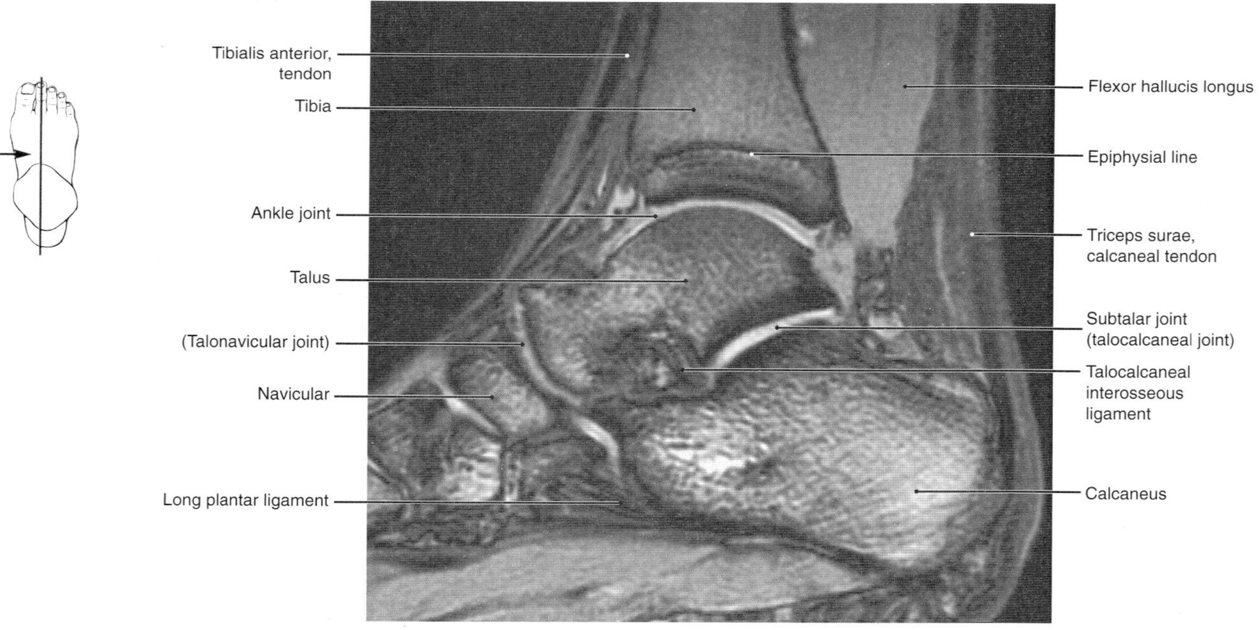
Tibialis anterior, tendon
Tibia
Flexor hallucis longus
Epiphysial line
Ankle joint
Triceps surae, calcaneal tendon
Talus
Subtalar joint (talocalcaneal joint)
(Talonavicular joint)
Talocalcaneal interosseous ligament
Navicular
Long plantar ligament
Calcaneus

Figure 456.2 MRI Showing the Ankle, Subtalar, and Talonavicular Joints
NOTE: This image is taken through the longitudinal axis of the foot.

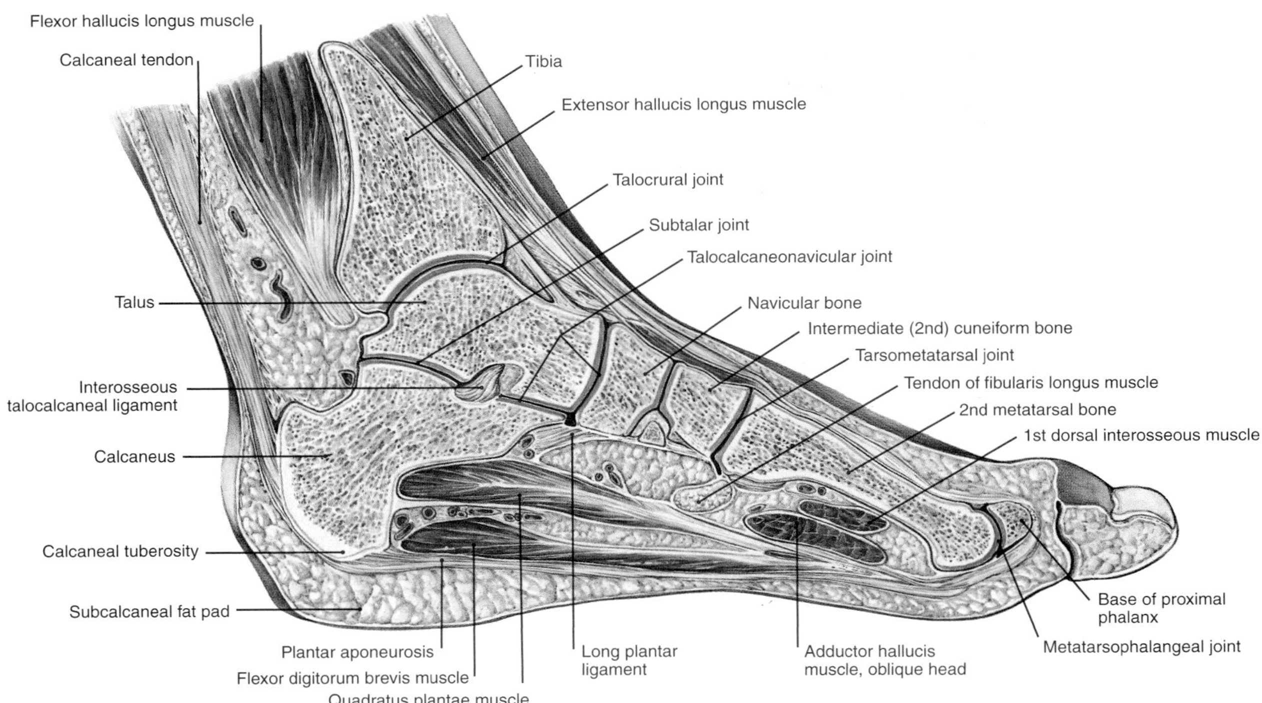
Flexor hallucis longus muscle
Calcaneal tendon
Tibia
Extensor hallucis longus muscle
Talocrural joint
Subtalar joint
Talocalcaneonavicular joint
Talus
Navicular bone
Intermediate (2nd) cuneiform bone
Tarsometatarsal joint
Interosseous talocalcaneal ligament
Tendon of fibularis longus muscle
2nd metatarsal bone
1st dorsal interosseous muscle
Calcaneus
Calcaneal tuberosity
Subcalcaneal fat pad
Base of proximal phalanx
Metatarsophalangeal joint
Plantar aponeurosis
Flexor digitorum brevis muscle
Quadratus plantae muscle
Long plantar ligament
Adductor hallucis muscle, oblique head

Figure 457.1 Sagittal Section of Foot Showing Talocrural, Subtalar, and Talocalcaneonavicular Joints

NOTE: (1) This sagittal section, viewed from the medial aspect, cuts through the trochlea, neck, and head of the talus.

(2) The **talocalcaneonavicular joint** anteriorly is of clinical significance because the weight of the body tends to push the head of the talus downward between the navicular and calcaneus. This results in flat feet.

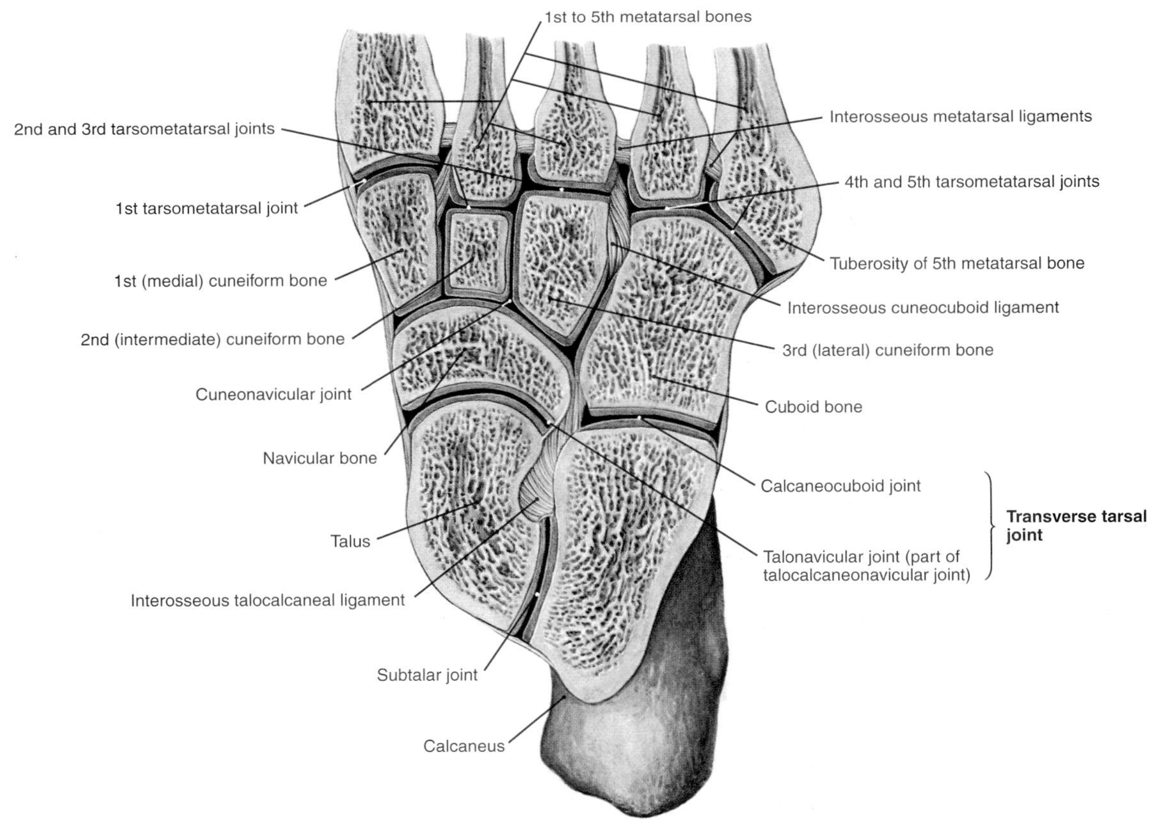
1st to 5th metatarsal bones
2nd and 3rd tarsometatarsal joints
Interosseous metatarsal ligaments
4th and 5th tarsometatarsal joints
1st tarsometatarsal joint
1st (medial) cuneiform bone
Tuberosity of 5th metatarsal bone
Interosseous cuneocuboid ligament
2nd (intermediate) cuneiform bone
3rd (lateral) cuneiform bone
Cuneonavicular joint
Cuboid bone
Navicular bone
Calcaneocuboid joint
Transverse tarsal joint
Talus
Talonavicular joint (part of talocalcaneonavicular joint)
Interosseous talocalcaneal ligament
Subtalar joint
Calcaneus

Figure 457.2 Intertarsal and Tarsometatarsal Joints (Horizontal Section of the Right Foot)

NOTE: The **transverse tarsal (midtarsal) joint** extends across the foot and actually is formed by two separate joint cavities, the **calcaneocuboid joint** laterally and the **talonavicular** part of the talocalcaneonavicular joint medially. These two joints allow some eversion and inversion movements of the foot.

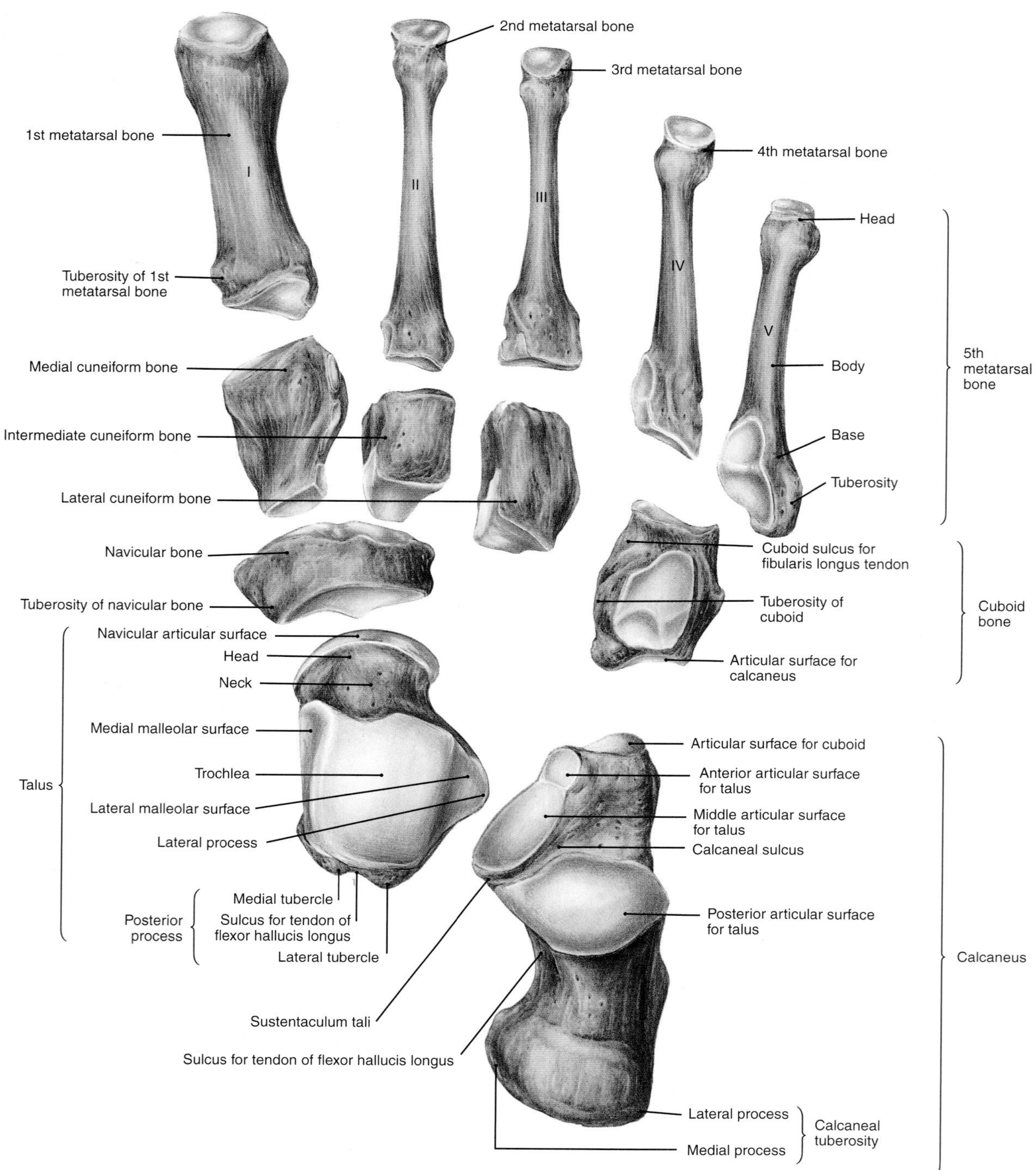
2nd metatarsal bone
3rd metatarsal bone
1st metatarsal bone
I
II
III
4th metatarsal bone
Head
IV
Tuberosity of 1st metatarsal bone
V
Medial cuneiform bone
Body
5th metatarsal bone
Intermediate cuneiform bone
Base
Tuberosity
Lateral cuneiform bone
Navicular bone
Cuboid sulcus for fibularis longus tendon
Tuberosity of navicular bone
Tuberosity of cuboid
Cuboid bone
Navicular articular surface
Head
Articular surface for calcaneus
Neck
Medial malleolar surface
Articular surface for cuboid
Anterior articular surface for talus
Trochlea
Talus
Lateral malleolar surface
Middle articular surface for talus
Lateral process
Calcaneal sulcus
Medial tubercle
Posterior articular surface for talus
Posterior process
Sulcus for tendon of flexor hallucis longus
Lateral tubercle
Calcaneus
Sustentaculum tali
Sulcus for tendon of flexor hallucis longus
Lateral process
Calcaneal tuberosity
Medial process

Figure 458 Tarsal and Metatarsal Bones of the Right Foot

NOTE: (1) In this dorsal view (except for the cuboid bone, which has been rotated so that its medial surface is presented dorsally) are depicted the **seven tarsal bones** and the **five metatarsal bones;** the phalanges are not shown.

(2) The tarsal bones, although homologues of the carpal bones, are of greater size and strength than the bones of the wrist because they function to support the weight of the body in standing.

(3) Of the seven tarsal bones, the **talus** and **calcaneus** comprise the proximal row and the **three cuneiforms** and the **cuboid** the distal row. Interposed between the talus and the cuneiforms medially is the **navicular bone,** while the calcaneus and cuboid articulate directly.

(4) The **five metatarsal bones** interconnect the tarsal bones with the phalanges (not shown), and they are numbered from medial to lateral. The medial cuneiform articulates distally with the first metatarsal, the intermediate cuneiform with the second metatarsal, and the lateral cuneiform with the third metatarsal. The cuboid articulates distally with both the fourth and fifth metatarsal bones.

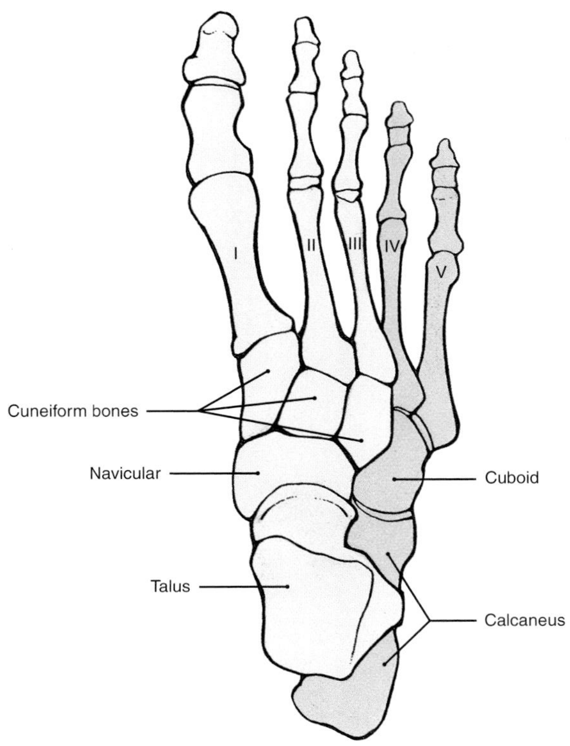

I
II
III
IV
V
Cuneiform bones
Navicular
Cuboid
Talus
Calcaneus

Figure 459.1 Longitudinal Arches of the Foot (Dorsal View)

NOTE: The **medial longitudinal arch** consists of the talus, navicular, three cuneiform bones, three medial metatarsal bones, and the phalanges of the large toe and those of the second and third toes.

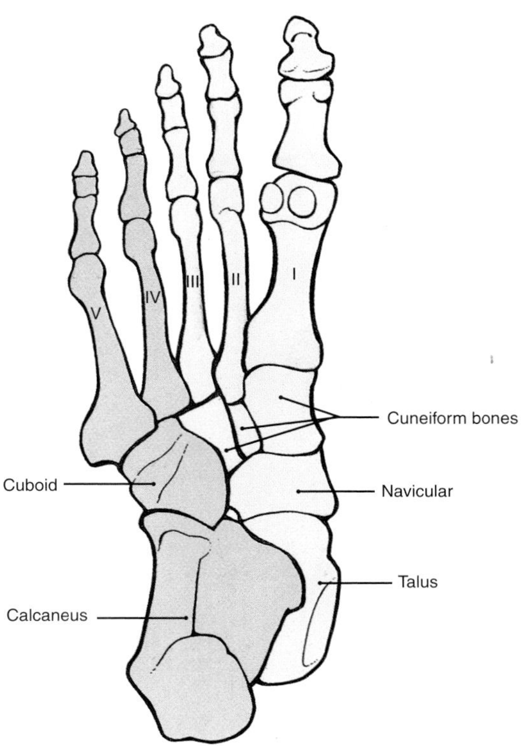

I
II
III
IV
V
Cuneiform bones
Navicular
Cuboid
Talus
Calcaneus

Figure 459.2 Longitudinal Arches of the Foot (Plantar View)

NOTE: The **lateral longitudinal arch consists** of the calcaneus and cuboid bones, the two lateral metatarsal bones, and the phalanges of the fourth and fifth toes.

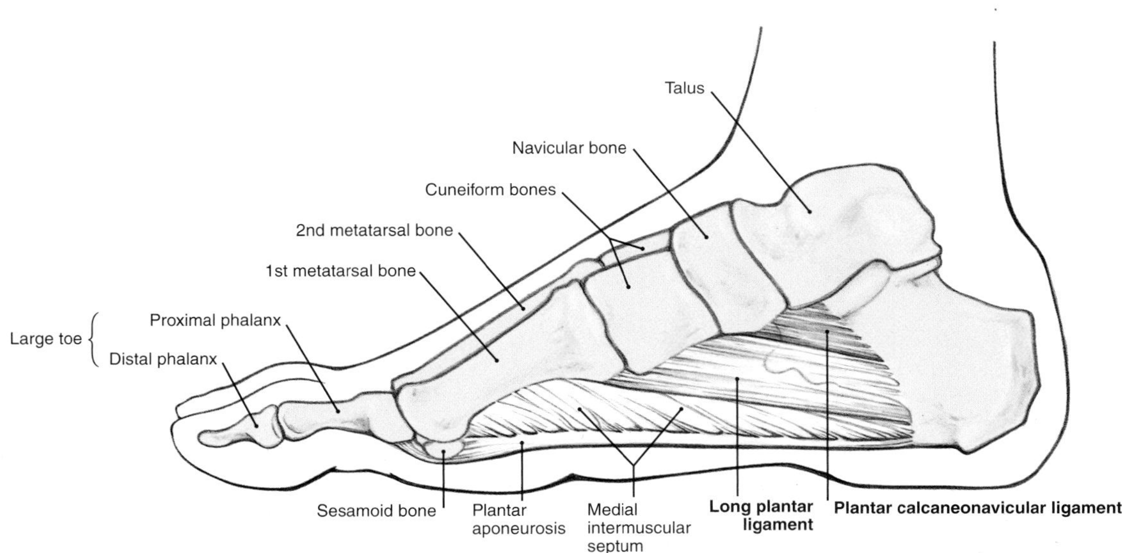

Talus
Navicular bone
Cuneiform bones
2nd metatarsal bone
1st metatarsal bone
Large toe
Proximal phalanx
Distal phalanx
Sesamoid bone
Plantar aponeurosis
Medial intermuscular septum
Long plantar ligament
Plantar calcaneonavicular ligament

Figure 459.3 Longitudinal Arch of the Foot: Underlying Support Structures

NOTE: (1) The medial longitudinal arch of the foot is formed by the calcaneus, talus, navicular, three cuneiform, and the medial three metatarsal bones. Observe the arched nature of the medial margin of the foot.

(2) The integrity of the medial longitudinal arch depends on structures underlying the talocalcaneonavicular septum, but much more important are the **long plantar ligament** and especially the **plantar calcaneonavicular ligament.**

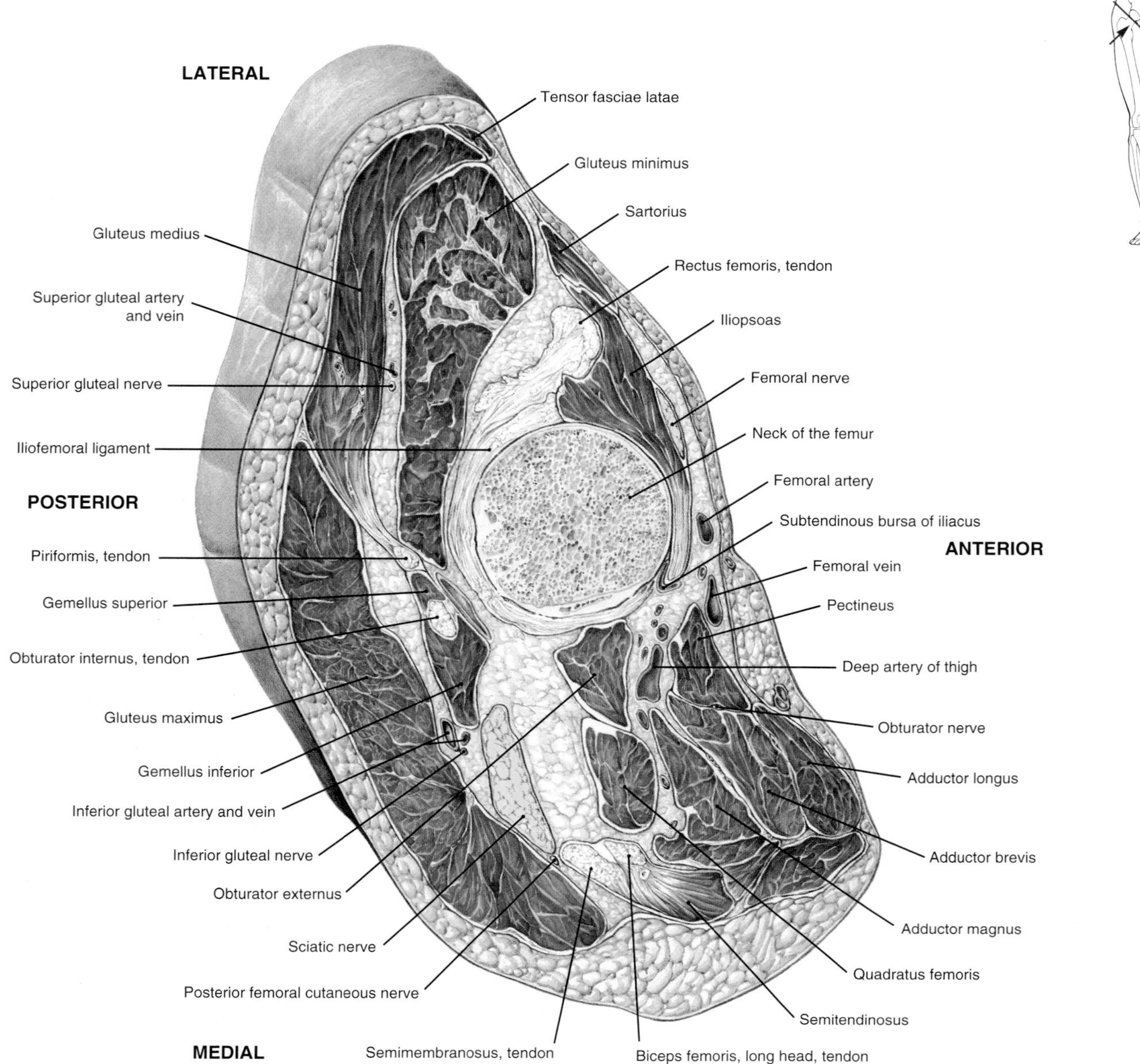
LATERAL
Tensor fasciae latae
Gluteus minimus
Sartorius
Gluteus medius
Rectus femoris, tendon
Superior gluteal artery and vein
Iliopsoas
Superior gluteal nerve
Femoral nerve
Iliofemoral ligament
Neck of the femur
POSTERIOR
Femoral artery
Subtendinous bursa of iliacus
ANTERIOR
Piriformis, tendon
Femoral vein
Gemellus superior
Pectineus
Obturator internus, tendon
Deep artery of thigh
Gluteus maximus
Obturator nerve
Gemellus inferior
Adductor longus
Inferior gluteal artery and vein
Inferior gluteal nerve
Adductor brevis
Obturator externus
Adductor magnus
Sciatic nerve
Quadratus femoris
Posterior femoral cutaneous nerve
Semitendinosus
MEDIAL
Semimembranosus, tendon
Biceps femoris, long head, tendon

Figure 460 Cross Section through the Superior Aspect of the Right Thigh

NOTE: (1) This section is through the femoral neck. See the tendon of the rectus femoris and the iliofemoral ligament. Observe the gluteus maximus, gluteus medius, and gluteus minimus along with the tendon of the obturator internus and the gemellus superior and gemellus inferior in the **gluteal region.**

(2) The sartorius, iliopsoas, pectineus, and femoral vessels and nerves in the **anterior thigh.** Observe the obturator externus located deep to the quadratus femoris, and note the adductor magnus, longus, and brevis in the **medial thigh.**

(3) The biceps femoris, semimembranosus, tendon of the semitendinosus and the **sciatic nerve** in the **posterior thigh.**

CLINICAL NOTES from Prof. Constantine P. Karakousis, Professor of Surgery, University of Buffalo, Buffalo, N.Y, (by personal communication):

(4) "In a medial compartment resection of the thigh due to sarcoma, resection of the adductor magnus may be required, and it should be kept in mind that as soon as the insertion of the adductor magnus to the linea aspera is divided, directly behind the medial portion of the adductor magnus lies the **sciatic nerve,** which is subject to injury unless some care is exercised."

(5) "The **sciatic nerve** lies between the ischial tuberosity and the greater trochanter, being lateral to the hamstring muscles. As it descends to the midthigh, the sciatic nerve assumes a position between the biceps femoris (long head) and the semitendinosus–semimembranosus muscles. For sarcomas in the buttocks, a longitudinal or slightly oblique incision is preferable to an incision along the fibers of the gluteus maximus. Such an incision can extend from the crest of the ilium to midway between the ischial tuberosity and the greater trochanter into the upper thigh. This provides an early exposure of the sciatic nerve below the lowermost fibers of the gluteus maximus and, therefore, resection of the gluteus maximus and any other gluteal muscles can be done safely by visualizing the sciatic nerve from this more distal point to the site where the nerve leaves the pelvis below the piriformis."

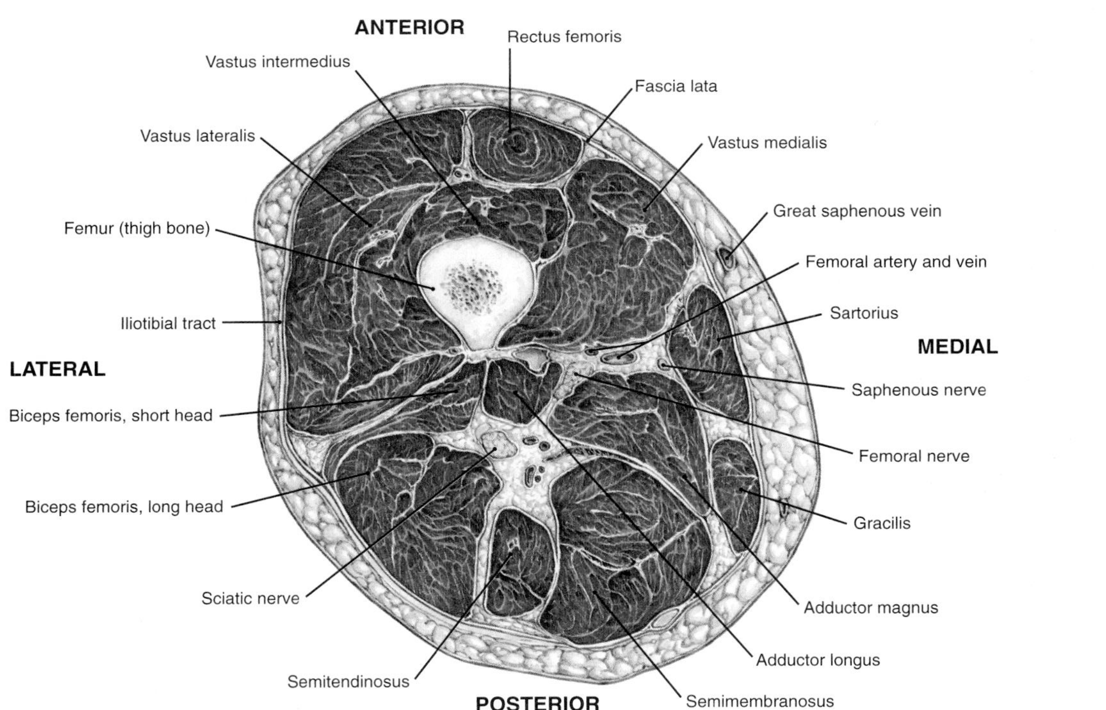
ANTERIOR
Rectus femoris
Vastus intermedius
Fascia lata
Vastus lateralis
Vastus medialis
Great saphenous vein
Femur (thigh bone)
Femoral artery and vein
Sartorius
Iliotibial tract
MEDIAL
LATERAL
Saphenous nerve
Biceps femoris, short head
Femoral nerve
Biceps femoris, long head
Gracilis
Sciatic nerve
Adductor magnus
Adductor longus
Semitendinosus
POSTERIOR
Semimembranosus

Figure 461.1 Cross Section through the Middle of the Right Thigh Viewed From the Distal Aspect

NOTE: (1) Compare this figure with the MRI seen in Figure 461.2.

(2) The **posterior** group of structures: biceps femoris, semitendinosus, semimembranosus, and the **sciatic nerve.**

(3) The **medial** structures: gracilis, adductor magnus, and adductor longus (the adductor brevis is more superior to this section).

(4) The **anterior** structures: four heads of the quadriceps muscle: rectus femoris, vastus lateralis, vastus intermedius, and vastus medialis.

CLINICAL NOTES from Professor Constantine P. Karakousis, Professor of Surgery, University of Buffalo, Buffalo, N.Y. (personal communication):

(5) "The bulk of the motor branches of the femoral nerve in the proximal groin deviate in an inferolateral direction along the branches of the lateral femoral circumflex artery and vein in a course between the rectus femoris, vastus intermedius, and vastus lateralis. A slender branch of the femoral nerve, however, remains outside the musculature until it reaches the middle of the vastus medialis, where it enters the muscle to provide its motor supply."

(6) "The difference in the course of the branch to vastus medialis as compared to the branches to the other heads of the quadriceps is useful in performing a modified anterior compartment resection of the anterior thigh for suitable cases of sarcoma, providing the tumor can adequately be resected, since it could potentially preserve the extensor action at the knee."

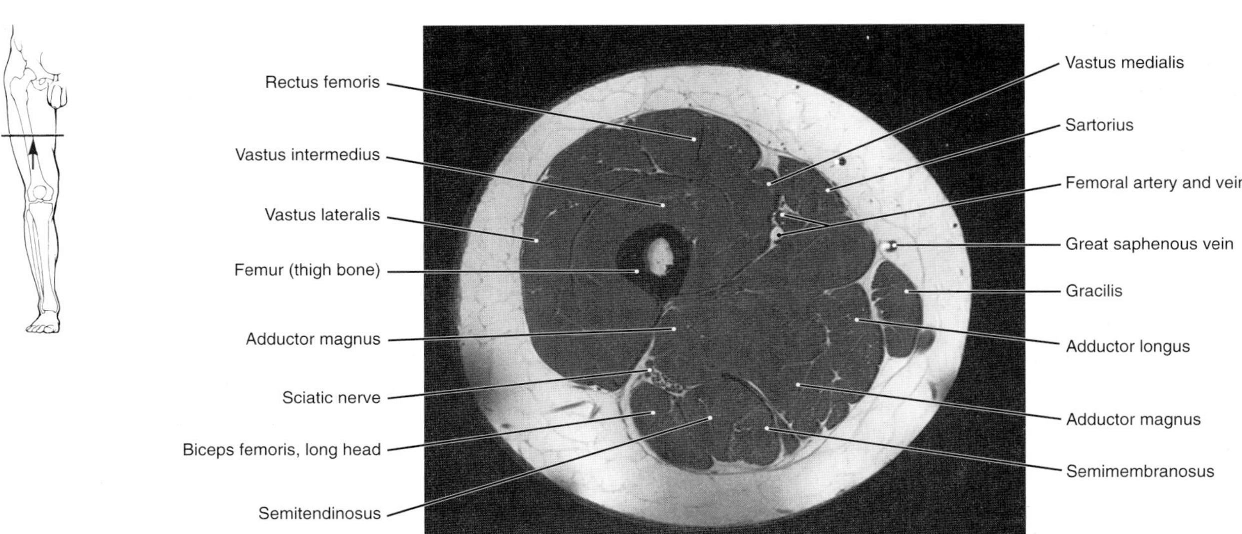
Rectus femoris
Vastus intermedius
Vastus lateralis
Femur (thigh bone)
Adductor magnus
Sciatic nerve
Biceps femoris, long head
Semitendinosus
Vastus medialis
Sartorius
Femoral artery and vein
Great saphenous vein
Gracilis
Adductor longus
Adductor magnus
Semimembranosus

Figure 461.2 MRI Near the Middle of the Right Thigh

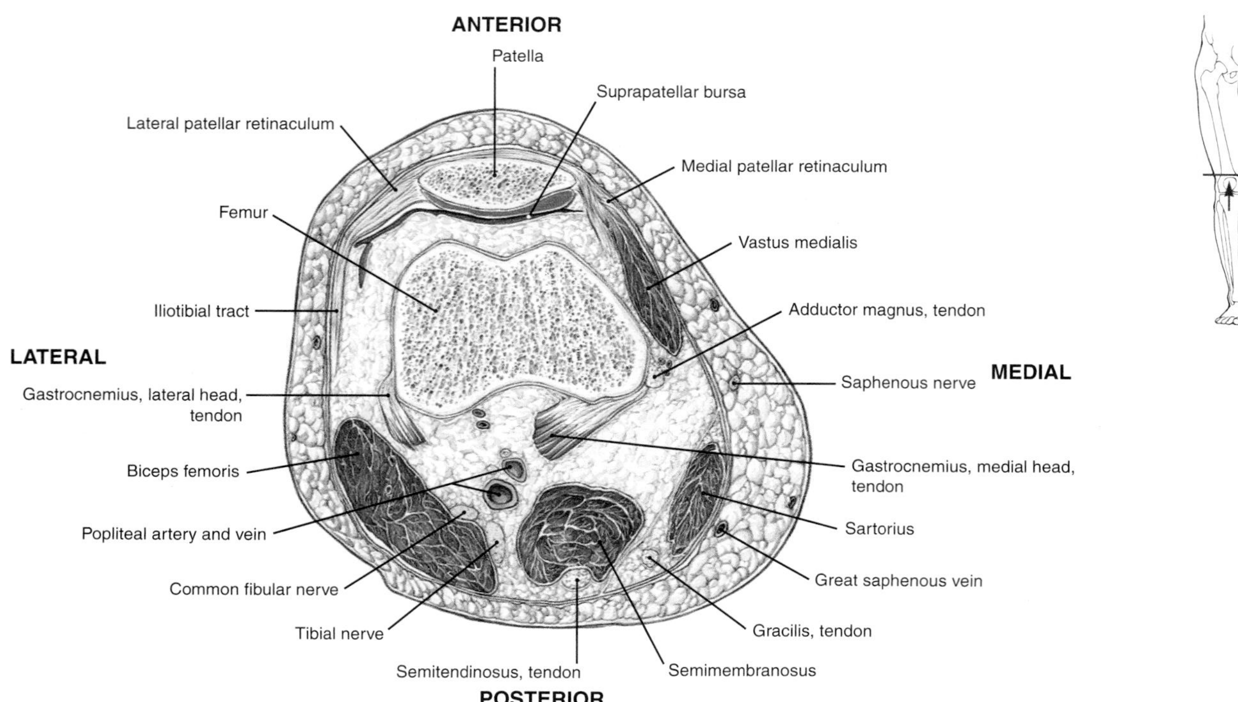
ANTERIOR
Patella
Suprapatellar bursa
Lateral patellar retinaculum
Medial patellar retinaculum
Femur
Vastus medialis
Iliotibial tract
Adductor magnus, tendon
LATERAL
Saphenous nerve
MEDIAL
Gastrocnemius, lateral head, tendon
Biceps femoris
Gastrocnemius, medial head, tendon
Popliteal artery and vein
Sartorius
Common fibular nerve
Great saphenous vein
Tibial nerve
Gracilis, tendon
Semitendinosus, tendon
Semimembranosus
POSTERIOR

Figure 462.1 Cross Section of the Inferior Thigh at the Level of the Popliteal Fossa Viewed from the Distal Aspect

NOTE: (1) Compare this figure with the MRI seen in Figure 462.2.

(2) In this cross section through the inferior aspect of the right femur, see the **popliteal vessels, tibial nerve,** and **common fibular** (common peroneal) **nerve** in the popliteal fossa posterior to the femur. Observe that the nerves are superficial (i.e., more posterior) to the vessels and that the artery is most deeply located and the vein is between the nerves and the artery.

(3) The patella and the suprapatellar bursa are anterior to the femur and the lateral patellar retinaculum and the iliotibial tract are lateral to the femur.

(4) Posteriorly, identify the two heads of the gastrocnemius muscle, the inferior parts of the "hamstring muscles" (biceps femoris, tendon of the semitendinosus and semimembranosus muscles), the two superior ends of the gastrocnemius muscle, and the sartorius muscle (that has coursed around the thigh to the medial aspect of the knee at this level).

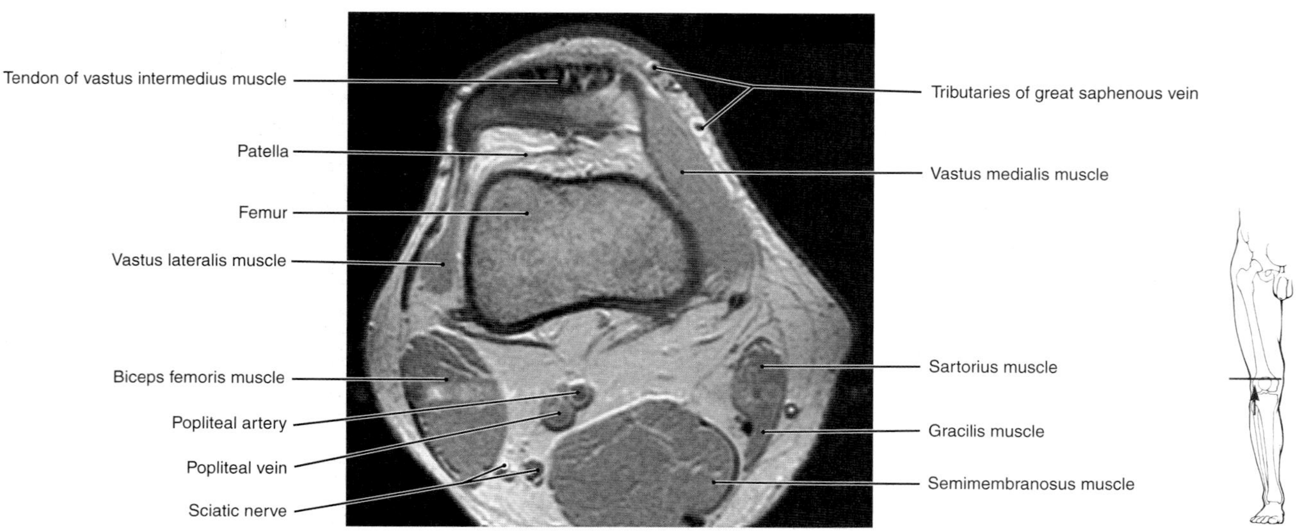
Tendon of vastus intermedius muscle
Patella
Femur
Vastus lateralis muscle
Biceps femoris muscle
Popliteal artery
Popliteal vein
Sciatic nerve
Tributaries of great saphenous vein
Vastus medialis muscle
Sartorius muscle
Gracilis muscle
Semimembranosus muscle

Figure 462.2 MRI: Cross Section through the Distal Part of the Right Thigh

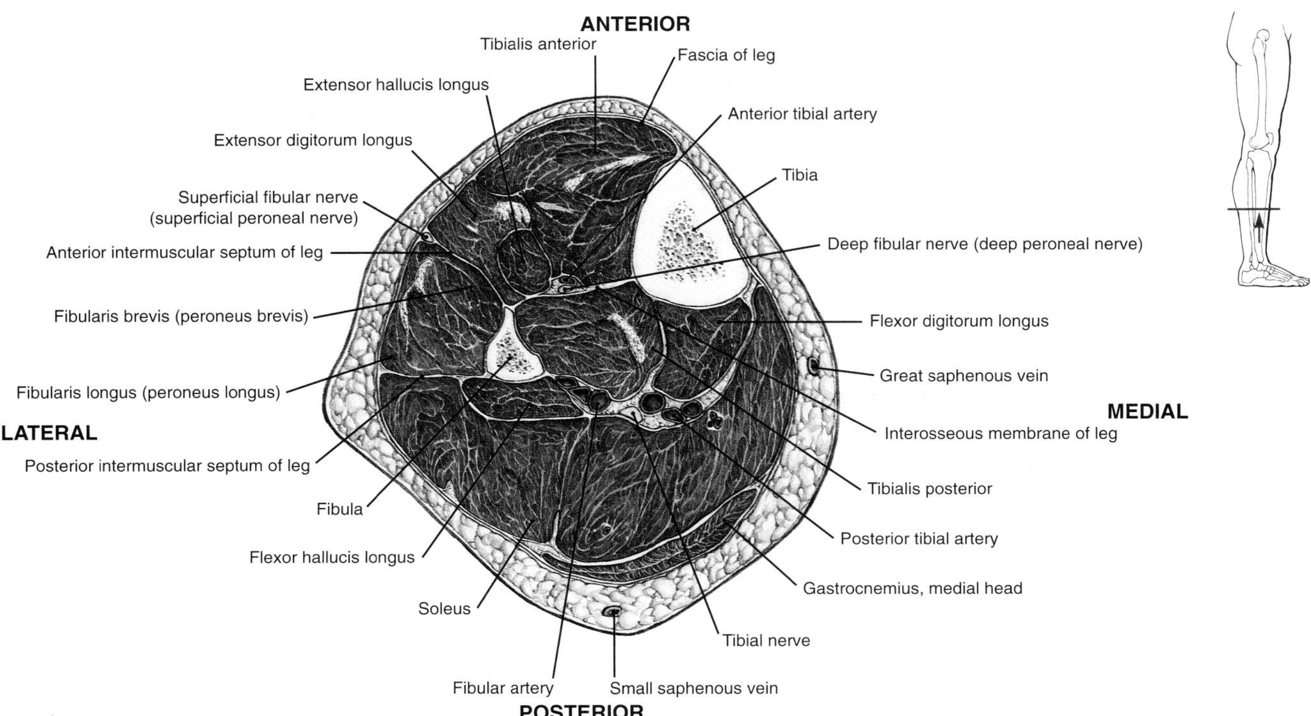
ANTERIOR
Tibialis anterior
Fascia of leg
Extensor hallucis longus
Anterior tibial artery
Extensor digitorum longus
Tibia
Superficial fibular nerve
(superficial peroneal nerve)
Anterior intermuscular septum of leg
Deep fibular nerve (deep peroneal nerve)
Fibularis brevis (peroneus brevis)
Flexor digitorum longus
Great saphenous vein
Fibularis longus (peroneus longus)
MEDIAL
LATERAL
Interosseous membrane of leg
Posterior intermuscular septum of leg
Tibialis posterior
Fibula
Posterior tibial artery
Flexor hallucis longus
Gastrocnemius, medial head
Soleus
Tibial nerve
Fibular artery
Small saphenous vein
POSTERIOR

Figure 463.1 Cross Section through the Middle of the Right Leg

NOTE: (1) The tibia, fibula, and interosseous membrane (that interconnects the bones) and the intermuscular septa divide the leg into **anterior, lateral,** and **posterior compartments.**

(2) The **tibialis anterior, extensor hallucis longus, extensor digitorum longus, deep fibular nerve** (from the common fibular nerve), and **anterior tibial artery** are all located in the **anterior compartment.**

(3) The **fibularis longus, fibularis brevis** (peroneal longus and brevis), and **superficial fibular nerve** (from the common fibular nerve) that supply the two muscles are all located in the lateral compartment.

(4) The **posterior compartment** contains **superficial and deep parts.**

(5) The **superficial part** of the posterior compartment contains the **gastrocnemius muscle,** the **soleus muscle,** and the **tendon of the plantaris muscle** (this latter structure is not shown in this figure; see Fig. 416).

(6) The **deep part** of the posterior compartment contains the **flexor digitorum longus, tibialis posterior,** and **flexor hallucis longus** muscles.

(7) The **posterior tibial artery** (and **vein**), the **fibular artery** (a branch of the posterior tibial) and **vein,** and the **posterior tibial nerve** course in the plane between the superficial and deep posterior compartment structures.

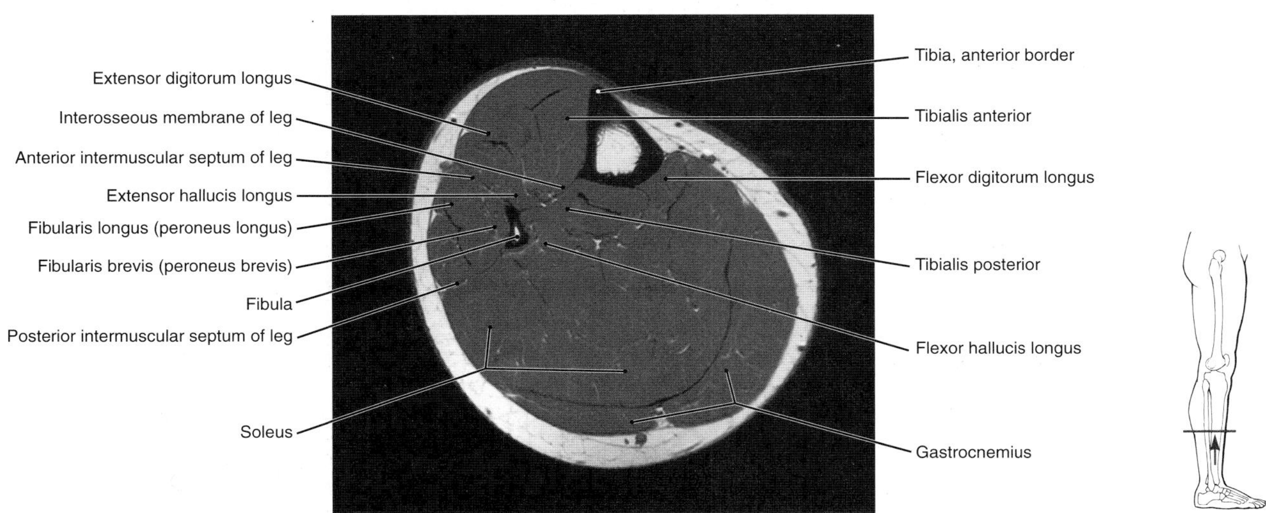
Extensor digitorum longus
Interosseous membrane of leg
Anterior intermuscular septum of leg
Extensor hallucis longus
Fibularis longus (peroneus longus)
Fibularis brevis (peroneus brevis)
Fibula
Posterior intermuscular septum of leg
Soleus
Tibia, anterior border
Tibialis anterior
Flexor digitorum longus
Tibialis posterior
Flexor hallucis longus
Gastrocnemius

Figure 463.2 MRI: Cross Section through the Middle of the Right Leg

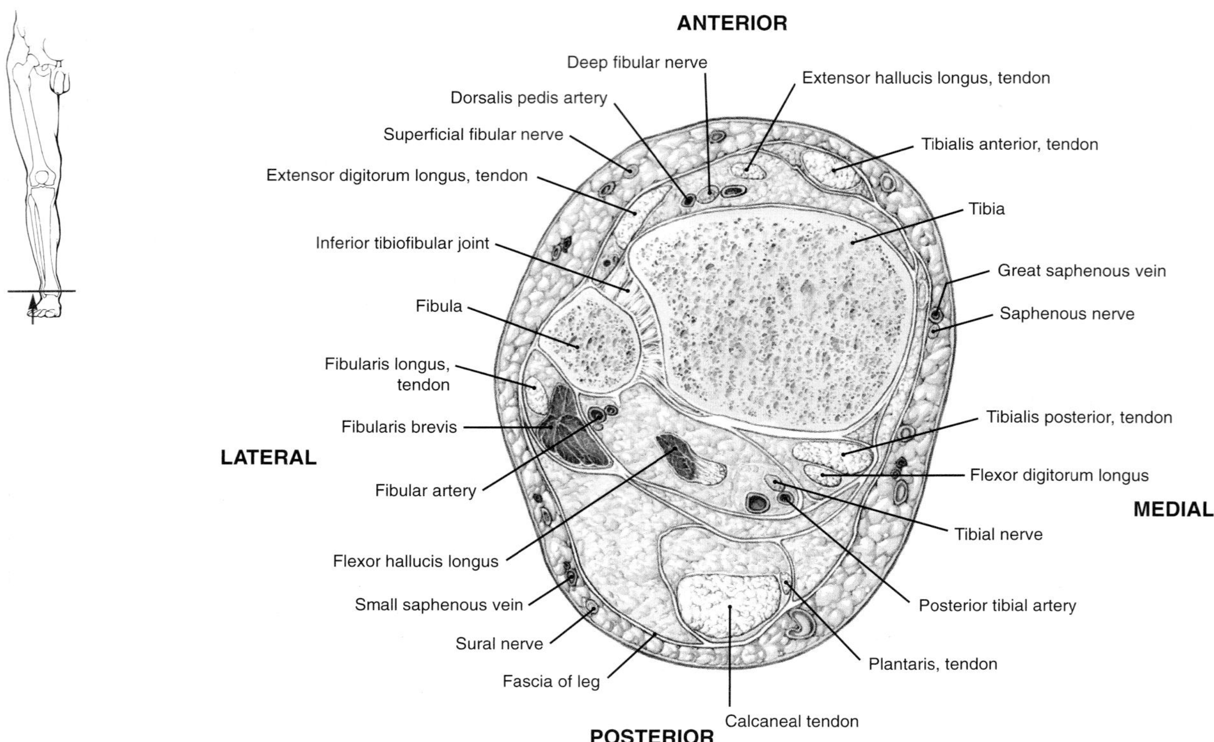
ANTERIOR
Deep fibular nerve
Dorsalis pedis artery
Superficial fibular nerve
Extensor digitorum longus, tendon
Inferior tibiofibular joint
Fibula
Fibularis longus, tendon
Fibularis brevis
LATERAL
Fibular artery
Flexor hallucis longus
Small saphenous vein
Sural nerve
Fascia of leg
POSTERIOR
Calcaneal tendon
Plantaris, tendon
Posterior tibial artery
Tibial nerve
MEDIAL
Flexor digitorum longus
Tibialis posterior, tendon
Saphenous nerve
Great saphenous vein
Tibia
Tibialis anterior, tendon
Extensor hallucis longus, tendon

Figure 464.1 Cross Section through the Right Leg Just Proximal to the Malleoli

NOTE: (1) The **anterior compartment** tendons, the superficial and deep fibular nerves, and the dorsalis pedis artery anterior to the tibia.

(2) The fibula, tendon of the fibularis longus, and the fibularis brevis muscle in the **lateral compartment.**

(3) The flexor hallucis longus, tendons of the tibialis posterior and flexor digitorum longus, the tibial nerve, the posterior tibial artery and its branch, and the fibular artery are all in the **deep part** of the **posterior compartment.**

(4) The calcaneal tendon and the small tendon of the plantaris muscle in the superficial part of the posterior compartment.

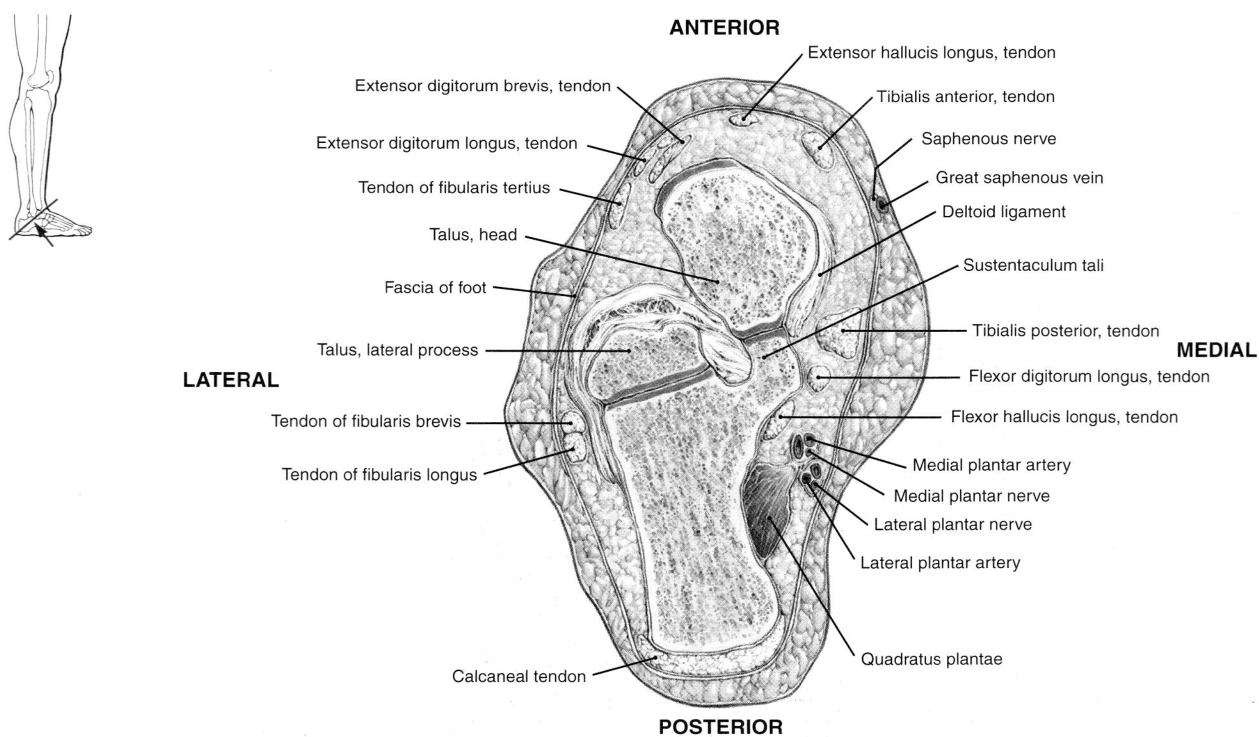
ANTERIOR
Extensor hallucis longus, tendon
Extensor digitorum brevis, tendon
Tibialis anterior, tendon
Extensor digitorum longus, tendon
Saphenous nerve
Great saphenous vein
Tendon of fibularis tertius
Deltoid ligament
Talus, head
Sustentaculum tali
Fascia of foot
Tibialis posterior, tendon
Talus, lateral process
MEDIAL
LATERAL
Flexor digitorum longus, tendon
Tendon of fibularis brevis
Flexor hallucis longus, tendon
Tendon of fibularis longus
Medial plantar artery
Medial plantar nerve
Lateral plantar nerve
Lateral plantar artery
Quadratus plantae
Calcaneal tendon
POSTERIOR

Figure 464.2 Oblique Section through the Calcaneus and Talus of the Right Foot

NOTE: The sustentaculum tali deep to the talus and the tendons of the leg descending anterior, lateral, and medial to the bony structures.

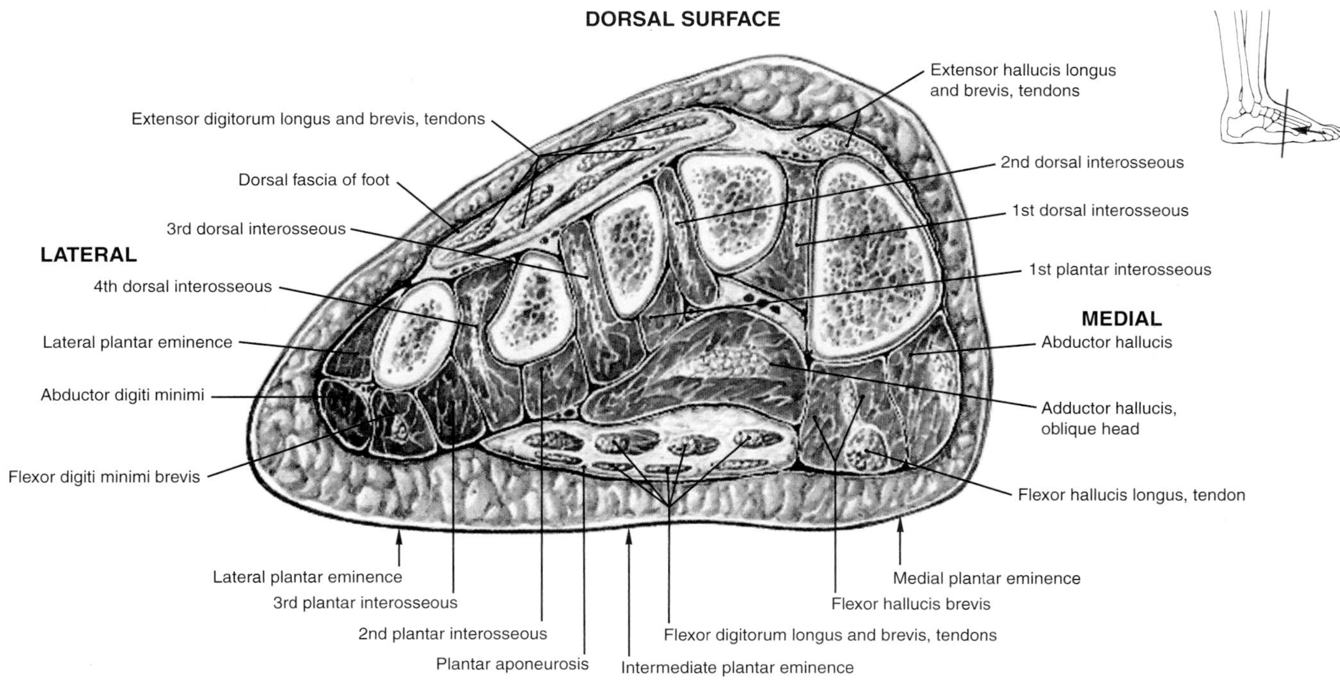
DORSAL SURFACE
Extensor hallucis longus and brevis, tendons
Extensor digitorum longus and brevis, tendons
2nd dorsal interosseous
Dorsal fascia of foot
1st dorsal interosseous
3rd dorsal interosseous
LATERAL
1st plantar interosseous
4th dorsal interosseous
MEDIAL
Abductor hallucis
Lateral plantar eminence
Abductor digiti minimi
Adductor hallucis, oblique head
Flexor digiti minimi brevis
Flexor hallucis longus, tendon
Lateral plantar eminence
Medial plantar eminence
3rd plantar interosseous
Flexor hallucis brevis
2nd plantar interosseous
Flexor digitorum longus and brevis, tendons
Plantar aponeurosis
Intermediate plantar eminence
PLANTAR SURFACE

Figure 465.1 Frontal Section through the Metatarsal Bones of the Right Foot

NOTE: (1) Compare this figure with Figure 465.2, and identify the metatarsal bones and the plantar and dorsal interosseous muscles.

(2) The abductor hallucis, flexor hallucis brevis, and tendon of the flexor hallucis longus on the medial side of plantar aspect of the foot.

(3) The tendons of the extensor digitorum longus and brevis muscles on the dorsum of the foot.

(4) The plantar aponeurosis and the tendons of the flexors digitorum longus and brevis on the plantar aspect of the foot; just dorsal to these is located the adductor hallucis.

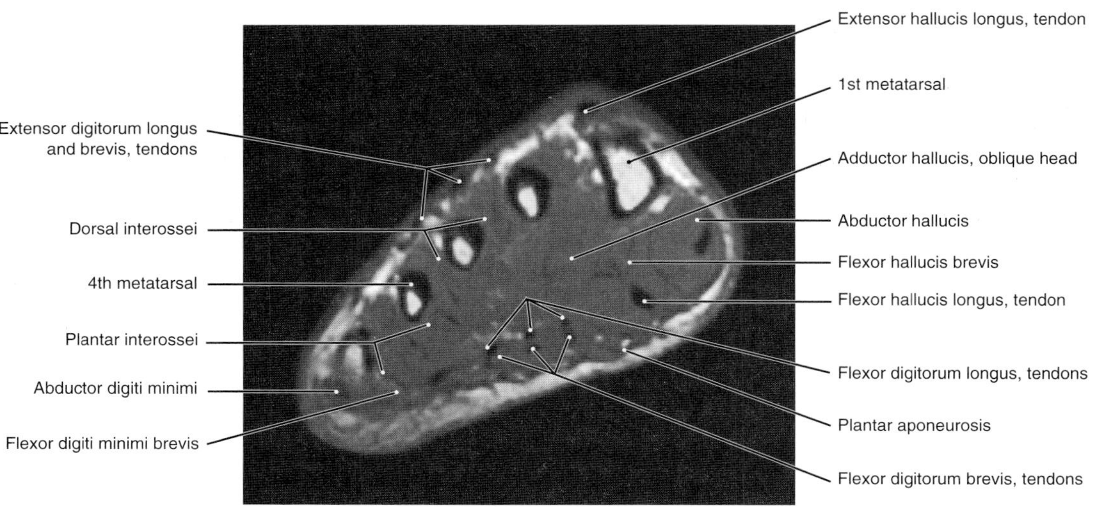
Extensor hallucis longus, tendon
1st metatarsal
Extensor digitorum longus and brevis, tendons
Adductor hallucis, oblique head
Abductor hallucis
Dorsal interossei
Flexor hallucis brevis
4th metatarsal
Flexor hallucis longus, tendon
Plantar interossei
Flexor digitorum longus, tendons
Abductor digiti minimi
Plantar aponeurosis
Flexor digiti minimi brevis
Flexor digitorum brevis, tendons

Figure 465.2 MRI through the Metatarsal Bones of the Right Foot

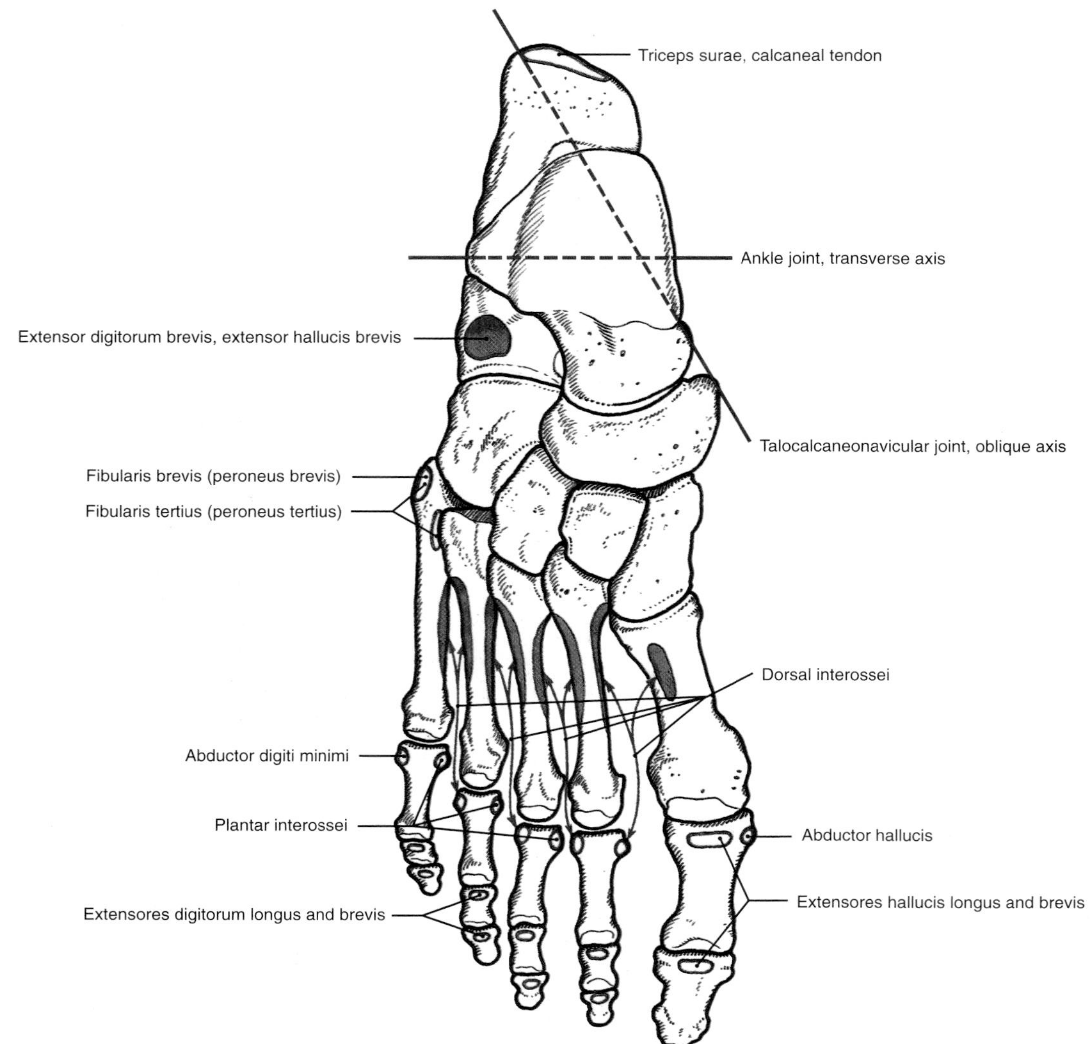
Triceps surae, calcaneal tendon
Ankle joint, transverse axis
Extensor digitorum brevis, extensor hallucis brevis
Talocalcaneonavicular joint, oblique axis
Fibularis brevis (peroneus brevis)
Fibularis tertius (peroneus tertius)
Dorsal interossei
Abductor digiti minimi
Plantar interossei
Abductor hallucis
Extensores hallucis longus and brevis
Extensores digitorum longus and brevis

Figure 466.1 Muscle Origins and Insertions Shown on the Bones of the Right Foot
NOTE: The origins are shown as solid red areas and the insertions as uncolored (circled areas).

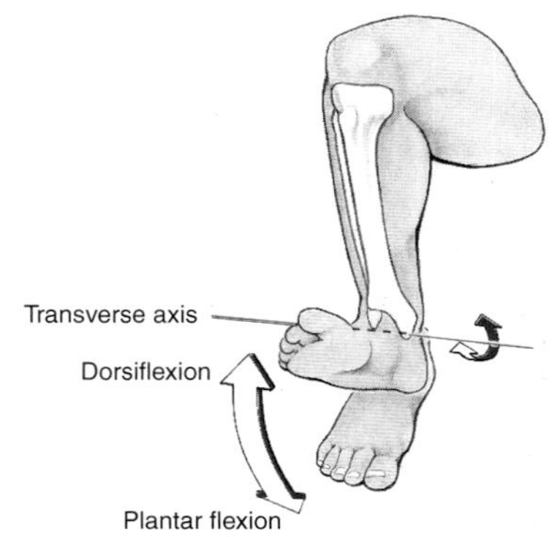
Transverse axis
Dorsiflexion
Plantar flexion

Figure 466.2 Movements of the Foot through the Transverse Axis of the Ankle (Talocrural) Joint
NOTE: These actions occur at the joint between the calcaneus and the tibia and fibula.

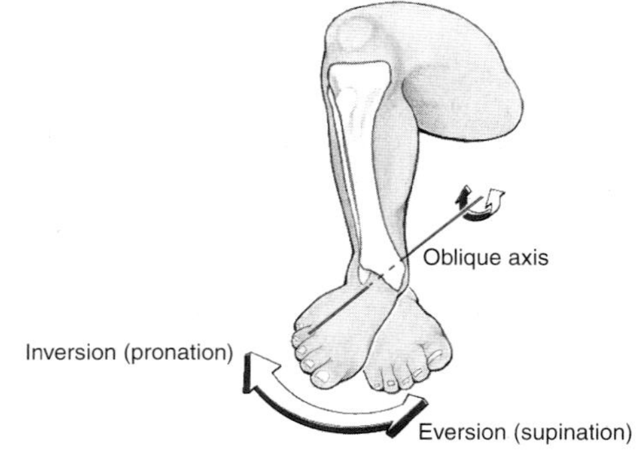
Oblique axis
Inversion (pronation)
Eversion (supination)

Figure 466.3 Movements of the Foot along the Oblique Axis
NOTE: The greater part of inversion and eversion occur at the subtalar joint.

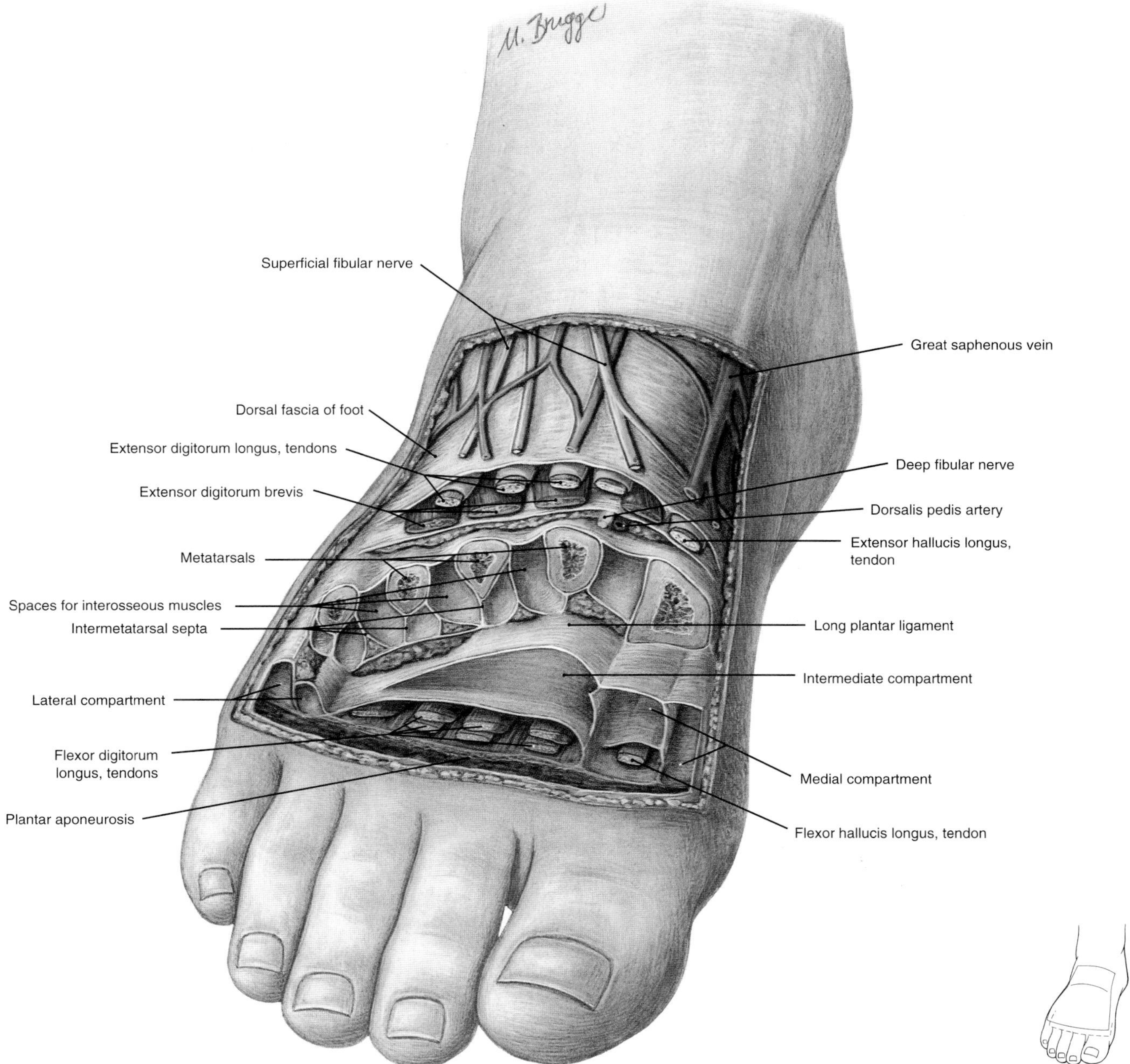
Superficial fibular nerve
Great saphenous vein
Dorsal fascia of foot
Extensor digitorum longus, tendons
Deep fibular nerve
Extensor digitorum brevis
Dorsalis pedis artery
Extensor hallucis longus, tendon
Metatarsals
Spaces for interosseous muscles
Intermetatarsal septa
Long plantar ligament
Intermediate compartment
Lateral compartment
Flexor digitorum longus, tendons
Medial compartment
Plantar aponeurosis
Flexor hallucis longus, tendon

Figure 467 Compartments of the Foot Shown by a Frontal Section at the Midmetatarsal Level

NOTE COMPARTMENTS SEQUENTIALLY FROM DORSAL TO PLANTAR SIDES:

(1) The superficial fibular nerve and superficial veins at the subcutaneous level on the foot dorsum.

(2) The extensor digitorum longus and extensor hallucis longus tendons and the bellies of the **extensor** digitorum brevis muscle of the foot dorsum. On the plantar aspect of these, observe the deep fibular nerve and dorsalis pedis artery.

(3) The metatarsal bones and the spaces for the dorsal and plantar interosseous muscles.

(4) On the plantar aspect of the metatarsal bones and interosseous muscles are the lateral, intermediate, and medial compartments that contain the intrinsic muscles on the plantar aspect of the foot (see Fig. 424).

The muscles of the **medial compartment** include the abductor hallucis, and the flexor hallucis brevis, and just deep to these is the tendon of the flexor hallucis longus muscle.

The muscles of the **intermediate compartment** include the transverse and oblique heads of the adductor hallucis, and just on the plantar aspect of these are the quadratus plantae muscle, the tendons of the flexor digitorum longus muscle and the lumbrical muscles.

The muscles of the **lateral compartment** are the opponens, flexor, and abductor digiti minimi muscles.

THE NECK AND HEAD

7

PLATES

• THE CRANIAL NERVES •

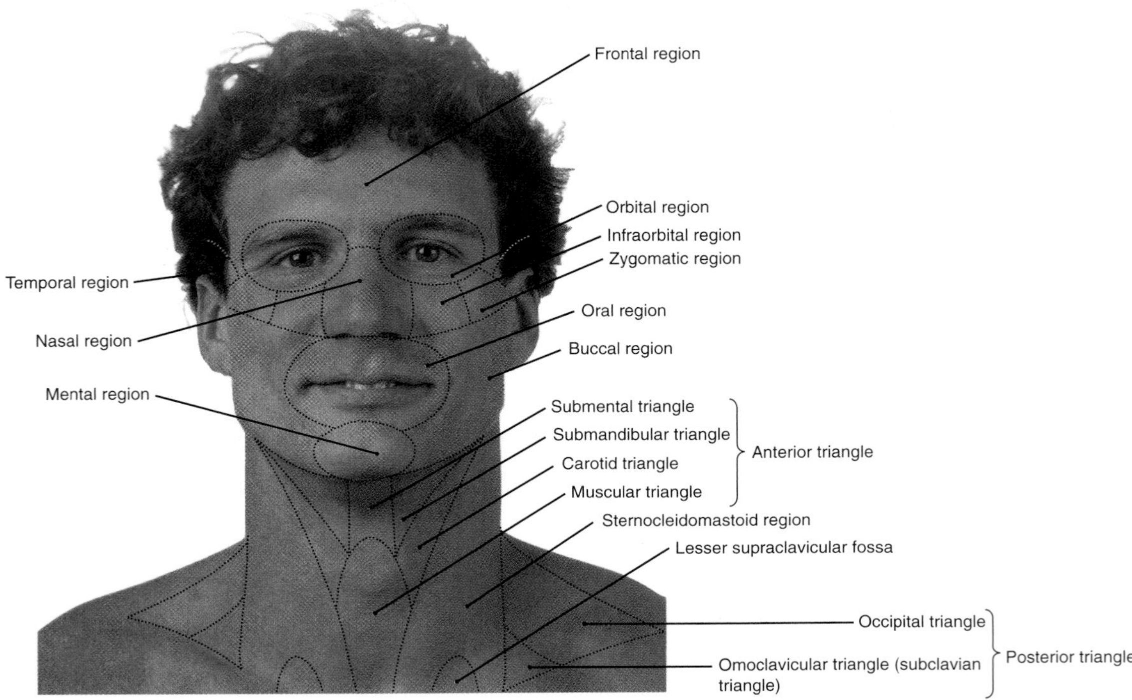
Frontal region
Orbital region
Infraorbital region
Zygomatic region
Temporal region
Nasal region
Oral region
Buccal region
Mental region
Submental triangle
Submandibular triangle
Carotid triangle
Muscular triangle
Anterior triangle
Sternocleidomastoid region
Lesser supraclavicular fossa
Occipital triangle
Omoclavicular triangle (subclavian triangle)
Posterior triangle

Figure 468.1 **Regions of the Head and Neck (Anterior Aspect)**

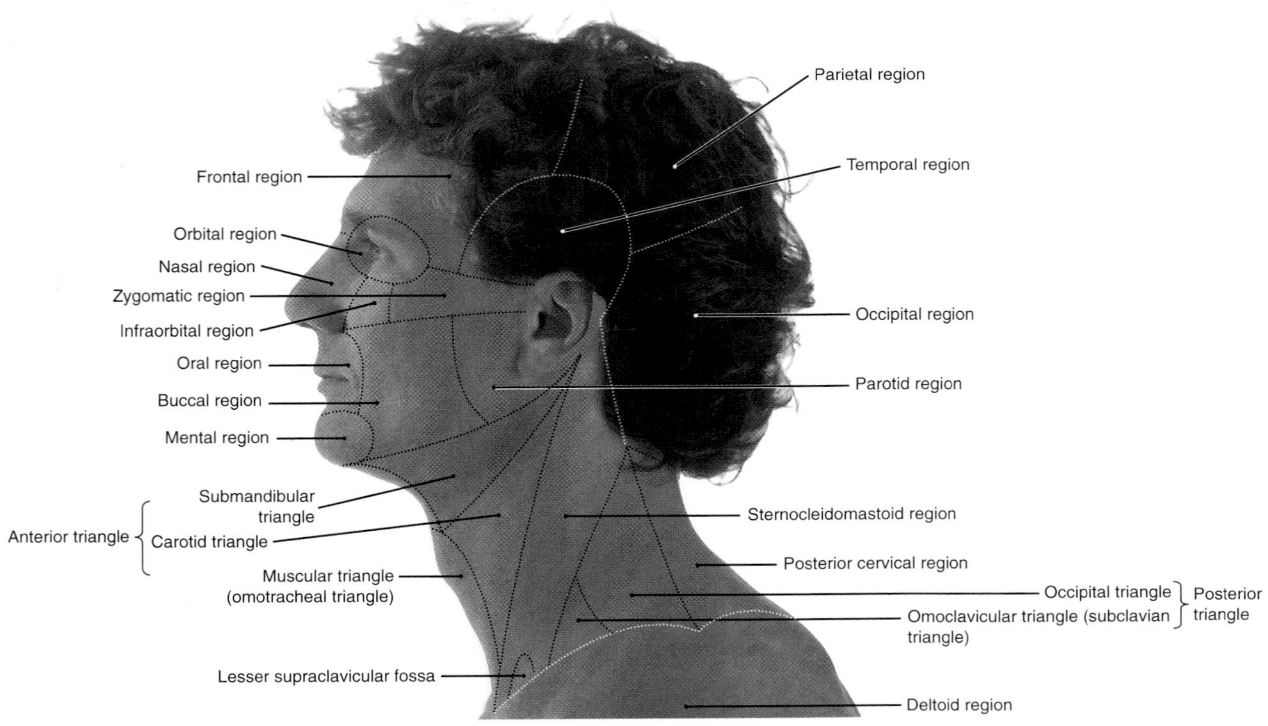
Parietal region
Frontal region
Temporal region
Orbital region
Nasal region
Zygomatic region
Infraorbital region
Occipital region
Oral region
Parotid region
Buccal region
Mental region
Submandibular triangle
Anterior triangle
Carotid triangle
Sternocleidomastoid region
Posterior cervical region
Muscular triangle (omotracheal triangle)
Occipital triangle
Omoclavicular triangle (subclavian triangle)
Posterior triangle
Lesser supraclavicular fossa
Deltoid region

Figure 468.2 **Regions of the Head and Neck (Lateral Aspect)**

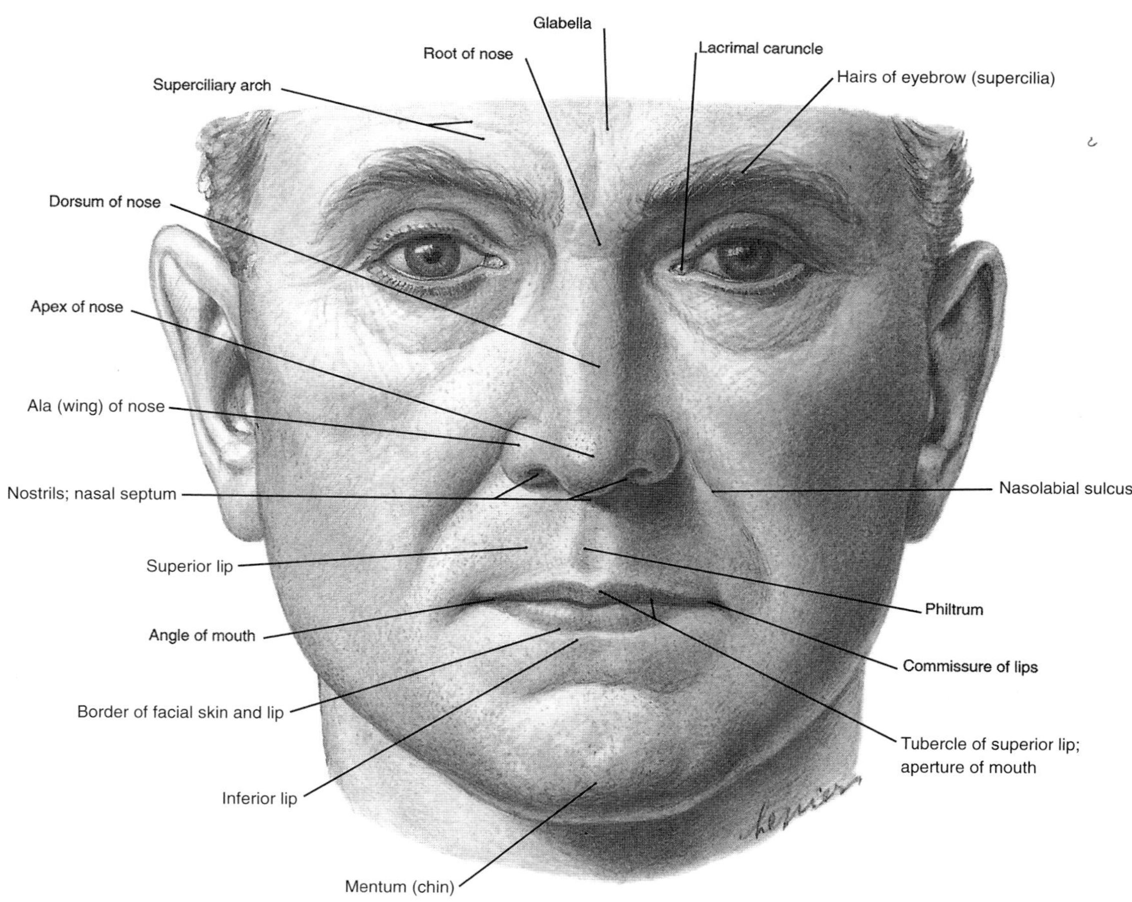
Glabella
Root of nose
Lacrimal caruncle
Hairs of eyebrow (supercilia)
Superciliary arch
Dorsum of nose
Apex of nose
Ala (wing) of nose
Nostrils; nasal septum
Nasolabial sulcus
Superior lip
Philtrum
Angle of mouth
Commissure of lips
Border of facial skin and lip
Tubercle of superior lip;
aperture of mouth
Inferior lip
Mentum (chin)

Figure 469.1 **Surface Features of the Anterior Face**

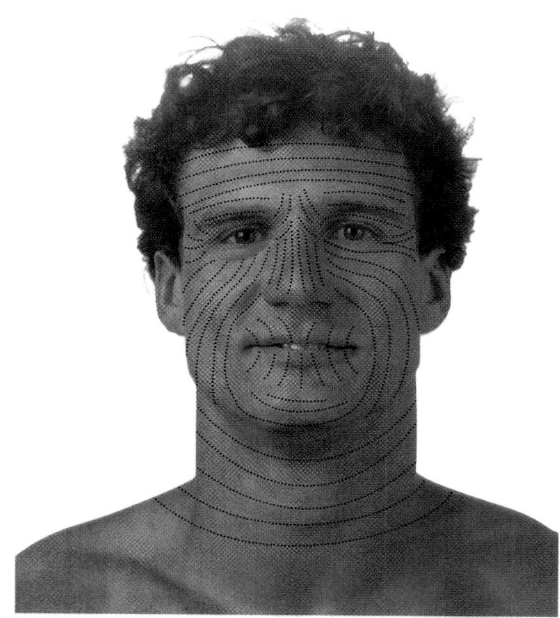

Figure 469.2 **Tension Lines of the Skin of the Head and Neck (Anterior Aspect)**

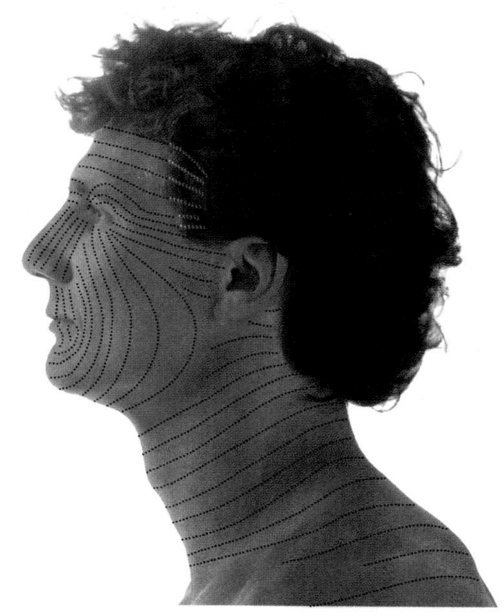

Figure 469.3 **Tension Lines of the Skin of the Head and Neck (Lateral Aspect)**

NOTE: For optimal healing, incision lines in the skin should be made along the lines of tension (Langer's lines).

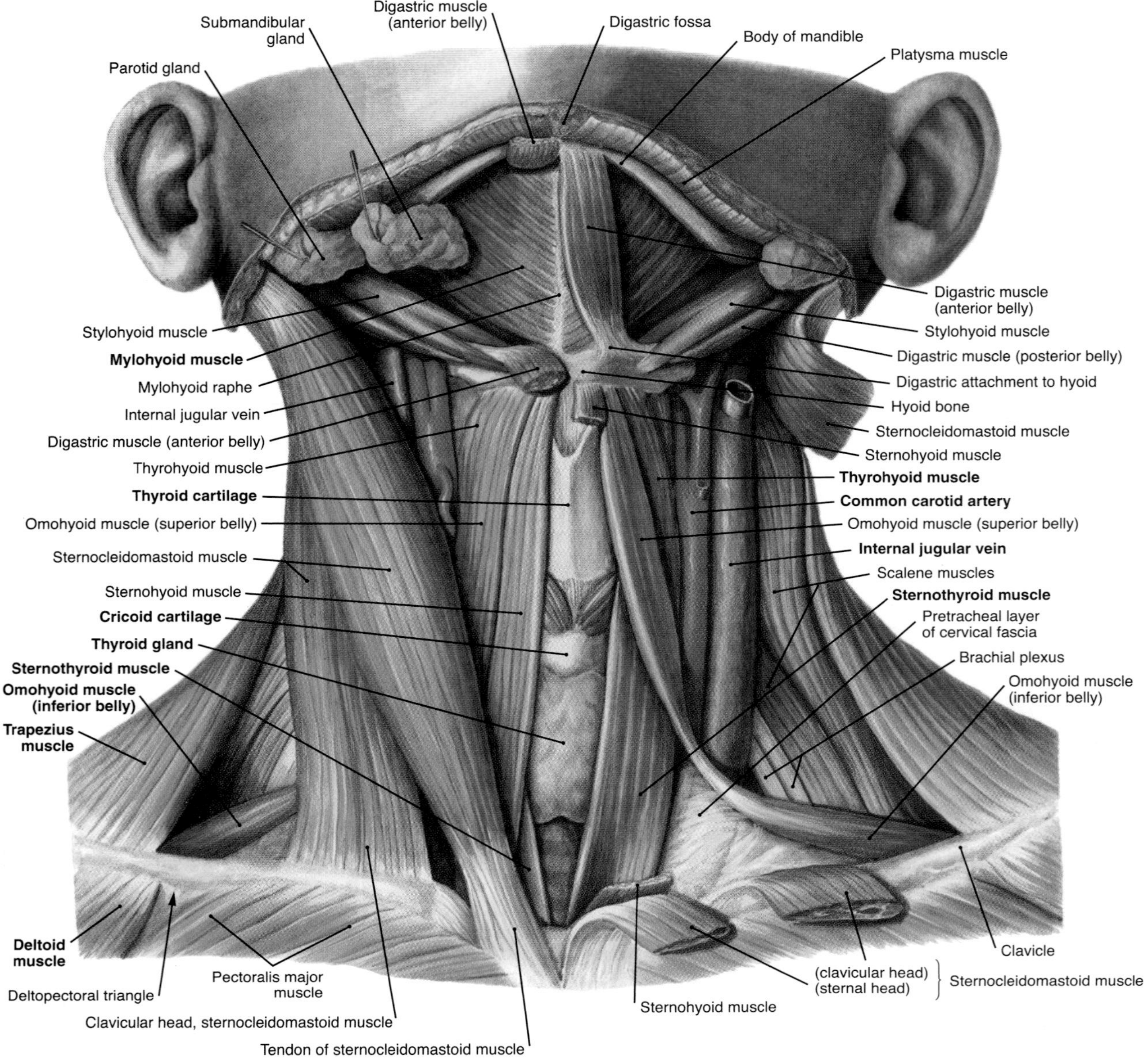

Submandibular gland
Digastric muscle (anterior belly)
Digastric fossa
Body of mandible
Platysma muscle
Parotid gland
Stylohyoid muscle
Mylohyoid muscle
Mylohyoid raphe
Internal jugular vein
Digastric muscle (anterior belly)
Thyrohyoid muscle
Thyroid cartilage
Omohyoid muscle (superior belly)
Sternocleidomastoid muscle
Sternohyoid muscle
Cricoid cartilage
Thyroid gland
Sternothyroid muscle
Omohyoid muscle (inferior belly)
Trapezius muscle
Digastric muscle (anterior belly)
Stylohyoid muscle
Digastric muscle (posterior belly)
Digastric attachment to hyoid
Hyoid bone
Sternocleidomastoid muscle
Sternohyoid muscle
Thyrohyoid muscle
Common carotid artery
Omohyoid muscle (superior belly)
Internal jugular vein
Scalene muscles
Sternothyroid muscle
Pretracheal layer of cervical fascia
Brachial plexus
Omohyoid muscle (inferior belly)
Deltoid muscle
Deltopectoral triangle
Pectoralis major muscle
Clavicular head, sternocleidomastoid muscle
Tendon of sternocleidomastoid muscle
Sternohyoid muscle
(clavicular head)
(sternal head)
Sternocleidomastoid muscle
Clavicle

Figure 470: **Anterior View of the Musculature of the Neck**

NOTE: (1) The right superior belly of the digastric muscle was removed and the submandibular gland elevated to show the mylohyoid muscle. On the left side (reader's right), the sternocleidomastoid and sternohyoid muscles have been transected and the submandibular gland removed.

(2) Observe the relationship of the strap muscles to the thyroid gland and realize that below the thyroid gland and above the suprasternal notch, the trachea lies immediately under the skin.

INFRAHYOID MUSCLES OF THE NECK

Muscle	Origin	Insertion	Innervation	Action
Sternohyoid	Manubrium of sternum and the medial end of the clavicle	Body of hyoid bone	Ansa cervicalis (C1, C2, C3)	Depresses the hyoid bone after food is swallowed
Sternothyroid	Posterior surface of the manubrium of the sternum	Oblique line on the lamina of the thyroid cartilage	Ansa cervicalis (C1, C2, C3)	Depresses the hyoid bone and the larynx
Thyrohyoid	Oblique line on the lamina of the thyroid cartilage	Lower border of the greater horn of the hyoid bone	Fibers from the C1 spinal nerve that course for a short distance with the hypoglossal nerve XII	Depresses the hyoid bone or elevates the larynx
Omohyoid	Upper border of the scapula near the suprascapular notch	Lower border of the body of the hyoid bone	Ansa cervicalis (C1, C2, C3)	Depresses and helps stabilize the hyoid bone

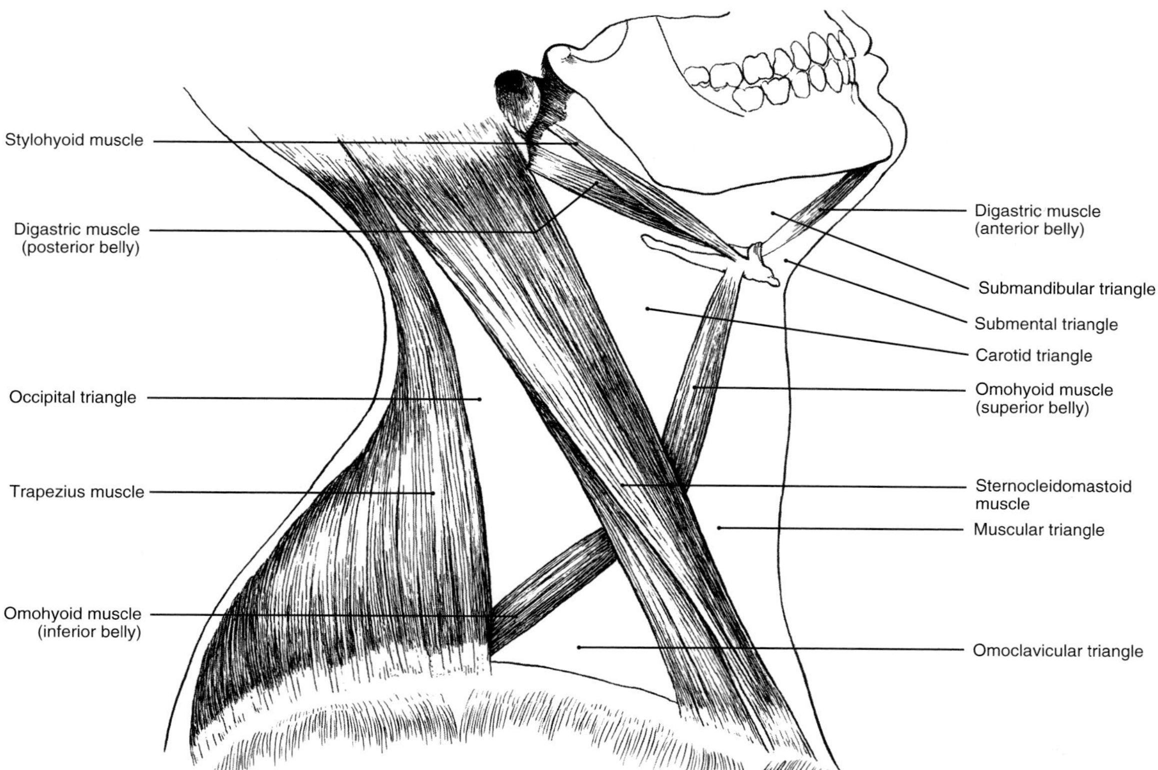
Stylohyoid muscle
Digastric muscle (posterior belly)
Occipital triangle
Trapezius muscle
Omohyoid muscle (inferior belly)
Digastric muscle (anterior belly)
Submandibular triangle
Submental triangle
Carotid triangle
Omohyoid muscle (superior belly)
Sternocleidomastoid muscle
Muscular triangle
Omoclavicular triangle

Figure 471.1 Triangles of the Neck (Lateral View)

NOTE: The triangles of the neck are useful in describing the location of cervical organs and other structures. The entire area anterior to the sternocleidomastoid muscle is called the **anterior triangle,** while the area posterior to this muscle is the **posterior triangle.**

Muscle	Origin	Insertion	Innervation	Action
Sternocleido-mastoid	**Sternal head:** Upper part of the ventral surface of the manubrium of the sternum. **Clavicular head:** Upper border and anterior surface of the medial third of the clavicle	Lateral surface of the mastoid process and the lateral half of the superior nuchal line	Motor fibers: Accessory nerve. Sensory fibers: Anterior rami of C2 and C3 nerves.	When one side acts: Bends the head laterally toward the shoulder of the same side; rotates the head, turning the face upward, directing it to the opposite side. When both sides act: Flexes the head and neck

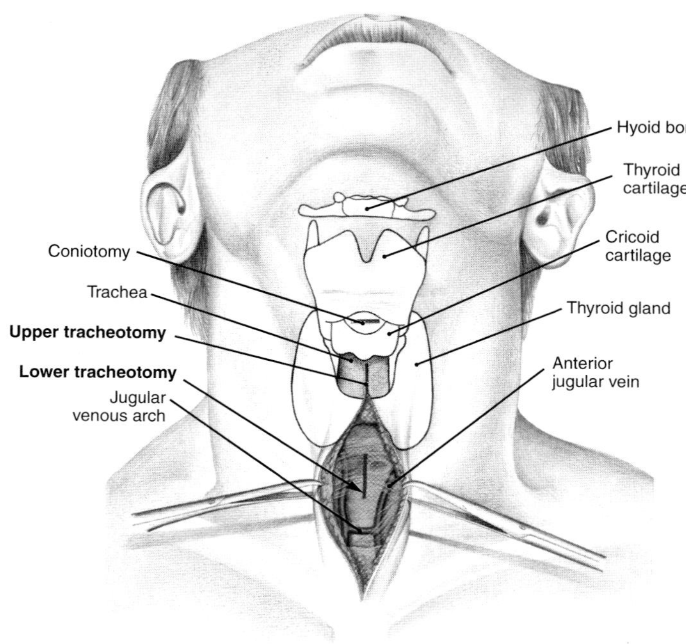
Hyoid bone
Thyroid cartilage
Cricoid cartilage
Thyroid gland
Anterior jugular vein
Coniotomy
Trachea
Upper tracheotomy
Lower tracheotomy
Jugular venous arch

Figure 471.2 Projection of Larynx and Trachea Showing Sites for Entry into the Respiratory Pathway

NOTE: (1) The hyoid bone, laryngeal cartilages (thyroid and cricoid), thyroid gland, and tracheal region of the anterior neck are projected to the surface, as are three sites where entrance into the respiratory tract may be achieved readily (in red).

(2) The upper transverse incision cuts through the cricothyroid ligament and conus elasticus and can be called a **cricothyrotomy** or **coniotomy,** while the **upper tracheotomy** and **lower tracheotomy** can be made in the trachea above or below the thyroid gland.

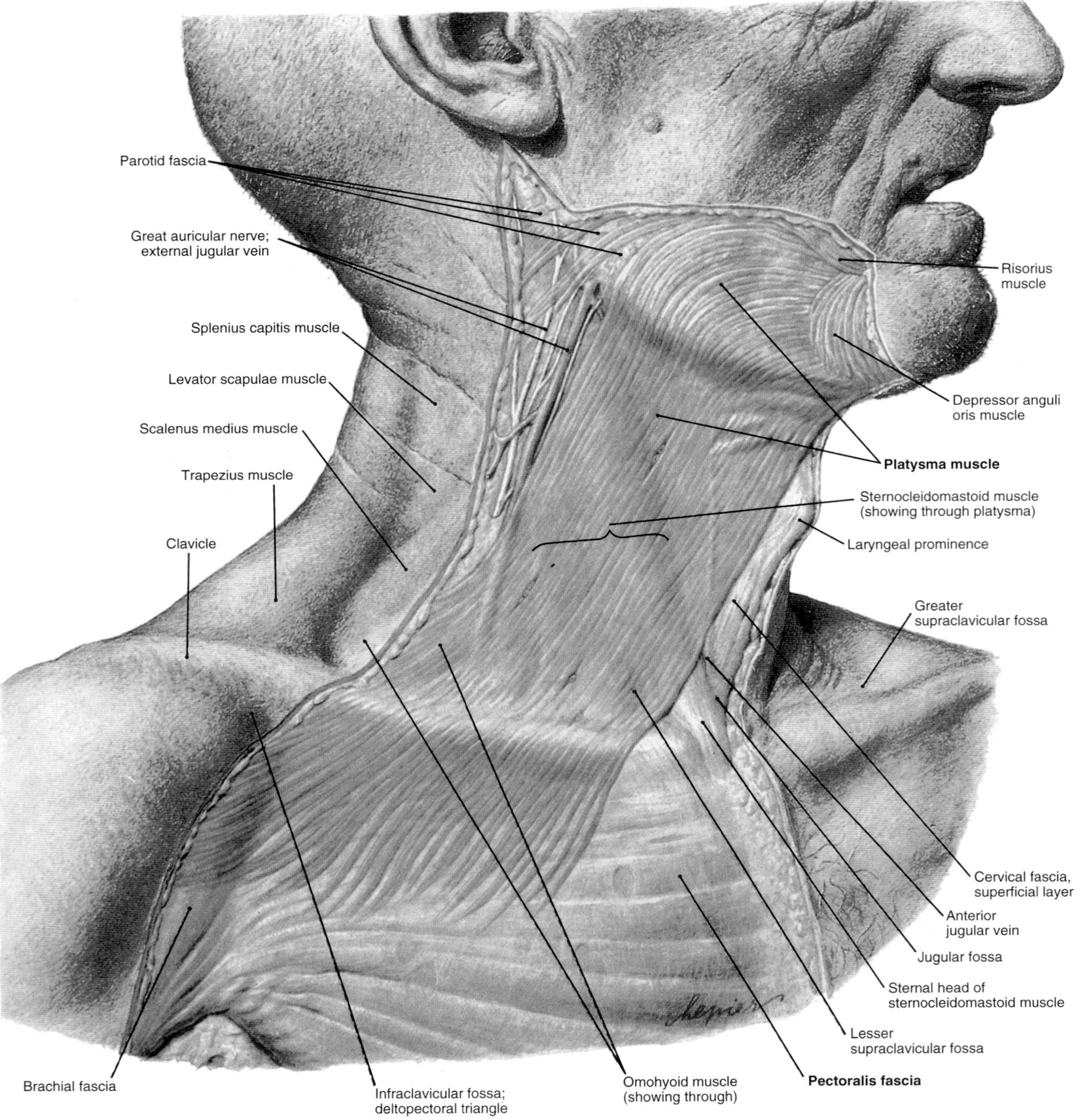
Parotid fascia
Great auricular nerve; external jugular vein
Splenius capitis muscle
Levator scapulae muscle
Scalenus medius muscle
Trapezius muscle
Clavicle
Risorius muscle
Depressor anguli oris muscle
Platysma muscle
Sternocleidomastoid muscle (showing through platysma)
Laryngeal prominence
Greater supraclavicular fossa
Cervical fascia, superficial layer
Anterior jugular vein
Jugular fossa
Sternal head of sternocleidomastoid muscle
Lesser supraclavicular fossa
Pectoralis fascia
Brachial fascia
Infraclavicular fossa; deltopectoral triangle
Omohyoid muscle (showing through)

Figure 472 **Right Platysma Muscle and Pectoral Fascia**

NOTE: (1) The **platysma muscle** is a broad, thin quadrangular muscle located in the superficial fascia; it extends from the angle of the mouth and chin downward across the clavicle to the upper part of the thorax and anterior shoulder.

(2) The platysma is considered one of the muscles of facial expression, many of which do not attach to bony structures, but arise and insert within the superficial fascia.

(3) Upon concentration, the platysma tends to depress the angle of the mouth and wrinkle the skin of the neck, thereby participating in the formation of facial expressions of anxiety, sadness, dissatisfaction, and suffering.

(4) Similar to other muscles of facial expression, the platysma is innervated by the **facial nerve** (**cervical branch**), the 7th cranial nerve (VII).

(5) Overlying the pectoralis major is the well-developed pectoralis fascia, which extends from the midline in the thorax laterally to the axilla. Observe the external jugular vein and great auricular nerve exposed in the upper lateral aspect of the neck.

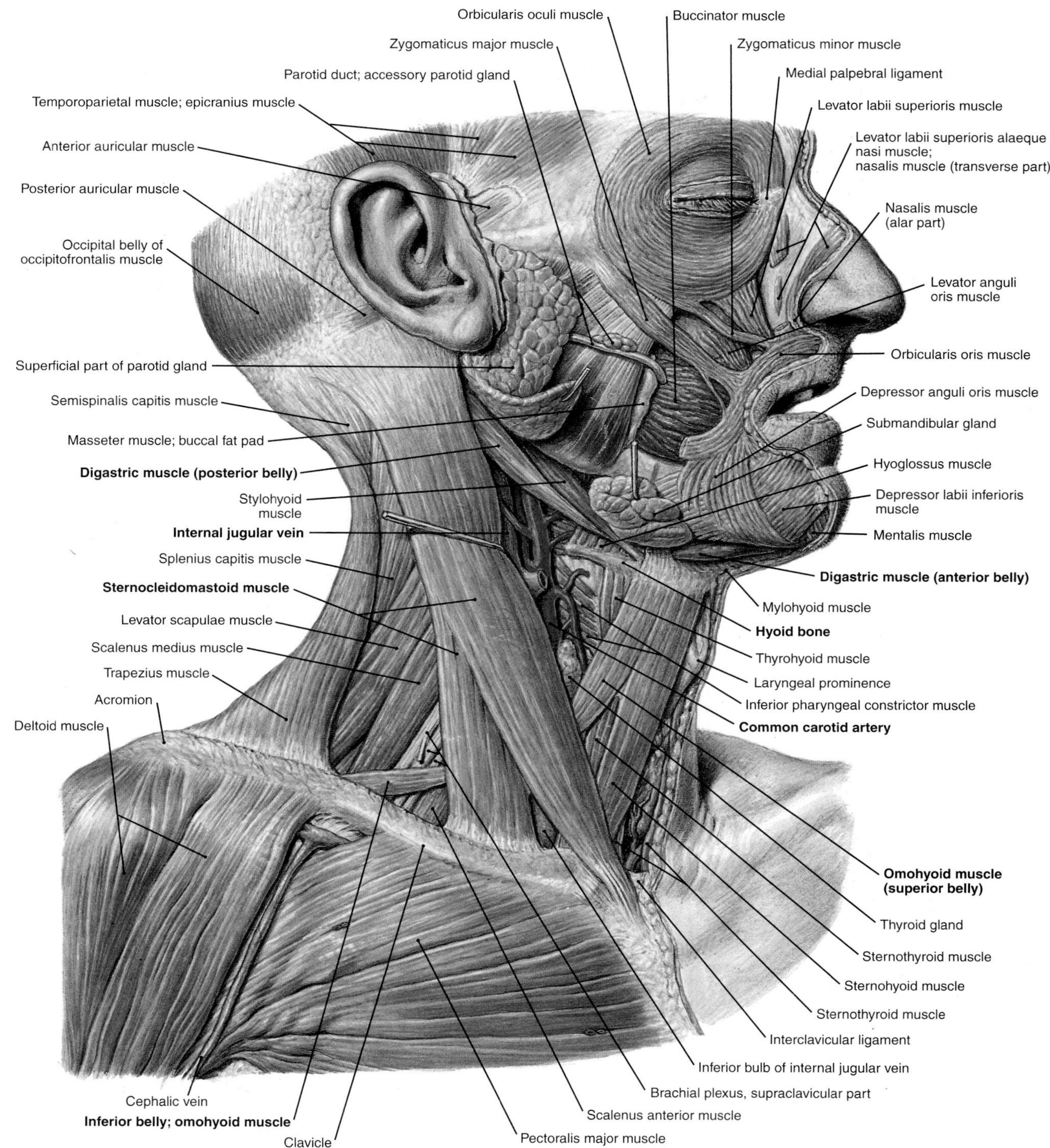
Orbicularis oculi muscle
Buccinator muscle
Zygomaticus major muscle
Zygomaticus minor muscle
Parotid duct; accessory parotid gland
Medial palpebral ligament
Temporoparietal muscle; epicranius muscle
Levator labii superioris muscle
Anterior auricular muscle
Levator labii superioris alaeque nasi muscle; nasalis muscle (transverse part)
Posterior auricular muscle
Nasalis muscle (alar part)
Occipital belly of occipitofrontalis muscle
Levator anguli oris muscle
Superficial part of parotid gland
Orbicularis oris muscle
Semispinalis capitis muscle
Depressor anguli oris muscle
Masseter muscle; buccal fat pad
Submandibular gland
Digastric muscle (posterior belly)
Hyoglossus muscle
Stylohyoid muscle
Depressor labii inferioris muscle
Internal jugular vein
Mentalis muscle
Splenius capitis muscle
Digastric muscle (anterior belly)
Sternocleidomastoid muscle
Mylohyoid muscle
Levator scapulae muscle
Hyoid bone
Scalenus medius muscle
Thyrohyoid muscle
Trapezius muscle
Laryngeal prominence
Acromion
Inferior pharyngeal constrictor muscle
Deltoid muscle
Common carotid artery
Omohyoid muscle (superior belly)
Thyroid gland
Sternothyroid muscle
Sternohyoid muscle
Sternothyroid muscle
Interclavicular ligament
Inferior bulb of internal jugular vein
Brachial plexus, supraclavicular part
Cephalic vein
Scalenus anterior muscle
Inferior belly; omohyoid muscle
Clavicle
Pectoralis major muscle

Figure 473 Anterior and Posterior Triangles of the Neck

NOTE: (1) The **anterior triangle** of the neck is bounded by the midline of the neck, the anterior border of the sternocleidomastoid muscle and the mandible. This area is further subdivided by the superior belly of the omohyoid muscle and the two bellies of the digastric into:

(a) **Muscular triangle** (midline, superior belly of omohyoid, and sternocleidomastoid).
(b) **Carotid triangle** (superior belly of omohyoid, sternocleidomastoid muscle, and posterior belly of digastric).
(c) **Submandibular triangle** (anterior and posterior bellies of digastric, and the inferior margin of the mandible).
(d) **Submental triangle** (midline, anterior belly of digastric, and hyoid bone).

(2) The **posterior triangle** of the neck is bounded by the posterior border of the sternocleidomastoid muscle, the trapezius, and the clavicle. This area is further subdivided into the **occipital triangle** above and the **omoclavicular triangle** below by the inferior belly of the omohyoid.

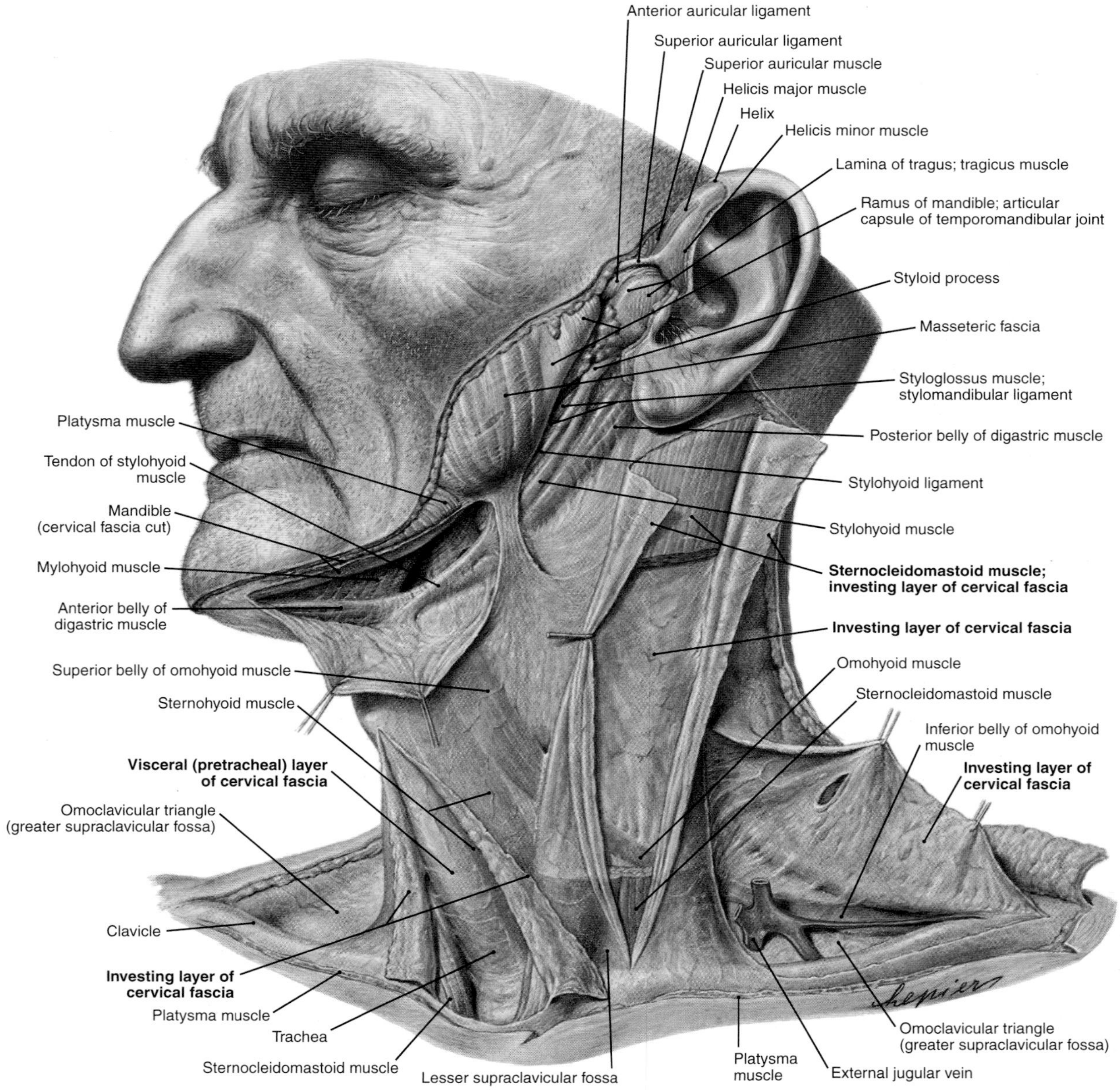

Anterior auricular ligament
Superior auricular ligament
Superior auricular muscle
Helicis major muscle
Helix
Helicis minor muscle
Lamina of tragus; tragicus muscle
Ramus of mandible; articular capsule of temporomandibular joint
Styloid process
Masseteric fascia
Styloglossus muscle; stylomandibular ligament
Posterior belly of digastric muscle
Stylohyoid ligament
Stylohyoid muscle
Sternocleidomastoid muscle; investing layer of cervical fascia
Investing layer of cervical fascia
Omohyoid muscle
Sternocleidomastoid muscle
Inferior belly of omohyoid muscle
Investing layer of cervical fascia
Platysma muscle
Tendon of stylohyoid muscle
Mandible (cervical fascia cut)
Mylohyoid muscle
Anterior belly of digastric muscle
Superior belly of omohyoid muscle
Sternohyoid muscle
Visceral (pretracheal) layer of cervical fascia
Omoclavicular triangle (greater supraclavicular fossa)
Clavicle
Investing layer of cervical fascia
Platysma muscle
Trachea
Sternocleidomastoid muscle
Lesser supraclavicular fossa
Platysma muscle
External jugular vein
Omoclavicular triangle (greater supraclavicular fossa)

Figure 474.1 External Investing and Pretracheal Fascial Layers of the Neck
NOTE: The **external investing layer** of deep fascia surrounds the sternocleidomastoid muscle, while the **pretracheal layer** of deep fascia is located deep to the investing layer and encloses the strap muscles.

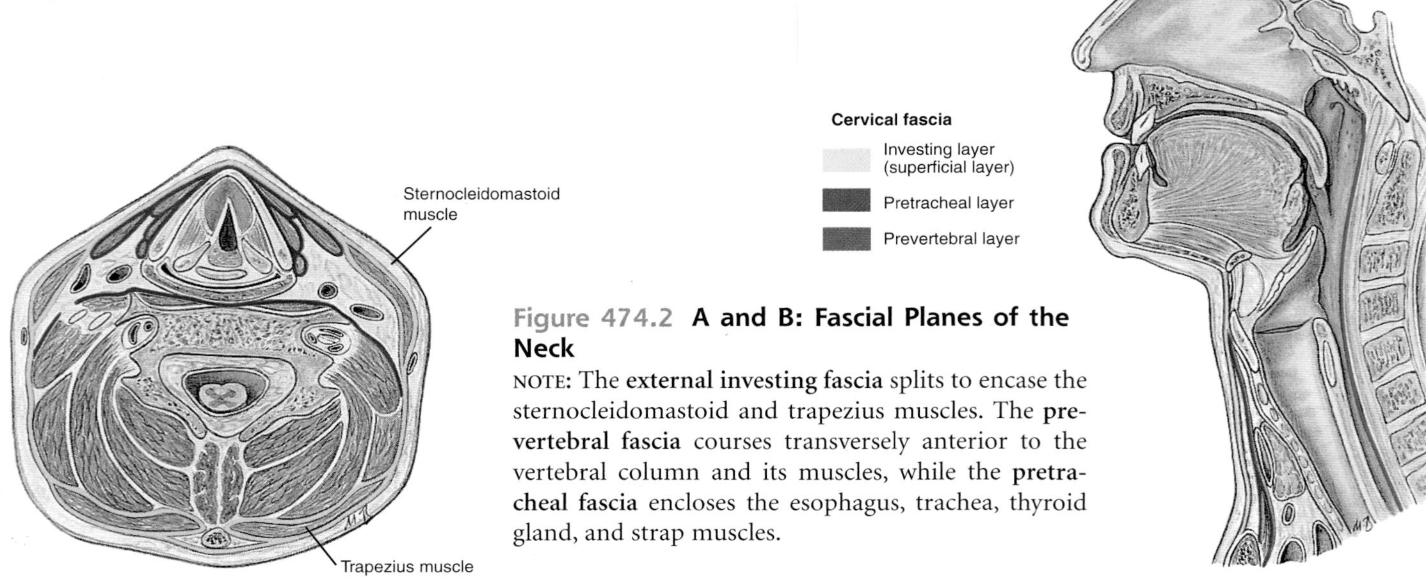
Cervical fascia
Investing layer (superficial layer)
Pretracheal layer
Prevertebral layer
Sternocleidomastoid muscle
Trapezius muscle
A Transverse section
B Median section

Figure 474.2 A and B: Fascial Planes of the Neck
NOTE: The **external investing fascia** splits to encase the sternocleidomastoid and trapezius muscles. The **prevertebral fascia** courses transversely anterior to the vertebral column and its muscles, while the **pretracheal fascia** encloses the esophagus, trachea, thyroid gland, and strap muscles.

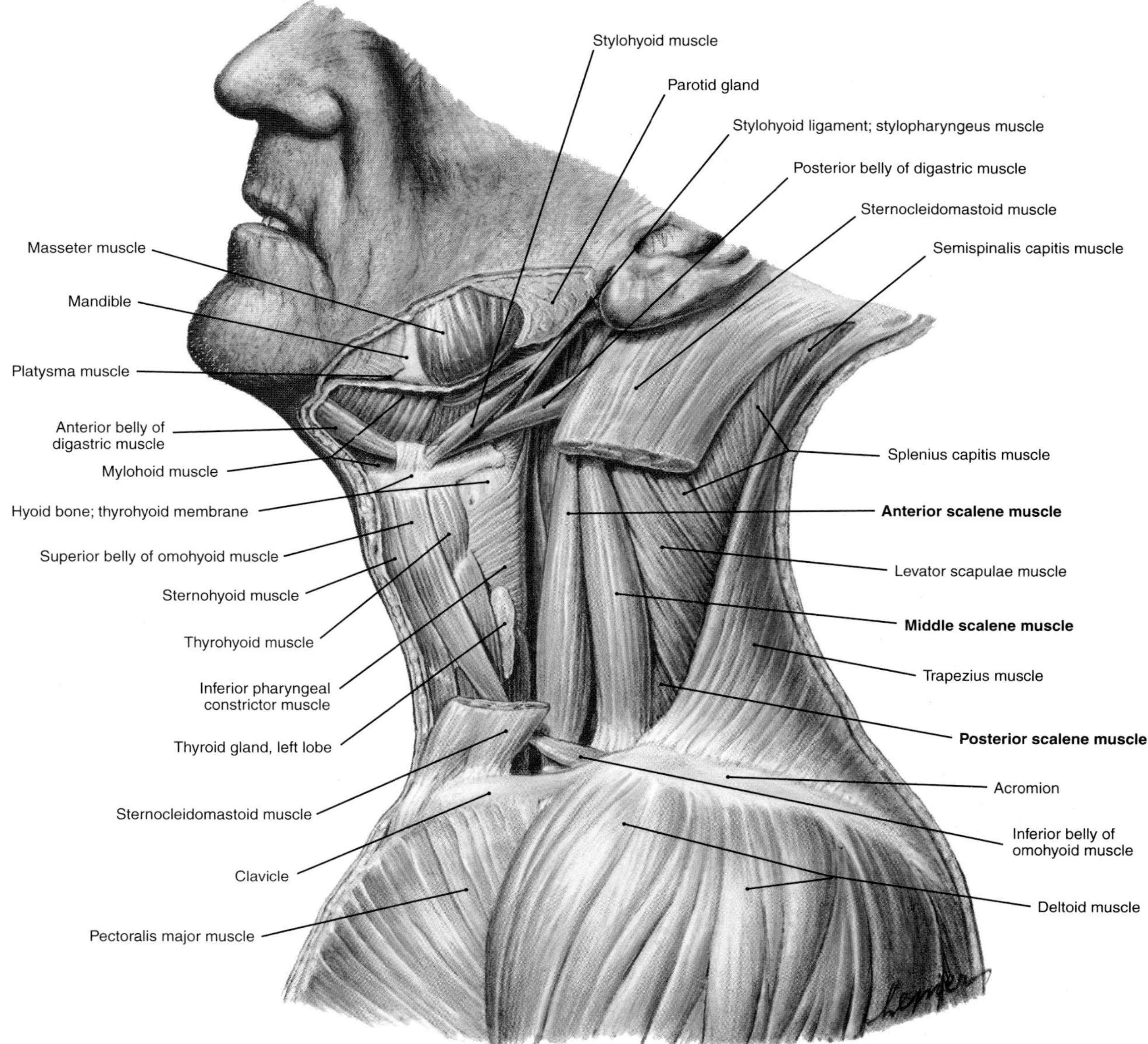
Stylohyoid muscle
Parotid gland
Stylohyoid ligament; stylopharyngeus muscle
Posterior belly of digastric muscle
Sternocleidomastoid muscle
Semispinalis capitis muscle
Masseter muscle
Mandible
Platysma muscle
Anterior belly of digastric muscle
Mylohoid muscle
Hyoid bone; thyrohyoid membrane
Superior belly of omohyoid muscle
Sternohyoid muscle
Thyrohyoid muscle
Inferior pharyngeal constrictor muscle
Thyroid gland, left lobe
Sternocleidomastoid muscle
Clavicle
Pectoralis major muscle
Splenius capitis muscle
Anterior scalene muscle
Levator scapulae muscle
Middle scalene muscle
Trapezius muscle
Posterior scalene muscle
Acromion
Inferior belly of omohyoid muscle
Deltoid muscle

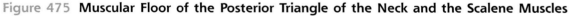

Figure 475 **Muscular Floor of the Posterior Triangle of the Neck and the Scalene Muscles**

MUSCLES OF THE POSTERIOR TRIANGLE OF THE NECK

LEVATOR SCAPULAE described on **Plate 334**
SEMISPINALIS CAPITIS described on **Plate 336**

Muscle	Origin	Insertion	Innervation	Action
Anterior scalene	By four tendons, each one from the transverse processes of the third, fourth, fifth, and sixth cervical vertebrae	Onto the scalene tubercle of the first rib	Anterior rami of the fourth, fifth, and sixth cervical spinal nerves	When neck is fixed: elevates the first rib. When first rib is fixed: Bends neck forward and laterally, and rotates it to the opposite side.
Middle scalene	Transverse processes of C2 to C7 vertebrae (often also from the atlas)	Superior surface of first rib between the tubercle and groove for subclavian artery	Anterior rami of the third through the eighth cervical nerves	Same as anterior scalene muscle
Posterior scalene	Transverse processes of fourth, fifth, and sixth cervical vertebrae	Outer surface of the second rib	Anterior rami of the C6, C7 and C8 spinal nerves	Raises the second rib; or, bends and rotates the neck
Splenius capitis	Caudal half of the ligamentum nuchae; spinous processes of C7, and upper 4 thoracic vertebrae	Lateral third of the superior nuchal line and onto the mastoid process of the temporal bone	Dorsal rami of the middle cervical spinal nerves	Laterally flexes head; rotates . head and neck to same side; when both muscles act they extend head and neck

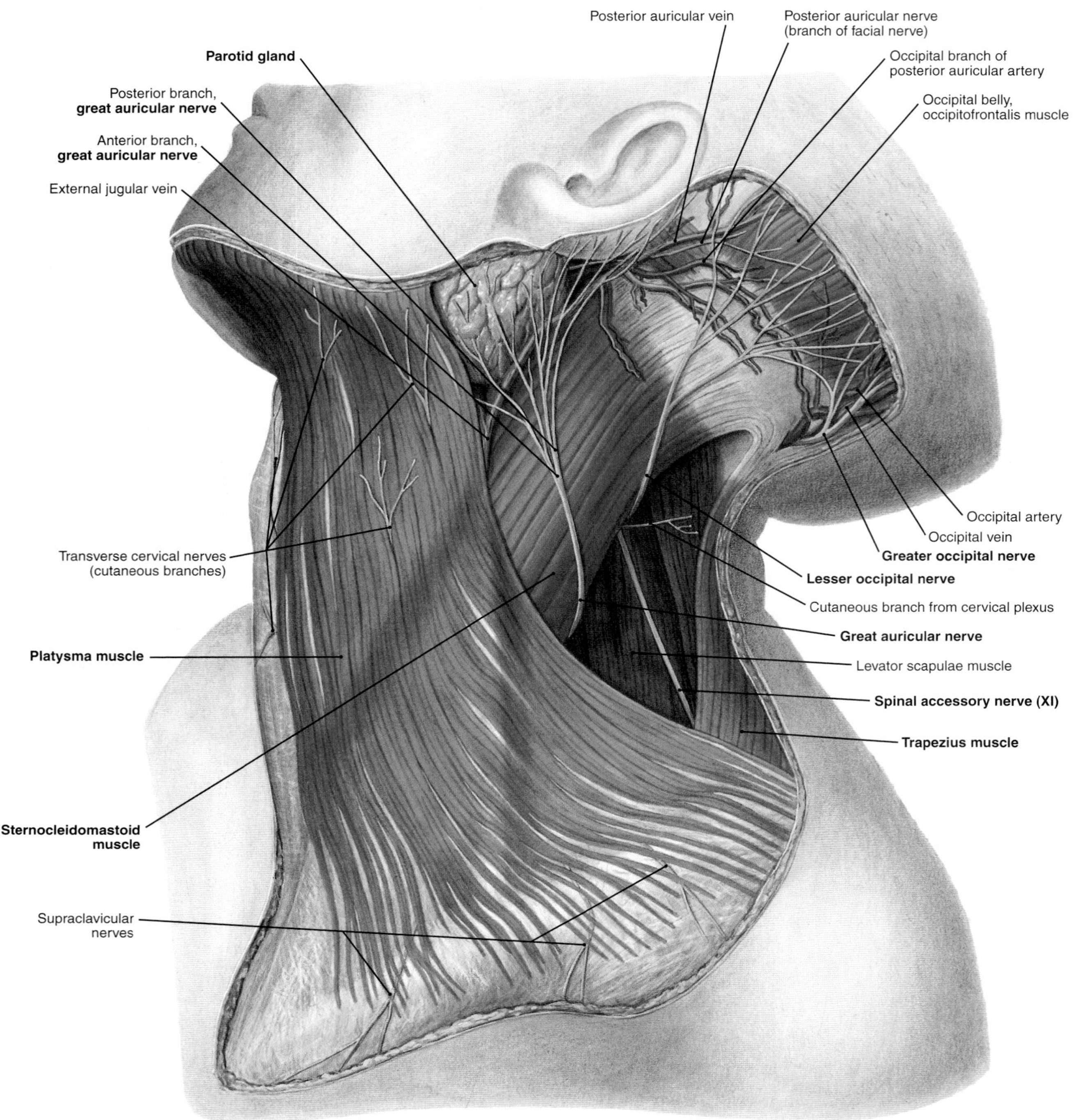

Posterior auricular vein
Posterior auricular nerve (branch of facial nerve)
Parotid gland
Occipital branch of posterior auricular artery
Posterior branch, great auricular nerve
Occipital belly, occipitofrontalis muscle
Anterior branch, great auricular nerve
External jugular vein
Occipital artery
Occipital vein
Greater occipital nerve
Transverse cervical nerves (cutaneous branches)
Lesser occipital nerve
Cutaneous branch from cervical plexus
Great auricular nerve
Platysma muscle
Levator scapulae muscle
Spinal accessory nerve (XI)
Trapezius muscle
Sternocleidomastoid muscle
Supraclavicular nerves

Figure 476 Nerves and Blood Vessels of the Neck, Stage 1: Platysma Layer

NOTE: (1) The skin has been removed from both the anterior and posterior triangle areas to reveal the platysma muscle. Observe the cutaneous branches of the **transverse cervical nerves,** derived from the cervical plexus and penetrating through the platysma and superficial fascia to reach the skin of the anterolateral aspect of the neck.

(2) Four other nerves: the **great auricular** (C2, C3); the **lesser occipital** (C2); the **greater occipital** (C2); and the **accessory** (XI).

(3) After it has supplied the sternocleidomastoid muscle, the accessory nerve (XI) descends in the posterior triangle to reach the trapezius muscle, which it also supplies.

(4) The **supraclavicular nerves.** These descend in the neck under cover of the deep fascia and platysma muscle. They become superficial just above the clavicle and then cross that bone at the medial, intermediate, and lateral supraclavicular nerves (see also, Fig. 477). They derive from the third and fourth cervical nerves, and supply skin over the clavicle, the upper trunk (down to the second rib), and the shoulder from the acromion laterally to the midline anteriorly.

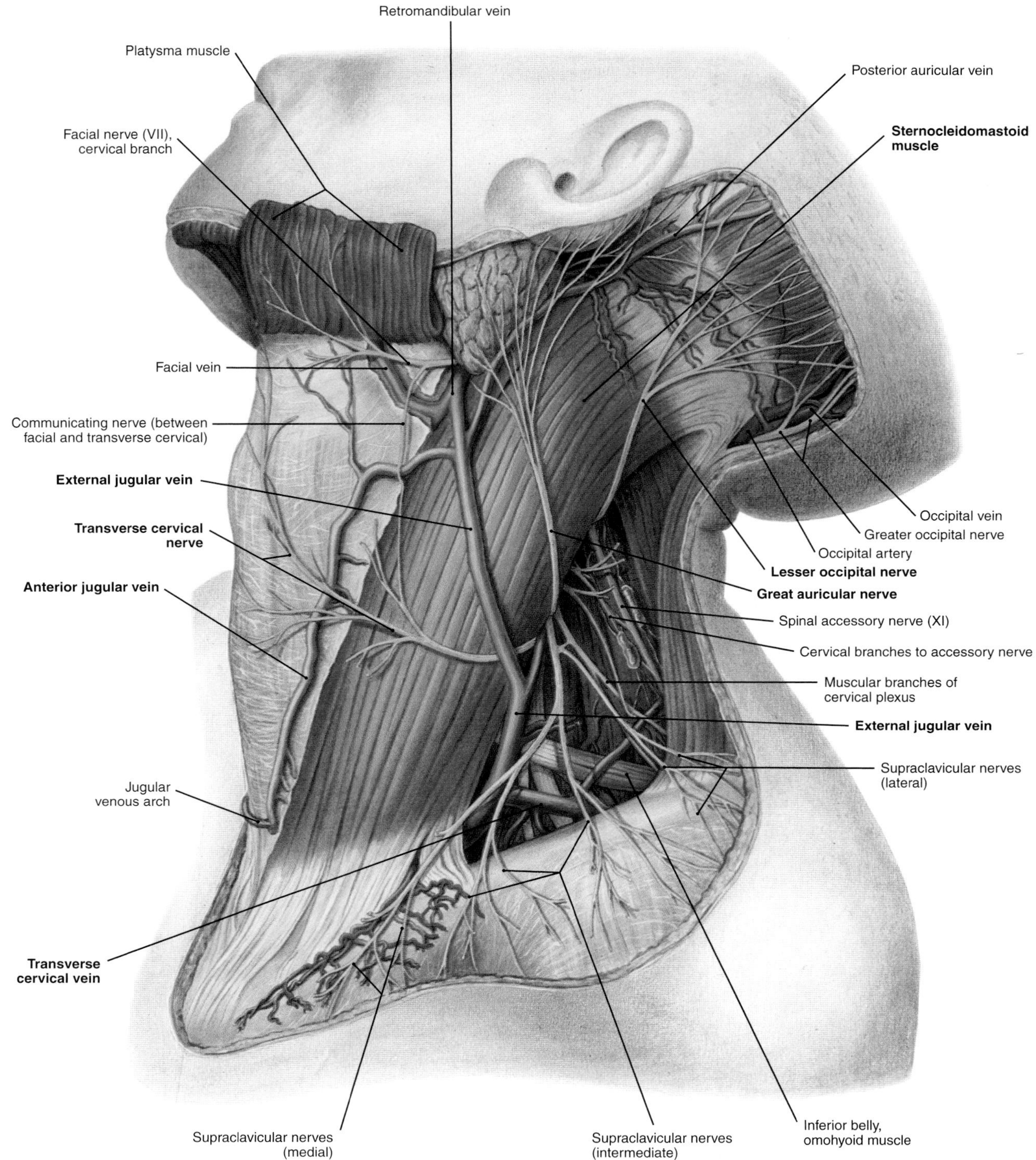
Retromandibular vein
Platysma muscle
Posterior auricular vein
Facial nerve (VII), cervical branch
Sternocleidomastoid muscle
Facial vein
Communicating nerve (between facial and transverse cervical)
External jugular vein
Transverse cervical nerve
Anterior jugular vein
Occipital vein
Greater occipital nerve
Occipital artery
Lesser occipital nerve
Great auricular nerve
Spinal accessory nerve (XI)
Cervical branches to accessory nerve
Muscular branches of cervical plexus
External jugular vein
Supraclavicular nerves (lateral)
Jugular venous arch
Transverse cervical vein
Supraclavicular nerves (medial)
Supraclavicular nerves (intermediate)
Inferior belly, omohyoid muscle

Figure 477 Nerves and Blood Vessels of the Neck, Stage 2: Sternocleidomastoid Layer

NOTE: (1) With the platysma muscle reflected upward, the full extent of the sternocleidomastoid muscle is exposed.

(2) The nerves of the cervical plexus diverge at the posterior border of the sternocleidomastoid muscle: the **great auricular** and **lesser occipital** ascend to the head, the **transverse cervical** (transverse colli) course across the neck, while the **supraclavicular nerves** descend over the clavicle.

(3) The **external jugular vein,** formed by the junction of the **retromandibular** and **posterior auricular veins.** The external jugular crosses the sternocleidomastoid muscle obliquely and receives tributaries from the anterior jugular, posterior external jugular (not shown), transverse cervical and suprascapular vein (not shown) before it ends in the subclavian vein.

(4) The cervical branch of the **facial (VII) nerve** supplying the inner surface of the platysma muscle with motor innervation.

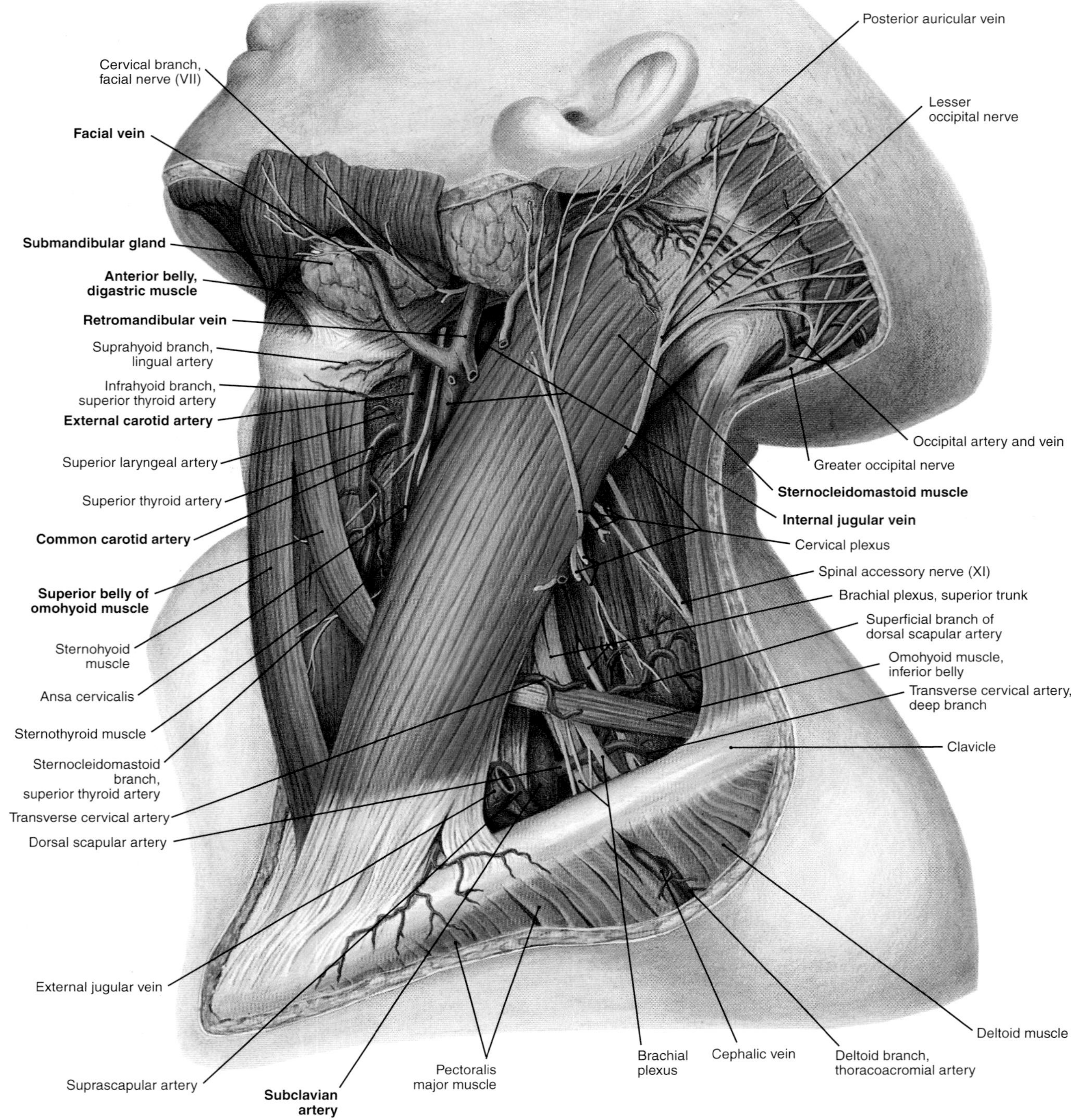
Cervical branch, facial nerve (VII)
Facial vein
Submandibular gland
Anterior belly, digastric muscle
Retromandibular vein
Suprahyoid branch, lingual artery
Infrahyoid branch, superior thyroid artery
External carotid artery
Superior laryngeal artery
Superior thyroid artery
Common carotid artery
Superior belly of omohyoid muscle
Sternohyoid muscle
Ansa cervicalis
Sternothyroid muscle
Sternocleidomastoid branch, superior thyroid artery
Transverse cervical artery
Dorsal scapular artery
External jugular vein
Suprascapular artery
Subclavian artery
Pectoralis major muscle
Brachial plexus
Cephalic vein
Deltoid branch, thoracoacromial artery
Deltoid muscle
Posterior auricular vein
Lesser occipital nerve
Occipital artery and vein
Greater occipital nerve
Sternocleidomastoid muscle
Internal jugular vein
Cervical plexus
Spinal accessory nerve (XI)
Brachial plexus, superior trunk
Superficial branch of dorsal scapular artery
Omohyoid muscle, inferior belly
Transverse cervical artery, deep branch
Clavicle

Figure 478 Nerves and Blood Vessels of the Neck, Stage 3: The Anterior Triangle

NOTE: (1) With the investing layer of fascia removed, the outlines of the muscular, carotid, and submandibular triangles within the anterior region of the neck are revealed.

(2) The infrahyoid (strap) muscles, which cover the thyroid gland and the lateral aspect of the larynx in the **muscular triangle.** This is bounded by the sternocleidomastoid, the midline, and the superior belly of the digastric muscle.

(3) The carotid vessels and internal jugular vein can be seen in the **carotid triangle,** which is bounded by the superior belly of the omohyoid, posterior belly of the digastric (not labeled), and the sternocleidomastoid.

(4) With the platysma muscle cut and reflected upward, the submandibular gland is seen in the **submandibular triangle,** between the anterior and posterior bellies of the digastric and the inferior border of the mandible.

(5) The spinal accessory nerve descending in the posterior triangle from beneath the sternocleidomastoid, which it supplies, to reach the trapezius muscle (not labeled), which it also supplies with motor innervation.

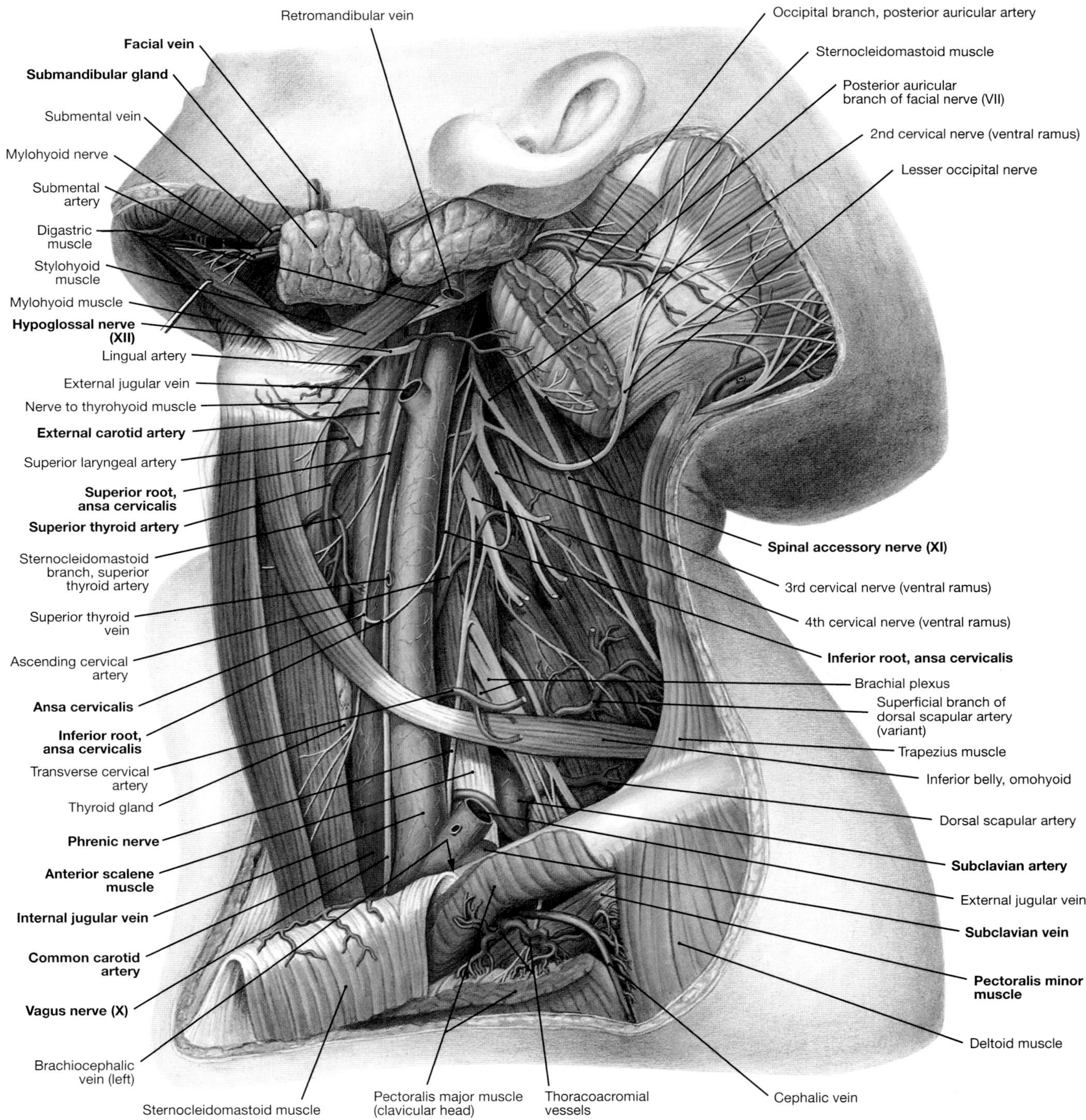
Retromandibular vein
Facial vein
Submandibular gland
Submental vein
Mylohyoid nerve
Submental artery
Digastric muscle
Stylohyoid muscle
Mylohyoid muscle
Hypoglossal nerve (XII)
Lingual artery
External jugular vein
Nerve to thyrohyoid muscle
External carotid artery
Superior laryngeal artery
Superior root, ansa cervicalis
Superior thyroid artery
Sternocleidomastoid branch, superior thyroid artery
Superior thyroid vein
Ascending cervical artery
Ansa cervicalis
Inferior root, ansa cervicalis
Transverse cervical artery
Thyroid gland
Phrenic nerve
Anterior scalene muscle
Internal jugular vein
Common carotid artery
Vagus nerve (X)
Brachiocephalic vein (left)
Sternocleidomastoid muscle
Pectoralis major muscle (clavicular head)
Thoracoacromial vessels
Cephalic vein
Occipital branch, posterior auricular artery
Sternocleidomastoid muscle
Posterior auricular branch of facial nerve (VII)
2nd cervical nerve (ventral ramus)
Lesser occipital nerve
Spinal accessory nerve (XI)
3rd cervical nerve (ventral ramus)
4th cervical nerve (ventral ramus)
Inferior root, ansa cervicalis
Brachial plexus
Superficial branch of dorsal scapular artery (variant)
Trapezius muscle
Inferior belly, omohyoid
Dorsal scapular artery
Subclavian artery
External jugular vein
Subclavian vein
Pectoralis minor muscle
Deltoid muscle

Figure 479 **Nerves and Blood Vessels of the Neck, Stage 4: Large Vessels**

NOTE: (1) The sternocleidomastoid and the superficial veins and nerves have been removed to expose the **carotid arteries, internal jugular vein, omohyoid muscle, vagus nerve,** and **ansa cervicalis.**

(2) Superiorly, the facial vein has been cut and the submandibular gland has been elevated, thereby exposing the **hypoglossal nerve** (XII).

(3) Nerve fibers, originating from C1 and traveling for a short distance with the hypoglossal nerve, leave that nerve to descend in the neck. They form the **superior root of the ansa cervicalis** and are joined by other descending fibers from C2 and C3, which are called the **inferior root of the ansa cervicalis.** The ansa cervicalis supplies motor innervation for a number of the strap muscles.

(4) The **common carotid artery, internal jugular vein,** and **vagus nerve.** These form a vertically oriented neurovascular bundle in the neck that is normally surrounded by the carotid sheath of deep fascia. The common carotid artery bifurcates at about the level of the hyoid bone to form the **external** and **internal carotid arteries.**

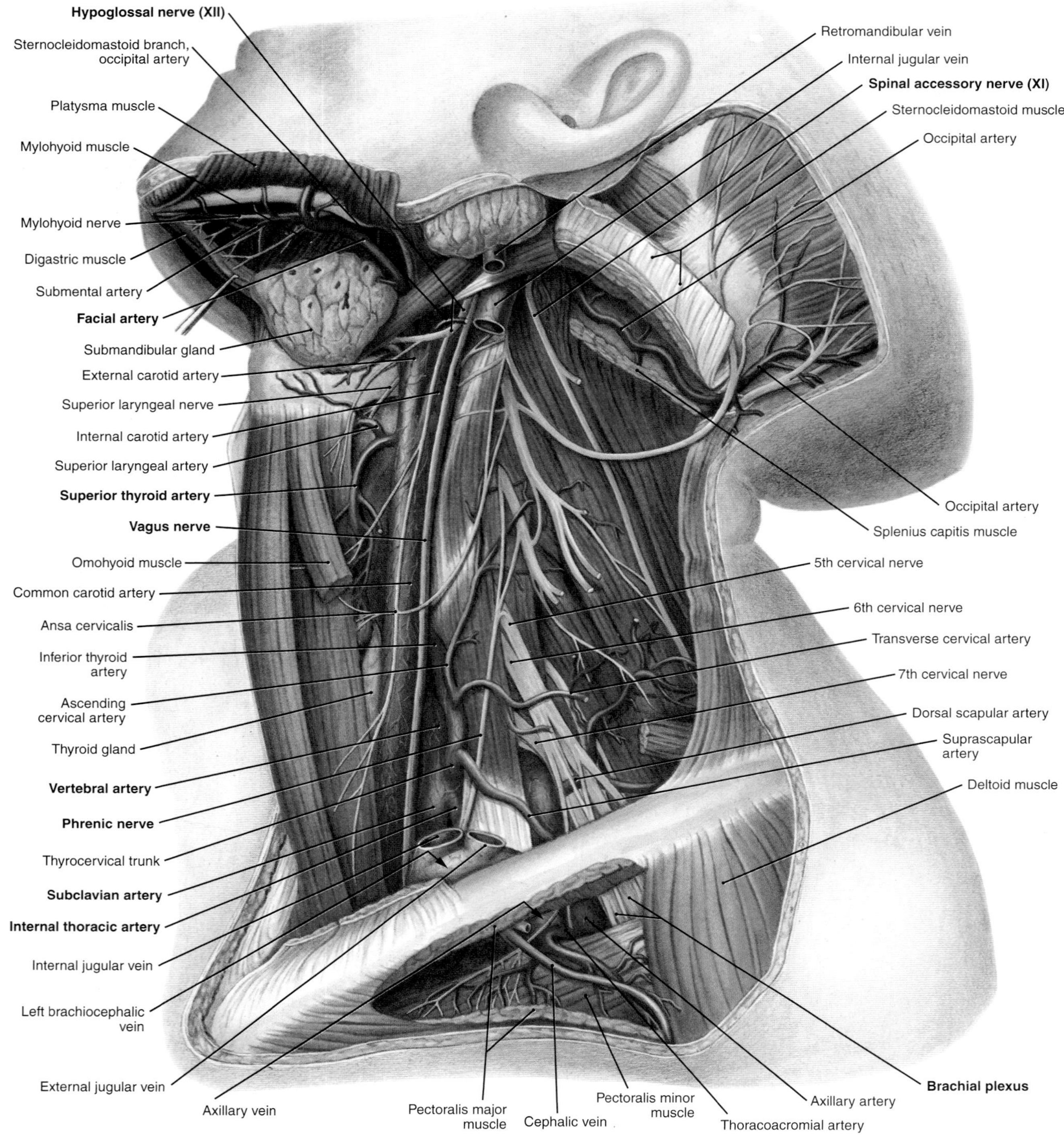
Hypoglossal nerve (XII)
Sternocleidomastoid branch, occipital artery
Platysma muscle
Mylohyoid muscle
Mylohyoid nerve
Digastric muscle
Submental artery
Facial artery
Submandibular gland
External carotid artery
Superior laryngeal nerve
Internal carotid artery
Superior laryngeal artery
Superior thyroid artery
Vagus nerve
Omohyoid muscle
Common carotid artery
Ansa cervicalis
Inferior thyroid artery
Ascending cervical artery
Thyroid gland
Vertebral artery
Phrenic nerve
Thyrocervical trunk
Subclavian artery
Internal thoracic artery
Internal jugular vein
Left brachiocephalic vein
External jugular vein
Axillary vein
Pectoralis major muscle
Cephalic vein
Pectoralis minor muscle
Thoracoacromial artery
Axillary artery
Brachial plexus
Retromandibular vein
Internal jugular vein
Spinal accessory nerve (XI)
Sternocleidomastoid muscle
Occipital artery
Occipital artery
Splenius capitis muscle
5th cervical nerve
6th cervical nerve
Transverse cervical artery
7th cervical nerve
Dorsal scapular artery
Suprascapular artery
Deltoid muscle

Figure 480 Nerves and Blood Vessels of the Neck, Stage 5: Subclavian Artery

NOTE: (1) With the internal and external jugular veins removed, the subclavian artery is exposed as it ascends from the thorax and loops within the subclavian triangle of the neck to descend beneath the clavicle into the axilla. Observe its **vertebral, thyrocervical,** and **internal thoracic** branches.

(2) The **transverse cervical artery** is a branch of the thyrocervical trunk from the subclavian.

(3) The **vagus nerve** coursing with the internal and common carotid arteries, and the **phrenic nerve** descending in the neck along the surface of the anterior scalene muscle.

(4) The **superior thyroid, facial** and **occipital** branches of the external carotid artery. The occipital artery courses posteriorly, deep to the sternocleidomastoid and splenius capitis muscles, and it becomes superficial on the posterior aspect of the scalp.

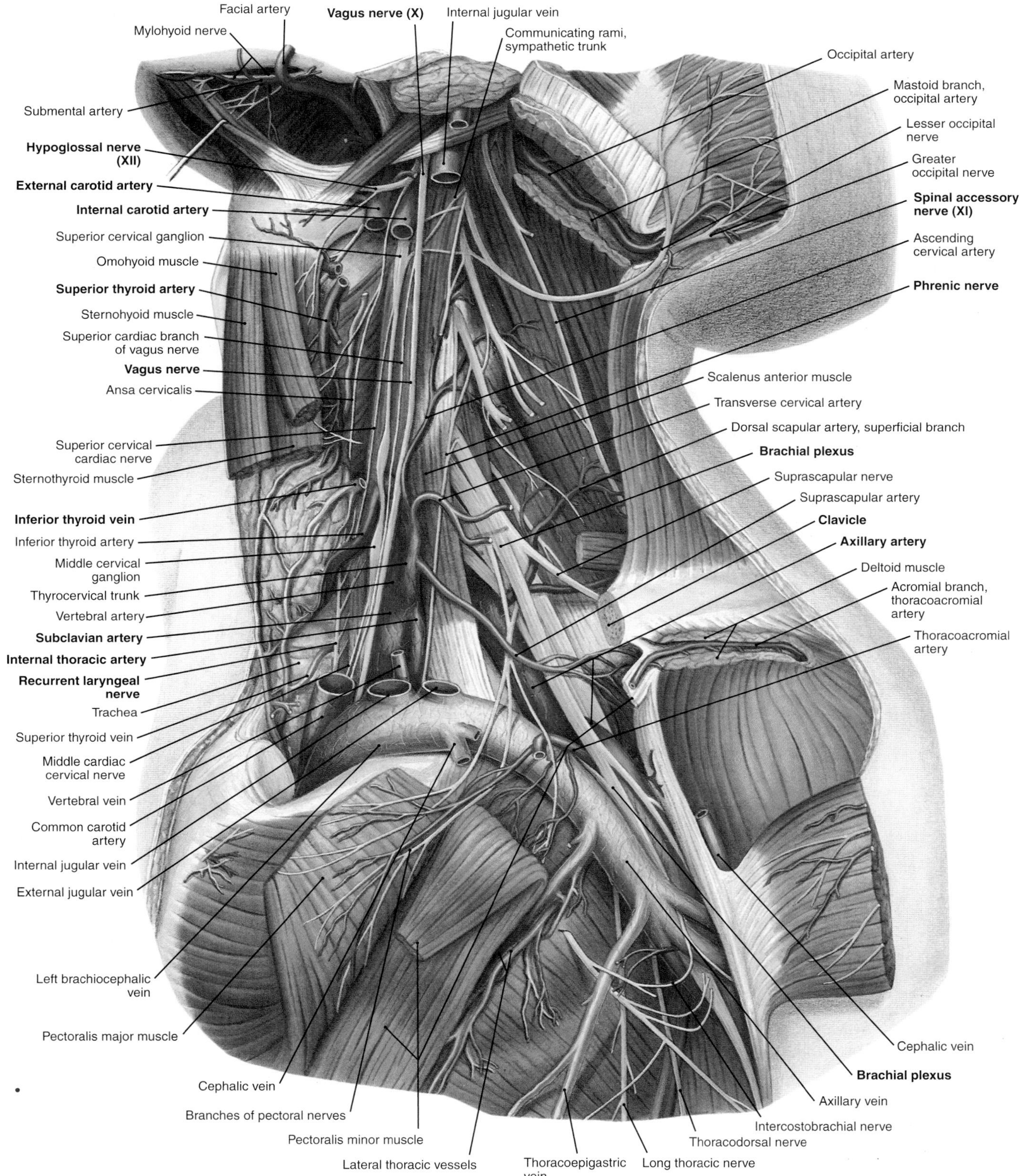
Facial artery
Mylohyoid nerve
Vagus nerve (X)
Internal jugular vein
Communicating rami, sympathetic trunk
Occipital artery
Mastoid branch, occipital artery
Lesser occipital nerve
Greater occipital nerve
Spinal accessory nerve (XI)
Ascending cervical artery
Phrenic nerve
Submental artery
Hypoglossal nerve (XII)
External carotid artery
Internal carotid artery
Superior cervical ganglion
Omohyoid muscle
Superior thyroid artery
Sternohyoid muscle
Superior cardiac branch of vagus nerve
Vagus nerve
Ansa cervicalis
Superior cervical cardiac nerve
Sternothyroid muscle
Inferior thyroid vein
Inferior thyroid artery
Middle cervical ganglion
Thyrocervical trunk
Vertebral artery
Subclavian artery
Internal thoracic artery
Recurrent laryngeal nerve
Trachea
Superior thyroid vein
Middle cardiac cervical nerve
Vertebral vein
Common carotid artery
Internal jugular vein
External jugular vein
Scalenus anterior muscle
Transverse cervical artery
Dorsal scapular artery, superficial branch
Brachial plexus
Suprascapular nerve
Suprascapular artery
Clavicle
Axillary artery
Deltoid muscle
Acromial branch, thoracoacromial artery
Thoracoacromial artery
Left brachiocephalic vein
Pectoralis major muscle
Cephalic vein
Branches of pectoral nerves
Pectoralis minor muscle
Lateral thoracic vessels
Thoracoepigastric vein
Long thoracic nerve
Thoracodorsal nerve
Intercostobrachial nerve
Axillary vein
Brachial plexus
Cephalic vein

Figure 481 Nerves and Blood Vessels of the Neck, Stage 6: Brachial Plexus

NOTE: (1) With the carotid arteries, jugular veins, and clavicle removed, the roots and trunks of the **brachial plexus** are exposed as they divide into cords that surround the axillary artery in the axilla.

(2) The **sympathetic trunk** lying deep to the carotid arteries and coursing with the vagus nerve and the superior cardiac branch of the vagus nerve.

(3) The **thyroid gland, superior** and **inferior thyroid arteries,** and the **thyroid veins**. Note also the proximity of the **recurrent laryngeal nerve** to the thyroid gland.

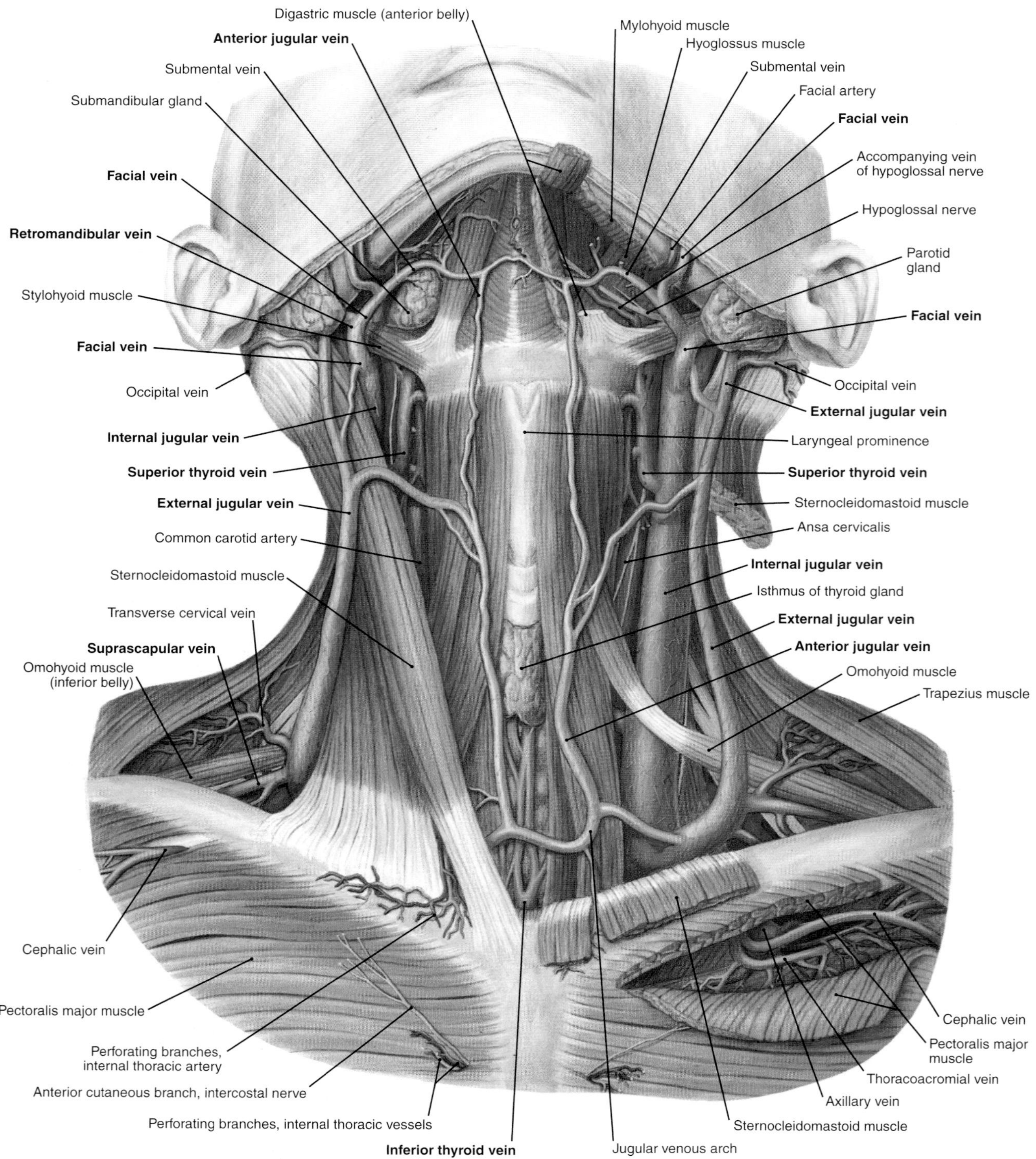
Digastric muscle (anterior belly)
Anterior jugular vein
Submental vein
Submandibular gland
Facial vein
Retromandibular vein
Stylohyoid muscle
Facial vein
Occipital vein
Internal jugular vein
Superior thyroid vein
External jugular vein
Common carotid artery
Sternocleidomastoid muscle
Transverse cervical vein
Suprascapular vein
Omohyoid muscle (inferior belly)
Cephalic vein
Pectoralis major muscle
Perforating branches, internal thoracic artery
Anterior cutaneous branch, intercostal nerve
Perforating branches, internal thoracic vessels
Inferior thyroid vein
Jugular venous arch
Mylohyoid muscle
Hyoglossus muscle
Submental vein
Facial artery
Facial vein
Accompanying vein of hypoglossal nerve
Hypoglossal nerve
Parotid gland
Facial vein
Occipital vein
External jugular vein
Laryngeal prominence
Superior thyroid vein
Sternocleidomastoid muscle
Ansa cervicalis
Internal jugular vein
Isthmus of thyroid gland
External jugular vein
Anterior jugular vein
Omohyoid muscle
Trapezius muscle
Cephalic vein
Pectoralis major muscle
Thoracoacromial vein
Axillary vein
Sternocleidomastoid muscle

Figure 482 Veins of the Neck and Infraclavicular Region

NOTE: (1) The **jugular system of veins** consists of anterior, external, and internal jugular veins, all shown on the left side, where the sternocleidomastoid muscle was removed.

(2) The **anterior jugular** descends close to the midline, is frequently small, and drains laterally into the external jugular. The **external jugular** courses along the surface of the sternocleidomastoid muscle. It forms within the parotid gland and enlarges because of its occipital, retromandibular, and posterior auricular tributaries. The external jugular flows into the subclavian vein after it receives tributaries from the scapular and clavicular regions.

(3) The **internal jugular** is large and collects blood from the brain, face, and neck. At its junction with the subclavian, the **brachiocephalic vein** is formed.

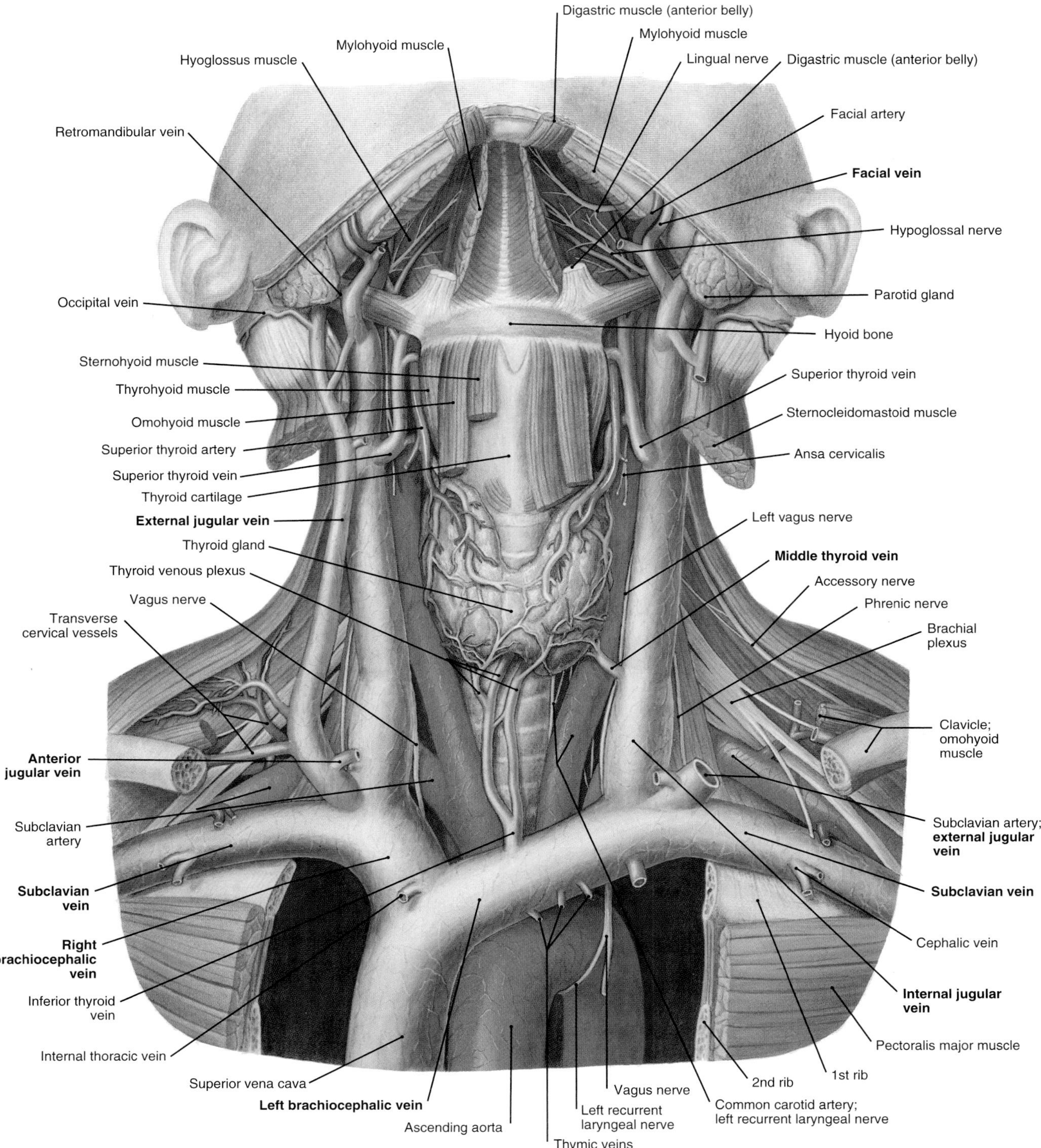
Digastric muscle (anterior belly)
Mylohyoid muscle
Mylohyoid muscle
Hyoglossus muscle
Lingual nerve
Digastric muscle (anterior belly)
Facial artery
Retromandibular vein
Facial vein
Hypoglossal nerve
Parotid gland
Occipital vein
Hyoid bone
Superior thyroid vein
Sternohyoid muscle
Thyrohyoid muscle
Sternocleidomastoid muscle
Omohyoid muscle
Superior thyroid artery
Ansa cervicalis
Superior thyroid vein
Thyroid cartilage
External jugular vein
Left vagus nerve
Thyroid gland
Middle thyroid vein
Thyroid venous plexus
Accessory nerve
Vagus nerve
Phrenic nerve
Transverse cervical vessels
Brachial plexus
Clavicle; omohyoid muscle
Anterior jugular vein
Subclavian artery
Subclavian artery; external jugular vein
Subclavian vein
Subclavian vein
Right brachiocephalic vein
Cephalic vein
Inferior thyroid vein
Internal jugular vein
Pectoralis major muscle
Internal thoracic vein
1st rib
2nd rib
Superior vena cava
Vagus nerve
Left brachiocephalic vein
Left recurrent laryngeal nerve
Common carotid artery; left recurrent laryngeal nerve
Ascending aorta
Thymic veins

Figure 483 Deep Arteries and Veins of the Neck and Great Vessels of the Thorax

NOTE: (1) The sternocleidomastoid and strap muscles have been removed from the neck, thereby exposing the carotid arteries, internal jugular veins, and thyroid gland.

(2) The middle portion of the anterior thoracic wall has been resected to show the aortic arch and its branches, the brachiocephalic veins and their tributaries, the superior vena cava and the vagus nerves.

(3) In the submandibular region, the mylohyoid and anterior digastric muscles have been cut, revealing the lingual and hypoglossal nerves.

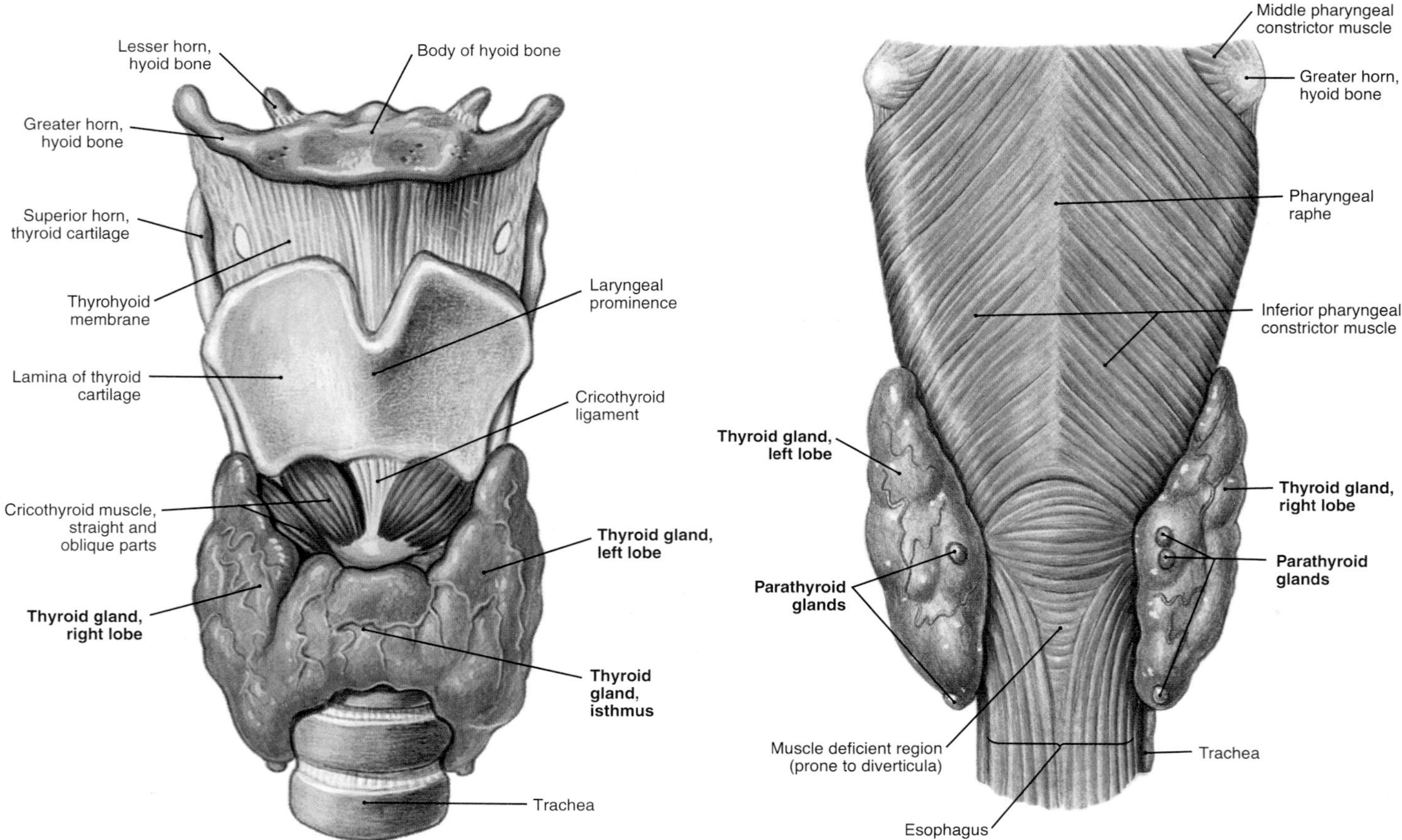
Lesser horn, hyoid bone
Body of hyoid bone
Greater horn, hyoid bone
Superior horn, thyroid cartilage
Thyrohyoid membrane
Laryngeal prominence
Lamina of thyroid cartilage
Cricothyroid ligament
Cricothyroid muscle, straight and oblique parts
Thyroid gland, left lobe
Thyroid gland, right lobe
Thyroid gland, isthmus
Trachea
Middle pharyngeal constrictor muscle
Greater horn, hyoid bone
Pharyngeal raphe
Inferior pharyngeal constrictor muscle
Thyroid gland, left lobe
Thyroid gland, right lobe
Parathyroid glands
Parathyroid glands
Muscle deficient region (prone to diverticula)
Trachea
Esophagus

Figure 484.1 Ventral View of Thyroid Gland Showing Relation to Larynx and Trachea

Figure 484.2 Dorsal View of Thyroid Gland Showing Relation to Pharynx and Parathyroids

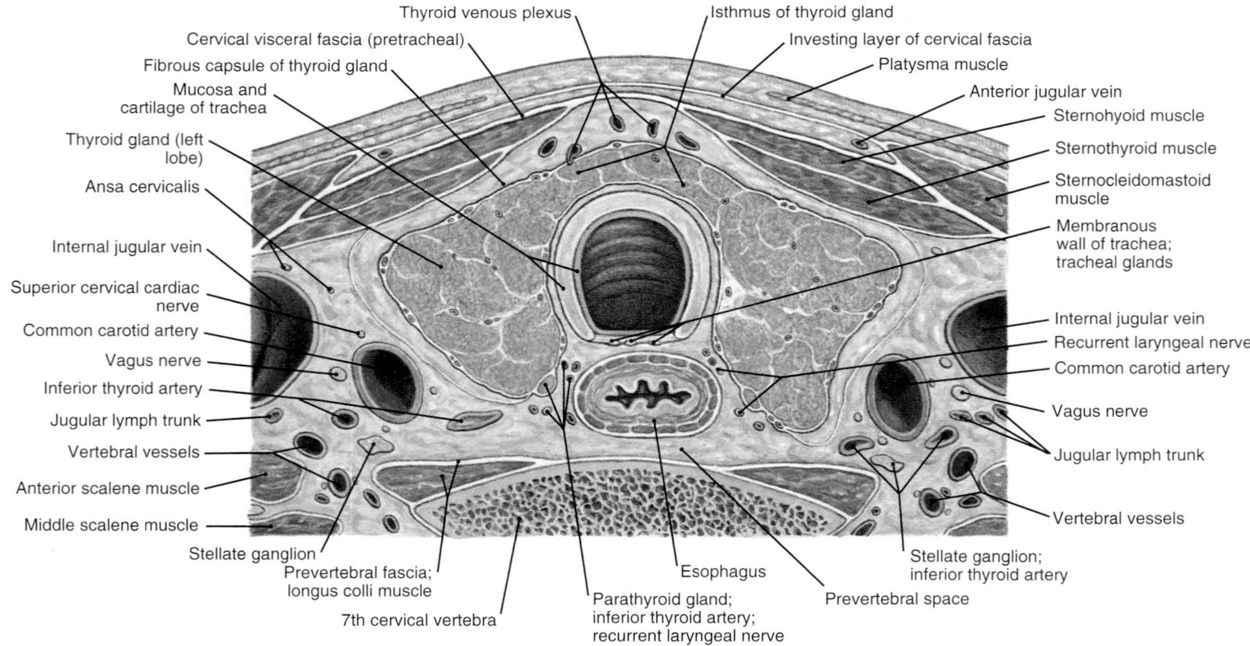
Thyroid venous plexus
Isthmus of thyroid gland
Cervical visceral fascia (pretracheal)
Investing layer of cervical fascia
Fibrous capsule of thyroid gland
Platysma muscle
Mucosa and cartilage of trachea
Anterior jugular vein
Sternohyoid muscle
Thyroid gland (left lobe)
Sternothyroid muscle
Ansa cervicalis
Sternocleidomastoid muscle
Membranous wall of trachea; tracheal glands
Internal jugular vein
Superior cervical cardiac nerve
Internal jugular vein
Common carotid artery
Recurrent laryngeal nerve
Vagus nerve
Common carotid artery
Inferior thyroid artery
Vagus nerve
Jugular lymph trunk
Vertebral vessels
Jugular lymph trunk
Anterior scalene muscle
Middle scalene muscle
Vertebral vessels
Stellate ganglion
Prevertebral fascia; longus colli muscle
Esophagus
Stellate ganglion; inferior thyroid artery
7th cervical vertebra
Parathyroid gland; inferior thyroid artery; recurrent laryngeal nerve
Prevertebral space

Figure 484.3 Cross Section of the Anterior Neck at the Level of the C7 Vertebra

NOTE: Observe the relationship of the isthmus and lobes of the thyroid gland to the trachea. Also observe the location of the parathyroid glands, the recurrent laryngeal nerves, and the inferior thyroid arteries along the posteromedial border of the thyroid gland.

Figure 485.1 Scintiscan of the Thyroid Gland ▶

NOTE: (1) A scintiscan (scintigram, scintigraph, or gamma image) is the visual representation of the distribution in an entire body (whole-body scan) or in an organ of a gamma-emitting radioactive substance as detected by as scintillation scanner or gamma camera.

(2) Radioactive iodine (^{123}I) and technetium-99m (^{99m} Tc) have excellent properties for imaging the thyroid gland, and the latter radionuclide was used to obtain this image 35 minutes after injection.

(3) This technique is used to detect thyroid nodules and tumors of thyroid glandular tissue in the bed of the thyroid and throughout the body as a follow-up technique after the removal of a thyroid cancer.

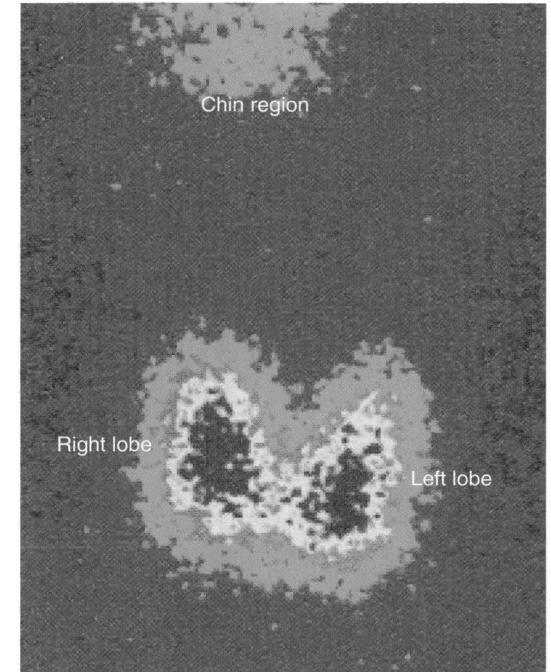
Chin region
Right lobe
Left lobe

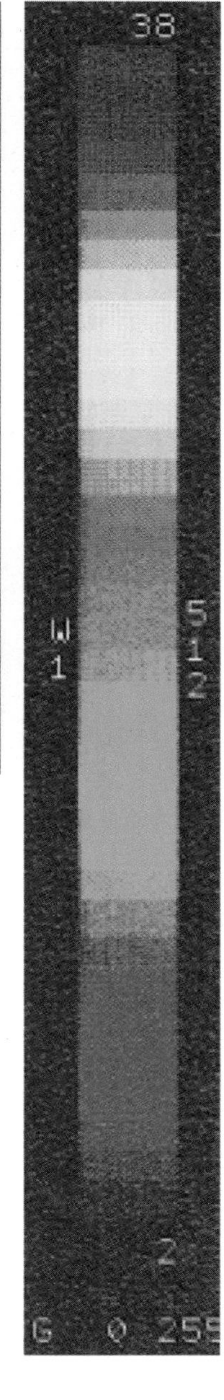
38
W
1
5
1
2
2
G
0
255

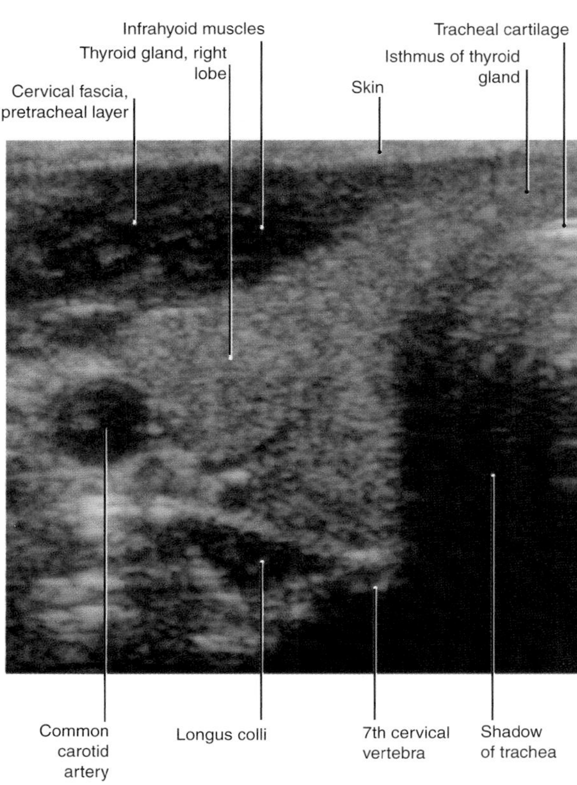
Infrahyoid muscles
Thyroid gland, right lobe
Cervical fascia, pretracheal layer
Skin
Tracheal cartilage
Isthmus of thyroid gland
Common carotid artery
Longus colli
7th cervical vertebra
Shadow of trachea

▲ **Figure 485.2 Ultrasound Scan of the Thyroid Gland**

NOTE: This is a horizontal ultrasound scan with the sound being administered in a ventrodorsal direction.

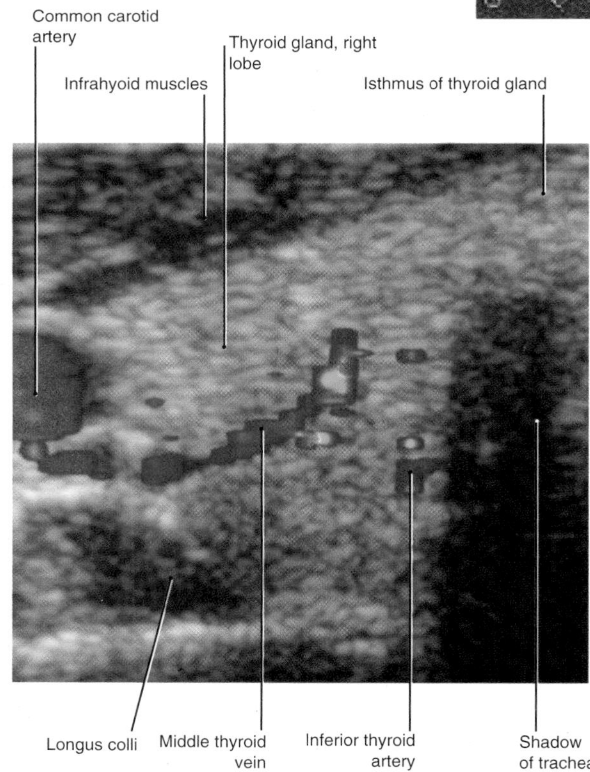
Common carotid artery
Thyroid gland, right lobe
Infrahyoid muscles
Isthmus of thyroid gland
Longus colli
Middle thyroid vein
Inferior thyroid artery
Shadow of trachea

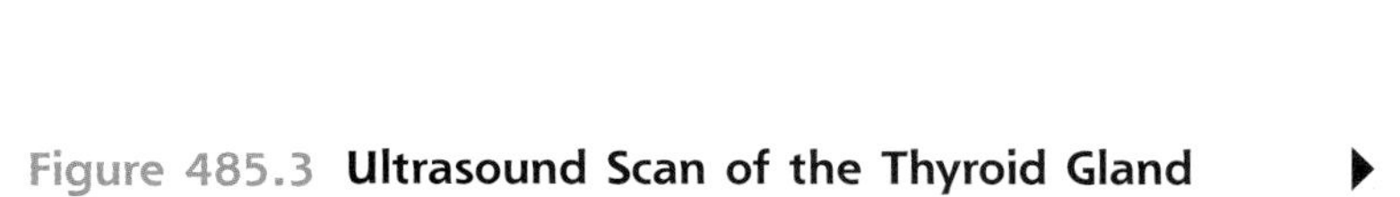

Figure 485.3 Ultrasound Scan of the Thyroid Gland ▶

NOTE: This scan shows the direction of blood flow; (color flow Doppler sonogram)

RED = toward the transducer (arteries)

BLUE = away from the transducer (veins)

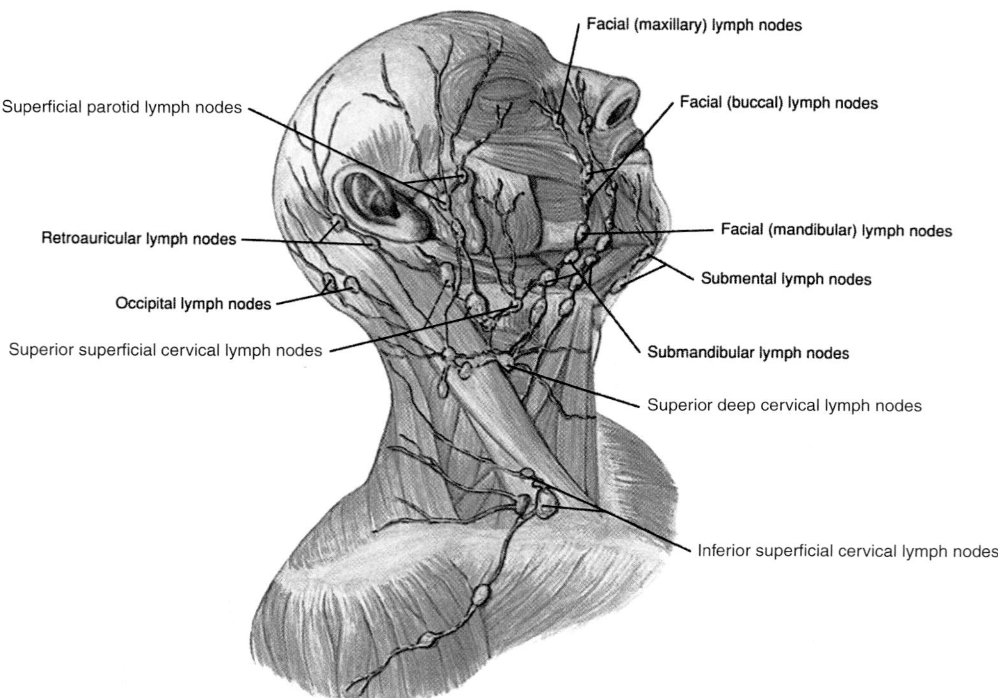
Facial (maxillary) lymph nodes
Superficial parotid lymph nodes
Facial (buccal) lymph nodes
Retroauricular lymph nodes
Facial (mandibular) lymph nodes
Submental lymph nodes
Occipital lymph nodes
Superior superficial cervical lymph nodes
Submandibular lymph nodes
Superior deep cervical lymph nodes
Inferior superficial cervical lymph nodes

Figure 486.1 **Superficial Lymph Nodes and Vessels of the Head and Neck**

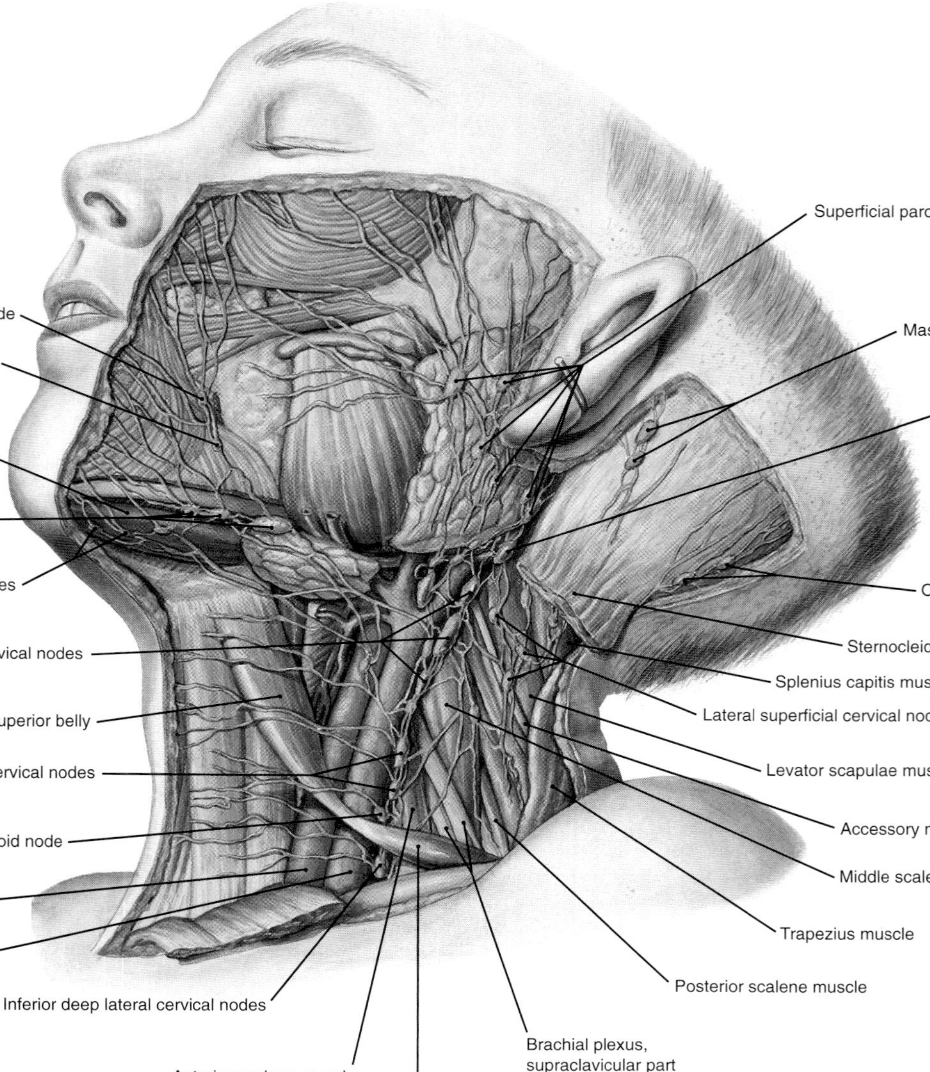

Superficial parotid nodes
Buccinator node
Mastoid nodes
Facial nodes
Jugulodigastric node
Digastric muscle, anterior belly
Submandibular nodes
Submental nodes
Occipital nodes
Sternocleidomastoid muscle
Superior deep lateral cervical nodes
Splenius capitis muscle
Lateral superficial cervical nodes
Omohyoid muscle, superior belly
Levator scapulae muscle
Inferior deep lateral cervical nodes
Accessory nerve [XI]
Jugulo-omohyoid node
Middle scalene muscle
Common carotid artery
Trapezius muscle
Internal jugular vein
Posterior scalene muscle
Inferior deep lateral cervical nodes
Brachial plexus, supraclavicular part
Anterior scalene muscle
Omohyoid muscle, inferior belly

Figure 486.2 **Superficial Nodes of the Face and Neck in an 8-Year-Old Boy**

NOTE: The platysma muscle has been removed and the sternocleidomastoid muscle has been sectioned.

Anterior cervical nodes
External jugular vein
Middle scalene muscle
Splenius cervicis muscle
Sternocleidomastoid muscle
Levator scapulae muscle
Omohyoid muscle, superior belly
Lateral supraclavicular nerves
Lateral cervical nodes
Clavicle
Transverse cervical artery and vein
Trapezius muscle
Suprascapular nerve
Anterior cervical nodes
Deltoid muscle
Suprascapular artery and vein
Anterior scalene muscle
Pectoralis minor muscle
Sternohyoid muscle
Left jugular lymph trunk
Cephalic vein
Lateral cervical node
Subscapular nodes
Internal jugular vein
Pectoralis major muscle
Radial nerve
Thoracic duct, cervical part
Musculocutaneous nerve
Anterior jugular vein
Posterior humeral circumflex artery
Jugular venous arch
Brachial vein
Sternoclavicular joint
Cephalic vein
Ulnar nerve
External jugular vein
Lateral axillary nodes
Left subclavian trunk
Medial brachial cutaneous nerve
Subclavian artery
Brachial vein
Subclavius muscle
Intercostal nodes
Pectoralis major muscle
2nd rib
Long thoracic nerve
Pectoralis minor muscle
Deltopectoral nodes
Axillary vein
Serratus anterior muscle
Superior thoracic artery
Pectoral nodes
T2 nerve
Lateral thoracic artery and vein
Central axillary nodes

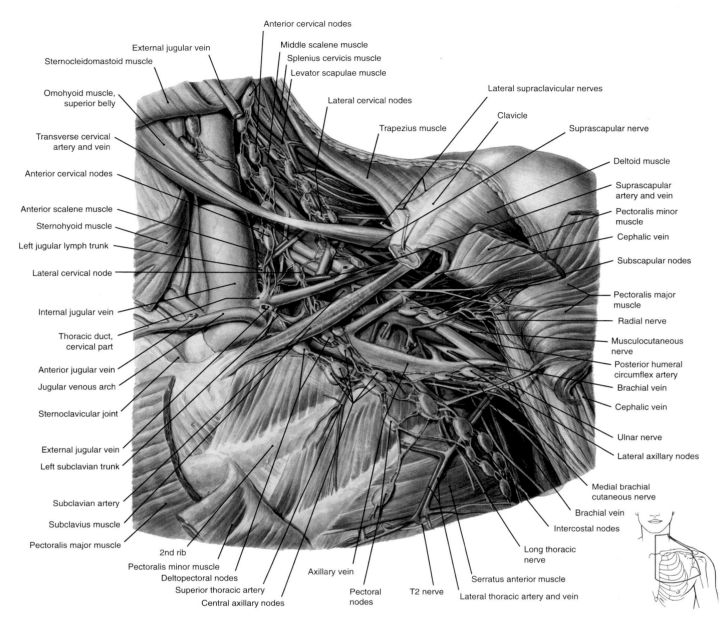

Figure 487.1 Lymph Nodes in the Deep Cervical and Axillary Regions
NOTE: Most of the clavicle and pectoralis muscles have been removed.

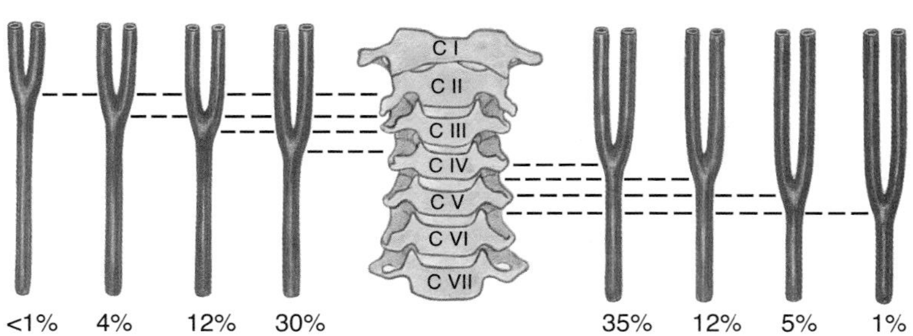
C I
C II
C III
C IV
C V
C VI
C VII
<1%
4%
12%
30%
35%
12%
5%
1%

Figure 487.2 Variations in the Vertebral Level for the Bifurcation of the Common Carotid Artery

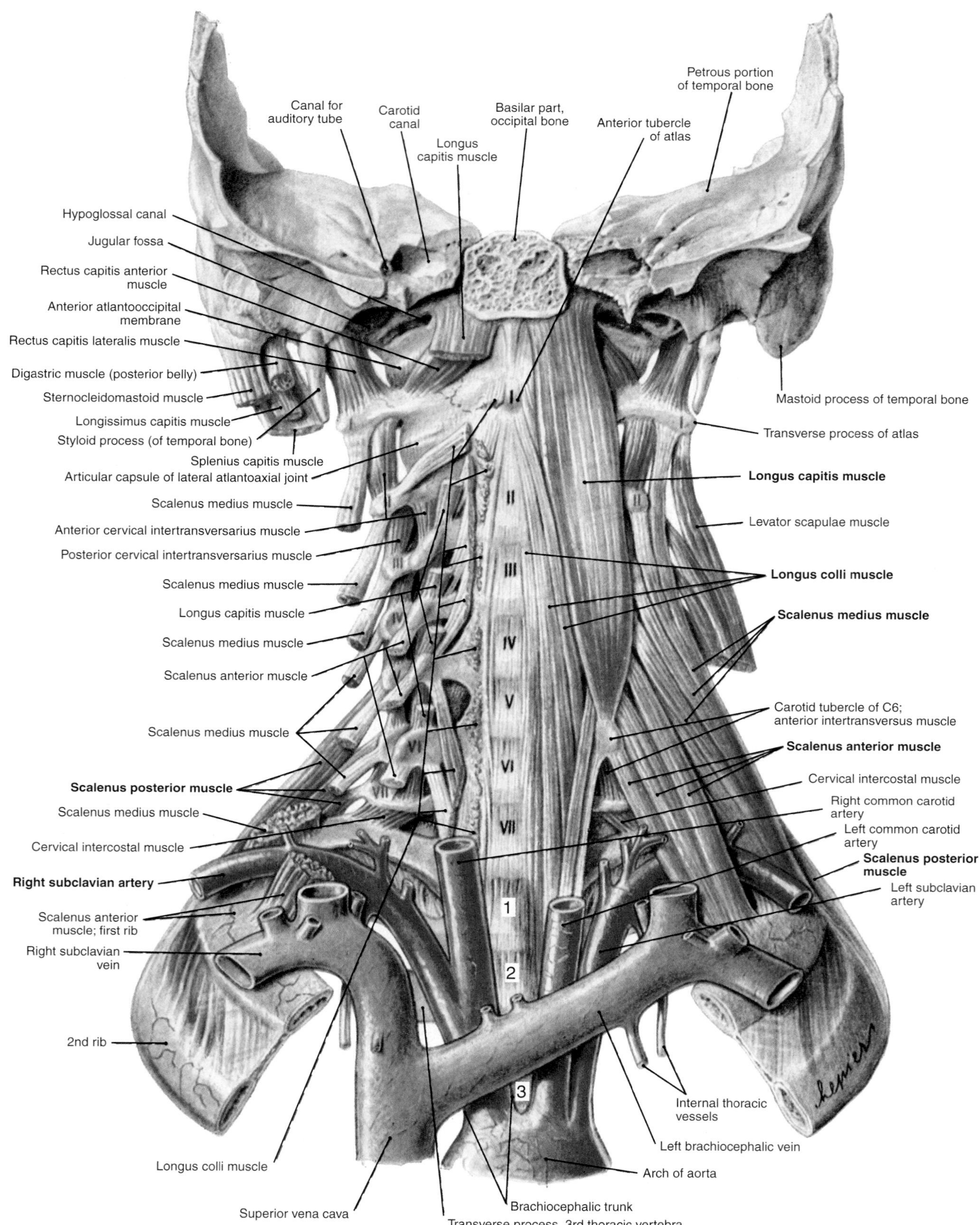
Canal for auditory tube
Carotid canal
Longus capitis muscle
Basilar part, occipital bone
Anterior tubercle of atlas
Petrous portion of temporal bone
Hypoglossal canal
Jugular fossa
Rectus capitis anterior muscle
Anterior atlantooccipital membrane
Rectus capitis lateralis muscle
Digastric muscle (posterior belly)
Sternocleidomastoid muscle
Longissimus capitis muscle
Styloid process (of temporal bone)
Splenius capitis muscle
Articular capsule of lateral atlantoaxial joint
Scalenus medius muscle
Anterior cervical intertransversarius muscle
Posterior cervical intertransversarius muscle
Scalenus medius muscle
Longus capitis muscle
Scalenus medius muscle
Scalenus anterior muscle
Scalenus medius muscle
Scalenus posterior muscle
Scalenus medius muscle
Cervical intercostal muscle
Right subclavian artery
Scalenus anterior muscle; first rib
Right subclavian vein
2nd rib
Longus colli muscle
Superior vena cava
Mastoid process of temporal bone
Transverse process of atlas
Longus capitis muscle
Levator scapulae muscle
Longus colli muscle
Scalenus medius muscle
Carotid tubercle of C6; anterior intertransversus muscle
Scalenus anterior muscle
Cervical intercostal muscle
Right common carotid artery
Left common carotid artery
Scalenus posterior muscle
Left subclavian artery
Internal thoracic vessels
Left brachiocephalic vein
Arch of aorta
Brachiocephalic trunk
Transverse process, 3rd thoracic vertebra
I
II
III
IV
V
VI
VII
1
2
3

Figure 488 Prevertebral Region and Root of the Neck (Anterior View)

NOTE: (1) On the specimen's right, the longus colli, longus capitis, and scalene muscles have been removed, exposing the transverse processes of the cervical vertebrae onto which these muscles are seen to attach.

(2) There are two long (longus colli and longus capitis) and two short (rectus capitis anterior and lateralis) prevertebral muscles. These flex the head and neck forward and bend the head and neck laterally.

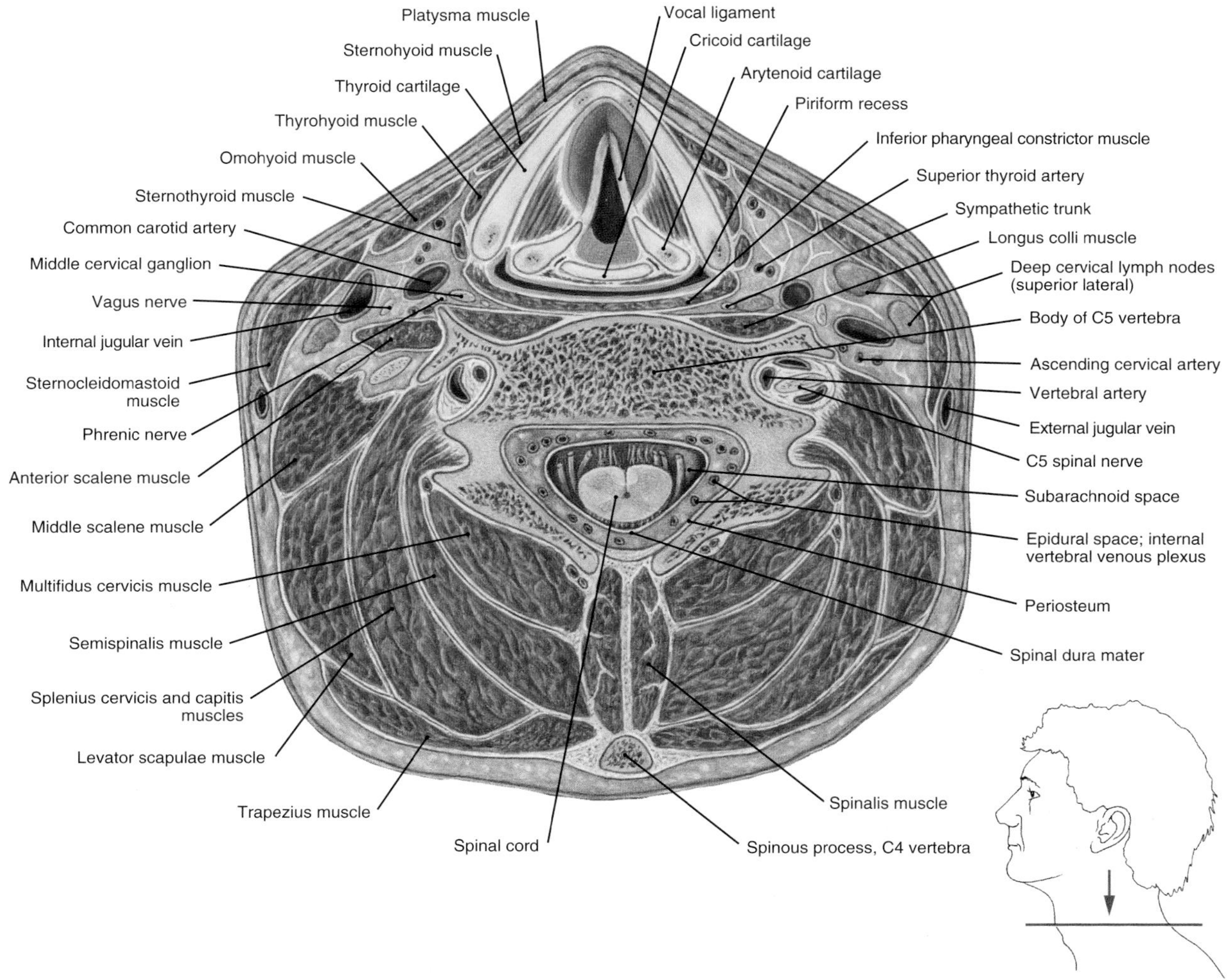

Platysma muscle
Sternohyoid muscle
Thyroid cartilage
Thyrohyoid muscle
Omohyoid muscle
Sternothyroid muscle
Common carotid artery
Middle cervical ganglion
Vagus nerve
Internal jugular vein
Sternocleidomastoid muscle
Phrenic nerve
Anterior scalene muscle
Middle scalene muscle
Multifidus cervicis muscle
Semispinalis muscle
Splenius cervicis and capitis muscles
Levator scapulae muscle
Trapezius muscle
Spinal cord
Vocal ligament
Cricoid cartilage
Arytenoid cartilage
Piriform recess
Inferior pharyngeal constrictor muscle
Superior thyroid artery
Sympathetic trunk
Longus colli muscle
Deep cervical lymph nodes (superior lateral)
Body of C5 vertebra
Ascending cervical artery
Vertebral artery
External jugular vein
C5 spinal nerve
Subarachnoid space
Epidural space; internal vertebral venous plexus
Periosteum
Spinal dura mater
Spinalis muscle
Spinous process, C4 vertebra

Figure 489 **Cross Section of the Neck at the C5 Vertebral Level**

ANTERIOR VERTEBRAL MUSCLES

Muscle	Origin	Insertion	Innervation	Action
		Superior Oblique Part		
Longus colli	Anterior tubercles of transverse processes of third, fourth, and fifth cervical vertebrae	Tubercle of the anterior arch of the atlas	Ventral rami of the C2 to C6 spinal nerves	
		Inferior Oblique Part		
	Anterior surface of the bodies of the first two or three thoracic vertebrae	Anterior tubercles of the transverse processes of the fifth and sixth cervical vertebrae		Weak flexor of the neck; slightly rotates and bends neck laterally
		Vertical Part		
	Anterolateral surfaces of the last 3 cervical and upper 3 thoracic vertebrae	Anterior surfaces of the bodies of second, third and fourth cervical vertebrae		
Longus capitis	By tendinous slips from the transverse processes of the third, fourth, fifth, and sixth cervical vertebrae	Inferior surface of the basilar part of the occipital bone	Branches from the anterior rami of C1, C2, and C3 nerves	Flexes the head and the upper cervical spine
Rectus capitis anterior	Anterior surface of the lateral mass of the atlas and its transverse process	Inferior surface of the basilar part of the occipital bone	Fibers from the anterior rami of C1 and C2	Flexes the head and helps stabilize the atlantooccipital joint
Rectus capitis lateralis	Superior surface of the transverse process of the atlas	Inferior surface of the jugular process of the occipital bone	Anterior rami of the C1 and C2 nerves	Bends the head laterally to the same side

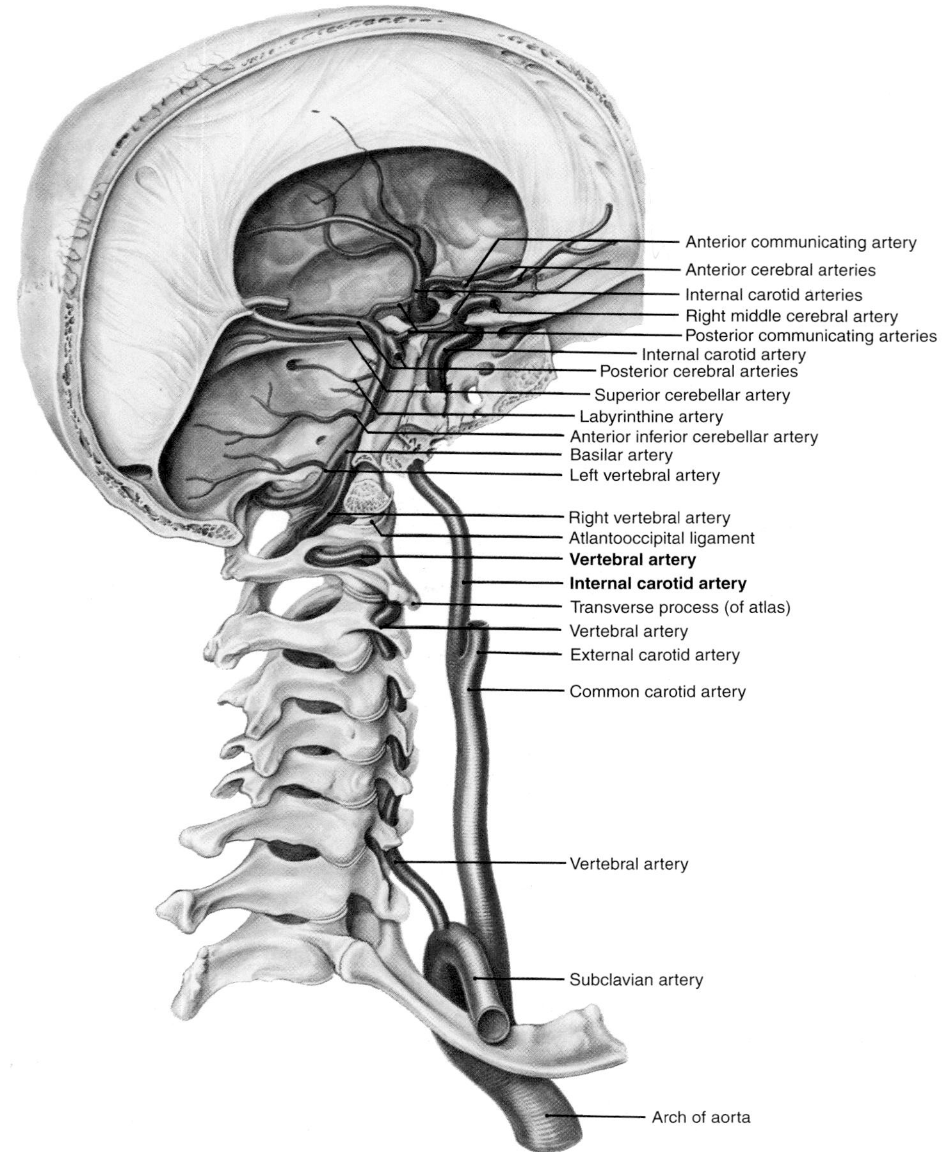
Anterior communicating artery
Anterior cerebral arteries
Internal carotid arteries
Right middle cerebral artery
Posterior communicating arteries
Internal carotid artery
Posterior cerebral arteries
Superior cerebellar artery
Labyrinthine artery
Anterior inferior cerebellar artery
Basilar artery
Left vertebral artery
Right vertebral artery
Atlantooccipital ligament
Vertebral artery
Internal carotid artery
Transverse process (of atlas)
Vertebral artery
External carotid artery
Common carotid artery
Vertebral artery
Subclavian artery
Arch of aorta

Figure 490.1 Vertebral and Internal Carotid Arteries

NOTE: (1) Both the internal carotid and the vertebral arteries ascend in the neck to enter the cranial cavity to supply blood to the brain. Although the vertebral arteries give off some spinal and muscular branches in the neck prior to entering the skull, the internal carotid arteries do not have branches in the neck.

(2) The origin of the **vertebral artery** from the subclavian ascends in the neck through the foramina in the transverse processes of the cervical vertebrae.

(3) The two vertebral arteries join to form the **basilar artery**. This vessel courses along the ventral aspect of the brainstem.

(4) The **internal carotid artery** begins at the bifurcation of the common carotid and ascends to its entrance in the carotid canal in the petrous part of the temporal bone. After a somewhat tortuous course, it enters the cranial cavity.

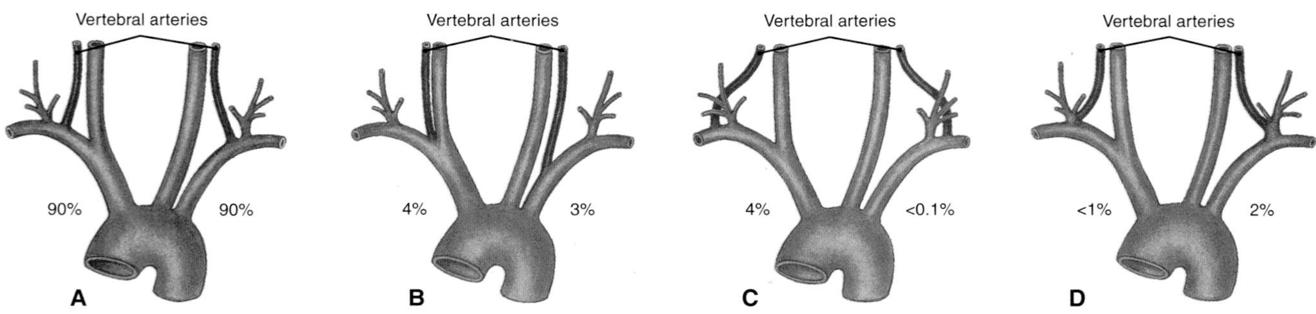
Vertebral arteries
90%
90%
A
Vertebral arteries
4%
3%
B
Vertebral arteries
4%
<0.1%
C
Vertebral arteries
<1%
2%
D

Figure 490.2 Variations (and Percentages) in the Origin of the Vertebral Arteries

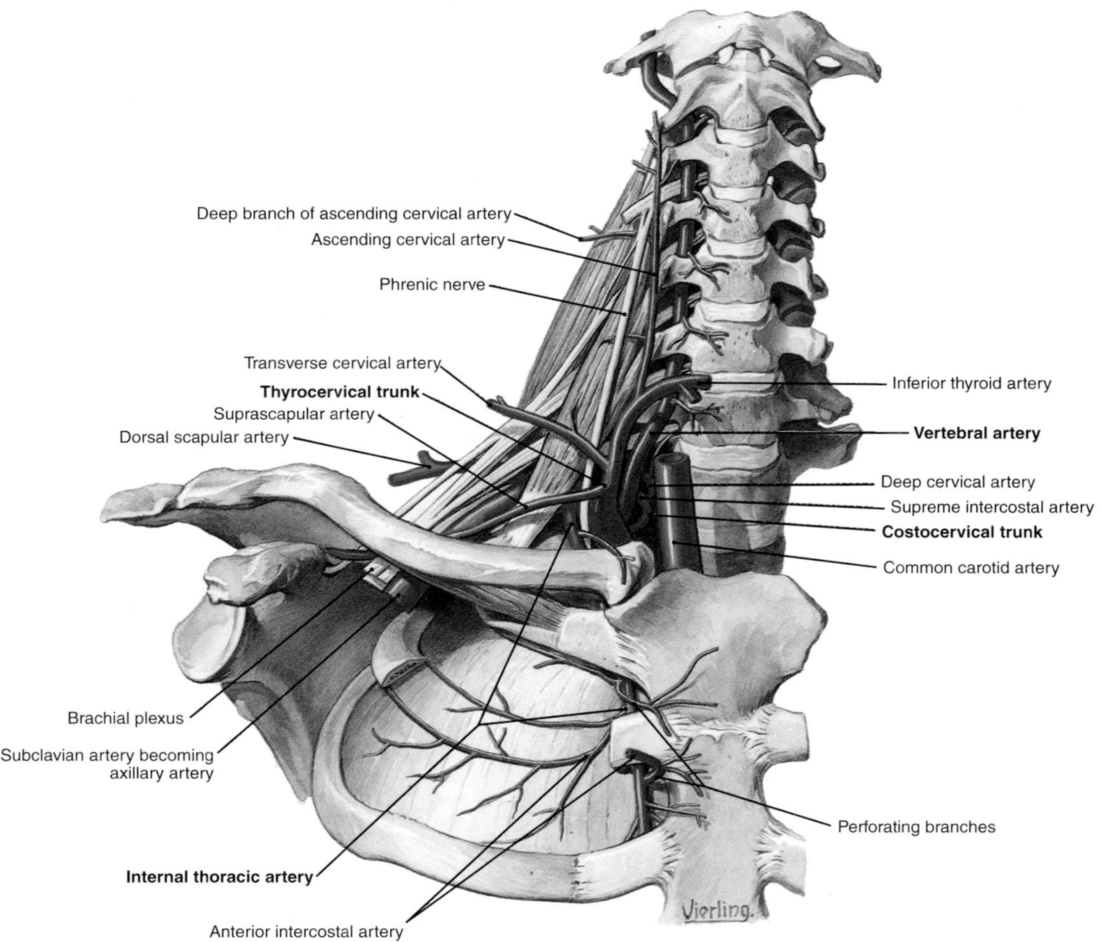
Deep branch of ascending cervical artery
Ascending cervical artery
Phrenic nerve
Transverse cervical artery
Thyrocervical trunk
Suprascapular artery
Dorsal scapular artery
Inferior thyroid artery
Vertebral artery
Deep cervical artery
Supreme intercostal artery
Costocervical trunk
Common carotid artery
Brachial plexus
Subclavian artery becoming axillary artery
Perforating branches
Internal thoracic artery
Anterior intercostal artery
Vierling

Figure 491.1 **Right Subclavian Artery and Its Branches**

NOTE: (1) The right subclavian artery arises from the brachiocephalic trunk, although on the left it branches from the aorta. It ascends into the root of the neck, arches laterally, and then descends between the first rib and clavicle to become the axillary artery.

(2) The subclavian artery generally has four major branches and sometimes five. These are the **vertebral artery**, the **internal thoracic artery**, the **thyrocervical trunk**, and the **costocervical trunk**.

(3) In about 40% of bodies, there is also a **dorsal scapular artery** arising directly from the subclavian. Thus, in this region there is considerable variation in the origin of vessels such as the suprascapular artery, the transverse cervical artery, and this latter vessel's superficial and deep branches, the superficial cervical artery and the descending scapular artery. (For a complete description of these vessels see: Clemente CD, ed. Gray's anatomy of the human body, 30th ed. Philadelphia: Lea & Febiger, 1985:703–709.)

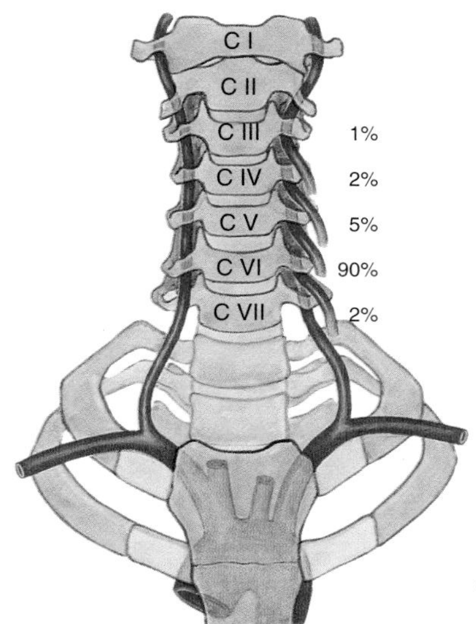
C I
C II
C III
C IV
C V
C VI
C VII
1%
2%
5%
90%
2%

Figure 491.2 **Variations in the Level of Entry of the Vertebral Artery into the Transverse Foramina of Cervical Vertebrae**

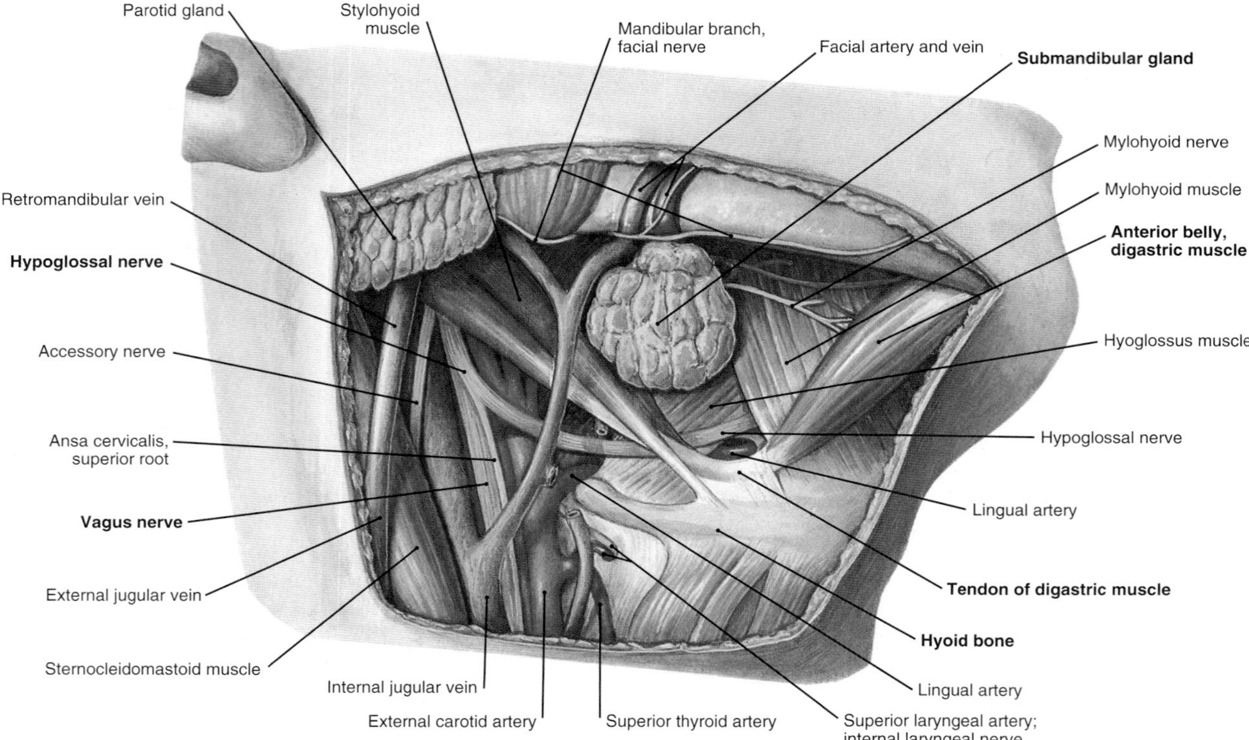
Parotid gland
Stylohyoid muscle
Mandibular branch, facial nerve
Facial artery and vein
Submandibular gland
Mylohyoid nerve
Mylohyoid muscle
Anterior belly, digastric muscle
Hyoglossus muscle
Hypoglossal nerve
Lingual artery
Tendon of digastric muscle
Hyoid bone
Lingual artery
Superior laryngeal artery; internal laryngeal nerve
Superior thyroid artery
External carotid artery
Internal jugular vein
Sternocleidomastoid muscle
External jugular vein
Vagus nerve
Ansa cervicalis, superior root
Accessory nerve
Hypoglossal nerve
Retromandibular vein

Figure 492.1 Right Submandibular Triangle and Submandibular Gland

NOTE: The **submandibular triangle** is bounded by the two bellies of the digastric muscle and by the lower border of the mandible. The floor of the triangle is formed by the mylohyoid and hyoglossus muscles, between which the **hypoglossal nerve** enters the oral cavity.

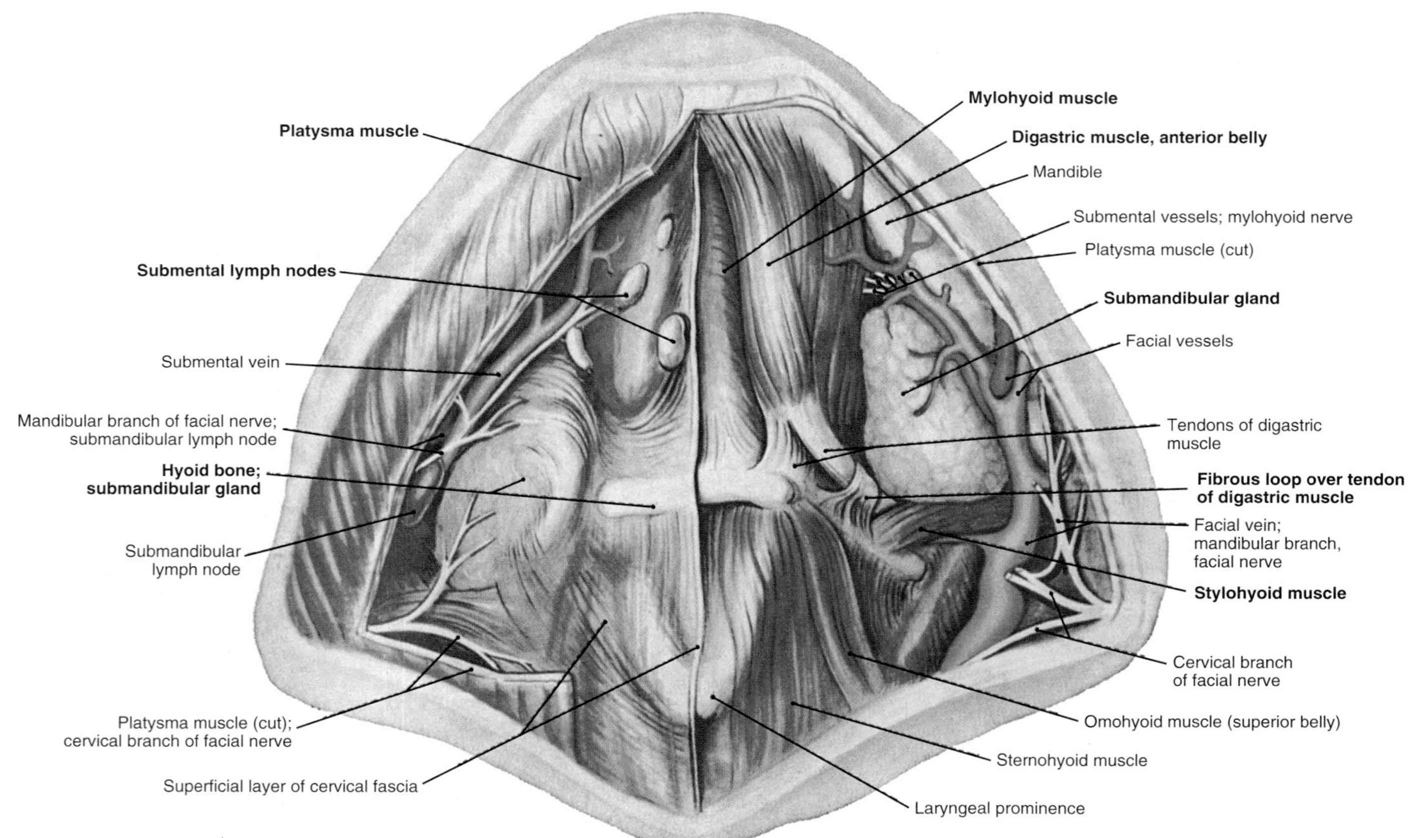
Platysma muscle
Mylohyoid muscle
Digastric muscle, anterior belly
Mandible
Submental vessels; mylohyoid nerve
Platysma muscle (cut)
Submental lymph nodes
Submandibular gland
Facial vessels
Submental vein
Mandibular branch of facial nerve; submandibular lymph node
Tendons of digastric muscle
Hyoid bone; submandibular gland
Fibrous loop over tendon of digastric muscle
Facial vein; mandibular branch, facial nerve
Submandibular lymph node
Stylohyoid muscle
Cervical branch of facial nerve
Platysma muscle (cut); cervical branch of facial nerve
Omohyoid muscle (superior belly)
Sternohyoid muscle
Superficial layer of cervical fascia
Laryngeal prominence

Figure 492.2 Submandibular and Submental Regions (Dissection Stages 1 [Reader's Left] and 2)

NOTE: In dissection **Stage 1**, the superficial fascia with the platysma has been opened, showing the submandibular gland and lymph nodes. In **Stage 2** (reader's right), the superficial layer of cervical fascia has been opened, showing the digastric, mylohyoid, and stylohyoid muscles.

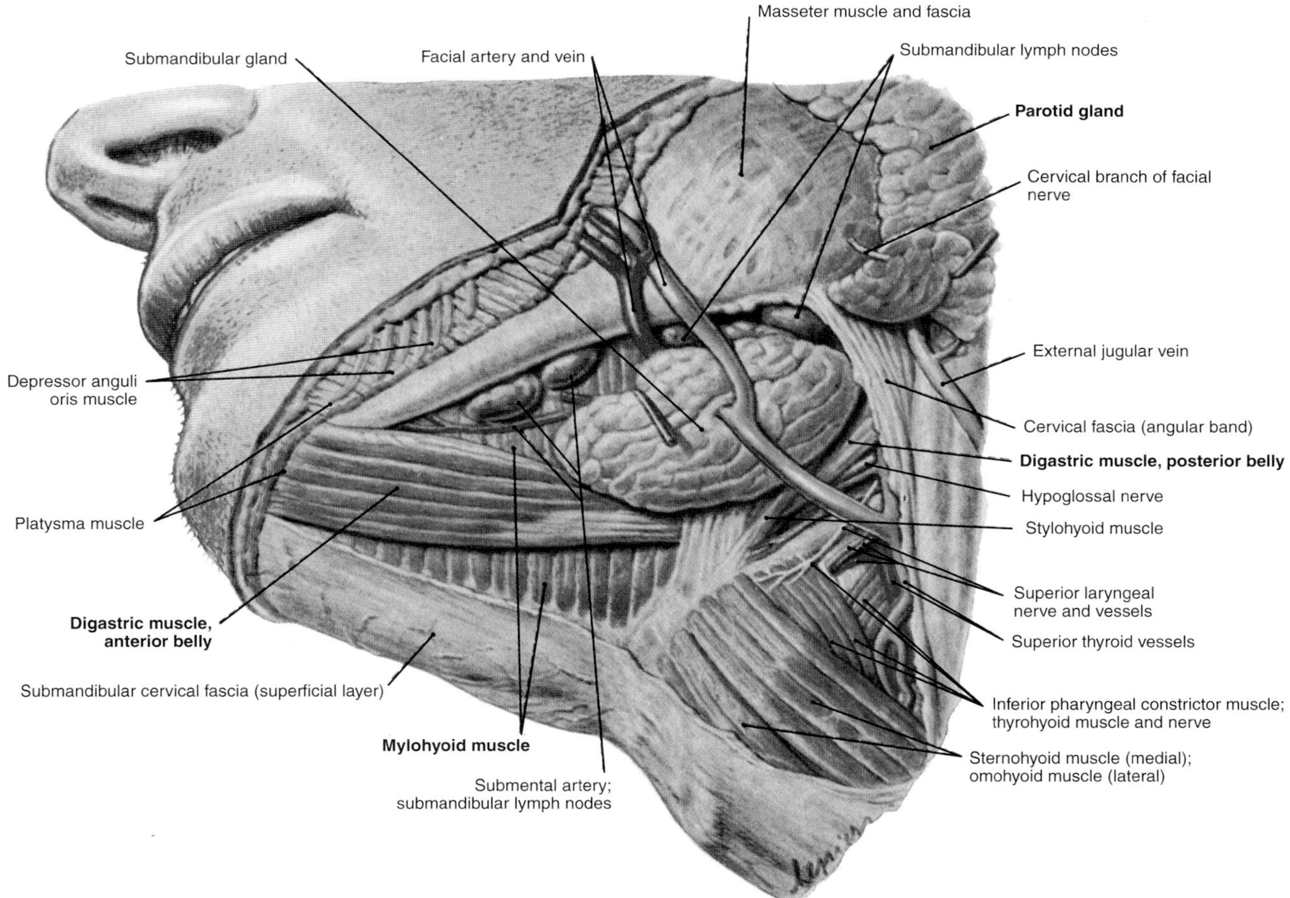
Masseter muscle and fascia
Submandibular gland
Facial artery and vein
Submandibular lymph nodes
Parotid gland
Cervical branch of facial nerve
Depressor anguli oris muscle
External jugular vein
Cervical fascia (angular band)
Digastric muscle, posterior belly
Hypoglossal nerve
Platysma muscle
Stylohyoid muscle
Superior laryngeal nerve and vessels
Digastric muscle, anterior belly
Superior thyroid vessels
Submandibular cervical fascia (superficial layer)
Inferior pharyngeal constrictor muscle; thyrohyoid muscle and nerve
Mylohyoid muscle
Sternohyoid muscle (medial); omohyoid muscle (lateral)
Submental artery; submandibular lymph nodes

Figure 493.1 Left Submandibular Triangle and Submandibular Gland (Viewed from Below)
NOTE: Crossing the submandibular triangle are the **anterior facial vein** and the **facial artery.** Observe also, the **submandibular** and **parotid glands** and the **submandibular lymph nodes.**

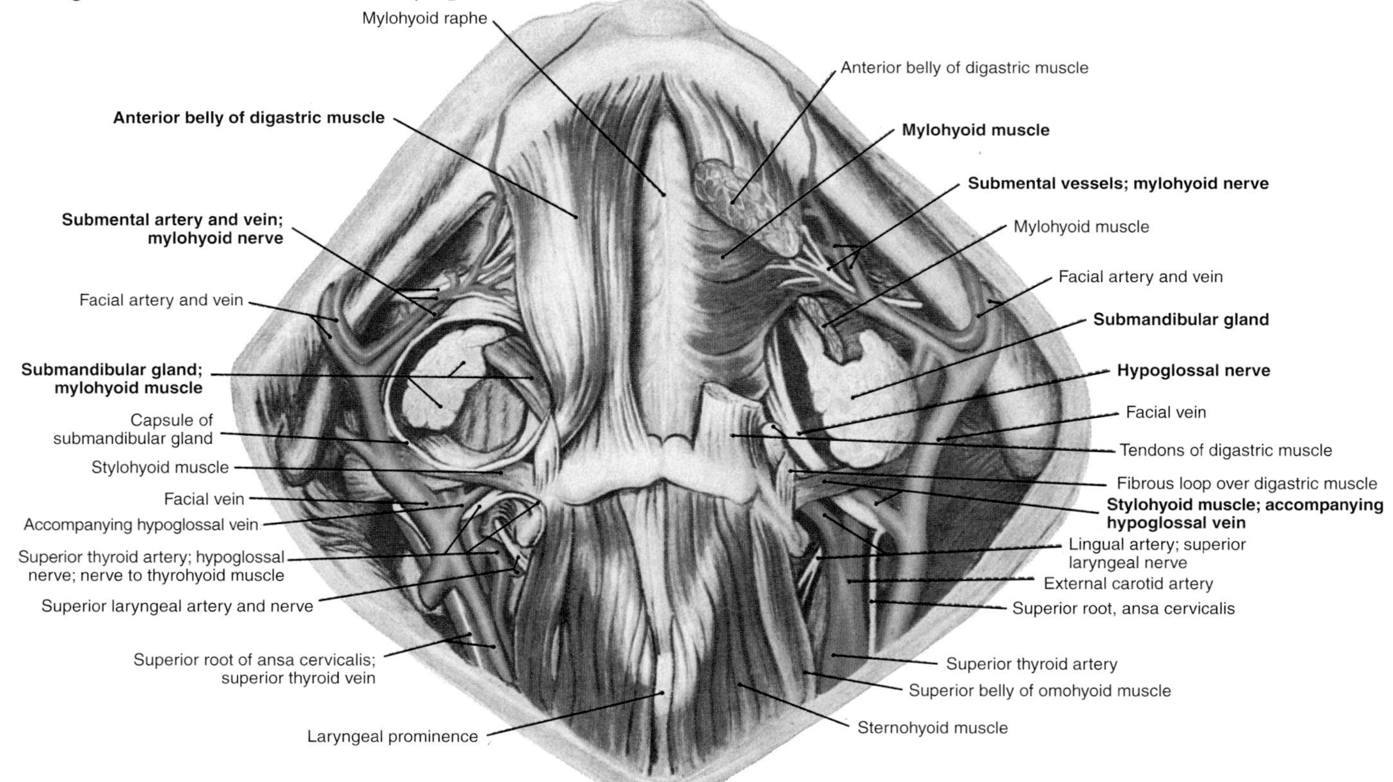
Mylohyoid raphe
Anterior belly of digastric muscle
Anterior belly of digastric muscle
Mylohyoid muscle
Submental vessels; mylohyoid nerve
Submental artery and vein; mylohyoid nerve
Mylohyoid muscle
Facial artery and vein
Facial artery and vein
Submandibular gland
Submandibular gland; mylohyoid muscle
Hypoglossal nerve
Facial vein
Capsule of submandibular gland
Tendons of digastric muscle
Stylohyoid muscle
Fibrous loop over digastric muscle
Facial vein
Stylohyoid muscle; accompanying hypoglossal vein
Accompanying hypoglossal vein
Lingual artery; superior laryngeal nerve
Superior thyroid artery; hypoglossal nerve; nerve to thyrohyoid muscle
External carotid artery
Superior laryngeal artery and nerve
Superior root, ansa cervicalis
Superior root of ansa cervicalis; superior thyroid vein
Superior thyroid artery
Superior belly of omohyoid muscle
Sternohyoid muscle
Laryngeal prominence

Figure 493.2 Submandibular and Submental Regions (Dissection Stages 3 [Reader's Left] and 4)
NOTE: In dissection **Stage** 3 much of the submandibular gland has been removed, revealing the **submental nerve** and the **mylohyoid nerve.** In **Stage** 4 (reader's right), the anterior digastric nerve and part of the mylohyoid nerve were removed, exposing the **hypoglossal nerve** and **accompanying vein.**

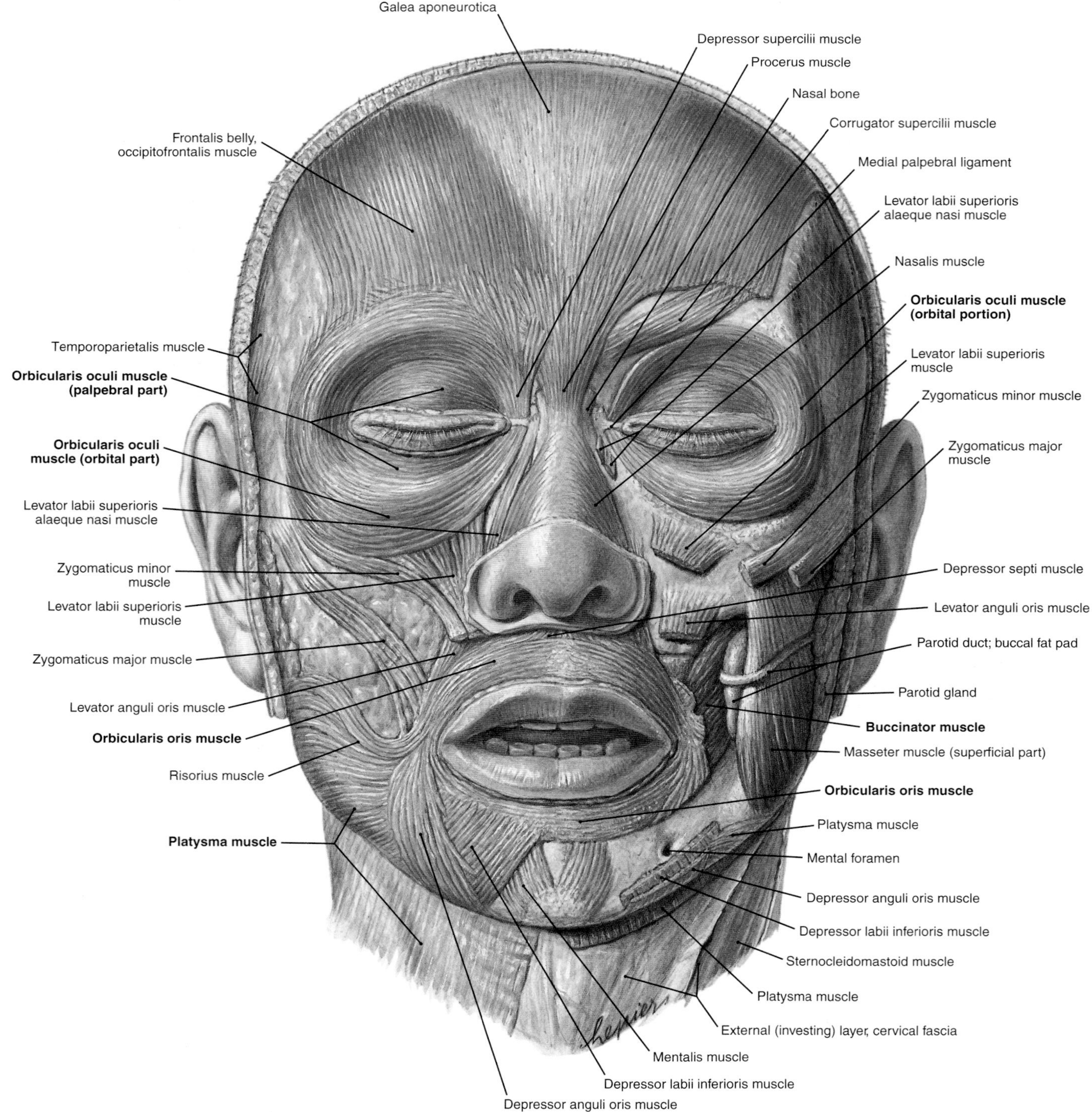
Galea aponeurotica
Depressor supercilii muscle
Procerus muscle
Nasal bone
Corrugator supercilii muscle
Medial palpebral ligament
Levator labii superioris alaeque nasi muscle
Nasalis muscle
Orbicularis oculi muscle (orbital portion)
Levator labii superioris muscle
Zygomaticus minor muscle
Zygomaticus major muscle
Depressor septi muscle
Levator anguli oris muscle
Parotid duct; buccal fat pad
Parotid gland
Buccinator muscle
Masseter muscle (superficial part)
Orbicularis oris muscle
Platysma muscle
Mental foramen
Depressor anguli oris muscle
Depressor labii inferioris muscle
Sternocleidomastoid muscle
Platysma muscle
External (investing) layer, cervical fascia
Mentalis muscle
Depressor labii inferioris muscle
Depressor anguli oris muscle
Frontalis belly, occipitofrontalis muscle
Temporoparietalis muscle
Orbicularis oculi muscle (palpebral part)
Orbicularis oculi muscle (orbital part)
Levator labii superioris alaeque nasi muscle
Zygomaticus minor muscle
Levator labii superioris muscle
Zygomaticus major muscle
Levator anguli oris muscle
Orbicularis oris muscle
Risorius muscle
Platysma muscle

Figure 494 Muscles of Facial Expression (Anterior View)

NOTE: (1) The muscles of facial expression are located within the layers of superficial fascia. Having developed from the mesoderm of the **second branchial arch,** they are innervated by the nerve of that arch, the seventh cranial or **facial nerve.**

(2) Facial muscles may be grouped into: (a) muscles of the **scalp,** (b) muscles of the **external ear,** (c) muscles of the **eyelid,** (d) the **nasal muscles,** and (e) the **oral muscles**. The borders of some facial muscles are not easily defined. The **platysma muscle** also belongs to the facial group, even though it extends over the neck.

(3) The circular muscles surrounding the eyes (**orbicularis oculi**) and the mouth (**orbicularis oris**) assist in closure of the orbital and oral apertures, and thus contribute to functions such as closing the eyes and the ingestion of liquids and food.

(4) Since facial muscles respond to thoughts and emotions, they aid in communication.

(5) The **buccinator muscles** are flat and are situated on the lateral aspects of the oral cavity. They assist in mastication by pressing the cheeks against the teeth, preventing food from accumulating in the oral vestibule.

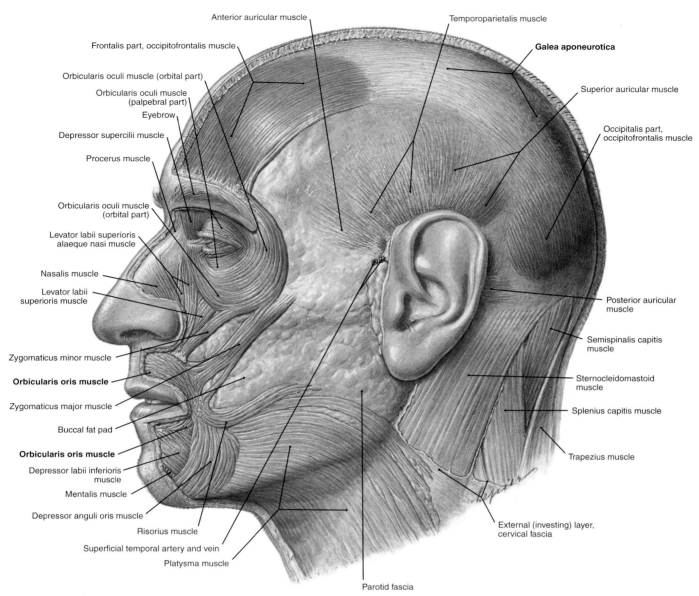

Anterior auricular muscle
Temporoparietalis muscle
Frontalis part, occipitofrontalis muscle
Galea aponeurotica
Orbicularis oculi muscle (orbital part)
Orbicularis oculi muscle (palpebral part)
Eyebrow
Superior auricular muscle
Depressor supercilii muscle
Occipitalis part, occipitofrontalis muscle
Procerus muscle
Orbicularis oculi muscle (orbital part)
Levator labii superioris alaeque nasi muscle
Nasalis muscle
Levator labii superioris muscle
Posterior auricular muscle
Semispinalis capitis muscle
Zygomaticus minor muscle
Orbicularis oris muscle
Sternocleidomastoid muscle
Zygomaticus major muscle
Splenius capitis muscle
Buccal fat pad
Orbicularis oris muscle
Trapezius muscle
Depressor labii inferioris muscle
Mentalis muscle
Depressor anguli oris muscle
Risorius muscle
External (investing) layer, cervical fascia
Superficial temporal artery and vein
Platysma muscle
Parotid fascia

Figure 495.1 **Muscles of Facial Expression and the Superficial Posterior Cervical Muscles**

NOTE: (1) The **frontalis** and **occipitalis** portions of the occipitofrontalis muscle are continuous with an epicranial aponeurosis called the **galea aponeurotica.**

(2) The **orbicularis oculi** consists of orbital, palpebral, and lacrimal (not shown) portions.

(3) Into the **orbicularis oris** merge a number of facial muscles in a somewhat radial manner.

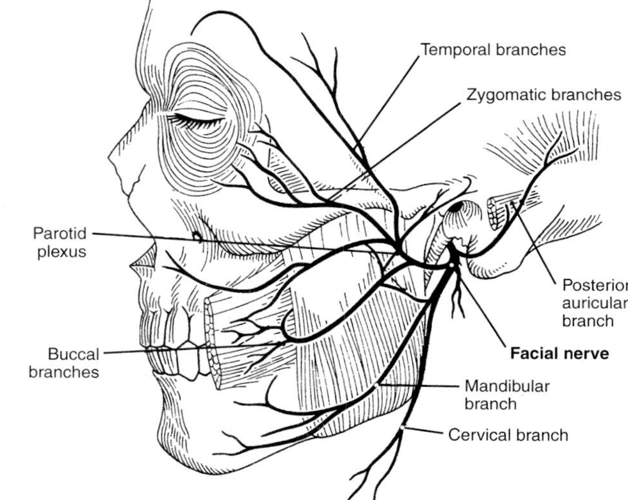
Temporal branches
Zygomatic branches
Parotid plexus
Posterior auricular branch
Facial nerve
Buccal branches
Mandibular branch
Cervical branch

Figure 495.2 **Branches of the Facial Nerve Supplying the Superficial Facial Muscles** ▶

NOTE: All the muscles of facial expression are innervated by branches of the seventh cranial nerve, the **facial nerve.** These branches are the **temporal, zygomatic, buccal, mandibular, cervical,** and **posterior auricular nerves.**

SUPRAHYOID MUSCLES

Muscle	Origin	Insertion	Innervation	Action
Digastric	Anterior belly: Digastric fossa on inner aspect of lower border of mandible. Posterior belly: Mastoid notch of the temporal bone.	Ends by an intermediate tendon between the two bellies that attaches to the hyoid bone	Anterior belly: Mylohyoid branch of trigeminal nerve (V). Posterior belly: Digastric branch of the facial nerve (VII).	Opens the mouth by depressing the mandible; elevates the hyoid bone
Stylohyoid	Posterior and lateral surface of styloid process of temporal bone	Body of the hyoid bone near the greater horn	Stylohyoid branch of the facial nerve (VII)	Elevates, fixes, and retracts the hyoid bone
Mylohyoid The two mylohyoid muscles form the floor of the oral cavity.	Entire length of the mylohyoid line of the mandible	Posterior fibers: Into body of the hyoid bone. Middle and anterior fibers: The median raphe between the muscles of both sides.	Mylohyoid branch of the trigeminal nerve (V)	During swallowing, both muscles raise floor of mouth, elevate the hyoid bone, and depress the mandible in opening the mouth.
Geniohyoid	Inferior mental spine on the inner surface of the symphysis menti	Anterior surface of the body of hyoid bone	First cervical nerve carried along the hypoglossal nerve	Elevates and draws hyoid bone forward; when hyoid is fixed, it retracts and depresses mandible.

SUPERFICIAL MUSCLES OF THE FACE AND HEAD
MUSCLES OF THE SCALP

Muscle	Origin	Insertion	Innervation	Action
Occipitofrontalis	Occipital belly: Lateral two-thirds of superior nuchal line on occipital bone and mastoid part of temporal bone	Into the galea aponeurotica	Posterior auricular branch of the facial nerve (VII)	Draws scalp back; raises eye brow and wrinkles forehead in expression of surprise
	Frontal belly: Fibers continuous with those of procerus medially and orbicularis oculi laterally	Into the galea aponeurotica	Temporal branch of the facial nerve (VII)	
Temporoparietalis	From temporal fascia above and in front of auricle of ear	Onto the temporal fascia and skin on the side of the head	Temporal branch of the facial nerve (VII)	Tightens the scalp and draws back the skin of the temples

EXTRINSIC MUSCLES OF THE EAR

Muscle	Origin	Insertion	Innervation	Action
Anterior auricular	Anterior part of the temporal fascia	Onto the spine of the helix	Temporal branch of the facial nerve (VII)	Draws auricle of ear forward and upward (minimal action)
Superior auricular	Epicranial aponeurosis on the side of the head	Upper part of the cranial surface of auricle of ear	Temporal branch of the facial nerve (VII)	Draws the auricle of the ear upward (minimal action)
Posterior auricular	Mastoid process of the temporal bone	Medial surface of auricle at convexity of concha	Posterior auricular branch of the facial nerve (VII)	Draws the auricle backward (minimal action)

MUSCLES OF EYELIDS

Muscle	Origin	Insertion	Innervation	Action
Orbicularis oculi: Palpebral part	Medial palpebral ligament	Cross the eyelids and interlace to form the lateral palpebral raphe	Temporal and zygomatic branches of the facial facial nerve (VII)	Closes the eyelids gently as in sleeping and blinking
Orbital part	Nasal part of frontal bone; frontal process of the maxilla; medial palpebral ligament	Forms ellipse around orbit without being interrupted on the lateral side	Temporal and zygomatic branches of the facial nerve (VII)	Closes the eyelids when a more forceful contraction is necessary, as in winking one eye
Corrugator supercilii	Medial end of the superciliary arch	Deep surface of the skin above the middle of the supraorbital margin	Temporal branch of the facial nerve (VII)	Draws the eyebrow medially and down

SUPERFICIAL MUSCLES OF THE FACE AND HEAD (CONT.)
MUSCLES OF THE NOSE

Muscle	Origin	Insertion	Innervation	Action
Procerus	From fascia over the lower of the nasal bone	Into the skin of the lower part of the forehead between eyebrows	Buccal branch of the facial nerve (VII)	Draws down the medial angle of eyebrow such as in frowning or concentration
Nasalis	Transverse part: From the maxilla lateral to the nasal notch.	Ascends to bridge of nose; meshes with opposite insertion	Buccal branch of the facial nerve (VII)	Compresses the nasal aperture
	Alar part: From the maxilla above the lateral incisor tooth.	Attaches to the cartilaginous ala of the nose	Buccal branch of the facial nerve (VII)	Assists in opening the nasal aperture in deep inspiration
Depressor septi	From the maxilla above the medial incisor	Into the mobile part of the nasal septum	Buccal branch of the facial nerve (VII)	Assists alar part of nasalis muscle in widening nares

MUSCLES OF THE MOUTH

Muscle	Origin	Insertion	Innervation	Action
Levator labii superioris	Along lower part of orbit from maxilla and zygomatic bones	Upper lip between levators anguli oris and labii superioris alaeque nasi	Buccal branch of the facial nerve (VII)	Raises the upper lip and carries it forward
Levator labii superioris alaeque nasi	Upper part of the frontal process of the maxilla	Inserts by two slips: into alar cartilage and into upper lip with levator labii superioris	Buccal branch of the facial nerve (VII)	Raises the upper lip and dilates the nostril
Levator anguli oris	Canine fossa of the maxilla just below the infraorbital foramen	Into angle of mouth merging with orbicularis oris, depressor anguli oris, and zygomaticus major	Buccal branch of the facial nerve (VII)	Raises the angle of the mouth and forms the nasolabial furrow
Zygomaticus minor	Lateral surface of the zygomatic bone	Upper lip between levator labii superioris and zygomaticus major	Buccal branch of the facial nerve (VII)	Elevates the upper lip and helps form the nasolabial furrow
Zygomaticus major	From the zygomatic bone in front of the zygomatico-temporal suture	Into angle of mouth with levator and depressor anguli oris and orbicularis oris muscles	Buccal branch of the facial nerve (VII)	Draws the angle of the mouth upward and backward as in laughing
Risorius	From parotid fascia over masseter muscle	Into the skin at the angle of the mouth	Buccal branch of the facial nerve (VII)	Retracts the angle of the mouth
Depressor labii inferioris	Oblique line of mandible between symphysis menti and the mental foramen	Into lower lip and at midline blending with muscle from other side	Mandibular branch of the facial nerve (VII)	Draws the lower lip downward and a bit laterally
Depressor anguli oris	From oblique line of mandible, lateral and below depressor labii inferioris	Into the angle of the mouth blending with orbicularis oris and risorius	Mandibular branch of the facial nerve (VII)	Draws angle of mouth down and laterally as in expression of sadness
Mentalis	From the incisive fossa of the mandible	Into the skin of the chin	Mandibular branch of the facial nerve (VII)	Raises and protrudes lower lip; wrinkles chin in expression of doubt or disdain
Orbicularis oris	Fibers derived from other facial muscles (buccinator, levators, and depressors of lips and angles, zygomatic muscles) pass into lips; also some intrinsic muscle fibers make up orbicularis oris	Several strata of muscle fibers form a sphincter-like muscle with fibers that decussate at the angles of the mouth	Buccal branch of the facial nerve (VII)	Closes the lips, and its deep fibers can press the lips against the teeth; also it protrudes the lips and is important in speech
Buccinator	Alveolar processes of mandible and maxilla opposite upper and lower molar teeth; posteriorly, it arises from the pterygo-mandibular raphe opposite superior constrictor	Fibers course forward to blend into the formation of the orbicularis oris, decussating at the angles of the mouth	Buccal branch of the facial nerve (VII)	Compresses the cheeks during chewing; also compresses the distended cheeks as in blowing a horn

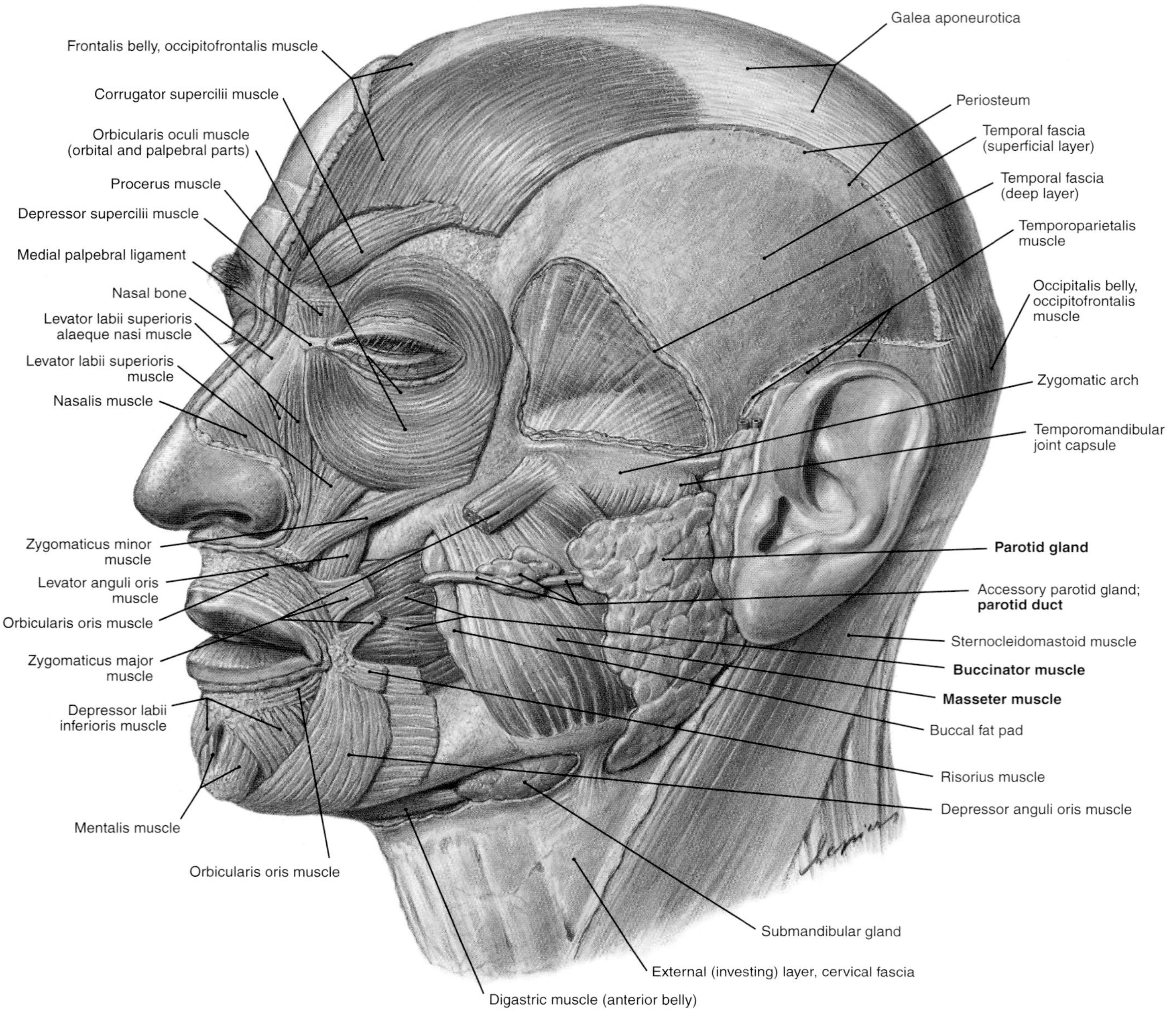

Frontalis belly, occipitofrontalis muscle
Corrugator supercilii muscle
Orbicularis oculi muscle (orbital and palpebral parts)
Procerus muscle
Depressor supercilii muscle
Medial palpebral ligament
Nasal bone
Levator labii superioris alaeque nasi muscle
Levator labii superioris muscle
Nasalis muscle
Zygomaticus minor muscle
Levator anguli oris muscle
Orbicularis oris muscle
Zygomaticus major muscle
Depressor labii inferioris muscle
Mentalis muscle
Orbicularis oris muscle
Galea aponeurotica
Periosteum
Temporal fascia (superficial layer)
Temporal fascia (deep layer)
Temporoparietalis muscle
Occipitalis belly, occipitofrontalis muscle
Zygomatic arch
Temporomandibular joint capsule
Parotid gland
Accessory parotid gland; **parotid duct**
Sternocleidomastoid muscle
Buccinator muscle
Masseter muscle
Buccal fat pad
Risorius muscle
Depressor anguli oris muscle
Submandibular gland
External (investing) layer, cervical fascia
Digastric muscle (anterior belly)

Figure 498.1 Parotid Gland and Duct and the Masseter Muscle

NOTE: (1) The **parotid gland** extends from the zygomatic arch to below the angle of the mandible. It lies anterior to the ear and superficial to the **masseter muscle.** It is enclosed in a tight fascial sheath, and its duct courses medially across the face to enter the oral cavity through the fibers of the **buccinator muscle.**

(2) The masseter muscle extends from the zygomatic bone to the ramus, angle, and body of the mandible. It elevates the mandible (closes the mouth) and is supplied by the trigeminal nerve.

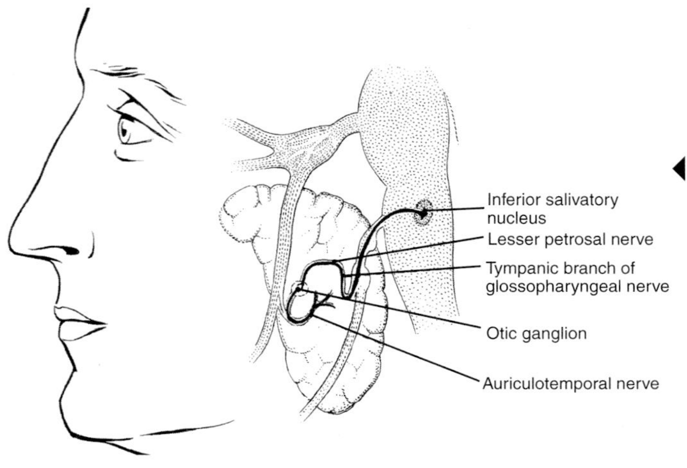
Inferior salivatory nucleus
Lesser petrosal nerve
Tympanic branch of glossopharyngeal nerve
Otic ganglion
Auriculotemporal nerve

Figure 498.2 Parasympathetic Innervation of the Parotid Gland

NOTE: (1) Preganglionic parasympathetic fibers that innervate the parotid gland emerge from the brainstem in the ninth (glossopharyngeal) nerve.

(2) These fibers then travel along the **tympanic nerve** to the middle ear, and then form the **lesser petrosal nerve** that joins the **otic ganglion.**

(3) Postganglionic fibers then travel within the **auriculotemporal nerve** to reach the parotid gland.

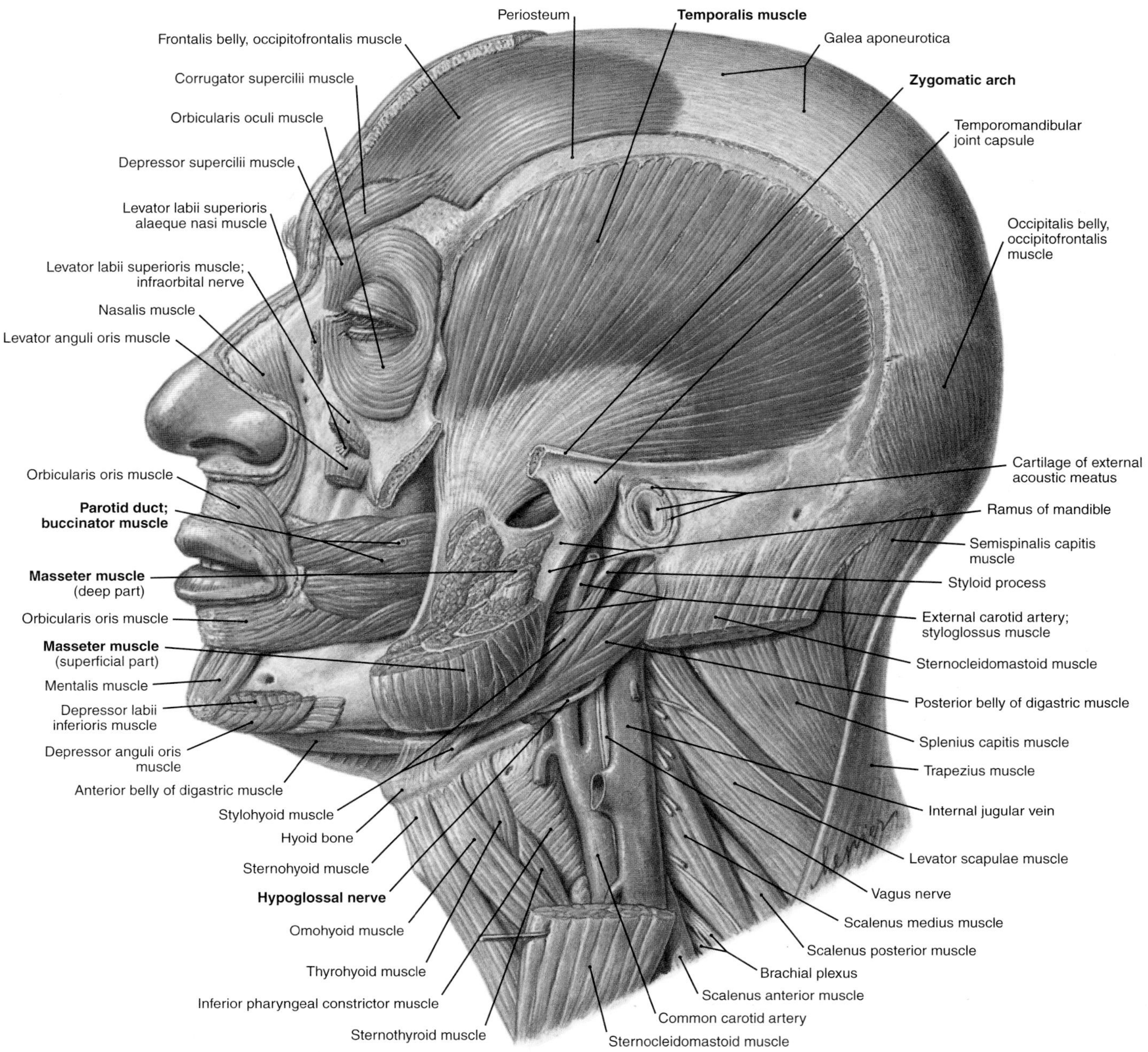

Periosteum
Temporalis muscle
Frontalis belly, occipitofrontalis muscle
Galea aponeurotica
Corrugator supercilii muscle
Zygomatic arch
Orbicularis oculi muscle
Temporomandibular joint capsule
Depressor supercilii muscle
Levator labii superioris alaeque nasi muscle
Occipitalis belly, occipitofrontalis muscle
Levator labii superioris muscle; infraorbital nerve
Nasalis muscle
Levator anguli oris muscle
Cartilage of external acoustic meatus
Orbicularis oris muscle
Ramus of mandible
Parotid duct; buccinator muscle
Semispinalis capitis muscle
Masseter muscle (deep part)
Styloid process
Orbicularis oris muscle
External carotid artery; styloglossus muscle
Masseter muscle (superficial part)
Sternocleidomastoid muscle
Mentalis muscle
Posterior belly of digastric muscle
Depressor labii inferioris muscle
Splenius capitis muscle
Depressor anguli oris muscle
Trapezius muscle
Anterior belly of digastric muscle
Internal jugular vein
Stylohyoid muscle
Hyoid bone
Levator scapulae muscle
Sternohyoid muscle
Vagus nerve
Hypoglossal nerve
Scalenus medius muscle
Omohyoid muscle
Scalenus posterior muscle
Brachial plexus
Thyrohyoid muscle
Scalenus anterior muscle
Inferior pharyngeal constrictor muscle
Common carotid artery
Sternothyroid muscle
Sternocleidomastoid muscle

Figure 499.1 **Temporalis and Buccinator Muscles**

NOTE: (1) The external ear and zygomatic arch have been removed, along with most of the masseter muscle to demonstrate the origin of the temporalis muscle from the temporal fossa and its insertion on the coronoid process of the mandible. Similar to the masseter, the temporalis is innervated by the mandibular branch of the trigeminal nerve.

(2) The various fiber bundles of the buccinator muscle as they extend directly into the orbicularis oris at both the upper and lower lips. Similar to the other facial muscles, the buccinator is supplied by the facial nerve (VII, buccal branch).

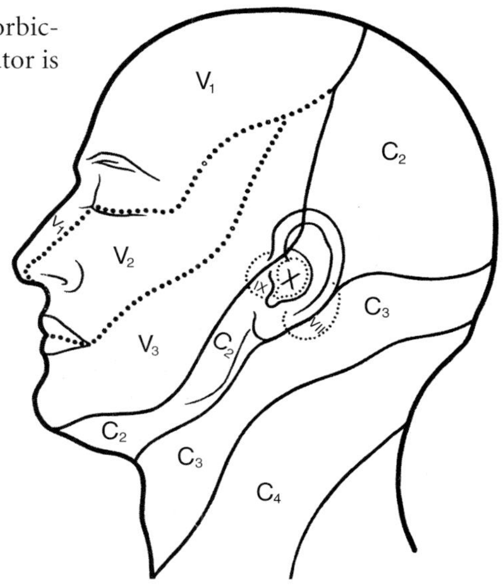
V_1
C_2
V_2
X
IX
C_3
VII
V_3
C_2
C_2
C_3
C_4

Figure 499.2 **Cutaneous Nerve Patterns (Dermatomes) of the Head and Neck** ▶

NOTE: (1) The anterior and lateral surfaces of the head and face are supplied by the divisions of the trigeminal nerve.

(2) The posterior and lateral surfaces of the head and neck are supplied by the cervical nerves. Small areas of skin around the car are innervated by the facial (VII), glossopharyngeal (IX), and vagus (X) nerves.

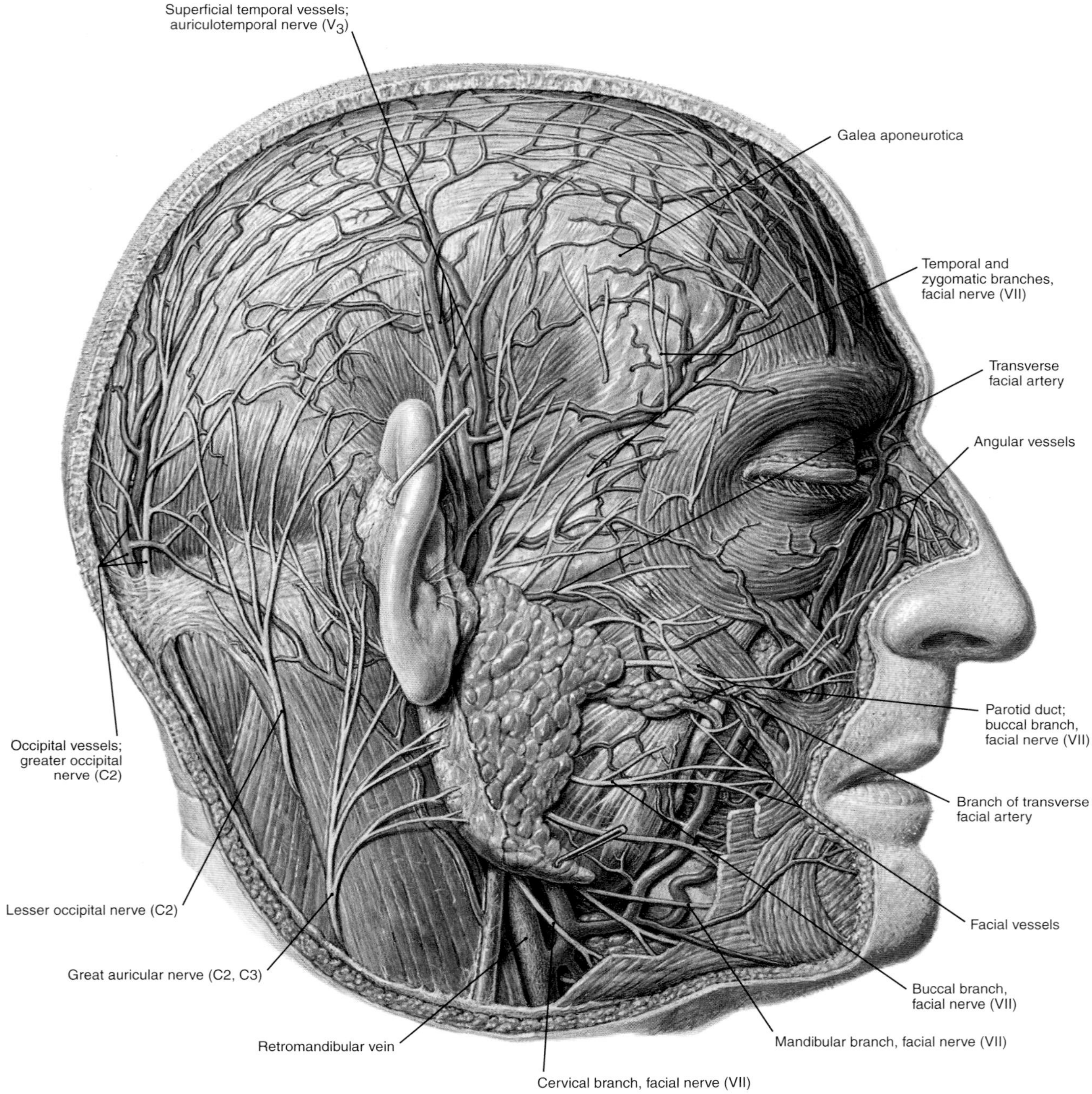
Superficial temporal vessels; auriculotemporal nerve (V_3)
Galea aponeurotica
Temporal and zygomatic branches, facial nerve (VII)
Transverse facial artery
Angular vessels
Parotid duct; buccal branch, facial nerve (VII)
Branch of transverse facial artery
Facial vessels
Buccal branch, facial nerve (VII)
Mandibular branch, facial nerve (VII)
Cervical branch, facial nerve (VII)
Retromandibular vein
Great auricular nerve (C2, C3)
Lesser occipital nerve (C2)
Occipital vessels; greater occipital nerve (C2)

Figure 500 Superficial Dissection of the Face: Vessels and Nerves (Dissection 1)

NOTE: (1) in this dissection the capsule of the parotid gland has been opened to reveal the substance of the gland and the branches of the **facial nerve** that emerge from under its borders. These cross the face to supply the muscles of facial expression (see Fig. 501) for a more complete view of the facial branches.

(2) The cervical nerves. The **greater occipital nerve** is a sensory nerve from the *posterior* primary ramus of C2, and it courses upward with the occipital vessels to supply the posterior scalp. The **lesser occipital** (**C2**) and **great auricular** (**C2, C3**) **nerves** are from the anterior primary rami and are also sensory nerves. They supply the posterolateral neck region and the lateral scalp behind the ear.

(3) The course of the **facial artery and vein** is partially covered by the muscles of facial expression. These vessels have been exposed to demonstrate their ascent lateral to the nose to reach the medial side of the orbit where they are called the **angular artery and vein.**

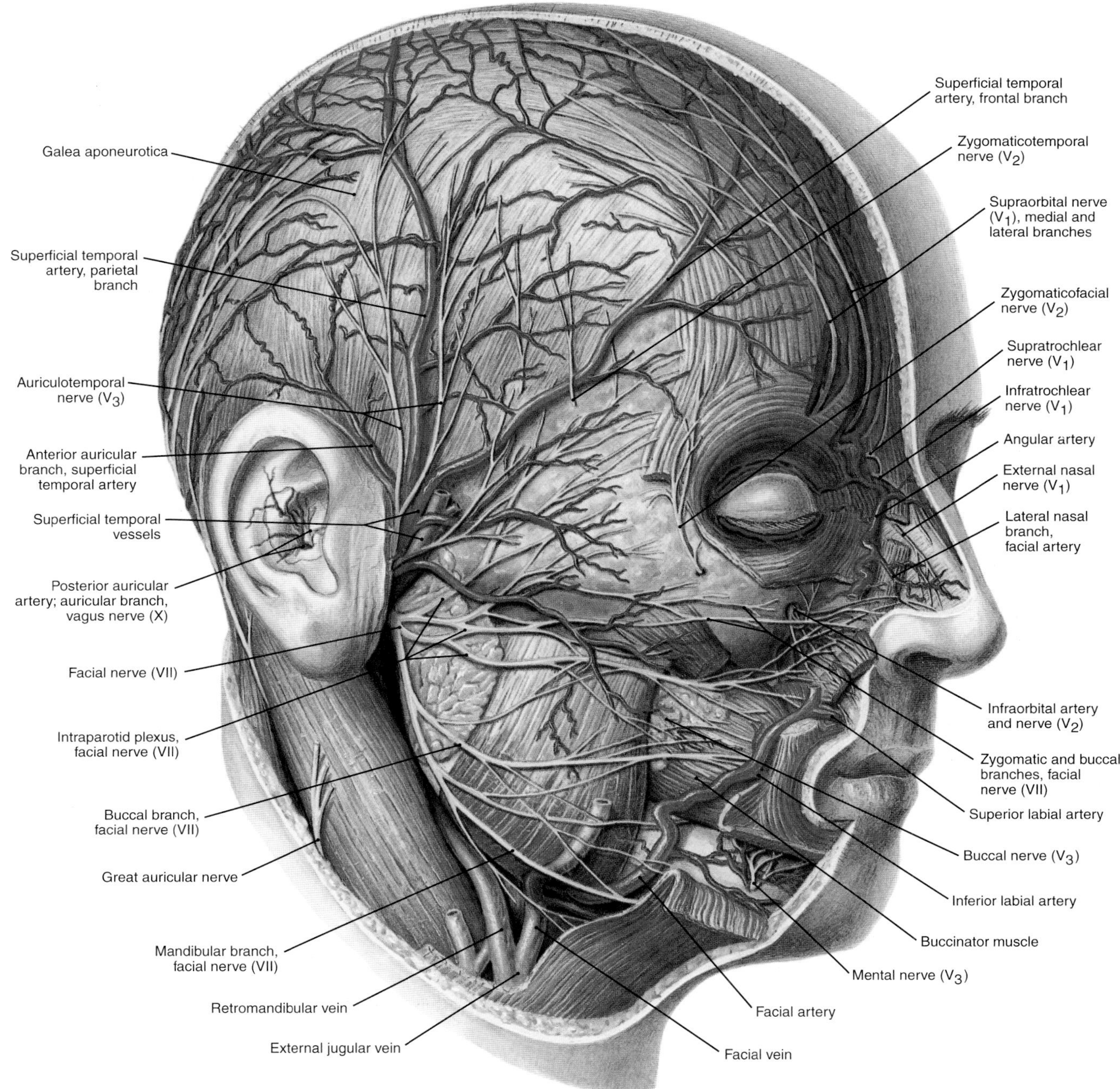
Galea aponeurotica
Superficial temporal artery, parietal branch
Auriculotemporal nerve (V_3)
Anterior auricular branch, superficial temporal artery
Superficial temporal vessels
Posterior auricular artery; auricular branch, vagus nerve (X)
Facial nerve (VII)
Intraparotid plexus, facial nerve (VII)
Buccal branch, facial nerve (VII)
Great auricular nerve
Mandibular branch, facial nerve (VII)
Retromandibular vein
External jugular vein
Superficial temporal artery, frontal branch
Zygomaticotemporal nerve (V_2)
Supraorbital nerve (V_1), medial and lateral branches
Zygomaticofacial nerve (V_2)
Supratrochlear nerve (V_1)
Infratrochlear nerve (V_1)
Angular artery
External nasal nerve (V_1)
Lateral nasal branch, facial artery
Infraorbital artery and nerve (V_2)
Zygomatic and buccal branches, facial nerve (VII)
Superior labial artery
Buccal nerve (V_3)
Inferior labial artery
Buccinator muscle
Mental nerve (V_3)
Facial artery
Facial vein

Figure 501 **Superficial Dissection of the Face: Vessels and Nerves (Dissection 2)**

NOTE: (1) The superficial part of the parotid gland has been removed to show the branches of the **facial nerve,** which emerge from the substance of the gland. Identify the **temporal, zygomatic, buccal, mandibular,** and **cervical** branches. The **posterior auricular** branch is not shown.

(2) The superficial sensory branches of the **trigeminal nerve:**

(a) From the **ophthalmic division:** the supraorbital, supratrochlear, the ascending and descending branches of the infratrochlear, and the external nasal.

(b) From the **maxillary division:** the zygomaticotemporal, zygomaticofacial and the infraorbital.

(c) From the **mandibular division:** the buccal, mental, and auriculotemporal.

(3) The general distribution of **superficial temporal artery**. Observe also the course of the **facial artery** across the face to become the **angular artery.** Among other structures, the facial artery supplies the chin and the upper and lower lips and it anastomoses with vessels emerging from the orbit.

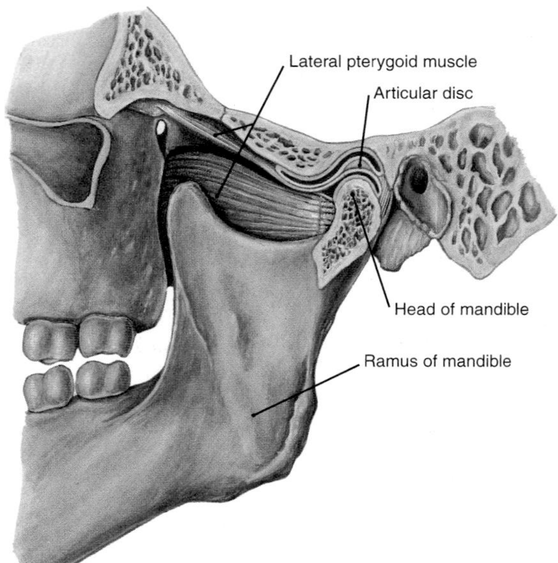
Lateral pterygoid muscle
Articular disc
Head of mandible
Ramus of mandible

Figure 502.1 Lateral Pterygoid Muscle (Lateral View)

NOTE: (1) The **lateral pterygoid muscle** arises by two heads, a **superior** from the greater wing of the sphenoid bone and an **inferior** from the lateral surface of the lateral pterygoid plate of the sphenoid.

(2) The two heads insert posteriorly on the neck of the condyle of the mandible and the articular disc of the temporomandibular joint. The lateral pterygoid muscle opens and protracts the mandible and also moves it from side to side.

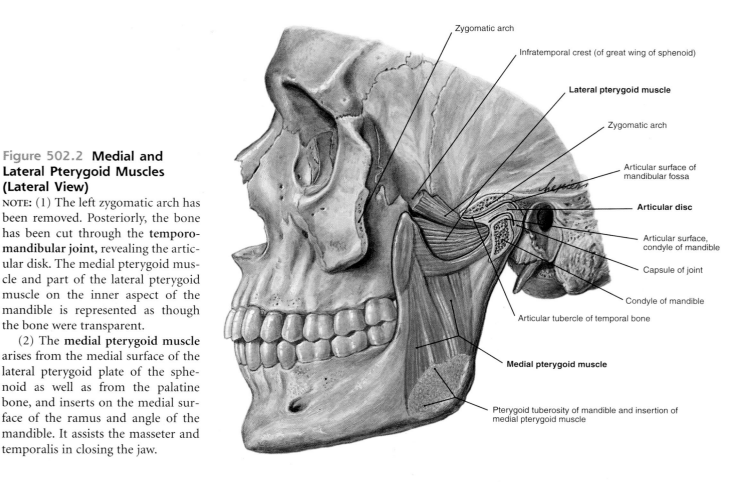

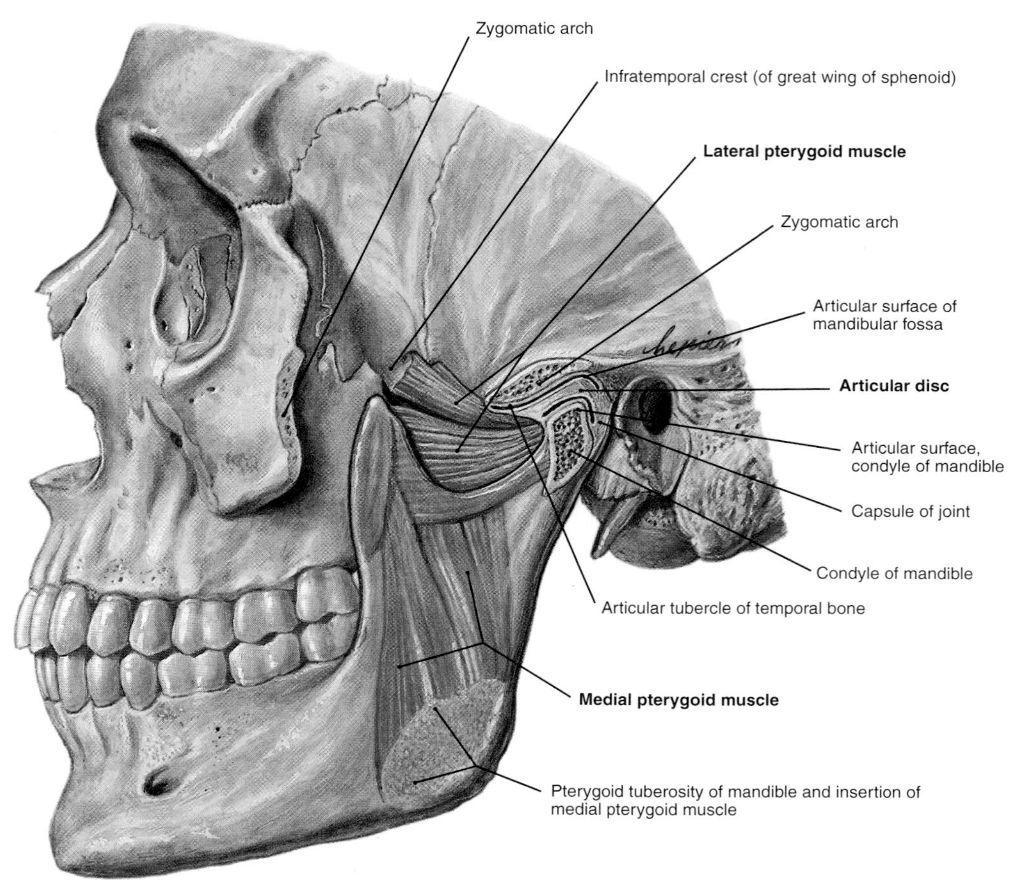
Zygomatic arch
Infratemporal crest (of great wing of sphenoid)
Lateral pterygoid muscle
Zygomatic arch
Articular surface of mandibular fossa
Articular disc
Articular surface, condyle of mandible
Capsule of joint
Condyle of mandible
Articular tubercle of temporal bone
Medial pterygoid muscle
Pterygoid tuberosity of mandible and insertion of medial pterygoid muscle

Figure 502.2 Medial and Lateral Pterygoid Muscles (Lateral View)

NOTE: (1) The left zygomatic arch has been removed. Posteriorly, the bone has been cut through the **temporomandibular joint,** revealing the articular disk. The medial pterygoid muscle and part of the lateral pterygoid muscle on the inner aspect of the mandible is represented as though the bone were transparent.

(2) The **medial pterygoid muscle** arises from the medial surface of the lateral pterygoid plate of the sphenoid as well as from the palatine bone, and inserts on the medial surface of the ramus and angle of the mandible. It assists the masseter and temporalis in closing the jaw.

MUSCLES OF MASTICATION

Muscle	Origin	Insertion	Innervation	Action
Masseter	Zygomatic surface of maxilla and the zygomatic arch	Lateral surface of ramus of mandible and the coronoid process of mandible	Masseteric branch of mandibular nerve	Closes the jaw by elevating the mandible
Temporalis	Temporal fossa and deep surface of the temporal fascia	Medial surface of anterior border of coronoid process; anterior border of ramus of mandible	Deep temporal branches of the mandibular nerve	Elevates mandible and closes the jaw; posterior fibers retract mandible

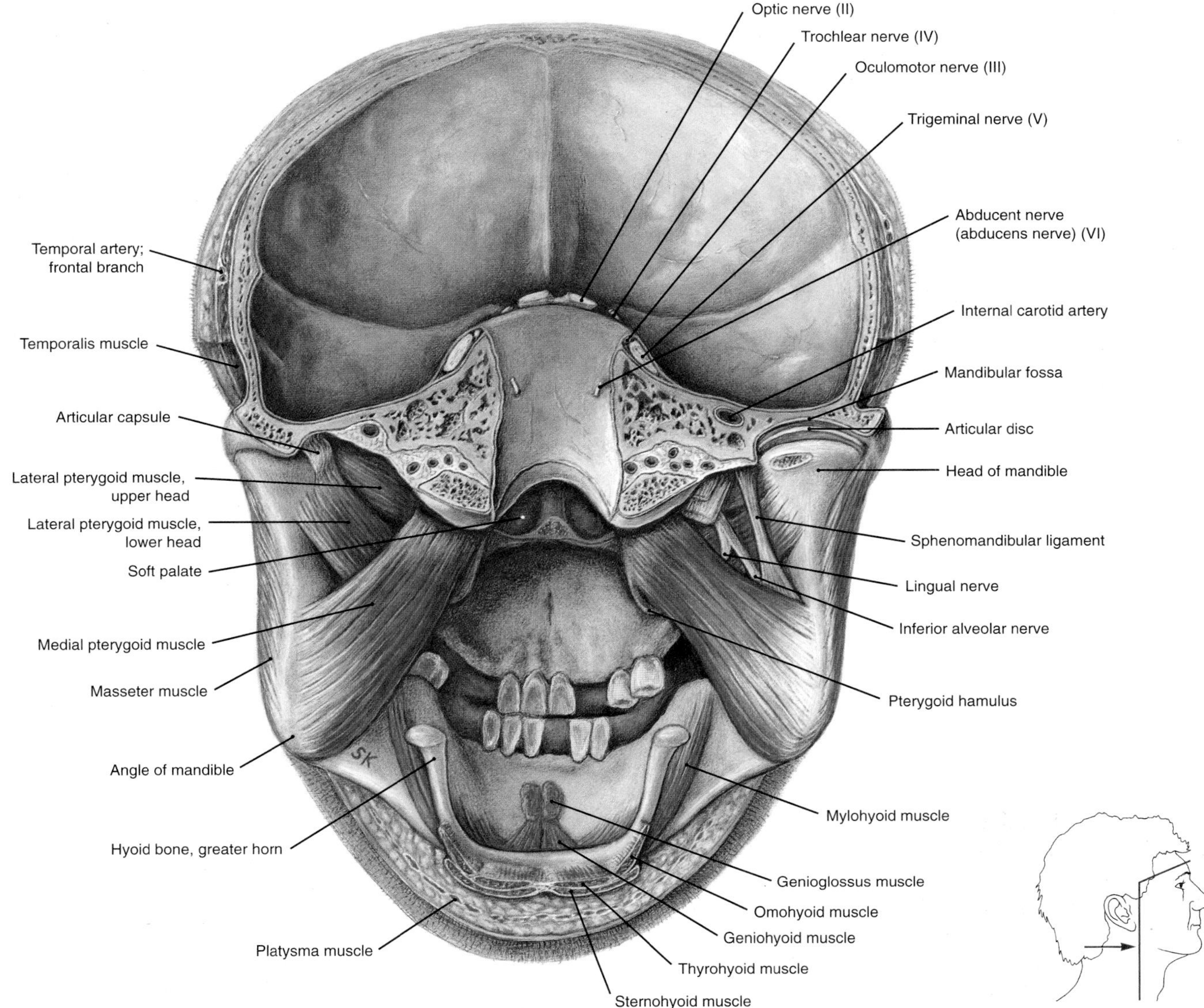
Optic nerve (II)
Trochlear nerve (IV)
Oculomotor nerve (III)
Trigeminal nerve (V)
Abducent nerve (abducens nerve) (VI)
Internal carotid artery
Mandibular fossa
Articular disc
Head of mandible
Sphenomandibular ligament
Lingual nerve
Inferior alveolar nerve
Pterygoid hamulus
Mylohyoid muscle
Genioglossus muscle
Omohyoid muscle
Geniohyoid muscle
Thyrohyoid muscle
Sternohyoid muscle
Temporal artery; frontal branch
Temporalis muscle
Articular capsule
Lateral pterygoid muscle, upper head
Lateral pterygoid muscle, lower head
Soft palate
Medial pterygoid muscle
Masseter muscle
Angle of mandible
Hyoid bone, greater horn
Platysma muscle

Figure 503 **Pterygoid, Mylohyoid, and Geniohyoid Muscles as Seen from Below and Behind**

NOTE: (1) A muscular sling is formed around the ramus of mandible to its angle by the insertions of the **medial pterygoid** (seen on the right) and **masseter muscles** (seen on the left). The medial pterygoid muscle descends to attach along the medial aspect of the mandible, while the masseter courses down to insert on the outer aspect of the jaw.

(2) The fibers of the lateral pterygoid (right side) course principally in the horizontal plane. The **mylohyoid** and **geniohyoid muscles** attach the mandible to the hyoid bone. Other muscles shown are the **tensor** and **levator veli palatini muscles.**

MUSCLES OF MASTICATION (Cont.)

Muscle	Origin	Insertion	Innervation	Action
Lateral pterygoid	**Superior head:** Infratemporal crest and lateral surface of greater wing of sphenoid bone. Inferior head: Lateral surface of lateral pterygoid plate of sphenoid.	Neck of condyle of mandible; articular disk and capsule of temporomandibular joint	Lateral pterygoid branch of mandibular nerve	Opens mouth by drawing condyle and disk forward.. Acting together: protrudes mandible. Acting alternately: grinding action.
Medial pterygoid	**Deep head:** Medial surface of lateral pterygoid plate of sphenoid; pyramidal process of palatine bone. Superficial head: Pyramidal process of palatine bone; tuberosity of maxilla.	Lower and posterior part of medial surface of ramus and angle of mandible	Medial pterygoid branch of mandibular nerve	Elevates mandible closing jaw. Acting together: protrudes mandible Acting alone: protrudes one side. Acting alternately: grinding action.

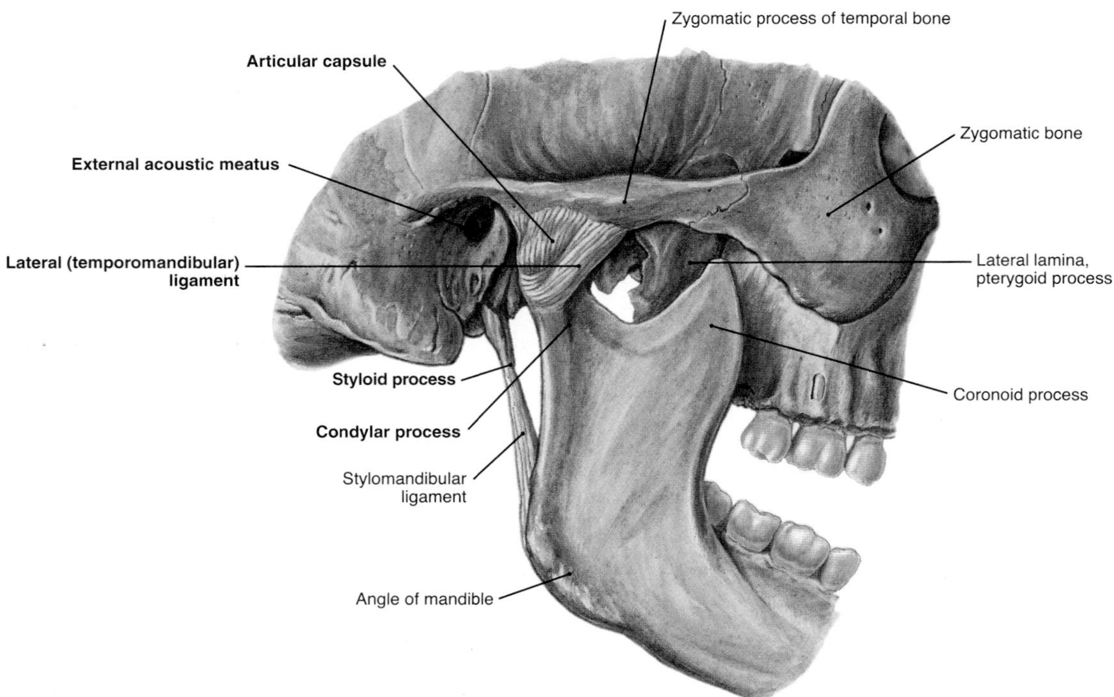
Zygomatic process of temporal bone
Articular capsule
Zygomatic bone
External acoustic meatus
Lateral (temporomandibular) ligament
Lateral lamina, pterygoid process
Coronoid process
Styloid process
Condylar process
Stylomandibular ligament
Angle of mandible

Figure 504.1 Right Temporomandibular Joint (Lateral View)

NOTE: (1) The articular capsule and the **lateral** (temporomandibular) **ligament** extend between the zygomatic process of the temporal bone above to the neck of the condylar process of the mandibular ramus below.

(2) The articular capsule is a loose sac that is fused anteriorly and laterally with the **lateral ligament.** Note also, the **stylomandibular ligament** extending from the tip of the styloid process to the angle and posterior border of the mandible.

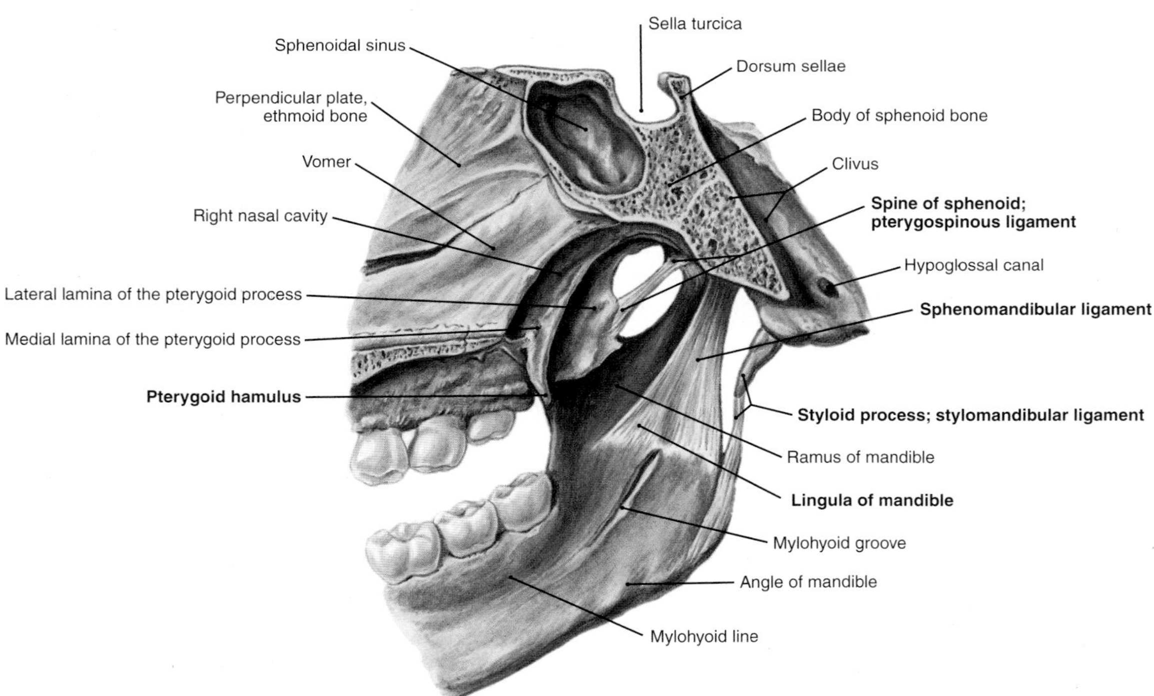
Sella turcica
Sphenoidal sinus
Dorsum sellae
Perpendicular plate, ethmoid bone
Body of sphenoid bone
Vomer
Clivus
Right nasal cavity
Spine of sphenoid; pterygospinous ligament
Hypoglossal canal
Lateral lamina of the pterygoid process
Sphenomandibular ligament
Medial lamina of the pterygoid process
Pterygoid hamulus
Styloid process; stylomandibular ligament
Ramus of mandible
Lingula of mandible
Mylohyoid groove
Angle of mandible
Mylohyoid line

Figure 504.2 Right Temporomandibular Region (Medial View)

NOTE: Medial to the temporomandibular joint, the **pterygospinous ligament** extends from the sphenoidal spine to the posterior margin of the lateral pterygoid plate. The **sphenomandibular ligament** descends from the sphenoidal spine to the lingula of the mandible.

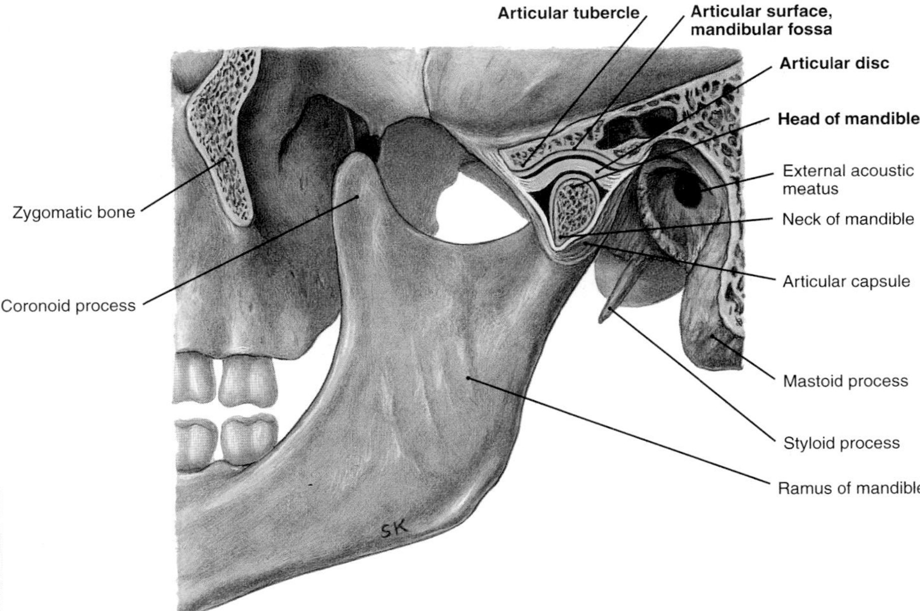
Articular tubercle
Articular surface, mandibular fossa
Articular disc
Head of mandible
External acoustic meatus
Neck of mandible
Articular capsule
Mastoid process
Styloid process
Ramus of mandible
Zygomatic bone
Coronoid process

Figure 505.1 Sagittal Section of the Temporomandibular Joint with the Jaw Closed

NOTE: (1) An **articular disk** is interposed between the mandibular fossa of the temporal bone and the mandibular condyle, creating two joint cavities.

(2) With the jaw closed, the head of the condyle of the mandible and the articular disk lie totally within the mandibular fossa.

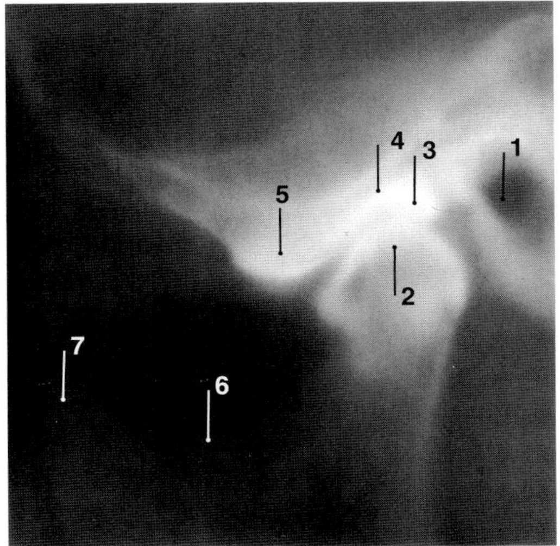
1
2
3
4
5
6
7

Figure 505.2 Arthrograph of the Temporomandibular Joint with the Jaw Closed

Fig. 505.2 and 505.4

1. External acoustic meatus
2. Condylar process
3. Articular disk
4. Mandibular fossa, temporal bone
5. Articular tubercle, temporal bone
6. Mandibular notch
7. Coronoid process

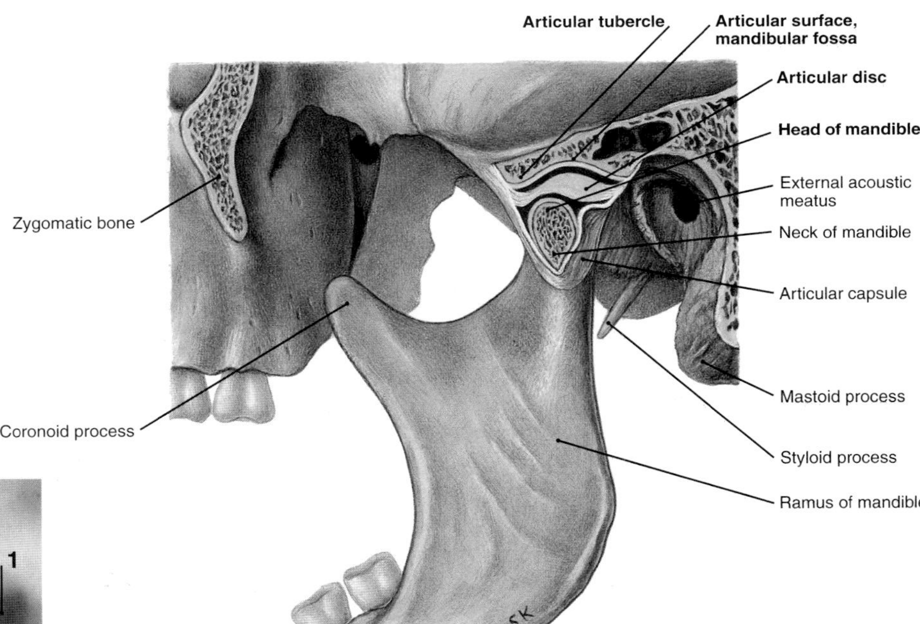
Articular tubercle
Articular surface, mandibular fossa
Articular disc
Head of mandible
External acoustic meatus
Neck of mandible
Articular capsule
Mastoid process
Styloid process
Ramus of mandible
Zygomatic bone
Coronoid process

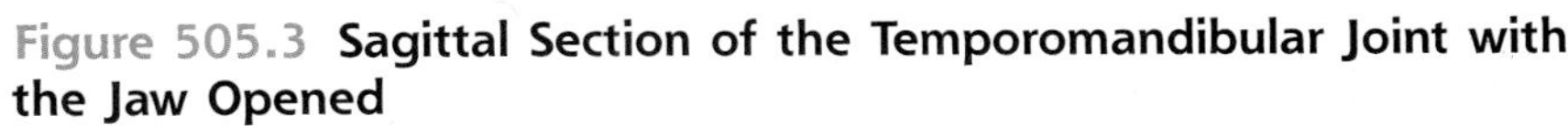

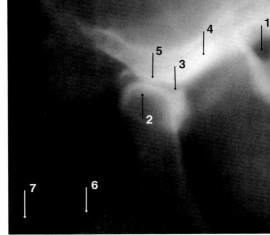

Figure 505.3 Sagittal Section of the Temporomandibular Joint with the Jaw Opened

NOTE: When the jaw is opened, the condyle **glides forward** within the joint capsule to lie opposite the **articular tubercle** of the temporal bone.

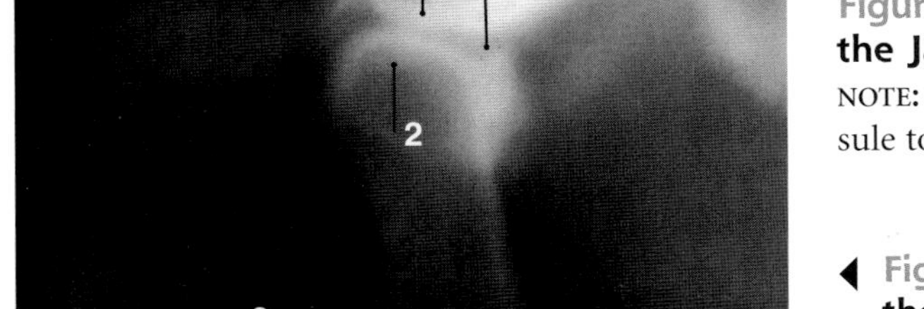
1
2
3
4
5
6
7

Figure 505.4 Arthrograph of the Temporomandibular Joint with the Jaw Opened

NOTE: The mandibular condyle moves forward significantly when the jaw is opened. In Figs. 505.2 and 505.4 compare the distance between the condyle (2) and the external acoustic meatus (1).

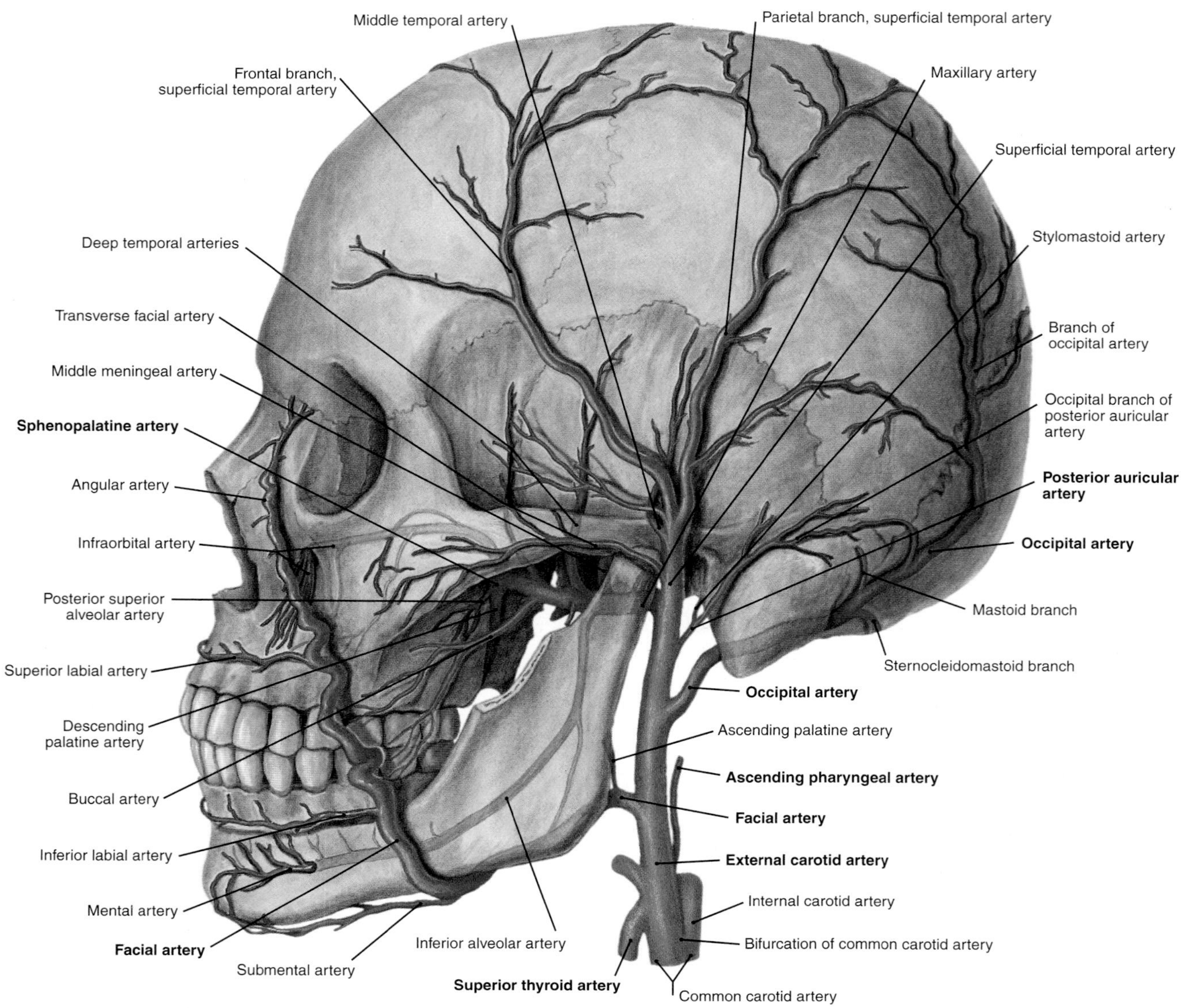
Middle temporal artery
Parietal branch, superficial temporal artery
Frontal branch, superficial temporal artery
Maxillary artery
Superficial temporal artery
Deep temporal arteries
Stylomastoid artery
Transverse facial artery
Branch of occipital artery
Middle meningeal artery
Occipital branch of posterior auricular artery
Sphenopalatine artery
Angular artery
Posterior auricular artery
Infraorbital artery
Occipital artery
Posterior superior alveolar artery
Mastoid branch
Superior labial artery
Sternocleidomastoid branch
Occipital artery
Descending palatine artery
Ascending palatine artery
Ascending pharyngeal artery
Buccal artery
Facial artery
Inferior labial artery
External carotid artery
Internal carotid artery
Mental artery
Bifurcation of common carotid artery
Facial artery
Inferior alveolar artery
Submental artery
Superior thyroid artery
Common carotid artery

Figure 506 External Carotid Artery and Its Branches

NOTE: (1) The **external carotid artery** branches from the common carotid and is the principal artery that supplies the anterior neck, the face, the scalp, the walls of the **oral** and **nasal cavities,** the bones of the skull and the dura mater, but not the orbit or brain.

(2) Its main branches from inferior to superior are:

(a) The **superior thyroid,** which courses downward to supply the thyroid gland. It also supplies the sternocleidomastoid and infrahyoid muscles and the inner aspect of the larynx by way of the **superior laryngeal artery.**

(b) The **ascending pharyngeal,** which ascends to supply the pharyngeal constrictor muscles and other small branches to the prevertebral muscles, middle ear, and dura mater.

(c) The **lingual,** which is the principal artery of the tongue. It also gives branches to suprahyoid muscles and the sublingual gland.

(d) The **facial,** which ascends to supply the anteromedial aspect of the face. It also gives branches to the palatine tonsil, the submandibular gland, and on the face, to both lips and the nose. It ends as the **angular artery,** which anastomoses with the infraorbital.

(e) The **occipital,** which courses to the back of the head to supply the scalp. On its way it sends branches to the sternocleidomastoid and other muscles and to the dura mater.

(f) The **posterior auricular,** which courses behind the external ear. It helps supply the scalp, the middle ear, and the external auricle.

(g) The **superficial temporal,** which supplies the side of the head and gives off the **transverse facial artery,** which courses across the face.

(h) The **maxillary,** which is the principal artery of the deep face. It has three parts and many branches. It supplies the tympanic membrane, gives rise to the **middle meningeal artery,** supplies the muscles of mastication, all lower and some upper teeth, the infraorbital region, the hard and soft palate, and the walls of the nasal cavity.

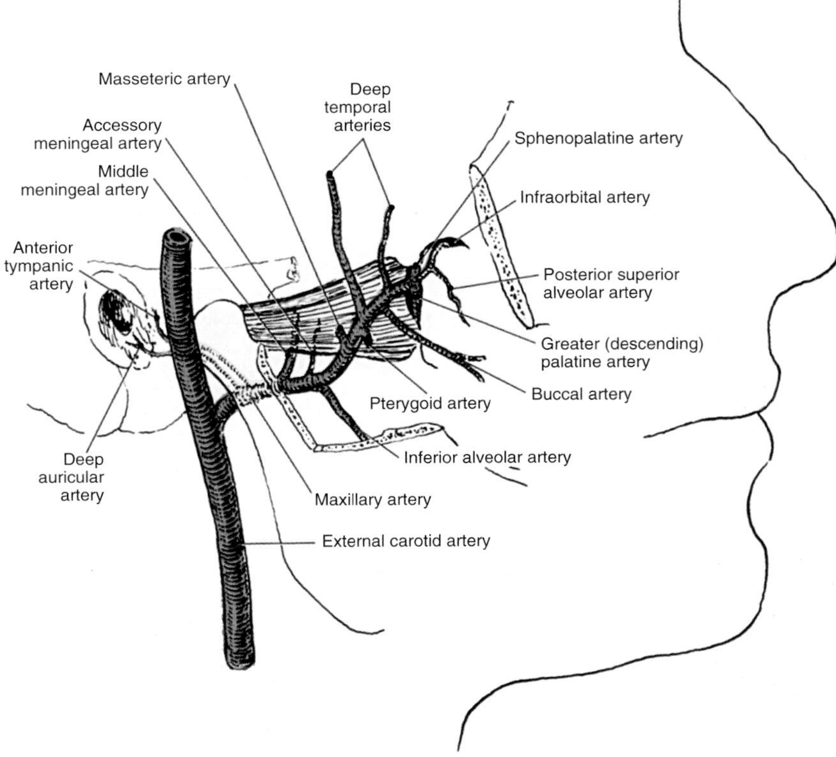
Masseteric artery
Deep temporal arteries
Accessory meningeal artery
Middle meningeal artery
Sphenopalatine artery
Infraorbital artery
Anterior tympanic artery
Posterior superior alveolar artery
Greater (descending) palatine artery
Buccal artery
Pterygoid artery
Deep auricular artery
Inferior alveolar artery
Maxillary artery
External carotid artery

Figure 507.1 Branches of the Maxillary Artery (after J.C.B. Grant)

NOTE: Branches from the maxillary artery are given off from all three parts of the vessel: from the first part: **anterior tympanic, deep auricular, middle and accessory meningeal,** and **inferior alveolar;** from the second part: **masseteric, deep temporal, pterygoid,** and **buccal;** from the third part: **sphenopalatine, infraorbital, greater (descending) palatine, posterior superior alveolar,** and **the artery of the pterygoid canal.**

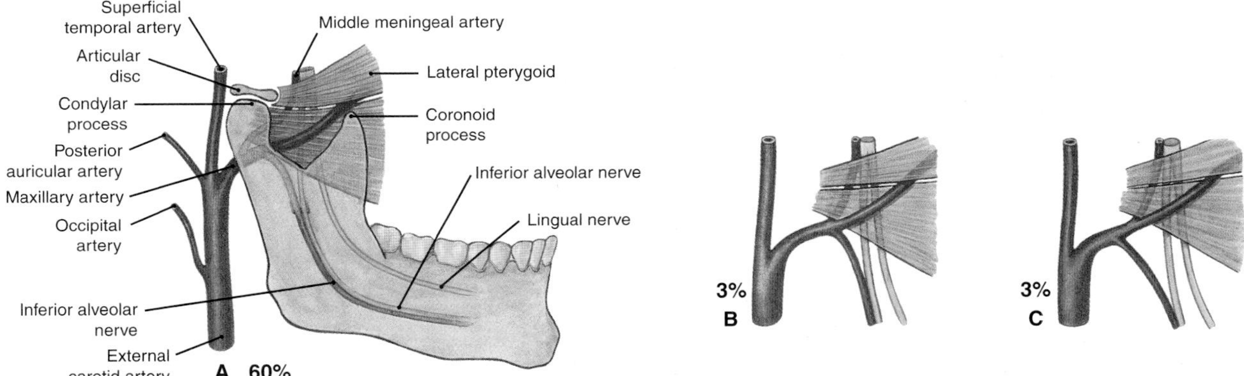
Superficial temporal artery
Articular disc
Condylar process
Posterior auricular artery
Maxillary artery
Occipital artery
Inferior alveolar nerve
External carotid artery
Middle meningeal artery
Lateral pterygoid
Coronoid process
Inferior alveolar nerve
Lingual nerve
A 60%
3% B
3% C

Figure 507.2 Variations in the Maxillary Artery Passing Lateral to the Lateral Pterygoid Muscle

NOTE: The maxillary artery courses lateral (superficial) to the lateral pterygoid muscle in about two-thirds of the cases. In 60% of these cadavers (A), the middle meningeal artery arises proximal to the inferior alveolar artery. In 3% of these cadavers (B), the middle meningeal artery arises opposite the inferior alveolar artery. In 3% of these cadavers (C), the middle meningeal artery arises distal to the inferior alveolar artery.

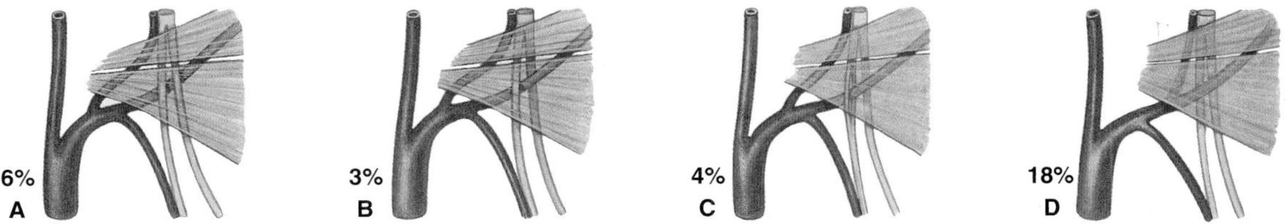
6% A
3% B
4% C
18% D

Figure 507.3 Variations in the Maxillary Artery Passing Medial to the Lateral Pterygoid Muscle

NOTE: The maxillary artery courses medial to the lateral pterygoid muscle in about 31 to 33% of cadavers. In A, the maxillary artery courses medial to the lingual and inferior alveolar nerves in 6%; in B, the maxillary artery courses between the lingual and inferior alveolar nerves in 3%; in C, the maxillary artery courses through a loop in the inferior alveolar nerve in 4%; in D, the maxillary artery gives origin to the middle meningeal artery distal to the inferior alveolar artery.

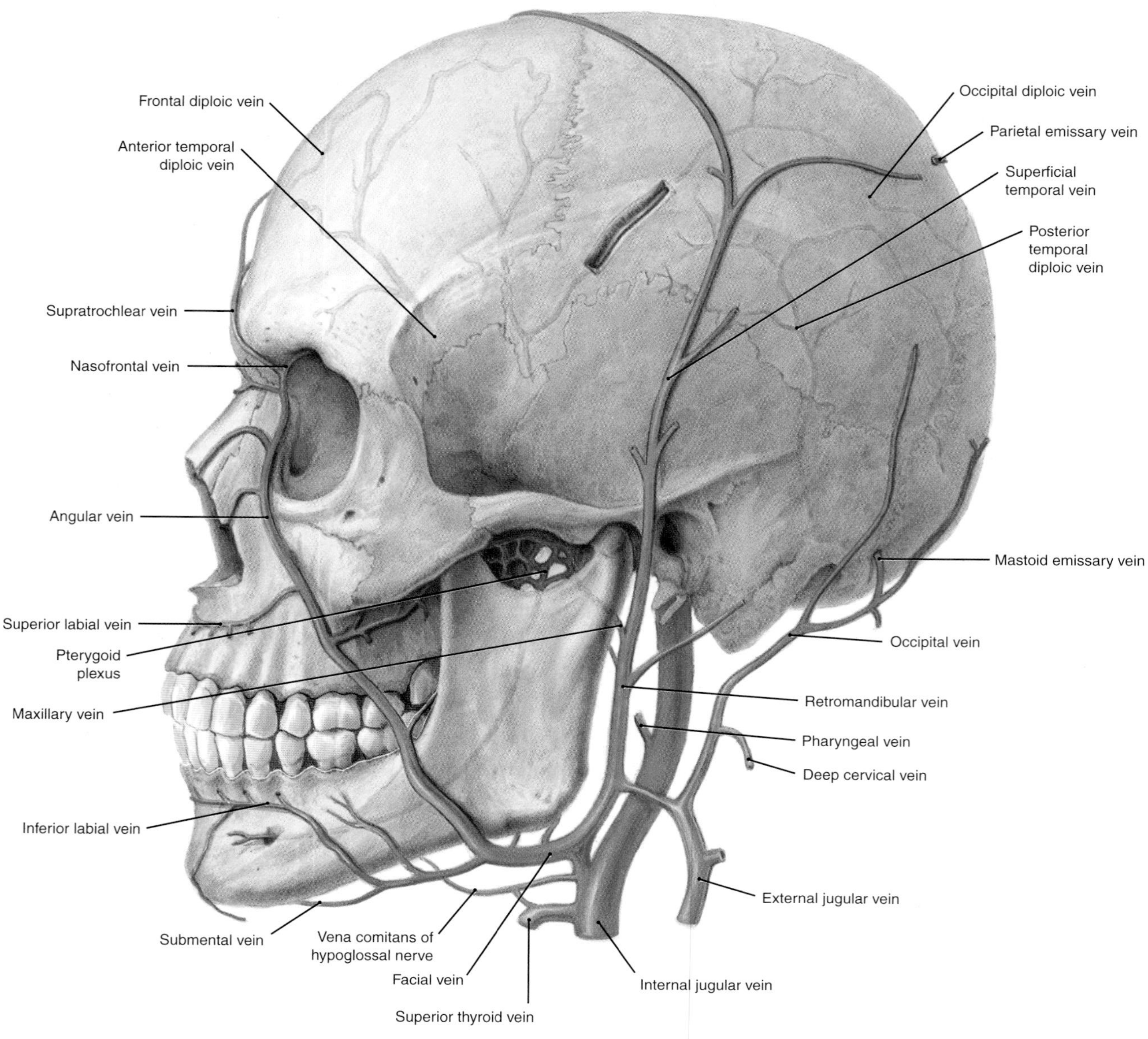
Frontal diploic vein
Anterior temporal diploic vein
Supratrochlear vein
Nasofrontal vein
Angular vein
Superior labial vein
Pterygoid plexus
Maxillary vein
Inferior labial vein
Submental vein
Vena comitans of hypoglossal nerve
Facial vein
Superior thyroid vein
Internal jugular vein
External jugular vein
Deep cervical vein
Pharyngeal vein
Retromandibular vein
Occipital vein
Mastoid emissary vein
Posterior temporal diploic vein
Superficial temporal vein
Parietal emissary vein
Occipital diploic vein

Figure 508 Principal Superficial Veins of the Face and Head, Showing Connections to Deeper Veins

NOTE: (1) The **angular vein** is formed at the root of the nose and courses inferolaterally to become the **facial vein.** The angular-facial trunk communicates by way of deeper vessels with the **cavernous sinus** within the cranial cavity and with **pterygoid plexus** of veins in the infratemporal fossa.

(2) The **superficial temporal vein,** which drains the lateral aspect of the superficial head and the **maxillary vein,** which drains the deep face. They join to form the **retromandibular vein.**

(3) The **occipital vein,** which forms on the posterolateral aspect of the scalp and which courses downward into the **external jugular vein.** The diploic veins and the various emissary veins (condylar, mastoid, and parietal veins) interconnect the superficial veins with the **dural sinuses.**

(4) Within the cranial cavity, the **sigmoid sinus,** draining most of the other dural sinuses, terminates at the jugular foramen. Just below this foramen, the sigmoid sinus becomes the **internal jugular vein,** which descends in the neck to the thorax.

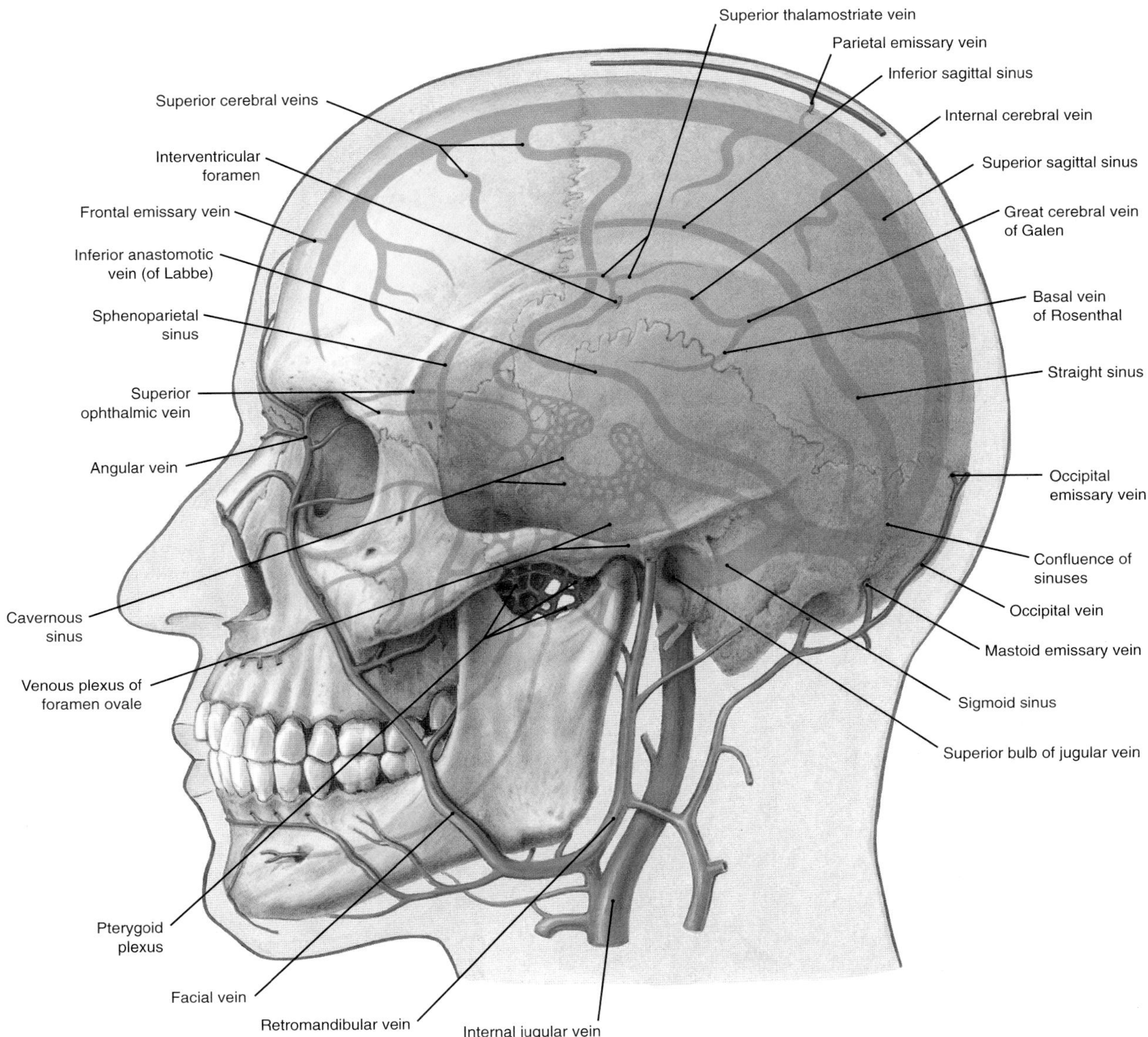
Superior thalamostriate vein
Parietal emissary vein
Inferior sagittal sinus
Superior cerebral veins
Internal cerebral vein
Interventricular foramen
Superior sagittal sinus
Frontal emissary vein
Great cerebral vein of Galen
Inferior anastomotic vein (of Labbe)
Basal vein of Rosenthal
Sphenoparietal sinus
Straight sinus
Superior ophthalmic vein
Angular vein
Occipital emissary vein
Confluence of sinuses
Cavernous sinus
Occipital vein
Mastoid emissary vein
Venous plexus of foramen ovale
Sigmoid sinus
Superior bulb of jugular vein
Pterygoid plexus
Facial vein
Retromandibular vein
Internal jugular vein

Figure 509 **Internal Jugular Vein and Its Extracranial Tributaries**

NOTE: (1) The superficial face is drained by the **angular vein** and the **superior** and **inferior labial** veins. These flow into the large facial vein that descends obliquely adjacent to the facial (not shown) artery (see Fig. 510).

(2) The internal jugular vein forms at the base of the skull. Within the skull, blood in the **sigmoid sinus** drains through the jugular foramen, and as the sigmoid sinus emerges from the jugular foramen in the neck it becomes the **internal jugular vein.**

(3) Within the skull, observe the confluence of sinuses. This large venous channel receives blood from the **superior sagittal sinus,** the **straight sinus,** and **the inferior anastomotic vein** (of Labbé).

(4) The **cavernous sinus** and its communications with the ophthalmic veins of the orbit and the pterygoid plexus of veins in the deep face.

(5) The many emissary veins passing through the skull and forming many connections between the dural sinuses and the veins on the exterior of the skull

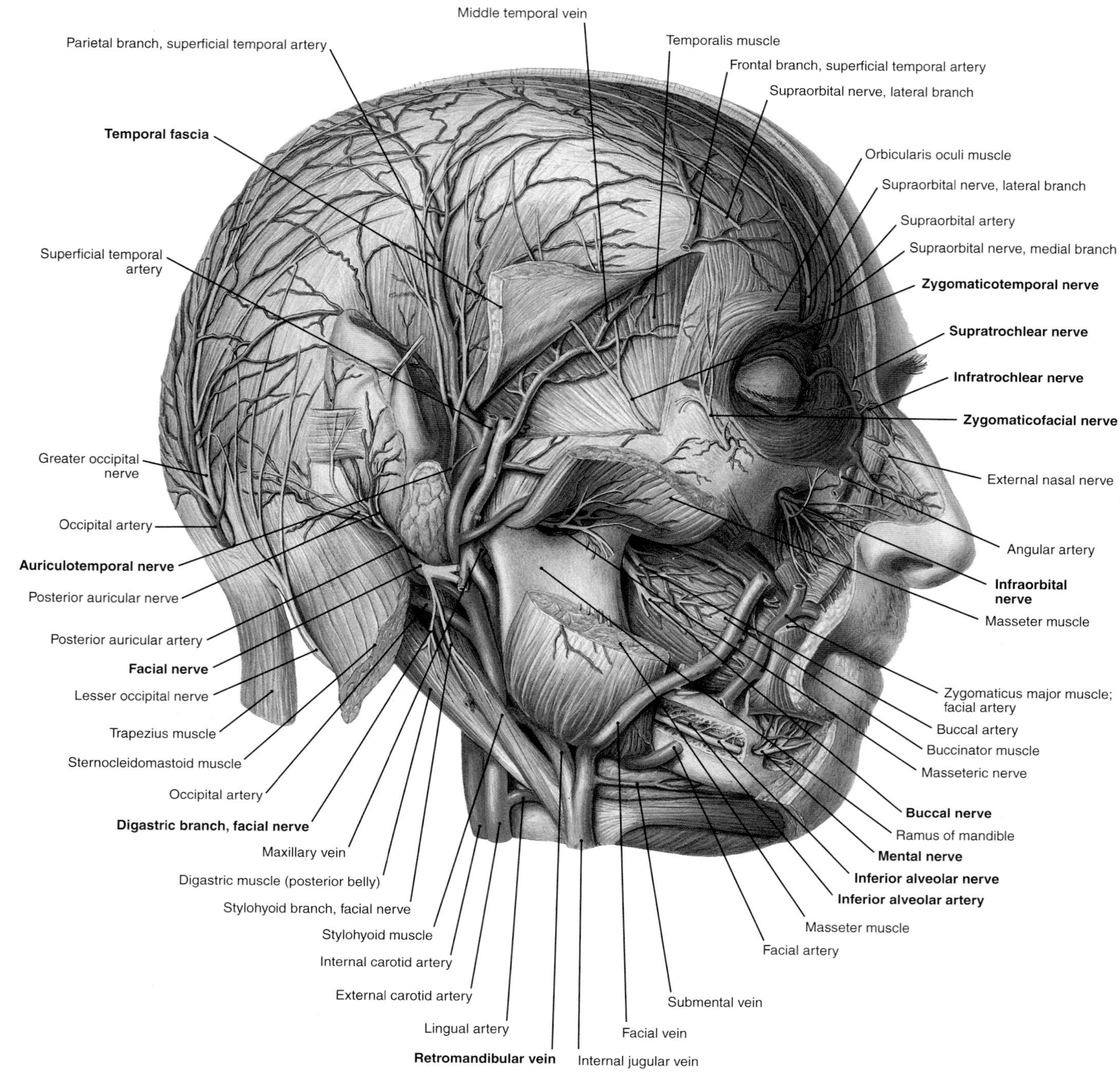
Middle temporal vein
Parietal branch, superficial temporal artery
Temporalis muscle
Frontal branch, superficial temporal artery
Supraorbital nerve, lateral branch
Temporal fascia
Orbicularis oculi muscle
Supraorbital nerve, lateral branch
Supraorbital artery
Superficial temporal artery
Supraorbital nerve, medial branch
Zygomaticotemporal nerve
Supratrochlear nerve
Infratrochlear nerve
Zygomaticofacial nerve
Greater occipital nerve
External nasal nerve
Occipital artery
Angular artery
Auriculotemporal nerve
Infraorbital nerve
Posterior auricular nerve
Masseter muscle
Posterior auricular artery
Facial nerve
Zygomaticus major muscle; facial artery
Lesser occipital nerve
Buccal artery
Trapezius muscle
Buccinator muscle
Sternocleidomastoid muscle
Masseteric nerve
Occipital artery
Buccal nerve
Digastric branch, facial nerve
Ramus of mandible
Maxillary vein
Mental nerve
Digastric muscle (posterior belly)
Inferior alveolar nerve
Stylohyoid branch, facial nerve
Inferior alveolar artery
Stylohyoid muscle
Masseter muscle
Internal carotid artery
Facial artery
External carotid artery
Submental vein
Lingual artery
Facial vein
Retromandibular vein
Internal jugular vein

Figure 510 Vessels and Nerves of the Deep Face (Dissection 1)

NOTE: (1) The temporal fascia has been cut and partially reflected. The superficial muscles on the side of the face and the parotid gland have been removed. The main trunk of the facial nerve has been cut and its branches across the face removed. The masseter muscle was severed and reflected upward to show the masseteric artery and nerve.

(2) The following are branches of the **trigeminal nerve:**

(a) **Ophthalmic division:** supraorbital, supratrochlear, infratrochlear, and external nasal branches.

(b) **Maxillary division**: zygomaticotemporal, zygomaticofacial, and infraorbital branches.

(c) **Mandibular division:** auriculotemporal, masseteric, buccal, inferior alveolar, and mental branches.

(3) The posterior auricular, digastric, and stylohyoid branches of the facial nerve, arise from the facial nerve trunk prior to its division within the parotid gland.

(4) The anastomosis of arteries above and at the medial aspect of the orbit. The vessels involved include the frontal branch of the superficial temporal, the supraorbital, supratrochlear, and angular arteries and their branches.

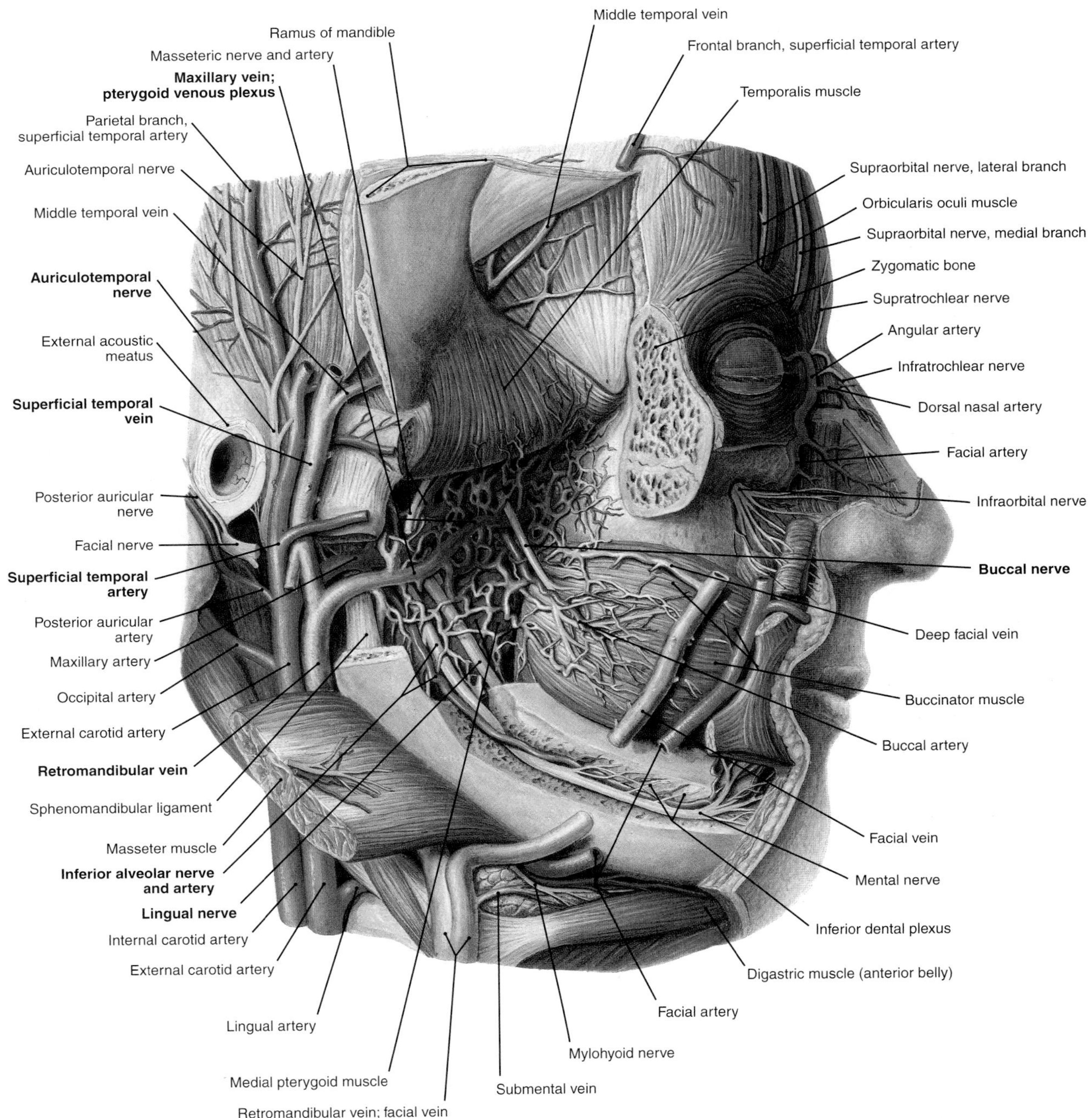
Middle temporal vein
Ramus of mandible
Frontal branch, superficial temporal artery
Masseteric nerve and artery
Maxillary vein; pterygoid venous plexus
Temporalis muscle
Parietal branch, superficial temporal artery
Auriculotemporal nerve
Supraorbital nerve, lateral branch
Orbicularis oculi muscle
Middle temporal vein
Supraorbital nerve, medial branch
Zygomatic bone
Auriculotemporal nerve
Supratrochlear nerve
Angular artery
External acoustic meatus
Infratrochlear nerve
Superficial temporal vein
Dorsal nasal artery
Facial artery
Posterior auricular nerve
Infraorbital nerve
Facial nerve
Buccal nerve
Superficial temporal artery
Posterior auricular artery
Deep facial vein
Maxillary artery
Occipital artery
Buccinator muscle
External carotid artery
Buccal artery
Retromandibular vein
Sphenomandibular ligament
Facial vein
Masseter muscle
Mental nerve
Inferior alveolar nerve and artery
Lingual nerve
Inferior dental plexus
Internal carotid artery
External carotid artery
Digastric muscle (anterior belly)
Facial artery
Lingual artery
Mylohyoid nerve
Medial pterygoid muscle
Submental vein
Retromandibular vein; facial vein

Figure 511 Infratemporal Region of the Deep Face (Dissection 2)

NOTE: (1) The zygomatic arch has been cut and reflected upward along with the insertion of the temporalis muscle. A portion of the mandible has also been removed to show the course of the **maxillary vein** and **artery** deep to the mandible. The branches of the artery in the infratemporal region can better be seen in Figure 512.

(2) The maxillary vein forms from the **pterygoid plexus** of veins, which lies adjacent to the pterygoid muscles and which anastomoses with the facial vein by way of the **deep facial vein.** This plexus also anastomoses with the cavernous sinus through communicating veins in the foramen lacerum and foramen ovale and by way of the inferior ophthalmic vein.

(3) The body of the mandible has been opened to expose the inferior alveolar artery and nerve.

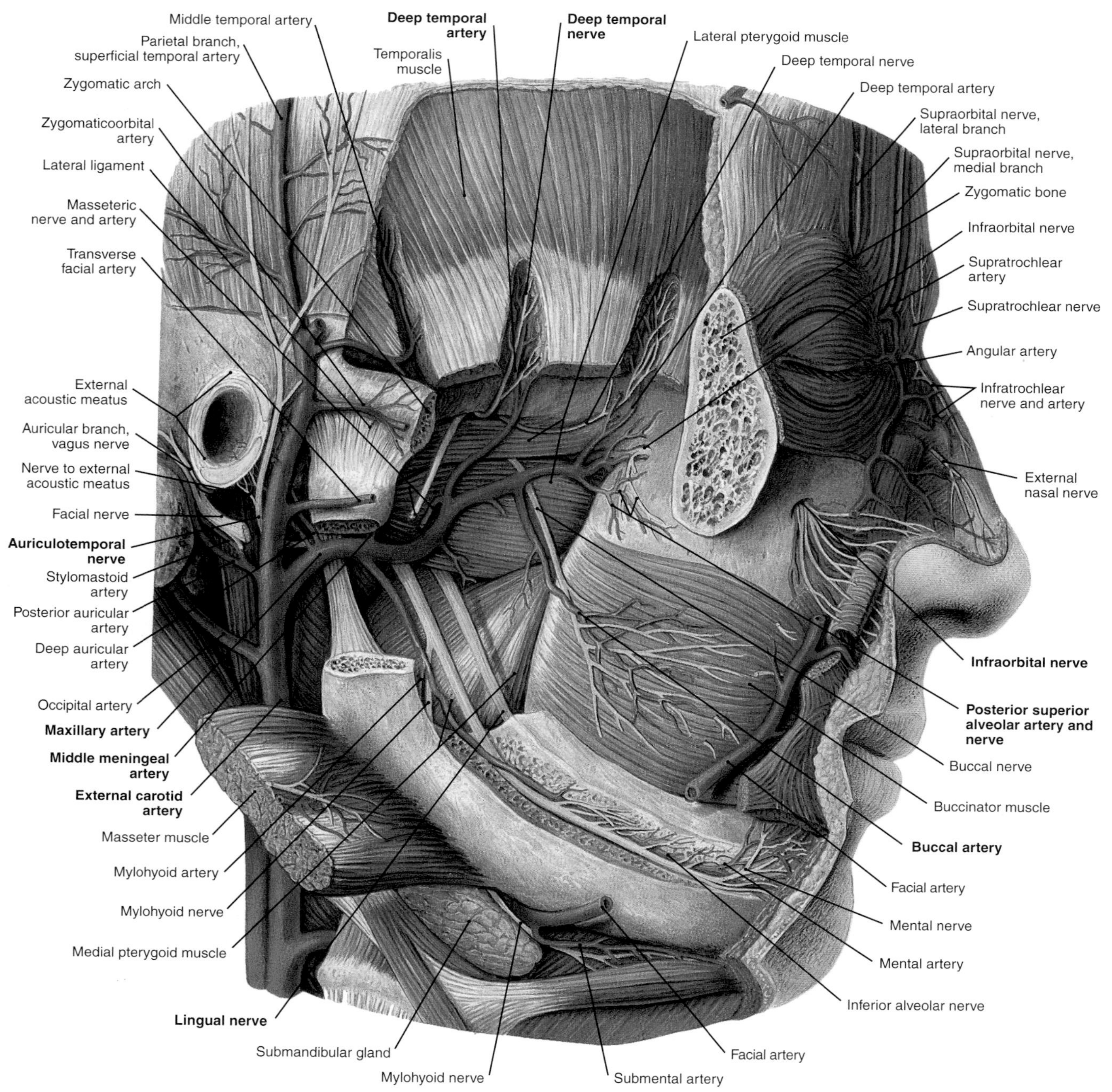
Middle temporal artery
Parietal branch, superficial temporal artery
Zygomatic arch
Zygomaticoorbital artery
Lateral ligament
Masseteric nerve and artery
Transverse facial artery
External acoustic meatus
Auricular branch, vagus nerve
Nerve to external acoustic meatus
Facial nerve
Auriculotemporal nerve
Stylomastoid artery
Posterior auricular artery
Deep auricular artery
Occipital artery
Maxillary artery
Middle meningeal artery
External carotid artery
Masseter muscle
Mylohyoid artery
Mylohyoid nerve
Medial pterygoid muscle
Lingual nerve
Submandibular gland
Mylohyoid nerve
Submental artery
Facial artery
Deep temporal artery
Temporalis muscle
Deep temporal nerve
Lateral pterygoid muscle
Deep temporal nerve
Deep temporal artery
Supraorbital nerve, lateral branch
Supraorbital nerve, medial branch
Zygomatic bone
Infraorbital nerve
Supratrochlear artery
Supratrochlear nerve
Angular artery
Infratrochlear nerve and artery
External nasal nerve
Infraorbital nerve
Posterior superior alveolar artery and nerve
Buccal nerve
Buccinator muscle
Buccal artery
Facial artery
Mental nerve
Mental artery
Inferior alveolar nerve

Figure 512 **Infratemporal Region of the Deep Face: Maxillary Artery (Dissection 3)**

NOTE: (1) The **infratemporal fossa** has been opened laterally to show the pterygoid muscles, the maxillary artery and its branches, and some of the branches of the mandibular division of the trigeminal nerve.

(2) In this dissection, the following branches of the **maxillary artery** are shown: (a) deep auricular, (b) anterior tympanic, (c) inferior alveolar, (d) middle meningeal, (e) masseteric (cut), (f) deep temporal, (g) pterygoid (not labeled), (h) buccal, (i) posterior superior alveolar, and (j) infraorbital. **NOT** shown in this view are the descending palatine branch, the artery of the pterygoid canal, and the pharyngeal and sphenopalatine branches.

(3) The following are branches of the **mandibular division** of the **trigeminal nerve:** (a) auriculotemporal, (b) lingual, (c) inferior alveolar, (d) mylohyoid, (e) masseteric, (f) deep temporal, and (g) buccal. Observe the course of the inferior alveolar nerve, accompanied by the inferior alveolar artery within the mandible.

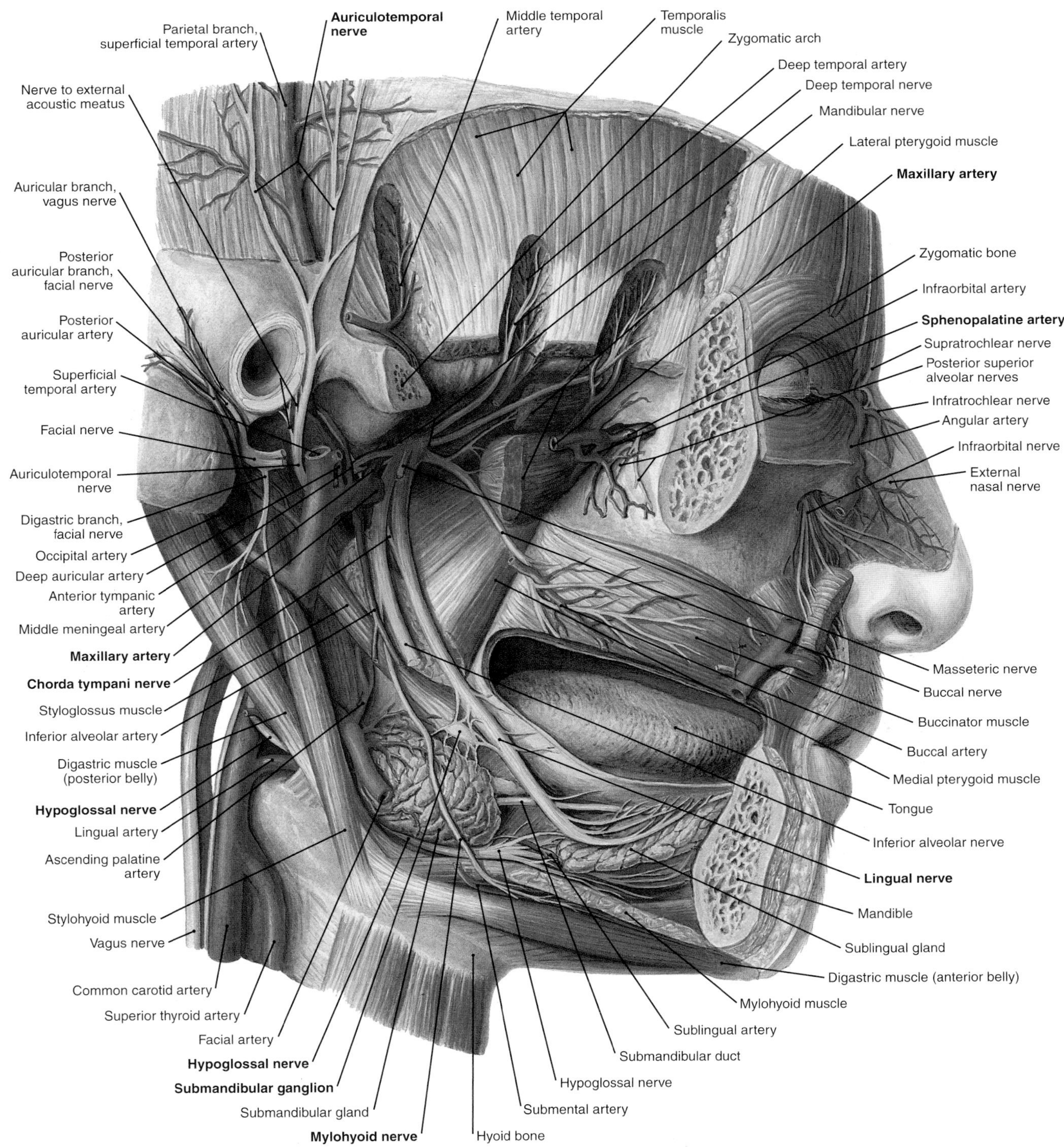
Parietal branch, superficial temporal artery
Auriculotemporal nerve
Middle temporal artery
Temporalis muscle
Zygomatic arch
Deep temporal artery
Deep temporal nerve
Mandibular nerve
Lateral pterygoid muscle
Maxillary artery
Nerve to external acoustic meatus
Auricular branch, vagus nerve
Posterior auricular branch, facial nerve
Posterior auricular artery
Superficial temporal artery
Facial nerve
Auriculotemporal nerve
Digastric branch, facial nerve
Occipital artery
Deep auricular artery
Anterior tympanic artery
Middle meningeal artery
Maxillary artery
Chorda tympani nerve
Styloglossus muscle
Inferior alveolar artery
Digastric muscle (posterior belly)
Hypoglossal nerve
Lingual artery
Ascending palatine artery
Stylohyoid muscle
Vagus nerve
Common carotid artery
Superior thyroid artery
Facial artery
Hypoglossal nerve
Submandibular ganglion
Submandibular gland
Mylohyoid nerve
Hyoid bone
Submental artery
Hypoglossal nerve
Submandibular duct
Sublingual artery
Mylohyoid muscle
Digastric muscle (anterior belly)
Sublingual gland
Mandible
Lingual nerve
Inferior alveolar nerve
Tongue
Medial pterygoid muscle
Buccal artery
Buccinator muscle
Buccal nerve
Masseteric nerve
Zygomatic bone
Infraorbital artery
Sphenopalatine artery
Supratrochlear nerve
Posterior superior alveolar nerves
Infratrochlear nerve
Angular artery
Infraorbital nerve
External nasal nerve

Figure 513 Infratemporal Region of the Deep Face: Mandibular Nerve Branches (Dissection 4)

NOTE: (1) The zygomatic arch, much of the right mandible, and the lateral pterygoid muscle have been removed in this dissection. Also, a portion of the maxillary artery has been cut away, along with the distal part of the inferior alveolar nerve beyond the point where the mylohyoid nerve branches.

(2) The **lingual nerve** coursing to the tongue. High in the infratemporal fossa, the **chorda tympani nerve** (a branch of the facial) joins the lingual. The chorda tympani carries both special sensory **taste** fibers from the anterior two-thirds of the tongue and **preganglionic parasympathetic** fibers from the facial to the **submandibular ganglion.**

(3) The distal part of the maxillary artery as it courses toward the sphenopalatine foramen. After giving off the infraorbital artery, the sphenopalatine branch enters the nasal cavity through the foramen and serves as the principal vessel to the nasal mucosa.

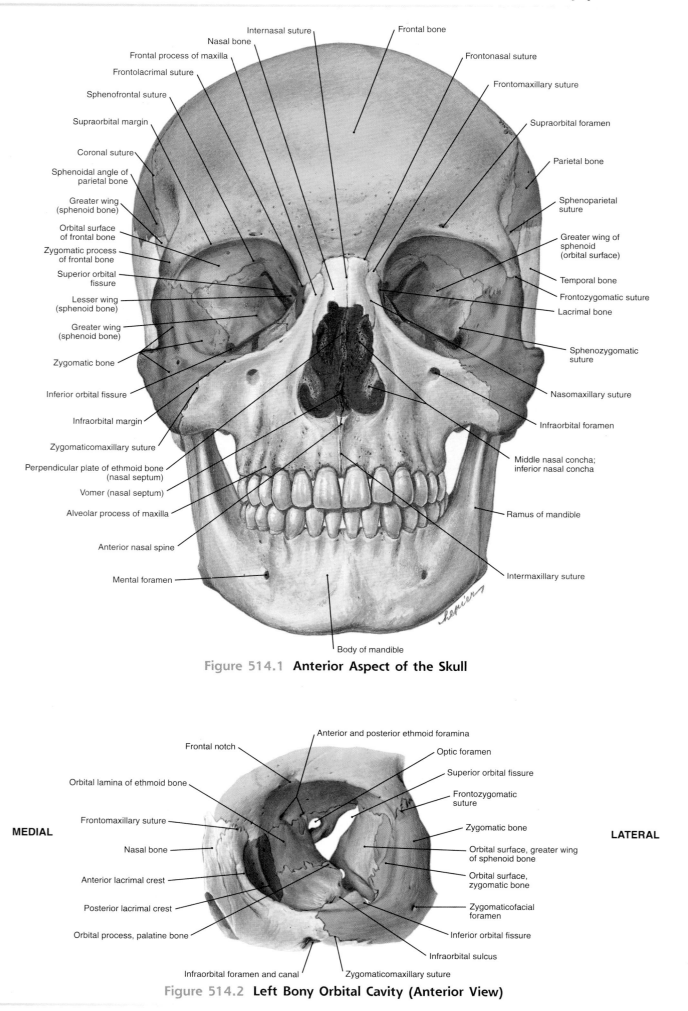

Internasal suture
Nasal bone
Frontal process of maxilla
Frontolacrimal suture
Sphenofrontal suture
Supraorbital margin
Coronal suture
Sphenoidal angle of parietal bone
Greater wing (sphenoid bone)
Orbital surface of frontal bone
Zygomatic process of frontal bone
Superior orbital fissure
Lesser wing (sphenoid bone)
Greater wing (sphenoid bone)
Zygomatic bone
Inferior orbital fissure
Infraorbital margin
Zygomaticomaxillary suture
Perpendicular plate of ethmoid bone (nasal septum)
Vomer (nasal septum)
Alveolar process of maxilla
Anterior nasal spine
Mental foramen
Frontal bone
Frontonasal suture
Frontomaxillary suture
Supraorbital foramen
Parietal bone
Sphenoparietal suture
Greater wing of sphenoid (orbital surface)
Temporal bone
Frontozygomatic suture
Lacrimal bone
Sphenozygomatic suture
Nasomaxillary suture
Infraorbital foramen
Middle nasal concha; inferior nasal concha
Ramus of mandible
Intermaxillary suture
Body of mandible

Figure 514.1 **Anterior Aspect of the Skull**

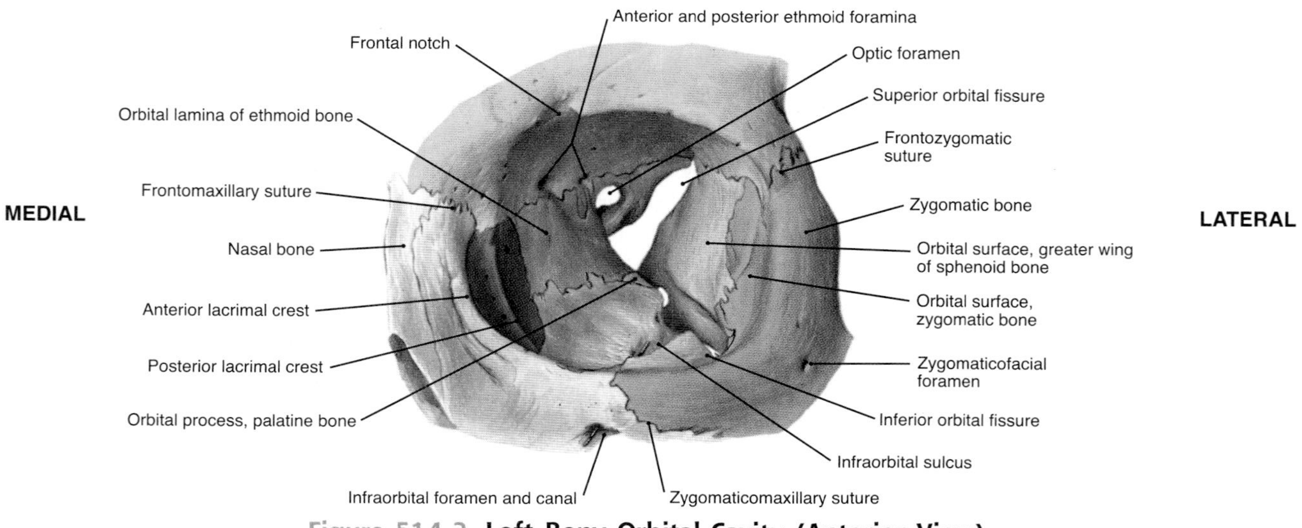
MEDIAL
LATERAL
Frontal notch
Anterior and posterior ethmoid foramina
Optic foramen
Superior orbital fissure
Frontozygomatic suture
Orbital lamina of ethmoid bone
Frontomaxillary suture
Nasal bone
Anterior lacrimal crest
Posterior lacrimal crest
Orbital process, palatine bone
Zygomatic bone
Orbital surface, greater wing of sphenoid bone
Orbital surface, zygomatic bone
Zygomaticofacial foramen
Inferior orbital fissure
Infraorbital sulcus
Infraorbital foramen and canal
Zygomaticomaxillary suture

Figure 514.2 **Left Bony Orbital Cavity (Anterior View)**

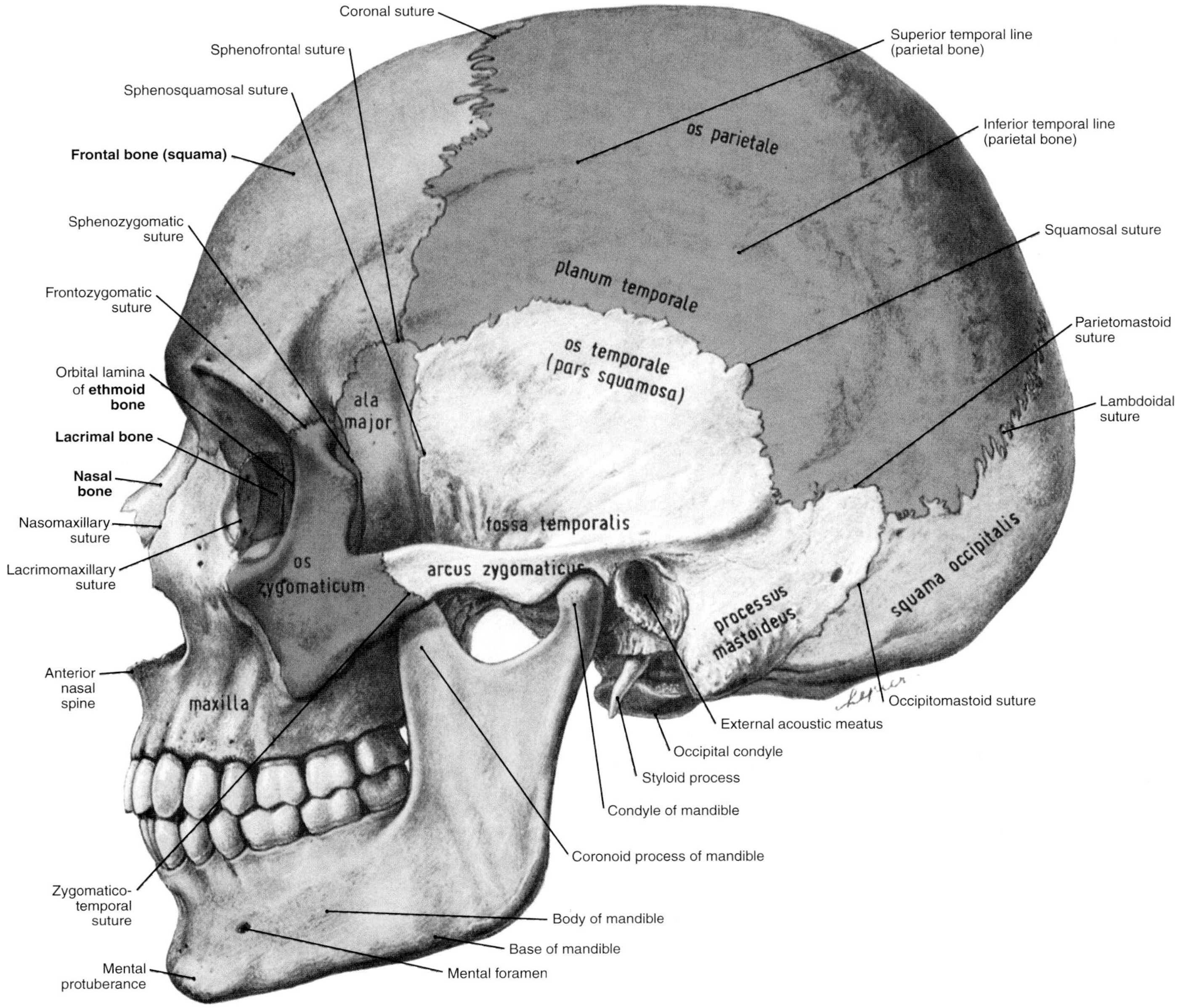

Coronal suture
Sphenofrontal suture
Sphenosquamosal suture
Frontal bone (squama)
Sphenozygomatic suture
Frontozygomatic suture
Orbital lamina of **ethmoid bone**
Lacrimal bone
Nasal bone
Nasomaxillary suture
Lacrimomaxillary suture
Anterior nasal spine
Zygomatico-temporal suture
Mental protuberance
os parietale
planum temporale
os temporale (pars squamosa)
ala major
fossa temporalis
arcus zygomaticus
os zygomaticum
maxilla
processus mastoideus
squama occipitalis
Superior temporal line (parietal bone)
Inferior temporal line (parietal bone)
Squamosal suture
Parietomastoid suture
Lambdoidal suture
Occipitomastoid suture
External acoustic meatus
Occipital condyle
Styloid process
Condyle of mandible
Coronoid process of mandible
Body of mandible
Base of mandible
Mental foramen

Figure 515.1 **Lateral Aspect of the Skull**

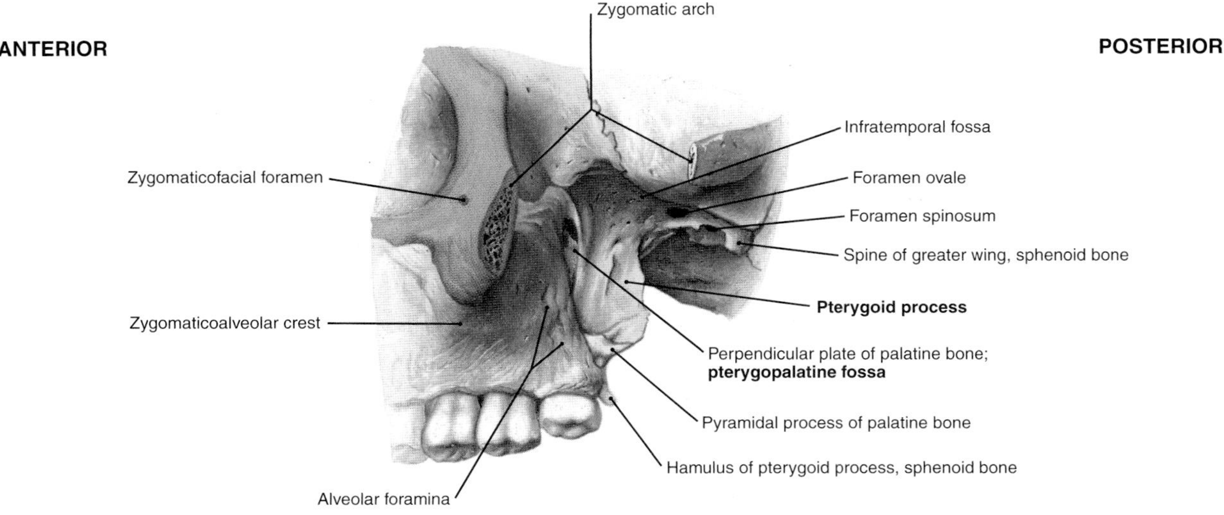
ANTERIOR
POSTERIOR
Zygomatic arch
Infratemporal fossa
Foramen ovale
Foramen spinosum
Spine of greater wing, sphenoid bone
Zygomaticofacial foramen
Pterygoid process
Zygomaticoalveolar crest
Perpendicular plate of palatine bone; pterygopalatine fossa
Pyramidal process of palatine bone
Hamulus of pterygoid process, sphenoid bone
Alveolar foramina

Figure 515.2 **Inferolateral Aspect of the Skull with the Zygomatic Arch Removed**

NOTE: The pterygopalatine fossa and the pterygoid process of the sphenoid bone.

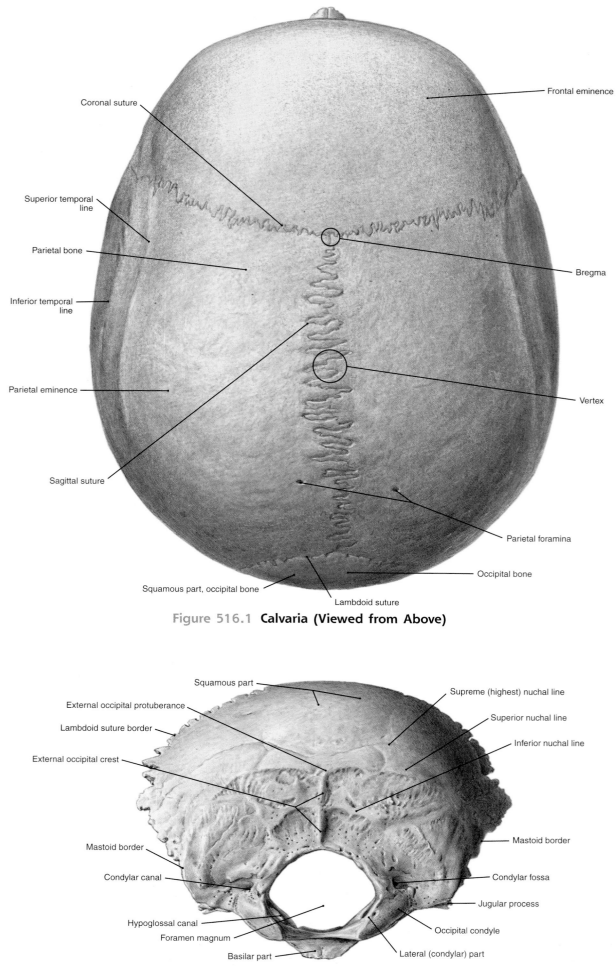

Frontal eminence
Coronal suture
Superior temporal line
Parietal bone
Bregma
Inferior temporal line
Parietal eminence
Vertex
Sagittal suture
Parietal foramina
Occipital bone
Squamous part, occipital bone
Lambdoid suture

Figure 516.1 **Calvaria (Viewed from Above)**

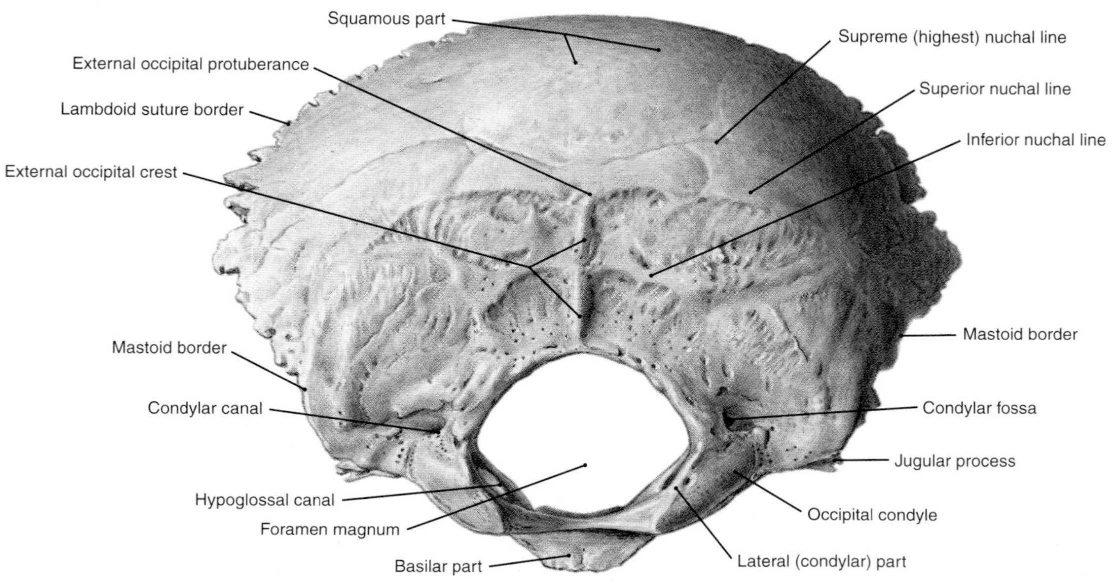
Squamous part
Supreme (highest) nuchal line
External occipital protuberance
Superior nuchal line
Lambdoid suture border
Inferior nuchal line
External occipital crest
Mastoid border
Mastoid border
Condylar canal
Condylar fossa
Jugular process
Hypoglossal canal
Occipital condyle
Foramen magnum
Basilar part
Lateral (condylar) part

Figure 516.2 **Occipital Bone from Behind Showing Some Posterior Features of the Skull**

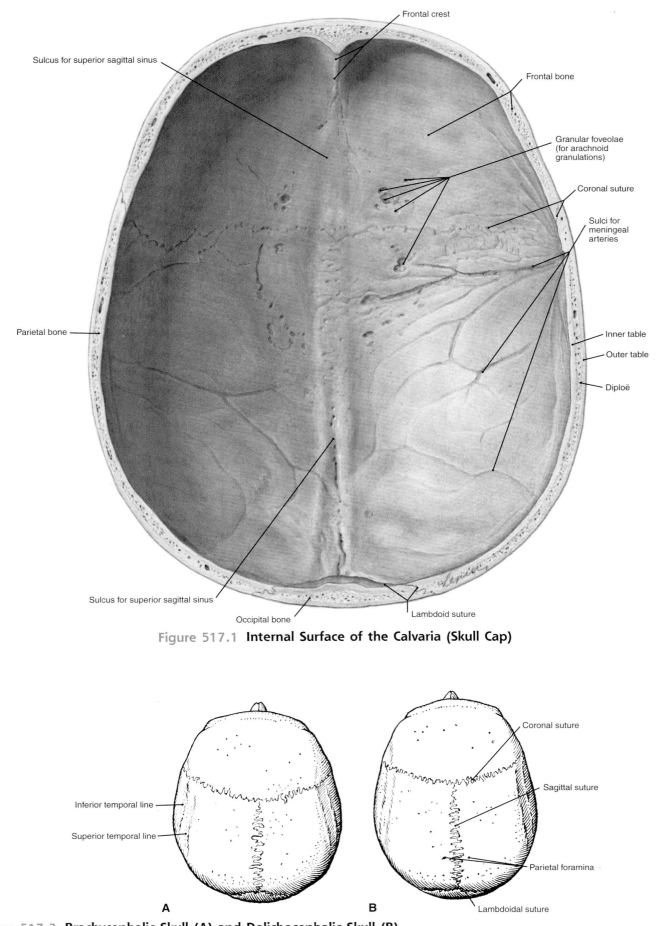

Frontal crest
Sulcus for superior sagittal sinus
Frontal bone
Granular foveolae (for arachnoid granulations)
Coronal suture
Sulci for meningeal arteries
Parietal bone
Inner table
Outer table
Diploë
Sulcus for superior sagittal sinus
Occipital bone
Lambdoid suture

Figure 517.1 **Internal Surface of the Calvaria (Skull Cap)**

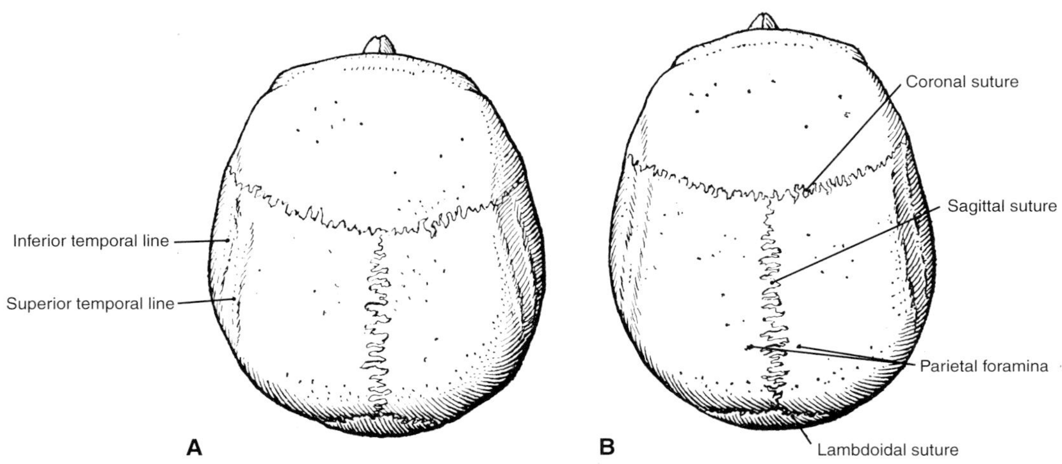
Coronal suture
Sagittal suture
Inferior temporal line
Superior temporal line
Parietal foramina
A
B
Lambdoidal suture

Figure 517.2 **Brachycephalic Skull (A) and Dolichocephalic Skull (B)**

NOTE: Skulls are classified by comparing their width to their length. When the greatest width exceeds 80% of the length, the skull is more round and called **brachycephalic** (A). When the width is less than 75% of length, the more oblong skull is called **dolichocephalic** (B). When the comparison is between 75% and 80%, the skull is classified as **mesaticephalic**.

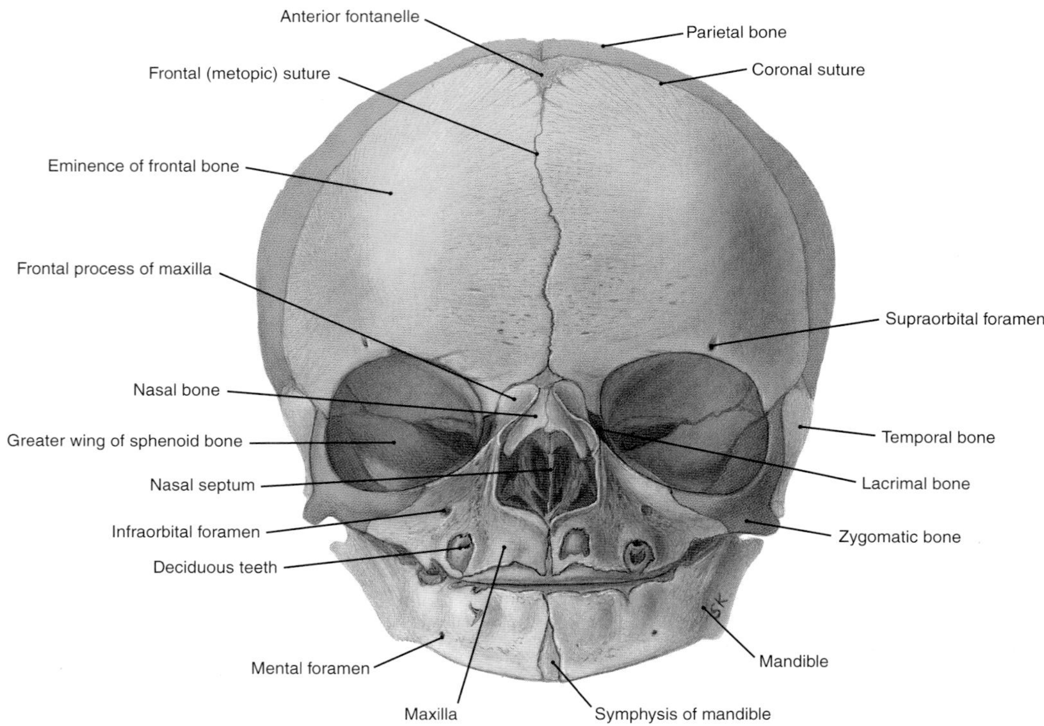
Anterior fontanelle
Parietal bone
Coronal suture
Frontal (metopic) suture
Eminence of frontal bone
Frontal process of maxilla
Supraorbital foramen
Nasal bone
Greater wing of sphenoid bone
Temporal bone
Nasal septum
Lacrimal bone
Infraorbital foramen
Zygomatic bone
Deciduous teeth
Mental foramen
Mandible
Maxilla
Symphysis of mandible

Figure 518.1 Skull at Birth (Frontal View)

NOTE: (1) The bones that enclose the cranial cavity (neurocranium) include the **frontal, parietal, occipital, temporal** and **sphenoid bones,** and the **cribriform plate** of the **ethmoid bone.**

(2) The bones that form the face and hard palate and enclose the nasal cavity are the **mandible, maxilla, zygomatic, lacrimal, nasal** and **palatine bones, inferior concha,** most of the **ethmoid bone,** and the **vomer.**

(3) The skull at birth is large in comparison to the size of the rest of the body because of the precocious growth of the brain; the facial bones, however, are still not well developed.

(4) The maxilla and mandible are rudimentary at birth and the teeth have yet to erupt. In addition, the maxillary sinuses and nasal cavity are small, as are the frontal, ethmoid and sphenoid sinuses.

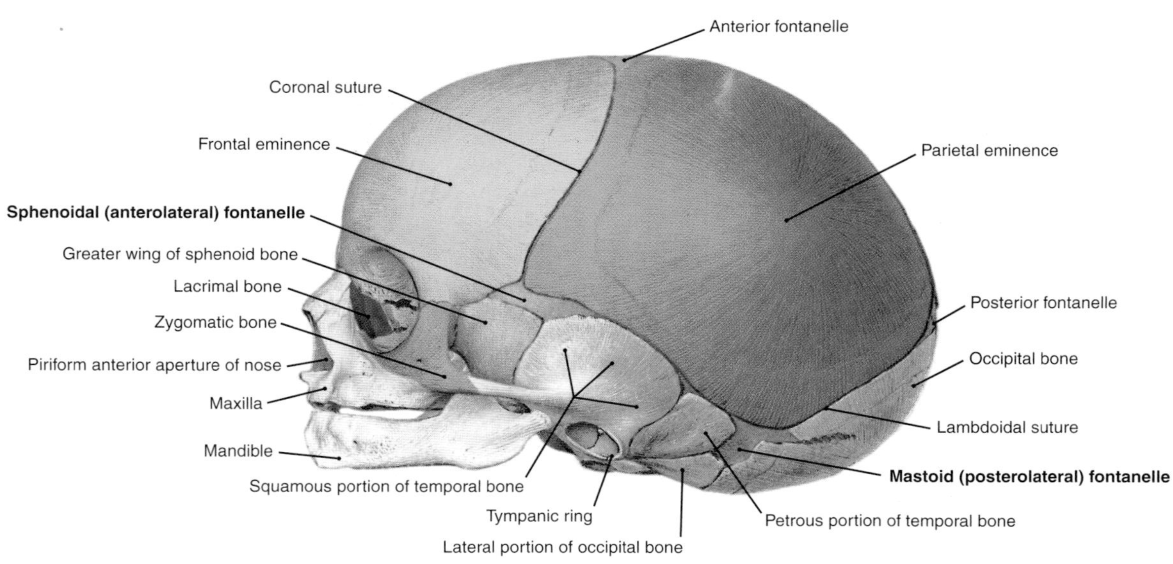
Anterior fontanelle
Coronal suture
Frontal eminence
Parietal eminence
Sphenoidal (anterolateral) fontanelle
Greater wing of sphenoid bone
Lacrimal bone
Posterior fontanelle
Zygomatic bone
Piriform anterior aperture of nose
Occipital bone
Maxilla
Lambdoidal suture
Mandible
Mastoid (posterolateral) fontanelle
Squamous portion of temporal bone
Tympanic ring
Petrous portion of temporal bone
Lateral portion of occipital bone

Figure 518.2 Skull at Birth (Lateral View)

NOTE: (1) Ossification of the maturing **flat bones of the skull** is accomplished by the intramembranous process of bone formation. At birth this process is incomplete, thereby leaving soft membranous sites between the growing bones. Bones forming the base of the cranial cavity develop by ossification in cartilage.

(2) The incompletely ossified nature of the skull just prior to birth is of some benefit, however, since the mobility of the bones permits changes in skull shape, as may be required during the birth process.

(3) The **sphenoidal** (or anterolateral) fontanelle located at the pterion and the **mastoid** (or posterolateral) found at the asterion.

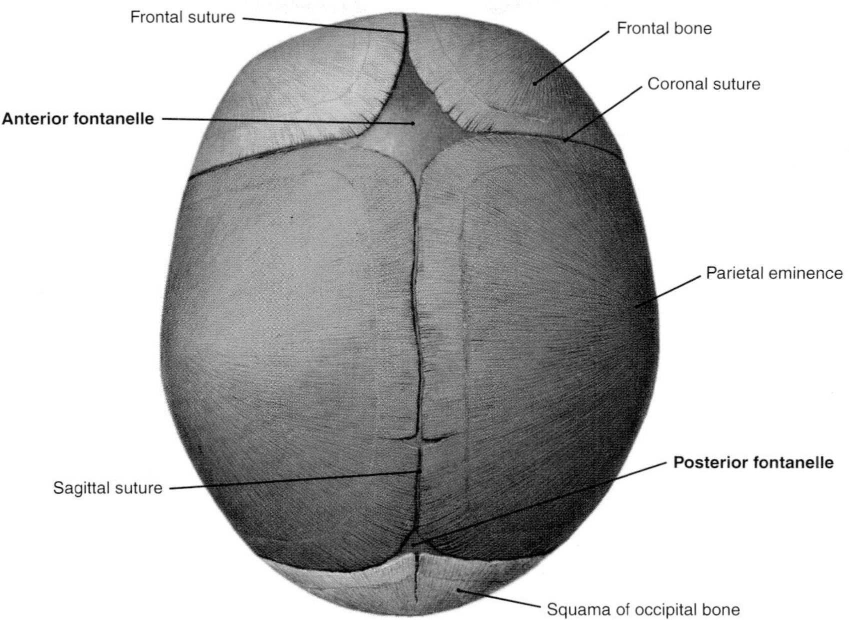
Frontal suture
Frontal bone
Coronal suture
Anterior fontanelle
Parietal eminence
Posterior fontanelle
Sagittal suture
Squama of occipital bone

Figure 519.1 **Skull at Birth (Seen from Above)**

NOTE: (1) The soft sites on the skull of the newborn infant are called **fontanelles.** From this superior view can be seen the **anterior** and **posterior fontanelles.**

(2) The largest of the fontanelles at birth is the **anterior fontanelle** located at the bregma and interconnecting the frontal and parietal bones. It is approximately diamond-shaped and is situated at the junction of the coronal and sagittal sutures.

(3) Following the sagittal suture to its junction with the occipital bone will locate the **posterior fontanelle** (at the lambda). This is generally triangular in shape and is small at birth.

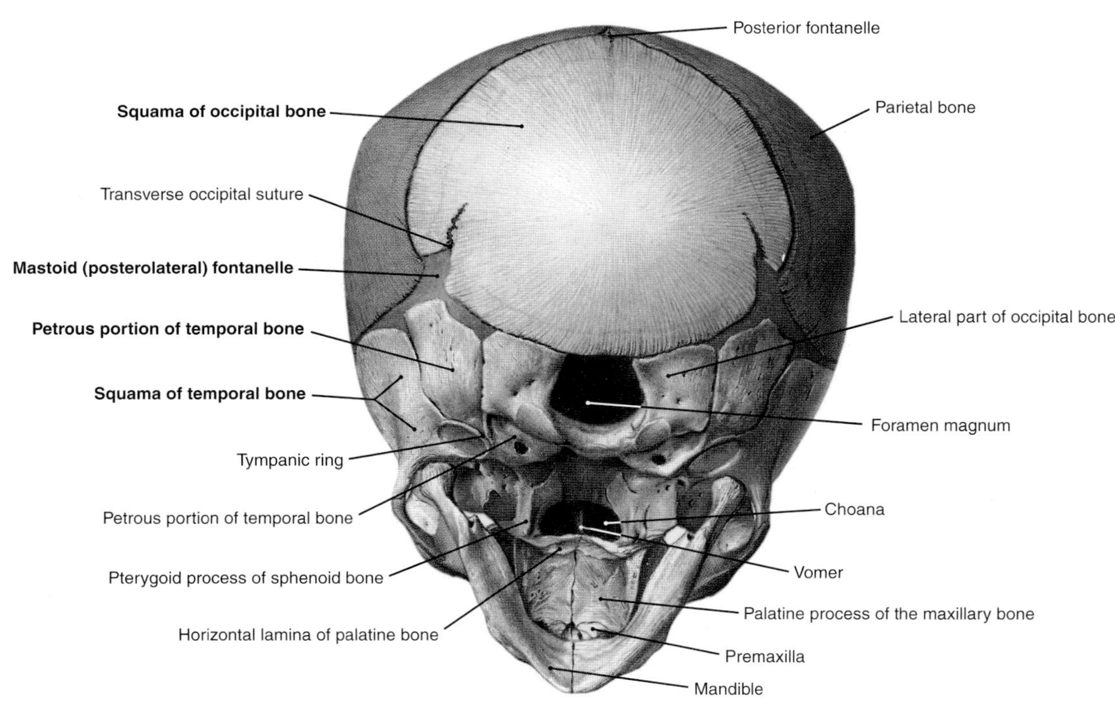
Posterior fontanelle
Squama of occipital bone
Parietal bone
Transverse occipital suture
Mastoid (posterolateral) fontanelle
Petrous portion of temporal bone
Lateral part of occipital bone
Squama of temporal bone
Foramen magnum
Tympanic ring
Petrous portion of temporal bone
Choana
Pterygoid process of sphenoid bone
Vomer
Palatine process of the maxillary bone
Horizontal lamina of palatine bone
Premaxilla
Mandible

Figure 519.2 **Skull at Birth (Posteroinferior View)**

NOTE: (1) The separate ossification of the petrous and squamous portions of the temporal bone as well as the basilar and squamous parts of the occipital bone.

(2) The **mastoid** (posterolateral) **fontanelles** are found at the articulation of the occipital, temporal, and parietal bones.

(3) Growth and ossification of the bones that encase the brain are more precocious than the bones that form the facial skeleton. Facial bones continue growth through puberty. This differential accounts for the marked differences in facial features seen in a 4- or 5-year-old child with that same person at 15 or 16 years of age.

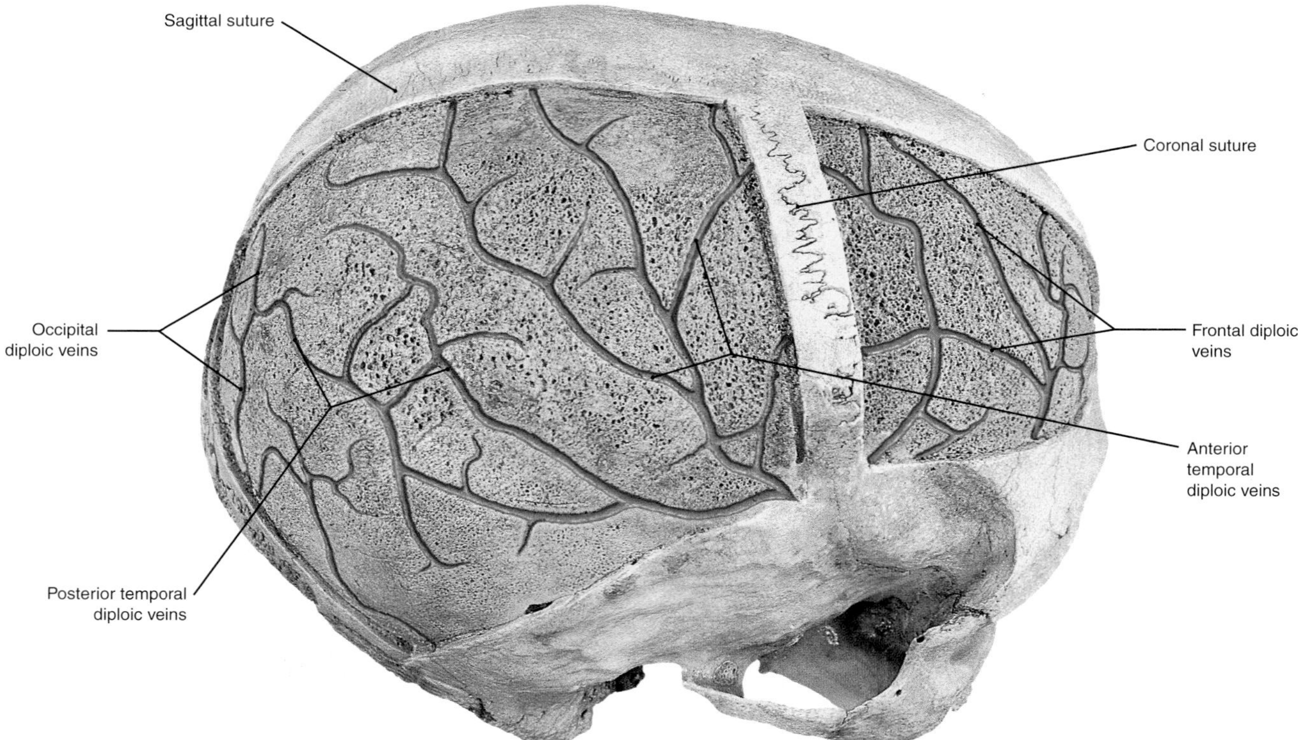
Sagittal suture
Coronal suture
Occipital diploic veins
Frontal diploic veins
Anterior temporal diploic veins
Posterior temporal diploic veins

Figure 520.1 **Diploic Veins**

NOTE: (1) Removing the outermost table of compact bone reveals a more spongy layer of bone. Within this latter layer course venous channels called the **diploic veins.** These veins communicate with the scalp on the exterior and the dural sinuses within the skull.

(2) The diploic veins are named according to their location: **frontal, temporal**, and **occipital.**

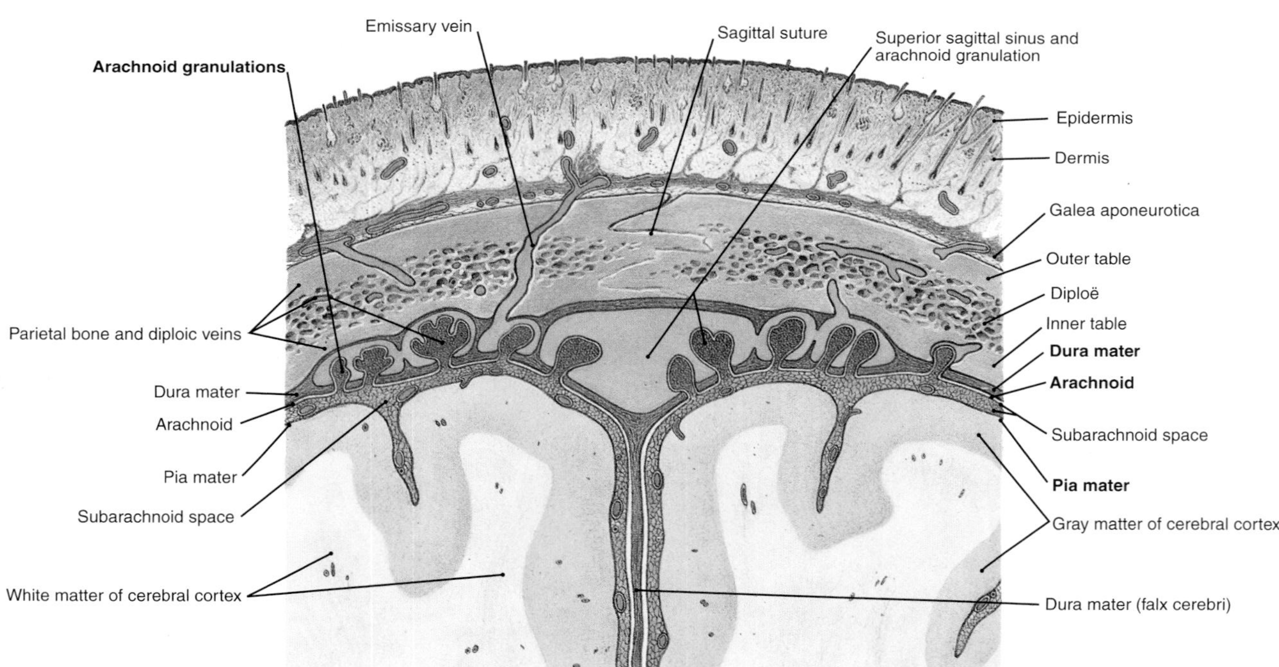
Emissary vein
Sagittal suture
Superior sagittal sinus and arachnoid granulation
Arachnoid granulations
Epidermis
Dermis
Galea aponeurotica
Outer table
Diploë
Inner table
Dura mater
Arachnoid
Parietal bone and diploic veins
Dura mater
Arachnoid
Subarachnoid space
Pia mater
Pia mater
Subarachnoid space
Gray matter of cerebral cortex
White matter of cerebral cortex
Dura mater (falx cerebri)

Figure 520.2 **Scalp, Skull, Meninges, and Brain**

NOTE: (1) This is a frontal section through the cranium and upper cerebrum and shows the bony and soft coverings of the brain. The veins and dural sinuses are colored in blue while the bone is light brown.

(2) Superficial to the dura mater, arachnoid, and pia mater that encase the neural tissue of the brain are found the bony skull and the layers of the scalp.

(3) The **arachnoid granulations.** Tufts of arachnoid (sometime called arachnoid villi) lie next to the endothelium of the sinuses and allow passage of the cerebrospinal fluid from the subarachnoid space into the venous system.

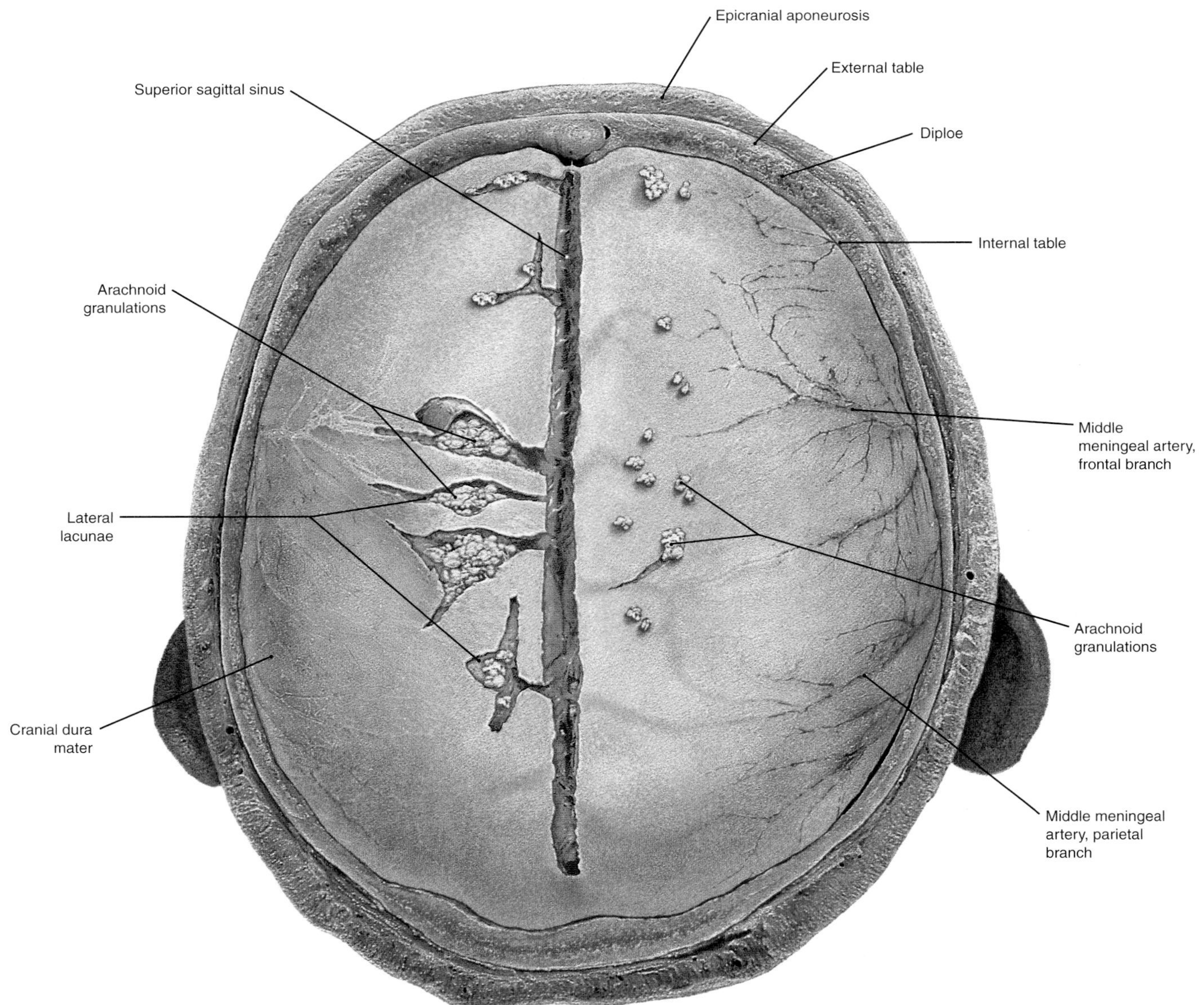
Epicranial aponeurosis
External table
Superior sagittal sinus
Diploe
Internal table
Arachnoid granulations
Middle meningeal artery, frontal branch
Lateral lacunae
Arachnoid granulations
Cranial dura mater
Middle meningeal artery, parietal branch

Figure 521 **Surface of the Dura Mater with the Superior Sagittal Sinus Opened (Viewed from Above)**

NOTE: (1) The skull cap (also called the **calvaria**) has been removed, leaving the **dura mater** intact. The dura is a two-layered structure (an inner **meningeal layer** and an outer **periosteal layer**), but these layers are inseparably fused throughout much of their expanse. In this dissection the "two layers" were stripped from the skull as a single membrane.

(2) In some regions, the meningeal and periosteal layers are separated to form the cavities for the **venous sinuses** in the dura mater. In this dissection the longitudinally oriented **superior sagittal sinus** has been opened, as have a number of lateral venous lacunae that communicate with this sinus.

(3) The **arachnoid granulations.** These are elevated bulbous protrusions of the arachnoid into the dura mater and, since they grow from infancy through childhood, they eventually form pits on the inner surface of the skull (see Fig. 517.1).

(4) The projections from the arachnoid are called **arachnoid villi** and appear as diverticula of the subarachnoid space into the venous sinuses. Cerebrospinal fluid passes from the subarachnoid space through the arachnoid villi into the venous blood of the dural sinus (see also Fig. 520.2).

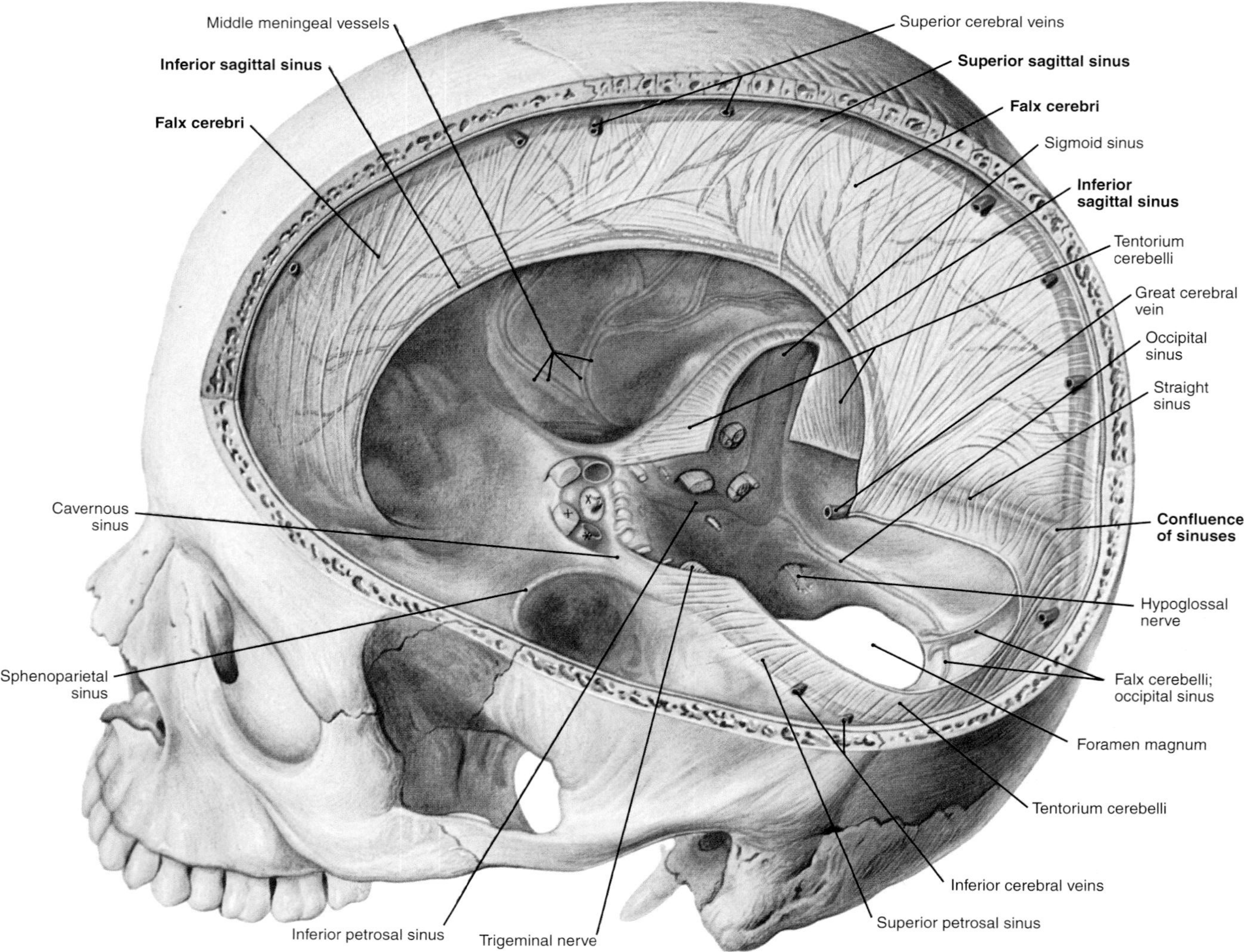
Middle meningeal vessels
Inferior sagittal sinus
Falx cerebri
Superior cerebral veins
Superior sagittal sinus
Falx cerebri
Sigmoid sinus
Inferior sagittal sinus
Tentorium cerebelli
Great cerebral vein
Occipital sinus
Straight sinus
Cavernous sinus
Confluence of sinuses
Hypoglossal nerve
Sphenoparietal sinus
Falx cerebelli; occipital sinus
Foramen magnum
Tentorium cerebelli
Inferior cerebral veins
Superior petrosal sinus
Inferior petrosal sinus
Trigeminal nerve

Figure 522 **Intracranial Dura Mater and the Dural Sinuses**

NOTE: (1) With the skull opened and the brain removed, the reflections of the dura mater are exposed. The sinuses are colored blue, the arteries red. Most of the left **tentorium cerebelli** and part of the right were cut away to open the posterior cranial fossa.

(2) The six **unpaired sinuses:** the **superior** and **inferior sagittal sinuses**, the **occipital sinus**, and the **straight sinuses.** Two other unpaired sinuses (not labeled) at the base of the skull are the **intercavernous** and **basilar sinuses.** These can be seen in Fig. 523.

(3) The six **paired sinuses: transverse, sigmoid, superior** and **inferior petrosal, cavernous,** and **sphenoparietal.** The dural sinuses consist of spaces between the two layers of dura, which drain the cerebral blood, returning it to the **internal jugular vein.**

(4) The **sphenoparietal sinuses** course near the posterior margin of the lesser wings of the sphenoid bone and help form the boundary between the anterior and middle cranial fossae. Similarly, the **superior petrosal sinuses** course along the superior margins of the petrous parts of the temporal bone at the boundary between the middle and posterior cranial fossae.

(5) The sickle-shaped **falx cerebri.** This double-layered, midline reflection of dura mater extends from the crista galli anteriorly to the tentorium cerebelli posteriorly. It also extends vertically between the two cerebral hemispheres. Within the layers of the falx, observe the **superior** and **inferior sagittal sinuses** and the **straight sinus,** all of which flow into the **transverse sinus** or the **confluence of sinuses.**

(6) The **tentorium cerebelli** is a tent-like reflection of dura mater that forms a partition between the occipital lobes of the cerebral cortex and the cerebellum. The **falx cerebelli** extends vertically between the two cerebellar hemispheres.

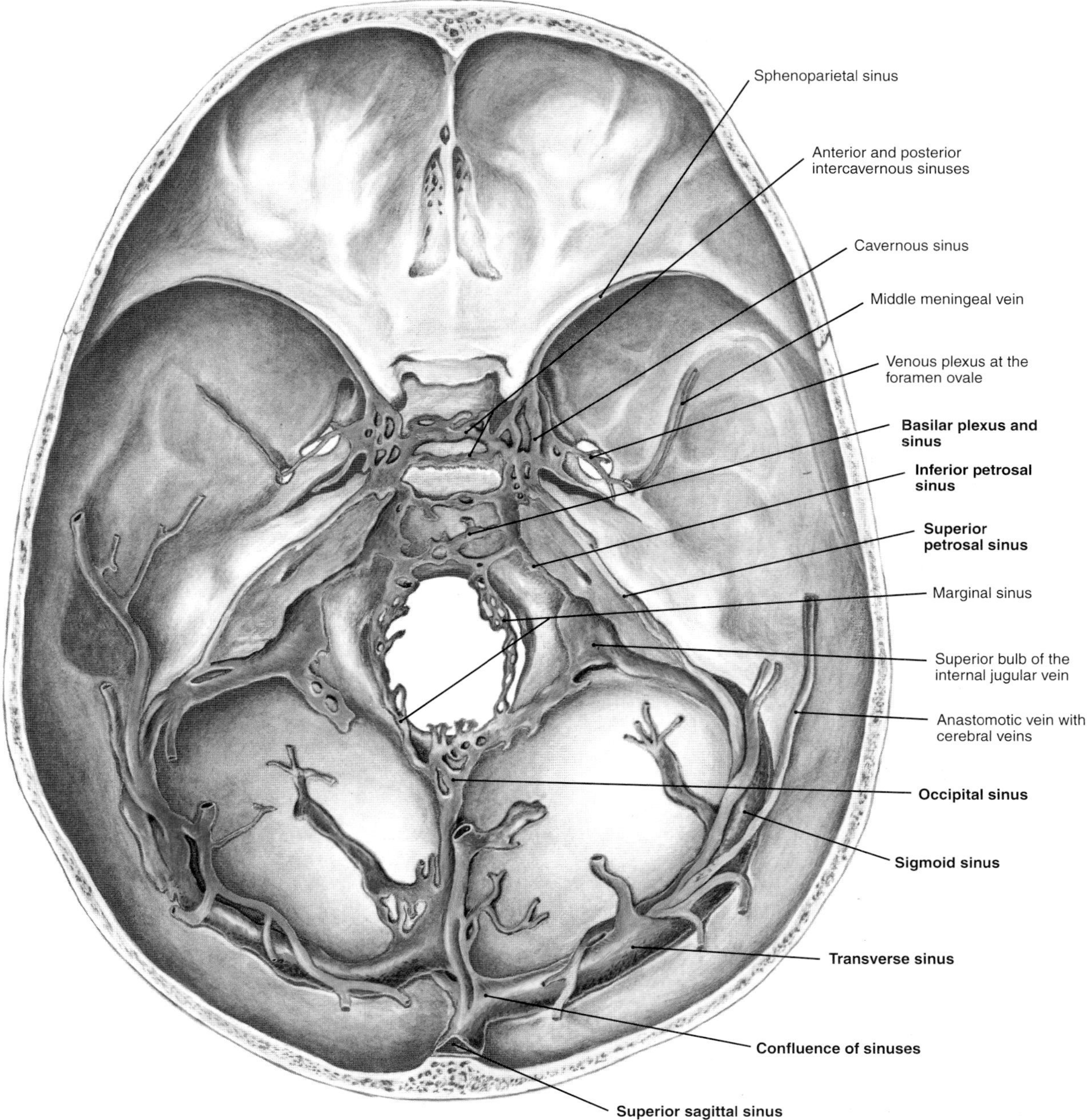
Sphenoparietal sinus
Anterior and posterior intercavernous sinuses
Cavernous sinus
Middle meningeal vein
Venous plexus at the foramen ovale
Basilar plexus and sinus
Inferior petrosal sinus
Superior petrosal sinus
Marginal sinus
Superior bulb of the internal jugular vein
Anastomotic vein with cerebral veins
Occipital sinus
Sigmoid sinus
Transverse sinus
Confluence of sinuses
Superior sagittal sinus

Figure 523 **Dural Sinuses at the Base of the Cranial Cavity Seen from Above**

NOTE: (1) The falx cerebri and the tentorium cerebelli and other dural reflections at the base of the cranial cavity have been removed to expose the venous sinuses from above.

(2) On both sides, the **transverse sinus** courses laterally from the **confluence of sinuses** and then continues as the **sigmoid sinus.** Just above the jugular foramen, the sigmoid sinus enlarges as the **superior bulb of the internal jugular vein.** Below the jugular foramen it becomes the **internal jugular vein** (see Fig. 509).

(3) Venous blood also flows to the transverse-sigmoid sinus from the **occipital sinus** and the **superior** and **inferior petrosal sinuses.** In addition, the **cavernous, intercavernous,** and **basilar sinuses** adjacent to the body of the sphenoid bone and the basilar part of the occipital bone also drain posteriorly and laterally into the sigmoid sinus at the jugular foramen.

(4) Anastomoses between these internal sinuses and the external veins occur through the various foramina, such as the superior orbital fissure (with the ophthalmic veins) and through the foramen lacerum and the foramen ovale (with the pterygoid plexus of veins). Other anastomoses occur with the cerebral, meningeal, and emissary veins.

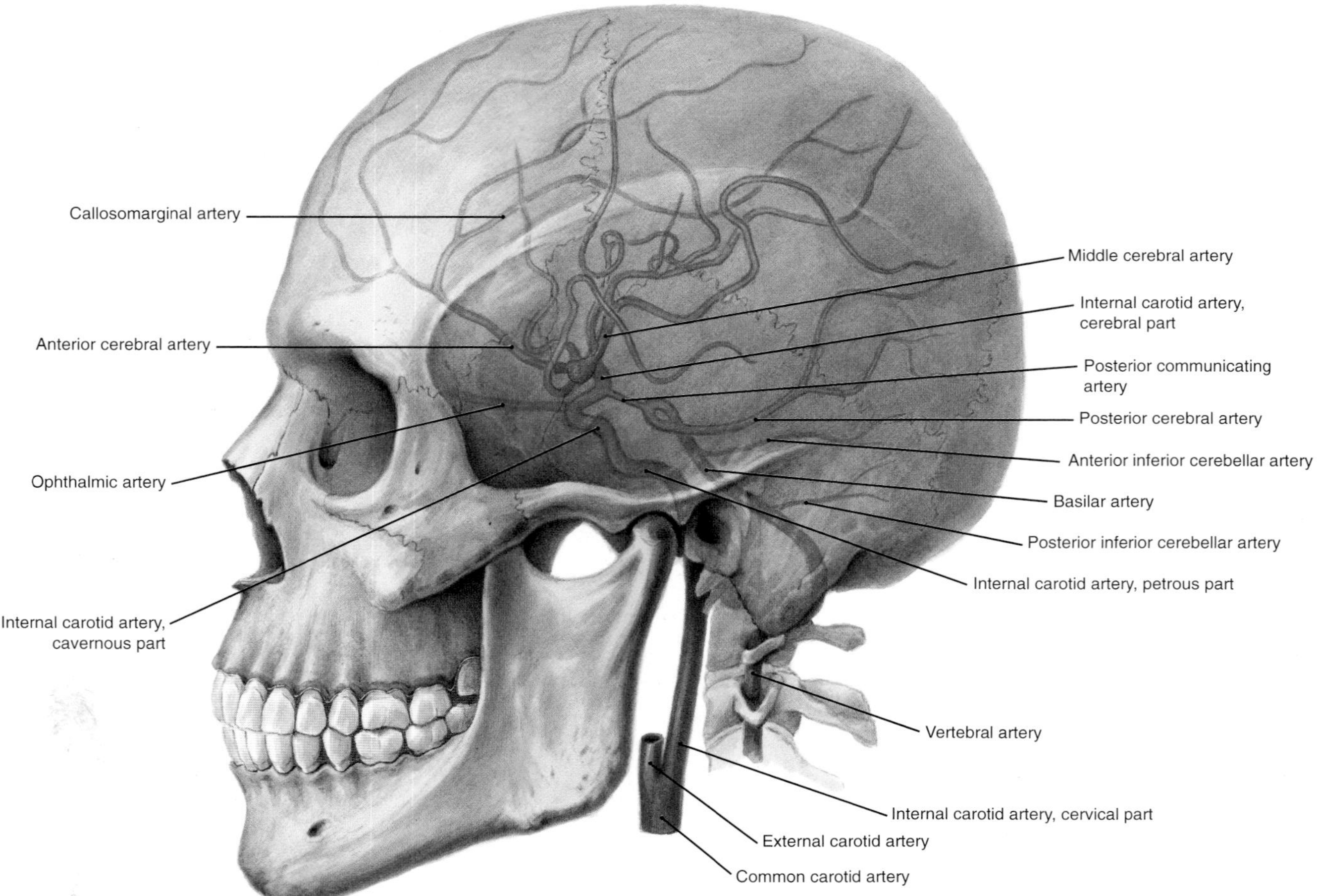
Callosomarginal artery
Anterior cerebral artery
Ophthalmic artery
Internal carotid artery, cavernous part
Middle cerebral artery
Internal carotid artery, cerebral part
Posterior communicating artery
Posterior cerebral artery
Anterior inferior cerebellar artery
Basilar artery
Posterior inferior cerebellar artery
Internal carotid artery, petrous part
Vertebral artery
Internal carotid artery, cervical part
External carotid artery
Common carotid artery

Figure 524.1 **Internal Carotid and Vertebral Arteries: Intracerebral Branches**
NOTE: The direct branches off of the internal carotid artery in the skull are the ophthalmic arteries; the anterior and middle cerebral arteries; and the posterior communicating branch to the circle of Willis.

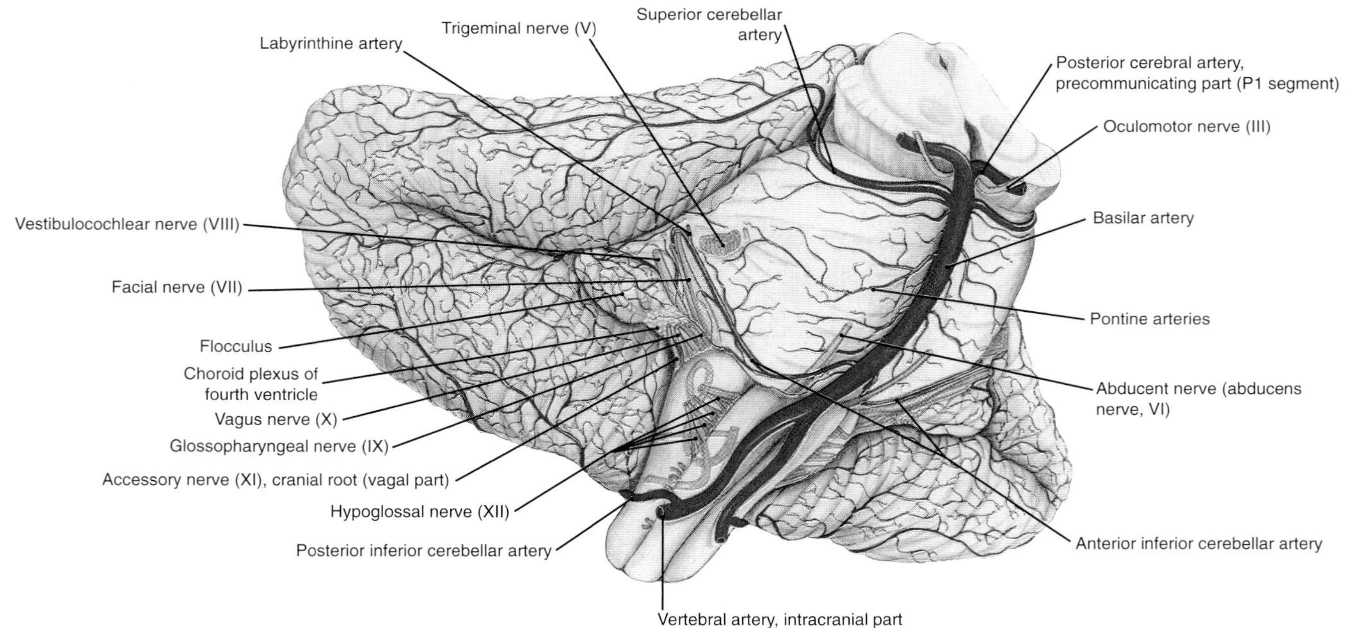
Labyrinthine artery
Trigeminal nerve (V)
Superior cerebellar artery
Posterior cerebral artery, precommunicating part (P1 segment)
Oculomotor nerve (III)
Vestibulocochlear nerve (VIII)
Basilar artery
Facial nerve (VII)
Pontine arteries
Flocculus
Choroid plexus of fourth ventricle
Abducent nerve (abducens nerve, VI)
Vagus nerve (X)
Glossopharyngeal nerve (IX)
Accessory nerve (XI), cranial root (vagal part)
Hypoglossal nerve (XII)
Posterior inferior cerebellar artery
Anterior inferior cerebellar artery
Vertebral artery, intracranial part

Figure 524.2 **Basilar Artery and Its Branches**
NOTE: The two vertebral arteries join to form the **basilar artery**, which ascends on the ventral surface of the brainstem. These vessels supply the cerebellum, medulla oblongata, pons, and posterior aspect of the cerebral cortex. The vertebral arteries also send descending branches to supply the spinal cord.

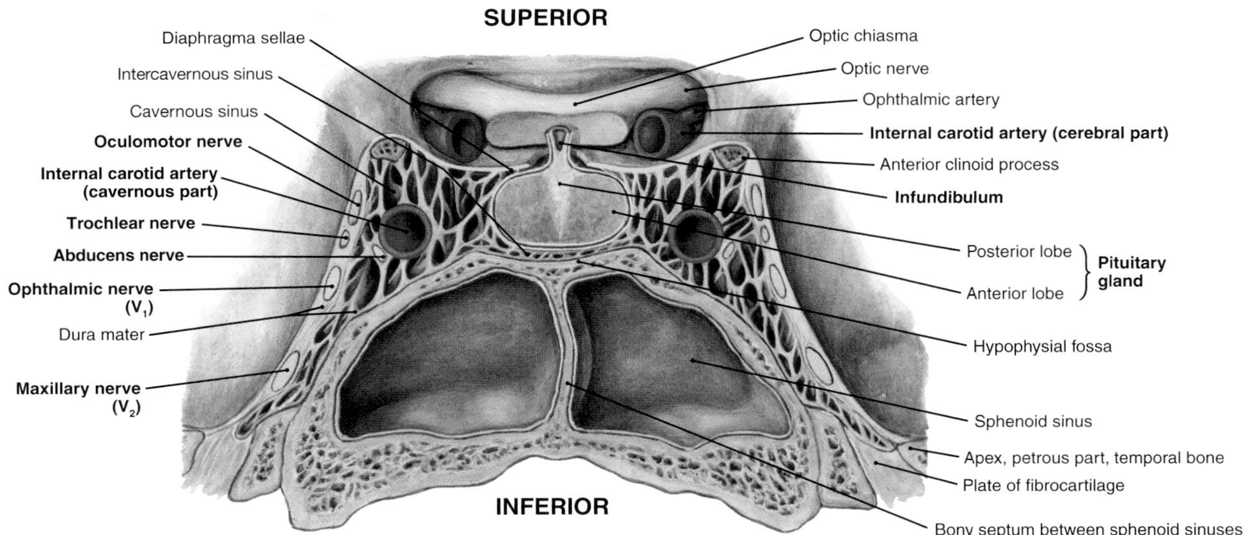
SUPERIOR
Diaphragma sellae
Intercavernous sinus
Cavernous sinus
Oculomotor nerve
Internal carotid artery (cavernous part)
Trochlear nerve
Abducens nerve
Ophthalmic nerve (V_1)
Dura mater
Maxillary nerve (V_2)
Optic chiasma
Optic nerve
Ophthalmic artery
Internal carotid artery (cerebral part)
Anterior clinoid process
Infundibulum
Posterior lobe
Anterior lobe
Pituitary gland
Hypophysial fossa
Sphenoid sinus
Apex, petrous part, temporal bone
Plate of fibrocartilage
Bony septum between sphenoid sinuses
INFERIOR

Figure 525.1 **Frontal Section through the Cavernous Sinus and Base of the Skull Showing the Internal Carotid Artery**

NOTE: (1) This is an anterior view of the cavernous sinus and shows the internal carotid artery (which is seen to have turned back on itself) and the oculomotor, trochlear, V_2, V_3, and abducens nerves all within the cavernous sinus.

(2) Upon traversing the carotid canal, the internal carotid artery courses anteriorly, medially, and superiorly to enter the cavernous sinus.

(3) **Within the sinus,** the artery initially courses forward (medial to the abducens nerve and the sphenoid bone, as shown in this figure). The vessel then curves superiorly and then posteriorly in a U-shaped manner and pierces the dura mater medial to the anterior clinoid process. At this site the **ophthalmic artery** branches from the main stem.

(4) The internal carotid artery then gives off the **anterior** and **middle cerebral arteries,** as shown in Figure 525.2.

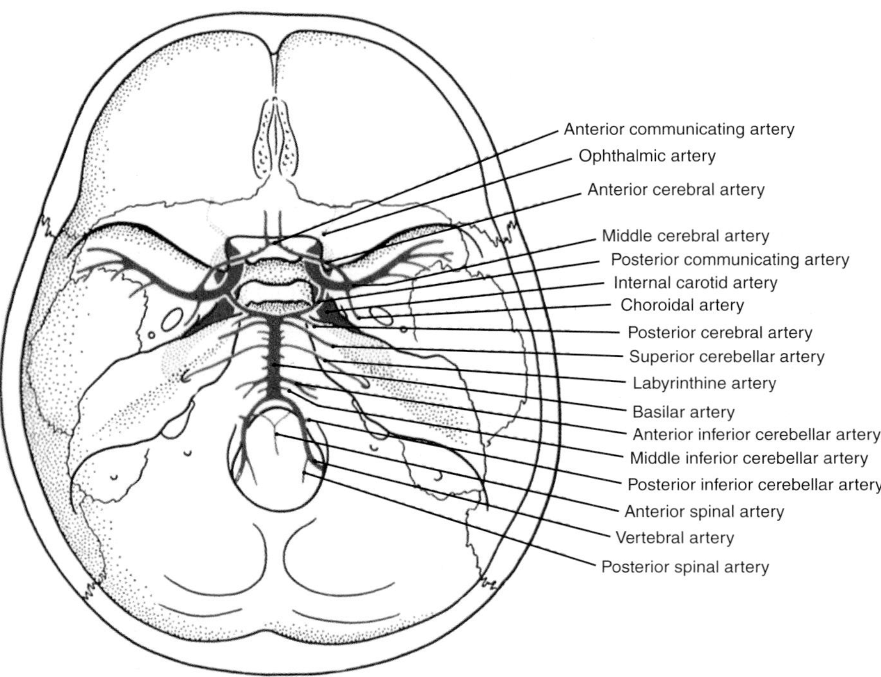
Anterior communicating artery
Ophthalmic artery
Anterior cerebral artery
Middle cerebral artery
Posterior communicating artery
Internal carotid artery
Choroidal artery
Posterior cerebral artery
Superior cerebellar artery
Labyrinthine artery
Basilar artery
Anterior inferior cerebellar artery
Middle inferior cerebellar artery
Posterior inferior cerebellar artery
Anterior spinal artery
Vertebral artery
Posterior spinal artery

Figure 525.2 **Cerebral Part of the Internal Carotid Artery and Other Vessels at the Base of the Brain**

NOTE: The two internal carotid arteries (cerebral parts) and the basilar artery (formed by the two vertebral arteries) give rise to all the named vessels in this figure (see also Fig. 526.2).

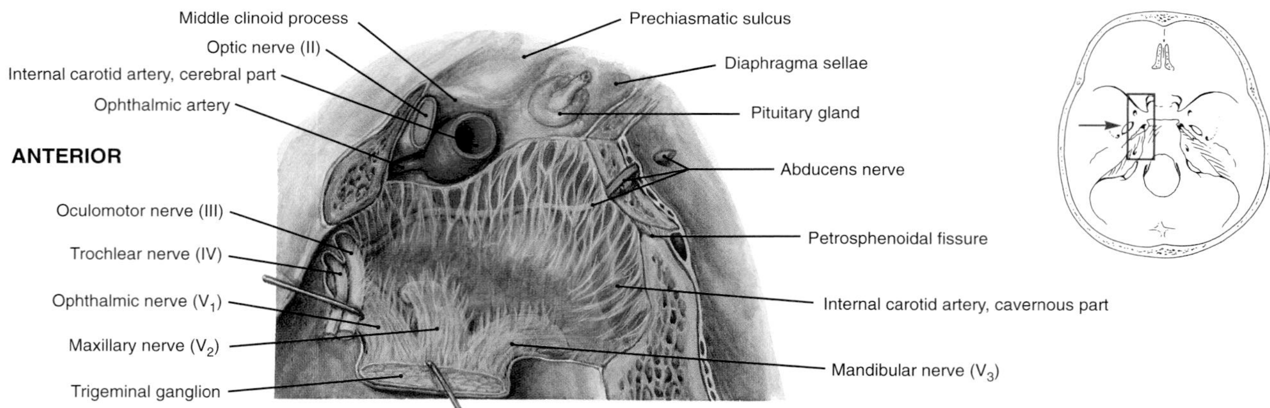
Middle clinoid process
Optic nerve (II)
Internal carotid artery, cerebral part
Ophthalmic artery
ANTERIOR
Oculomotor nerve (III)
Trochlear nerve (IV)
Ophthalmic nerve (V_1)
Maxillary nerve (V_2)
Trigeminal ganglion
Prechiasmatic sulcus
Diaphragma sellae
Pituitary gland
Abducens nerve
Petrosphenoidal fissure
Internal carotid artery, cavernous part
Mandibular nerve (V_3)

Figure 526.1 Internal Carotid Artery within the Cavernous Sinus

NOTE: The lateral dural wall of the cavernous sinus has been removed and the trigeminal ganglion has been pulled laterally. Observe the loop formed by the internal carotid artery before entering the base of the skull and the ophthalmic artery branching anteriorly to enter the orbit in the optic canal with the optic nerve.

Anterior communicating artery
Optic chiasma
Lateral frontobasal artery
Anterior cerebral artery
Subcallosal region
Middle cerebral artery
Insula
Middle cerebral artery
Temporal lobe
Anterior choroidal artery
Posterior perforated substance
Posterior cerebral artery
Superior cerebellar artery
Basilar artery
Abducens nerve (VI)
Hypoglossal nerve (XII)
Vertebral artery
Anterior spinal artery
Olfactory bulb
Medial frontobasal artery
Olfactory tract
Optic nerve (II)
Internal carotid artery
Posterior communicating artery
Oculomotor nerve (III)
Posterior cerebral artery
Superior cerebellar artery
Trigeminal nerve (V)
Labyrinthine artery
Facial nerve (VII)
Vestibulocochlear nerve (VIII)
Choroid plexus of fourth ventricle
Glossopharyngeal nerve (IX)
Anterior inferior cerebellar artery
Hemisphere of cerebellum
Vagus nerve (X)
Accessory nerve (XI)
Posterior inferior cerebellar artery
Spinal cord

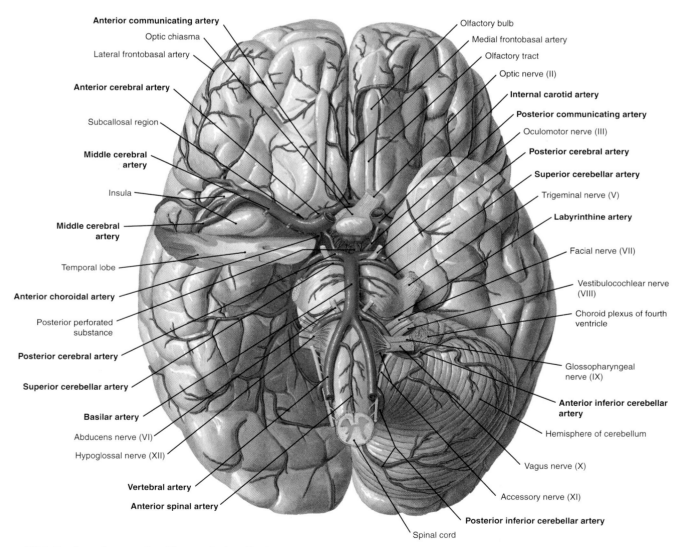

Figure 526.2 Arteries at the Base of the Brain

NOTE: (1) Branches of the **vertebral arteries** form the anterior spinal artery medially and the posterior inferior cerebellar arteries *laterally.*

(2) The **basilar artery** is formed near the pontomedullary junction and gives off the anterior inferior cerebellar, labyrinthine, pontine (not labeled), superior cerebellar, and posterior cerebral arteries successively as it ascends.

(3) The **internal carotid arteries** connect with the posterior cerebral by way of the posterior communicating arteries, and then give off the middle and anterior and cerebral arteries. The anterior cerebral arteries are joined by the anterior communicating artery.

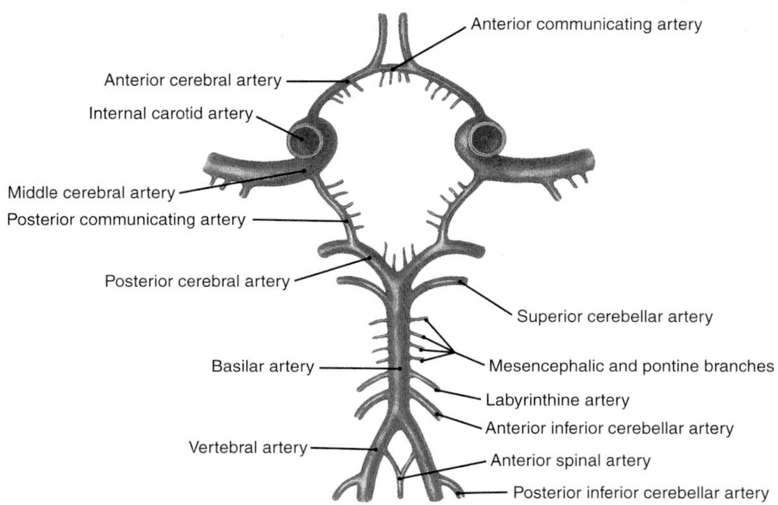
Anterior communicating artery
Anterior cerebral artery
Internal carotid artery
Middle cerebral artery
Posterior communicating artery
Posterior cerebral artery
Superior cerebellar artery
Mesencephalic and pontine branches
Basilar artery
Labyrinthine artery
Anterior inferior cerebellar artery
Vertebral artery
Anterior spinal artery
Posterior inferior cerebellar artery

Figure 527.1 **Circle of Willis**

NOTE: The circle of Willis is formed by the **posterior cerebral, posterior communicating, internal carotid, anterior cerebral,** and **anterior communicating arteries.**

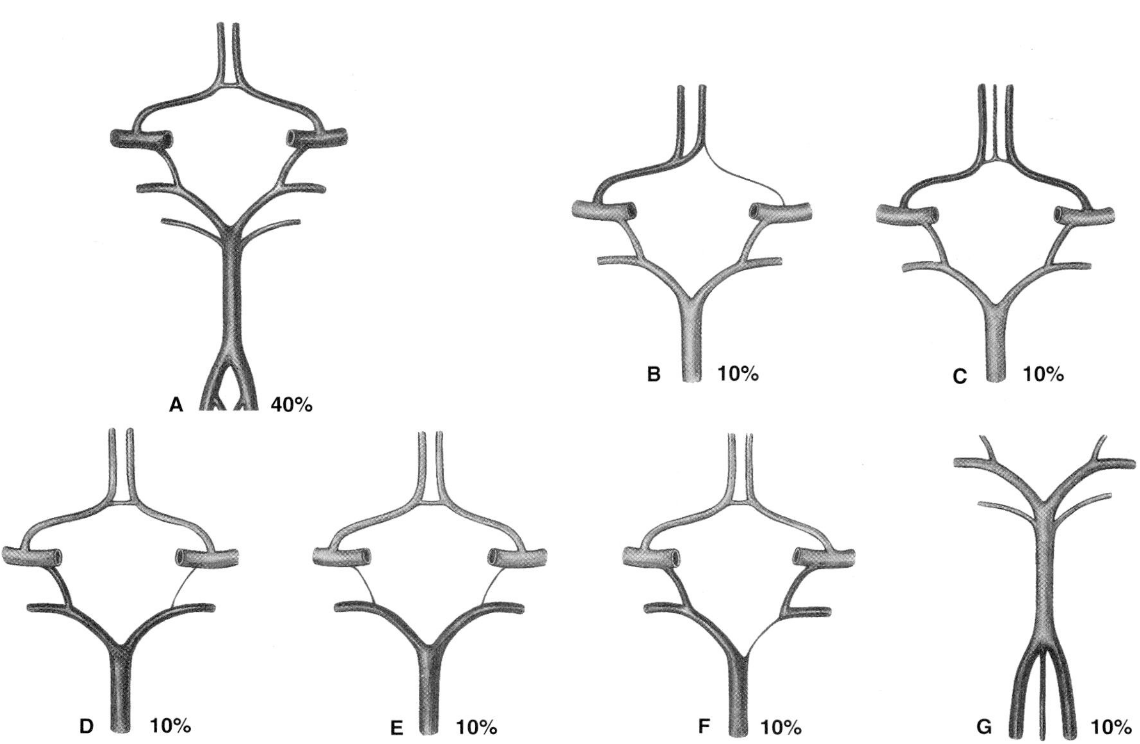
A 40%
B 10%
C 10%
D 10%
E 10%
F 10%
G 10%

Figure 527.2 **Variations in the Formation of the Circle of Willis**

NOTE: Only about 40% of cadavers show the "normal" pattern of formation seen in **A.**

A shows the "normal" textbook pattern.

B shows a narrow anterior cerebral artery on one side.

C shows a small branch coursing forward from the anterior communicating artery.

D shows a narrow posterior communicating artery on one side.

E shows narrow posterior communicating arteries on both sides.

F shows a narrow posterior cerebral artery on one side. The posterior cerebral on the side with the anomaly is substituted for by a continuation of the posterior communicating artery of that same side.

G shows a low junction of the two vertebral arteries in the formation of the basilar artery.

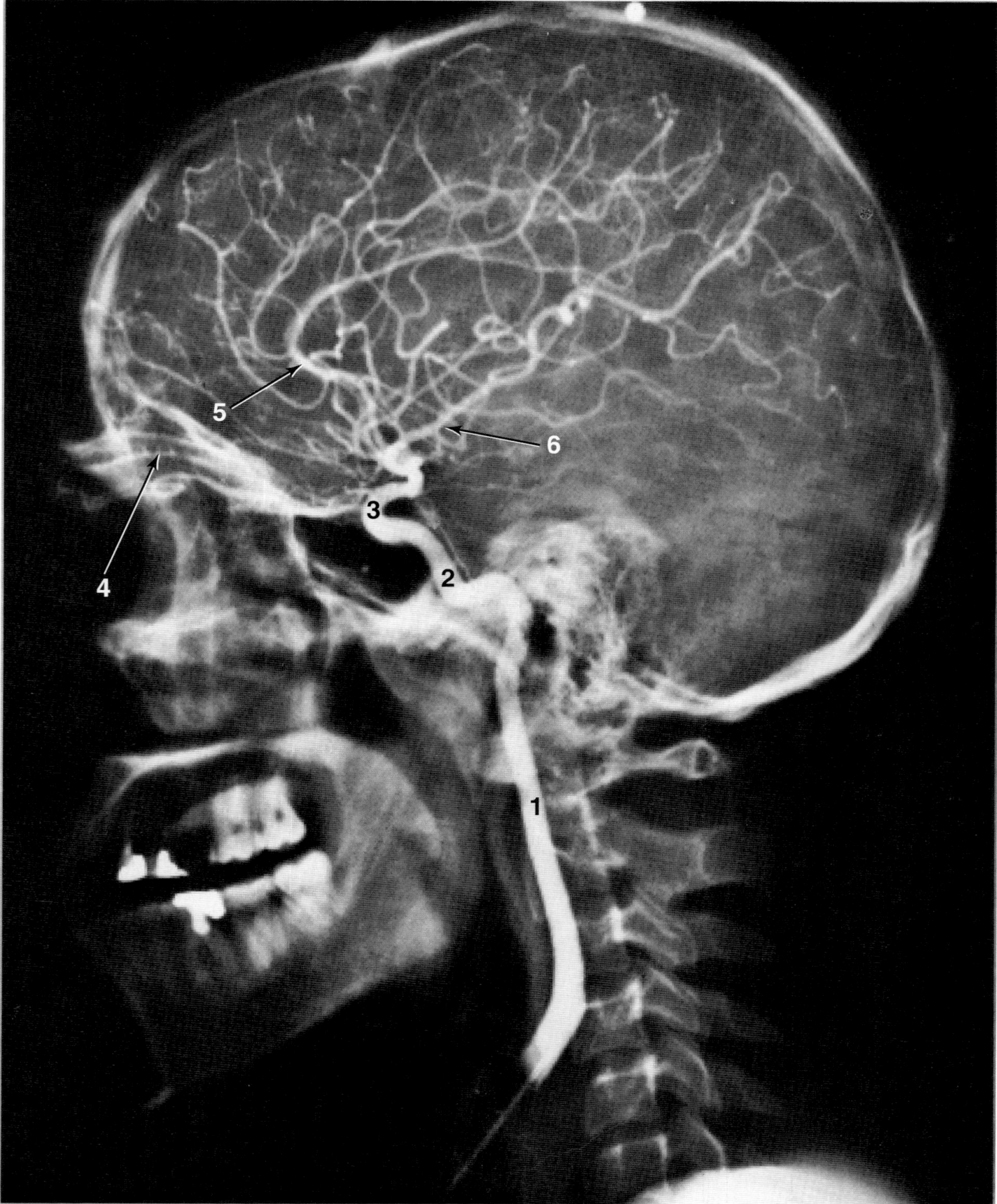
5
6
3
2
4
1

Figure 528 Carotid Arteriogram (Lateral View)

NOTE: (1) This is a lateral view of a left carotid arteriogram showing the internal carotid artery and its **cervical, petrous**, and **cavernous** parts before entering the cranial cavity as the **cerebral** part.

(2) The cervical part courses in the carotid canal, while the cavernous part courses through the cavernous sinus.

(3) The ophthalmic artery is a branch of the internal carotid artery that enters the orbital cone posteriorly. Also note the anterior and middle cerebral arteries that branch from the anterior end of the circle of Willis.

(From Wicke, 6th ed.)

1. Internal carotid artery (cervical part)
2. Internal carotid artery (petrous part)
3. Internal carotid artery (cavernous part)
4. Ophthalmic artery
5. Anterior cerebral artery
6. Middle cerebral artery

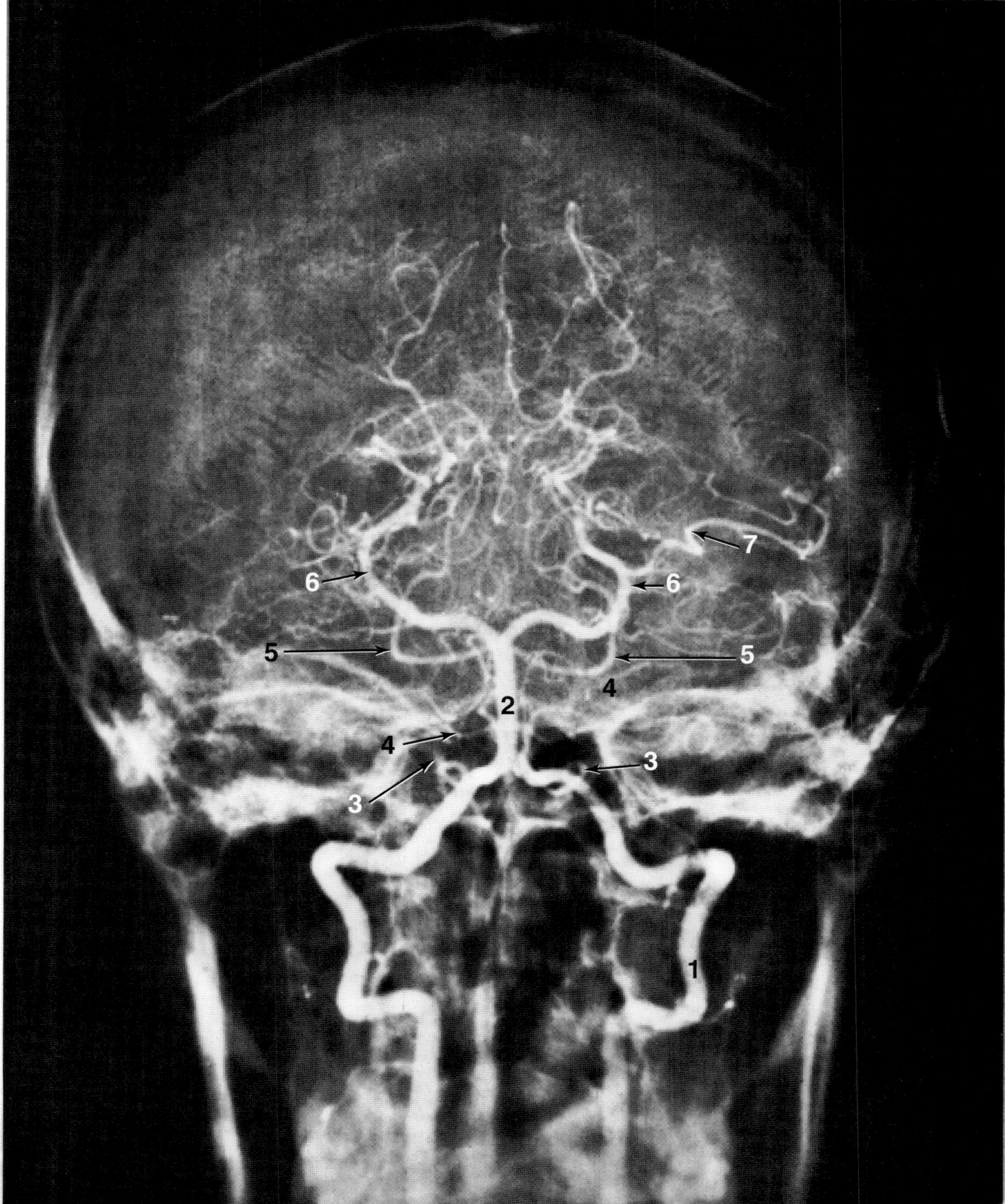
6
6
7
5
5
4
2
4
3
3
1

Figure 529 **Vertebral Arteriogram (Posterior View)**

NOTE: (1) The two vertebral arteries ascend in the neck through foramina in the transverse processes of the first six cervical vertebrae. Above the atlas the arteries bend medially and lie in a groove on the superior surface of the atlas.

(2) The two vessels perforate the atlantaloccipito membrane and join on the ventral surface of the medulla oblongata to form the **basilar artery.** This vessel ascends along the pons and finally terminates as it divides into the two **posterior cerebral arteries.**

(3) On their ascent, the vertebral and basilar arteries supply the cerebellum, the medulla, and pons and also give off the branches that form the **anterior spinal artery.**

(From Wicke, 6th ed.)

1. Vertebral artery
2. Basilar artery
3. Posterior inferior cerebellar artery
4. Anterior inferior cerebellar artery
5. Superior cerebellar artery
6. Posterior cerebral artery (sometimes referred to as the artery of sight)
7. Occipital branch of the posterior cerebral artery

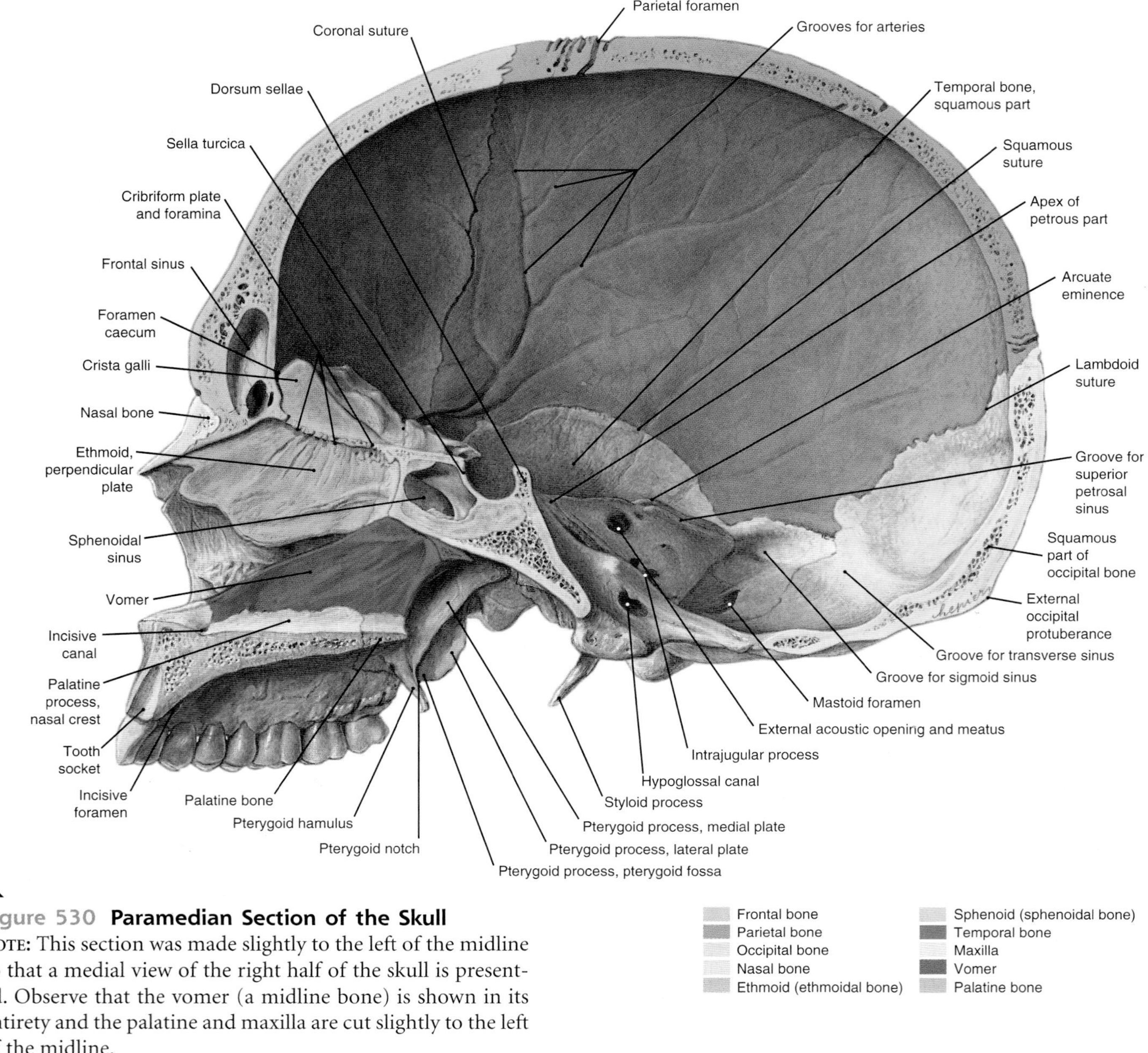
Parietal foramen
Coronal suture
Grooves for arteries
Dorsum sellae
Temporal bone, squamous part
Sella turcica
Squamous suture
Cribriform plate and foramina
Apex of petrous part
Frontal sinus
Arcuate eminence
Foramen caecum
Crista galli
Lambdoid suture
Nasal bone
Ethmoid, perpendicular plate
Groove for superior petrosal sinus
Sphenoidal sinus
Squamous part of occipital bone
Vomer
External occipital protuberance
Incisive canal
Groove for transverse sinus
Palatine process, nasal crest
Groove for sigmoid sinus
Mastoid foramen
Tooth socket
External acoustic opening and meatus
Intrajugular process
Incisive foramen
Palatine bone
Hypoglossal canal
Styloid process
Pterygoid hamulus
Pterygoid process, medial plate
Pterygoid notch
Pterygoid process, lateral plate
Pterygoid process, pterygoid fossa
Frontal bone
Parietal bone
Occipital bone
Nasal bone
Ethmoid (ethmoidal bone)
Sphenoid (sphenoidal bone)
Temporal bone
Maxilla
Vomer
Palatine bone

▲

Figure 530 Paramedian Section of the Skull

NOTE: This section was made slightly to the left of the midline so that a medial view of the right half of the skull is presented. Observe that the vomer (a midline bone) is shown in its entirety and the palatine and maxilla are cut slightly to the left of the midline.

Figure 531 Base of the Skull: Internal Aspect (Superior View)

NOTE: There are important structures that traverse the foramina at the base of the skull.

(1) **Anterior cranial fossa:**
- (a) **Foramen cecum:** a small vein
- (b) **Cribriform plate:** filaments of olfactory receptor neurons to the olfactory bulb
- (c) **Anterior ethmoid foramen:** anterior ethmoidal vessels and nerve
- (d) **Posterior ethmoid foramen:** posterior ethmoidal vessels and nerve

(2) **Middle cranial fossa:**
- (a) **Optic foramen:** optic nerve; ophthalmic artery
- (b) **Superior orbital fissure:** oculomotor nerve; trochlear nerve; ophthalmic nerve; abducens nerve; sympathetic nerve fibers; superior ophthalmic vein; orbital branch of middle meningeal artery; dural recurrent branch of the lacrimal artery
- (c) **Foramen rotundum:** maxillary nerve

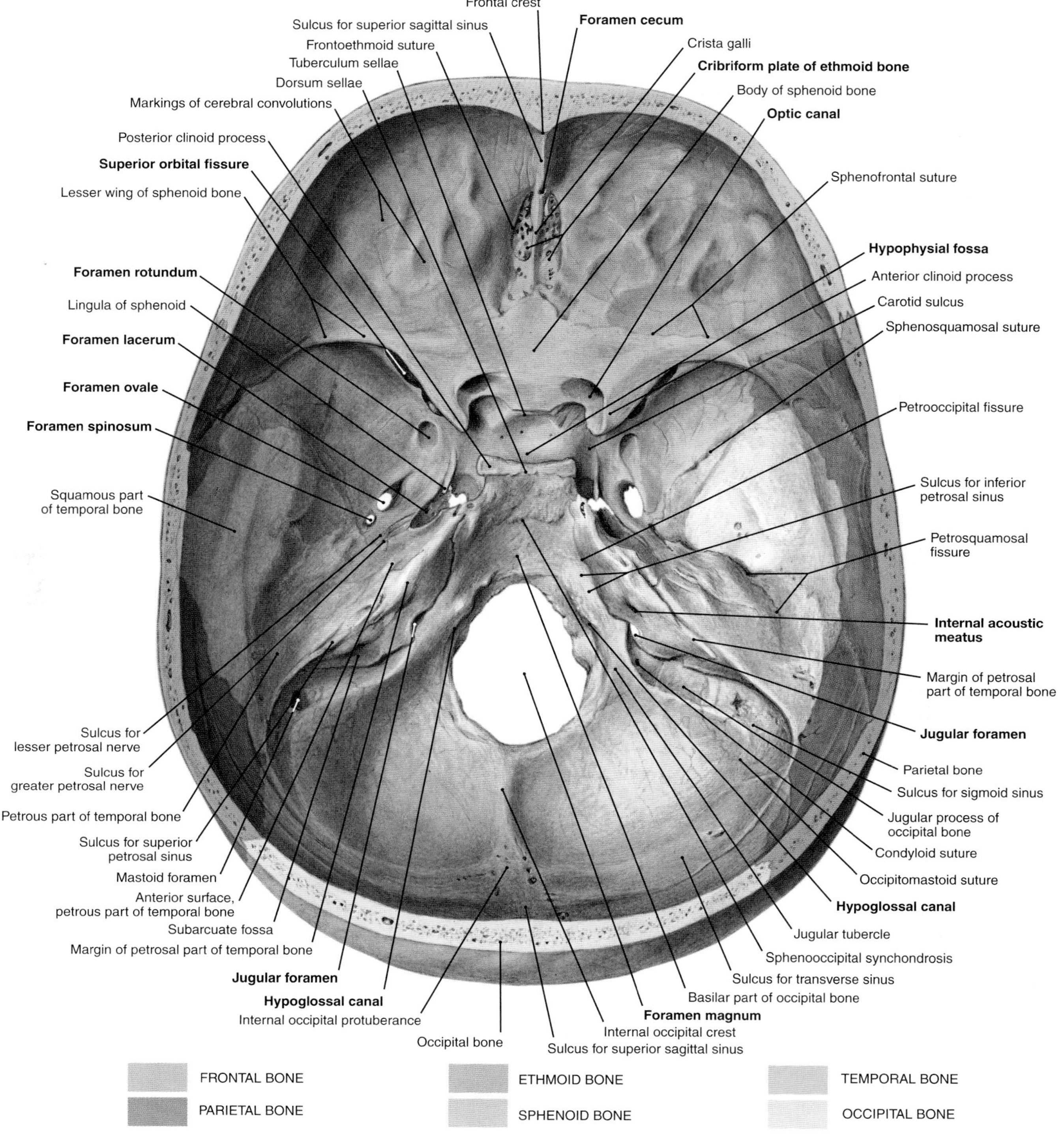

Frontal crest
Sulcus for superior sagittal sinus
Foramen cecum
Frontoethmoid suture
Crista galli
Tuberculum sellae
Cribriform plate of ethmoid bone
Dorsum sellae
Body of sphenoid bone
Markings of cerebral convolutions
Optic canal
Posterior clinoid process
Superior orbital fissure
Lesser wing of sphenoid bone
Sphenofrontal suture
Hypophysial fossa
Foramen rotundum
Anterior clinoid process
Lingula of sphenoid
Carotid sulcus
Sphenosquamosal suture
Foramen lacerum
Foramen ovale
Petrooccipital fissure
Foramen spinosum
Squamous part of temporal bone
Sulcus for inferior petrosal sinus
Petrosquamosal fissure
Internal acoustic meatus
Margin of petrosal part of temporal bone
Jugular foramen
Sulcus for lesser petrosal nerve
Sulcus for greater petrosal nerve
Parietal bone
Sulcus for sigmoid sinus
Petrous part of temporal bone
Jugular process of occipital bone
Sulcus for superior petrosal sinus
Condyloid suture
Mastoid foramen
Occipitomastoid suture
Anterior surface, petrous part of temporal bone
Hypoglossal canal
Subarcuate fossa
Jugular tubercle
Margin of petrosal part of temporal bone
Sphenooccipital synchondrosis
Jugular foramen
Sulcus for transverse sinus
Hypoglossal canal
Basilar part of occipital bone
Internal occipital protuberance
Foramen magnum
Internal occipital crest
Occipital bone
Sulcus for superior sagittal sinus
FRONTAL BONE
PARIETAL BONE
ETHMOID BONE
SPHENOID BONE
TEMPORAL BONE
OCCIPITAL BONE

(d) **Foramen ovale:** mandibular nerve; accessory meningeal artery

(e) **Foramen spinosum:** middle meningeal artery; a recurrent dural branch of mandibular nerve

(f) **Foramen lacerum:** The internal carotid artery passes across the foramen above the fibrocartilaginous plate but does *not* traverse it. The nerve of the pterygoid canal emerges from the foramen to enter the pterygoid canal. The meningeal branch of the ascending pharyngeal artery actually traverses the foramen.

(3) **Posterior cranial fossa:**

(a) **Internal acoustic meatus:** facial nerve; vestibulocochlear nerve; labyrinthine artery

(b) **Jugular foramen:** sigmoid sinus, which becomes internal jugular vein; meningeal branches of occipital and ascending pharyngeal arteries; glossopharyngeal nerve; vagus nerve; accessory nerve

(c) **Hypoglossal canal:** hypoglossal nerve

(d) **Foramen magnum:** spinal cord; spinal part of accessory nerve; anterior and posterior spinal arteries; vertebral arteries; tectorial membrane

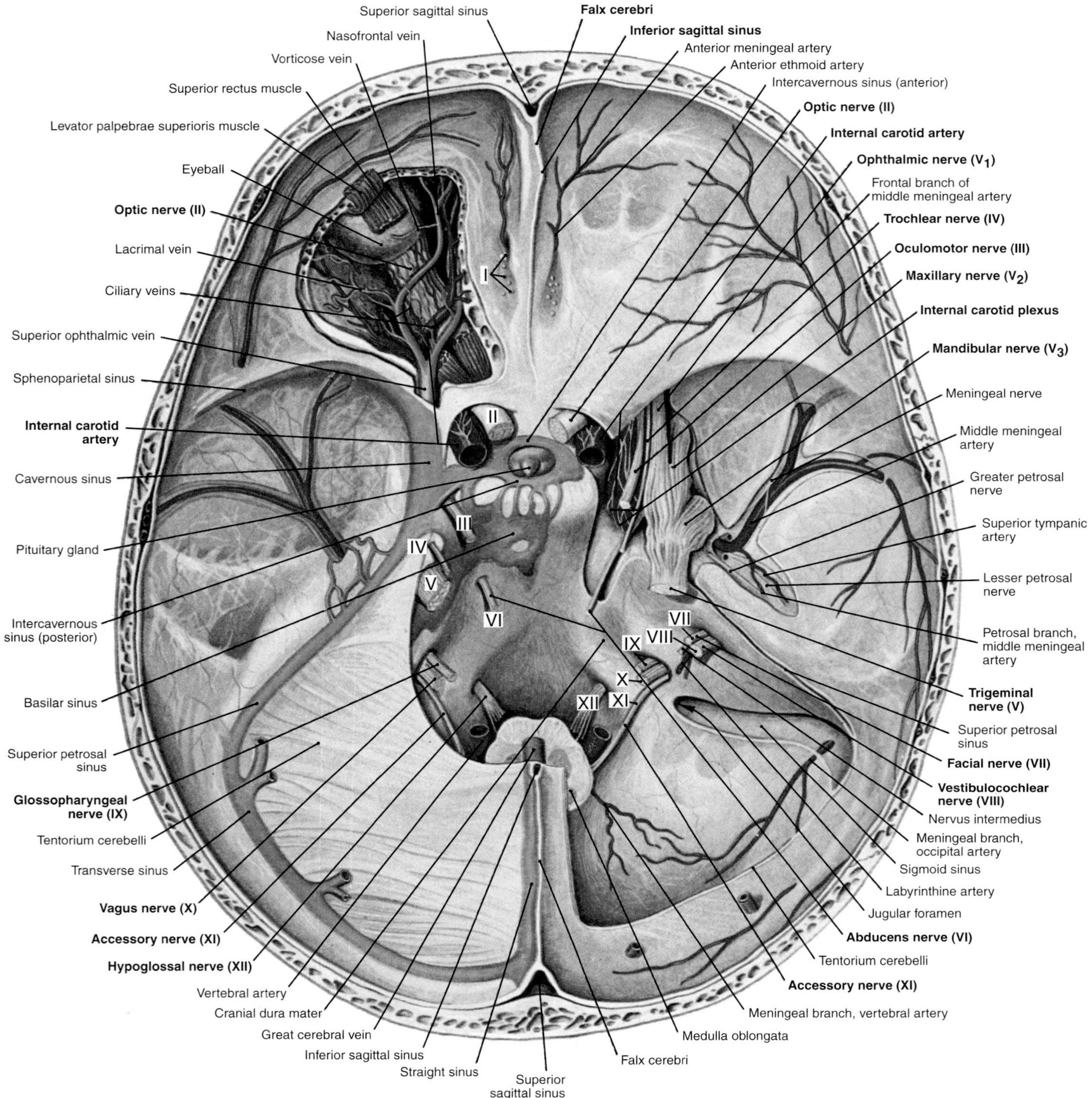
Superior sagittal sinus
Falx cerebri
Inferior sagittal sinus
Nasofrontal vein
Anterior meningeal artery
Vorticose vein
Anterior ethmoid artery
Superior rectus muscle
Intercavernous sinus (anterior)
Optic nerve (II)
Levator palpebrae superioris muscle
Internal carotid artery
Ophthalmic nerve (V_1)
Eyeball
Frontal branch of middle meningeal artery
Optic nerve (II)
Trochlear nerve (IV)
Lacrimal vein
Oculomotor nerve (III)
Maxillary nerve (V_2)
Ciliary veins
Internal carotid plexus
Superior ophthalmic vein
Mandibular nerve (V_3)
Sphenoparietal sinus
Meningeal nerve
Internal carotid artery
Middle meningeal artery
Cavernous sinus
Greater petrosal nerve
Superior tympanic artery
Pituitary gland
Lesser petrosal nerve
Intercavernous sinus (posterior)
Petrosal branch, middle meningeal artery
Basilar sinus
Trigeminal nerve (V)
Superior petrosal sinus
Superior petrosal sinus
Facial nerve (VII)
Glossopharyngeal nerve (IX)
Vestibulocochlear nerve (VIII)
Nervus intermedius
Tentorium cerebelli
Meningeal branch, occipital artery
Transverse sinus
Sigmoid sinus
Labyrinthine artery
Vagus nerve (X)
Jugular foramen
Accessory nerve (XI)
Abducens nerve (VI)
Hypoglossal nerve (XII)
Tentorium cerebelli
Accessory nerve (XI)
Vertebral artery
Cranial dura mater
Meningeal branch, vertebral artery
Great cerebral vein
Medulla oblongata
Inferior sagittal sinus
Falx cerebri
Straight sinus
Superior sagittal sinus
I
II
III
IV
V
VI
VII
VIII
IX
X
XI
XII

Figure 532 Base of the Cranial Cavity: Vessels, Nerves, and Dura Mater

NOTE: (1) The anterior, middle, and posterior **cranial fossae** in the floor of the cranial cavity. In the anterior fossae rest the **frontal lobes** of the brain, while the **temporal lobes** lie in the middle fossae and the **brainstem** and **cerebellum** rest in the posterior fossa.

(2) The dura mater and the orbital plate of the frontal bone have been removed to expose the left orbit from above. The **superior ophthalmic vein** drains posteriorly into the cavernous sinus and the **optic nerve** is seen to course from the orbit through the optic canal.

(3) The medial aspect of the middle fossa shows the cavernous sinus, the internal carotid artery, the third, fourth, fifth, and sixth cranial nerves coursing toward the orbit or the face and the middle meningeal artery traversing the foramen spinosum.

(4) The foramina for the last six pairs of cranial nerves in the posterior fossa. The 7th and 8th nerves pass through the internal acoustic meatus, while the 9th, 10th, and 11th nerves traverse the jugular foramen and the 12th nerve traverses at the hypoglossal canal.

Cranial Nerves II through VI in the Skull Base; Pituitary Gland

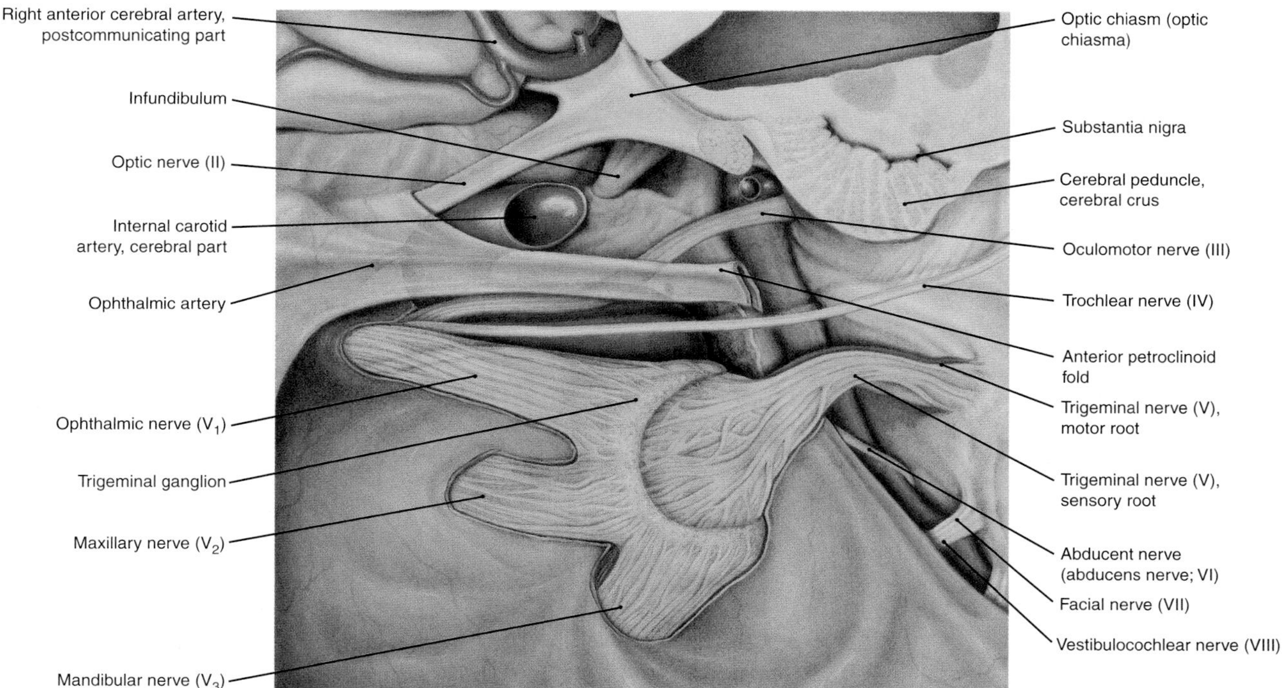
Right anterior cerebral artery, postcommunicating part
Infundibulum
Optic nerve (II)
Internal carotid artery, cerebral part
Ophthalmic artery
Ophthalmic nerve (V_1)
Trigeminal ganglion
Maxillary nerve (V_2)
Mandibular nerve (V_3)
Optic chiasm (optic chiasma)
Substantia nigra
Cerebral peduncle, cerebral crus
Oculomotor nerve (III)
Trochlear nerve (IV)
Anterior petroclinoid fold
Trigeminal nerve (V), motor root
Trigeminal nerve (V), sensory root
Abducent nerve (abducens nerve; VI)
Facial nerve (VII)
Vestibulocochlear nerve (VIII)

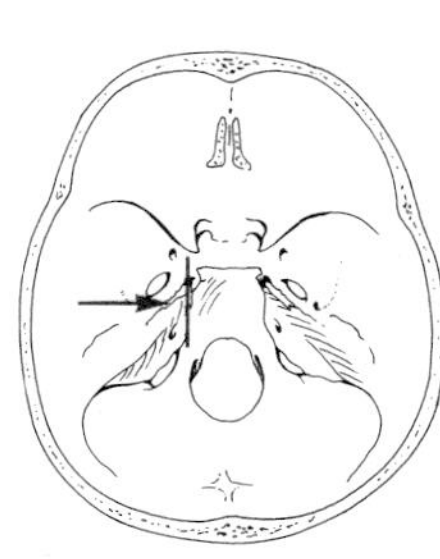

Figure 533.1 **Cranial Nerves II through VI Coursing from the Brainstem through Foramina in the Base of the Skull**

NOTE: (1) The **optic nerve** (II) courses through the optic canal in the body of the sphenoid bone (the ophthalmic branch of the internal carotid artery is not shown in this figure, since it arises deeper to this section, but it too passes through the optic canal).

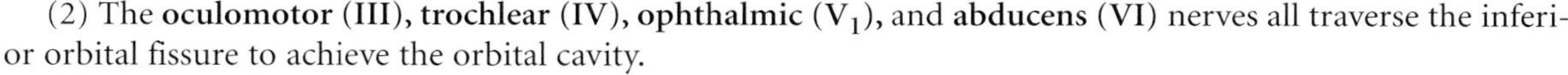

(2) The **oculomotor** (III), **trochlear** (IV), **ophthalmic** (V_1), and **abducens** (VI) nerves all traverse the inferior orbital fissure to achieve the orbital cavity.

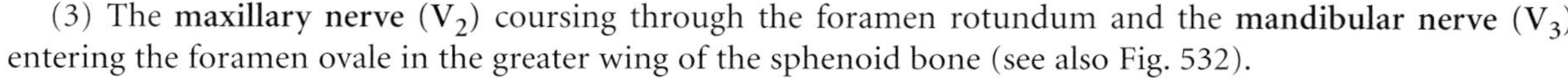

(3) The **maxillary nerve** (V_2) coursing through the foramen rotundum and the **mandibular nerve** (V_3) entering the foramen ovale in the greater wing of the sphenoid bone (see also Fig. 532).

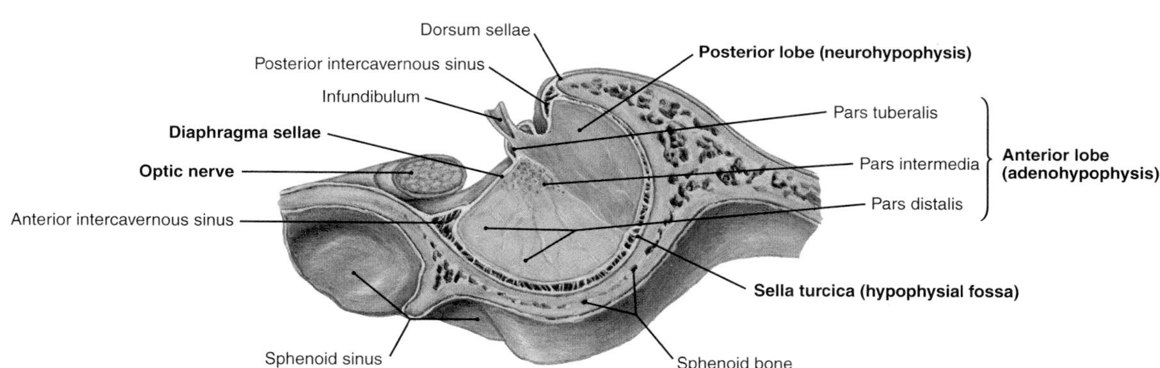
Dorsum sellae
Posterior intercavernous sinus
Infundibulum
Diaphragma sellae
Optic nerve
Anterior intercavernous sinus
Sphenoid sinus
Posterior lobe (neurohypophysis)
Pars tuberalis
Pars intermedia
Pars distalis
Anterior lobe (adenohypophysis)
Sella turcica (hypophysial fossa)
Sphenoid bone

Figure 533.2 **Median Sagittal Section through the Pituitary Gland and the Sella Turcica of the Sphenoid Bone**

NOTE: The **sella turcica** (hypophysial fossa) in the sphenoid bone is lined and covered (**diaphragma sellae**) by dura mater. The anterior and posterior lobes form a single organ that lies below and slightly behind the optic chiasma.

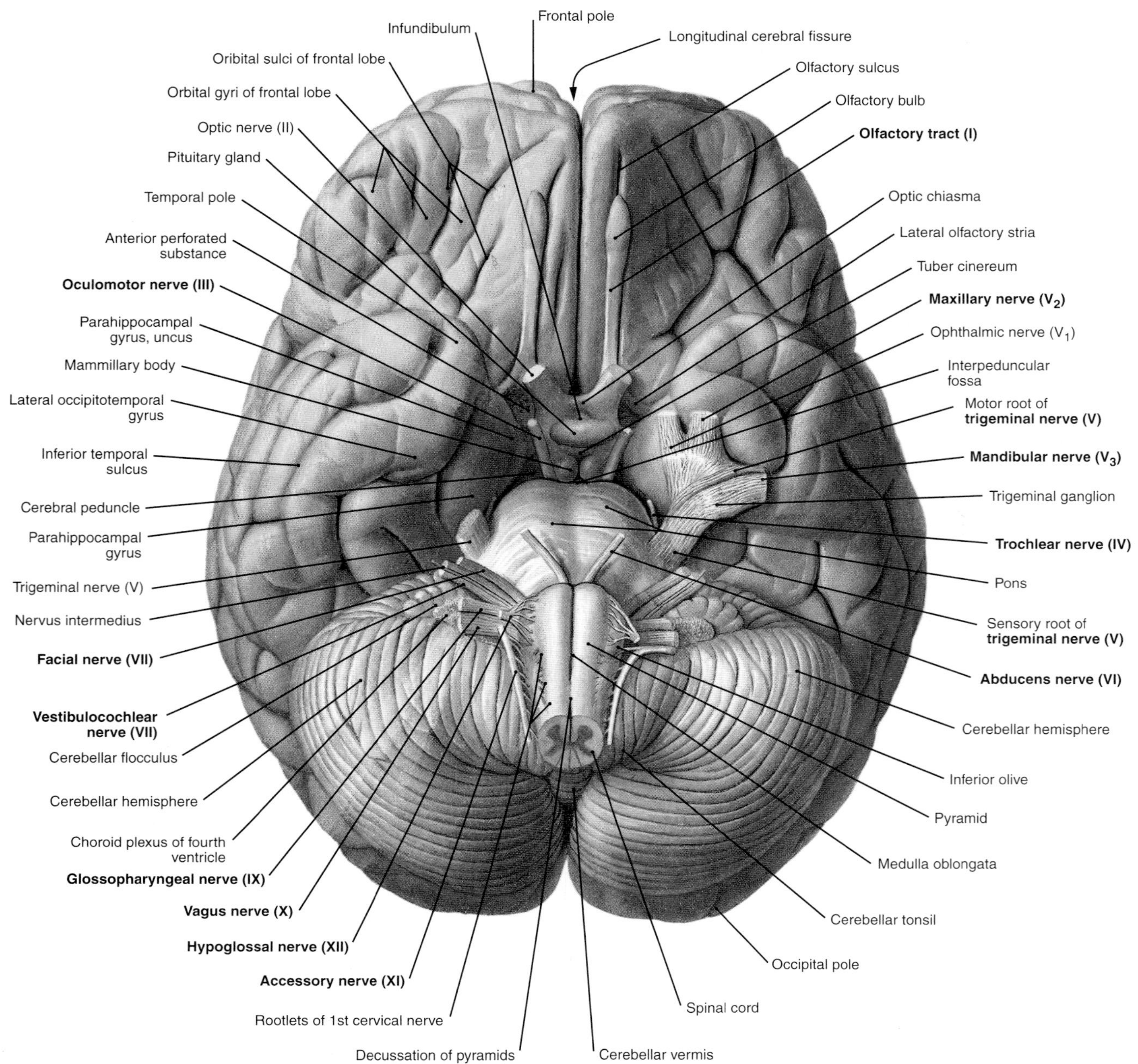
Frontal pole
Infundibulum
Longitudinal cerebral fissure
Oribital sulci of frontal lobe
Olfactory sulcus
Orbital gyri of frontal lobe
Olfactory bulb
Optic nerve (II)
Olfactory tract (I)
Pituitary gland
Temporal pole
Optic chiasma
Anterior perforated substance
Lateral olfactory stria
Tuber cinereum
Oculomotor nerve (III)
Maxillary nerve (V_2)
Parahippocampal gyrus, uncus
Ophthalmic nerve (V_1)
Mammillary body
Interpeduncular fossa
Lateral occipitotemporal gyrus
Motor root of trigeminal nerve (V)
Inferior temporal sulcus
Mandibular nerve (V_3)
Trigeminal ganglion
Cerebral peduncle
Parahippocampal gyrus
Trochlear nerve (IV)
Trigeminal nerve (V)
Pons
Nervus intermedius
Sensory root of trigeminal nerve (V)
Facial nerve (VII)
Abducens nerve (VI)
Vestibulocochlear nerve (VII)
Cerebellar hemisphere
Cerebellar flocculus
Inferior olive
Cerebellar hemisphere
Pyramid
Choroid plexus of fourth ventricle
Medulla oblongata
Glossopharyngeal nerve (IX)
Vagus nerve (X)
Cerebellar tonsil
Hypoglossal nerve (XII)
Occipital pole
Accessory nerve (XI)
Spinal cord
Rootlets of 1st cervical nerve
Decussation of pyramids
Cerebellar vermis

Figure 534 Ventral View of the Brain Showing the Origins of the Cranial Nerves

NOTE: (1) The cranial nerves attach to the base of the brain. The **olfactory tracts** and **optic nerves** (I and II) subserve receptors of special sense in the nose and eye, and as cranial nerve trunks, attach to the base of the forebrain in contrast to all other cranial nerves that attach to the midbrain, pons, or medulla of the brainstem.

(2) The **oculomotor** (III), **trochlear** (IV), and **abducens** (VI) **nerves** are motor nerves to the extraocular muscles. The **trigeminal nerve** (V) is the largest of the cranial nerves, and the **trochlear** is the smallest. The abducens nerve attaches to the brainstem at the junction of the pons and medulla (pontomedullary junction) medial to the attachments of the **facial** (VII) and **vestibulocochlear** (VIII) **nerves.**

(3) The **glossopharyngeal** (IX) and **vagus** (X) **nerves** emerge from the medulla laterally in a line comparable to the spinal and medullary parts of the **accessory nerve** (XI). In contrast, the **hypoglossal nerve** (XII) rootlets emerge from the ventral medulla in a line consistent with the ventral rootlets of the cervical nerves of the spinal cord.

(4) The cranial nerves are of the utmost importance as signposts in localizing disorders both inside and outside the cranial cavity. The functions of most cranial nerves are tested in each complete physical examination performed by competent physicians.

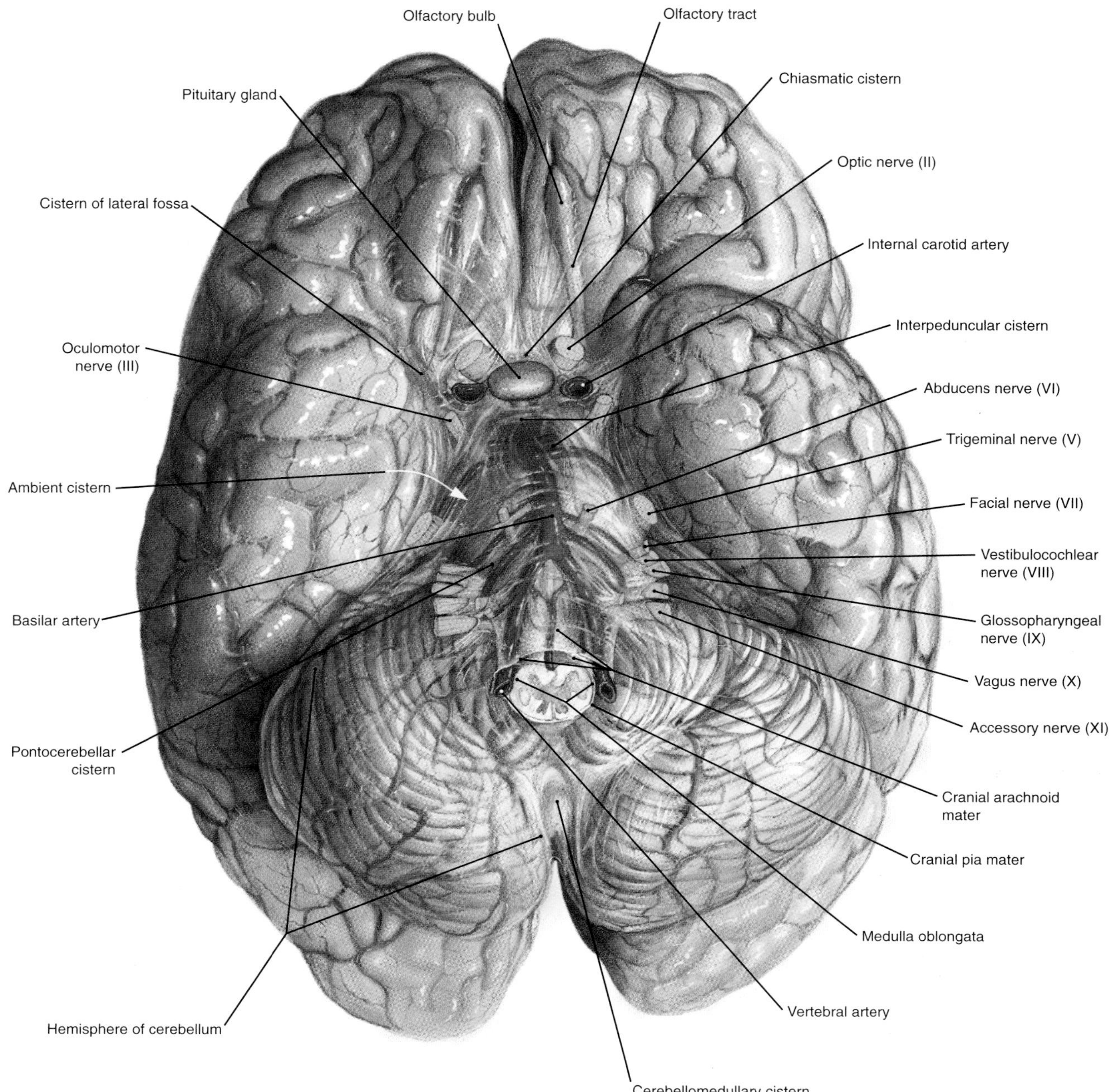
Olfactory bulb
Olfactory tract
Chiasmatic cistern
Pituitary gland
Optic nerve (II)
Cistern of lateral fossa
Internal carotid artery
Interpeduncular cistern
Oculomotor nerve (III)
Abducens nerve (VI)
Trigeminal nerve (V)
Ambient cistern
Facial nerve (VII)
Vestibulocochlear nerve (VIII)
Basilar artery
Glossopharyngeal nerve (IX)
Vagus nerve (X)
Accessory nerve (XI)
Pontocerebellar cistern
Cranial arachnoid mater
Cranial pia mater
Medulla oblongata
Vertebral artery
Hemisphere of cerebellum
Cerebellomedullary cistern

Figure 535 **Base of the Brain: Arteries and Cranial Nerves with the Arachnoid Mater Intact**

NOTE: (1) The dura mater has been completely removed from the brain, leaving intact the arachnoid mater and pia mater. Observe the vertebral arteries joining to form the basilar artery and, anteriorly, the internal carotid arteries severed upon entering the cranial cavity at the base of the brain.

(2) Between the arachnoid mater and the pia mater and the cerebral vessels is the **subarachnoid space,** within which is found the cerebrospinal fluid that is formed in the choroid plexuses. At certain sites the arachnoid mater separates from the pia mater to form pools of cerebrospinal fluid called **cisterns.**

(3) In this figure are seen the cisterns on the ventral aspect of the brainstem; however, they also are located on the dorsal aspect of the brainstem, especially between the cerebellum and the pons and medulla oblongata.

(4) Identify the following cisterns:

(a) The **cistern of the lateral fossa** extends between the orbital surface of the frontal lobe and the anteromedial surface of the temporal lobe. It contains the internal carotid artery.

(b) The **ambient cistern** (also called the **cistern of the great cerebral vein**) is located between the splenium of the corpus callosum and the rostral surface of the cerebellum. It contains the great cerebral vein and the pineal gland.

(c) The **pontocerebellar cistern** on the anterior surface of the pons containing the basilar artery. It communicates superiorly with the interpeduncular cistern and inferiorly with the subarachnoid space of the spinal cord.

(d) The large **cerebellomedullary cistern** (also called the **cisterna magna**) between the medulla oblongata and the inferior surface of the cerebellum.

(e) The **interpeduncular cistern** contains the circle of Willis; it also continues anteriorly as the **chiasmatic cistern** anterior to the pituitary gland and adjacent to the optic chiasma.

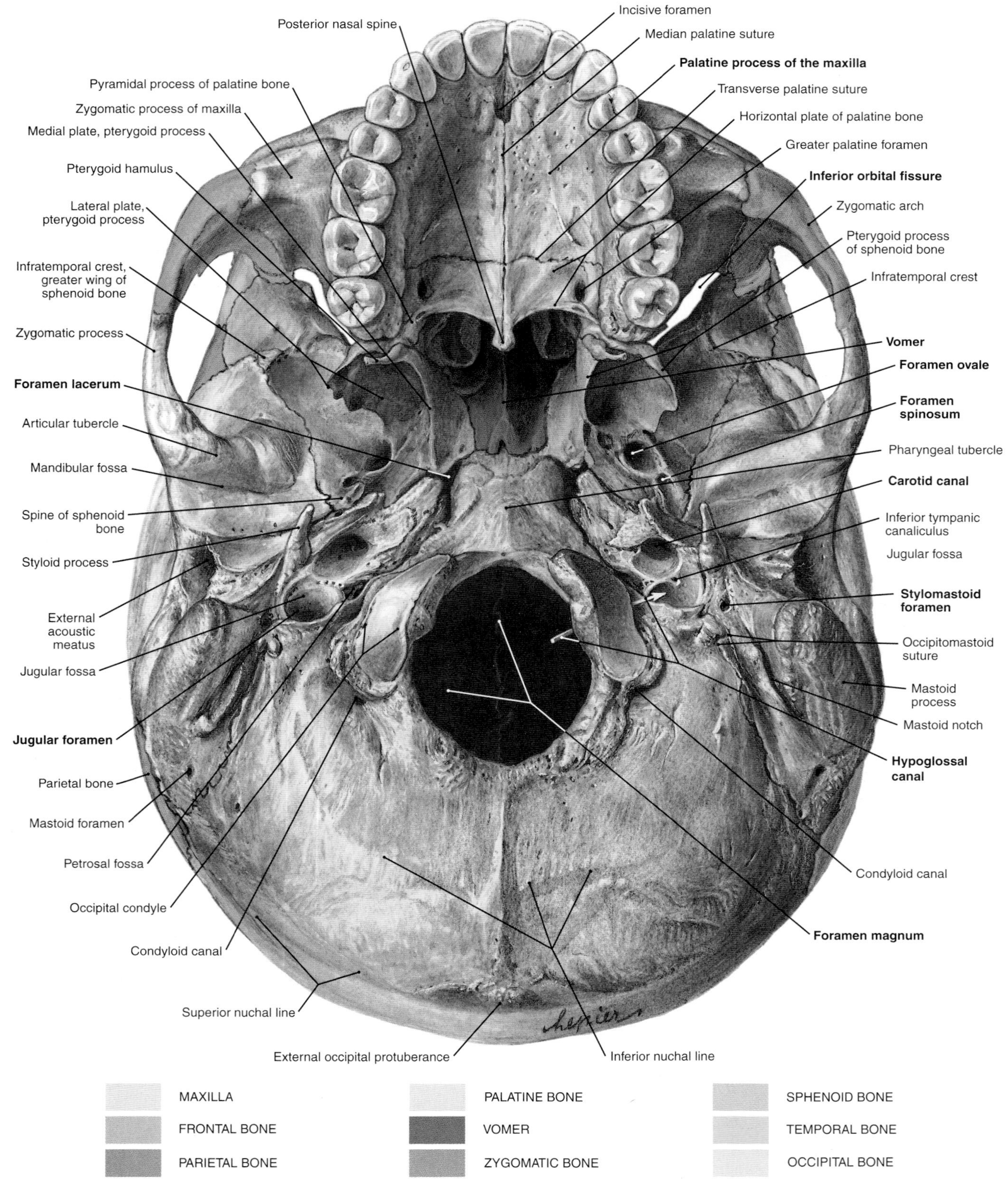
Incisive foramen
Posterior nasal spine
Median palatine suture
Palatine process of the maxilla
Pyramidal process of palatine bone
Transverse palatine suture
Zygomatic process of maxilla
Horizontal plate of palatine bone
Medial plate, pterygoid process
Greater palatine foramen
Pterygoid hamulus
Inferior orbital fissure
Lateral plate, pterygoid process
Zygomatic arch
Pterygoid process of sphenoid bone
Infratemporal crest, greater wing of sphenoid bone
Infratemporal crest
Zygomatic process
Vomer
Foramen ovale
Foramen lacerum
Foramen spinosum
Articular tubercle
Pharyngeal tubercle
Mandibular fossa
Carotid canal
Spine of sphenoid bone
Inferior tympanic canaliculus
Jugular fossa
Styloid process
Stylomastoid foramen
External acoustic meatus
Occipitomastoid suture
Jugular fossa
Mastoid process
Mastoid notch
Jugular foramen
Hypoglossal canal
Parietal bone
Mastoid foramen
Petrosal fossa
Condyloid canal
Occipital condyle
Foramen magnum
Condyloid canal
Superior nuchal line
External occipital protuberance
Inferior nuchal line
MAXILLA
PALATINE BONE
SPHENOID BONE
FRONTAL BONE
VOMER
TEMPORAL BONE
PARIETAL BONE
ZYGOMATIC BONE
OCCIPITAL BONE

Figure 536 Base of the Skull: External Aspect (Inferior View)

NOTE: (1) The posterior part of the base of the skull consists of the **occipital** and **temporal bones**. Anteriorly are the facial bones: the **maxilla, palatine, zygomatic,** and **vomer**. Interposed between these two groups of hones is the **sphenoid bone.**

(2) The bony palate is formed by the transverse processes of the two maxillae and the horizontal plates of the palatine bones.

(3) The medial and lateral plates of the pterygoid process of the sphenoid bone, behind which are the foramen ovale and foramen spinosum in the greater wings of the sphenoid.

(4) The **foramen lacerum, carotid canal, jugular foramen, styloid process** (of temporal bone), **hypoglossal canal** (arrow), and the **foramen magnum.**

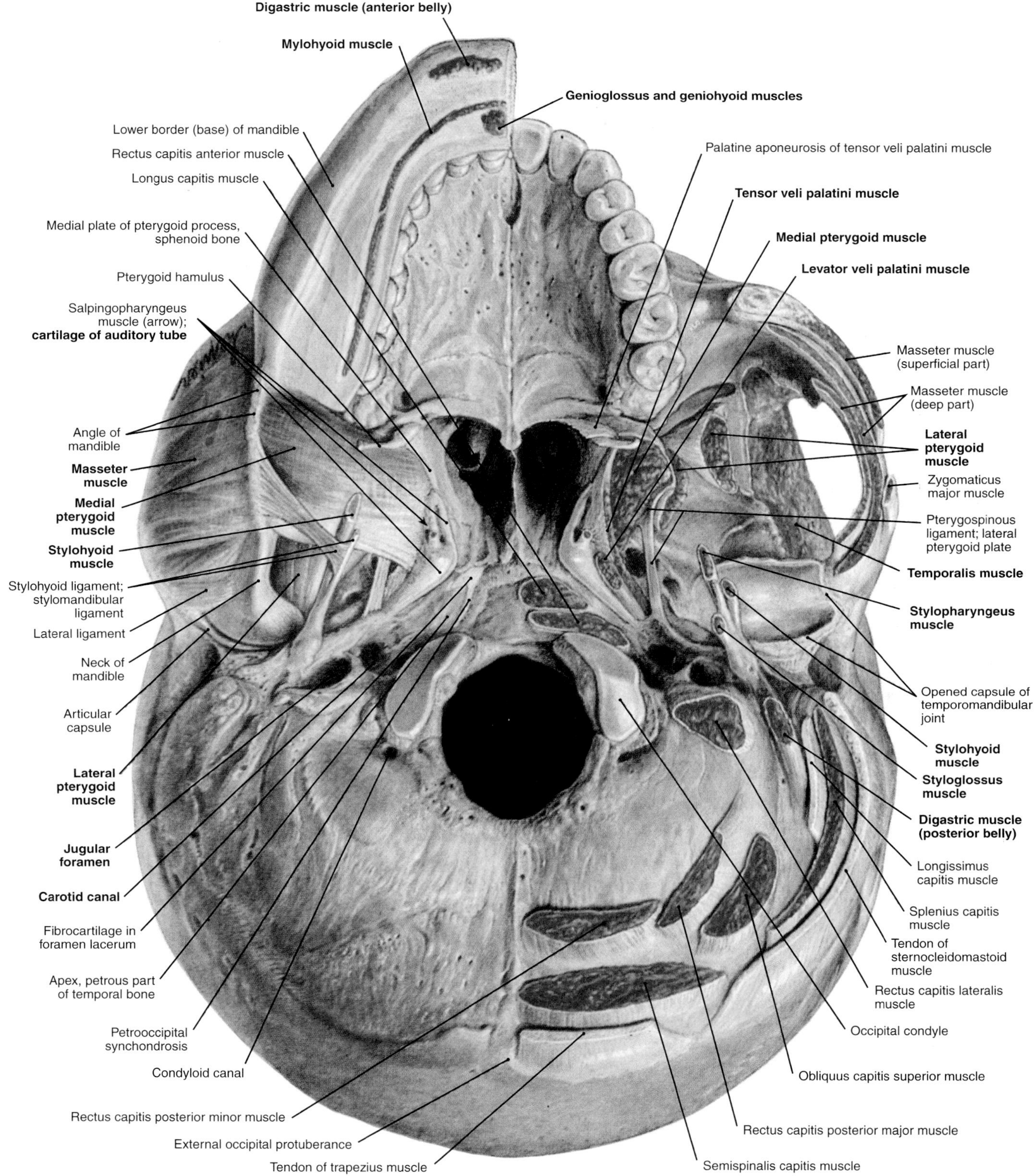
Digastric muscle (anterior belly)
Mylohyoid muscle
Genioglossus and geniohyoid muscles
Lower border (base) of mandible
Rectus capitis anterior muscle
Longus capitis muscle
Palatine aponeurosis of tensor veli palatini muscle
Tensor veli palatini muscle
Medial plate of pterygoid process, sphenoid bone
Medial pterygoid muscle
Levator veli palatini muscle
Pterygoid hamulus
Salpingopharyngeus muscle (arrow); cartilage of auditory tube
Masseter muscle (superficial part)
Masseter muscle (deep part)
Angle of mandible
Lateral pterygoid muscle
Masseter muscle
Zygomaticus major muscle
Medial pterygoid muscle
Pterygospinous ligament; lateral pterygoid plate
Stylohyoid muscle
Temporalis muscle
Stylohyoid ligament; stylomandibular ligament
Stylopharyngeus muscle
Lateral ligament
Neck of mandible
Opened capsule of temporomandibular joint
Articular capsule
Stylohyoid muscle
Styloglossus muscle
Lateral pterygoid muscle
Digastric muscle (posterior belly)
Jugular foramen
Longissimus capitis muscle
Carotid canal
Splenius capitis muscle
Fibrocartilage in foramen lacerum
Tendon of sternocleidomastoid muscle
Apex, petrous part of temporal bone
Rectus capitis lateralis muscle
Petrooccipital synchondrosis
Occipital condyle
Condyloid canal
Obliquus capitis superior muscle
Rectus capitis posterior minor muscle
Rectus capitis posterior major muscle
External occipital protuberance
Tendon of trapezius muscle
Semispinalis capitis muscle

Figure 537 Muscle Origins and Other Structures on the Base of the Skull

NOTE: (1) The left mandible and muscles of mastication (reader's right) have been removed. Observe the attachments of the superficial and deep parts of the **masseter muscle**, the **temporalis muscle**, the two heads of the **lateral pterygoid muscle** and the **medial pterygoid.**

(2) The **levator veli palatini muscle** arises from the inferior surface of the apex of the temporal bone, anterior to the opening of the carotid canal. The **tensor veli palatini muscle** lies lateral and anterior to the levator, and it arises from the scaphoid fossa at the base of the medial pterygoid plate, from the sphenoidal spine and from the lateral aspect of the cartilaginous auditory tube.

(3) The cartilage of the **auditory tube** opens inferomedially in the lateral wall of the nasopharynx.

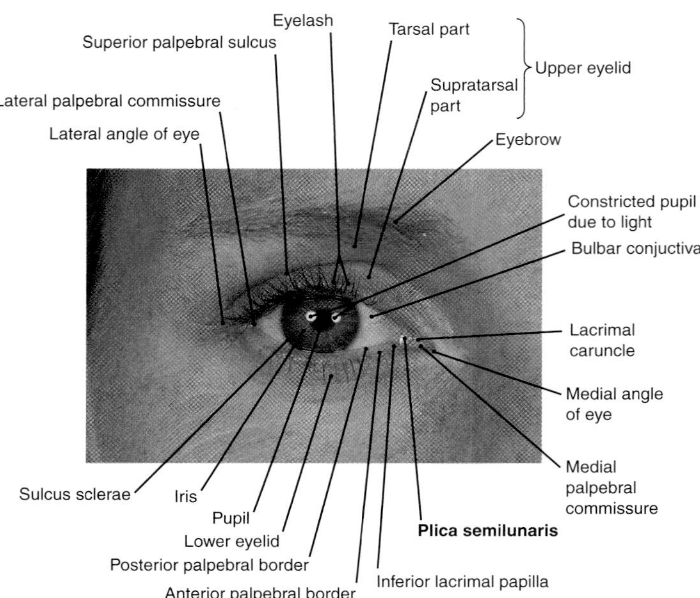
Eyelash
Superior palpebral sulcus
Tarsal part
Supratarsal part
Upper eyelid
Lateral palpebral commissure
Lateral angle of eye
Eyebrow
Constricted pupil due to light
Bulbar conjuctiva
Lacrimal caruncle
Medial angle of eye
Medial palpebral commissure
Sulcus sclerae
Iris
Pupil
Lower eyelid
Posterior palpebral border
Anterior palpebral border
Plica semilunaris
Inferior lacrimal papilla

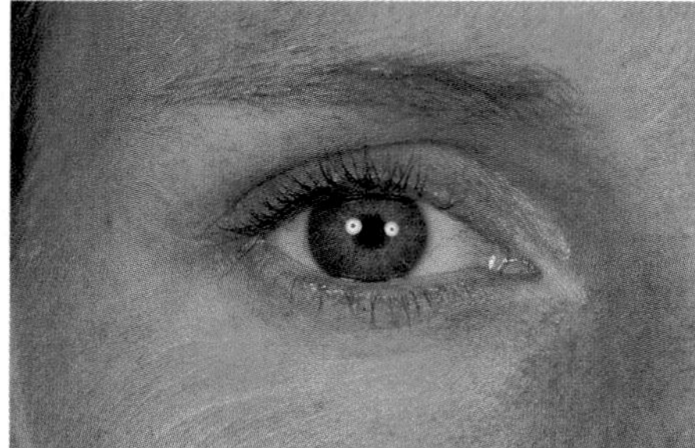

Figure 538.2 **Photograph of Living Eye Identical to Figure 538.1**

Figure 538.1 **Right Eye and Eyelids**

NOTE: (1) The eyeball, protected in front by two movable and thin **eyelids** or **palpebrae,** is covered by a transparent mucous membrane, the **conjunctiva,** which reflects along the inner surface of both eyelids as the **palpebral conjunctiva.**

(2) At the medial angle of the eye is located a small, reddish island of tissue called the **lacrimal caruncle.**

(3) The **pupil** is the opening in the **iris.** Constriction and dilation of the pupil is controlled autonomically. Parasympathetic fibers in the oculomotor nerve innervate the constrictor muscle of the pupil, while sympathetic fibers from the superior cervical ganglion supply the pupillary dilator muscle.

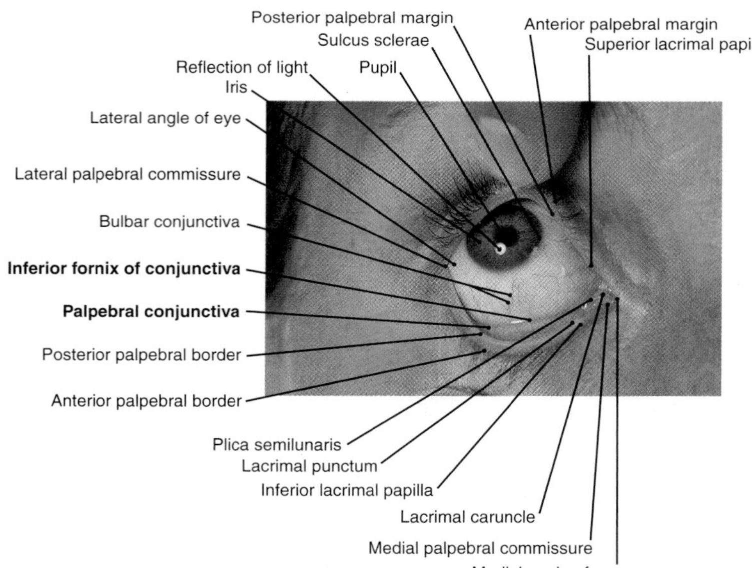
Posterior palpebral margin
Sulcus sclerae
Anterior palpebral margin
Superior lacrimal papilla
Reflection of light
Pupil
Iris
Lateral angle of eye
Lateral palpebral commissure
Bulbar conjunctiva
Inferior fornix of conjunctiva
Palpebral conjunctiva
Posterior palpebral border
Anterior palpebral border
Plica semilunaris
Lacrimal punctum
Inferior lacrimal papilla
Lacrimal caruncle
Medial palpebral commissure
Medial angle of eye

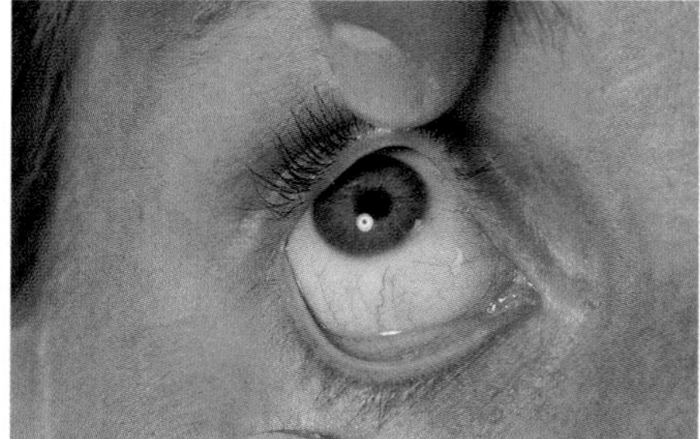

Figure 538.4 **Photograph of Living Eye Identical to Figure 538.3**

Figure 538.3 **Right Lower Eyelid and Medial Angle**

NOTE: (1) The right lower eyelid has been pulled downward to show the inner surface of the lower lid (i.e., the palpebral conjunctiva) and to enlarge the exposure of the medial angle (also called the **medial canthus**).

(2) The conjunctiva is highly vascular, and its bulbar part (over the eyeball) and inferior palpebral part (on the inner surface of the lower eyelid) are continuous along a line of reflection called the **inferior conjunctival fornix.** A similar reflection line, the **superior conjunctival fornix,** lies between the eyeball and the upper eyelid.

(3) When the medial angle is more completely exposed, a pair of small openings, the **lacrimal puncta,** can be found located above and below the lacrimal caruncle. These openings lead into small **lacrimal canals** through which tears enter the **lacrimal sac.**

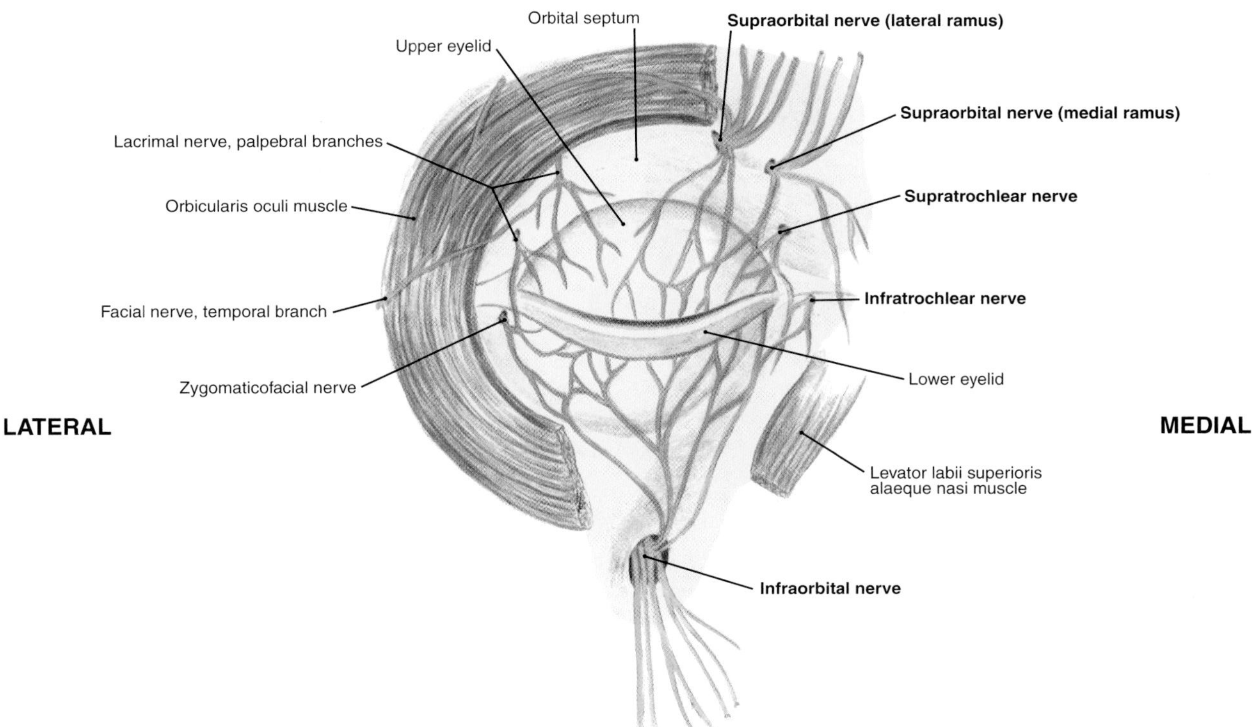
Orbital septum
Upper eyelid
Supraorbital nerve (lateral ramus)
Supraorbital nerve (medial ramus)
Lacrimal nerve, palpebral branches
Orbicularis oculi muscle
Supratrochlear nerve
Facial nerve, temporal branch
Infratrochlear nerve
Zygomaticofacial nerve
Lower eyelid
LATERAL
MEDIAL
Levator labii superioris alaeque nasi muscle
Infraorbital nerve

Figure 539.1 **Innervation of the Eyelids (Anterior View, Right Eye)**

NOTE: (1) The rich cutaneous innervation found around the anterior orbit is derived from the ophthalmic and maxillary divisions of the trigeminal nerve, which achieve the anterior orbital region through foramina in the frontal, zygomatic, and maxillary bones.

(2) Superomedially are found the large rami of the **supraorbital** branch of the frontal nerve (V_1), which emerges through the supraorbital foramen or notch. Also note the **supratrochlear** branch of the frontal nerve, which appears through a small foramen above the trochlea of the superior oblique muscle.

(3) The **infratrochlear nerve** is a terminal branch of the nasociliary nerve (V_1) that becomes superficial below the trochlea of the superior oblique. Along with palpebral branches of the **infraorbital nerve** (V_2), it sends fibers to the lower eyelid.

(4) The **lacrimal nerve** (V_1) superolaterally, supplying the upper eyelid; the **zygomaticofacial nerve** (V_2) to the lower eyelid and skin over the cheek bone; the **temporal branch of the facial nerve,** which is a motor nerve to the orbicularis oculi muscle.

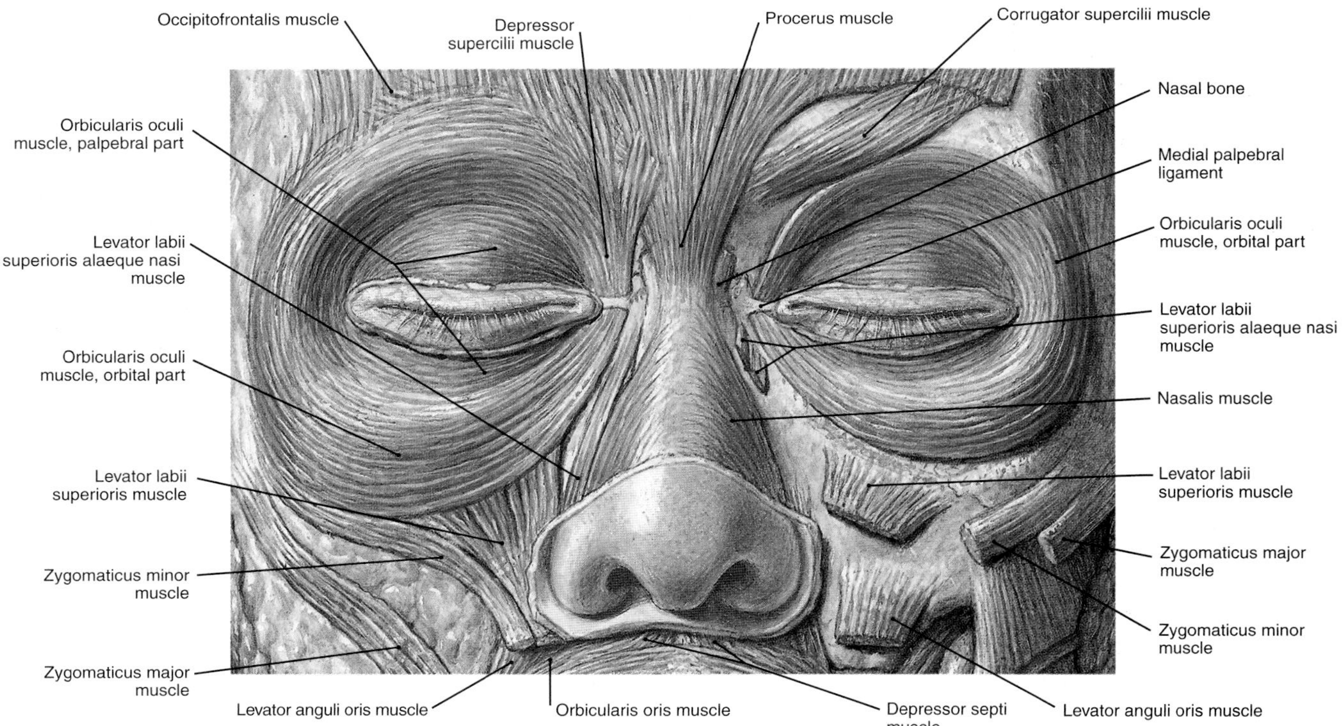
Occipitofrontalis muscle
Depressor supercilii muscle
Procerus muscle
Corrugator supercilii muscle
Nasal bone
Orbicularis oculi muscle, palpebral part
Medial palpebral ligament
Orbicularis oculi muscle, orbital part
Levator labii superioris alaeque nasi muscle
Levator labii superioris alaeque nasi muscle
Orbicularis oculi muscle, orbital part
Nasalis muscle
Levator labii superioris muscle
Levator labii superioris muscle
Zygomaticus major muscle
Zygomaticus minor muscle
Zygomaticus minor muscle
Zygomaticus major muscle
Levator anguli oris muscle
Orbicularis oris muscle
Depressor septi muscle
Levator anguli oris muscle

Figure 539.2 **Superficial Facial Muscles around the Orbit (Anterior View)**

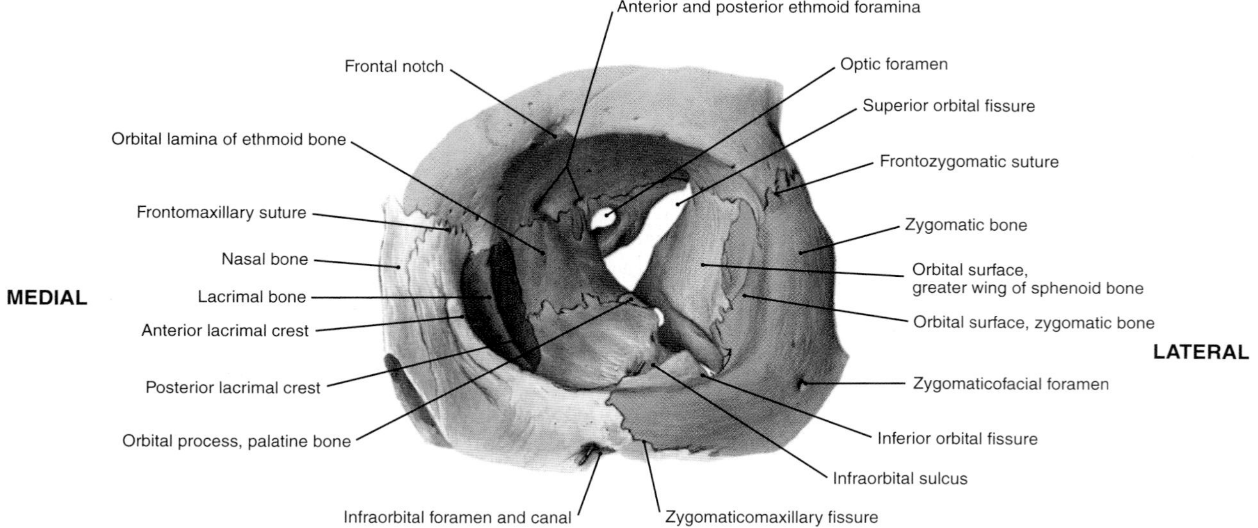
Anterior and posterior ethmoid foramina
Frontal notch
Optic foramen
Superior orbital fissure
Orbital lamina of ethmoid bone
Frontozygomatic suture
Frontomaxillary suture
Zygomatic bone
Nasal bone
Orbital surface, greater wing of sphenoid bone
MEDIAL
Lacrimal bone
Orbital surface, zygomatic bone
Anterior lacrimal crest
LATERAL
Posterior lacrimal crest
Zygomaticofacial foramen
Orbital process, palatine bone
Inferior orbital fissure
Infraorbital sulcus
Infraorbital foramen and canal
Zygomaticomaxillary fissure

Figure 540.1 **Bones That Form the Orbital Cavity (Left Side, Anterior View)**

NOTE: (1) The bony structure of the orbit is composed of parts of seven bones: the **maxilla, zygomatic, frontal, lacrimal, palatine, ethmoid,** and **sphenoid.**

(2) The **roof** of the orbit is formed by the orbital plate of the **frontal bone;** the **floor** consists of the orbital plate of the **maxilla,** the **palatine** and the **zygomatic bones;** the **medial wall** is thin and delicate and is formed by the frontal process of the **maxilla,** the orbital lamina of the **ethmoid** and the **lacrimal bone;** the strong **lateral wall** consists of the orbital processes of the **sphenoid** and **zygomatic bones.**

(3) The **optic foramen,** the **superior** and **inferior orbital fissures,** and the **anterior** and **posterior ethmoid foramina.**

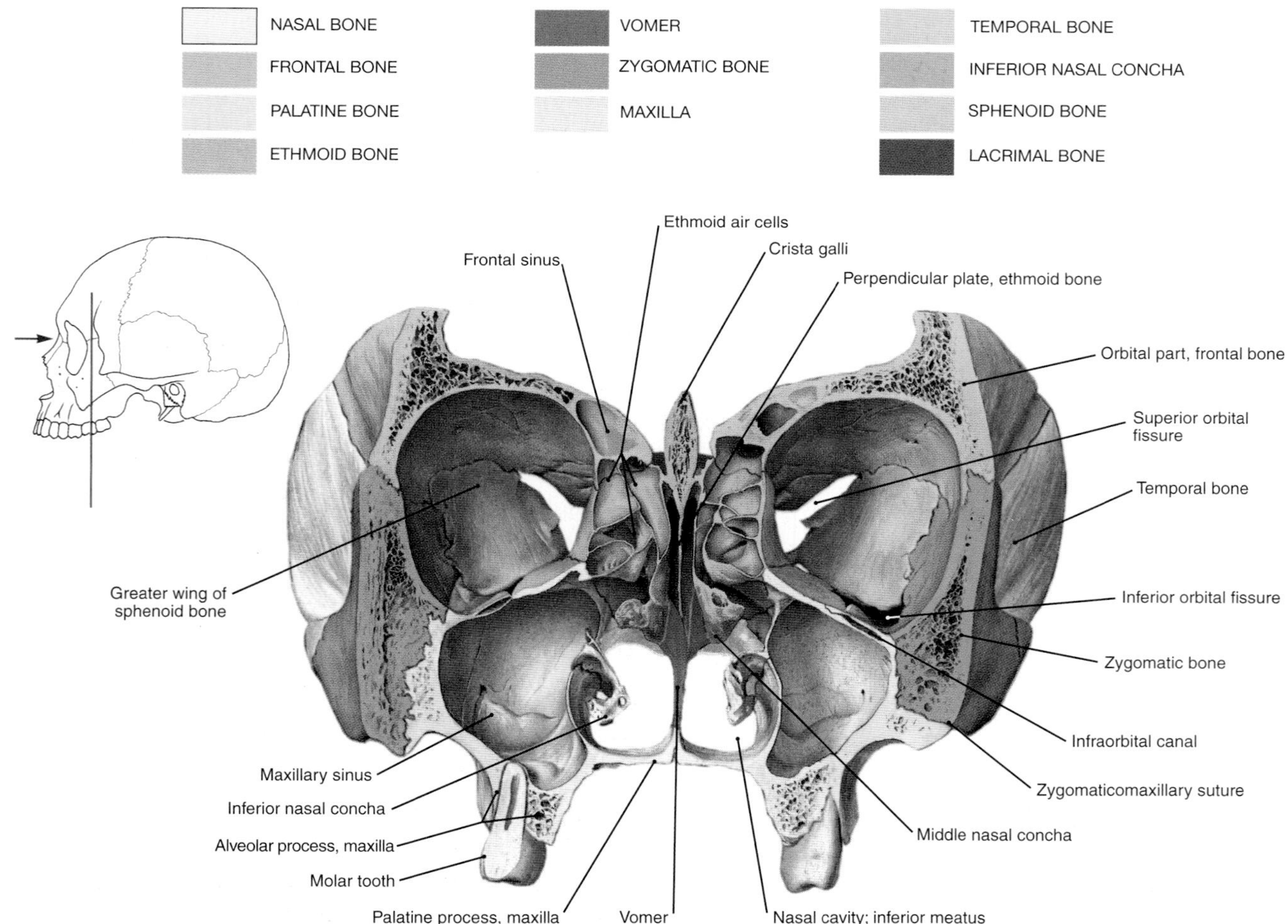
NASAL BONE
FRONTAL BONE
PALATINE BONE
ETHMOID BONE
VOMER
ZYGOMATIC BONE
MAXILLA
TEMPORAL BONE
INFERIOR NASAL CONCHA
SPHENOID BONE
LACRIMAL BONE
Ethmoid air cells
Crista galli
Frontal sinus
Perpendicular plate, ethmoid bone
Orbital part, frontal bone
Superior orbital fissure
Temporal bone
Greater wing of sphenoid bone
Inferior orbital fissure
Zygomatic bone
Infraorbital canal
Maxillary sinus
Zygomaticomaxillary suture
Inferior nasal concha
Middle nasal concha
Alveolar process, maxilla
Molar tooth
Palatine process, maxilla
Vomer
Nasal cavity; inferior meatus

Figure 540.2 **Frontal Section through the Orbital and Nasal Cavities and the Maxillary Sinus**

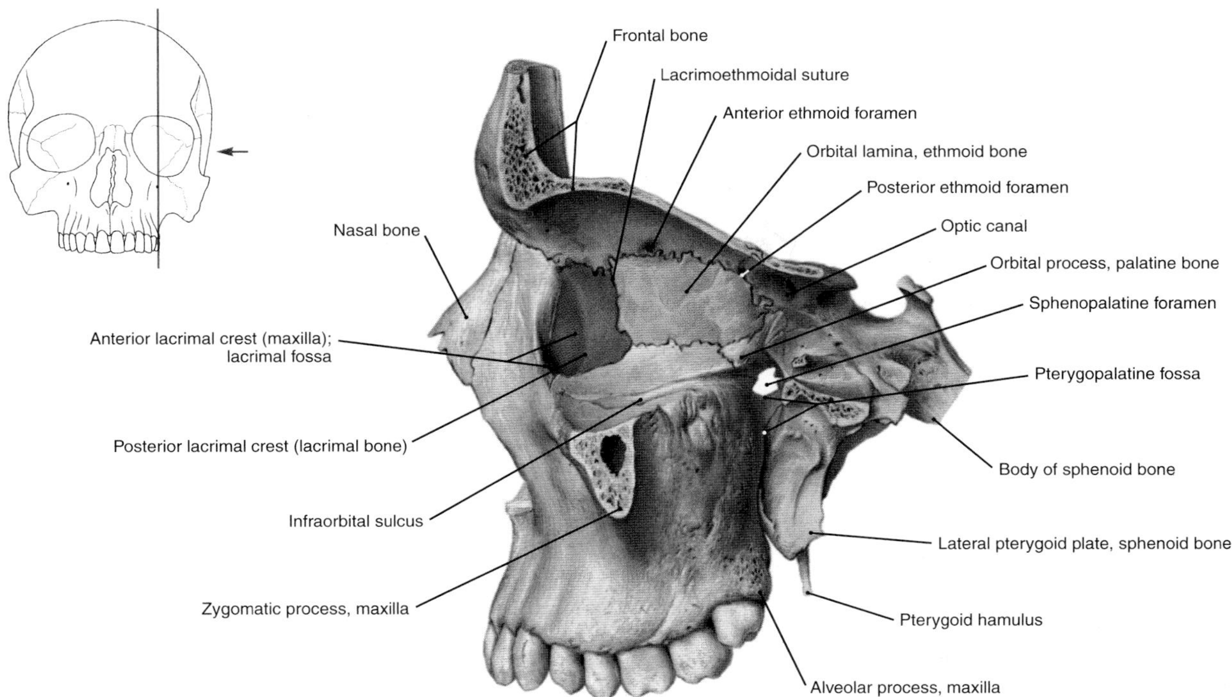
Frontal bone
Lacrimoethmoidal suture
Anterior ethmoid foramen
Orbital lamina, ethmoid bone
Posterior ethmoid foramen
Optic canal
Orbital process, palatine bone
Sphenopalatine foramen
Pterygopalatine fossa
Body of sphenoid bone
Lateral pterygoid plate, sphenoid bone
Pterygoid hamulus
Alveolar process, maxilla
Nasal bone
Anterior lacrimal crest (maxilla); lacrimal fossa
Posterior lacrimal crest (lacrimal bone)
Infraorbital sulcus
Zygomatic process, maxilla

Figure 541.1 Medial Wall of the Left Orbital Cavity and a Lateral View of the Pterygopalatine Fossa

NOTE: (1) Anteriorly on the thin medial wall of the orbital cavity is found the **lacrimal fossa** for the **lacrimal sac.** The fossa is limited in front by the anterior lacrimal crest of the maxilla and behind by the posterior lacrimal crest of the lacrimal bone.

(2) The medial wall is formed by the orbital lamina of the **ethmoid bone** and the **lacrimal bone.** The **maxilla** inferiorly and the **sphenoid** and **palatine bones** posteriorly also contribute to this wall. Observe also the **anterior** and **posterior ethmoidal foramina.**

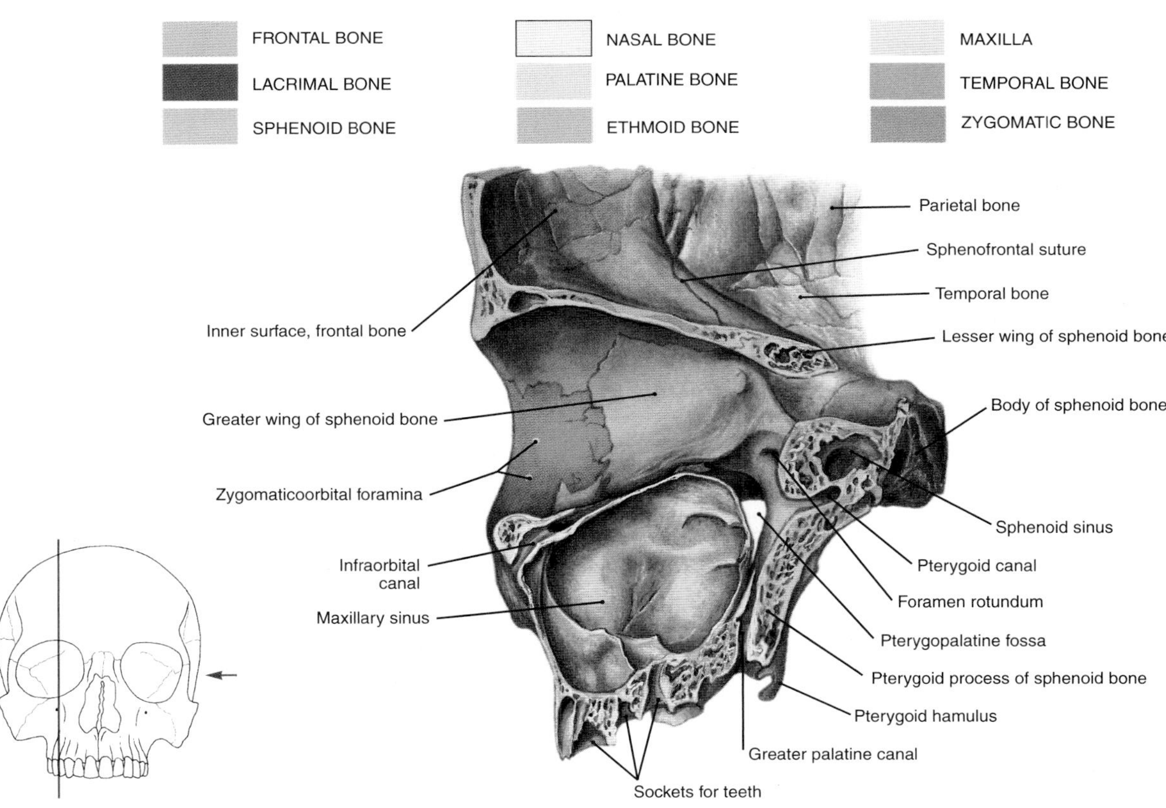
FRONTAL BONE
LACRIMAL BONE
SPHENOID BONE
NASAL BONE
PALATINE BONE
ETHMOID BONE
MAXILLA
TEMPORAL BONE
ZYGOMATIC BONE
Parietal bone
Sphenofrontal suture
Temporal bone
Lesser wing of sphenoid bone
Body of sphenoid bone
Sphenoid sinus
Pterygoid canal
Foramen rotundum
Pterygopalatine fossa
Pterygoid process of sphenoid bone
Pterygoid hamulus
Greater palatine canal
Sockets for teeth
Inner surface, frontal bone
Greater wing of sphenoid bone
Zygomaticoorbital foramina
Infraorbital canal
Maxillary sinus

Figure 541.2 Lateral Wall of the Right Orbital Cavity and a Medial View of the Pterygopalatine Fossa

NOTE: (1) The lateral wall of the orbit is formed by the orbital surface of the greater wing of the **sphenoid bone** and the frontal process of the **zygomatic bone.** Note the small zygomaticoorbital foramina through which course the **zygomaticofacial** and **zygomaticotemporal** branches of the maxillary nerve (sensory nerves).

(2) The **foramen rotundum** and the **infraorbital canal** for the **maxillary nerve.** Also note the **maxillary sinus** below the orbit and the **pterygopalatine fossa** and **greater palatine canal** behind the maxillary sinus and below the apex of the orbit.

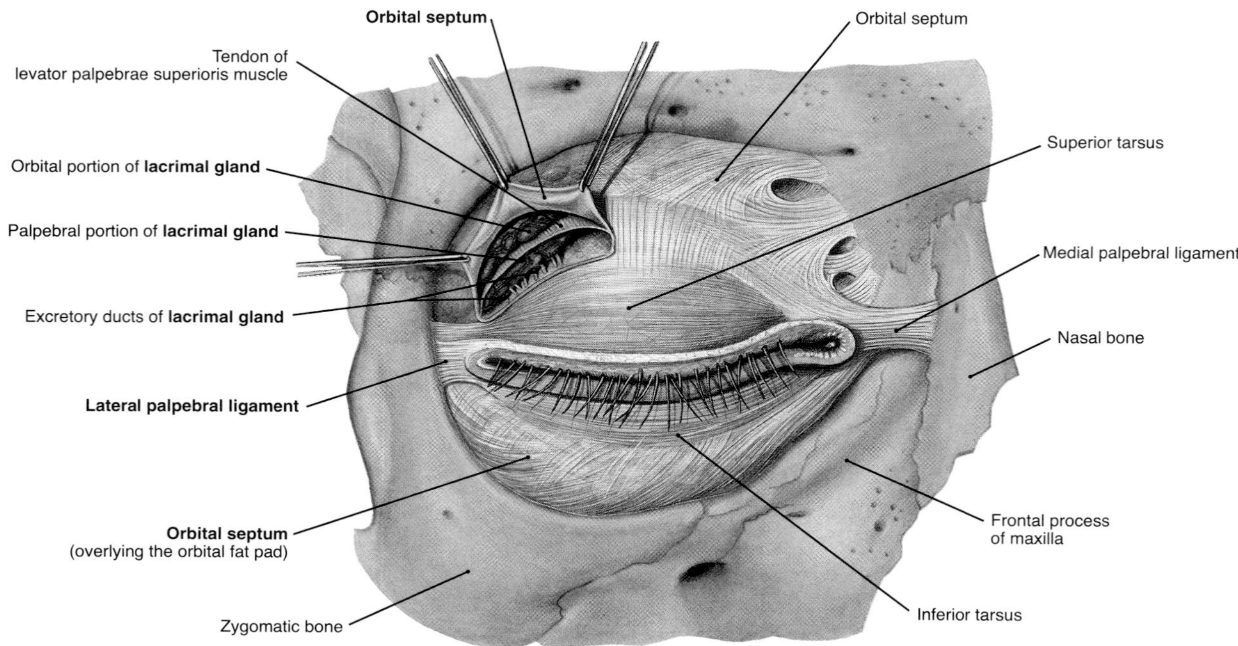
Orbital septum
Orbital septum
Tendon of
levator palpebrae superioris muscle
Superior tarsus
Orbital portion of lacrimal gland
Palpebral portion of lacrimal gland
Medial palpebral ligament
Excretory ducts of lacrimal gland
Nasal bone
Lateral palpebral ligament
Orbital septum
(overlying the orbital fat pad)
Frontal process
of maxilla
Zygomatic bone
Inferior tarsus

Figure 542.1 Orbital Septum, Lacrimal Gland, and Tarsi of the Right Eye

NOTE: (1) With the skin, superficial fascia, and orbicularis oculi muscle removed, the orbital septum has been exposed anteriorly. The septum attaches to the periosteum of the bone peripherally around the orbit and to the tarsi of the eyelids centrally.

(2) The lacrimal gland and its excretory ducts in the upper lateral aspect of the anterior orbit lying just beneath the orbital septum.

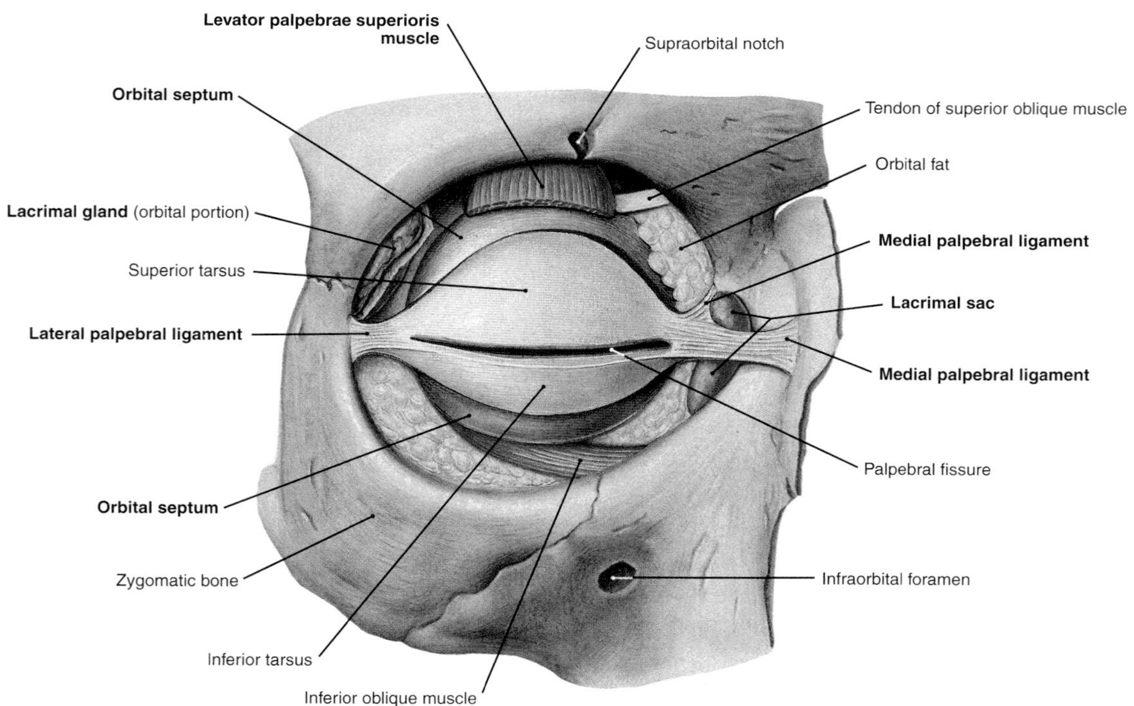
Levator palpebrae superioris
muscle
Supraorbital notch
Orbital septum
Tendon of superior oblique muscle
Orbital fat
Lacrimal gland (orbital portion)
Medial palpebral ligament
Superior tarsus
Lacrimal sac
Lateral palpebral ligament
Medial palpebral ligament
Palpebral fissure
Orbital septum
Zygomatic bone
Infraorbital foramen
Inferior tarsus
Inferior oblique muscle

Figure 542.2 Palpebral Ligaments and Tarsal Plates (Anterior View)

NOTE: (1) The superficial structures of the orbit have been removed along with the orbital septum and the tendon of the levator palpebrae superioris muscle.

(2) The lateral and medial margins of the tarsal plates are attached to the lateral and medial palpebral ligaments, which in turn are attached to bone. The medial ligament is located just anterior to the lacrimal sac.

(3) From this anterior view, both the tendon of the superior oblique muscle and the inferior oblique muscle can be visualized. Note also the location of the orbital portion of the lacrimal gland in the upper lateral part of the orbit.

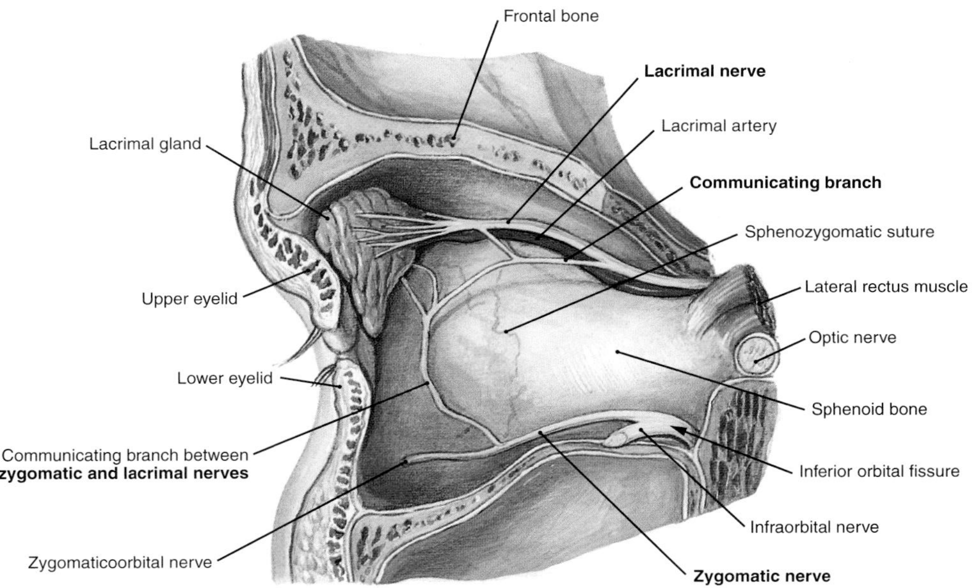
Frontal bone
Lacrimal nerve
Lacrimal artery
Lacrimal gland
Communicating branch
Sphenozygomatic suture
Upper eyelid
Lateral rectus muscle
Optic nerve
Lower eyelid
Sphenoid bone
Communicating branch between
zygomatic and lacrimal nerves
Inferior orbital fissure
Infraorbital nerve
Zygomaticoorbital nerve
Zygomatic nerve

Figure 543.1 **Innervation of the Lacrimal Gland**

NOTE: (1) The lacrimal gland is supplied by the lacrimal artery, which is a thin, tortuous branch of the ophthalmic artery that courses anteriorly in the orbital cavity.

(2) The lacrimal gland receives postganglionic parasympathetic fibers that are secretomotor in type. Preganglionic fibers are said to emerge from the brain in the nervus intermedius part of the facial nerve (VII). These fibers then synapse with the cell bodies of the post-ganglionic neurons in the pterygopalatine ganglion.

(3) The preganglionic parasympathetic fibers reach the pterygopalatine ganglion by way of the greater petrosal nerve, which then becomes part of the nerve of the pterygoid canal. The postganglionic fibers leave the ganglion and travel for a short distance with the zygomatic nerve, a branch of the infraorbital nerve. From this nerve, in the inferior part of the orbit, the parasympathetic fibers, by way of a communicating branch to the lacrimal nerve, travel to the lacrimal gland.

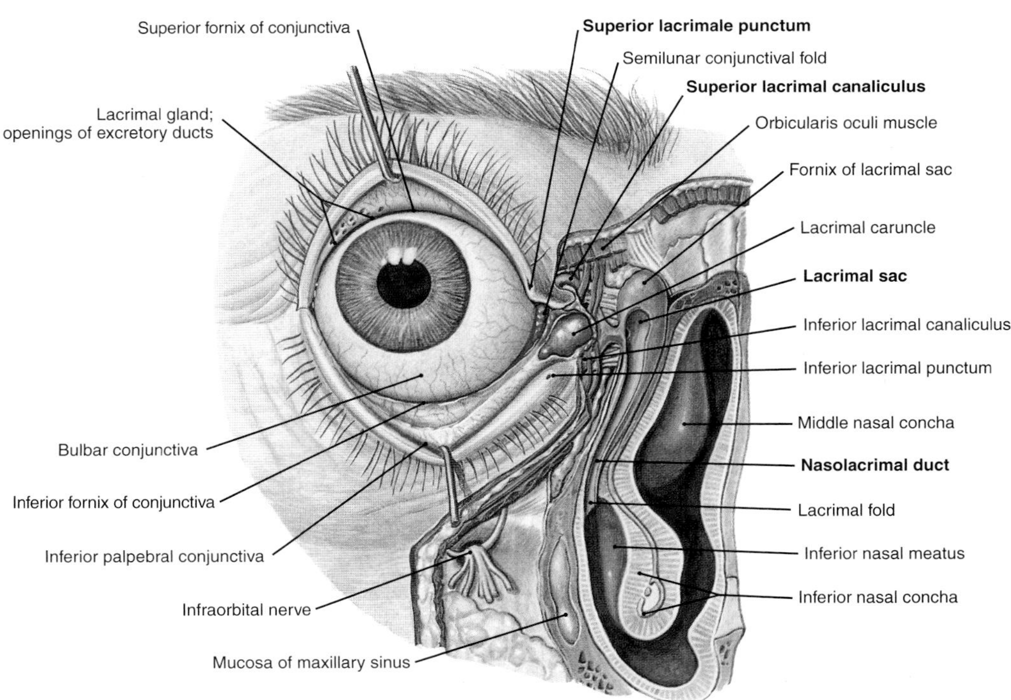
Superior fornix of conjunctiva
Superior lacrimale punctum
Semilunar conjunctival fold
Superior lacrimal canaliculus
Lacrimal gland;
openings of excretory ducts
Orbicularis oculi muscle
Fornix of lacrimal sac
Lacrimal caruncle
Lacrimal sac
Inferior lacrimal canaliculus
Inferior lacrimal punctum
Middle nasal concha
Bulbar conjunctiva
Nasolacrimal duct
Inferior fornix of conjunctiva
Lacrimal fold
Inferior palpebral conjunctiva
Inferior nasal meatus
Inferior nasal concha
Infraorbital nerve
Mucosa of maxillary sinus

Figure 543.2 **Lacrimal Canaliculi, Lacrimal Sac, and Nasolacrimal Duct**

NOTE: From the ducts of the lacrimal gland, tears moisten the surface of the eyeball and drain medially through the lacrimal canaliculi to the lacrimal sac and then descend to the nasal cavity by way of the nasolacrimal duct.

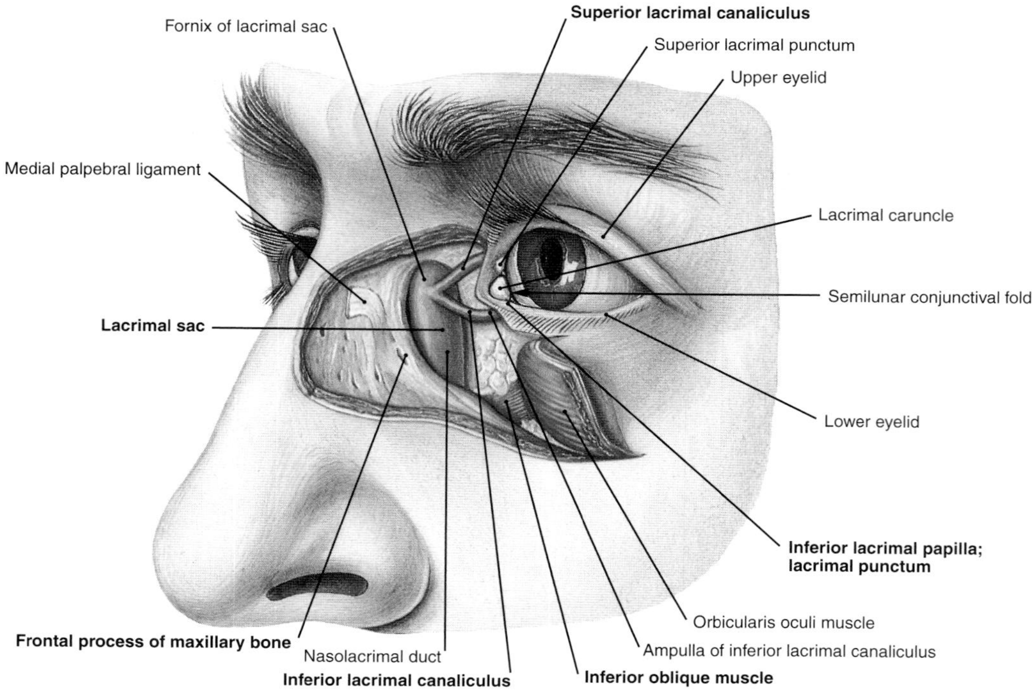
Fornix of lacrimal sac
Superior lacrimal canaliculus
Superior lacrimal punctum
Upper eyelid
Medial palpebral ligament
Lacrimal caruncle
Semilunar conjunctival fold
Lacrimal sac
Lower eyelid
Inferior lacrimal papilla; lacrimal punctum
Orbicularis oculi muscle
Frontal process of maxillary bone
Nasolacrimal duct
Ampulla of inferior lacrimal canaliculus
Inferior lacrimal canaliculus
Inferior oblique muscle

Figure 544.1 Lacrimal Canaliculi and Lacrimal Sac (Left Side, Superficial Dissection)

NOTE: (1) The skin and superficial fascia have been removed over the medial angle of the orbit. Observe the cut orbicularis oculi muscle and medial palpebral ligament. The latter structure is still attached to the frontal process of the maxilla.

(2) Severance of the medial palpebral ligament exposes the underlying lacrimal sac, which is located in a small fossa formed by the maxilla and lacrimal bone. This sac receives a lacrimal canaliculus from each eyelid, and each of these two ducts is about 1 cm long.

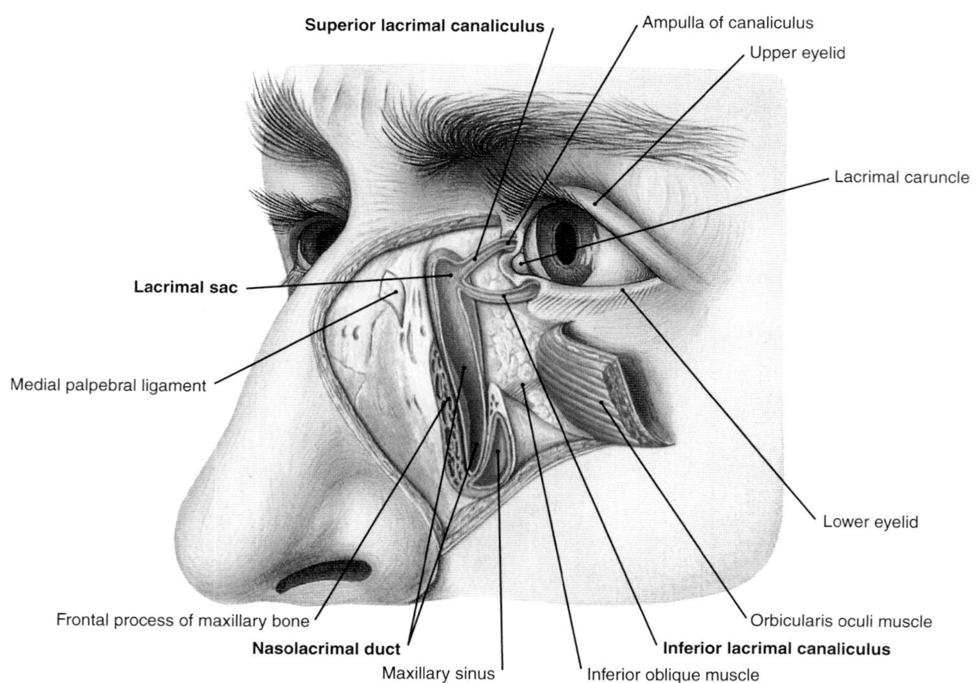
Superior lacrimal canaliculus
Ampulla of canaliculus
Upper eyelid
Lacrimal caruncle
Lacrimal sac
Medial palpebral ligament
Lower eyelid
Frontal process of maxillary bone
Orbicularis oculi muscle
Nasolacrimal duct
Inferior lacrimal canaliculus
Maxillary sinus
Inferior oblique muscle

Figure 544.2 Lacrimal Canaliculi, Lacrimal Sac, and Nasolacrimal Duct (Left Side, Deep Dissection)

NOTE: (1) At the medial edge of both eyelids are found single minute orifices (lacrimal puncta) of the lacrimal canaliculi, which lead from the eyelids to the lacrimal sac.

(2) The lacrimal sac forms the upper end of the nasolacrimal duct, which then extends about 2 cm into the inferior meatus of the nasal cavity.

(3) Lacrimal secretions pass across the surface of the eyeball toward the canaliculi and then are transported to the nasal cavity by the nasolacrimal duct. Excessive secretions, as in crying, roll over the edge of the lower eyelid as tears.

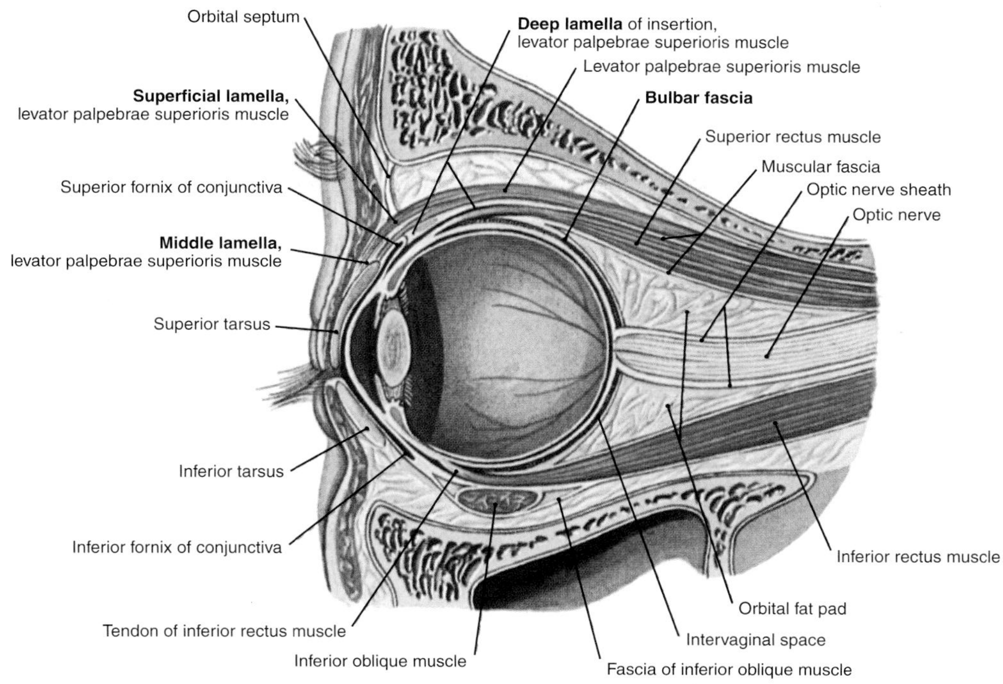
Orbital septum
Deep lamella of insertion, levator palpebrae superioris muscle
Levator palpebrae superioris muscle
Superficial lamella, levator palpebrae superioris muscle
Bulbar fascia
Superior rectus muscle
Muscular fascia
Superior fornix of conjunctiva
Optic nerve sheath
Optic nerve
Middle lamella, levator palpebrae superioris muscle
Superior tarsus
Inferior tarsus
Inferior fornix of conjunctiva
Inferior rectus muscle
Orbital fat pad
Tendon of inferior rectus muscle
Intervaginal space
Inferior oblique muscle
Fascia of inferior oblique muscle

Figure 545.1 Sagittal View of the Orbital Cavity and Eyeball

NOTE: (1) The **bulbar fascia** is a thin membrane that encloses the posterior three-fourths of the eyeball and separates the eyeball from the orbital fat and other contents of the orbital cavity.

(2) The bulbar fascia is prolonged over the bellies of the ocular muscles but then is pierced by the tendons of these muscles as they insert on the outer coat of the eyeball.

(3) The insertion of the **levator palpebrae superioris** is trilaminar. The superficial layer inserts into the upper eyelid, the middle layer into the superior tarsus, and the deep layer into the superior fornix of the conjunctiva.

(4) The palpebral **conjunctiva** is a thin transparent mucous membrane on the innermost aspect of the eyelid. At the conjunctival angle (fornix), it reflects over the eyeball as far as the sclerocorneal junction.

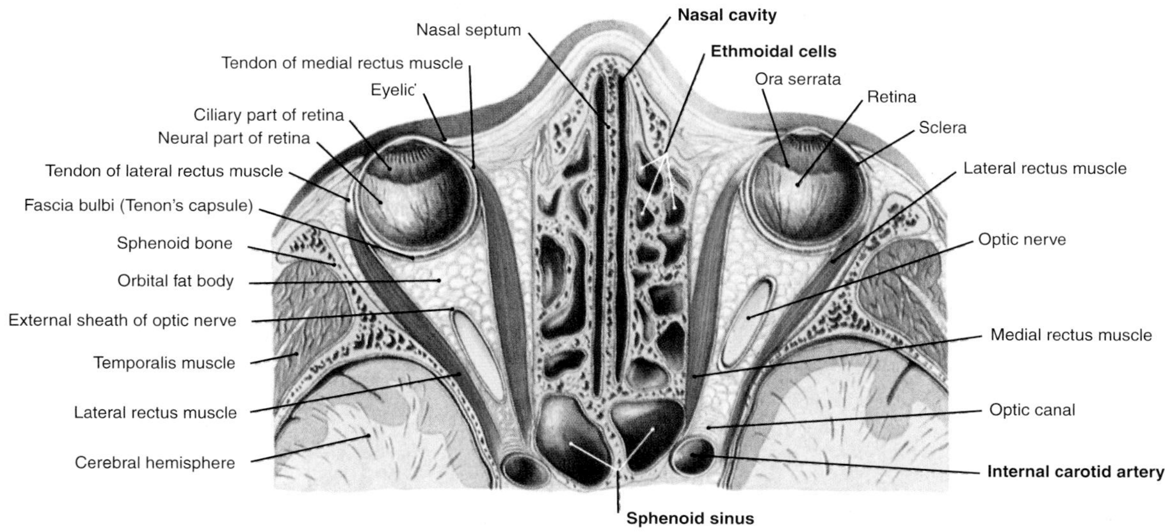
Nasal septum
Nasal cavity
Ethmoidal cells
Tendon of medial rectus muscle
Ora serrata
Eyelid
Retina
Ciliary part of retina
Sclera
Neural part of retina
Tendon of lateral rectus muscle
Lateral rectus muscle
Fascia bulbi (Tenon's capsule)
Sphenoid bone
Optic nerve
Orbital fat body
External sheath of optic nerve
Medial rectus muscle
Temporalis muscle
Lateral rectus muscle
Optic canal
Cerebral hemisphere
Internal carotid artery
Sphenoid sinus

Figure 545.2 Horizontal Section through Both Orbits at the Level of the Sphenoid Sinus

NOTE: (1) Between the orbital cavities is situated the **ethmoid bone,** containing the ethmoidal air sinuses (air cells). The vertically oriented perpendicular plate of the ethmoid serves as part of the nasal septum, and it subdivides the nasal cavity into two chambers.

(2) The posterior portion of the orbits are separated by the **sphenoid sinuses,** located within the body of the sphenoid bone. These sinuses frequently are not symmetrical.

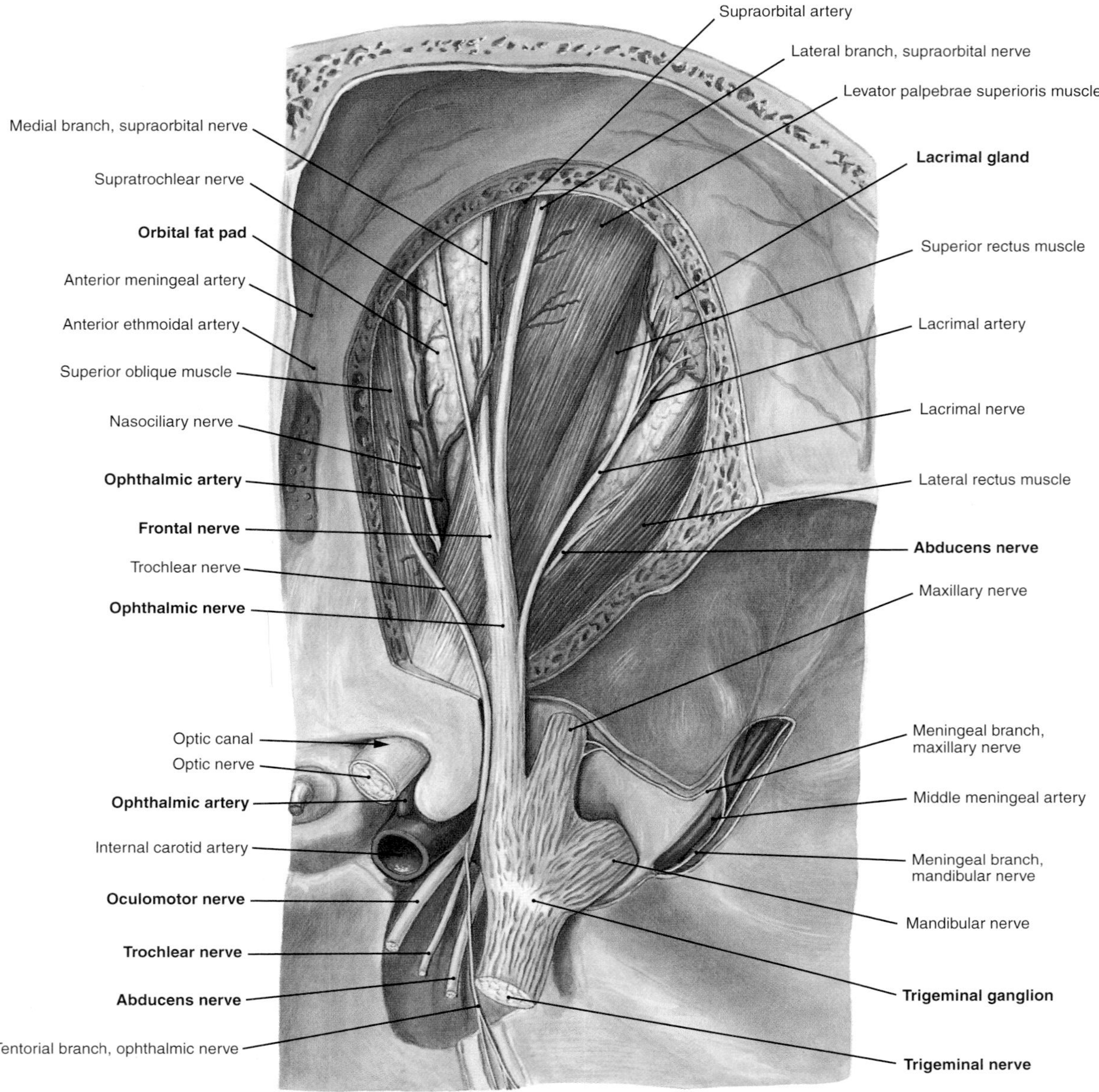
Supraorbital artery
Lateral branch, supraorbital nerve
Levator palpebrae superioris muscle
Medial branch, supraorbital nerve
Lacrimal gland
Supratrochlear nerve
Orbital fat pad
Superior rectus muscle
Anterior meningeal artery
Anterior ethmoidal artery
Lacrimal artery
Superior oblique muscle
Nasociliary nerve
Lacrimal nerve
Ophthalmic artery
Lateral rectus muscle
Frontal nerve
Abducens nerve
Trochlear nerve
Maxillary nerve
Ophthalmic nerve
Optic canal
Meningeal branch, maxillary nerve
Optic nerve
Ophthalmic artery
Middle meningeal artery
Internal carotid artery
Meningeal branch, mandibular nerve
Oculomotor nerve
Mandibular nerve
Trochlear nerve
Abducens nerve
Trigeminal ganglion
Tentorial branch, ophthalmic nerve
Trigeminal nerve

Figure 546 Nerves and Arteries of the Orbit (Stage 1), Superior View: Ophthalmic Nerve and Artery

NOTE: (1) The orbital plate of the frontal bone has been removed and the superior orbital fissure opened to expose the structures of the right orbit from above. The ophthalmic division of the trigeminal nerve divides into **lacrimal, frontal,** and **nasociliary branches.**

(2) The **lacrimal nerve** courses anteriorly and laterally in the orbit and accompanies the lacrimal branch of the ophthalmic artery to supply the lacrimal gland.

(3) The **frontal nerve** overlies the levator palpebrae superioris muscle and soon divides into a delicate **supratrochlear branch** and larger medial and lateral **supraorbital branches.** These course to the front of the orbit, where they emerge on the forehead.

(4) The **nasociliary nerve** crosses the orbit from lateral to medial, deep to the superior rectus muscle, and accompanies the ophthalmic artery for a short distance.

(5) The **trochlear nerve** enters the orbit medial to the ophthalmic nerve to supply the superior oblique muscle.

(6) The **optic nerve** leaves the orbit and enters the cranial cavity just medial to the internal carotid artery and the ophthalmic artery enters the orbit through the optic canal.

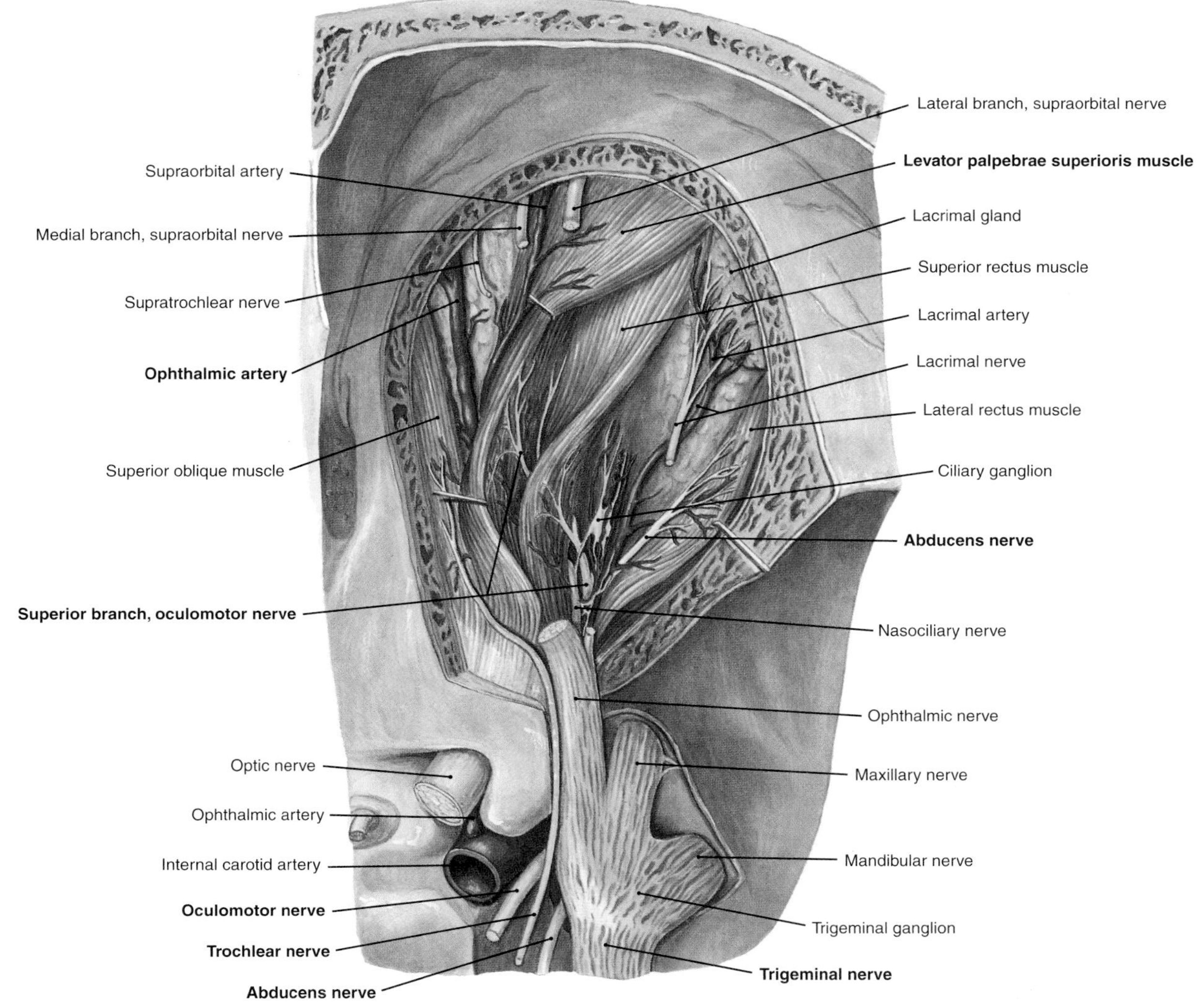
Lateral branch, supraorbital nerve
Levator palpebrae superioris muscle
Lacrimal gland
Superior rectus muscle
Lacrimal artery
Lacrimal nerve
Lateral rectus muscle
Ciliary ganglion
Abducens nerve
Nasociliary nerve
Ophthalmic nerve
Maxillary nerve
Mandibular nerve
Trigeminal ganglion
Trigeminal nerve
Supraorbital artery
Medial branch, supraorbital nerve
Supratrochlear nerve
Ophthalmic artery
Superior oblique muscle
Superior branch, oculomotor nerve
Optic nerve
Ophthalmic artery
Internal carotid artery
Oculomotor nerve
Trochlear nerve
Abducens nerve

Figure 547 **Nerves and Arteries of the Orbit (Stage 2), Superior View: Trochlear and Abducens Nerves**

NOTE: (1) With the right orbit opened from above, the ophthalmic division of the trigeminal nerve and its lacrimal, supratrochlear, and frontal branches have been cut. The levator palpebrae superioris and superior rectus muscles have been pulled medially to reveal their inferior surfaces, where filaments from the **superior branch of the oculomotor nerve** innervate the two muscles.

(2) The **nasociliary branch** of the ophthalmic nerve is still intact as it is seen turning medially deep to the superior rectus muscle. Note also that a fine communicating filament containing sensory fibers interconnects the ciliary ganglion and nasociliary nerve.

(3) The **trochlear nerve** supplies the superior oblique muscle along its upper surface. If this nerve is injured, a patient has difficulty turning the eyeball laterally and down; when asked to look inferolaterally, the affected eye rotates medially, resulting in double vision, or diplopia.

(4) The **abducens nerve** supplies the lateral rectus muscle along its medial surface. After emerging from the brainstem at the pontomedullary junction, this nerve follows a long course in the floor of the cranial cavity and enters the orbit through the superior orbital fissure.

(5) Injury to the abducens nerve produces a diminished ability to move the eyeball laterally. From the resulting medial or convergent gaze of the affected eyeball, the patient experiences diplopia (double vision).

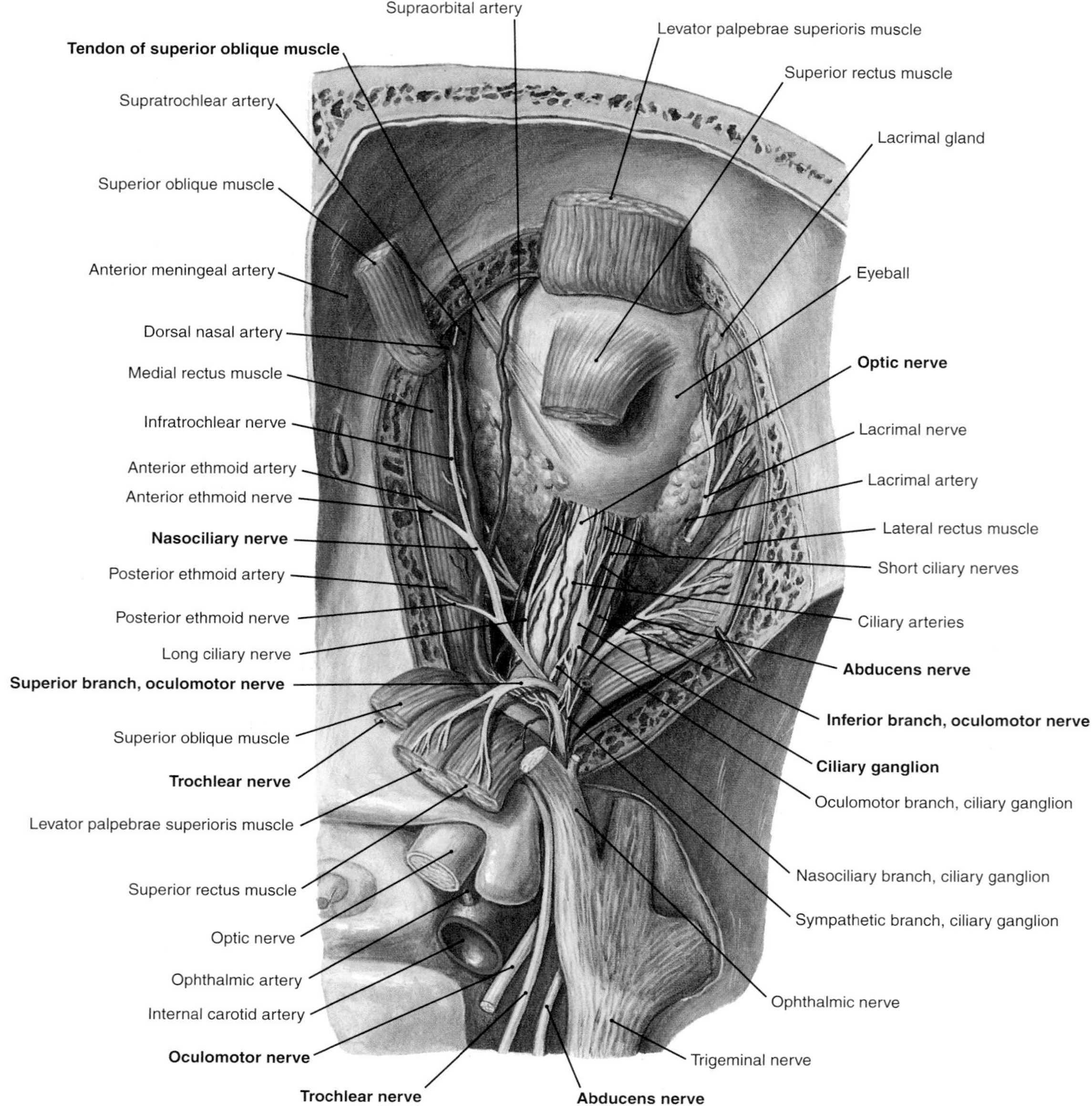
Supraorbital artery
Levator palpebrae superioris muscle
Tendon of superior oblique muscle
Superior rectus muscle
Supratrochlear artery
Lacrimal gland
Superior oblique muscle
Anterior meningeal artery
Eyeball
Dorsal nasal artery
Medial rectus muscle
Optic nerve
Infratrochlear nerve
Lacrimal nerve
Anterior ethmoid artery
Lacrimal artery
Anterior ethmoid nerve
Lateral rectus muscle
Nasociliary nerve
Short ciliary nerves
Posterior ethmoid artery
Posterior ethmoid nerve
Ciliary arteries
Long ciliary nerve
Abducens nerve
Superior branch, oculomotor nerve
Inferior branch, oculomotor nerve
Superior oblique muscle
Ciliary ganglion
Trochlear nerve
Oculomotor branch, ciliary ganglion
Levator palpebrae superioris muscle
Nasociliary branch, ciliary ganglion
Superior rectus muscle
Sympathetic branch, ciliary ganglion
Optic nerve
Ophthalmic artery
Ophthalmic nerve
Internal carotid artery
Oculomotor nerve
Trigeminal nerve
Trochlear nerve
Abducens nerve

Figure 548 **Nerves and Arteries of the Orbit (Stage 3), Superior View: Optic Nerve and Ciliary Ganglion**

NOTE: (1) With the levator palpebrae superioris, superior rectus, and superior oblique muscles cut and reflected, the **nasociliary nerve** and **ophthalmic artery** are seen crossing over the **optic nerve** from lateral to medial.

(2) The relationship to the optic nerve of the longitudinally oriented **long posterior ciliary arteries** (from the ophthalmic) and the **long ciliary nerves** (two or three branches from the nasociliary nerve).

(3) The **ciliary ganglion** lies lateral to the optic nerve. Its **parasympathetic root** comes from the oculomotor nerve and its **sensory root** from the nasociliary nerve. Postganglionic parasympathetic fibers reach the eyeball by the **short ciliary nerves.**

(4) Postganglionic parasympathetic nerve fibers supply the **sphincter of the pupil** and the muscle responsible for accommodation of the lens, the **ciliary muscle.**

(5) Some **sympathetic fibers** that arrive in the orbit along the ophthalmic artery also course through the ciliary ganglion. These are principally vasoconstrictor fibers to arteries that supply the eyeball. Sympathetic fibers that supply the **dilator of the pupil** course to the posterior pole of the eyeball by way of the **long ciliary nerves.**

(6) Although the supratrochlear nerve is derived from the frontal branch of the ophthalmic nerve, the **infratrochlear nerve** (as well as the **anterior** and **posterior ethmoid nerves**) is derived from the nasociliary branch of the ophthalmic nerve.

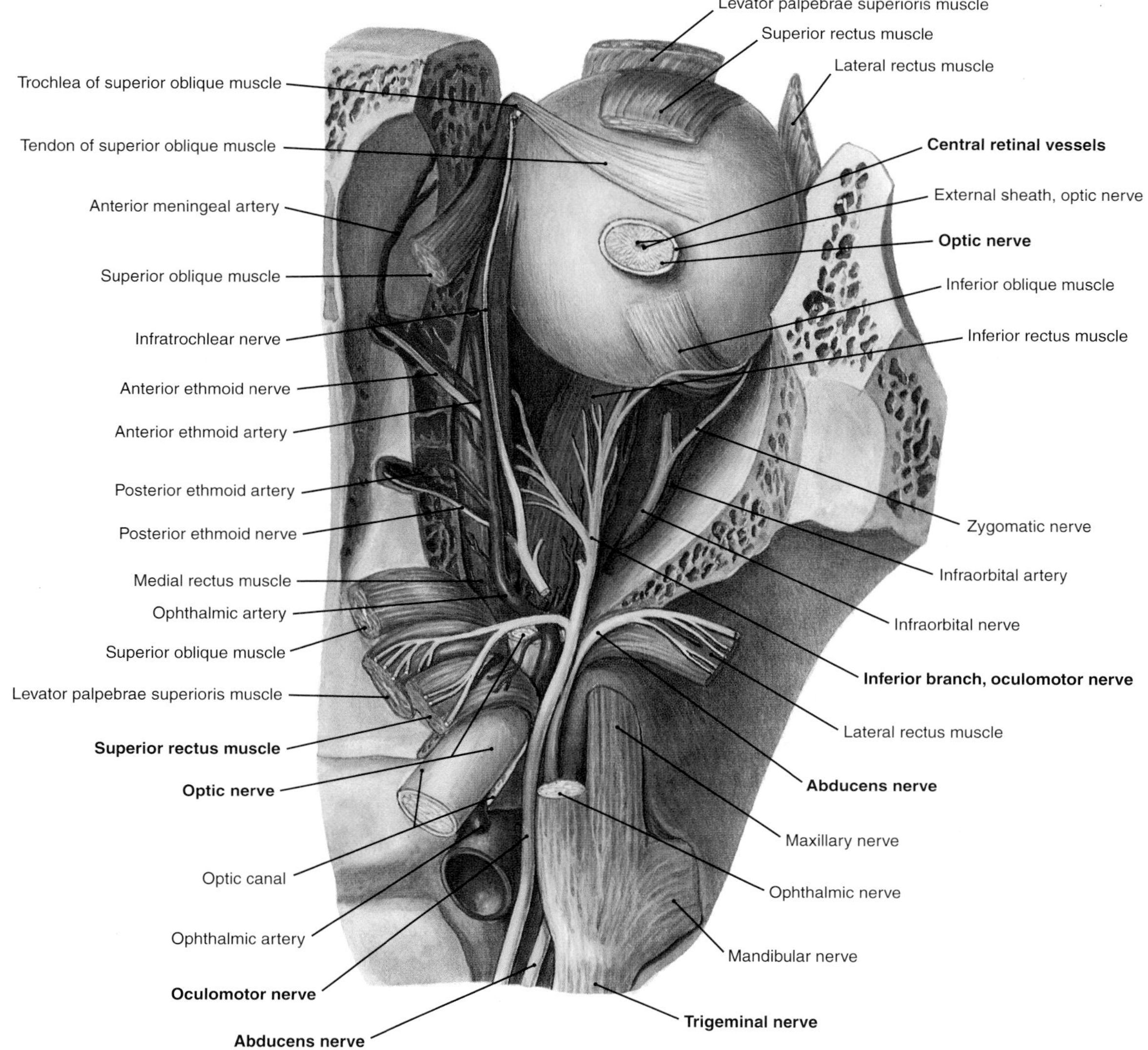
Levator palpebrae superioris muscle
Superior rectus muscle
Lateral rectus muscle
Trochlea of superior oblique muscle
Tendon of superior oblique muscle
Central retinal vessels
External sheath, optic nerve
Anterior meningeal artery
Optic nerve
Superior oblique muscle
Inferior oblique muscle
Infratrochlear nerve
Inferior rectus muscle
Anterior ethmoid nerve
Anterior ethmoid artery
Posterior ethmoid artery
Zygomatic nerve
Posterior ethmoid nerve
Infraorbital artery
Medial rectus muscle
Ophthalmic artery
Infraorbital nerve
Superior oblique muscle
Inferior branch, oculomotor nerve
Levator palpebrae superioris muscle
Lateral rectus muscle
Superior rectus muscle
Optic nerve
Abducens nerve
Maxillary nerve
Optic canal
Ophthalmic nerve
Ophthalmic artery
Mandibular nerve
Oculomotor nerve
Trigeminal nerve
Abducens nerve

Figure 549 **Nerves and Arteries of the Orbit (Stage 4), Superior View: Oculomotor Nerve (Inferior Branch)**

NOTE: (1) The levator palpebrae superioris, superior rectus, superior oblique, and lateral rectus muscles have been cut and reflected; the optic nerve has also been severed. The anterior half of the eyeball has been depressed and its posterior pole directed upward. Observe the **central retinal vessels**, as well as the insertions of the superior oblique and inferior oblique muscles.

(2) The **oculomotor nerve** courses through the superior orbital fissure and the common tendinous ring. It quickly gives off its **superior branch,** which courses upward in the orbit to supply the levator palpebrae superioris and superior rectus muscles. The **inferior branch** of the oculomotor nerve courses anteriorly in the deep part of the orbit to supply the inferior rectus, medial rectus, and inferior oblique muscles.

(3) The anterior and posterior ethmoid arteries and nerves and the infratrochlear nerve all located medially in the orbit. Note also the **infraorbital nerve** and **artery** in the infraorbital groove more laterally.

(4) The **ophthalmic artery** is the first branch of the internal carotid artery within the cranial cavity; it immediately enters the orbit through the optic canal with the optic nerve. Probably, the most important of the branches of the ophthalmic artery is the **central retinal artery**, which courses with its **vein** within the optic nerve.

(5) The central artery is the **only** source of blood to the neural retina and an increase in pressure on the posterior part of the orbital cavity or edema of the optic nerve caused by an inflammatory process can seriously compromise vision either by blockage of the artery or by diminishing the flow in the **central retinal vein.**

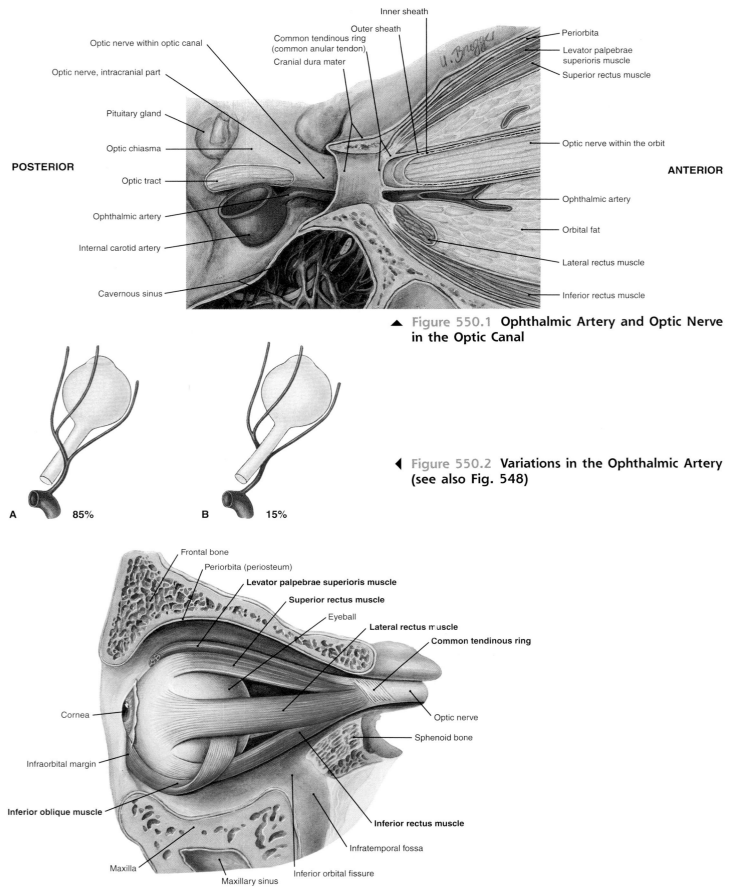

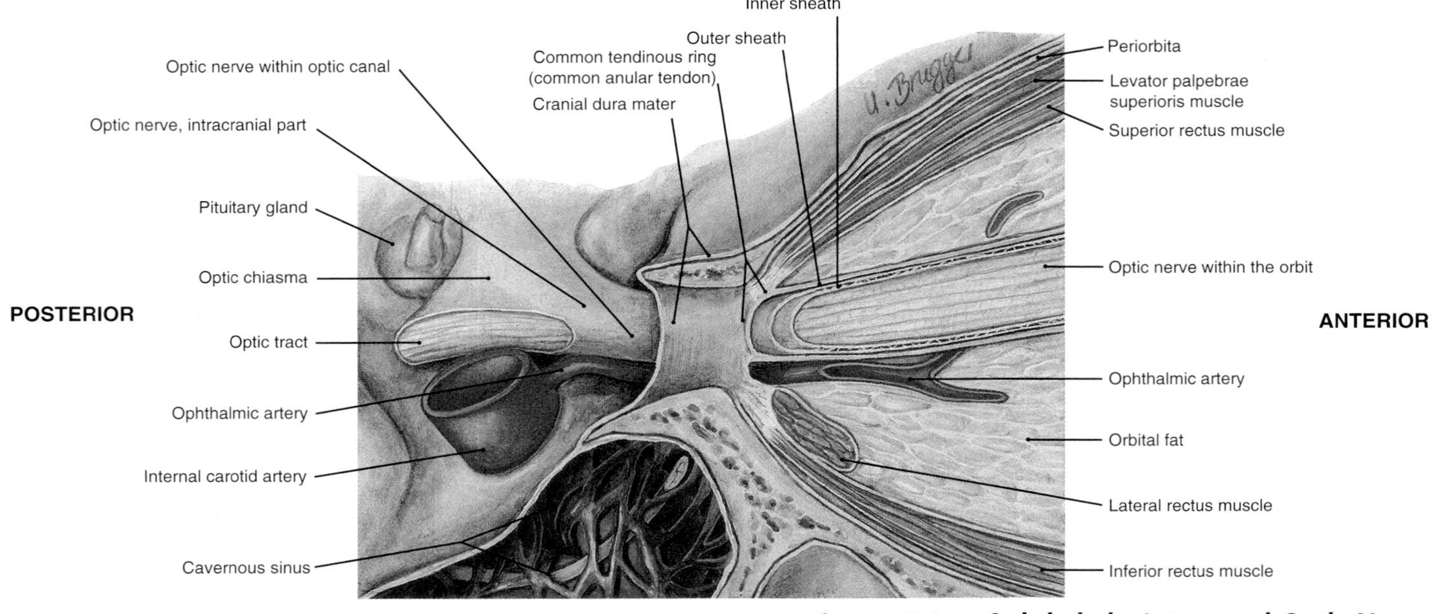
Inner sheath
Outer sheath
Common tendinous ring
(common anular tendon)
Cranial dura mater
Optic nerve within optic canal
Optic nerve, intracranial part
Pituitary gland
Optic chiasma
POSTERIOR
Optic tract
Ophthalmic artery
Internal carotid artery
Cavernous sinus
Periorbita
Levator palpebrae
superioris muscle
Superior rectus muscle
Optic nerve within the orbit
ANTERIOR
Ophthalmic artery
Orbital fat
Lateral rectus muscle
Inferior rectus muscle

▲ Figure 550.1 **Ophthalmic Artery and Optic Nerve in the Optic Canal**

A 85%

B 15%

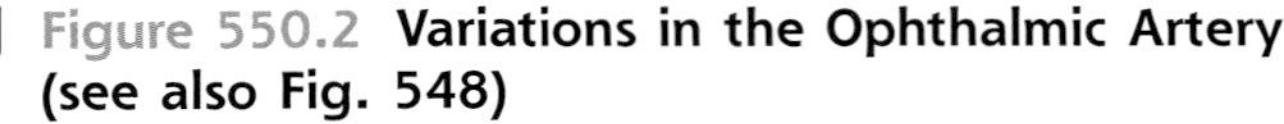

◀ Figure 550.2 **Variations in the Ophthalmic Artery (see also Fig. 548)**

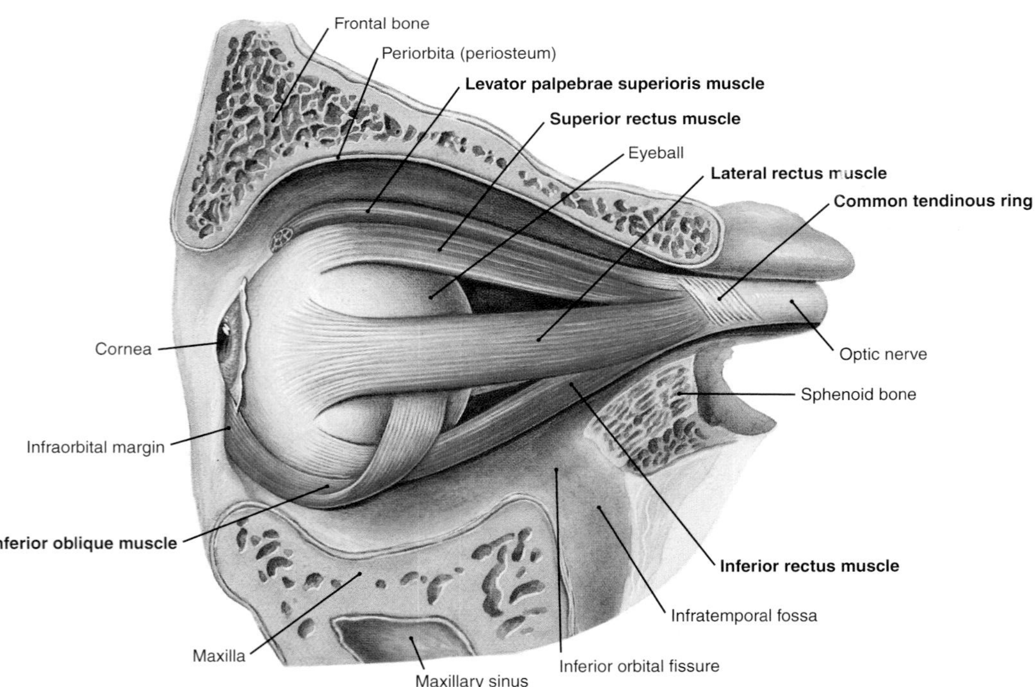
Frontal bone
Periorbita (periosteum)
Levator palpebrae superioris muscle
Superior rectus muscle
Eyeball
Lateral rectus muscle
Common tendinous ring
Optic nerve
Sphenoid bone
Cornea
Infraorbital margin
Inferior oblique muscle
Inferior rectus muscle
Infratemporal fossa
Maxilla
Inferior orbital fissure
Maxillary sinus

Figure 550.3 **Eye Muscles (Left Lateral View)**

NOTE: (1) With the lateral wall of the left orbit removed along with the bulbar fascia and eyelids, five of the seven extraocular muscles become exposed. Those evident from this view are the superior, lateral, and inferior rectus muscles, along with the levator palpebrae superioris and inferior oblique. Not seen are the superior rectus and superior oblique.

(2) Of the seven muscles, all except the levator palpebrae superioris and the inferior oblique take origin from the common tendinous ring that surrounds the optic nerve.

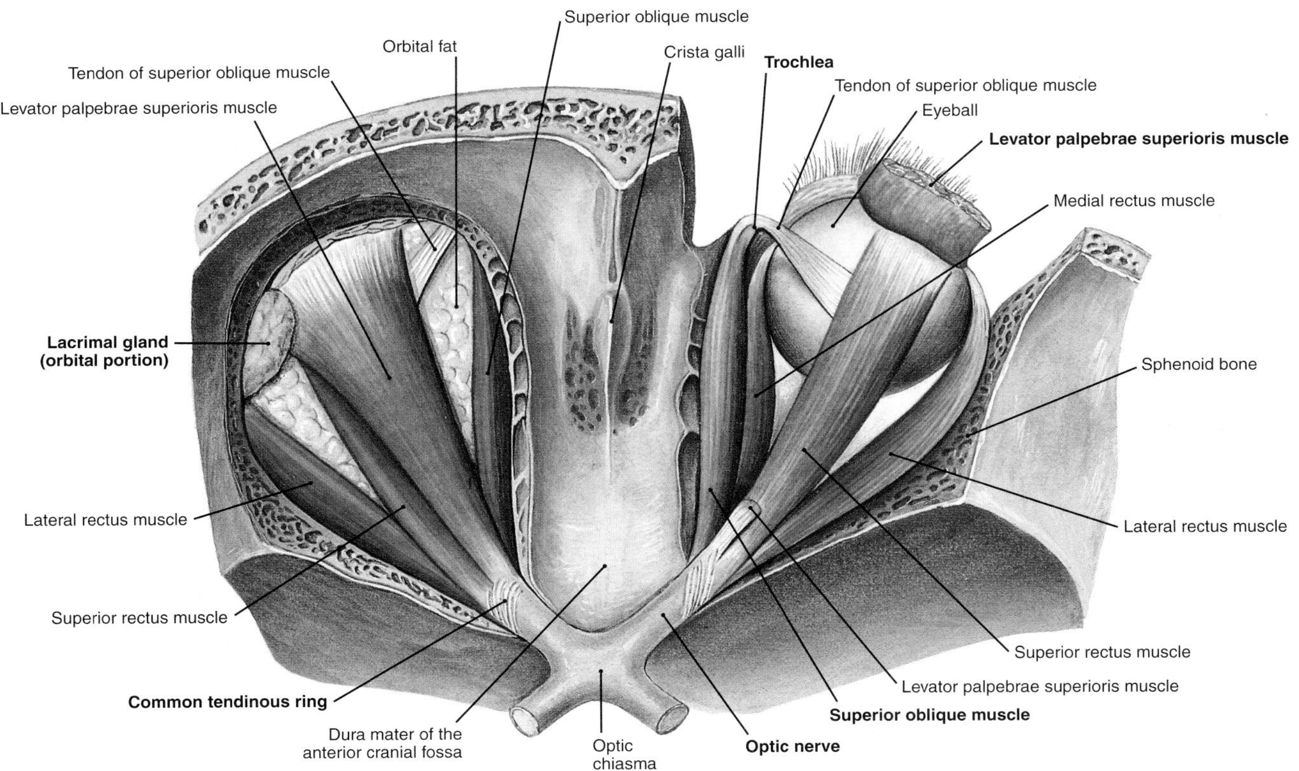
Superior oblique muscle
Orbital fat
Crista galli
Trochlea
Tendon of superior oblique muscle
Levator palpebrae superioris muscle
Tendon of superior oblique muscle
Eyeball
Levator palpebrae superioris muscle
Medial rectus muscle
Lacrimal gland (orbital portion)
Sphenoid bone
Lateral rectus muscle
Lateral rectus muscle
Superior rectus muscle
Superior rectus muscle
Levator palpebrae superioris muscle
Common tendinous ring
Superior oblique muscle
Dura mater of the anterior cranial fossa
Optic chiasma
Optic nerve

Figure 551.1 Muscles of the Orbital Cavity (Seen from above)

NOTE: (1) The orbital plates of the frontal bones have been removed from within the cranial cavity. On the left side, only the bony roof of the orbit has been opened and the muscles, orbital fat and lacrimal gland have been left intact.

(2) On the right side, the levator palpebrae superioris muscle has been resected and the orbital fat removed to expose the ocular muscles.

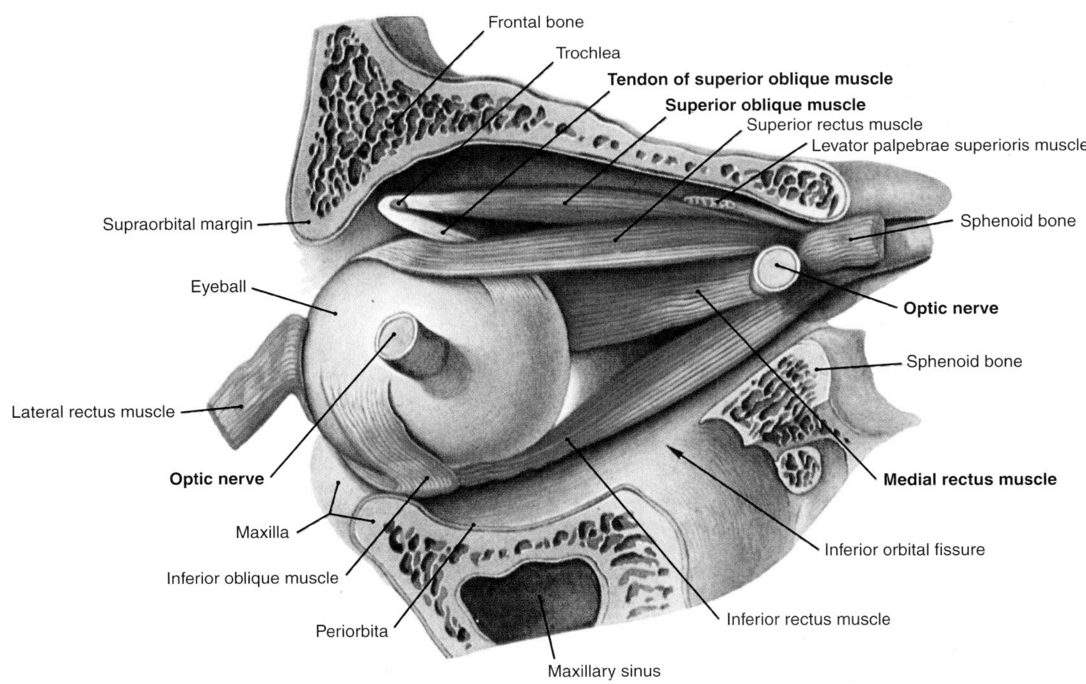
Frontal bone
Trochlea
Tendon of superior oblique muscle
Superior oblique muscle
Superior rectus muscle
Levator palpebrae superioris muscle
Supraorbital margin
Sphenoid bone
Eyeball
Optic nerve
Sphenoid bone
Lateral rectus muscle
Optic nerve
Medial rectus muscle
Maxilla
Inferior orbital fissure
Inferior oblique muscle
Periorbita
Inferior rectus muscle
Maxillary sinus

Figure 551.2 Eye Muscles, Left Lateral View (Lateral Rectus Muscle and Optic Nerve Cut)

NOTE: The eyeball has been rotated 90 degrees so that its posterior pole is directed laterally. This reveals to advantage the insertion of the inferior oblique muscle, and the superior oblique muscle and tendon as it bends around the trochlea to insert on the eyeball.

Superior rectus muscle
Tendon of superior oblique muscle
Pupil
Medial rectus muscle
Lateral rectus muscle
Ocular conjunctiva
Cornea
Inferior oblique muscle
Inferior rectus muscle

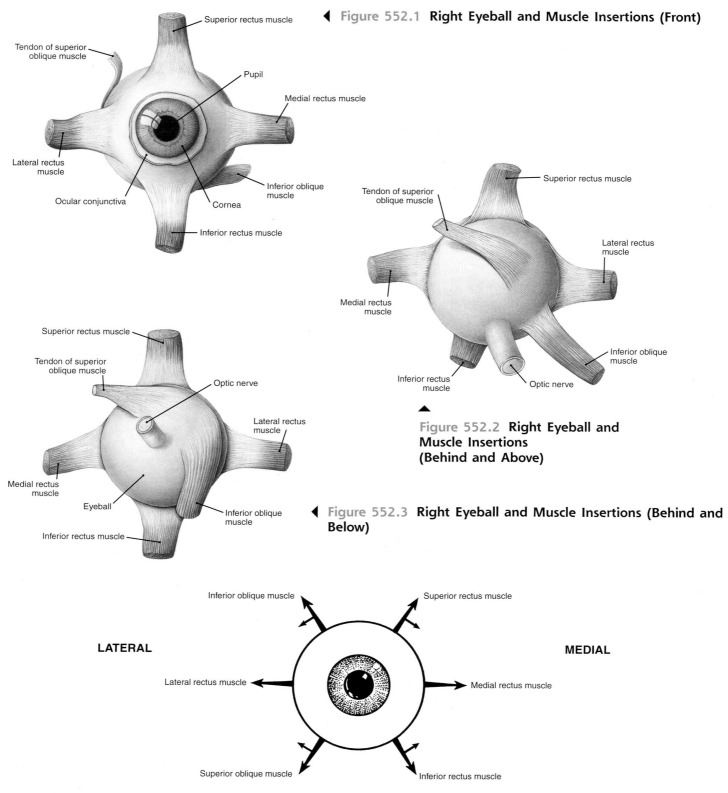

Figure 552.1 Right Eyeball and Muscle Insertions (Front)

Superior rectus muscle
Tendon of superior oblique muscle
Lateral rectus muscle
Medial rectus muscle
Inferior oblique muscle
Inferior rectus muscle
Optic nerve

Figure 552.2 Right Eyeball and Muscle Insertions (Behind and Above)

Superior rectus muscle
Tendon of superior oblique muscle
Optic nerve
Lateral rectus muscle
Medial rectus muscle
Eyeball
Inferior oblique muscle
Inferior rectus muscle

Figure 552.3 Right Eyeball and Muscle Insertions (Behind and Below)

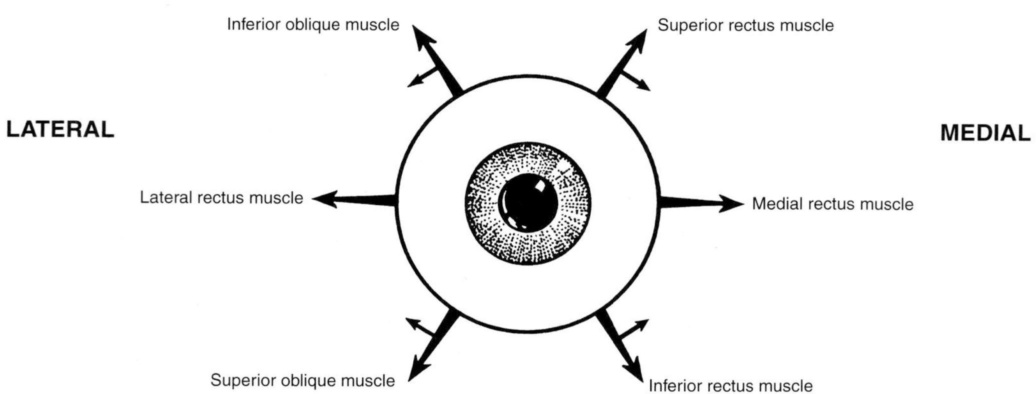
Inferior oblique muscle
Superior rectus muscle
LATERAL
MEDIAL
Lateral rectus muscle
Medial rectus muscle
Superior oblique muscle
Inferior rectus muscle

Figure 552.4 Schema of Extraocular Muscle Actions

NOTE:

(a) The **lateral rectus** *abducts* the eyeball only.
(b) The **superior oblique** *abducts, depresses*, and *medially rotates* the eyeball.
(c) The **inferior oblique** *abducts, elevates*, and *laterally rotates* the eyeball.
(d) The **medial rectus** *adducts* the eyeball only.
(e) The **inferior rectus** *adducts, depresses*, and *laterally rotates* the eyeball.
(f) The **superior rectus** *adducts, elevates*, and *medially rotates* the eyeball.

NOTE: The following muscle innervations:

(a) The **oculomotor nerve (III)**: levator palpebrae superioris, superior rectus, medial rectus, inferior rectus, inferior oblique muscles.
(b) The **trochlear nerve (IV)**: superior oblique muscle.
(c) The **abducens nerve (VI)**: lateral rectus muscle.

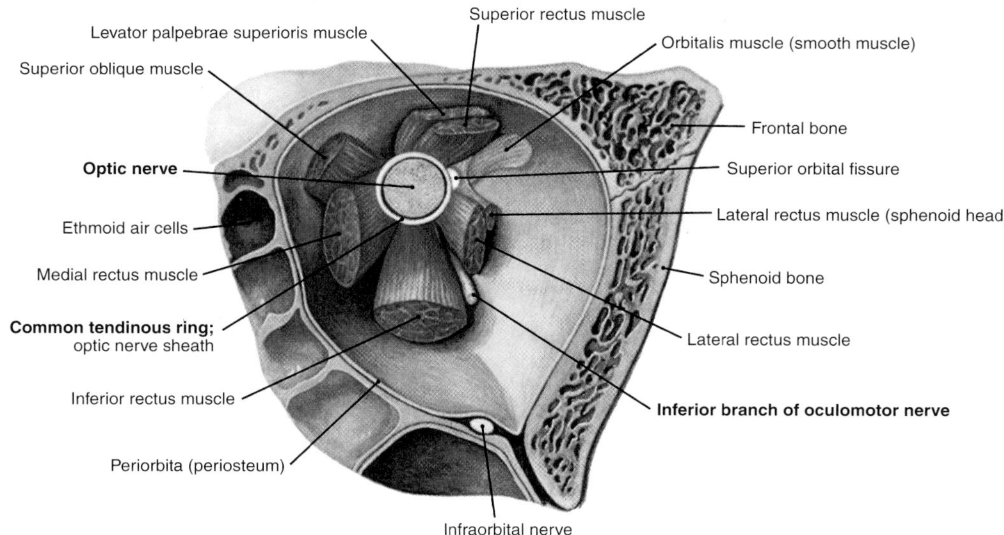
Superior rectus muscle
Levator palpebrae superioris muscle
Orbitalis muscle (smooth muscle)
Superior oblique muscle
Frontal bone
Optic nerve
Superior orbital fissure
Lateral rectus muscle (sphenoid head)
Ethmoid air cells
Medial rectus muscle
Sphenoid bone
Common tendinous ring; optic nerve sheath
Lateral rectus muscle
Inferior rectus muscle
Inferior branch of oculomotor nerve
Periorbita (periosteum)
Infraorbital nerve

Figure 553.1 **Origins of the Ocular Muscles, Apex of Left Orbit**

NOTE: (1) This anterior view of the apex of the left orbit shows the stumps of the ocular muscles, which have been cut close to their origins.

(2) The four rectus muscles arise from a tendinous ring surrounding the optic canal. The levator palpebrae superioris and superior oblique arise from the sphenoid bone close to the tendinous ring, while the inferior oblique (not shown here, see Fig. 542.2) arises from the orbital surface of the maxilla.

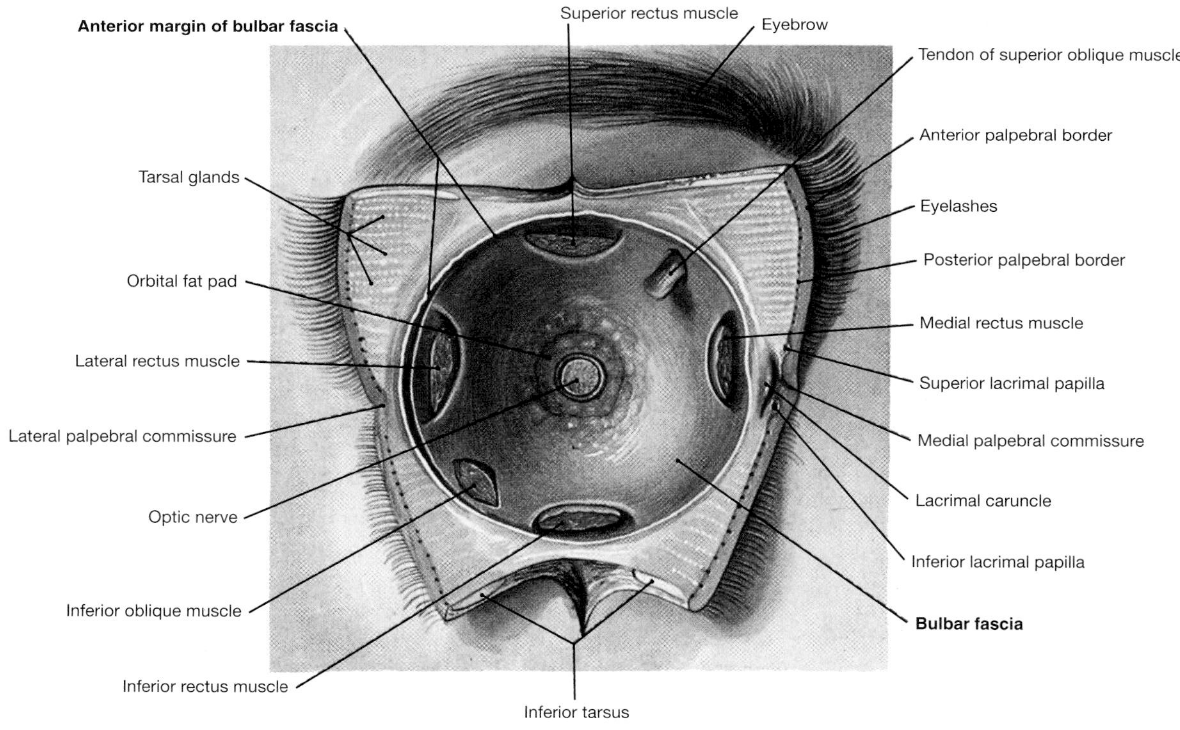
Anterior margin of bulbar fascia
Superior rectus muscle
Eyebrow
Tendon of superior oblique muscle
Anterior palpebral border
Tarsal glands
Eyelashes
Posterior palpebral border
Orbital fat pad
Medial rectus muscle
Lateral rectus muscle
Superior lacrimal papilla
Lateral palpebral commissure
Medial palpebral commissure
Lacrimal caruncle
Optic nerve
Inferior lacrimal papilla
Inferior oblique muscle
Bulbar fascia
Inferior rectus muscle
Inferior tarsus

Figure 553.2 **Bulbar Fascia (Capsule of Tenon), Right Eye**

NOTE: (1) Longitudinal incisions have been made down the middle of each eyelid and the flaps have been reflected to expose the orbital cavity anteriorly.

(2) The **optic nerve** has been severed at the optic disk, and the eyeball, along with the insertions of the ocular muscles, have been removed from the orbital cavity.

(3) The **bulbar fascia**, which envelops the posterior aspect of the eyeball (from the sclerocorneal junction to the optic nerve), has been left within the orbit. Observe how the bulbar fascia is perforated by the tendons of the ocular muscles. It is also pierced from behind by the ciliary vessels and nerves.

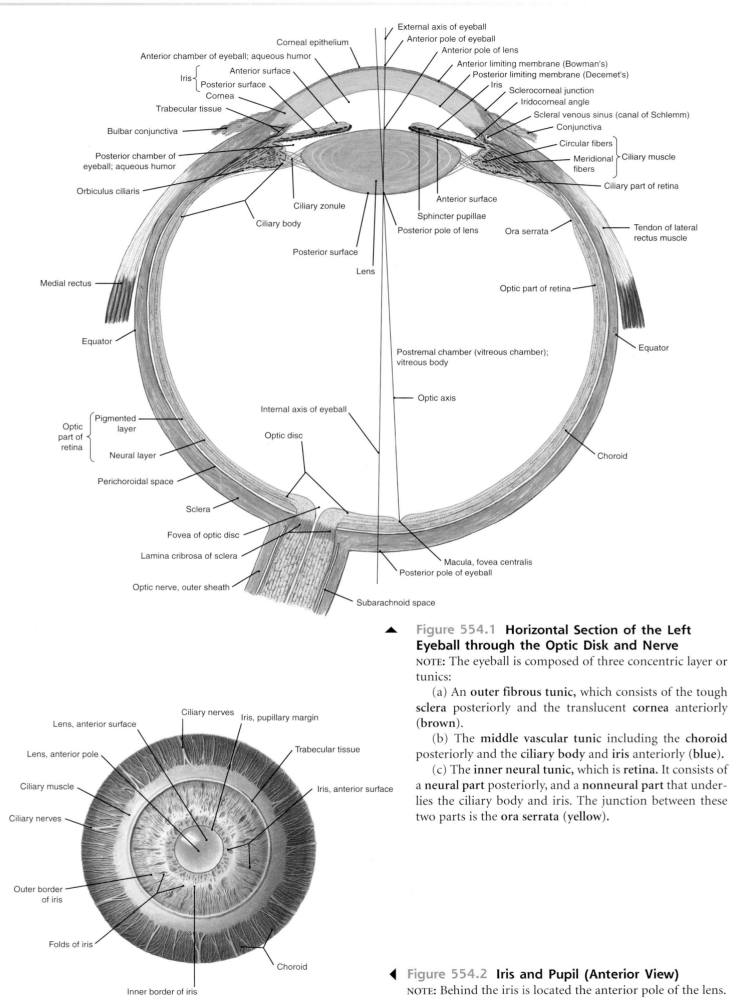

External axis of eyeball
Anterior pole of eyeball
Corneal epithelium
Anterior pole of lens
Anterior chamber of eyeball; aqueous humor
Anterior limiting membrane (Bowman's)
Iris { Anterior surface / Posterior surface
Posterior limiting membrane (Decemet's)
Iris
Cornea
Sclerocorneal junction
Trabecular tissue
Iridocorneal angle
Scleral venous sinus (canal of Schlemm)
Bulbar conjunctiva
Conjunctiva
Circular fibers
Meridional fibers
Ciliary muscle
Posterior chamber of eyeball; aqueous humor
Ciliary part of retina
Orbiculus ciliaris
Anterior surface
Ciliary zonule
Sphincter pupillae
Ciliary body
Posterior pole of lens
Ora serrata
Tendon of lateral rectus muscle
Posterior surface
Lens
Medial rectus
Optic part of retina
Equator
Equator
Postremal chamber (vitreous chamber); vitreous body
Optic axis
Internal axis of eyeball
Optic part of retina { Pigmented layer / Neural layer
Optic disc
Choroid
Perichoroidal space
Sclera
Fovea of optic disc
Lamina cribrosa of sclera
Macula, fovea centralis
Posterior pole of eyeball
Optic nerve, outer sheath
Subarachnoid space

Figure 554.1 Horizontal Section of the Left Eyeball through the Optic Disk and Nerve

NOTE: The eyeball is composed of three concentric layer or tunics:

(a) An **outer fibrous tunic,** which consists of the tough **sclera** posteriorly and the translucent **cornea** anteriorly **(brown).**

(b) The **middle vascular tunic** including the **choroid** posteriorly and the **ciliary body** and **iris** anteriorly **(blue).**

(c) The **inner neural tunic,** which is **retina.** It consists of a **neural part** posteriorly, and a **nonneural part** that underlies the ciliary body and iris. The junction between these two parts is the **ora serrata (yellow).**

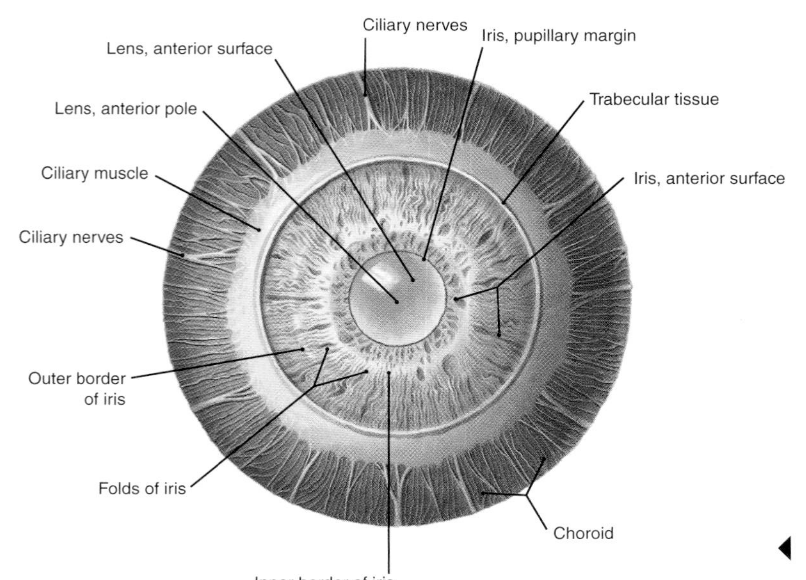
Ciliary nerves
Iris, pupillary margin
Lens, anterior surface
Trabecular tissue
Lens, anterior pole
Ciliary muscle
Iris, anterior surface
Ciliary nerves
Outer border of iris
Folds of iris
Choroid
Inner border of iris

Figure 554.2 Iris and Pupil (Anterior View)

NOTE: Behind the iris is located the anterior pole of the lens.

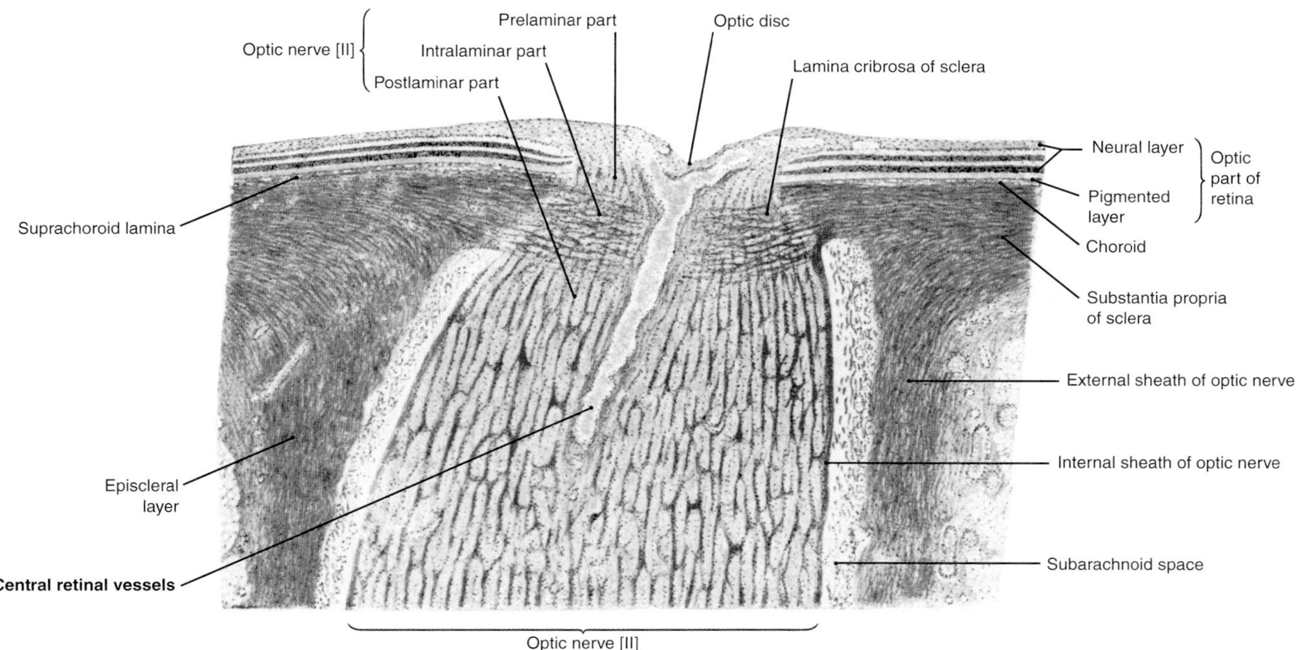
Optic nerve [II]
Prelaminar part
Intralaminar part
Postlaminar part
Optic disc
Lamina cribrosa of sclera
Neural layer
Pigmented layer
Optic part of retina
Choroid
Substantia propria of sclera
External sheath of optic nerve
Internal sheath of optic nerve
Subarachnoid space
Suprachoroid lamina
Episcleral layer
Central retinal vessels
Optic nerve [II]

Figure 555.1 Horizontal Section of the Optic Disk Region of the Eyeball

NOTE: The axons of the optic nerve leave the eyeball at the **optic disk,** or blind spot, where there are no visual receptors.

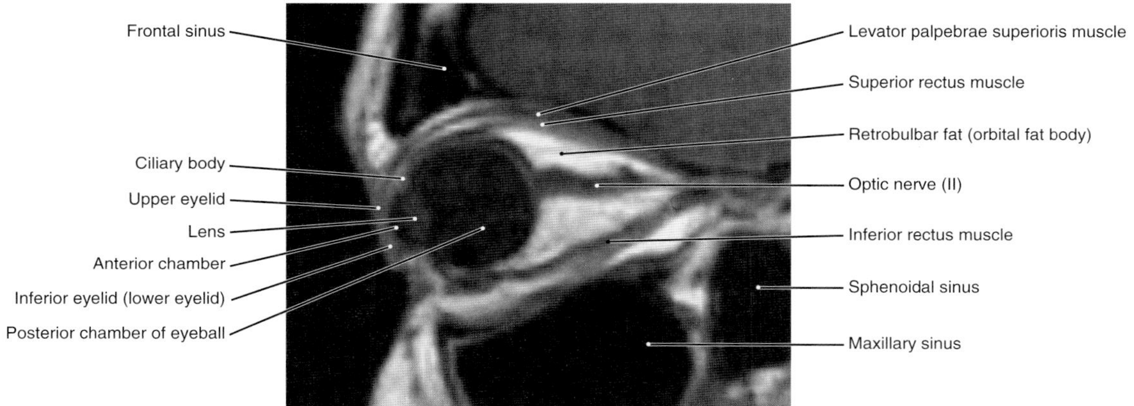
Frontal sinus
Ciliary body
Upper eyelid
Lens
Anterior chamber
Inferior eyelid (lower eyelid)
Posterior chamber of eyeball
Levator palpebrae superioris muscle
Superior rectus muscle
Retrobulbar fat (orbital fat body)
Optic nerve (II)
Inferior rectus muscle
Sphenoidal sinus
Maxillary sinus

Figure 555.2 Magnetic Resonance through the Right Orbit (Lateral Aspect)

NOTE: This is a sagittal section through the optic nerve.

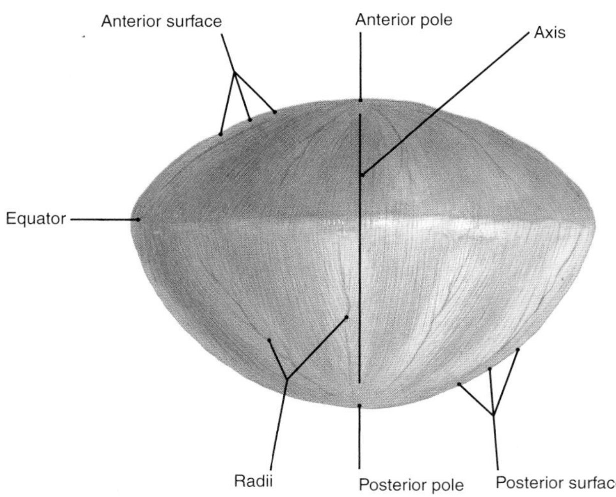
Anterior surface
Anterior pole
Axis
Equator
Radii
Posterior pole
Posterior surface

Figure 555.3 Lens

NOTE: The anteroposterior axis and the equator.

Cornea
Sinus venosus sclerae (canal of Schlemm)
Greater arterial circle of iris
Anterior conjunctival artery and vein
Anterior ciliary artery
Anterior ciliary artery
Lens
Lesser arterial circle of the iris
Ora serrata
Anterior ciliary vessels
Lateral rectus muscle
Long posterior ciliary artery
Retina
Retinal vessels
Choroid membrane
Vorticose vein
Capillary layer of choroid
Vascular layer of choroid (uvea)
Sclera
Episcleral artery and vein
Long posterior ciliary artery
Short posterior ciliary arteries
Central retinal artery and vein

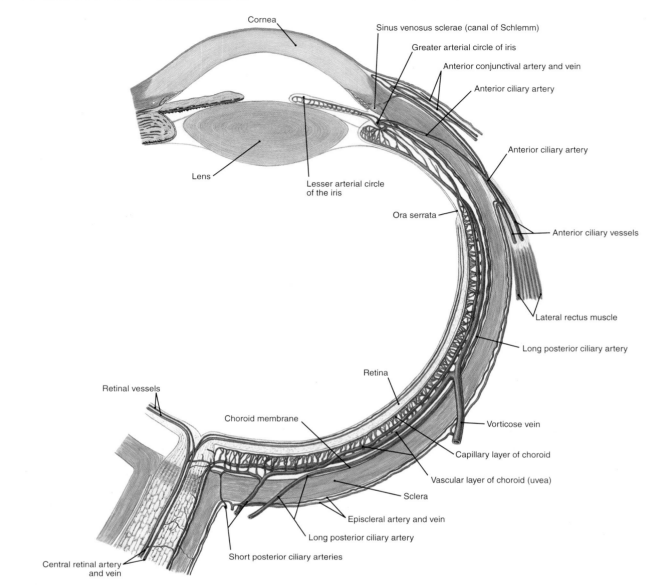

Figure 556.1 **Horizontal Section through the Eyeball Showing the Blood Supply to Its Three Layers**

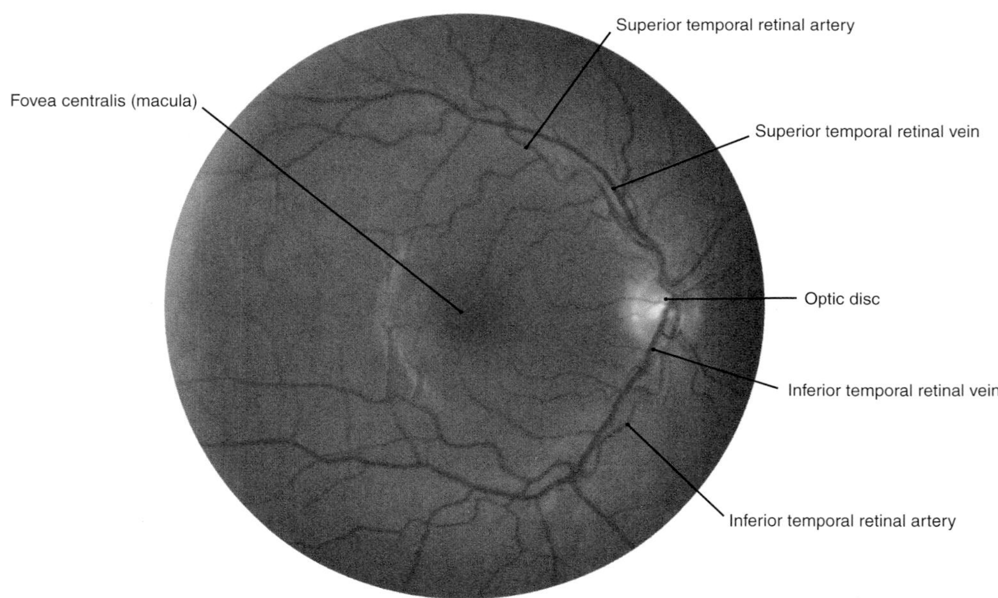
Superior temporal retinal artery
Fovea centralis (macula)
Superior temporal retinal vein
Optic disc
Inferior temporal retinal vein
Inferior temporal retinal artery

Figure 556.2 **Retina and Its Vessels as Seen with an Ophthalmoscope**

NOTE: This shows the fundus of the eye with the **retinal vessels** passing through the optic disc.

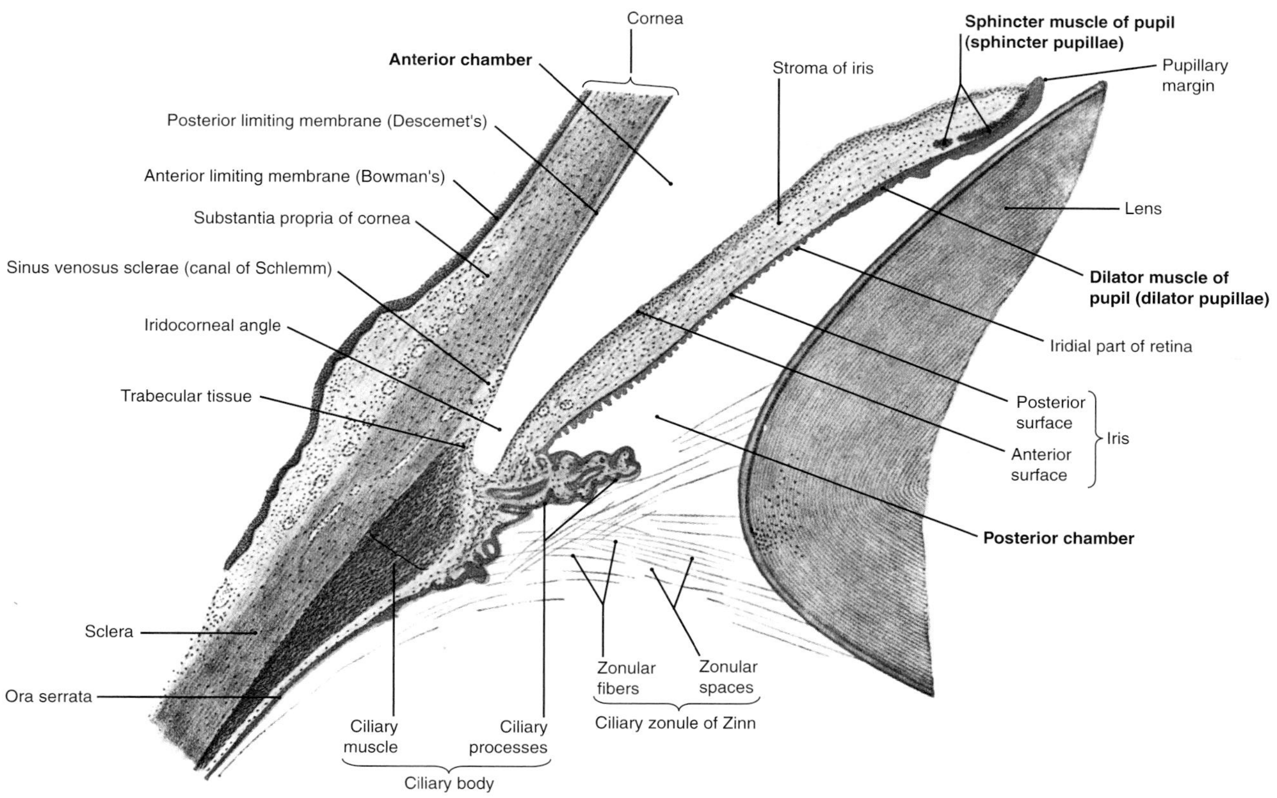
Cornea
Anterior chamber
Posterior limiting membrane (Descemet's)
Anterior limiting membrane (Bowman's)
Substantia propria of cornea
Sinus venosus sclerae (canal of Schlemm)
Iridocorneal angle
Trabecular tissue
Sclera
Ora serrata
Ciliary muscle
Ciliary processes
Ciliary body
Zonular fibers
Zonular spaces
Ciliary zonule of Zinn
Stroma of iris
Sphincter muscle of pupil (sphincter pupillae)
Pupillary margin
Lens
Dilator muscle of pupil (dilator pupillae)
Iridial part of retina
Posterior surface
Anterior surface
Iris
Posterior chamber

Figure 557.1 Horizontal Section through the Anterior Part of the Eyeball

NOTE: (1) The **iris** is the anterior continuation of the ciliary body and choroid, and it separates the anterior chamber from the posterior chamber.

(2) The **ciliary body** contains the **ciliary muscle,** and its fibers are oriented in radial, circular, and meridional (longitudinal) directions. When the eye needs to focus on a near object (accommodation), the ciliary muscle contracts, and this pulls the ciliary body and choroid forward, thereby relieving tension produced by the zonular fibers. The lens becomes thicker and increases its convexity. Parasympathetic fibers supply this muscle.

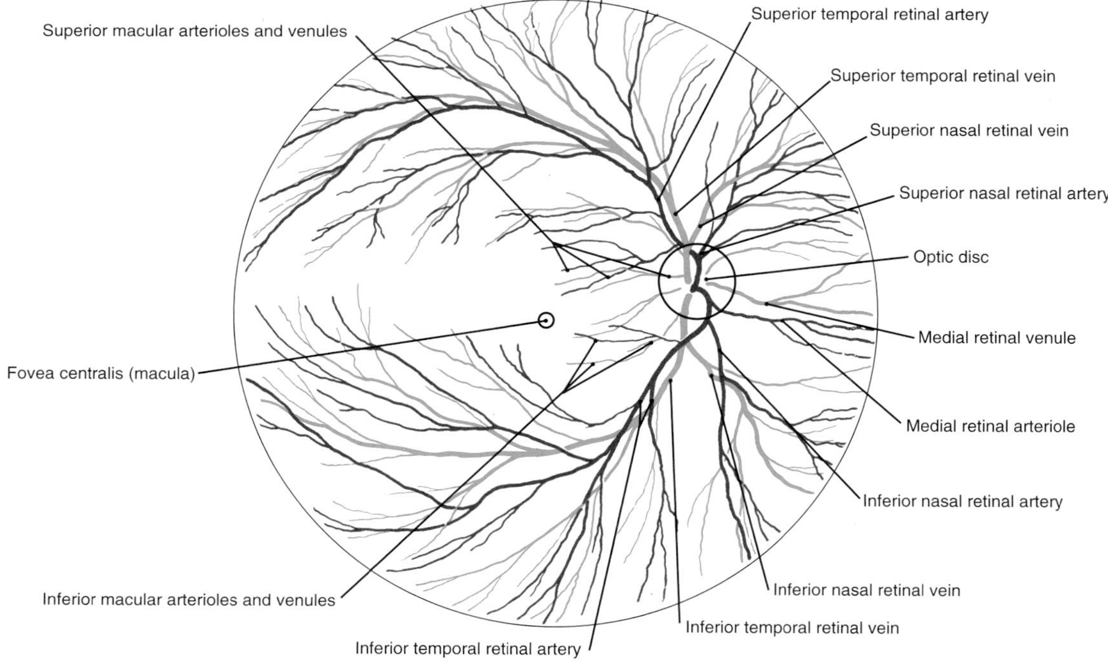
Superior macular arterioles and venules
Superior temporal retinal artery
Superior temporal retinal vein
Superior nasal retinal vein
Superior nasal retinal artery
Optic disc
Medial retinal venule
Fovea centralis (macula)
Medial retinal arteriole
Inferior nasal retinal artery
Inferior nasal retinal vein
Inferior macular arterioles and venules
Inferior temporal retinal vein
Inferior temporal retinal artery

Figure 557.2 Schematic Drawing of the Retinal Vessels

NOTE: The central retinal artery initially divides into **superior and inferior branches.** Each of these subdivide into **nasal and temporal branches,** supplying the four retinal quadrants.

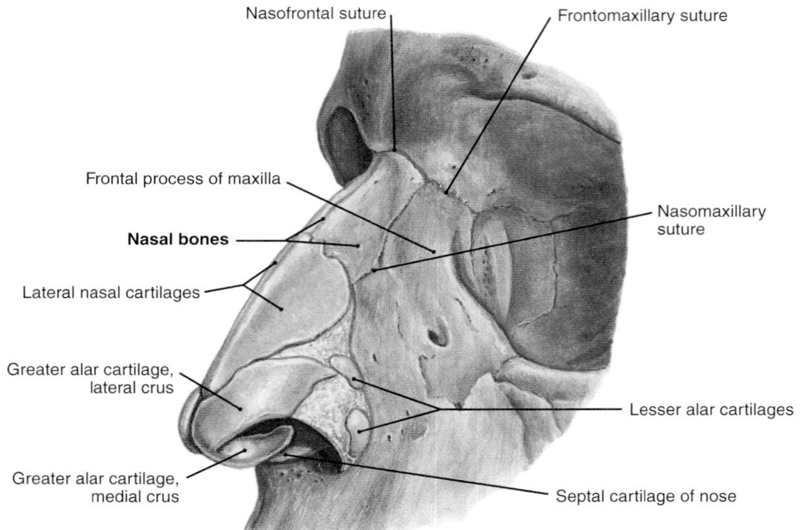
Nasofrontal suture
Frontomaxillary suture
Frontal process of maxilla
Nasal bones
Nasomaxillary suture
Lateral nasal cartilages
Greater alar cartilage, lateral crus
Lesser alar cartilages
Greater alar cartilage, medial crus
Septal cartilage of nose

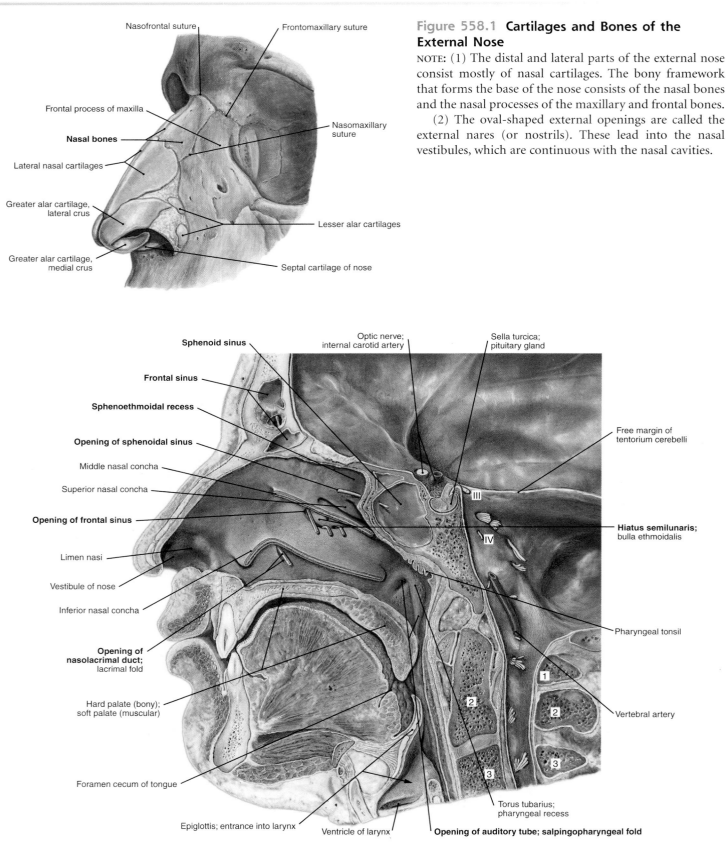

Figure 558.1 Cartilages and Bones of the External Nose

NOTE: (1) The distal and lateral parts of the external nose consist mostly of nasal cartilages. The bony framework that forms the base of the nose consists of the nasal bones and the nasal processes of the maxillary and frontal bones.

(2) The oval-shaped external openings are called the external nares (or nostrils). These lead into the nasal vestibules, which are continuous with the nasal cavities.

Sphenoid sinus
Optic nerve; internal carotid artery
Sella turcica; pituitary gland
Frontal sinus
Sphenoethmoidal recess
Free margin of tentorium cerebelli
Opening of sphenoidal sinus
Middle nasal concha
Superior nasal concha
III
Opening of frontal sinus
Hiatus semilunaris; bulla ethmoidalis
IV
Limen nasi
Vestibule of nose
Inferior nasal concha
Pharyngeal tonsil
Opening of nasolacrimal duct; lacrimal fold
1
Hard palate (bony); soft palate (muscular)
2
2
Vertebral artery
3
3
Foramen cecum of tongue
Torus tubarius; pharyngeal recess
Epiglottis; entrance into larynx
Ventricle of larynx
Opening of auditory tube; salpingopharyngeal fold

Figure 558.2 Lateral Wall of the Right Nasal Cavity Showing Openings of the Paranasal Air Sinuses and the Nasopharynx

NOTE: (1) This paramedian sagittal section of the head shows the right nasal cavity after the middle and inferior nasal conchae were removed. The nasal cavity communicates anteriorly with the exterior through the nostril and posteriorly with the nasopharynx.

(2) The openings of the paranasal sinuses and other structures:

(a) The **sphenoid sinus,** which drains into the **sphenoethmoid recess** above the superior concha.

(b) The **frontal** and **maxillary sinuses,** both of which open in a groove called the **hiatus semilunaris** in the middle meatus below the middle concha.

(c) The **nasolacrimal duct,** which opens into the inferior meatus below the inferior concha.

(d) The **auditory tube,** which opens into the nasopharynx just behind the inferior concha.

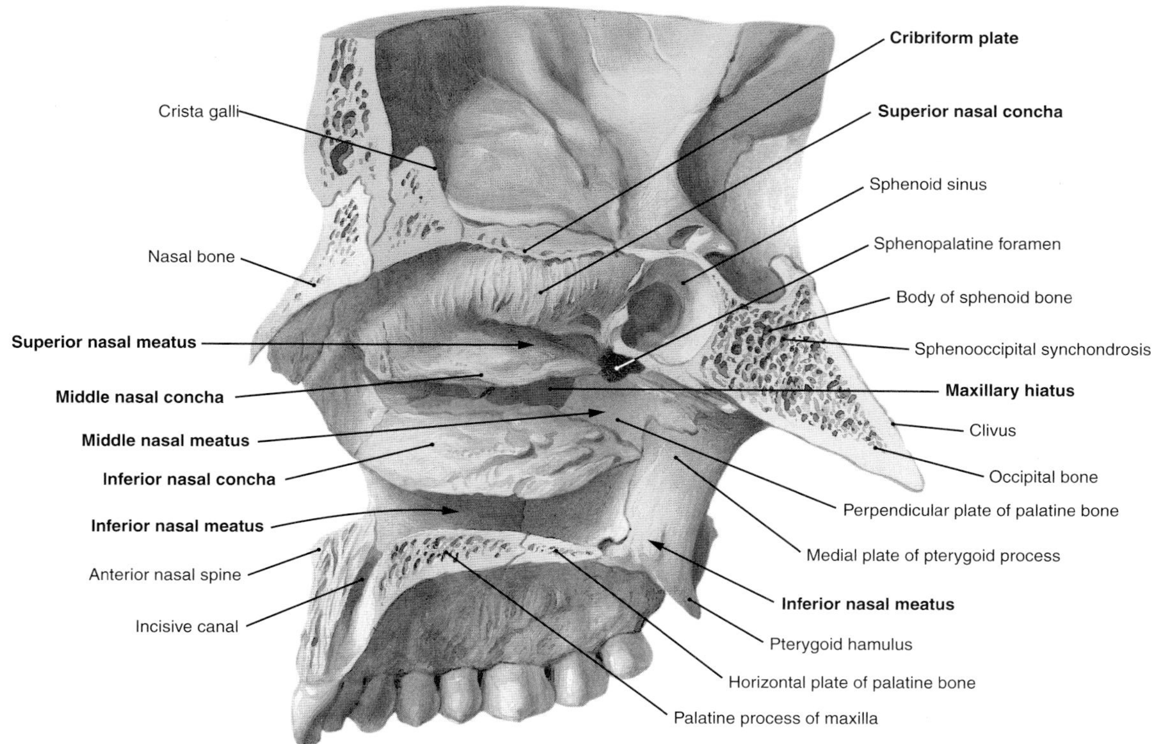
Crista galli
Nasal bone
Superior nasal meatus
Middle nasal concha
Middle nasal meatus
Inferior nasal concha
Inferior nasal meatus
Anterior nasal spine
Incisive canal
Cribriform plate
Superior nasal concha
Sphenoid sinus
Sphenopalatine foramen
Body of sphenoid bone
Sphenooccipital synchondrosis
Maxillary hiatus
Clivus
Occipital bone
Perpendicular plate of palatine bone
Medial plate of pterygoid process
Inferior nasal meatus
Pterygoid hamulus
Horizontal plate of palatine bone
Palatine process of maxilla

Figure 559.1 Bony Lateral Wall of the Right Nasal Cavity

NOTE: (1) The nasal septum has been removed and the mucosa stripped from the irregular lateral wall of the nasal cavity and the hard palate. Note also that in front of the nasal conchae are the **nasal bone** (gray) and the **maxilla,** and behind is the **perpendicular plate** of the **palatine bone** (blue).

(2) The **crista galli, cribriform plate,** and the **superior** and **middle nasal conchae** are all part of the **ethmoid bone** (light orange). Below these is the **inferior nasal concha,** which is a separate bone (gray). The bony floor of the nasal cavity is the hard palate, formed by the **palatine process** of the **maxilla** and the **horizontal plate** of the **palatine bone.**

(3) The arrows that follow the courses of the **superior, middle,** and **inferior meatuses,** each under its respective nasal concha. Note also the **sphenoid sinus,** the **sphenopalatine foramen,** and the opening of the maxillary sinus (**maxillary hiatus**).

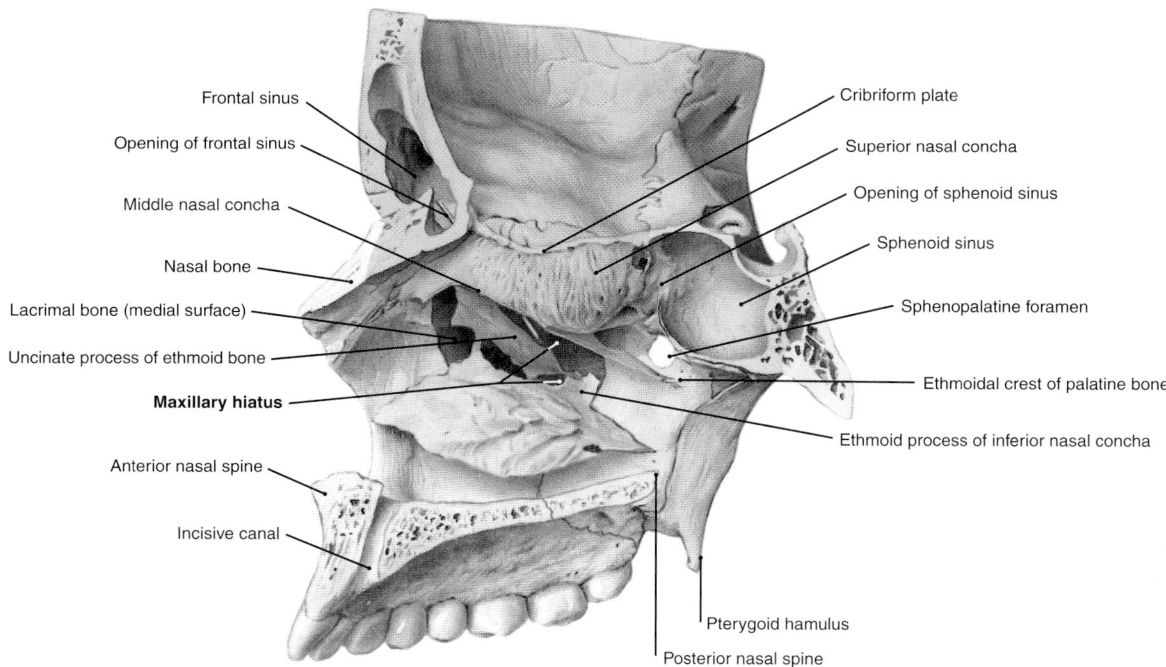
Frontal sinus
Opening of frontal sinus
Middle nasal concha
Nasal bone
Lacrimal bone (medial surface)
Uncinate process of ethmoid bone
Maxillary hiatus
Anterior nasal spine
Incisive canal
Cribriform plate
Superior nasal concha
Opening of sphenoid sinus
Sphenoid sinus
Sphenopalatine foramen
Ethmoidal crest of palatine bone
Ethmoid process of inferior nasal concha
Pterygoid hamulus
Posterior nasal spine

Figure 559.2 Bony Lateral Wall of the Right Nasal Cavity with the Middle Nasal Concha Removed

NOTE: More complete exposure of the **maxillary hiatus** and the bony structures deep to (lateral to) the middle nasal concha. Compare with Fig. 559.1.

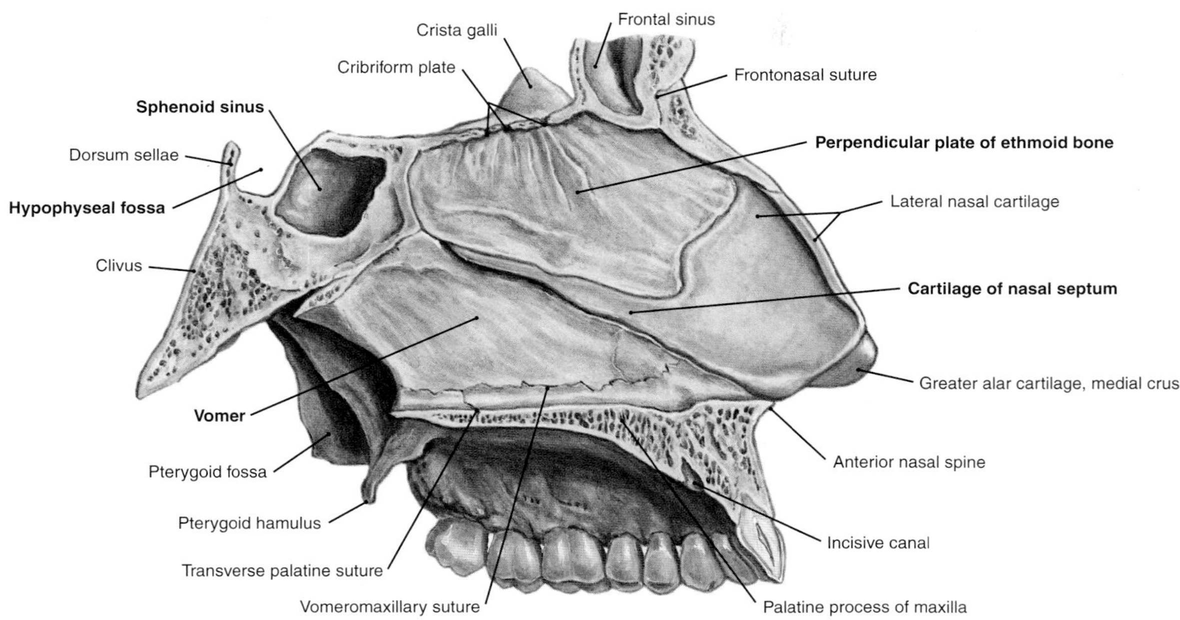
Crista galli
Frontal sinus
Cribriform plate
Frontonasal suture
Sphenoid sinus
Perpendicular plate of ethmoid bone
Dorsum sellae
Hypophyseal fossa
Lateral nasal cartilage
Clivus
Cartilage of nasal septum
Greater alar cartilage, medial crus
Vomer
Anterior nasal spine
Pterygoid fossa
Pterygoid hamulus
Incisive canal
Transverse palatine suture
Vomeromaxillary suture
Palatine process of maxilla

Figure 560.1 Nasal Septum: Structure and Blood Supply (Notes)

NOTE: (1) The skeletal structure of the nasal septum includes the **perpendicular plate of the ethmoid bone**, the **vomer bone**, and the **cartilage of the nasal septum.**

(2) The arteries of the septum include: superior and posterior—the **anterior and posterior ethmoid arteries** and the **posterior septal branches** of the **sphenopalatine artery;** inferior and anterior—the **septal branch** of the **superior labial artery,** which enters through the nostrils, and the **septal branch** of the **greater palatine artery,** which enters the nasal cavity by way of the incisive foramen.

(3) The **septal nerves** include: branches of the **anterior ethmoid nerve** (from the ophthalmic nerve), the **nasopalatine nerve** (from the maxillary nerve), and the **internal nasal branches** of the infraorbital nerves that enter the nasal cavities through the nostrils.

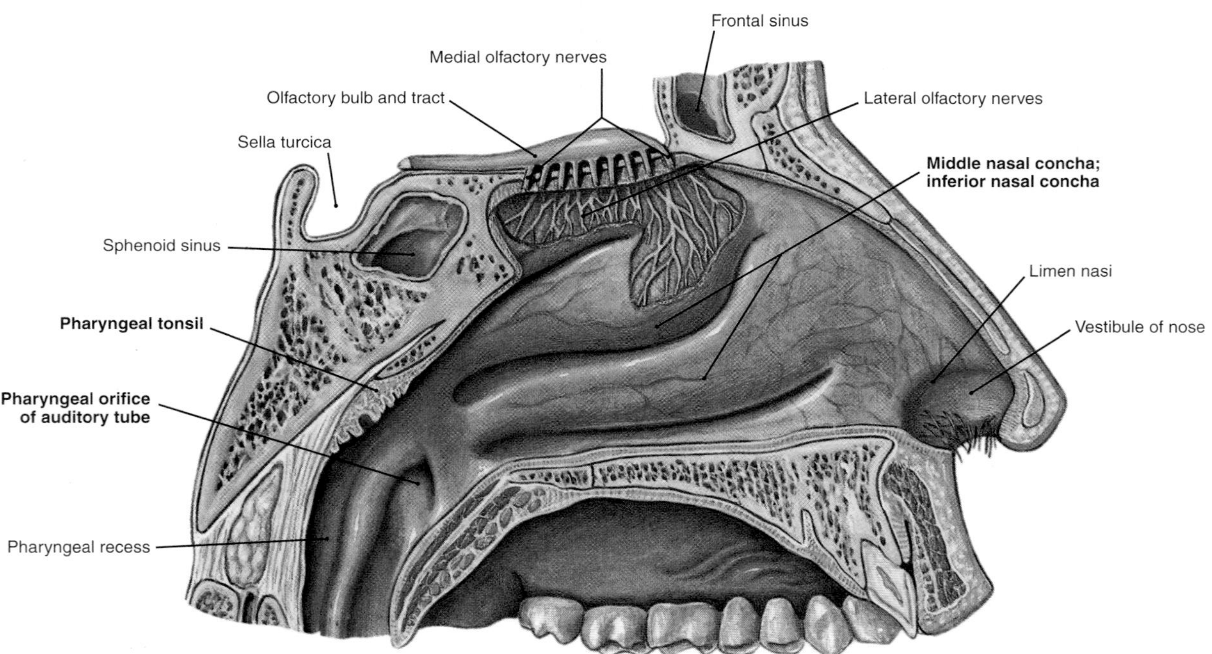
Frontal sinus
Medial olfactory nerves
Olfactory bulb and tract
Lateral olfactory nerves
Sella turcica
Middle nasal concha;
inferior nasal concha
Sphenoid sinus
Limen nasi
Pharyngeal tonsil
Vestibule of nose
Pharyngeal orifice
of auditory tube
Pharyngeal recess

Figure 560.2 Lateral Wall of the Left Nasal Cavity Showing the Olfactory Nerves

NOTE: The mucous membrane overlying the **lateral olfactory nerves** has been removed. The lateral wall of the nasal cavity is marked by the **superior, middle,** and **inferior nasal conchae.** Beneath each concha courses the corresponding nasal passage, or **meatus.**

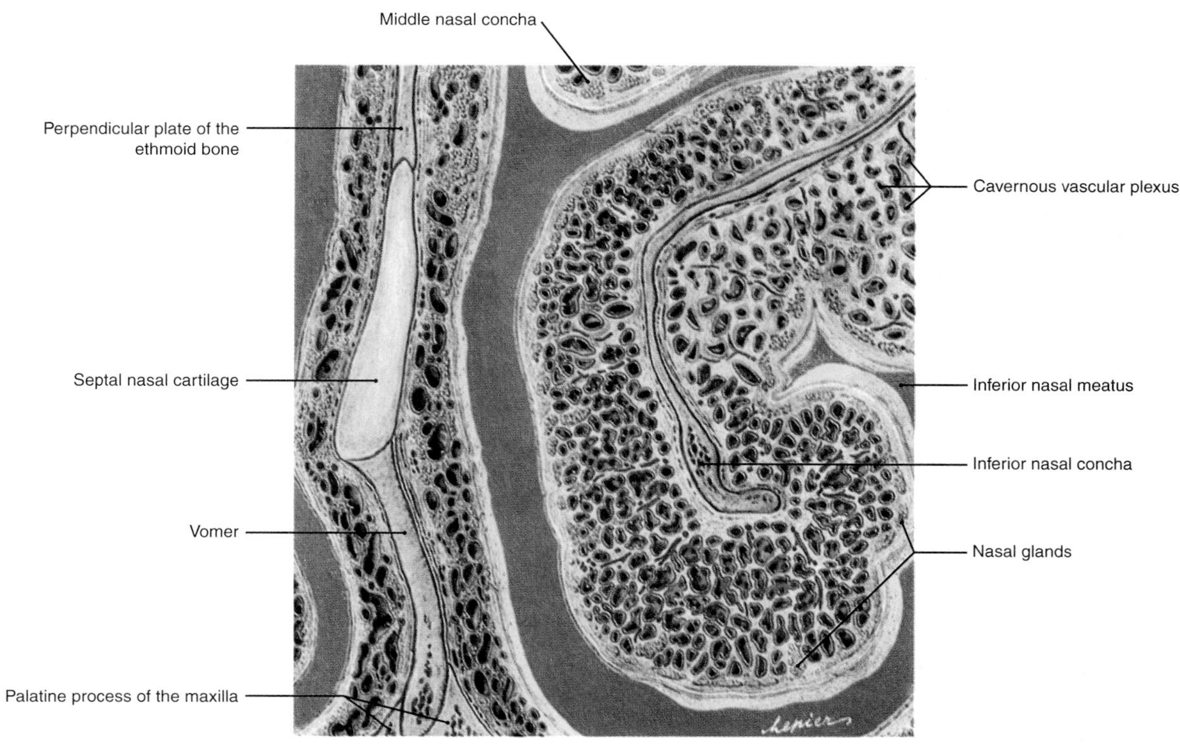
Middle nasal concha
Perpendicular plate of the ethmoid bone
Cavernous vascular plexus
Septal nasal cartilage
Inferior nasal meatus
Inferior nasal concha
Vomer
Nasal glands
Palatine process of the maxilla

Figure 561.1 **Macroscopic View of the Inferior Nasal Concha**

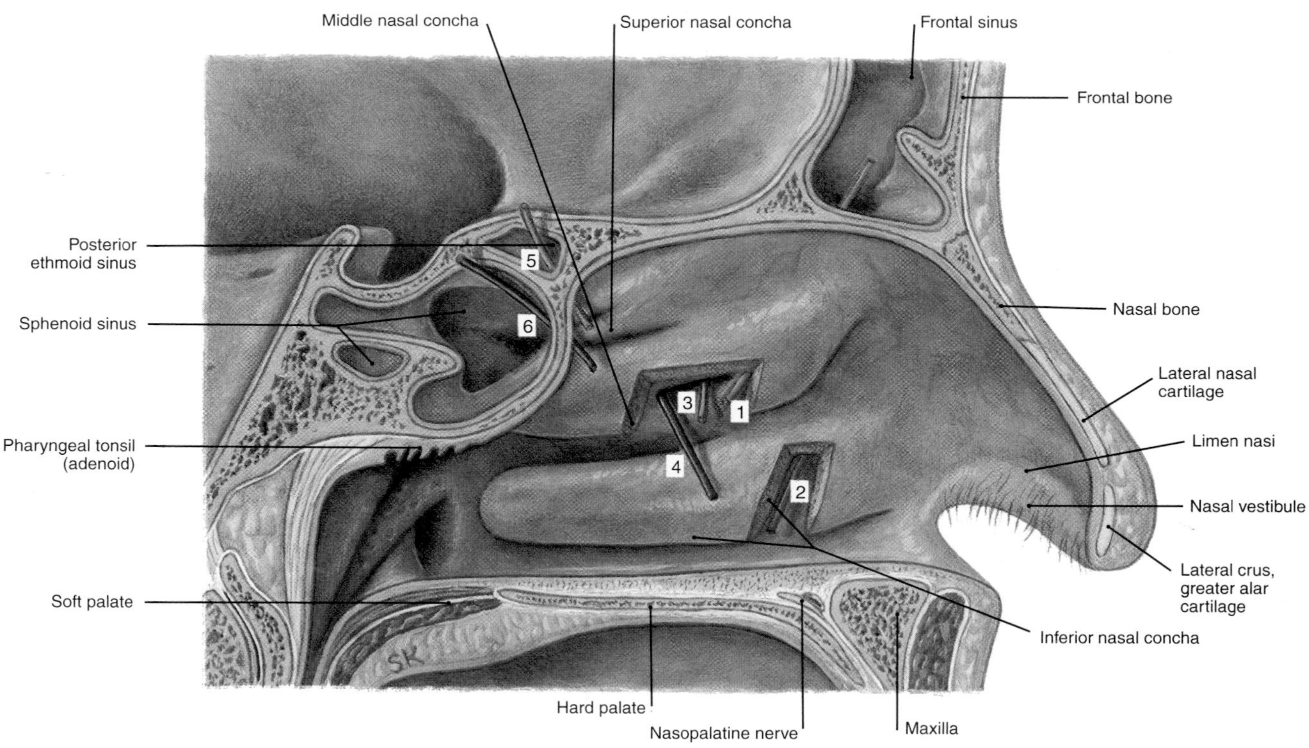
Middle nasal concha
Superior nasal concha
Frontal sinus
Frontal bone
Posterior ethmoid sinus
5
Sphenoid sinus
6
Nasal bone
Lateral nasal cartilage
3
1
Pharyngeal tonsil (adenoid)
Limen nasi
4
2
Nasal vestibule
Lateral crus, greater alar cartilage
Soft palate
Inferior nasal concha
Hard palate
Nasopalatine nerve
Maxilla

Figure 561.2 **Drainage Routes of the Paranasal Sinuses and the Nasolacrimal Duct**

NOTE: This drawing shows the left nasal cavity and variously colored probes emerging through orifices that drain into the nasal cavity. These are numbered as follows:

1. Frontal sinus
2. Nasolacrimal duct
3. Anterior ethmoid sinus
4. Maxillary sinus
5. Posterior ethmoid sinus
6. Sphenoid sinus

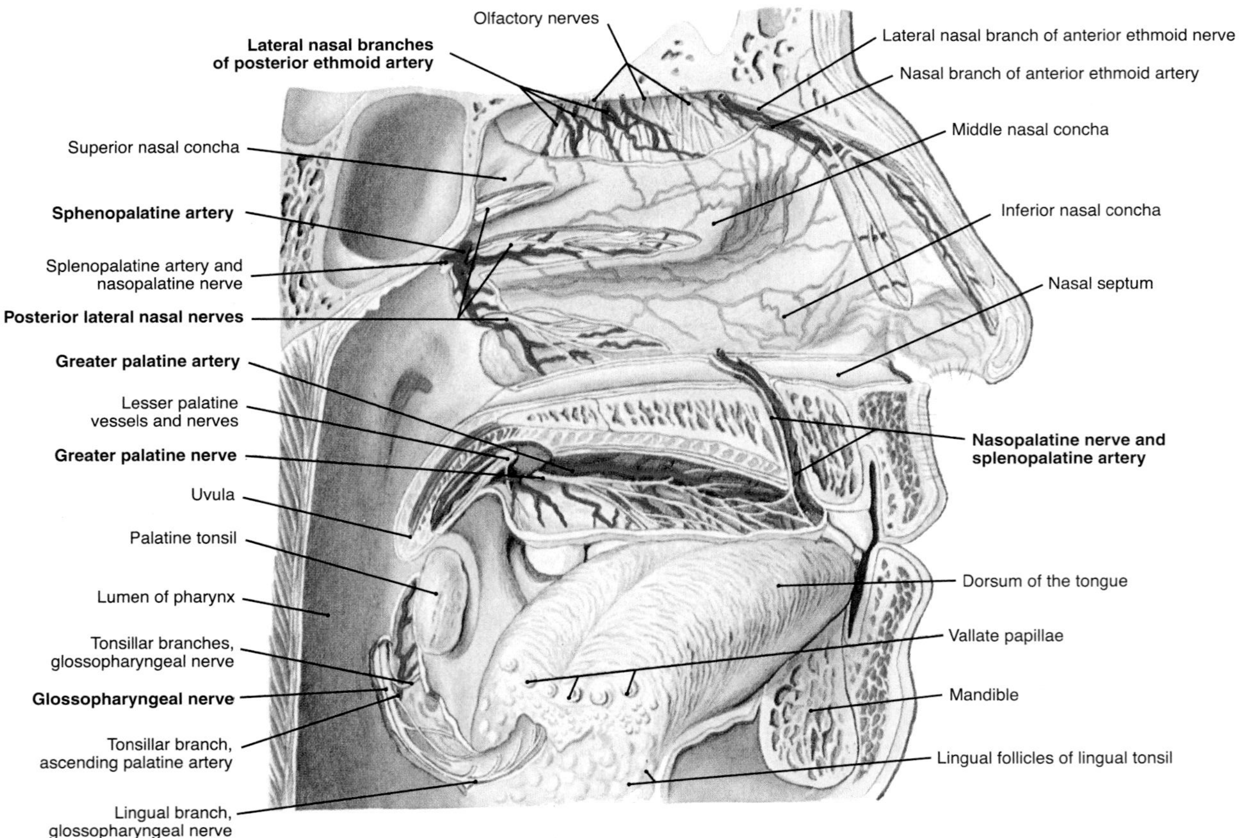
Olfactory nerves
Lateral nasal branches of posterior ethmoid artery
Lateral nasal branch of anterior ethmoid nerve
Nasal branch of anterior ethmoid artery
Superior nasal concha
Middle nasal concha
Sphenopalatine artery
Inferior nasal concha
Splenopalatine artery and nasopalatine nerve
Nasal septum
Posterior lateral nasal nerves
Greater palatine artery
Lesser palatine vessels and nerves
Nasopalatine nerve and splenopalatine artery
Greater palatine nerve
Uvula
Palatine tonsil
Dorsum of the tongue
Lumen of pharynx
Vallate papillae
Tonsillar branches, glossopharyngeal nerve
Glossopharyngeal nerve
Mandible
Tonsillar branch, ascending palatine artery
Lingual follicles of lingual tonsil
Lingual branch, glossopharyngeal nerve

Figure 562.1 **Nerves and Arteries of the Palate and Lateral Wall of the Nasal Cavity**

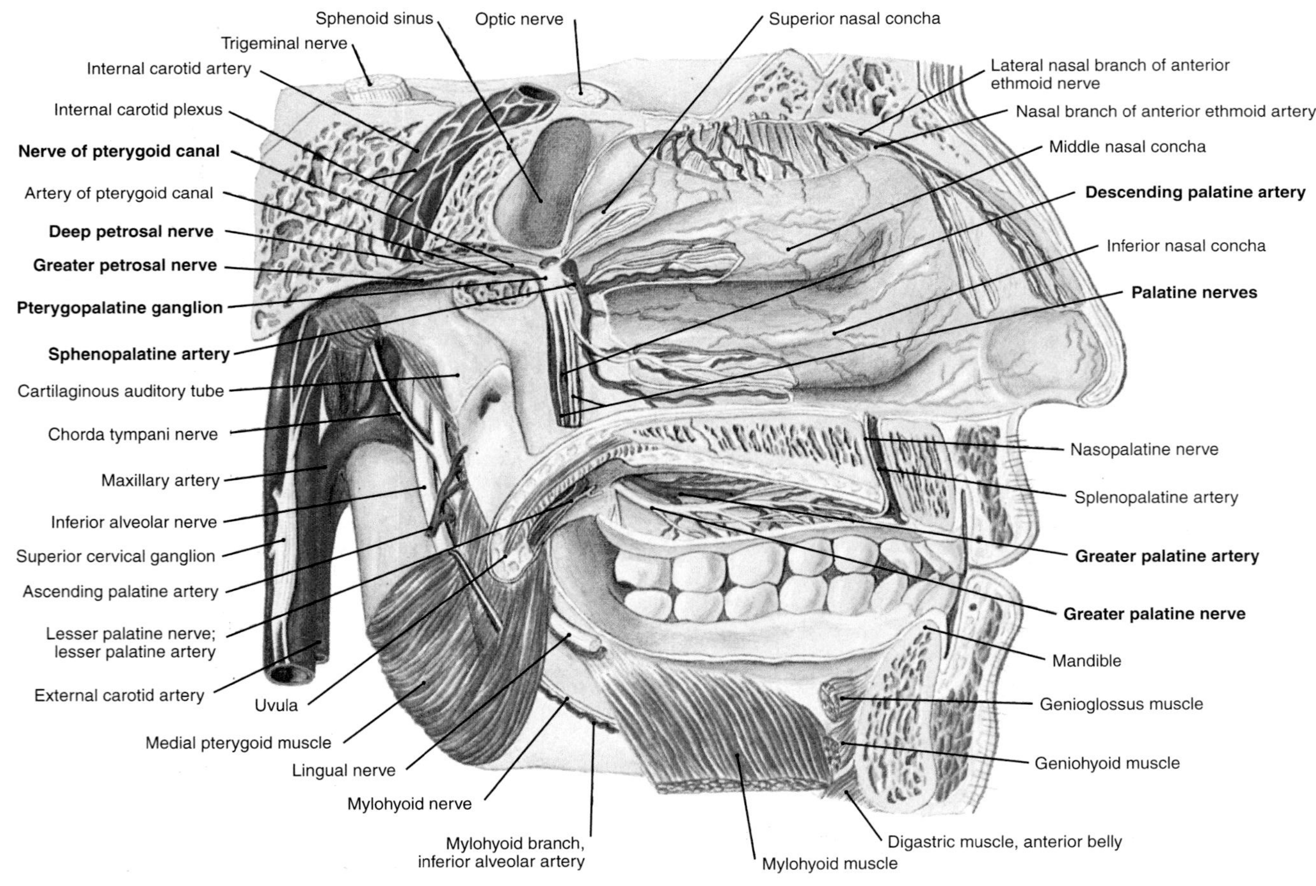
Sphenoid sinus
Optic nerve
Superior nasal concha
Trigeminal nerve
Internal carotid artery
Lateral nasal branch of anterior ethmoid nerve
Internal carotid plexus
Nasal branch of anterior ethmoid artery
Nerve of pterygoid canal
Middle nasal concha
Artery of pterygoid canal
Descending palatine artery
Deep petrosal nerve
Inferior nasal concha
Greater petrosal nerve
Palatine nerves
Pterygopalatine ganglion
Sphenopalatine artery
Cartilaginous auditory tube
Chorda tympani nerve
Nasopalatine nerve
Maxillary artery
Splenopalatine artery
Inferior alveolar nerve
Superior cervical ganglion
Greater palatine artery
Ascending palatine artery
Greater palatine nerve
Lesser palatine nerve; lesser palatine artery
Mandible
External carotid artery
Uvula
Genioglossus muscle
Medial pterygoid muscle
Geniohyoid muscle
Lingual nerve
Mylohyoid nerve
Mylohyoid branch, inferior alveolar artery
Digastric muscle, anterior belly
Mylohyoid muscle

Figure 562.2 **Pterygopalatine Ganglion and Its Branches**

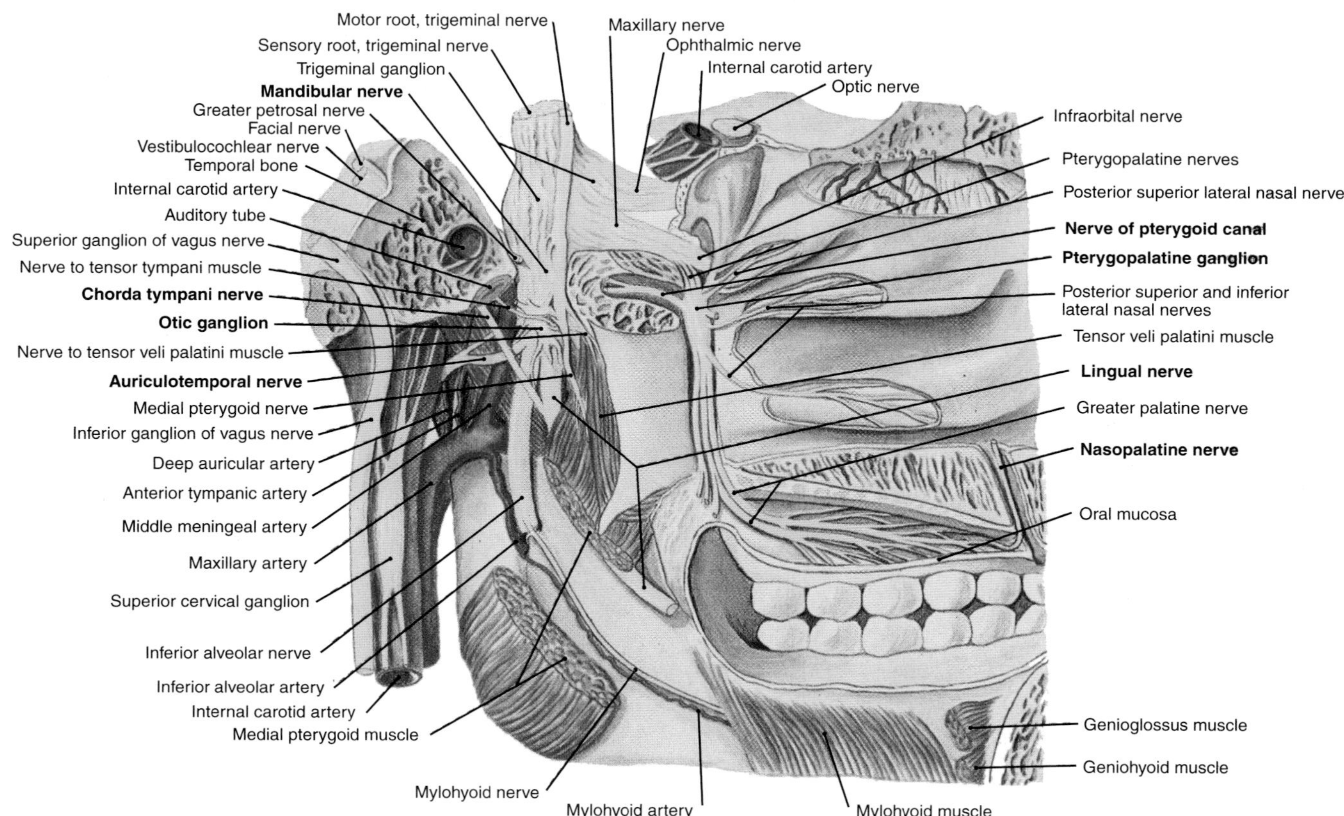
Motor root, trigeminal nerve
Sensory root, trigeminal nerve
Trigeminal ganglion
Mandibular nerve
Greater petrosal nerve
Facial nerve
Vestibulocochlear nerve
Temporal bone
Internal carotid artery
Auditory tube
Superior ganglion of vagus nerve
Nerve to tensor tympani muscle
Chorda tympani nerve
Otic ganglion
Nerve to tensor veli palatini muscle
Auriculotemporal nerve
Medial pterygoid nerve
Inferior ganglion of vagus nerve
Deep auricular artery
Anterior tympanic artery
Middle meningeal artery
Maxillary artery
Superior cervical ganglion
Inferior alveolar nerve
Inferior alveolar artery
Internal carotid artery
Medial pterygoid muscle
Mylohyoid nerve
Mylohyoid artery
Mylohyoid muscle
Maxillary nerve
Ophthalmic nerve
Internal carotid artery
Optic nerve
Infraorbital nerve
Pterygopalatine nerves
Posterior superior lateral nasal nerve
Nerve of pterygoid canal
Pterygopalatine ganglion
Posterior superior and inferior lateral nasal nerves
Tensor veli palatini muscle
Lingual nerve
Greater palatine nerve
Nasopalatine nerve
Oral mucosa
Genioglossus muscle
Geniohyoid muscle

Figure 563.1 Nerves of the Nasal and Oral Cavities and the Otic Ganglion

NOTE: The **chorda tympani nerve** joins the **lingual nerve,** and the **otic ganglion** lies just medial to the mandibular division of the trigeminal nerve below foramen ovale.

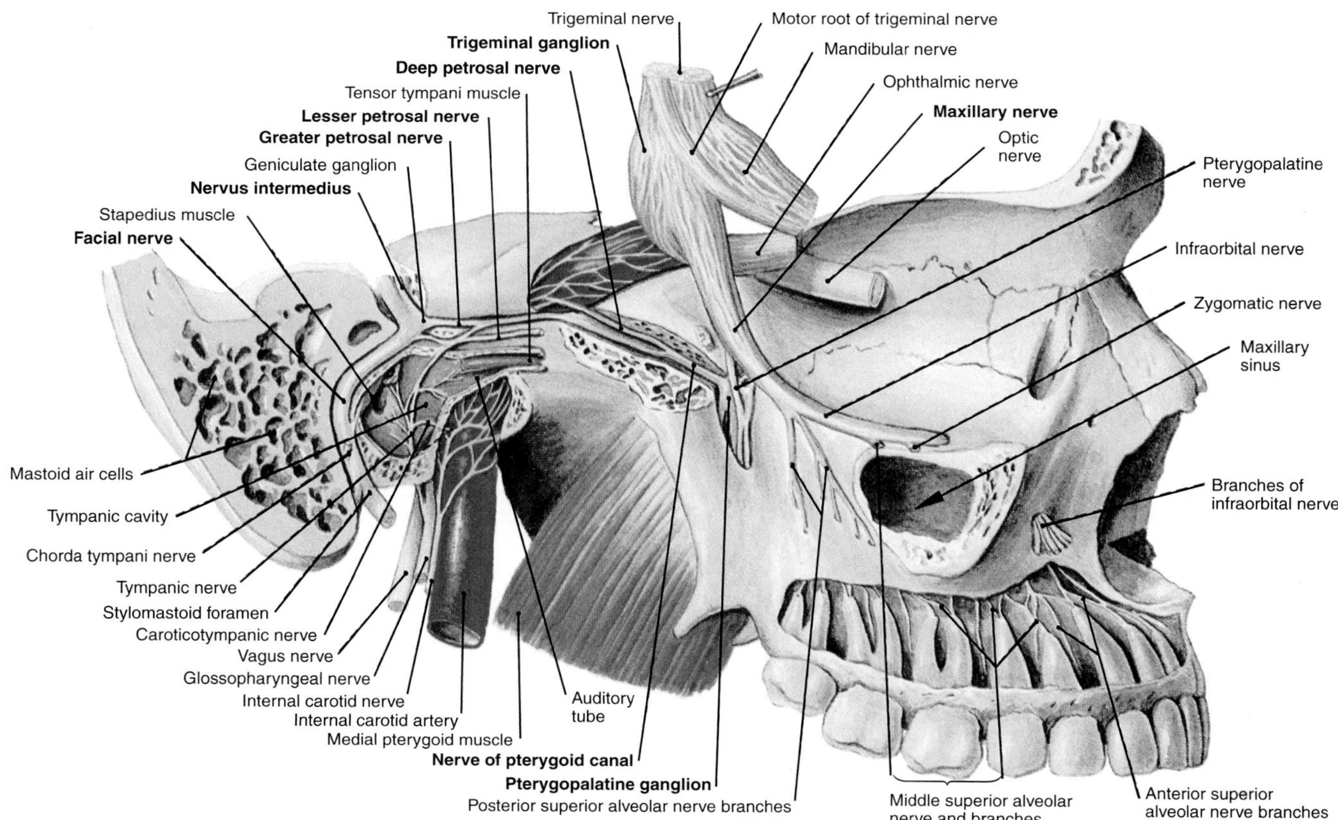
Trigeminal nerve
Trigeminal ganglion
Deep petrosal nerve
Tensor tympani muscle
Lesser petrosal nerve
Greater petrosal nerve
Geniculate ganglion
Nervus intermedius
Stapedius muscle
Facial nerve
Mastoid air cells
Tympanic cavity
Chorda tympani nerve
Tympanic nerve
Stylomastoid foramen
Caroticotympanic nerve
Vagus nerve
Glossopharyngeal nerve
Internal carotid nerve
Internal carotid artery
Medial pterygoid muscle
Auditory tube
Nerve of pterygoid canal
Pterygopalatine ganglion
Posterior superior alveolar nerve branches
Middle superior alveolar nerve and branches
Anterior superior alveolar nerve branches
Motor root of trigeminal nerve
Mandibular nerve
Ophthalmic nerve
Maxillary nerve
Optic nerve
Pterygopalatine nerve
Infraorbital nerve
Zygomatic nerve
Maxillary sinus
Branches of infraorbital nerve

Figure 563.2 Maxillary Nerve, Petrosal Nerves, and Facial Nerve

NOTE: The **nerve of the pterygoid canal** is formed by the union of the **deep petrosal nerve** (postganglionic sympathetic) and the **greater petrosal nerve** (sensory and preganglionic, VII, parasympathetic fibers). The **lesser petrosal nerve** carries preganglionic, IX, parasympathetic fibers to the **otic ganglion.**

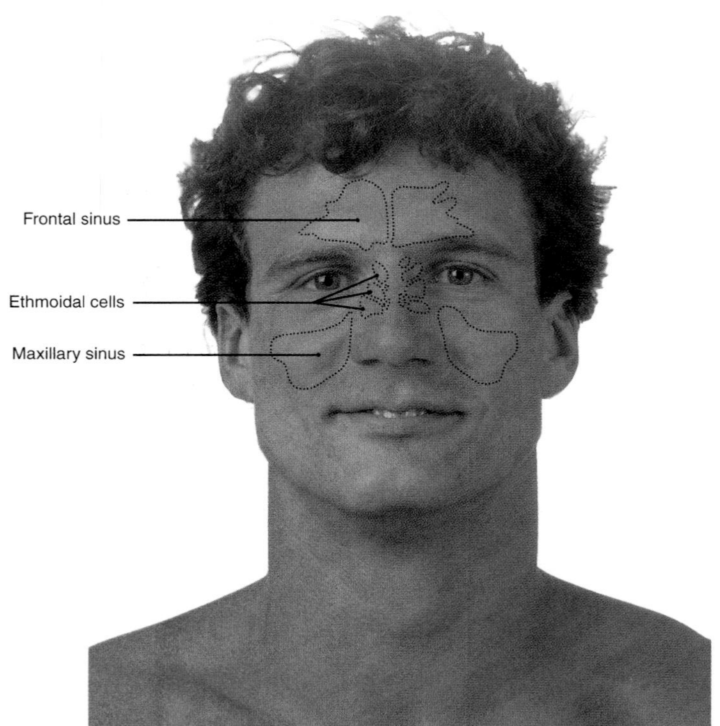
Frontal sinus
Ethmoidal cells
Maxillary sinus

Figure 564.1 Surface Projection of the Paranasal Sinuses onto the Anterior Aspect of the Face
NOTE: The sphenoid sinus is not shown in this figure.

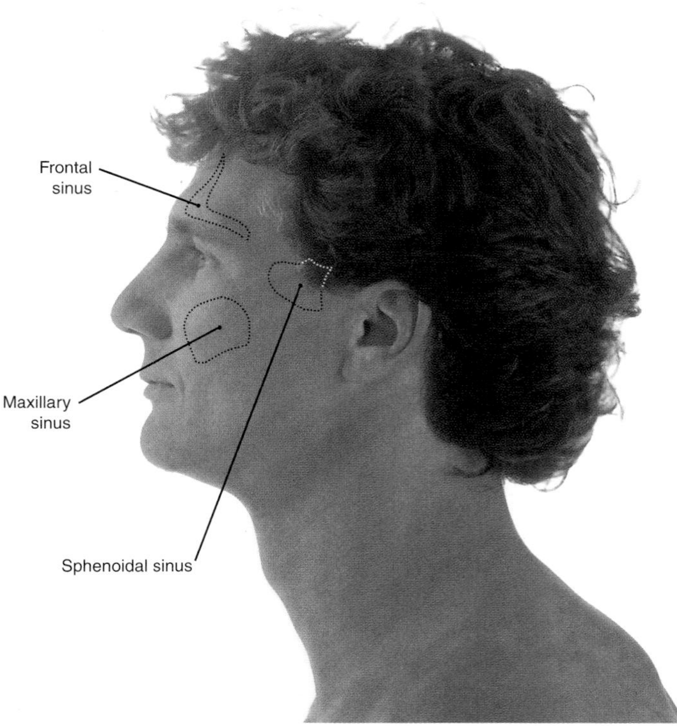
Frontal sinus
Maxillary sinus
Sphenoidal sinus

Figure 564.2 Surface Projection of the Paranasal Sinuses onto the Lateral Aspect of the Face
NOTE: The ethmoid sinuses are not shown in this figure.

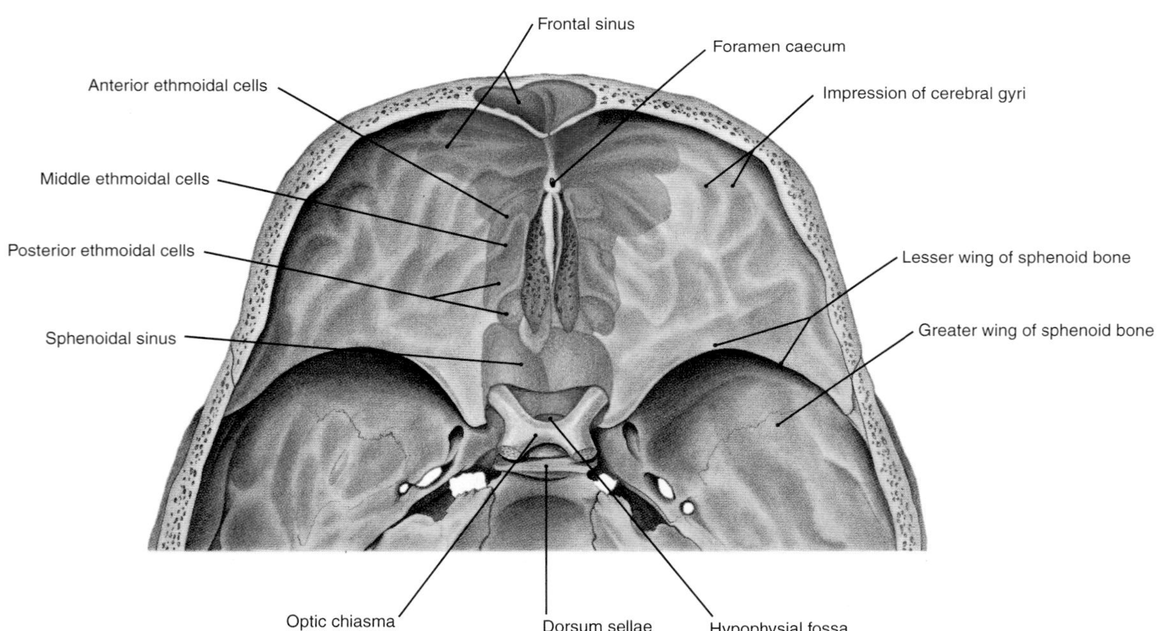
Frontal sinus
Foramen caecum
Anterior ethmoidal cells
Impression of cerebral gyri
Middle ethmoidal cells
Posterior ethmoidal cells
Lesser wing of sphenoid bone
Sphenoidal sinus
Greater wing of sphenoid bone
Optic chiasma
Dorsum sellae
Hypophysial fossa

Figure 564.3 Paranasal Sinuses Viewed from Above
NOTE: (1) The frontal anterior ethmoid, middle ethmoid, posterior ethmoid, and sphenoid sinuses are projected onto the base of the anterior cranial fossa; the maxillary sinus is not shown.

(2) The sinuses are named for the bones that contain them.

(3) The **frontal sinus** drains into the middle meatus of the nasal cavity through the ethmoidal infundibulum or the frontonasal duct; the **anterior ethmoid air cells** open into the ethmoidal infundibulum or the frontonasal duct, **the middle ethmoid cells** open onto the ethmoid bulla in the middle meatus, and the **posterior ethmoid air cells** open into the superior meatus; the **sphenoid sinus** opens into the sphenoethmoidal recess posterior to the superior concha.

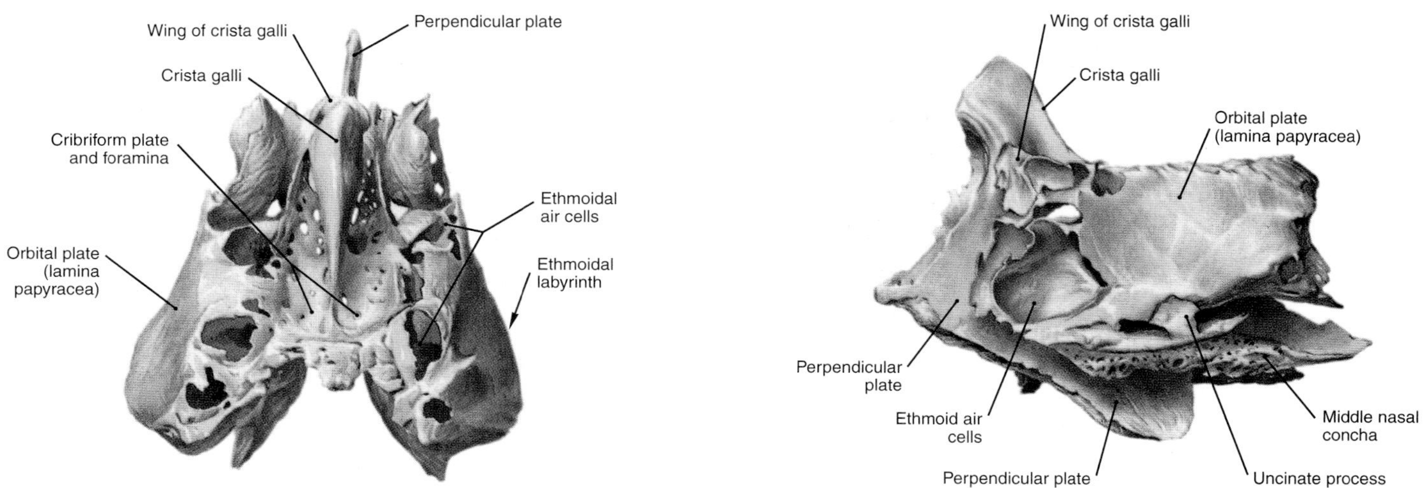
Wing of crista galli
Perpendicular plate
Crista galli
Cribriform plate and foramina
Ethmoidal air cells
Orbital plate (lamina papyracea)
Ethmoidal labyrinth
Wing of crista galli
Crista galli
Orbital plate (lamina papyracea)
Perpendicular plate
Ethmoid air cells
Middle nasal concha
Perpendicular plate
Uncinate process

Figure 565.1 Superior Surface of the Ethmoid Bone

Figure 565.2 Ethmoid Bone (Left Lateral View)

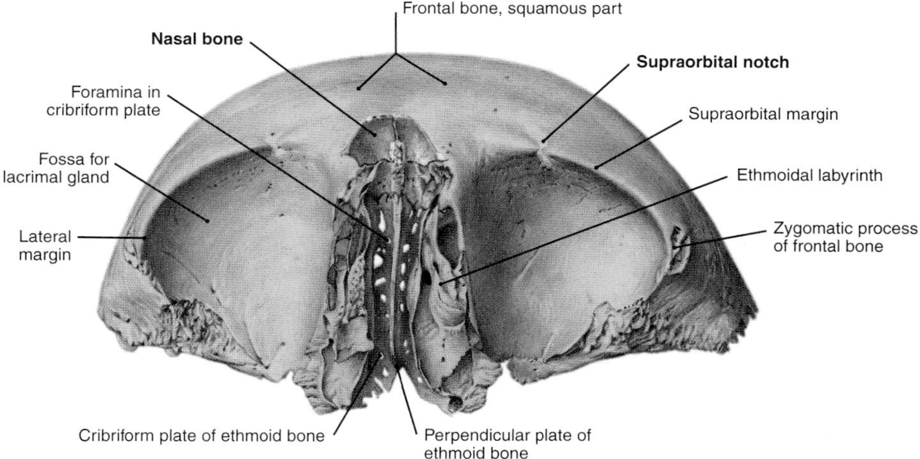
Frontal bone, squamous part
Nasal bone
Supraorbital notch
Foramina in cribriform plate
Supraorbital margin
Fossa for lacrimal gland
Ethmoidal labyrinth
Lateral margin
Zygomatic process of frontal bone
Cribriform plate of ethmoid bone
Perpendicular plate of ethmoid bone

Figure 565.3 Frontal, Ethmoid, and Nasal Bones Viewed from Above

NOTE: The cribriform plate of the ethmoid bone (orange color) extends laterally from the midline on both sides and it is perforated by many foramina. Through these foramina course the nerve fibers of the primary olfactory receptor cells.

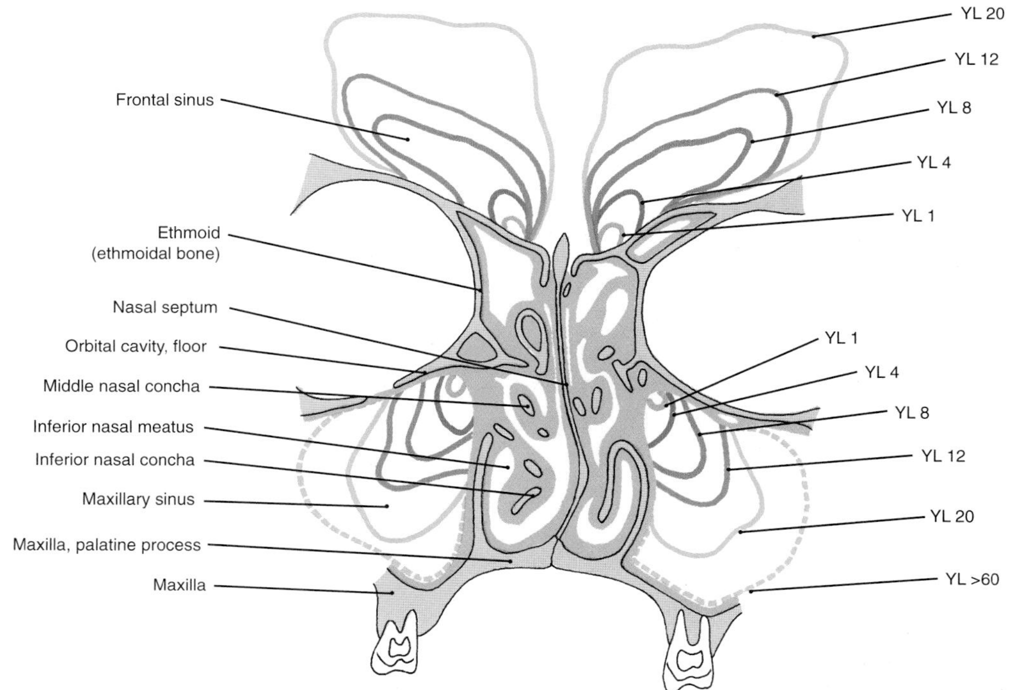
YL 20
YL 12
Frontal sinus
YL 8
YL 4
YL 1
Ethmoid (ethmoidal bone)
Nasal septum
YL 1
Orbital cavity, floor
YL 4
Middle nasal concha
YL 8
Inferior nasal meatus
Inferior nasal concha
YL 12
Maxillary sinus
YL 20
Maxilla, palatine process
Maxilla
YL >60

Figure 565.4 Enlargement of the Frontal and Maxillary Sinuses

NOTE: The growth of the frontal sinus is indicated from the 1st year of life (YL) to the 20th year, while the maxillary sinus is shown from the 1st year of life to the 20th year, and then at the 60th year.

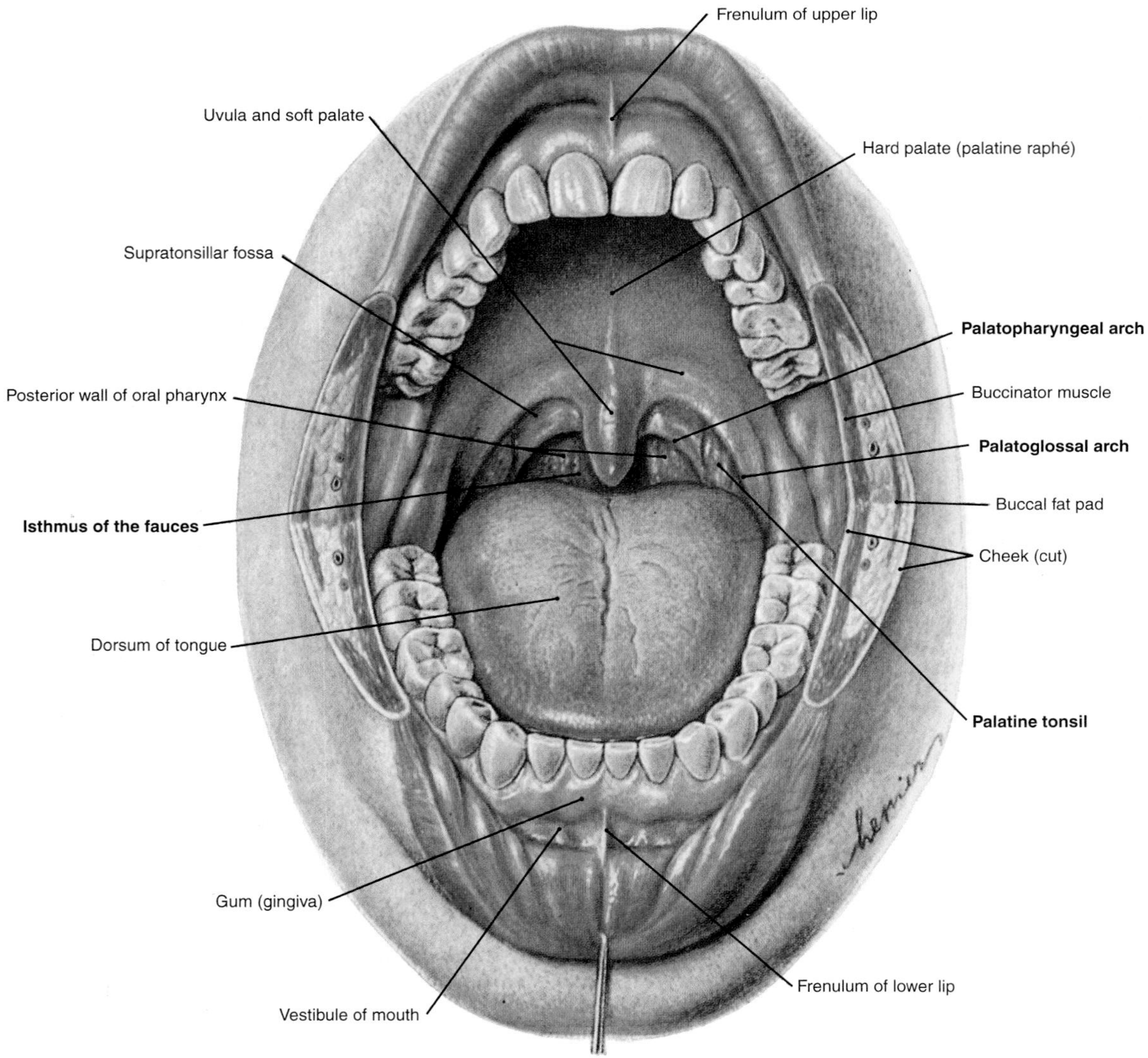
Frenulum of upper lip
Uvula and soft palate
Hard palate (palatine raphé)
Supratonsillar fossa
Palatopharyngeal arch
Buccinator muscle
Posterior wall of oral pharynx
Palatoglossal arch
Buccal fat pad
Isthmus of the fauces
Cheek (cut)
Dorsum of tongue
Palatine tonsil
Gum (gingiva)
Frenulum of lower lip
Vestibule of mouth

Figure 566.1 Oral Cavity

NOTE: (1) The position of the **palatine tonsils** located on each side of the oral cavity within fossae between the **palatoglossal** and **palatopharyngeal folds** (or **arches**).

(2) The passage between the oral cavity and the oral pharynx is called the **fauces.** This aperture or isthmus commences anteriorly at the palatoglossal arches on each side and is also bounded by the soft palate superiorly and the dorsum of the tongue inferiorly.

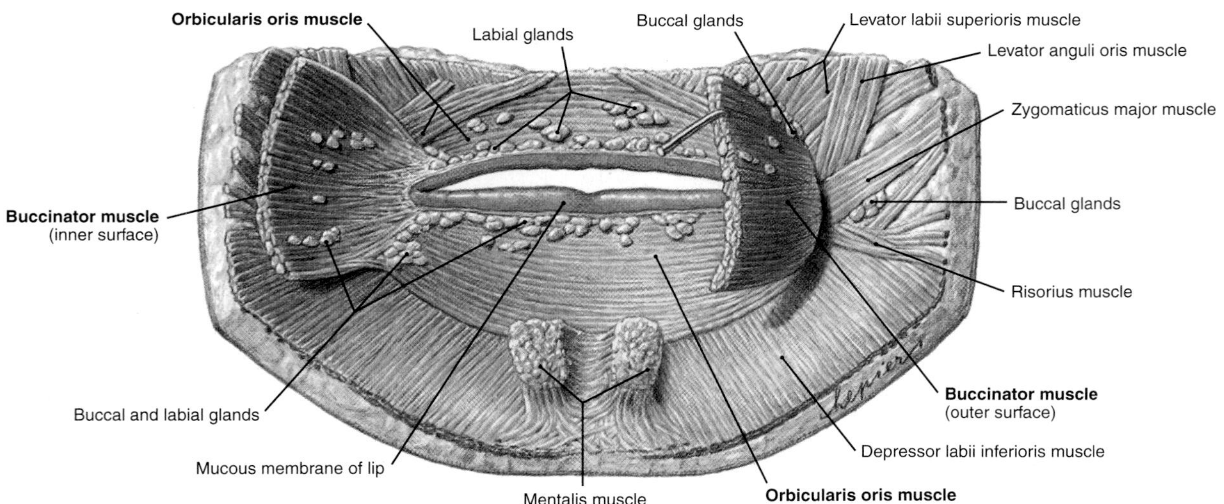
Orbicularis oris muscle
Labial glands
Buccal glands
Levator labii superioris muscle
Levator anguli oris muscle
Zygomaticus major muscle
Buccinator muscle
(inner surface)
Buccal glands
Risorius muscle
Buccinator muscle
(outer surface)
Buccal and labial glands
Depressor labii inferioris muscle
Mucous membrane of lip
Orbicularis oris muscle
Mentalis muscle

Figure 566.2 Lips Viewed from within the Oral Cavity

NOTE: The contour of the lips depends on the arrangement of the muscular bundles, which interlace at the labial margins. These include the elevators and depressors of the lips and their angles along with the **orbicularis oris** and **buccinator muscles.**

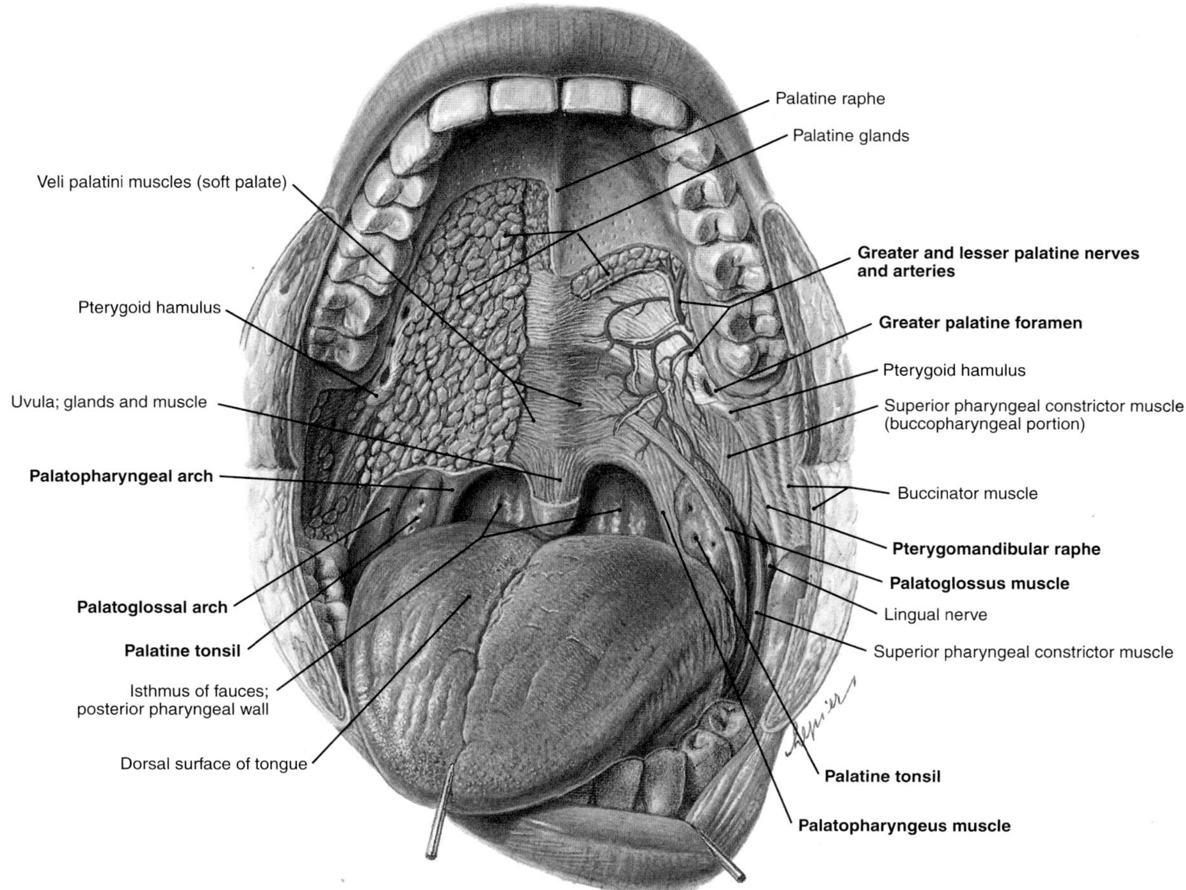
Palatine raphe
Palatine glands
Veli palatini muscles (soft palate)
Greater and lesser palatine nerves and arteries
Pterygoid hamulus
Greater palatine foramen
Pterygoid hamulus
Uvula; glands and muscle
Superior pharyngeal constrictor muscle (buccopharyngeal portion)
Palatopharyngeal arch
Buccinator muscle
Pterygomandibular raphe
Palatoglossus muscle
Palatoglossal arch
Lingual nerve
Palatine tonsil
Superior pharyngeal constrictor muscle
Isthmus of fauces; posterior pharyngeal wall
Dorsal surface of tongue
Palatine tonsil
Palatopharyngeus muscle

Figure 567.1 Palate: Muscular Folds and Glands

NOTE: The oral mucosa has been removed from both the hard and soft palate, revealing the palatal musculature, vessels, and glands. Observe the **palatoglossus** and **palatopharyngeus muscles,** along with the **greater** and **lesser palatine nerves** and **vessels.**

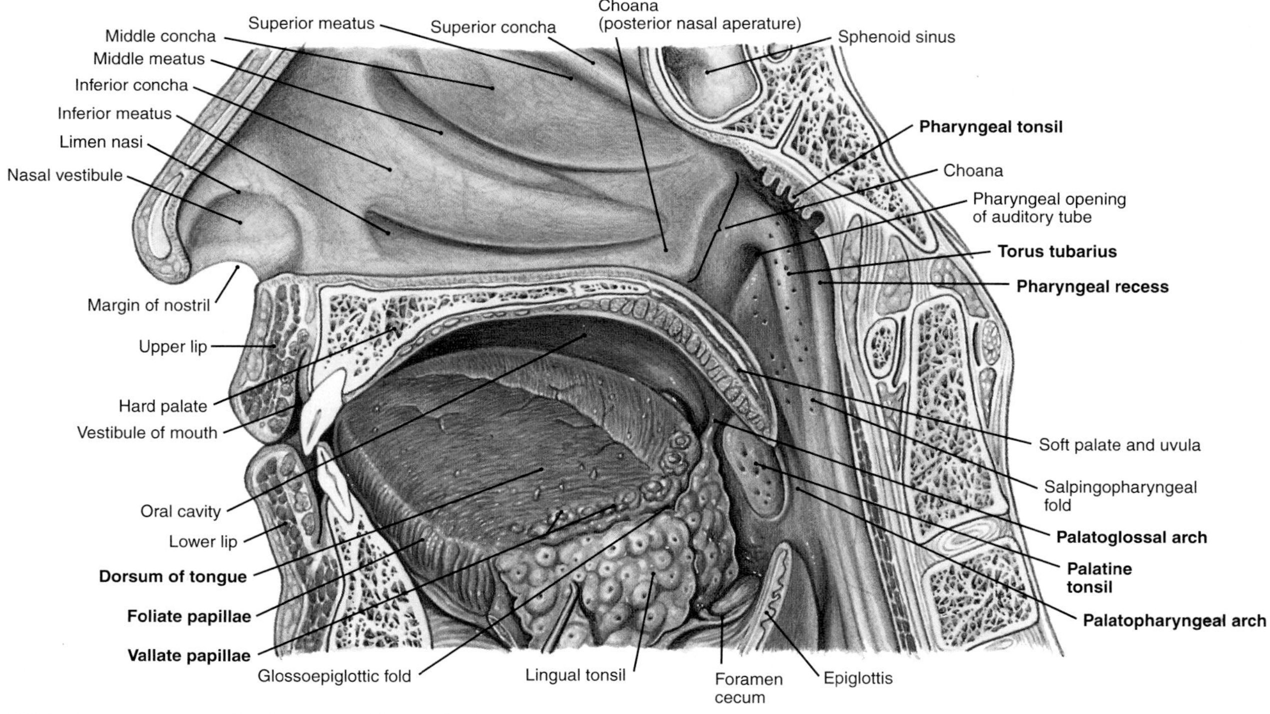
Choana (posterior nasal aperature)
Middle concha
Superior meatus
Superior concha
Sphenoid sinus
Middle meatus
Inferior concha
Inferior meatus
Pharyngeal tonsil
Limen nasi
Nasal vestibule
Choana
Pharyngeal opening of auditory tube
Torus tubarius
Pharyngeal recess
Margin of nostril
Upper lip
Hard palate
Vestibule of mouth
Soft palate and uvula
Salpingopharyngeal fold
Oral cavity
Lower lip
Palatoglossal arch
Palatine tonsil
Dorsum of tongue
Foliate papillae
Palatopharyngeal arch
Vallate papillae
Glossoepiglottic fold
Lingual tonsil
Foramen cecum
Epiglottis

Figure 567.2 Tongue, Palatine Tonsil, and the Oropharynx

NOTE: (1) In this sagittal view, the tongue has been deviated to demonstrate the right palatoglossal arch and right palatine tonsil. Observe the large **vallate papillae.**

(2) The opening of the **auditory tube** in the nasopharynx, behind which is a cartilaginous elevation of the tube called the **torus tubarius.** Note also the **pharyngeal tonsil (adenoid).**

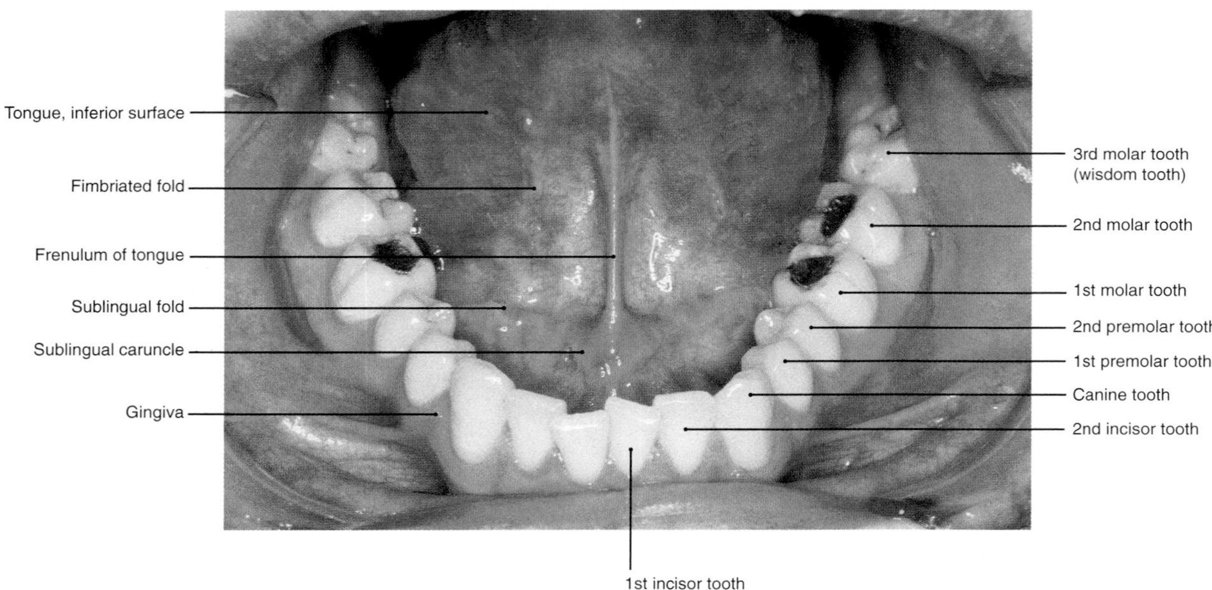
Tongue, inferior surface
Fimbriated fold
Frenulum of tongue
Sublingual fold
Sublingual caruncle
Gingiva
3rd molar tooth
(wisdom tooth)
2nd molar tooth
1st molar tooth
2nd premolar tooth
1st premolar tooth
Canine tooth
2nd incisor tooth
1st incisor tooth

Figure 568.1 Anterior Sublingual Region of the Oral Cavity

NOTE: (1) The mucous membrane covering the floor of the oral cavity continues over the inferior surface of the tongue and meets at the midline as an elevated fold called the **frenulum of the tongue.**

(2) The **sublingual folds.** Along these open the **ducts of the sublingual glands**, and at their anterior end on each side is an orifice for the **submandibular duct** called the **sublingual caruncle.**

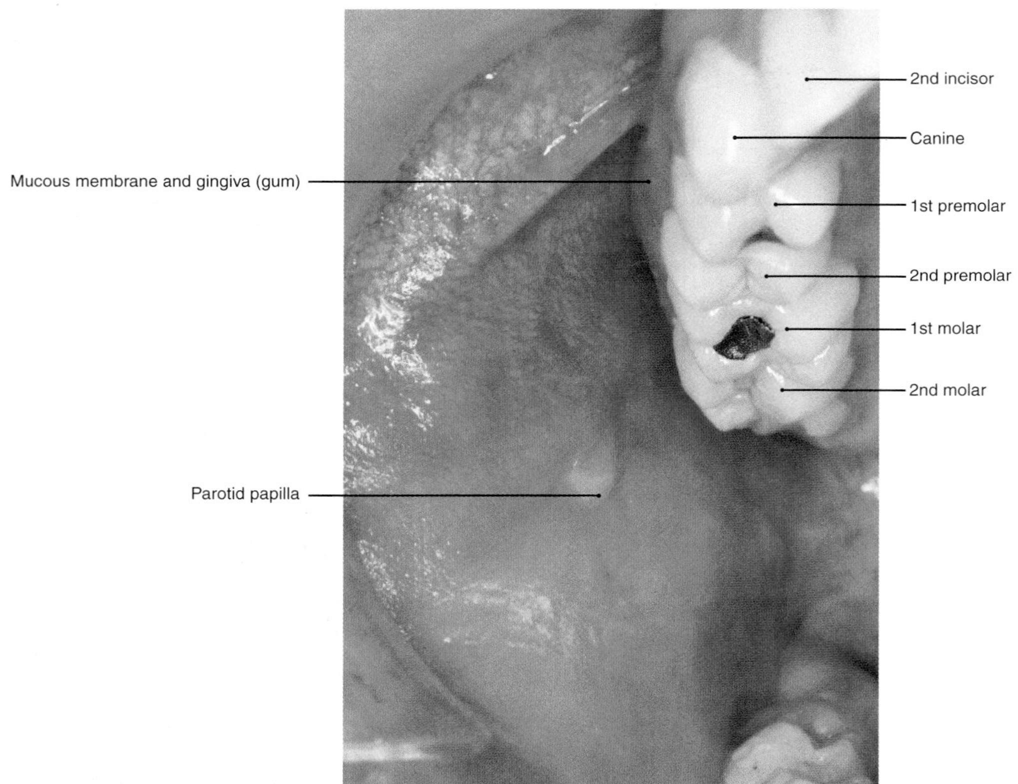
Mucous membrane and gingiva (gum)
Parotid papilla
2nd incisor
Canine
1st premolar
2nd premolar
1st molar
2nd molar

Figure 568.2 Orifice of the Parotid Duct

NOTE: The opening of the parotid duct (sometimes called Stensen's duct) in the oral cavity is marked by a small elevation called the parotid papilla, which is located opposite the upper (maxillary) second molar tooth.

Oral Cavity: Mouth (Anterior View); Muscular Floor (Sagittal Section)

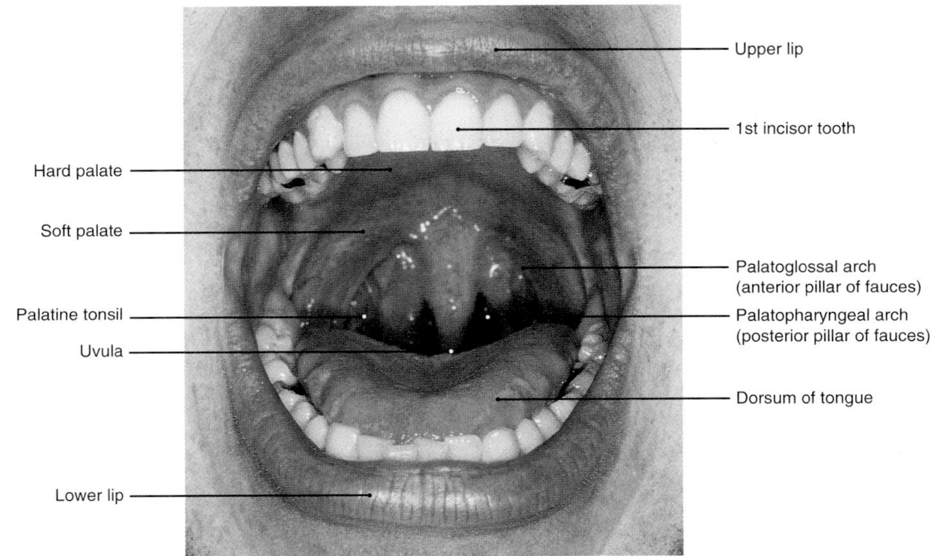
Upper lip
1st incisor tooth
Hard palate
Soft palate
Palatoglossal arch (anterior pillar of fauces)
Palatine tonsil
Palatopharyngeal arch (posterior pillar of fauces)
Uvula
Dorsum of tongue
Lower lip

Figure 569.1 Oral Cavity; Anterior View of the Palate and Dorsum of the Tongue

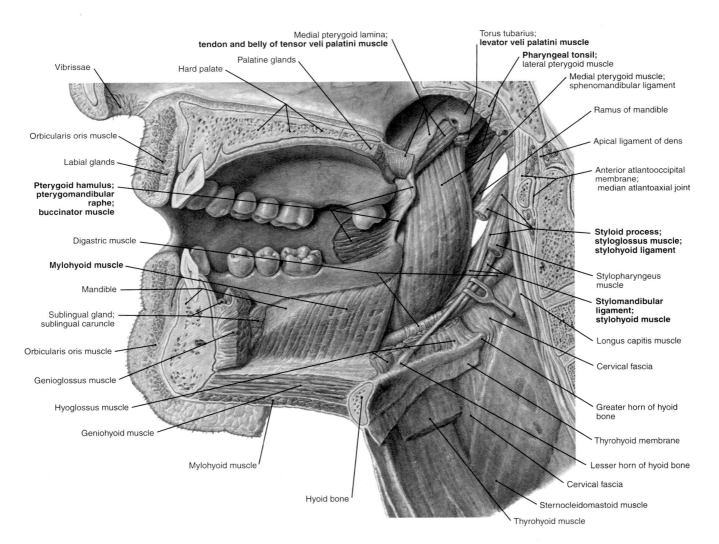

Medial pterygoid lamina;
tendon and belly of tensor veli palatini muscle
Torus tubarius;
levator veli palatini muscle
Palatine glands
Hard palate
Vibrissae
Pharyngeal tonsil;
lateral pterygoid muscle
Medial pterygoid muscle;
sphenomandibular ligament
Ramus of mandible
Orbicularis oris muscle
Apical ligament of dens
Labial glands
Anterior atlantooccipital membrane;
median atlantoaxial joint
Pterygoid hamulus; pterygomandibular raphe; buccinator muscle
Digastric muscle
Styloid process; styloglossus muscle; stylohyoid ligament
Mylohyoid muscle
Stylopharyngeus muscle
Mandible
Stylomandibular ligament; stylohyoid muscle
Sublingual gland;
sublingual caruncle
Longus capitis muscle
Orbicularis oris muscle
Cervical fascia
Genioglossus muscle
Greater horn of hyoid bone
Hyoglossus muscle
Geniohyoid muscle
Thyrohyoid membrane
Mylohyoid muscle
Lesser horn of hyoid bone
Cervical fascia
Hyoid bone
Sternocleidomastoid muscle
Thyrohyoid muscle

Figure 569.2 Paramedian Sagittal View of the Interior of the Right Oral Cavity and the Upper Neck (Muscles and Ligaments)

NOTE: In this dissection, the right half of the oral cavity was exposed and the mucous membrane removed from the floor of the mouth to reveal the **mylohyoid muscle.** Observe also the **pterygomandibular raphe** and **buccinator muscle.**

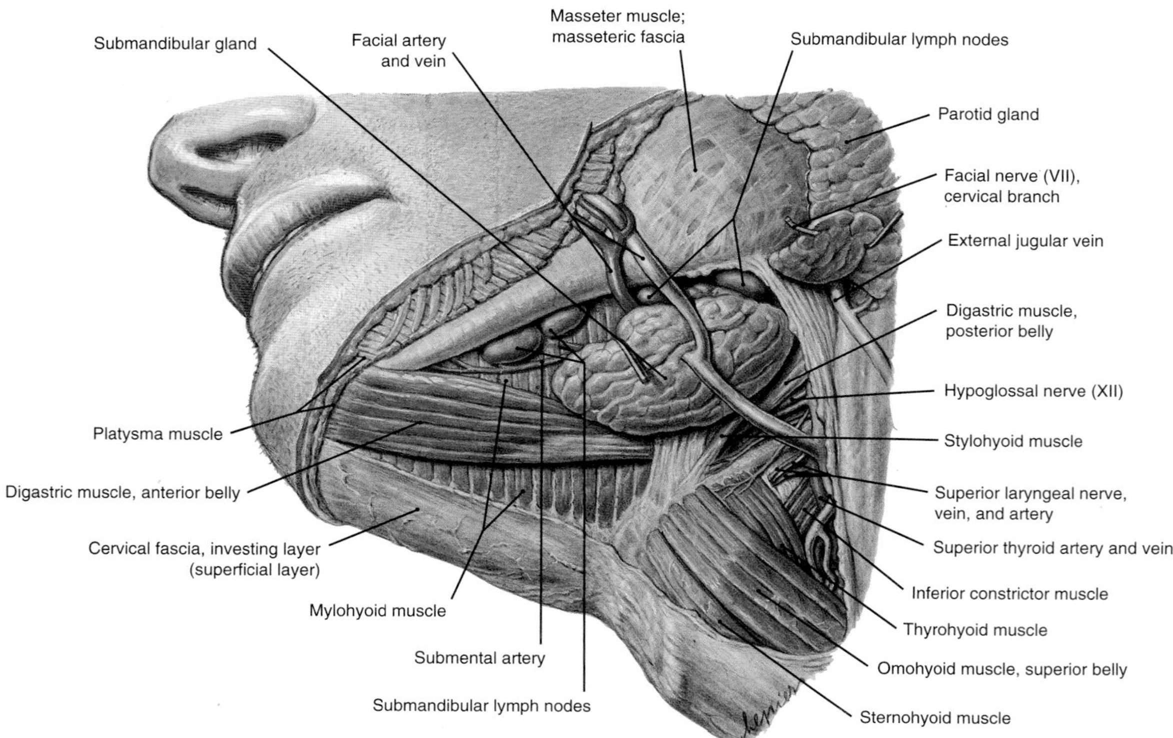
Submandibular gland
Facial artery and vein
Masseter muscle; masseteric fascia
Submandibular lymph nodes
Parotid gland
Facial nerve (VII), cervical branch
External jugular vein
Digastric muscle, posterior belly
Hypoglossal nerve (XII)
Stylohyoid muscle
Superior laryngeal nerve, vein, and artery
Superior thyroid artery and vein
Inferior constrictor muscle
Thyrohyoid muscle
Omohyoid muscle, superior belly
Sternohyoid muscle
Platysma muscle
Digastric muscle, anterior belly
Cervical fascia, investing layer (superficial layer)
Mylohyoid muscle
Submental artery
Submandibular lymph nodes

Figure 570.1 **Floor of the Oral Cavity: Intact and Viewed from the Submandibular Region in the Upper Neck**

NOTE: (1) The **submandibular** and **parotid glands** that produce saliva that is transported by secretory ducts to the oral cavity.

(2) The **submandibular triangle** bounded by the anterior and posterior bellies of the digastric muscle and the mandible.

(3) The **mylohyoid muscle** forming the largest part of the floor of the oral cavity. Compare this figure with Figs. 571.1 and 571.2.

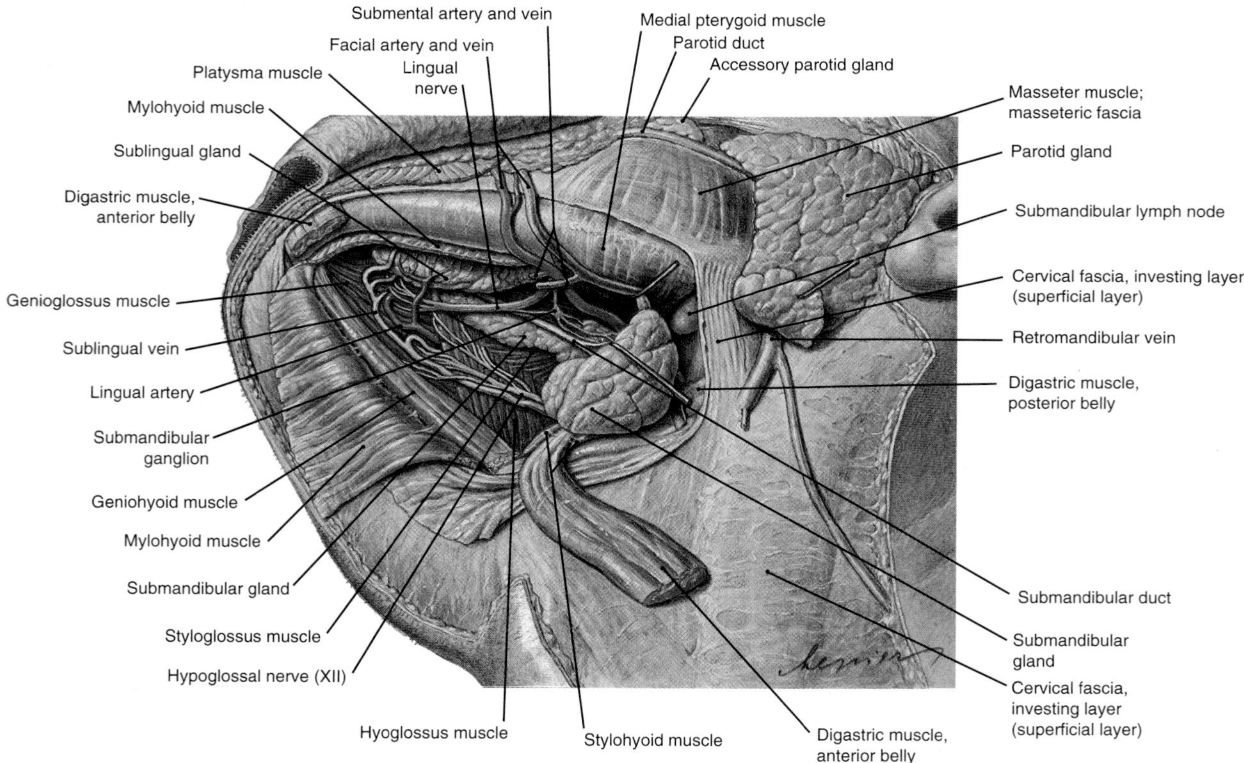
Submental artery and vein
Facial artery and vein
Lingual nerve
Platysma muscle
Mylohyoid muscle
Sublingual gland
Digastric muscle, anterior belly
Genioglossus muscle
Sublingual vein
Lingual artery
Submandibular ganglion
Geniohyoid muscle
Mylohyoid muscle
Submandibular gland
Styloglossus muscle
Hypoglossal nerve (XII)
Hyoglossus muscle
Stylohyoid muscle
Digastric muscle, anterior belly
Medial pterygoid muscle
Parotid duct
Accessory parotid gland
Masseter muscle; masseteric fascia
Parotid gland
Submandibular lymph node
Cervical fascia, investing layer (superficial layer)
Retromandibular vein
Digastric muscle, posterior belly
Submandibular duct
Submandibular gland
Cervical fascia, investing layer (superficial layer)

Figure 570.2 **Floor of the Oral Cavity: Opened Inferiorly from the Submandibular Region**

NOTE: (1) The anterior belly of the digastric and mylohyoid muscles have been reflected to reveal: the **sublingual gland, lingual nerve, submandibular ganglion** and **duct, hypoglossal nerve** and **vein,** and **lingual artery.**

(2) The hypoglossal nerve is the motor nerve to all tongue muscles *except* the palatoglossus. The lingual nerve supplies the anterior two-thirds of the tongue with general sensation.

(3) The three salivary glands are all shown in this figure: the **parotid gland** on the side of the face, the **submandibular gland** in the suprahyoid region, and the **sublingual gland,** which lies in its entirety within the oral cavity. Compare this figure with Figures 570.1, 571.1, and 571.2.

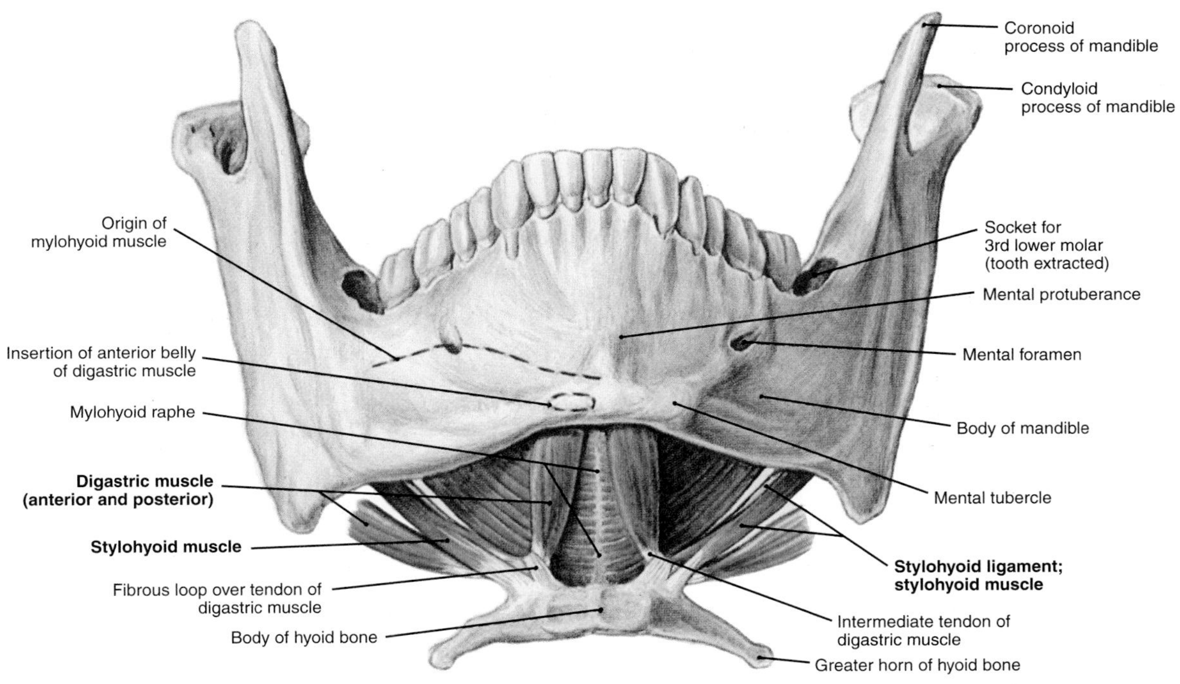
Coronoid process of mandible
Condyloid process of mandible
Origin of mylohyoid muscle
Socket for 3rd lower molar (tooth extracted)
Mental protuberance
Insertion of anterior belly of digastric muscle
Mental foramen
Mylohyoid raphe
Body of mandible
Digastric muscle (anterior and posterior)
Mental tubercle
Stylohyoid muscle
Stylohyoid ligament; stylohyoid muscle
Fibrous loop over tendon of digastric muscle
Intermediate tendon of digastric muscle
Body of hyoid bone
Greater horn of hyoid bone

Figure 571.1 **Suprahyoid Muscles and Floor of the Mouth (Viewed from Below)**

NOTE: (1) On the mandible are the inner attachments of the **mylohyoid muscle** (broken line) and the **anterior belly of the digastric muscle** (circle). Observe the attachments of the **mylohyoid, digastric,** and **stylohyoid muscles** and the **stylohyoid ligament** on the hyoid bone.

(2) The tendon between the anterior and posterior bellies of the digastric muscle is anchored by a fibrous loop to the hyoid bone.

(3) The stylohyoid muscle is supplied by the facial (or seventh) cranial nerve, as is the posterior belly of the digastric muscle. The action of the stylohyoid muscle is to retract and elevate the hyoid bone, thus, elongating the floor of the mouth.

(4) The two bellies of the digastric muscle also elevate the hyoid bone, while the mylohyoid muscle raises the floor of the mouth when swallowing and is capable of pushing the tongue upward in the mouth and protruding the tongue forward.

(5) In addition, the mylohyoid muscles depress the mandible in chewing, swallowing, sucking, and blowing air out of the mouth.

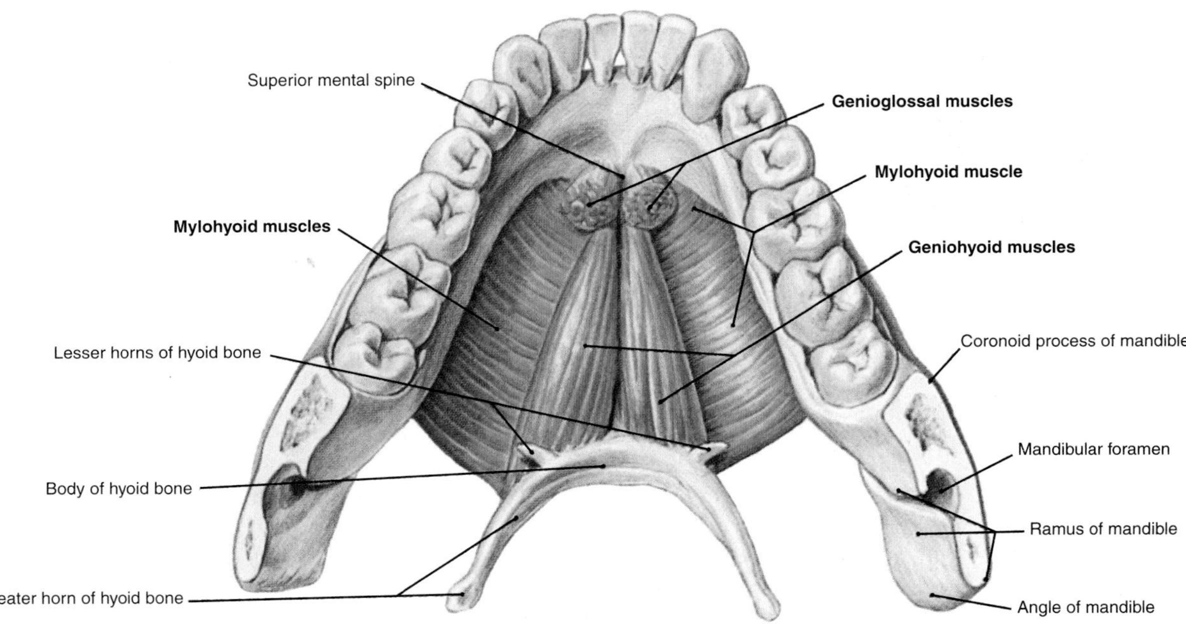
Superior mental spine
Genioglossal muscles
Mylohyoid muscle
Mylohyoid muscles
Geniohyoid muscles
Coronoid process of mandible
Lesser horns of hyoid bone
Mandibular foramen
Body of hyoid bone
Ramus of mandible
Greater horn of hyoid bone
Angle of mandible

Figure 571.2 **Mylohyoid and Geniohyoid Muscles (Viewed from Above)**

NOTE: The **mylohyoid** and **geniohyoid muscles** form the floor of the oral cavity. The mylohyoids arise along the mylohyoid lines of the mandible and insert into the median raphe, which extends from the hyoid bone to the symphysis menti. The genioglossal muscles have been severed near their origin.

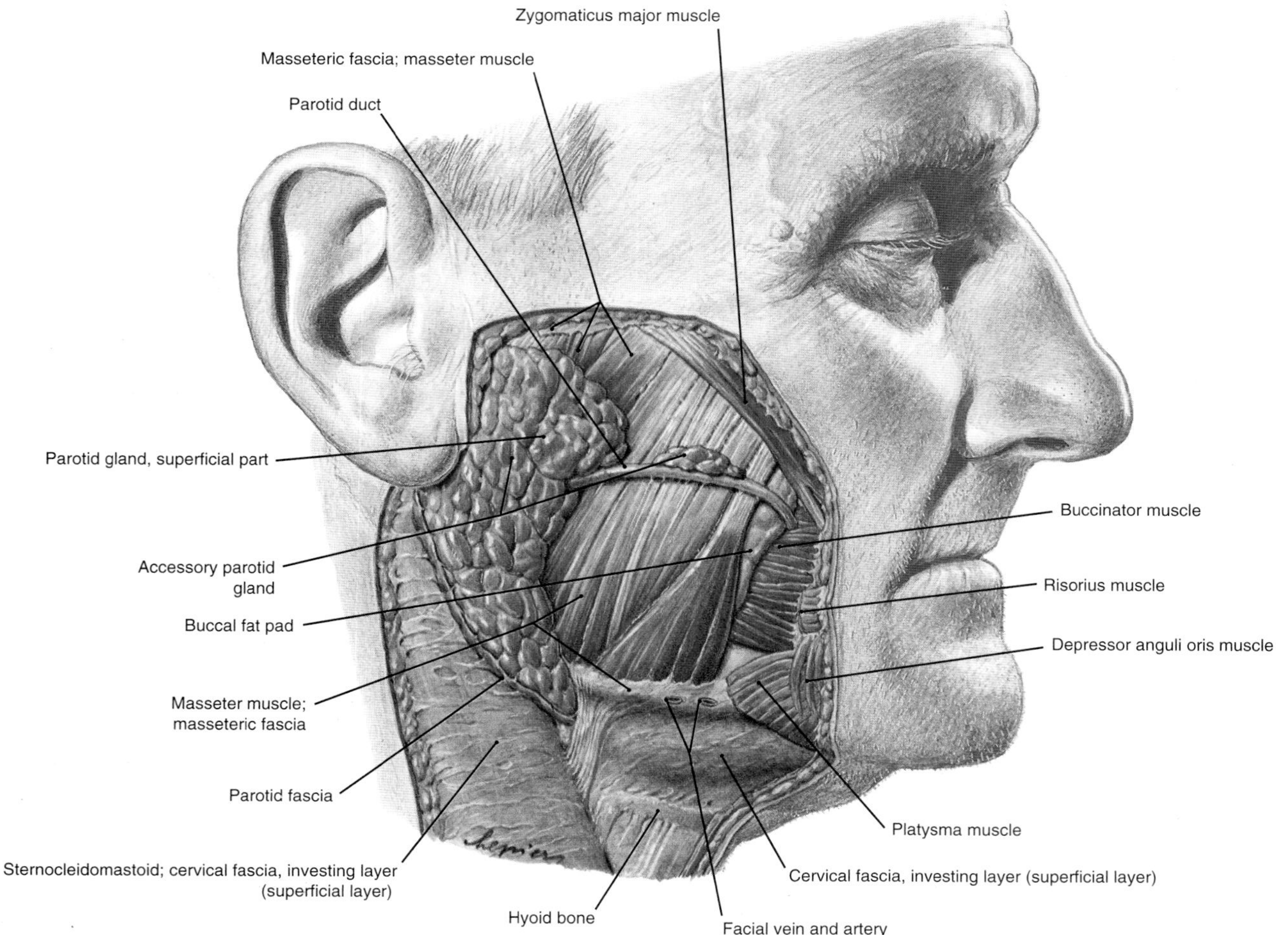
Zygomaticus major muscle
Masseteric fascia; masseter muscle
Parotid duct
Parotid gland, superficial part
Accessory parotid gland
Buccal fat pad
Masseter muscle; masseteric fascia
Parotid fascia
Sternocleidomastoid; cervical fascia, investing layer (superficial layer)
Hyoid bone
Facial vein and artery
Cervical fascia, investing layer (superficial layer)
Platysma muscle
Depressor anguli oris muscle
Risorius muscle
Buccinator muscle

Figure 572 **Lateral View of the Parotid Gland and an Accessory Parotid Gland Attached to the Parotid Duct**

PAROTID GLAND

DEVELOPMENT: Arises during the sixth week of gestation as an epithelial outgrowth from the mouth and forms a tube that grows backward toward the ear. The posterior part of the tube branches into lobes that become the gland, and it enmeshes the facial nerve. The tube remains as the **parotid duct,** which opens into the mouth opposite the second upper molar tooth.

ADULT GLAND: A serous gland, weighing about 25 g, on either side of the face in front of the ear. Located between the mandible and the sternocleidomastoid muscle.

ARTERIES: Branches of the external carotid artery as it passes behind the gland.

VEINS: Empty into the external jugular vein.

INNERVATION: *Sympathetic:* Postganglionic vasomotor fibers come from the superior cervical ganglion by way of the external carotid plexus. *Parasympathetic:* Preganglionic secretomotor fibers course in the **glossopharyngeal nerve** and then the **lesser petrosal nerve** to the **otic ganglion,** where they synapse. Postganglionic fibers course to the parotid gland by way of the **auriculotemporal nerve** (V).

LYMPH DRAINAGE: Superficial and deep parotid nodes drain into cervical lymph nodes.

SUBMANDIBULAR GLAND

DEVELOPMENT: Arises during the sixth week of gestation from an epithelial ridge in a groove between the tongue and the lower jaw. The caudal end of the ridge forms numerous branches that extend backward and ventrally beneath the mandible as glandular lobules. The main stalk, connected to the deep part of the gland persists as the **submandibular duct.**

ADULT GLAND: A seromucous gland of about 8 g on each side. The **superficial part** is the size of a walnut, and is located in the digastric triangle of the upper neck. The **deep part** extends above the mylohyoid muscle into the oral cavity. The **submandibular duct** extends forward from the deep part and opens at the **sublingual caruncle** at the side of the frenulum below the tongue.

ARTERIES: Submental branches of the **facial artery** in neck and of **lingual artery** in oral cavity.

VEINS: Drain into the facial and lingual veins and then into the **internal jugular vein.**

INNERVATION: *Sympathetic:* Postganglionic vasomotor fibers come from the superior cervical ganglion by way of the external carotid plexus. *Parasympathetic:* Preganglionic fibers course in the **nervus intermedius** part of the **facial nerve.** They travel to the **submandibular ganglion** by way of the **chorda tympani nerve** and then the **lingual nerve.** Postganglionic fibers from the ganglion **course directly** to the gland.

LYMPH DRAINAGE: Into submandibular nodes and then into upper and lower deep cervical nodes.

Figure 573.1 Submandibular and Sublingual Glands

NOTE: (1) With the tongue removed and the genioglossus and geniohyoid muscles cut, the submandibular and sublingual glands are exposed and their relationship to the inner aspect of the mandible is demonstrated.

(2) The submandibular duct measures about 5 cm and courses anteriorly between the sublingual gland and genioglossus muscle (cut). It opens in the floor of the mouth at the sublingual caruncle.

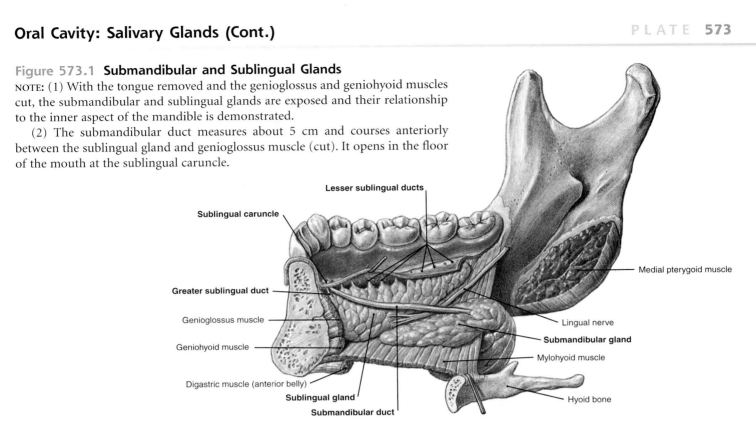

Lesser sublingual ducts
Sublingual caruncle
Medial pterygoid muscle
Greater sublingual duct
Genioglossus muscle
Lingual nerve
Submandibular gland
Geniohyoid muscle
Mylohyoid muscle
Digastric muscle (anterior belly)
Sublingual gland
Hyoid bone
Submandibular duct

SUBLINGUAL GLAND

DEVELOPMENT: Appears as a series of epithelial buds along the groove between the lower jaw and tongue during the eighth week of gestation, just lateral to the submandibular primordium. The buds enlarge and some of the more anterior ones join to form a duct that opens near the submandibular duct. The remaining buds open by separate ducts (8 to 10) in the floor of the mouth above the sublingual fold.

ADULT GLAND: A seromucous gland on each side (30% serous, 70% mucous) weighing about 4 g. It is narrow and flattened and located deep to the mucous membrane in the floor of the mouth. Its ducts (10 to 20) open in a line along the surface of the sublingual fold. Several anterior ducts join to form the main sublingual duct. This opens near the caruncle of the submandibular duct.

ARTERIES: **Sublingual branch** of the **lingual artery,** which anastomoses with the **submental branch** of the **facial artery.**

VEINS: Drain into lingual vein and then into internal jugular vein.

INNERVATION: Same as for the submandibular gland.

LYMPH DRAINAGE: Superficial and deep submandibular nodes and then into deep cervical nodes.

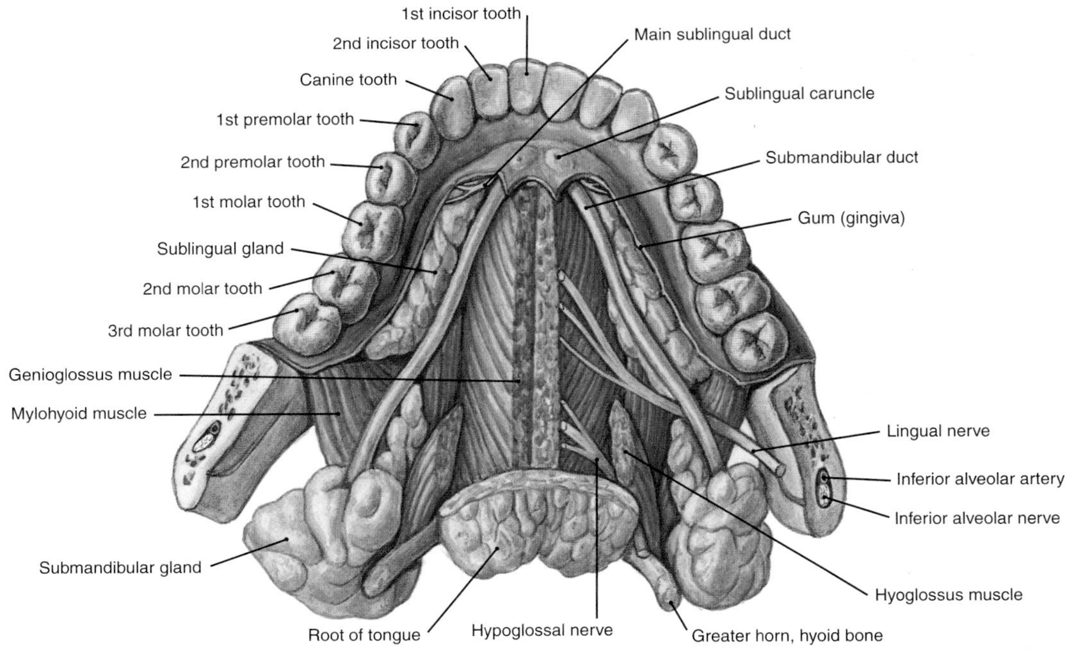
1st incisor tooth
2nd incisor tooth
Main sublingual duct
Canine tooth
Sublingual caruncle
1st premolar tooth
2nd premolar tooth
Submandibular duct
1st molar tooth
Gum (gingiva)
Sublingual gland
2nd molar tooth
3rd molar tooth
Genioglossus muscle
Mylohyoid muscle
Lingual nerve
Inferior alveolar artery
Inferior alveolar nerve
Submandibular gland
Hyoglossus muscle
Root of tongue
Hypoglossal nerve
Greater horn, hyoid bone

Figure 573.2 Salivary Glands in the Floor of the Oral Cavity (Seen from Above)

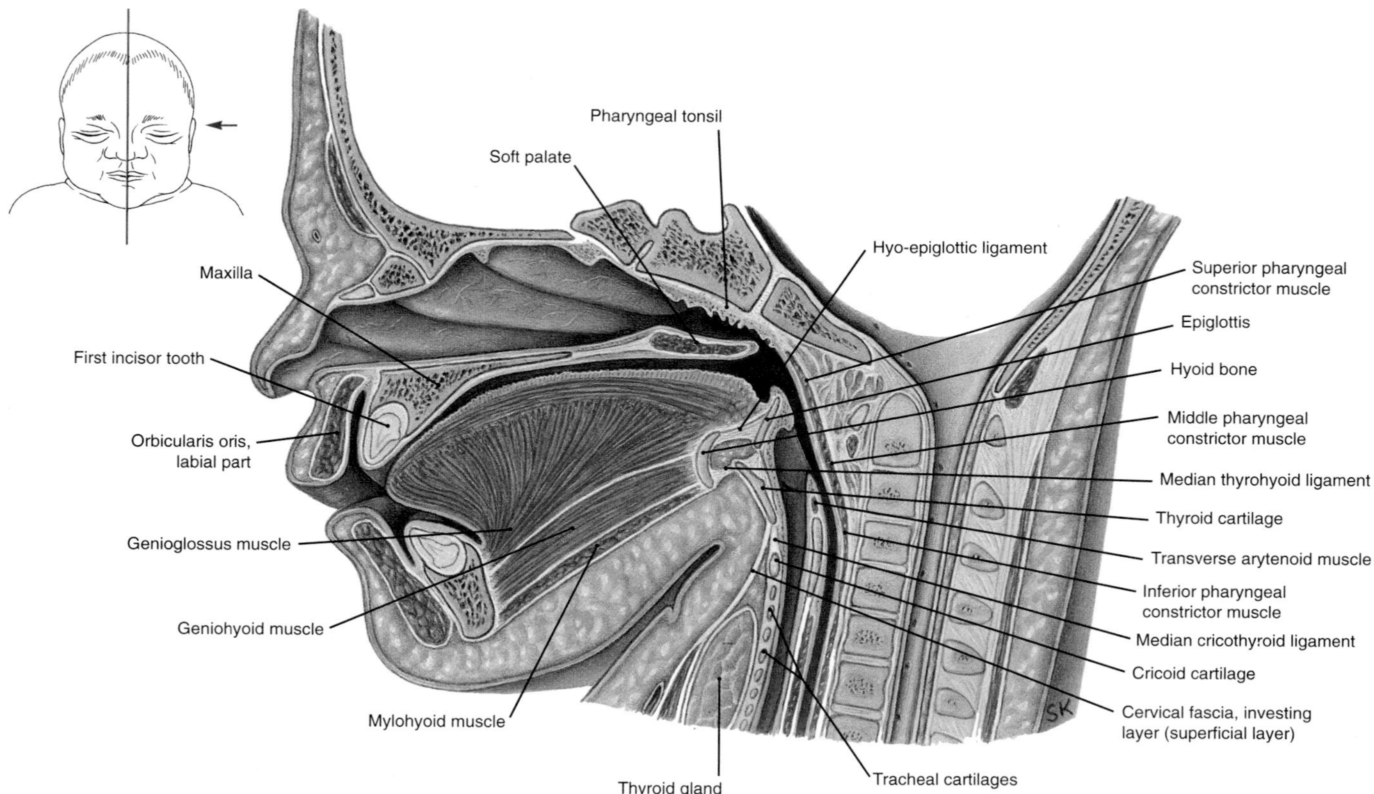
Pharyngeal tonsil
Soft palate
Hyo-epiglottic ligament
Maxilla
Superior pharyngeal constrictor muscle
Epiglottis
First incisor tooth
Hyoid bone
Middle pharyngeal constrictor muscle
Orbicularis oris, labial part
Median thyrohyoid ligament
Thyroid cartilage
Genioglossus muscle
Transverse arytenoid muscle
Inferior pharyngeal constrictor muscle
Geniohyoid muscle
Median cricothyroid ligament
Cricoid cartilage
Cervical fascia, investing layer (superficial layer)
Mylohyoid muscle
Thyroid gland
Tracheal cartilages

Figure 574.1 Median Section through the Head of a Newborn Child

NOTE: (1) The midline section of the tongue and its underlying muscles, the geniohyoid and the mylohyoid.

(2) In the newborn, the larynx is considerably higher than in the adult.

(3) The genioglossus muscle is shown in this figure and in Fig. 574.2.

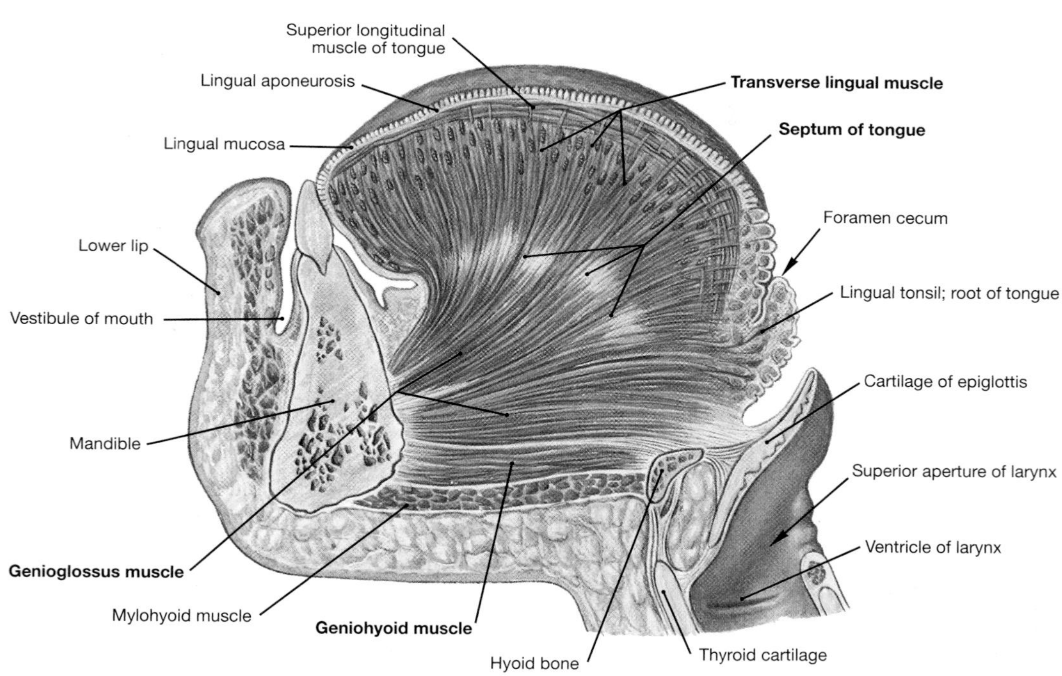
Superior longitudinal muscle of tongue
Lingual aponeurosis
Transverse lingual muscle
Septum of tongue
Lingual mucosa
Foramen cecum
Lower lip
Lingual tonsil; root of tongue
Vestibule of mouth
Cartilage of epiglottis
Mandible
Superior aperture of larynx
Ventricle of larynx
Genioglossus muscle
Mylohyoid muscle
Geniohyoid muscle
Hyoid bone
Thyroid cartilage

Figure 574.2 Genioglossus and Intrinsic Muscles of the Tongue

NOTE: (1) In this midsagittal section can be seen the median fibrous septum of the tongue and the **intrinsic** tongue musculature, which includes the longitudinal, transverse, and vertical muscles of the tongue.

(2) The **genioglossus** constitutes most of the tongue musculature, and its fibers radiate backward and upward in a fan-like manner from the uppermost of the mental spines (genial tubercles) on the inner surface of the mandible, just above the origin of the geniohyoid muscle.

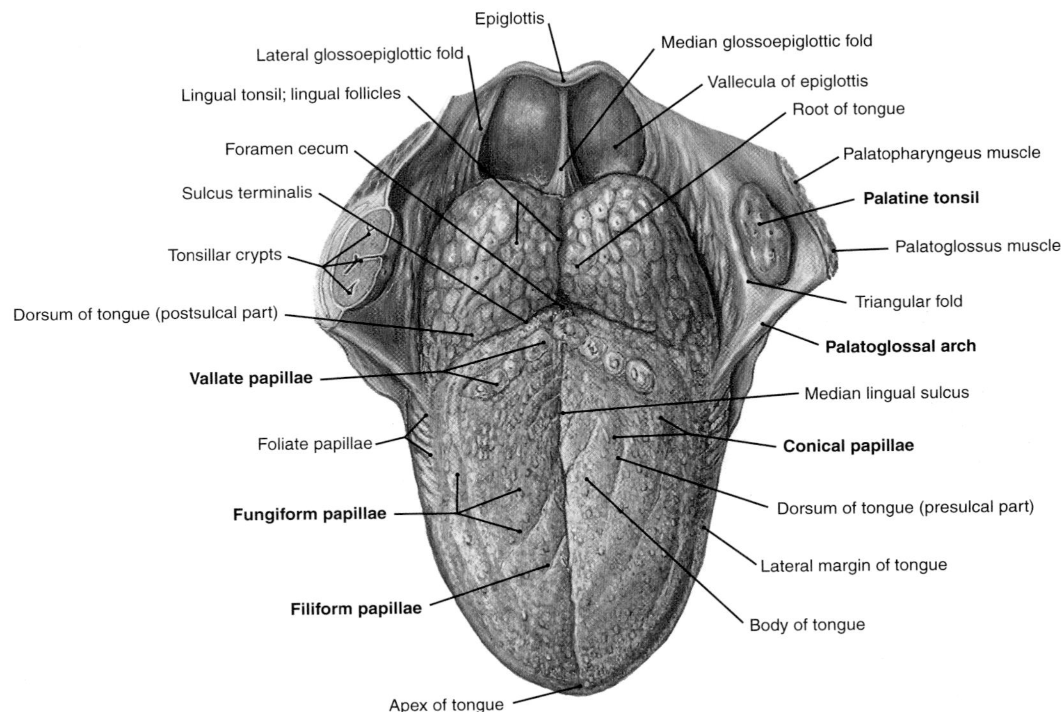

Epiglottis
Lateral glossoepiglottic fold
Median glossoepiglottic fold
Lingual tonsil; lingual follicles
Vallecula of epiglottis
Root of tongue
Foramen cecum
Palatopharyngeus muscle
Sulcus terminalis
Palatine tonsil
Tonsillar crypts
Palatoglossus muscle
Triangular fold
Dorsum of tongue (postsulcal part)
Palatoglossal arch
Vallate papillae
Median lingual sulcus
Foliate papillae
Conical papillae
Fungiform papillae
Dorsum of tongue (presulcal part)
Lateral margin of tongue
Filiform papillae
Body of tongue
Apex of tongue

Figure 575.1 **Dorsal Surface of the Tongue**

NOTE: (1) The dorsum of the tongue is marked by numerous elevations called papillae. These serve as location sites of receptors for the special sense of **taste.** Observe the inverted V-shaped group of large **vallate papillae.**

(2) The **fungiform papillae** are found principally at the sides and apex of the tongue. These are large, round, and deep red.

(3) The **filiform** (conical) **papillae.** These are small and arranged in rows that course parallel to the vallate papillae.

(4) The parallel vertical folds (about five in number) called the **foliate papillae** on the lateral border of the tongue just anterior to the palatoglossal arch. These are studded with taste receptors.

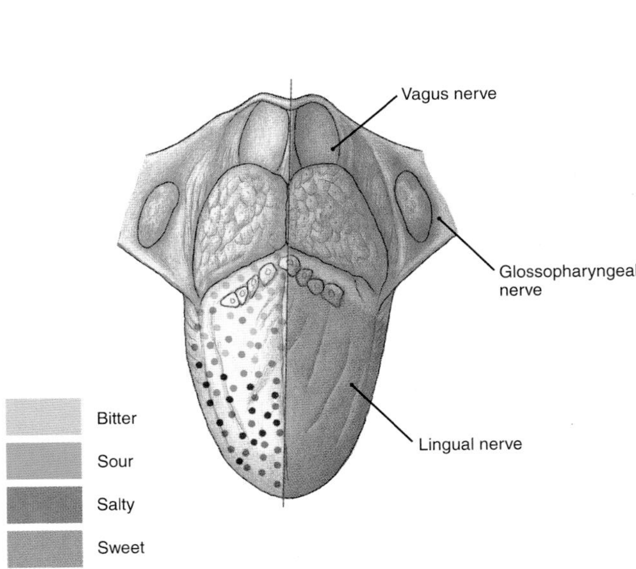

Vagus nerve
Glossopharyngeal nerve
Lingual nerve
Bitter
Sour
Salty
Sweet

Figure 575.2 **Innervation and Location of Taste Qualities on the Dorsum of the Tongue**

NOTE: On the right: fields of innervation by the **lingual, glossopharyngeal** and **vagus nerves.** On the left: Receptors for the basic tastes of **salt** and **sweet** are clustered anterior to those for **bitter** and **sour.**

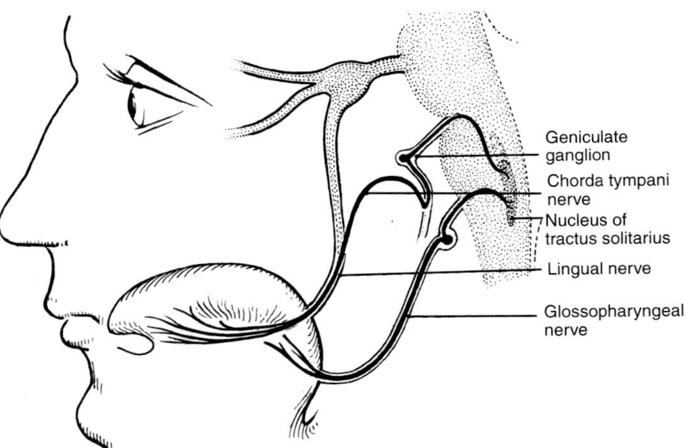

Geniculate ganglion
Chorda tympani nerve
Nucleus of tractus solitarius
Lingual nerve
Glossopharyngeal nerve

Figure 575.3 **Principal Pathways for Taste**

NOTE: (1) The two principal pathways for taste are along the **lingual nerve** to the **chorda tympani nerve** for the anterior two-thirds of the tongue and the **glossopharyngeal nerve** for the posterior third of the tongue.

(2) Two lesser pathways (not shown) are:

(a) From the epiglottis along the **internal laryngeal branch** of the **vagus,** and

(b) From the palate along the **palatine nerves** and the **nerve of the pterygoid canal** to the **greater petrosal nerve** and then the **nervus intermedius part** of the **facial nerve.**

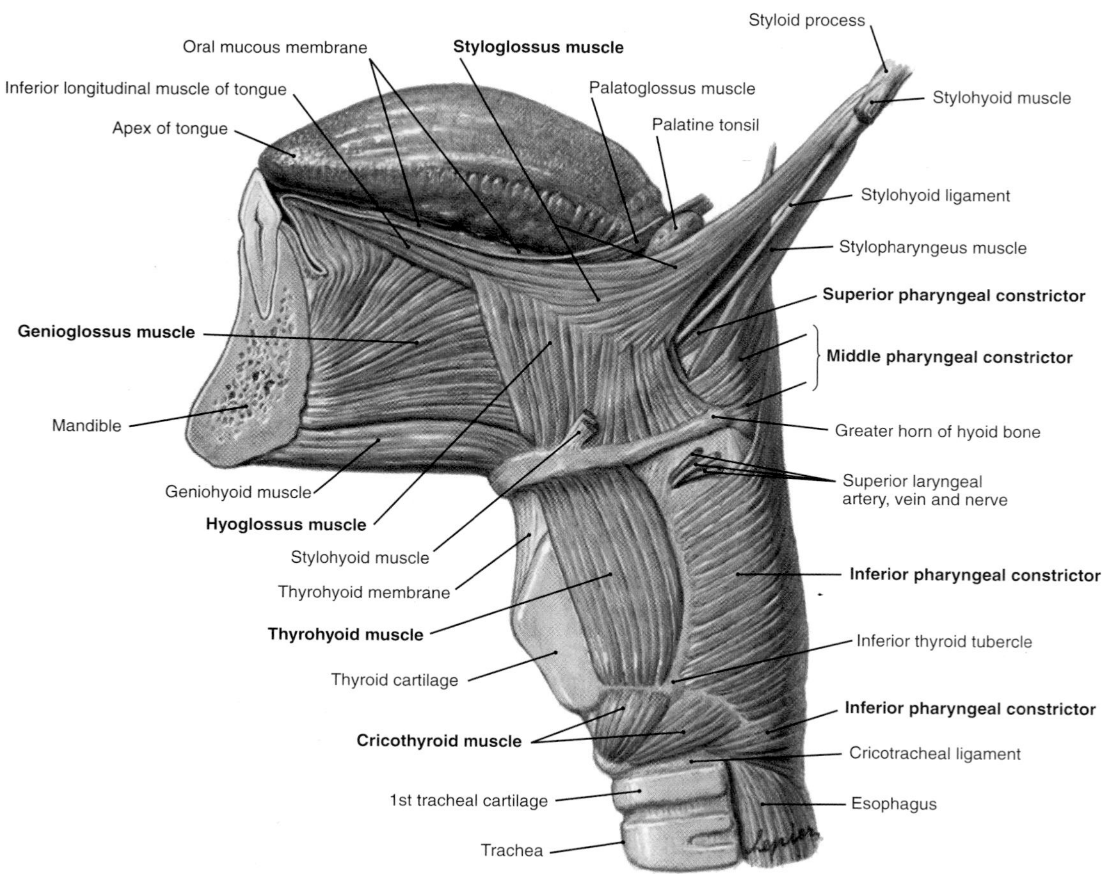
Styloid process
Oral mucous membrane
Styloglossus muscle
Inferior longitudinal muscle of tongue
Palatoglossus muscle
Stylohyoid muscle
Apex of tongue
Palatine tonsil
Stylohyoid ligament
Stylopharyngeus muscle
Superior pharyngeal constrictor
Genioglossus muscle
Middle pharyngeal constrictor
Mandible
Greater horn of hyoid bone
Superior laryngeal artery, vein and nerve
Geniohyoid muscle
Hyoglossus muscle
Stylohyoid muscle
Thyrohyoid membrane
Inferior pharyngeal constrictor
Thyrohyoid muscle
Inferior thyroid tubercle
Thyroid cartilage
Inferior pharyngeal constrictor
Cricothyroid muscle
Cricotracheal ligament
1st tracheal cartilage
Esophagus
Trachea

Figure 576.1 **Extrinsic Tongue Muscles; External Larynx and Pharynx (Lateral View 1)**
NOTE: The tongue is attached to the hyoid bone, the mandible, the styloid process, the soft palate, and the pharyngeal wall.

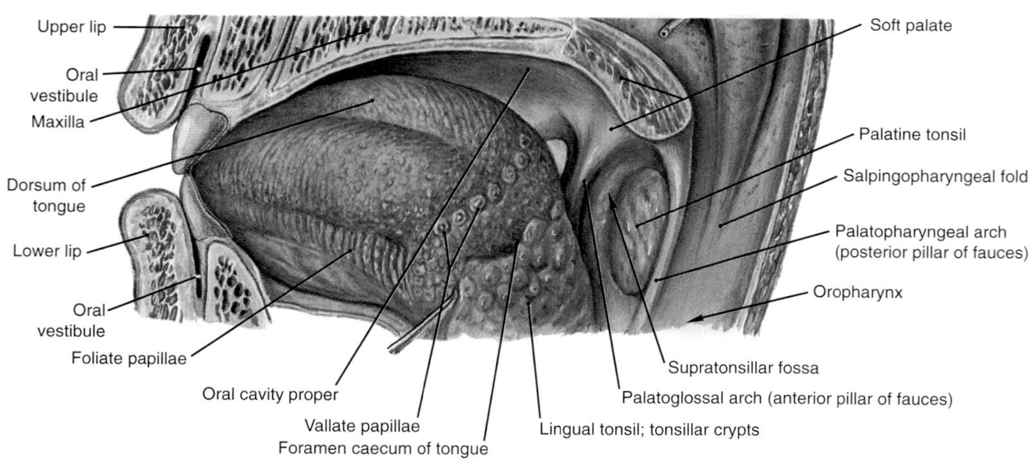
Upper lip
Soft palate
Oral vestibule
Maxilla
Palatine tonsil
Dorsum of tongue
Salpingopharyngeal fold
Lower lip
Palatopharyngeal arch (posterior pillar of fauces)
Oropharynx
Oral vestibule
Foliate papillae
Supratonsillar fossa
Oral cavity proper
Palatoglossal arch (anterior pillar of fauces)
Vallate papillae
Foramen caecum of tongue
Lingual tonsil; tonsillar crypts

Figure 576.2 **Paramedian Section of the Oral Cavity, Oral Pharynx, and Tongue**
NOTE: (1) The lingual tonsil covering the posterior third of the tongue. Observe also the vallate papillae located in a line between the anterior two-thirds of the tongue and the posterior third.

(2) The palatine tonsil in the tonsillar bed located between the palatoglossal and palatopharyngeal folds.

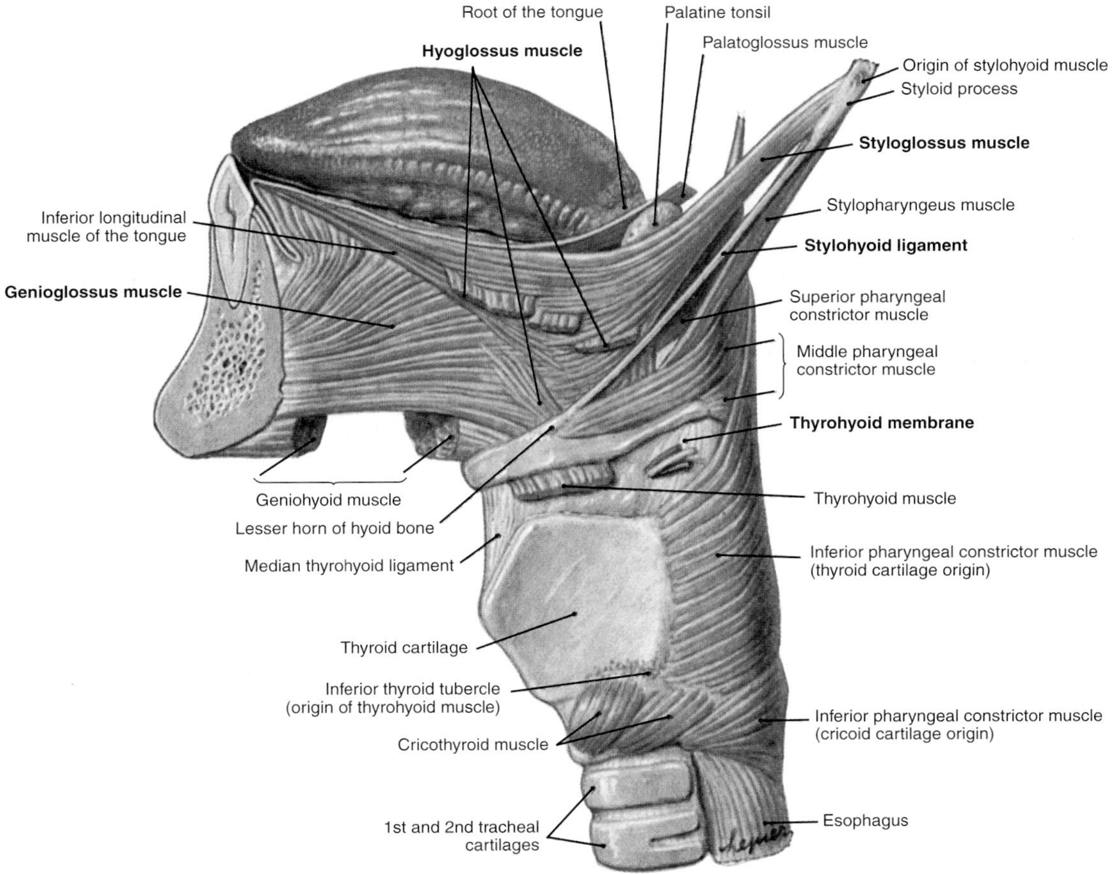
Root of the tongue
Palatine tonsil
Hyoglossus muscle
Palatoglossus muscle
Origin of stylohyoid muscle
Styloid process
Styloglossus muscle
Stylopharyngeus muscle
Stylohyoid ligament
Inferior longitudinal muscle of the tongue
Genioglossus muscle
Superior pharyngeal constrictor muscle
Middle pharyngeal constrictor muscle
Thyrohyoid membrane
Geniohyoid muscle
Lesser horn of hyoid bone
Thyrohyoid muscle
Median thyrohyoid ligament
Inferior pharyngeal constrictor muscle (thyroid cartilage origin)
Thyroid cartilage
Inferior thyroid tubercle (origin of thyrohyoid muscle)
Cricothyroid muscle
Inferior pharyngeal constrictor muscle (cricoid cartilage origin)
1st and 2nd tracheal cartilages
Esophagus

Figure 577.1 **Extrinsic Tongue Muscles; External Larynx and Pharynx (Lateral View 2)**

NOTE: (1) In this dissection, the hyoglossus muscle has been removed, revealing the attachments of the **stylohyoid ligament** and the **middle pharyngeal constrictor muscle** along the hyoid bone. The geniohyoid muscle has been cut and the thyrohyoid **muscle removed.**

(2) The blending of the fibers of the styloglossus, hyoglossus, and genioglossus at the base of the **tongue.**

(3) The penetration through the **thyrohyoid membrane** by the **superior laryngeal vessels** and **nerve.**

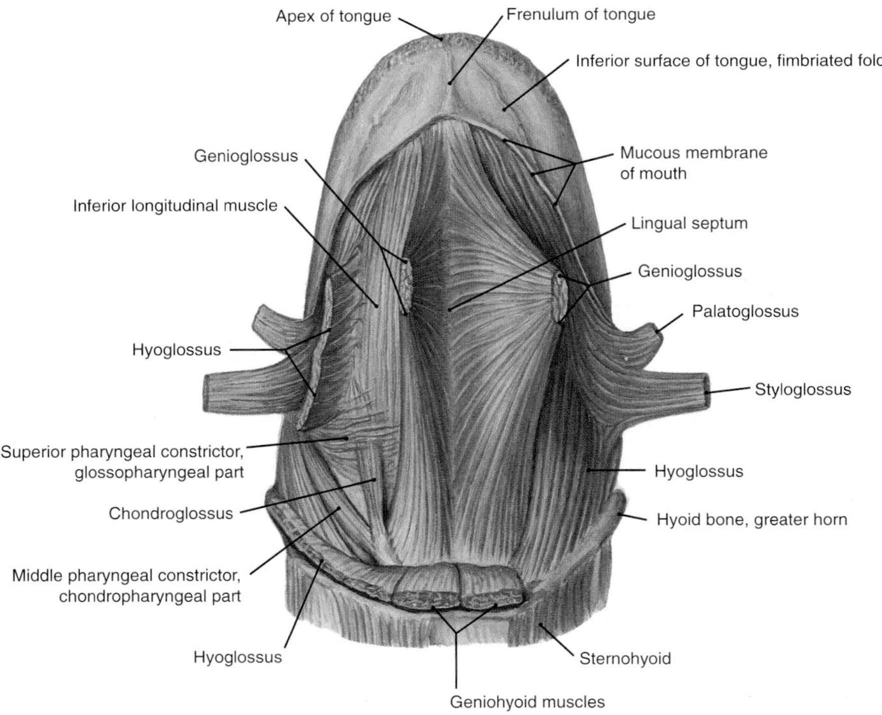
Apex of tongue
Frenulum of tongue
Inferior surface of tongue, fimbriated fold
Genioglossus
Mucous membrane of mouth
Inferior longitudinal muscle
Lingual septum
Genioglossus
Palatoglossus
Hyoglossus
Styloglossus
Superior pharyngeal constrictor, glossopharyngeal part
Hyoglossus
Chondroglossus
Hyoid bone, greater horn
Middle pharyngeal constrictor, chondropharyngeal part
Hyoglossus
Sternohyoid
Geniohyoid muscles

Figure 577.2 **Ventral View of the Muscles of the Tongue**

NOTE: The large genioglossus muscle detached from the mandible and the hyoglossus muscle inserting into the side of the tongue from its origin on the hyoid bone. Observe also the insertions of the palatoglossus and styloglossus muscles.

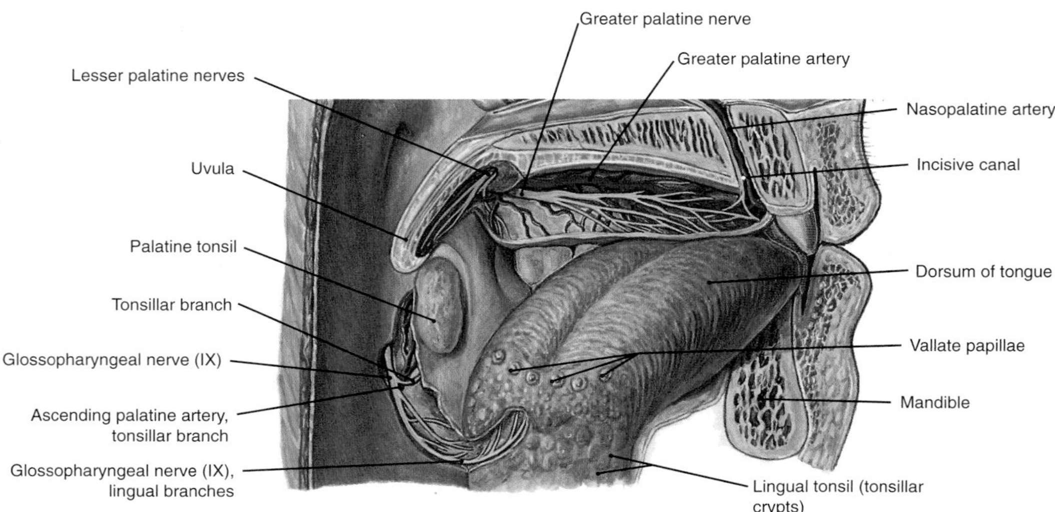
Greater palatine nerve
Greater palatine artery
Lesser palatine nerves
Nasopalatine artery
Uvula
Incisive canal
Palatine tonsil
Dorsum of tongue
Tonsillar branch
Vallate papillae
Glossopharyngeal nerve (IX)
Mandible
Ascending palatine artery, tonsillar branch
Glossopharyngeal nerve (IX), lingual branches
Lingual tonsil (tonsillar crypts)

Figure 578.1 Nerves and Arteries of the Posterior Tongue and Palate

NOTE: (1) The **glossopharyngeal nerve** supplies both general sensation and the special sense of taste to the posterior third of the tongue.

(2) The **greater palatine artery** and **nerve** supply the palate in the roof of the oral cavity and the **ascending** pharyngeal artery, one of several vessels that supply the palatine tonsil located in the oropharynx.

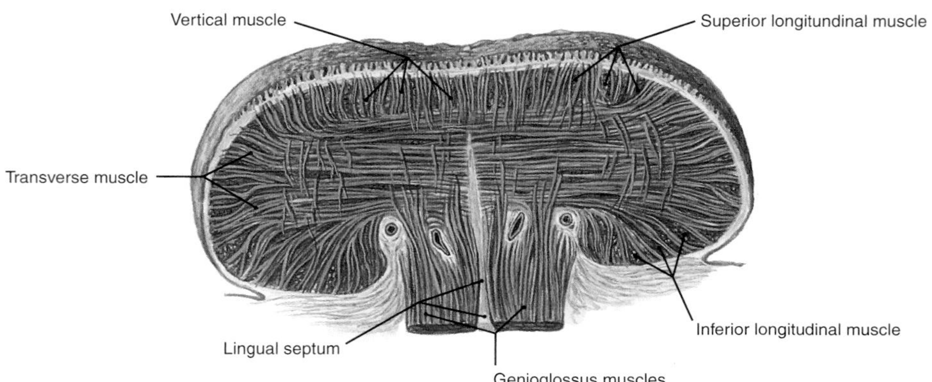
Vertical muscle
Superior longitundinal muscle
Transverse muscle
Inferior longitudinal muscle
Lingual septum
Genioglossus muscles

Figure 578.2 Transverse Section through the Middle of the Tongue (Anterior View)

NOTE: The transverse and vertical fibers of the intrinsic tongue muscles can best be seen in a transverse section. Observe, however, the cut longitudinal fibers both superiorly and inferiorly.

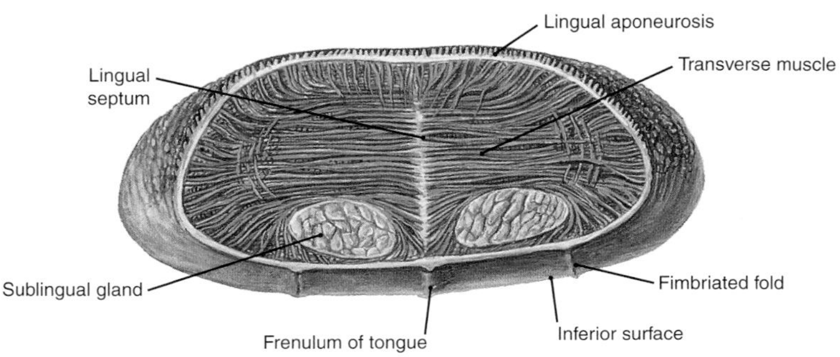
Lingual aponeurosis
Lingual septum
Transverse muscle
Sublingual gland
Fimbriated fold
Inferior surface
Frenulum of tongue

Figure 578.3 Transverse Section through the Tip of the Tongue

NOTE: The sublingual glands deep to the anterior part of the tongue.

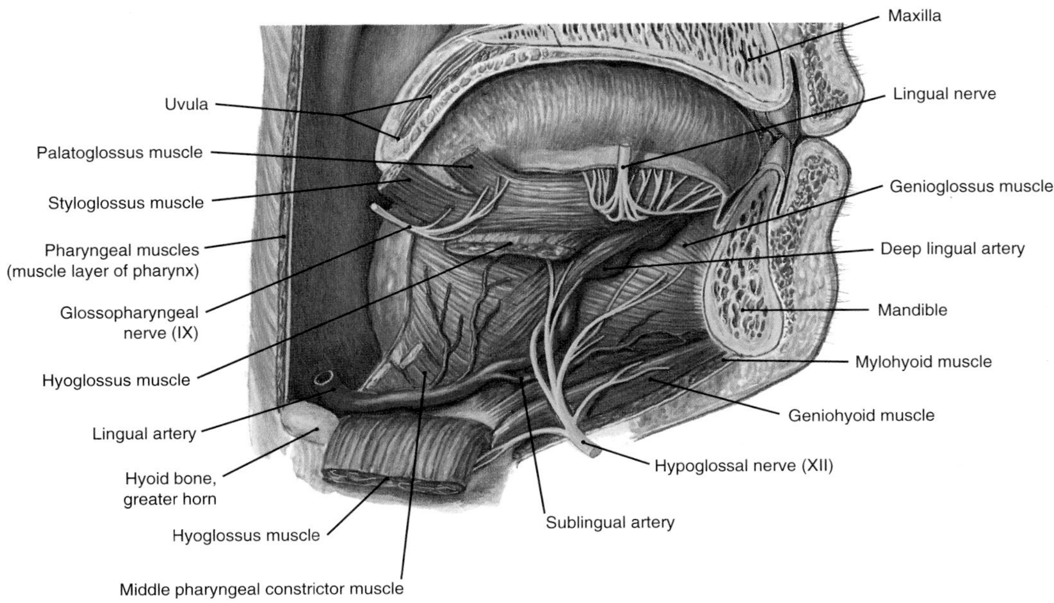
Maxilla
Lingual nerve
Uvula
Palatoglossus muscle
Styloglossus muscle
Genioglossus muscle
Pharyngeal muscles
(muscle layer of pharynx)
Deep lingual artery
Glossopharyngeal
nerve (IX)
Mandible
Mylohyoid muscle
Hyoglossus muscle
Geniohyoid muscle
Lingual artery
Hypoglossal nerve (XII)
Hyoid bone,
greater horn
Sublingual artery
Hyoglossus muscle
Middle pharyngeal constrictor muscle

Figure 579 **Opened Oral Cavity Showing the Tongue and Its Nerves and Arterial Supply**

NOTE: (1) The longitudinal and medial course of the **lingual artery**. Observe also the **lingual, glossopharyngeal,** and **hypoglossal nerves.**

(2) The **hypoglossal nerve** supplies the genioglossus, hyoglossus, and styloglossus muscles as well as all of the intrinsic muscles of the tongue.

(3) The **lingual nerve** is sensory to the anterior two-thirds of the tongue (both general sensation and taste, the latter by way of the **chorda tympani** nerve fibers), while the **glossopharyngeal nerve** supplies the posterior third of the tongue (both general sensation and taste).

(4) The **geniohyoid muscle** extending from the mental spine of the mandible (posterior to the symphysis menti) to the anterior surface of the hyoid bone.

(5) The **hyoglossus muscle** has been severed in order to show the forward course of the lingual artery.

EXTRINSIC MUSCLES OF THE TONGUE

Muscle	Origin	Insertion	Innervation	Action
Genioglossus	Upper part of the mental spine of mandible	In a fan-like manner along the ventral surface of tongue; anterior surface of body of hyoid bone	Hypoglossal nerve	Draws the tongue forward and protrudes the apex of the tongue
Hyoglossus	Entire length of the greater horn of hyoid bone and lateral part of body of hyoid bone	Into the side of tongue	Hypoglossal nerve	Depresses the tongue
Styloglossus	Styloid process of temporal bone and the stylohyoid ligament	Side and inferior aspect of the tongue	Hypoglossal nerve	Draws the tongue upward and backward
Palatoglossus	Oral surface of the palatine aponeurosis	Side and dorsum of the tongue	Pharyngeal branch of the vagus nerve (fibers emerge from brain in cranial part of accessory nerve [i.e., XI via X])	Elevates the posterior part of the tongue

In addition, the tongue contains longitudinal, transverse, and vertical muscles whose fibers commence and terminate within the tongue itself and, hence, are considered **intrinsic tongue muscles**. These are all supplied by the **hypoglossal nerve**.

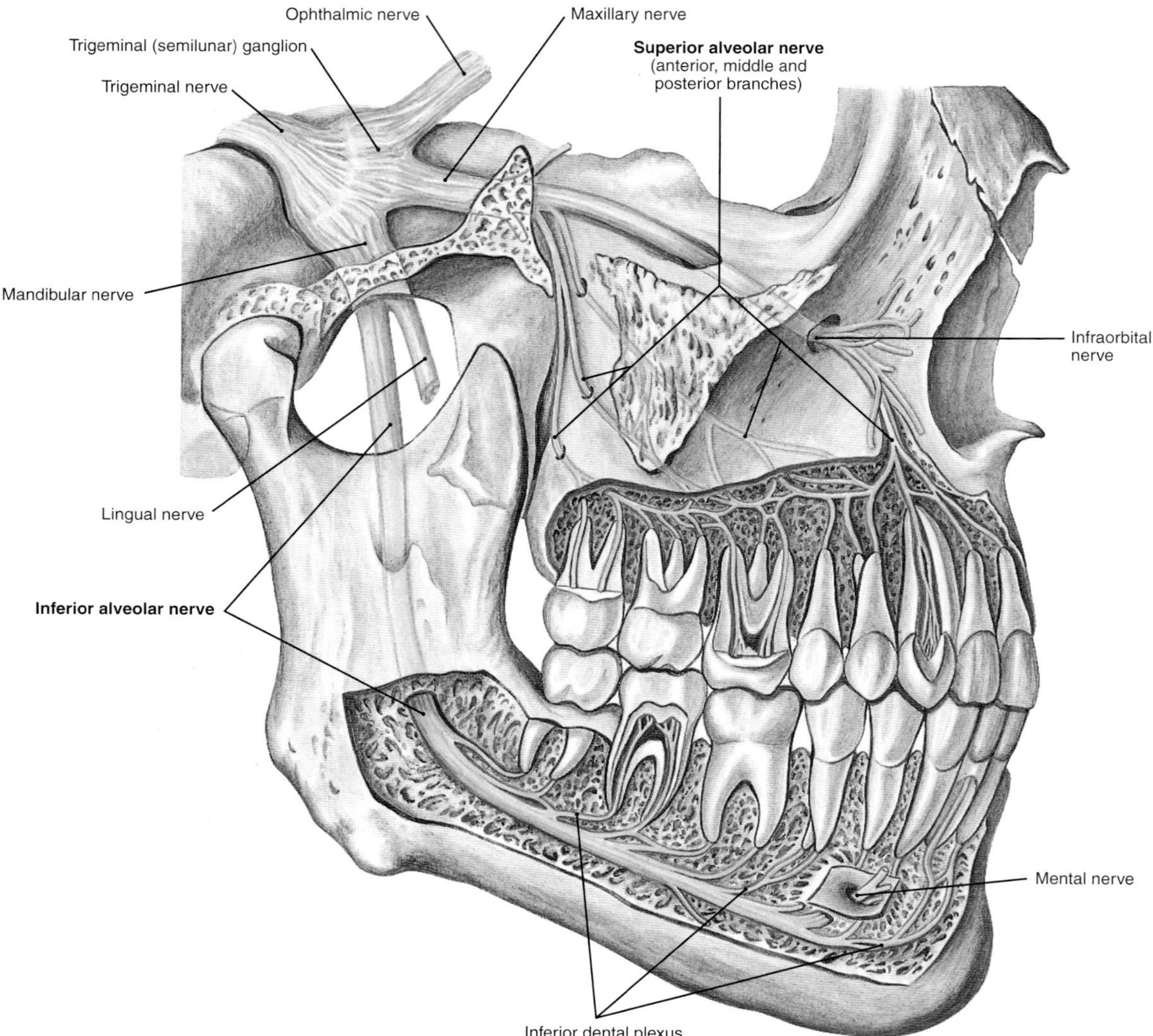
Ophthalmic nerve
Maxillary nerve
Trigeminal (semilunar) ganglion
Superior alveolar nerve
(anterior, middle and
posterior branches)
Trigeminal nerve
Mandibular nerve
Infraorbital
nerve
Lingual nerve
Inferior alveolar nerve
Mental nerve
Inferior dental plexus

Figure 580.1 **Superior Alveolar Nerves (Maxillary) and Inferior Alveolar Nerve (Mandibular) and Their Branches to the Upper and Lower Teeth**

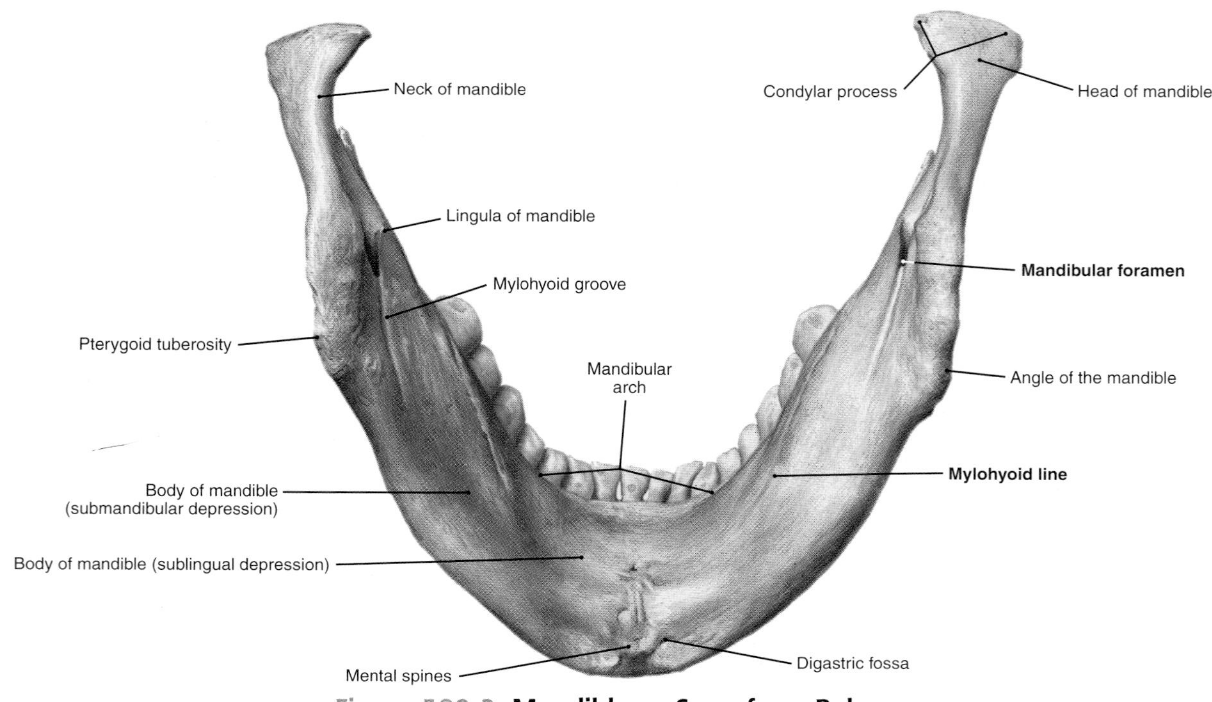
Neck of mandible
Condylar process
Head of mandible
Lingula of mandible
Mandibular foramen
Mylohyoid groove
Pterygoid tuberosity
Mandibular
arch
Angle of the mandible
Mylohyoid line
Body of mandible
(submandibular depression)
Body of mandible (sublingual depression)
Mental spines
Digastric fossa

Figure 580.2 **Mandible as Seen from Below**

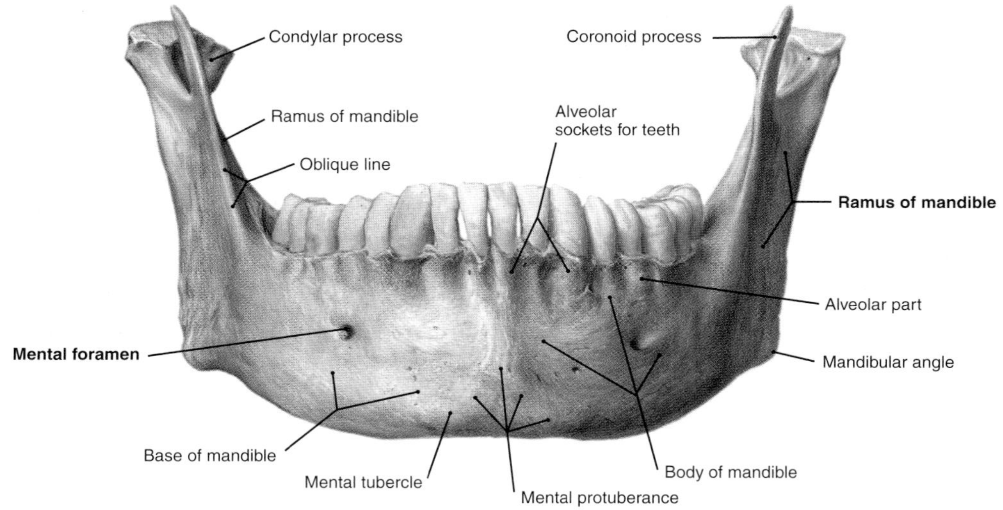
Condylar process
Coronoid process
Ramus of mandible
Alveolar sockets for teeth
Oblique line
Ramus of mandible
Alveolar part
Mental foramen
Mandibular angle
Base of mandible
Mental tubercle
Body of mandible
Mental protuberance

Figure 581.1 **Mandible as Seen from the Front**

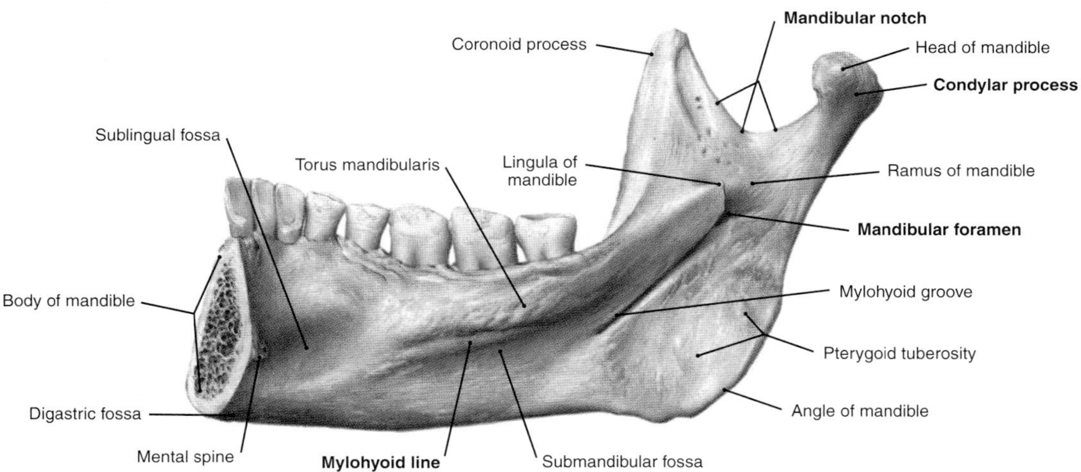
Mandibular notch
Coronoid process
Head of mandible
Condylar process
Sublingual fossa
Torus mandibularis
Lingula of mandible
Ramus of mandible
Mandibular foramen
Body of mandible
Mylohyoid groove
Pterygoid tuberosity
Digastric fossa
Angle of mandible
Mental spine
Mylohyoid line
Submandibular fossa

Figure 581.2 **Right Mandible (Inner Surface)**

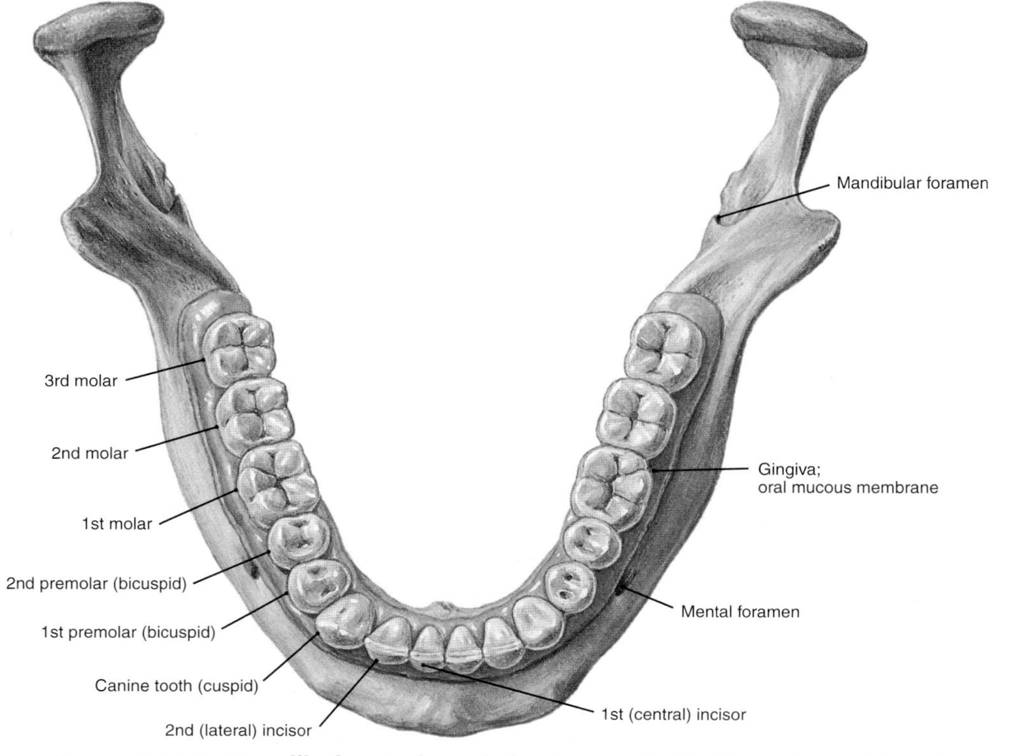
Mandibular foramen
3rd molar
2nd molar
Gingiva; oral mucous membrane
1st molar
2nd premolar (bicuspid)
Mental foramen
1st premolar (bicuspid)
Canine tooth (cuspid)
1st (central) incisor
2nd (lateral) incisor

Figure 581.3 **Mandibular Arch and the Lower Teeth (Seen from Above)**

2nd incisor (lateral)
1st incisor (medial)
Canine tooth
Incisive papilla
1st premolar
2nd premolar
Transverse palatine folds
1st molar
Hard palate
2nd molar
3rd molar
Palatine raphe
Soft palate
Openings of palatine glands
Palatoglossal arch
Palatopharyngeal arch
Uvula

Figure 582.1 Hard and Soft Palates and Upper Teeth (Seen from Below)

NOTE: The palate consists of an anterior **hard** region and a posterior **soft** region. Transverse ridges mark the anterior palatal surface, while a median palatal raphe extends from the incisive papilla to the uvula. The upper teeth are named similarly to the lower teeth.

Median palatine suture
Incisive foramen
Incisive bone (premaxilla)
Incisive bone (premaxilla)
Incisive suture
Palatine process of maxilla
Palatine spines
Palatine sulci
Zygomatic process of maxilla
Greater palatine foramen
Greater palatine foramen
Lesser palatine foramen
Pyramidal process of palatine bone
Horizontal part of palatine bone
Posterior nasal spine
Lateral pterygoid plate
Transverse palatine suture
Medial pterygoid plate

Figure 582.2 Bony Hard Palate and Upper Teeth (Seen from Below)

NOTE: The hard palate is formed principally by the palatine processes of the two maxillae and the horizontal laminae of the palatine bones.

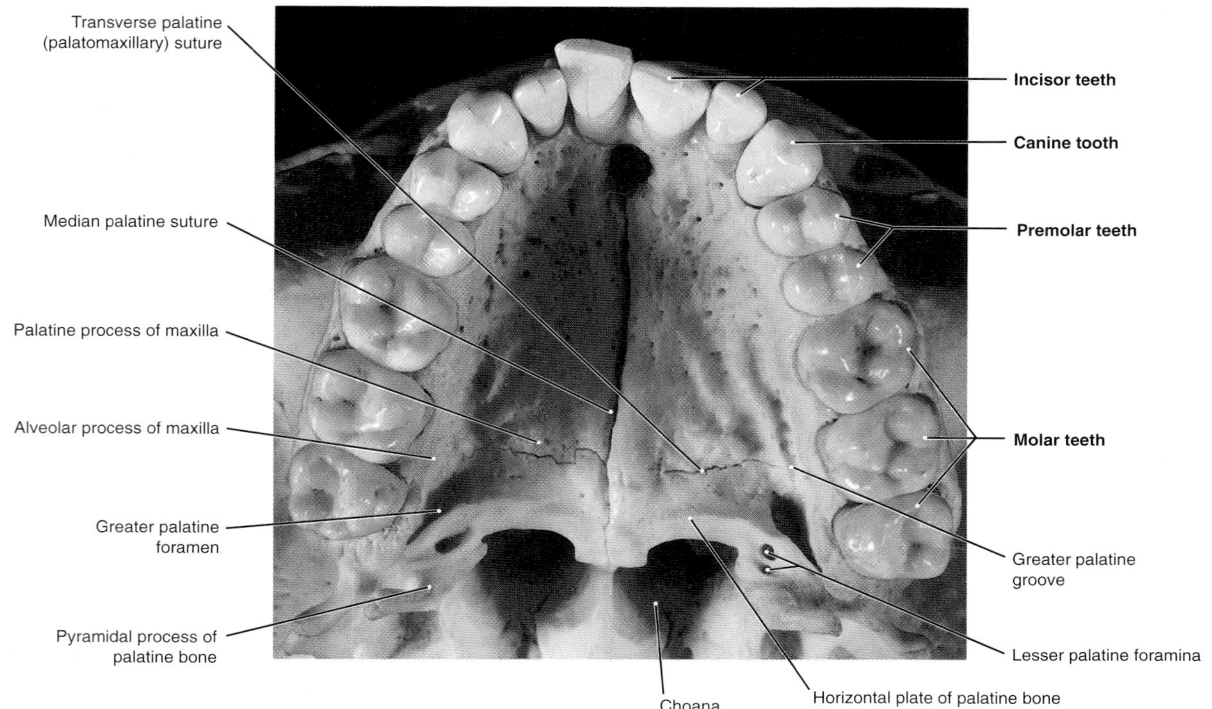
Transverse palatine (palatomaxillary) suture
Incisor teeth
Canine tooth
Premolar teeth
Median palatine suture
Palatine process of maxilla
Alveolar process of maxilla
Molar teeth
Greater palatine foramen
Greater palatine groove
Pyramidal process of palatine bone
Lesser palatine foramina
Choana
Horizontal plate of palatine bone

Figure 582.3 Photograph of the Bony Palate Showing the Maxillary Arch and Upper Teeth

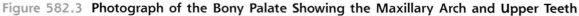

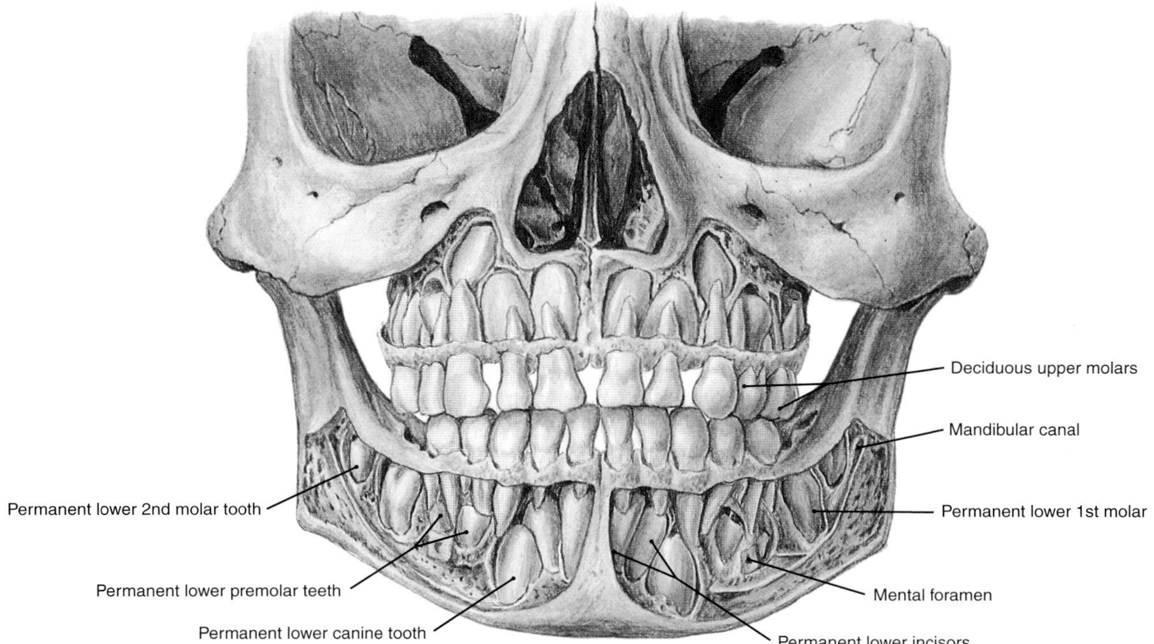
Deciduous upper molars
Mandibular canal
Permanent lower 2nd molar tooth
Permanent lower 1st molar
Permanent lower premolar teeth
Mental foramen
Permanent lower canine tooth
Permanent lower incisors

Figure 583.1 Facial Skeleton of a 5-Year-Old Child Showing Full Deciduous Dentition (20 Teeth)

NOTE: (1) The **deciduous teeth** are shown as white, whereas the rudiments of the **permanent teeth,** shown in blue, have been exposed by removing the outer walls of the alveolar processes of both maxillae and the mandible.

(2) All 20 deciduous teeth have erupted: eight incisors, four canines, and eight molars. Normally all deciduous teeth are replaced by the 12th year.

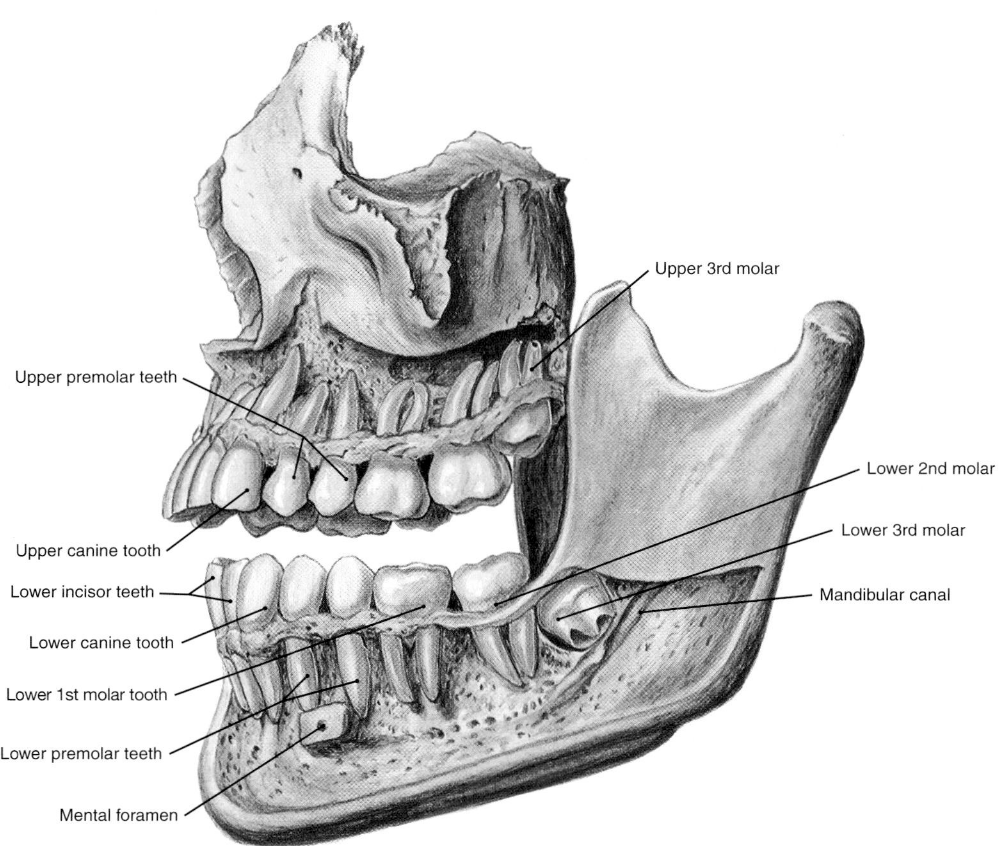
Upper 3rd molar
Upper premolar teeth
Lower 2nd molar
Lower 3rd molar
Upper canine tooth
Mandibular canal
Lower incisor teeth
Lower canine tooth
Lower 1st molar tooth
Lower premolar teeth
Mental foramen

Figure 583.2 Dentition of a 20-Year-Old Person, Seen from the Left Side

NOTE: (1) The roots of the permanent teeth have been exposed by removing the alveolar walls. All of the permanent teeth have erupted through the gums, with the exception of the lower third molar.

(2) The canines and incisors have but one root, as generally do the premolars, although the latter may have two roots. The first and second molars usually have three roots, whereas the smaller third molar may have less than three and may even be single-rooted.

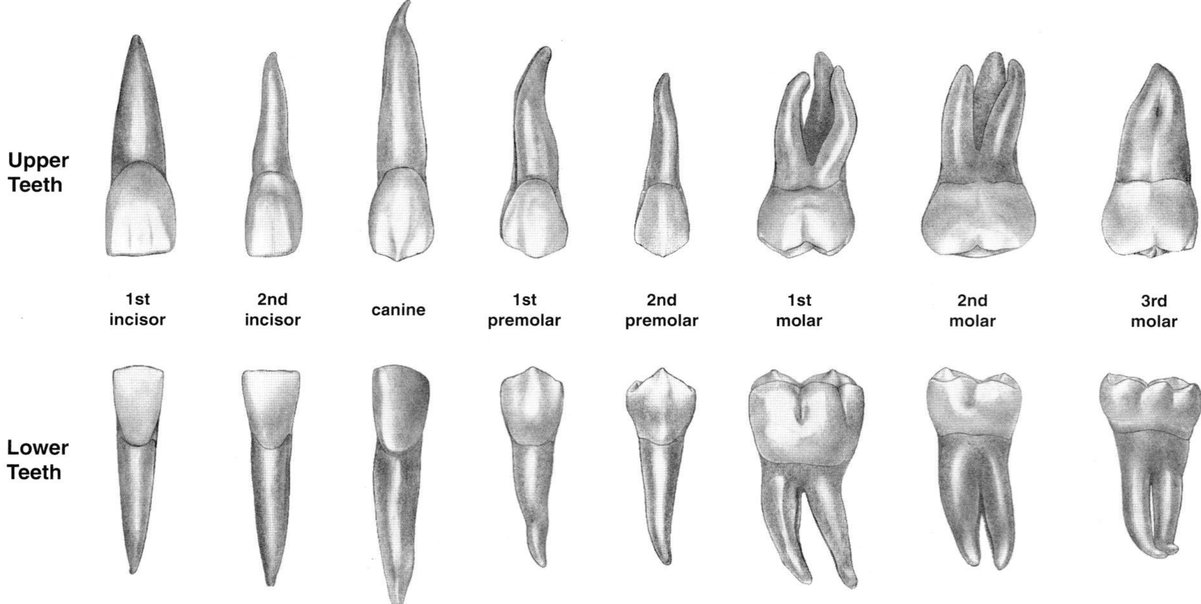
Upper Teeth
1st incisor
2nd incisor
canine
1st premolar
2nd premolar
1st molar
2nd molar
3rd molar
Lower Teeth

Figure 584.1 **Left Permanent Teeth (Vestibular Aspect)**

NOTE: (1) The **incisor teeth** have a sharp edge and a single root. Observe that the maxillary incisors are larger than the mandibular, and the roots of the maxillary incisors are rounded, while the roots of the mandibular incisors are flattened.

(2) The **canine tooth** is somewhat larger than the incisors, and it has a single cusp. It is also the longest of all the teeth.

(3) The **premolar teeth** each have a buccal and a palatal cusp (hence they are often called bicuspids). The upper first premolar usually has two roots and the upper second premolar usually has one root, but it may have two. Both lower premolars have a single root, but the root of the first lower premolar may be bifid.

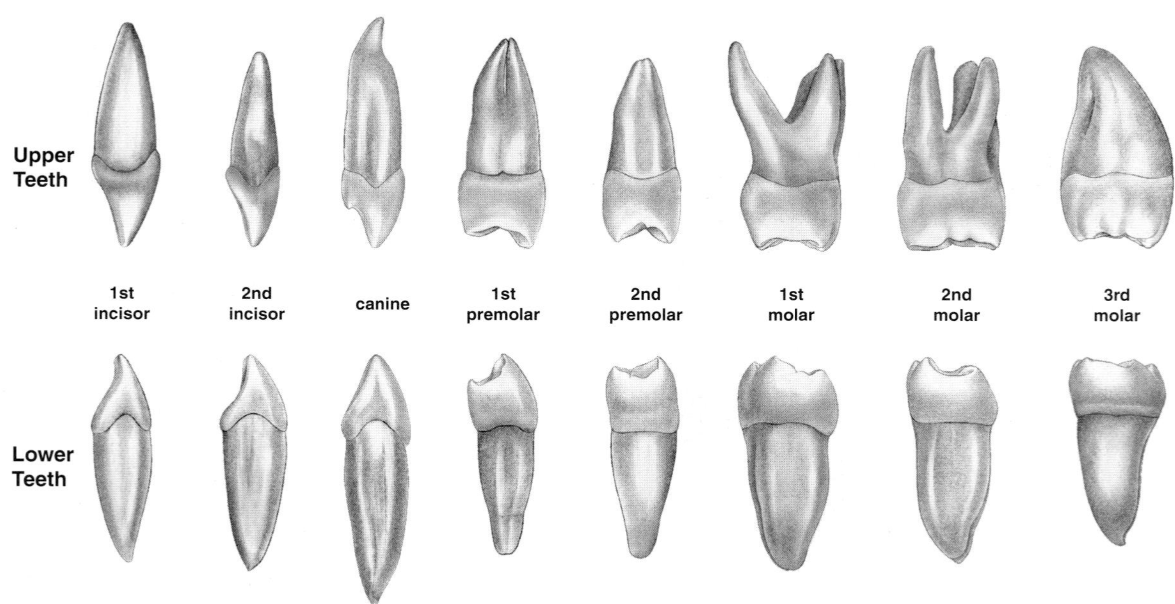
Upper Teeth
1st incisor
2nd incisor
canine
1st premolar
2nd premolar
1st molar
2nd molar
3rd molar
Lower Teeth

Figure 584.2 **Left Permanent Teeth (Medial Aspect)**

(4) The **molar teeth** decrease in size posteriorly. They have four or five cusps. The first and second molars generally have three roots, while the third molar (wisdom tooth) often may have only a single root.

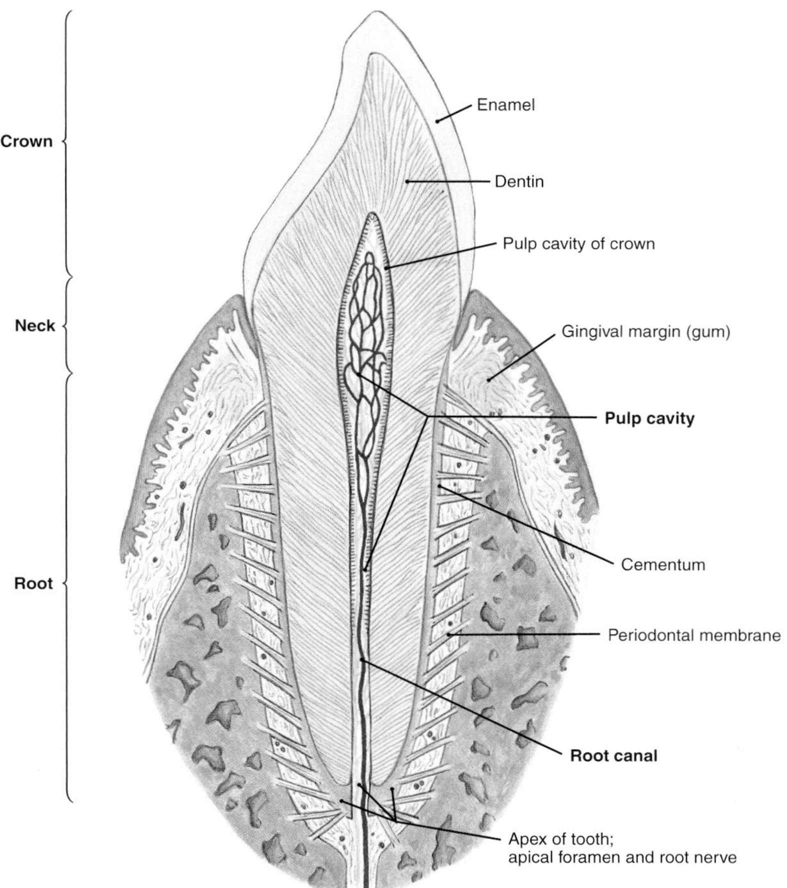
Crown
Neck
Root
Enamel
Dentin
Pulp cavity of crown
Gingival margin (gum)
Pulp cavity
Cementum
Periodontal membrane
Root canal
Apex of tooth;
apical foramen and root nerve

Figure 585.1 Longitudinal Section of the Tooth

NOTE: The crown of the tooth is covered with **enamel** and projects from the **gingiva,** or gum. The **root** is embedded within the alveolar bony **socket** and covered by a thin layer of **cementum.** The main portion of the tooth consists of **dentin,** which surrounds the **root canal** and **pulp cavity** containing the **dental artery** and **nerve.**

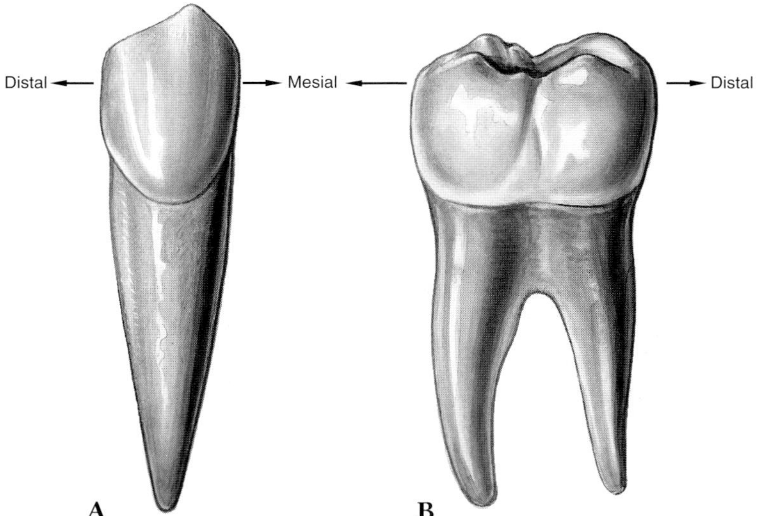
Distal
Mesial
Mesial
Distal
A
B

Figure 585.2. A, Right Lower Permanent Canine Tooth Seen from the Vestibular Surface. B, Left Lower Second Molar Tooth Seen from the Vestibular Surface

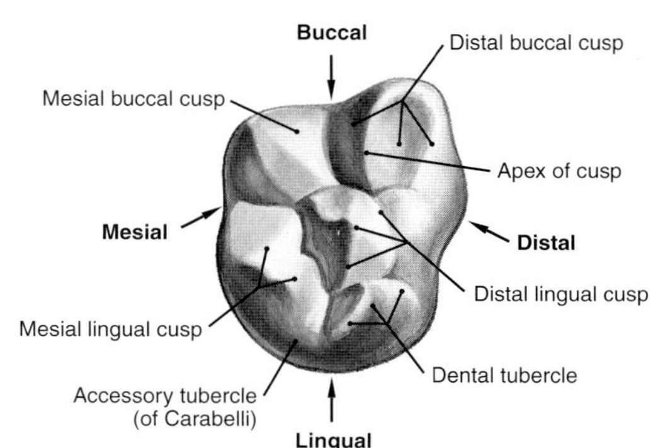
Buccal
Distal buccal cusp
Mesial buccal cusp
Apex of cusp
Mesial
Distal
Distal lingual cusp
Mesial lingual cusp
Dental tubercle
Accessory tubercle
(of Carabelli)
Lingual

Figure 585.3 Occlusal Surface of the Right Upper First Molar

NOTE: The upper first molar may have a fifth cusp, the tubercle of Carabelli on the mesiolingual surface of its crown.

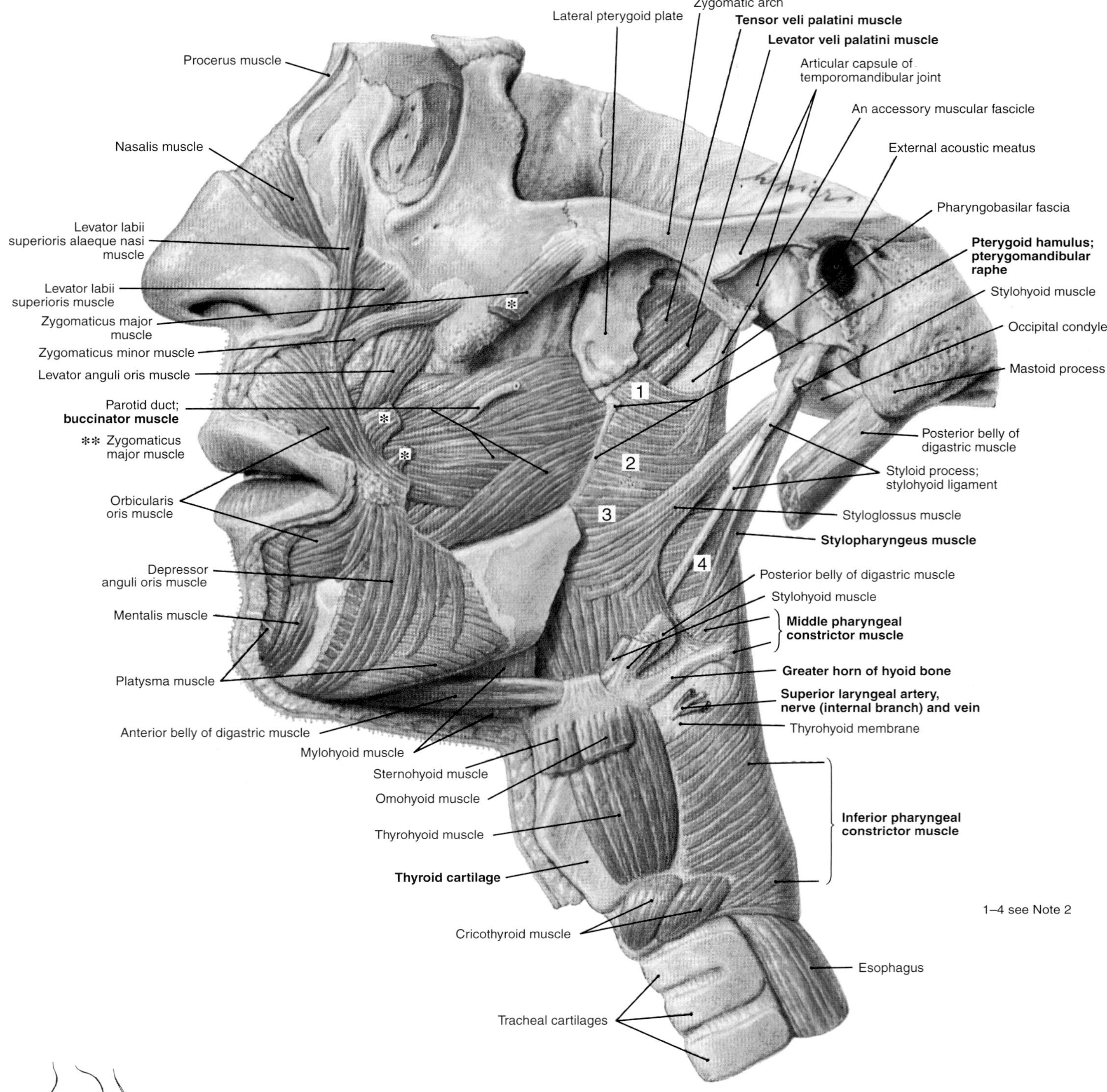
Zygomatic arch
Lateral pterygoid plate
Tensor veli palatini muscle
Levator veli palatini muscle
Articular capsule of temporomandibular joint
Procerus muscle
An accessory muscular fascicle
External acoustic meatus
Nasalis muscle
Pharyngobasilar fascia
Levator labii superioris alaeque nasi muscle
Pterygoid hamulus; pterygomandibular raphe
Levator labii superioris muscle
Stylohyoid muscle
Zygomaticus major muscle
Occipital condyle
Zygomaticus minor muscle
Mastoid process
Levator anguli oris muscle
Parotid duct; buccinator muscle
1
** Zygomaticus major muscle
Posterior belly of digastric muscle
2
Styloid process; stylohyoid ligament
Orbicularis oris muscle
3
Styloglossus muscle
Stylopharyngeus muscle
4
Depressor anguli oris muscle
Posterior belly of digastric muscle
Stylohyoid muscle
Mentalis muscle
Middle pharyngeal constrictor muscle
Platysma muscle
Greater horn of hyoid bone
Superior laryngeal artery, nerve (internal branch) and vein
Anterior belly of digastric muscle
Thyrohyoid membrane
Mylohyoid muscle
Sternohyoid muscle
Omohyoid muscle
Inferior pharyngeal constrictor muscle
Thyrohyoid muscle
Thyroid cartilage
1–4 see Note 2
Cricothyroid muscle
Esophagus
Tracheal cartilages

Figure 586.1 Muscles of the Pharynx and Face ▲

NOTE: (1) The tendinous **pterygomandibular raphe.** It extends between the pterygoid hamulus superiorly and the mylohyoid line of the mandible inferiorly and serves as a common site of origin for the **buccinator** and **superior pharyngeal constrictor.**

(2) The **superior constrictor** arises by four parts: (1) from the hamulus of the medial pterygoid plate; (2) from the pterygomandibular raphe; (3) from the mylohyoid line of the mandible; and (4) by certain fibers that blend with tongue muscles and emerge from the side of the tongue.

(3) The **middle constrictor** arises from the greater and lesser horns of the hyoid bone, while the larger and thicker **inferior constrictor** arises from the thyroid and cricoid cartilages.

Superior pharyngeal constrictor muscle
Stylopharyngeus muscle
Middle pharyngeal constrictor muscle
Inferior pharyngeal constrictor muscle
Cricothyroid muscle

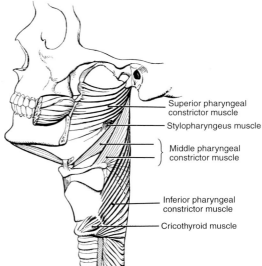

◀ **Figure 586.2 Diagram of the Origins of the Pharyngeal Constrictor Muscles**

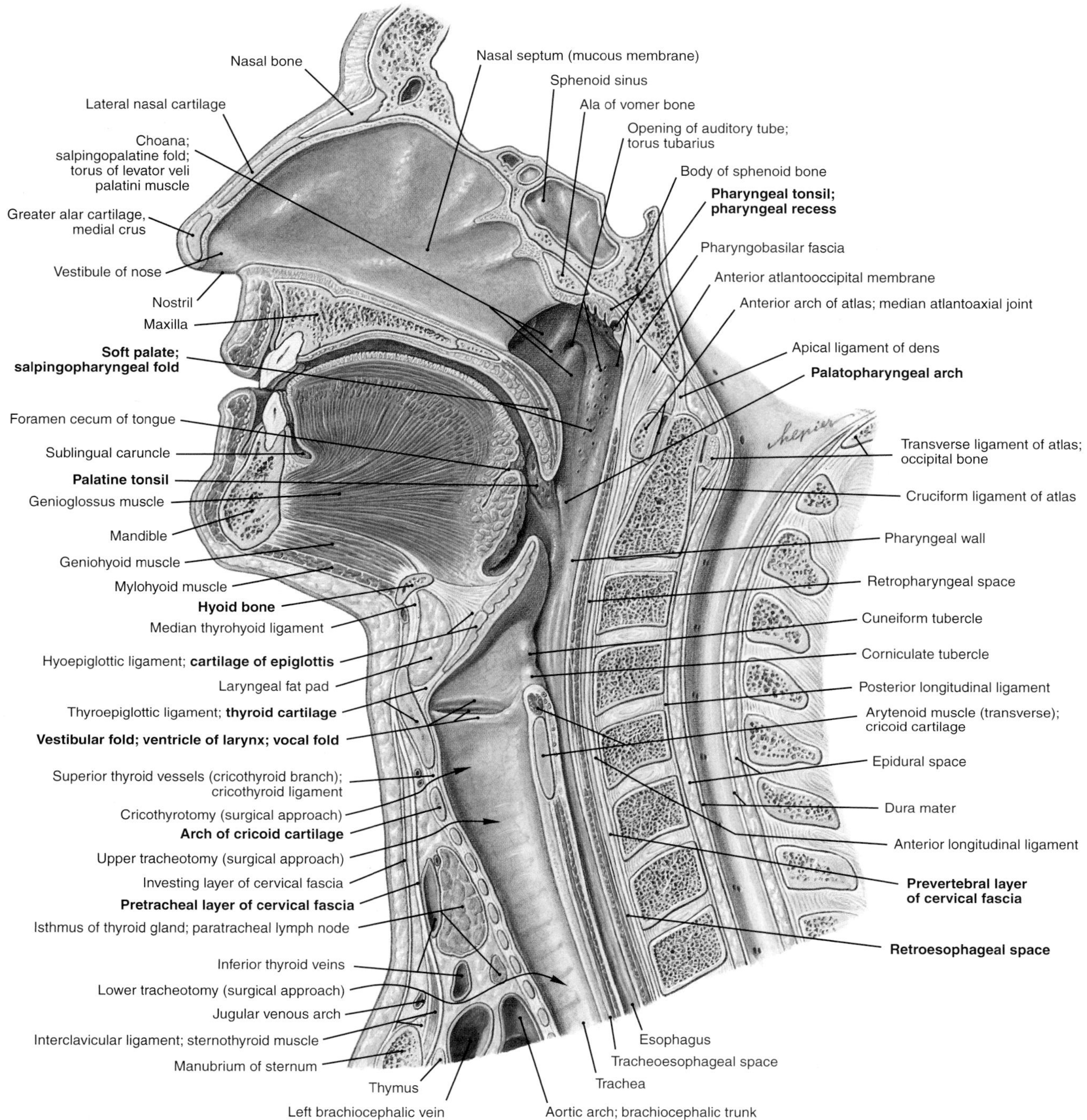
Nasal bone
Lateral nasal cartilage
Choana; salpingopalatine fold; torus of levator veli palatini muscle
Greater alar cartilage, medial crus
Vestibule of nose
Nostril
Maxilla
Soft palate; salpingopharyngeal fold
Foramen cecum of tongue
Sublingual caruncle
Palatine tonsil
Genioglossus muscle
Mandible
Geniohyoid muscle
Mylohyoid muscle
Hyoid bone
Median thyrohyoid ligament
Hyoepiglottic ligament; cartilage of epiglottis
Laryngeal fat pad
Thyroepiglottic ligament; thyroid cartilage
Vestibular fold; ventricle of larynx; vocal fold
Superior thyroid vessels (cricothyroid branch); cricothyroid ligament
Cricothyrotomy (surgical approach)
Arch of cricoid cartilage
Upper tracheotomy (surgical approach)
Investing layer of cervical fascia
Pretracheal layer of cervical fascia
Isthmus of thyroid gland; paratracheal lymph node
Inferior thyroid veins
Lower tracheotomy (surgical approach)
Jugular venous arch
Interclavicular ligament; sternothyroid muscle
Manubrium of sternum
Thymus
Left brachiocephalic vein
Aortic arch; brachiocephalic trunk
Trachea
Tracheoesophageal space
Esophagus
Nasal septum (mucous membrane)
Sphenoid sinus
Ala of vomer bone
Opening of auditory tube; torus tubarius
Body of sphenoid bone
Pharyngeal tonsil; pharyngeal recess
Pharyngobasilar fascia
Anterior atlantooccipital membrane
Anterior arch of atlas; median atlantoaxial joint
Apical ligament of dens
Palatopharyngeal arch
Transverse ligament of atlas; occipital bone
Cruciform ligament of atlas
Pharyngeal wall
Retropharyngeal space
Cuneiform tubercle
Corniculate tubercle
Posterior longitudinal ligament
Arytenoid muscle (transverse); cricoid cartilage
Epidural space
Dura mater
Anterior longitudinal ligament
Prevertebral layer of cervical fascia
Retroesophageal space

Figure 587 **Midsagittal Section of the Mouth, Pharynx, Larynx, and Other Head and Neck Viscera**

NOTE: (1) The closed oral cavity is occupied principally by the tongue. The posterior end of the oral cavity opens into the **oropharynx.** Superiorly, the posterior nasal cavities are continuous with the **nasopharynx,** whereas inferiorly the **laryngeal part of the pharynx** (between the levels of the epiglottis and cricoid cartilages) communicates with the larynx.

(2) The pharynx continues inferiorly as the **esophagus,** while the larynx becomes the **trachea** below the level of the cricoid cartilage.

(3) During **deglutition** (swallowing) food gets directed toward the posterior part of the oral cavity. The soft palate is then elevated and tensed (levator and tensor veli palatini muscles) thereby closing off the nasopharynx so that food enters the oropharynx. At the same time the larynx is drawn upward toward the epiglottis and the pharynx ascends as well. This action closes off the laryngeal orifice (aditus) and prevents food from entering the larynx.

(4) The arrows indicate surgical approaches to the airway (larynx and trachea).

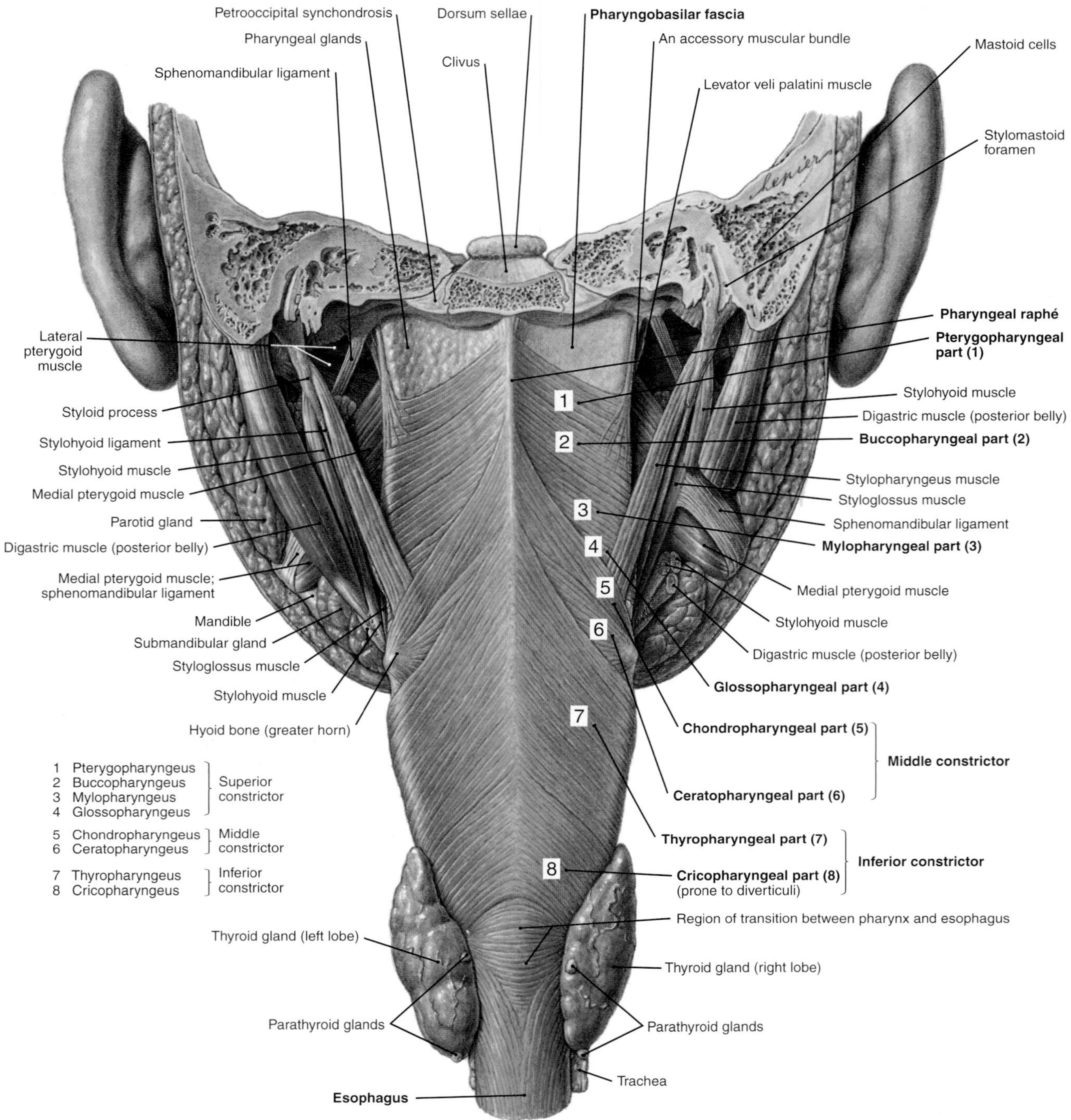
Petrooccipital synchondrosis
Dorsum sellae
Pharyngobasilar fascia
Pharyngeal glands
An accessory muscular bundle
Mastoid cells
Clivus
Sphenomandibular ligament
Levator veli palatini muscle
Stylomastoid foramen
Lateral pterygoid muscle
Pharyngeal raphé
Pterygopharyngeal part (1)
Stylohyoid muscle
Styloid process
Digastric muscle (posterior belly)
Stylohyoid ligament
Buccopharyngeal part (2)
Stylohyoid muscle
Stylopharyngeus muscle
Medial pterygoid muscle
Styloglossus muscle
Parotid gland
Sphenomandibular ligament
Digastric muscle (posterior belly)
Mylopharyngeal part (3)
Medial pterygoid muscle; sphenomandibular ligament
Medial pterygoid muscle
Mandible
Stylohyoid muscle
Submandibular gland
Digastric muscle (posterior belly)
Styloglossus muscle
Glossopharyngeal part (4)
Stylohyoid muscle
Hyoid bone (greater horn)
Chondropharyngeal part (5)
Middle constrictor
Ceratopharyngeal part (6)
Thyropharyngeal part (7)
Inferior constrictor
Cricopharyngeal part (8) (prone to diverticuli)
Region of transition between pharynx and esophagus
Thyroid gland (left lobe)
Thyroid gland (right lobe)
Parathyroid glands
Parathyroid glands
Trachea
Esophagus
1 Pterygopharyngeus
2 Buccopharyngeus
3 Mylopharyngeus
4 Glossopharyngeus
Superior constrictor
5 Chondropharyngeus
6 Ceratopharyngeus
Middle constrictor
7 Thyropharyngeus
8 Cricopharyngeus
Inferior constrictor

Figure 588 Dorsal View of the Pharyngeal Muscles

NOTE: (1) This posterior view of the pharynx was achieved by making a frontal transection through the petrous and mastoid parts of the temporal bone and through the body of the occipital bone. The styloid processes and their muscular attachments are left intact.

(2) The divisions of the **pharyngeal constrictors.** Their muscle fibers arise laterally to insert in a posterior raphe in the midline. The **superior constrictor** is divisible into four parts, while the **middle and inferior constrictors** are each divisible into two.

(3) Above the superior constrictor is found the fibrous **pharyngobasilar fascia,** which attaches to the basal portion of the occipital bone and to the temporal bones. Below the inferior constrictor, the pharynx is continuous with the muscular esophagus.

(4) The superior and middle constrictor muscles and the thyropharyngeal part of the inferior constrictor are innervated by the **pharyngeal branch of the vagus nerve.** These fibers have their cell bodies in the nucleus ambiguus in the medulla oblongata; they emerge from the brain in the rootlets of the bulbar part of the accessory nerve and then, by a communicating branch, join the vagus nerve.

(5) The cricopharyngeal part of the inferior constrictor is supplied by the recurrent laryngeal branch of the vagus nerve.

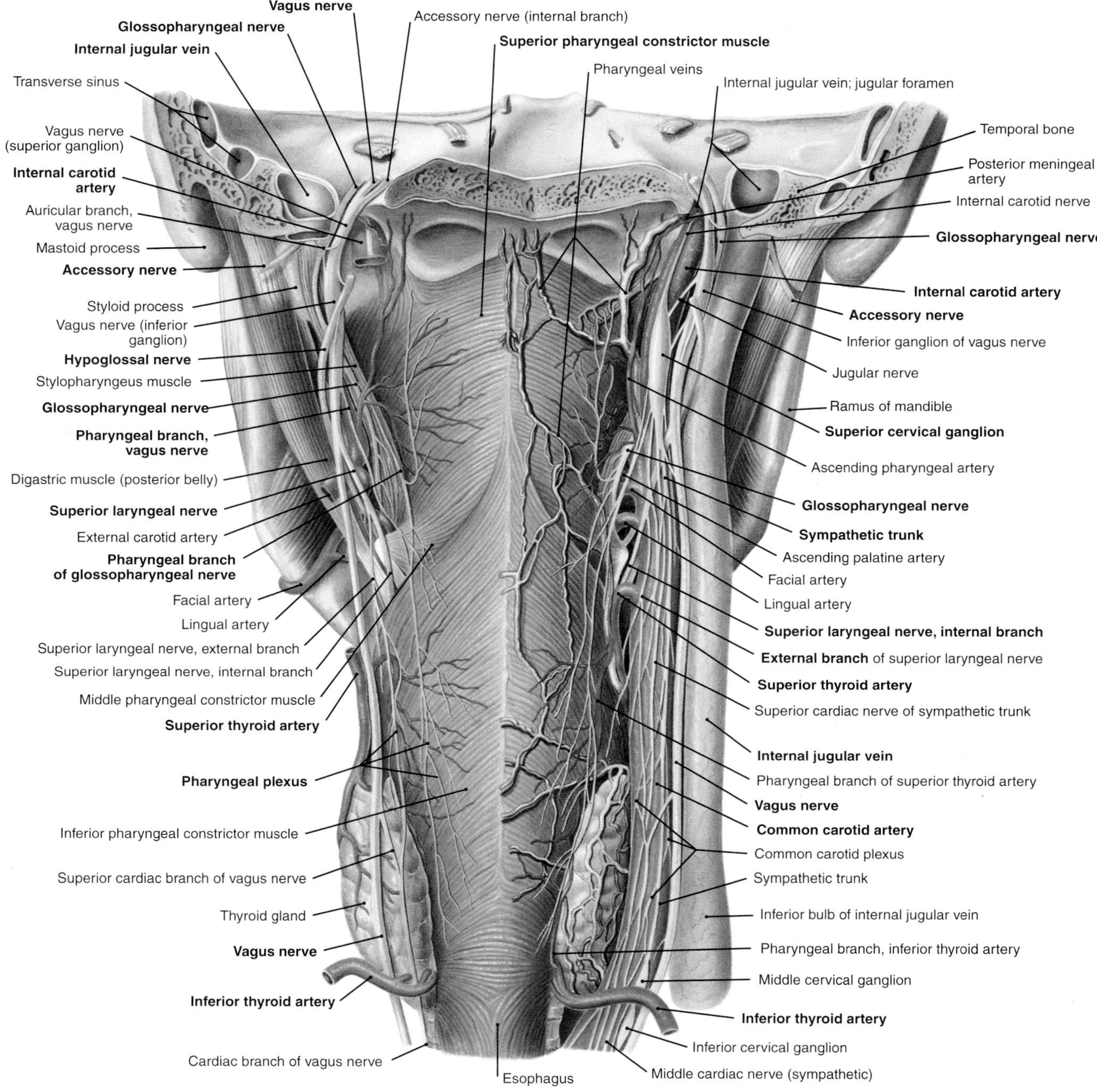
Vagus nerve
Glossopharyngeal nerve
Internal jugular vein
Accessory nerve (internal branch)
Superior pharyngeal constrictor muscle
Pharyngeal veins
Internal jugular vein; jugular foramen
Transverse sinus
Vagus nerve (superior ganglion)
Internal carotid artery
Auricular branch, vagus nerve
Mastoid process
Accessory nerve
Styloid process
Vagus nerve (inferior ganglion)
Hypoglossal nerve
Stylopharyngeus muscle
Glossopharyngeal nerve
Pharyngeal branch, vagus nerve
Digastric muscle (posterior belly)
Superior laryngeal nerve
External carotid artery
Pharyngeal branch of glossopharyngeal nerve
Facial artery
Lingual artery
Superior laryngeal nerve, external branch
Superior laryngeal nerve, internal branch
Middle pharyngeal constrictor muscle
Superior thyroid artery
Pharyngeal plexus
Inferior pharyngeal constrictor muscle
Superior cardiac branch of vagus nerve
Thyroid gland
Vagus nerve
Inferior thyroid artery
Cardiac branch of vagus nerve
Esophagus
Temporal bone
Posterior meningeal artery
Internal carotid nerve
Glossopharyngeal nerve
Internal carotid artery
Accessory nerve
Inferior ganglion of vagus nerve
Jugular nerve
Ramus of mandible
Superior cervical ganglion
Ascending pharyngeal artery
Glossopharyngeal nerve
Sympathetic trunk
Ascending palatine artery
Facial artery
Lingual artery
Superior laryngeal nerve, internal branch
External branch of superior laryngeal nerve
Superior thyroid artery
Superior cardiac nerve of sympathetic trunk
Internal jugular vein
Pharyngeal branch of superior thyroid artery
Vagus nerve
Common carotid artery
Common carotid plexus
Sympathetic trunk
Inferior bulb of internal jugular vein
Pharyngeal branch, inferior thyroid artery
Middle cervical ganglion
Inferior thyroid artery
Inferior cervical ganglion
Middle cardiac nerve (sympathetic)

Figure 589 Nerves and Vessels on the Dorsal and Lateral Walls of the Pharynx

NOTE: (1) The head has been split longitudinally. The pharynx, larynx, and facial structures were separated from the vertebral column and its associated muscles. This posterior view of the pharynx also shows the large nerves and blood vessels that course through the neck. On the right side, observe the **carotid artery, internal jugular vein, vagus nerve,** and the **sympathetic trunk.**

(2) On the left side are the **glossopharyngeal** and **hypoglossal nerves,** which were exposed by removing the carotid arteries and internal jugular vein. In addition to the jugular vein, the **jugular foramen** transmits the 9th, 10th, and 11th cranial nerves.

(3) The **thyroid gland** and its **superior and inferior thyroid arteries.** The superior and middle thyroid veins drain into the internal jugular vein, while the inferior thyroid veins (not shown) usually drain into the left brachiocephalic vein.

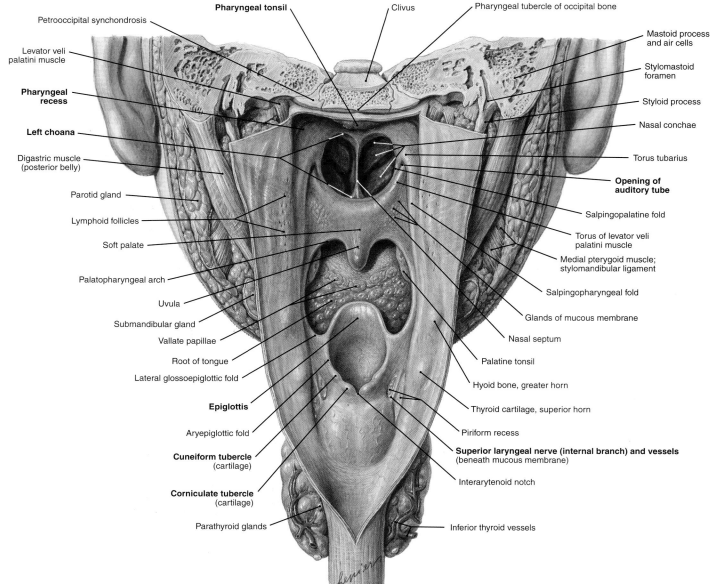

Pharyngeal tonsil
Clivus
Pharyngeal tubercle of occipital bone
Petrooccipital synchondrosis
Mastoid process and air cells
Levator veli palatini muscle
Stylomastoid foramen
Pharyngeal recess
Styloid process
Nasal conchae
Left choana
Torus tubarius
Digastric muscle (posterior belly)
Opening of auditory tube
Parotid gland
Salpingopalatine fold
Lymphoid follicles
Torus of levator veli palatini muscle
Soft palate
Medial pterygoid muscle; stylomandibular ligament
Palatopharyngeal arch
Salpingopharyngeal fold
Uvula
Glands of mucous membrane
Submandibular gland
Nasal septum
Vallate papillae
Root of tongue
Palatine tonsil
Lateral glossoepiglottic fold
Hyoid bone, greater horn
Epiglottis
Thyroid cartilage, superior horn
Aryepiglottic fold
Piriform recess
Cuneiform tubercle (cartilage)
Superior laryngeal nerve (internal branch) and vessels (beneath mucous membrane)
Interarytenoid notch
Corniculate tubercle (cartilage)
Parathyroid glands
Inferior thyroid vessels

Figure 590.1 Pharynx and Its Related Cavities (Dorsal)

NOTE: (1) The pharynx has been opened by a posterior longitudinal incision, thereby exposing its three parts: nasopharynx, oropharynx, and laryngopharynx. The **nasopharynx** lies above the soft palate, and it communicates with the nasal cavities by the choanae.

(2) The **oropharynx** communicates with the oral cavity through the isthmus of the fauces. It extends between the soft palate and the larynx.

(3) The **laryngopharynx** lies behind the larynx and is continuous below with the esophagus. The superior part of the laryngopharynx communicates with the larynx through the laryngeal inlet called the aditus.

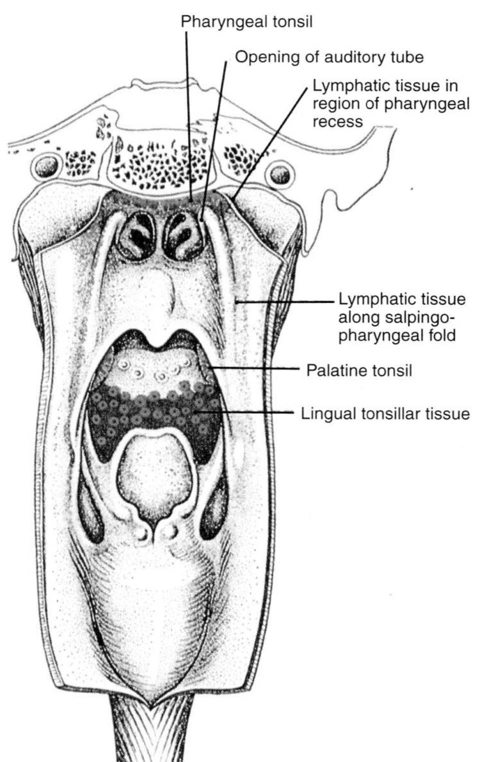
Pharyngeal tonsil
Opening of auditory tube
Lymphatic tissue in region of pharyngeal recess
Lymphatic tissue along salpingo-pharyngeal fold
Palatine tonsil
Lingual tonsillar tissue

Figure 590.2 Oronasopharyngeal Lymphatic Ring

NOTE: The lymphatic ring is shown in red. This circular accumulation of lymphatic tissue includes the lingual tonsil (which consists of lymphoid follicles on the posterior third of the tongue), the palatine tonsils, the pharyngeal tonsil, and more diffuse lymphoid tissue in the wall of the nasopharynx along the salpingopharyngeal fold.

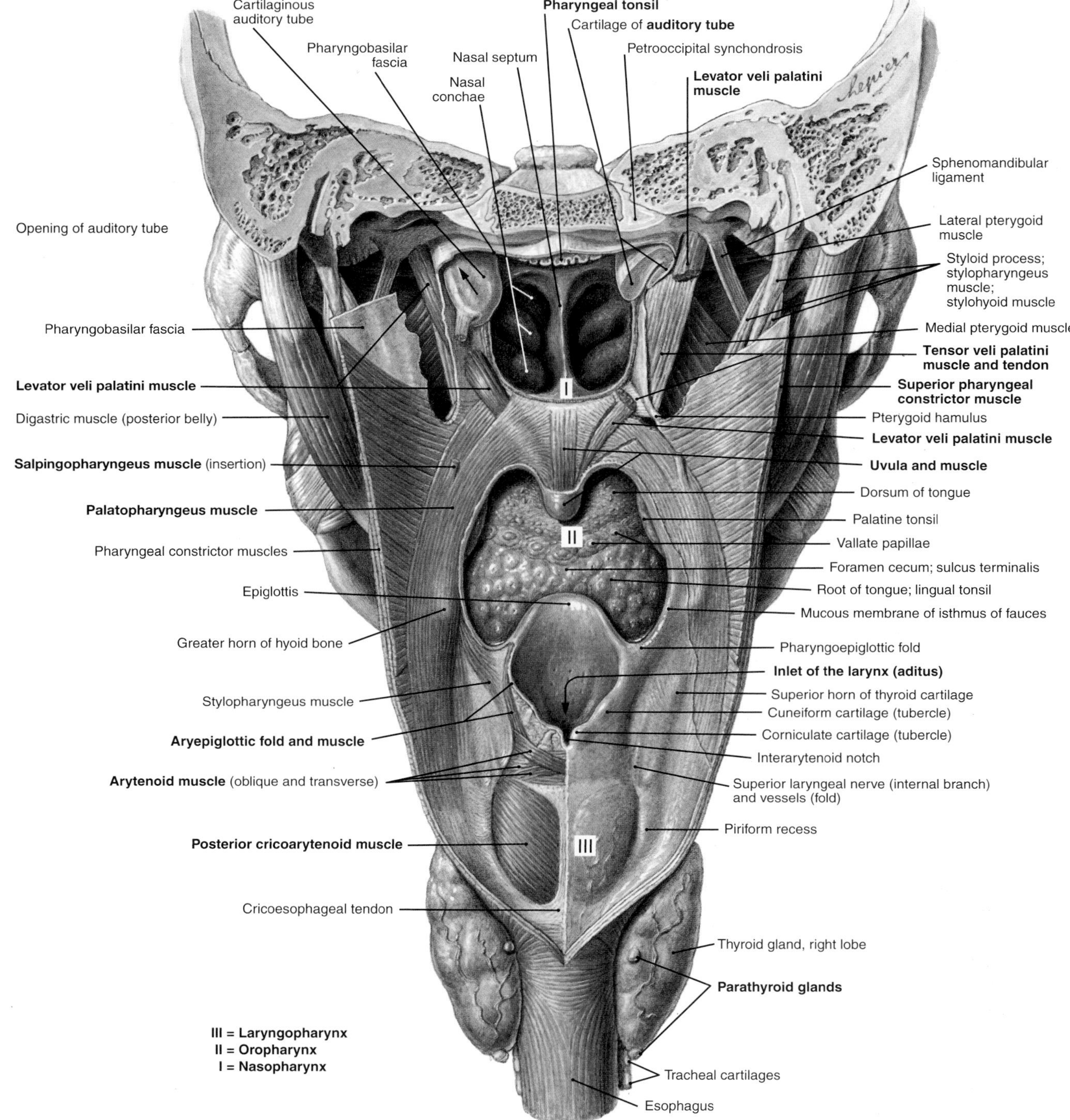
Cartilaginous auditory tube
Pharyngobasilar fascia
Nasal septum
Nasal conchae
Pharyngeal tonsil
Cartilage of auditory tube
Petrooccipital synchondrosis
Levator veli palatini muscle
Sphenomandibular ligament
Opening of auditory tube
Lateral pterygoid muscle
Styloid process; stylopharyngeus muscle; stylohyoid muscle
Pharyngobasilar fascia
Medial pterygoid muscle
Tensor veli palatini muscle and tendon
Levator veli palatini muscle
Superior pharyngeal constrictor muscle
Digastric muscle (posterior belly)
Pterygoid hamulus
Levator veli palatini muscle
Salpingopharyngeus muscle (insertion)
Uvula and muscle
Dorsum of tongue
Palatopharyngeus muscle
Palatine tonsil
Pharyngeal constrictor muscles
Vallate papillae
Foramen cecum; sulcus terminalis
Epiglottis
Root of tongue; lingual tonsil
Mucous membrane of isthmus of fauces
Greater horn of hyoid bone
Pharyngoepiglottic fold
Inlet of the larynx (aditus)
Superior horn of thyroid cartilage
Stylopharyngeus muscle
Cuneiform cartilage (tubercle)
Corniculate cartilage (tubercle)
Aryepiglottic fold and muscle
Interarytenoid notch
Arytenoid muscle (oblique and transverse)
Superior laryngeal nerve (internal branch) and vessels (fold)
Piriform recess
Posterior cricoarytenoid muscle
Cricoesophageal tendon
Thyroid gland, right lobe
Parathyroid glands
III = Laryngopharynx
II = Oropharynx
I = Nasopharynx
Tracheal cartilages
Esophagus
I
II
III

Figure 591 Muscles of the Soft Palate, Pharynx, and Posterior Larynx

NOTE: (1) This dissection is similar to that in Figure 590. The pharynx has been opened dorsally by a midline incision and the mucous membrane has been removed from the soft palate, pharynx, and left posterior larynx. On the right, a part of the levator veli **palatini muscle** has been removed to expose the adjacent **tensor veli palatini muscle.**

(2) The **muscles of the soft palate.** Both the muscle of the uvula and the levator veli palatini muscle are innervated by the pharyngeal branch of the vagus nerve, whereas the tensor veli palatini is supplied by the mandibular division of the trigeminal nerve.

(3) The **palatopharyngeus muscle** arises by two fascicles from the soft palate. The muscle fibers of these fascicles arise posterior and anterior to the insertion of the levator veli palatini muscle. The fascicles descend and merge and then insert into the posterior border of the thyroid cartilage and onto the adjacent pharyngeal wall.

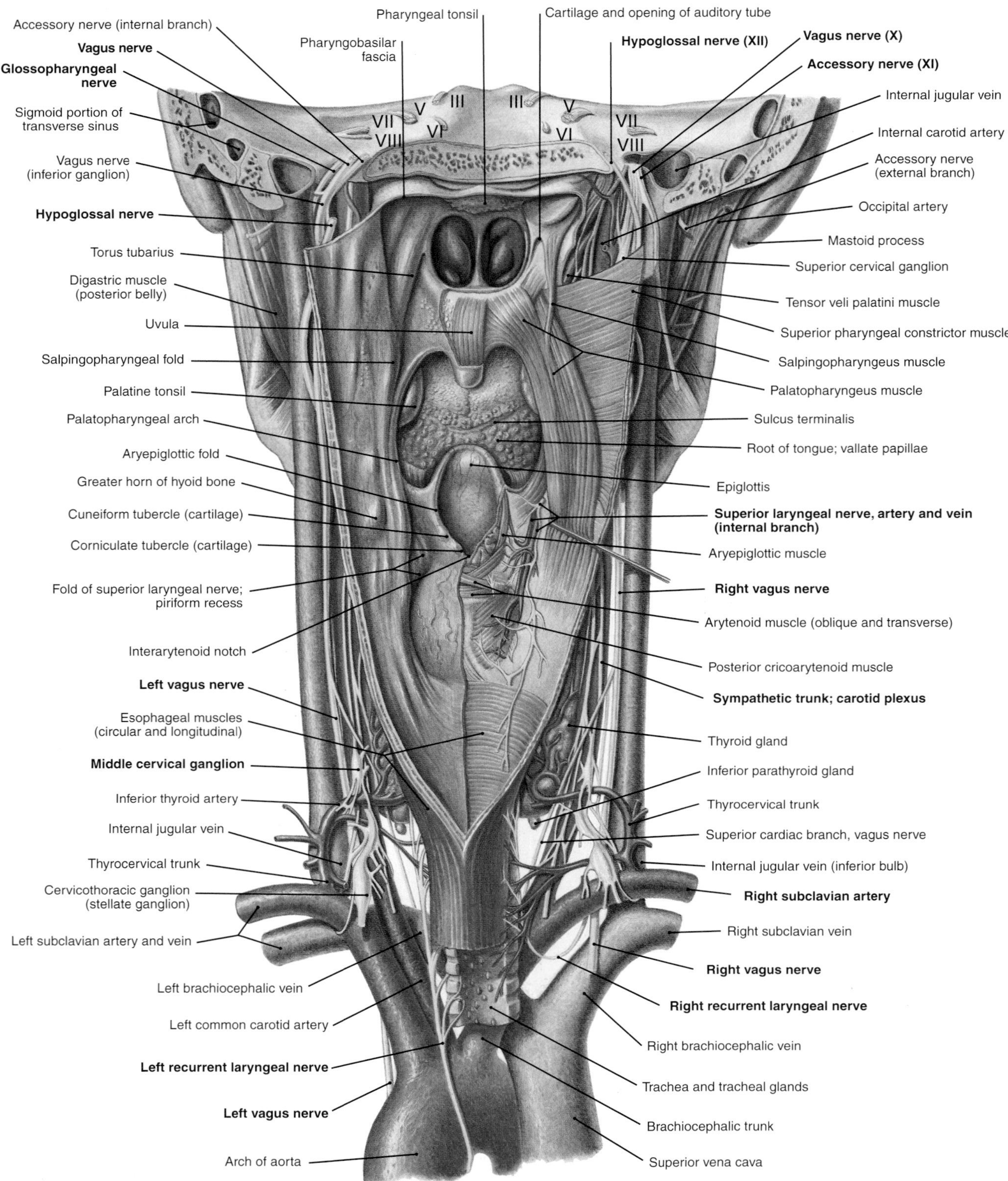
Accessory nerve (internal branch)
Vagus nerve
Glossopharyngeal nerve
Sigmoid portion of transverse sinus
Vagus nerve (inferior ganglion)
Hypoglossal nerve
Torus tubarius
Digastric muscle (posterior belly)
Uvula
Salpingopharyngeal fold
Palatine tonsil
Palatopharyngeal arch
Aryepiglottic fold
Greater horn of hyoid bone
Cuneiform tubercle (cartilage)
Corniculate tubercle (cartilage)
Fold of superior laryngeal nerve; piriform recess
Interarytenoid notch
Left vagus nerve
Esophageal muscles (circular and longitudinal)
Middle cervical ganglion
Inferior thyroid artery
Internal jugular vein
Thyrocervical trunk
Cervicothoracic ganglion (stellate ganglion)
Left subclavian artery and vein
Left brachiocephalic vein
Left common carotid artery
Left recurrent laryngeal nerve
Left vagus nerve
Arch of aorta
Pharyngobasilar fascia
Pharyngeal tonsil
Cartilage and opening of auditory tube
Hypoglossal nerve (XII)
Vagus nerve (X)
Accessory nerve (XI)
Internal jugular vein
Internal carotid artery
Accessory nerve (external branch)
Occipital artery
Mastoid process
Superior cervical ganglion
Tensor veli palatini muscle
Superior pharyngeal constrictor muscle
Salpingopharyngeus muscle
Palatopharyngeus muscle
Sulcus terminalis
Root of tongue; vallate papillae
Epiglottis
Superior laryngeal nerve, artery and vein (internal branch)
Aryepiglottic muscle
Right vagus nerve
Arytenoid muscle (oblique and transverse)
Posterior cricoarytenoid muscle
Sympathetic trunk; carotid plexus
Thyroid gland
Inferior parathyroid gland
Thyrocervical trunk
Superior cardiac branch, vagus nerve
Internal jugular vein (inferior bulb)
Right subclavian artery
Right subclavian vein
Right vagus nerve
Right recurrent laryngeal nerve
Right brachiocephalic vein
Trachea and tracheal glands
Brachiocephalic trunk
Superior vena cava
VII
VIII
V
III
VI

Figure 592 **Pharynx Opened from Behind: Cervical Viscera, Muscles, Vessels, and Nerves**

NOTE: (1) The nasal, oral, and laryngeal orifices communicate with the pharynx. Observe the **superior laryngeal artery, vein,** and **nerve (internal branch)** entering the larynx from above.

(2) The **recurrent laryngeal nerves** ascend to the larynx from the thorax. The left nerve courses around the arch of the aorta, while on the right side the recurrent laryngeal nerve curves around the subclavian artery.

(3) The **inferior cervical ganglion** at the level of the seventh cervical vertebra is fused with the first thoracic ganglion (in about 80% of cases). When fused, the joint ganglion is called the **stellate ganglion.**

Muscle Chart: Muscles of the Palate and Pharynx

MUSCLES OF THE PALATE

Muscle	Origin	Insertion	Innervation	Action
Musculus uvulae	Posterior nasal spine (palatine bone); palatine aponeurosis	Descends into the mucous membrane of the uvula	Pharyngeal branch of the vagus nerve	Pulls the uvula up and contracts the uvula on its own side
Tensor veli palatini	Scaphoid fossa of pterygoid process; cartilaginous part of auditory tube; spine of sphenoid	Tendon courses around the pterygoid hamulus and then inserts into the palatine aponeurosis	Branch of the mandibular division of the trigeminal nerve	Tenses the soft palate; acting singly, it pulls the soft palate to one side
Levator veli palatini	Inferior surface of temporal bone; cartilaginous part of auditory tube	Upper surface of the palatine aponeurosis	Pharyngeal branch of the vagus nerve	Elevates the soft palate
Palatoglossus	Oral surface of the palatine aponeurosis	Into the side of the tongue	Pharyngeal branch of the vagus nerve	Elevates root of tongue; two muscles together close off oral cavity from oropharynx
Palatopharyngeus	Posterior border of the hard palate; palatine aponeurosis	Posterior border of thyroid cartilage; lateral wall of pharynx	Pharyngeal branch of the vagus nerve	Pulls the pharynx upward during swallowing

MUSCLES OF THE PHARYNX

Superior pharyngeal constrictor	Pterygopharyngeal Part: Pterygoid hamulus of sphenoid bone	Pharyngobasilar fascia and the midline raphe		
	Buccopharyngeal Part: Pterygomandibular raphe	Posterior midline pharyngeal raphe	Motor fibers: Pharyngeal branch of vagus nerve (fibers originating in the medullary part of accessory nerve).	
	Mylopharyngeal Part: Mylohyoid line of mandible	Posterior midline pharyngeal raphe		The constrictor muscles act as sphincters of the pharynx and induce peristaltic waves during swallowing
	Glossopharyngeal part: A few fibers arise from the side of tongue	Posterior midline pharyngeal raphe	Sensory fibers of mucosa: Glossopharyngeal nerve and some trigeminal nerve fibers.	
Middle pharyngeal constrictor	Chondropharyngeal Part: Lesser horn of hyoid bone	Posterior midline pharyngeal raphe		
	Ceratopharyngeal Part: Greater horn of hyoid bone	Posterior midline pharyngeal raphe		
Inferior pharyngeal constrictor	Thyropharyngeal Part: Oblique line on the lamina of thyroid cartilage	Posterior midline pharyngeal raphe		
	Cricopharyngeal Part: Side of the cricoid cartilage	Posterior midline pharyngeal raphe	Cricopharyngeus: Recurrent laryngeal branch of vagus	
Stylopharyngeus	Medial side of base of styloid process	Lateral wall of pharynx between the superior and middle constrictors	Glossopharyngeal nerve	Elevates the lateral wall of the pharynx during swallowing and speech
Salpingopharyngeus	Inferior part of the cartilage of the auditory tube	Blends with the palatopharyngeus on the lateral wall of the pharynx	Pharyngeal branch of vagus nerve	Raises upper lateral wall of the pharynx
Palatopharyngeus	Described with the palatal muscles above			

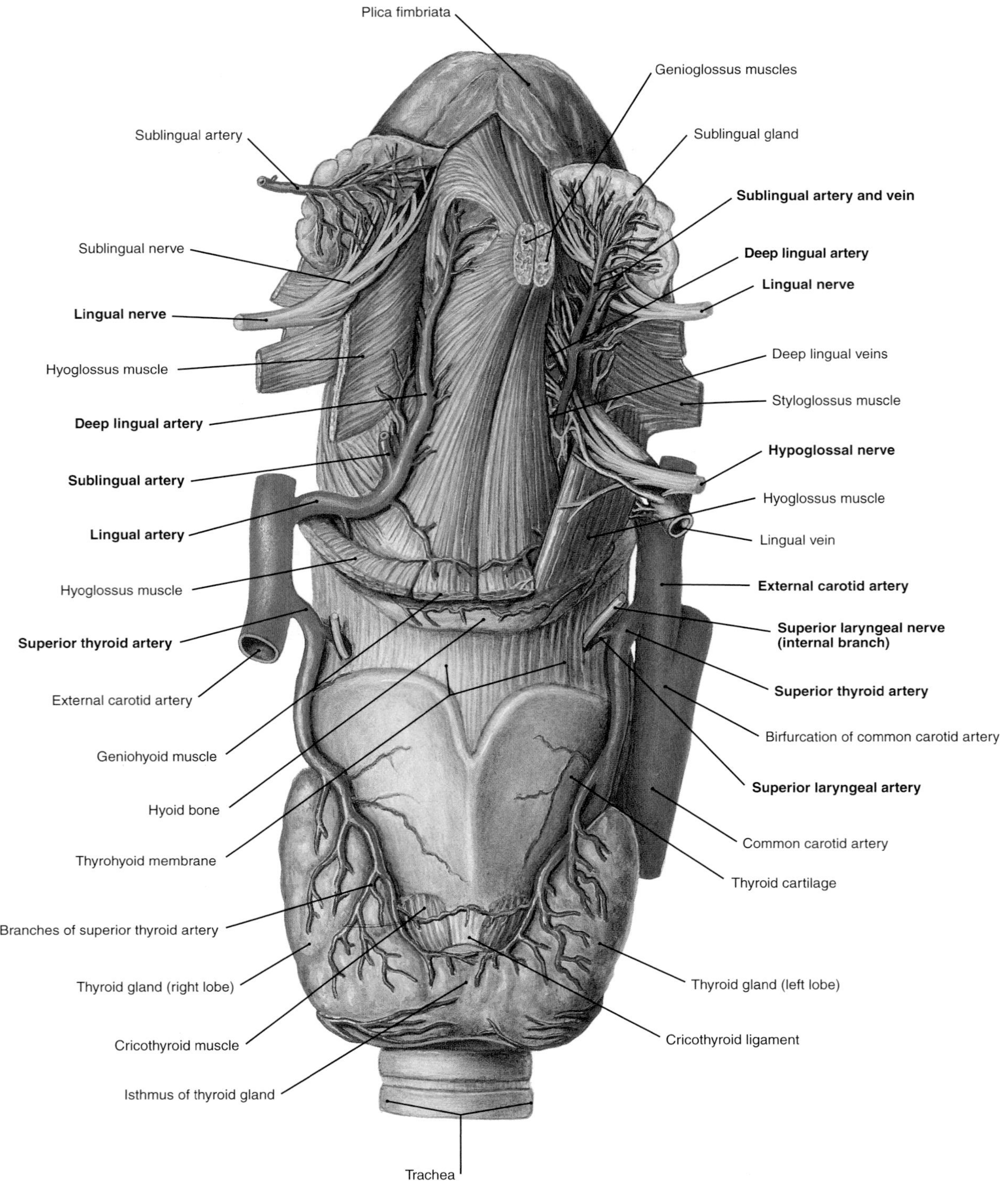
Plica fimbriata
Genioglossus muscles
Sublingual artery
Sublingual gland
Sublingual artery and vein
Sublingual nerve
Deep lingual artery
Lingual nerve
Lingual nerve
Hyoglossus muscle
Deep lingual veins
Styloglossus muscle
Deep lingual artery
Hypoglossal nerve
Sublingual artery
Hyoglossus muscle
Lingual artery
Lingual vein
Hyoglossus muscle
External carotid artery
Superior thyroid artery
Superior laryngeal nerve (internal branch)
External carotid artery
Superior thyroid artery
Birfurcation of common carotid artery
Geniohyoid muscle
Superior laryngeal artery
Hyoid bone
Common carotid artery
Thyrohyoid membrane
Thyroid cartilage
Branches of superior thyroid artery
Thyroid gland (right lobe)
Thyroid gland (left lobe)
Cricothyroid muscle
Cricothyroid ligament
Isthmus of thyroid gland
Trachea

Figure 594 Anterior View of Larynx, Tongue and Thyroid Gland, Vessels, and Nerves

NOTE: (1) The **superior thyroid arteries** descend to the thyroid gland. In their course, they give off the **superior laryngeal arteries,** which penetrate the thyrohyoid membrane to enter the interior of the larynx. They are accompanied by the **internal laryngeal branch** of the **superior laryngeal nerve.**

(2) The cranial and medial course of the **lingual artery** deep to the hyoglossus muscle and its suprahyoid (not labeled), sublingual, and deep lingual branches.

(3) The **lingual nerves** as they enter the tongue to supply its anterior two-thirds with general sensation. The motor nerve to the tongue is the **hypoglossal,** seen coursing along with its accompanying veins. It enters the base of the tongue just above the hyoid bone, passing anteriorly across the external carotid and lingual arteries.

(4) The **common carotid artery** bifurcates at about the level of the upper border of the thyroid cartilage. The lingual artery branches from the external carotid above the hyoid bone, while the superior laryngeal arises at the level of the thyrohyoid membrane.

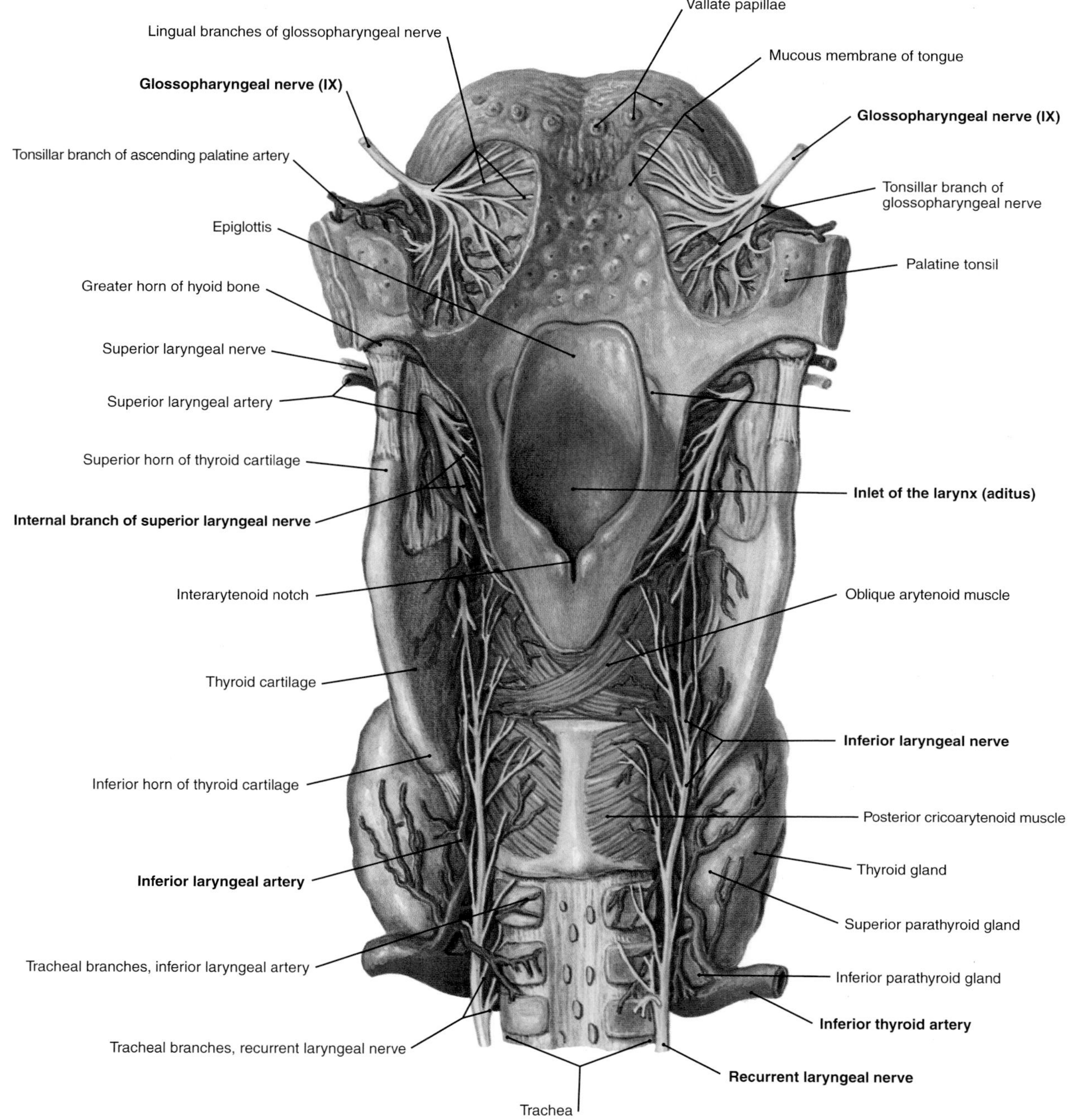
Vallate papillae
Lingual branches of glossopharyngeal nerve
Mucous membrane of tongue
Glossopharyngeal nerve (IX)
Glossopharyngeal nerve (IX)
Tonsillar branch of ascending palatine artery
Tonsillar branch of glossopharyngeal nerve
Epiglottis
Palatine tonsil
Greater horn of hyoid bone
Superior laryngeal nerve
Superior laryngeal artery
Superior horn of thyroid cartilage
Inlet of the larynx (aditus)
Internal branch of superior laryngeal nerve
Interarytenoid notch
Oblique arytenoid muscle
Thyroid cartilage
Inferior laryngeal nerve
Inferior horn of thyroid cartilage
Posterior cricoarytenoid muscle
Thyroid gland
Inferior laryngeal artery
Superior parathyroid gland
Tracheal branches, inferior laryngeal artery
Inferior parathyroid gland
Inferior thyroid artery
Tracheal branches, recurrent laryngeal nerve
Recurrent laryngeal nerve
Trachea

Figure 595 **Posterior View of the Larynx, Tongue and Thyroid Gland, Vessels, and Nerves**

NOTE: (1) The **glossopharyngeal nerves (IX)** enter the root or pharyngeal part of the tongue to supply the posterior third of the surface of the tongue with both general sensation and the special sense of taste. Note also the **tonsillar branch** of the **ascending palatine artery** (from facial artery) supplying the palatine tonsil.

(2) The course of the **internal branch** of the **superior laryngeal nerve.** It is sensory to the laryngeal mucous membrane on the interior of the larynx as far down as the vocal folds.

(3) The **recurrent laryngeal nerve** is the principal motor nerve to the larynx, and it supplies all of the laryngeal muscles *except* the cricothyroid muscle (which is supplied by the external branch of the superior laryngeal nerve). In addition, the recurrent laryngeal nerve supplies sensory innervation to the interior of the larynx below the vocal folds.

(4) The **important relationship** of the recurrent laryngeal nerves to the inferior thyroid artery and its inferior laryngeal branches. Observe also the proximity of the recurrent laryngeal nerves to the posterior aspect of the thyroid glands.

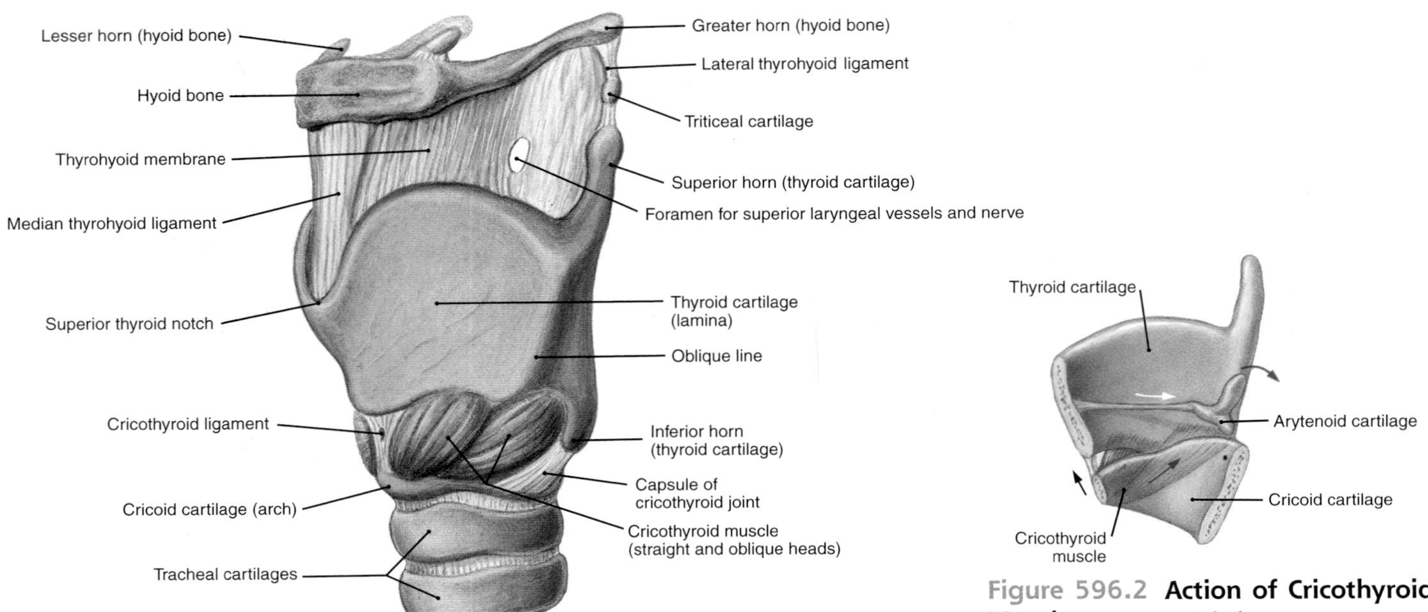
Lesser horn (hyoid bone)
Hyoid bone
Thyrohyoid membrane
Median thyrohyoid ligament
Superior thyroid notch
Cricothyroid ligament
Cricoid cartilage (arch)
Tracheal cartilages
Greater horn (hyoid bone)
Lateral thyrohyoid ligament
Triticeal cartilage
Superior horn (thyroid cartilage)
Foramen for superior laryngeal vessels and nerve
Thyroid cartilage (lamina)
Oblique line
Inferior horn (thyroid cartilage)
Capsule of cricothyroid joint
Cricothyroid muscle (straight and oblique heads)
Thyroid cartilage
Arytenoid cartilage
Cricoid cartilage
Cricothyroid muscle

Figure 596.2 Action of Cricothyroid Muscle: See NOTE 2 below.

Figure 596.1 Ventrolateral View of the Exterior Larynx and the Cricothyroid Muscle

NOTE: (1) The **cricothyroid muscle** consists of **straight** and **oblique** heads. The straight head is more vertical and inserts onto the lower border of the lamina of the thyroid cartilage, while the oblique head is more horizontal and inserts onto the inferior horn of the thyroid cartilage.

(2) The cricothyroid muscle tilts the anterior part of the cricoid cartilage upward. In so doing, the arytenoid cartilages (which are attached to the cricoid) are pulled dorsally. In addition, the thyroid cartilage is pulled forward and downward. These actions increase the distance between the arytenoid and thyroid cartilages, thereby increasing the tension of and elongating the vocal folds (see insert diagram above).

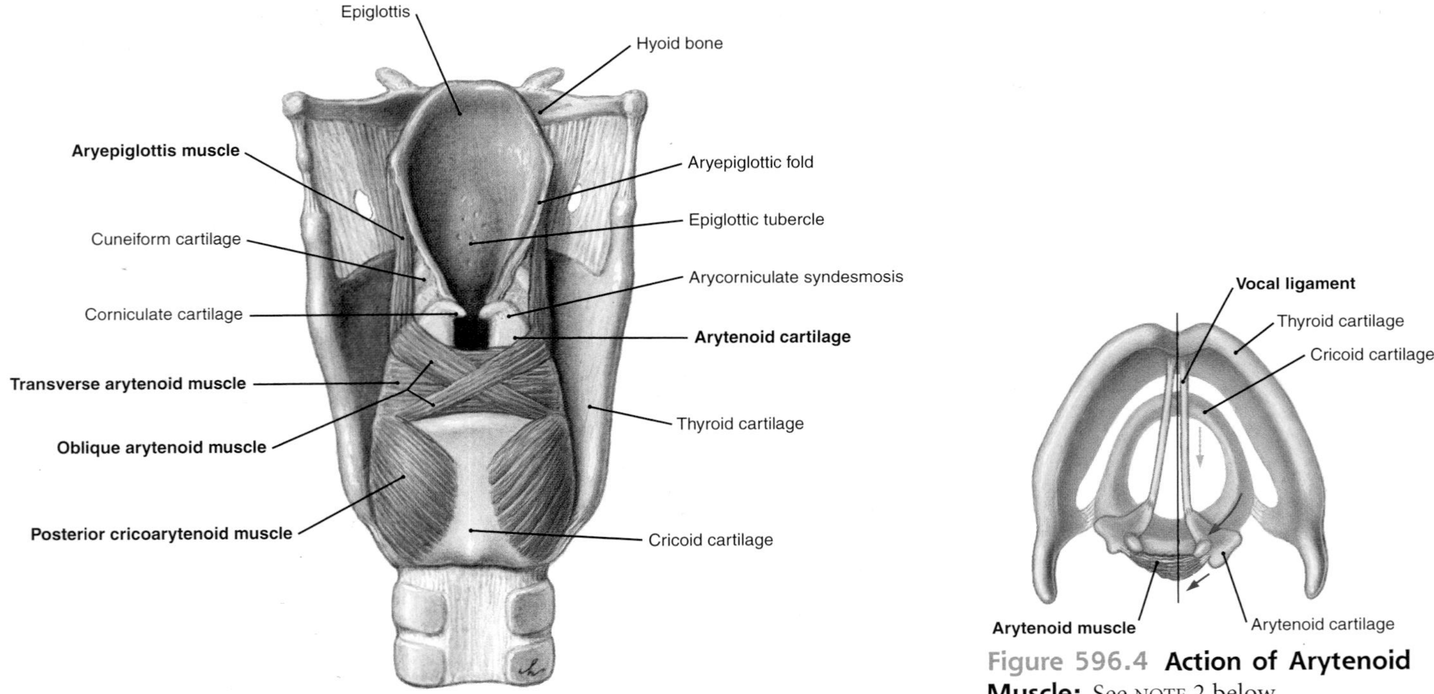
Epiglottis
Hyoid bone
Aryepiglottis muscle
Cuneiform cartilage
Corniculate cartilage
Transverse arytenoid muscle
Oblique arytenoid muscle
Posterior cricoarytenoid muscle
Aryepiglottic fold
Epiglottic tubercle
Arycorniculate syndesmosis
Arytenoid cartilage
Thyroid cartilage
Cricoid cartilage
Vocal ligament
Thyroid cartilage
Cricoid cartilage
Arytenoid muscle
Arytenoid cartilage

Figure 596.4 Action of Arytenoid Muscle: See NOTE 2 below.

Figure 596.3 Posterior View of the Larynx: Muscles

NOTE: (1) The **arytenoid muscle** consists of a **transverse portion** that spans the zone between the arytenoid cartilages, and an **oblique portion** that consists of muscular fascicles that cross posterior to the transverse fibers. Each of the fascicles of the oblique part extends from the base of the one arytenoid cartilage to the apex of the other cartilage. Some oblique fibers continue to the epiglottis as the **aryepiglottic muscle.**

(2) The transverse arytenoid approximates the arytenoid cartilages closing the posterior part of the rima glottis. The oblique arytenoid and the aryepiglottic muscles tend to close the inlet into the larynx by pulling the aryepiglottic folds together and approximating the arytenoid cartilages and epiglottis.

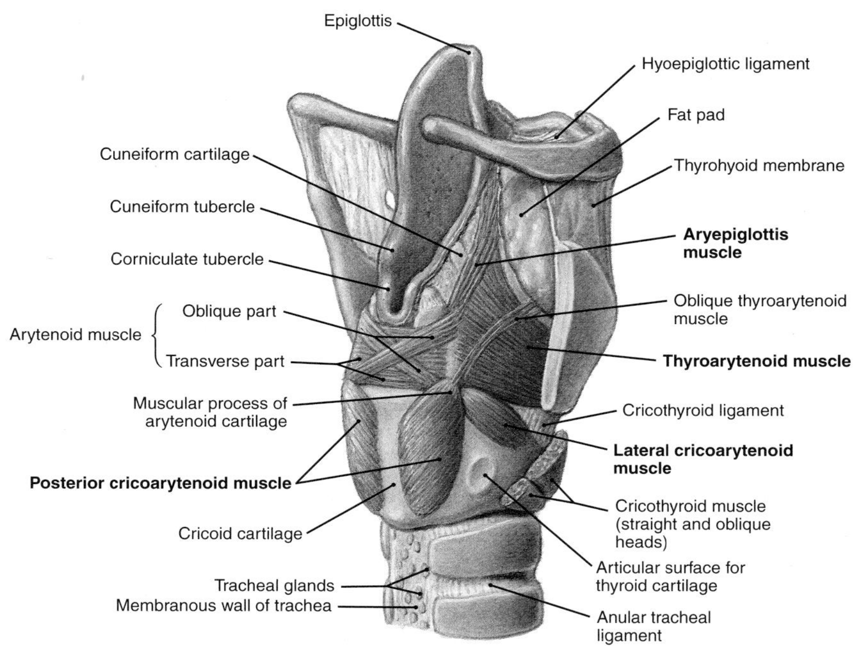
Epiglottis
Hyoepiglottic ligament
Fat pad
Thyrohyoid membrane
Cuneiform cartilage
Cuneiform tubercle
Corniculate tubercle
Aryepiglottis muscle
Arytenoid muscle
Oblique part
Transverse part
Oblique thyroarytenoid muscle
Thyroarytenoid muscle
Muscular process of arytenoid cartilage
Cricothyroid ligament
Lateral cricoarytenoid muscle
Posterior cricoarytenoid muscle
Cricothyroid muscle (straight and oblique heads)
Cricoid cartilage
Articular surface for thyroid cartilage
Tracheal glands
Membranous wall of trachea
Anular tracheal ligament

Figure 597.1 **Posterolateral View of the Laryngeal Muscles**

NOTE: (1) The right lamina of the thyroid cartilage and the thyrohyoid membrane have been partially cut away to expose the lateral cricoarytenoid and thyroarytenoid muscles.

(2) The **posterior cricoarytenoid muscle** extends from the lamina of the cricoid cartilage to the muscular process of the arytenoid cartilage, while the **lateral cricoarytenoid muscle** arises laterally from the arch of the cricoid cartilage and inserts with the posterior cricoarytenoid muscle onto the arytenoid cartilage.

(3) The posterior cricoarytenoids are the only **abductors** of the vocal folds, while the lateral cricoarytenoids act as antagonists, and **adduct** the vocal folds. The posterior muscle abducts by pulling the base of the arytenoid cartilages medially and posteriorly, while the lateral muscle adducts by pulling these same cartilages anteriorly and laterally.

(4) The **thyroarytenoid muscle** is a thin sheet of muscle radiating from the thyroid cartilage backward toward the arytenoid cartilage. Its upper fibers continue to the epiglottis and, joining the aryepiglottic fibers, become the **thyroepiglottic muscle.** Its deepest and most medial fibers form the **vocalis muscle** which is attached to the lateral aspect of the vocal fold. The thyroarytenoid muscles draw the arytenoid cartilages toward the thyroid cartilage and, thus shorten (relax) the vocal folds.

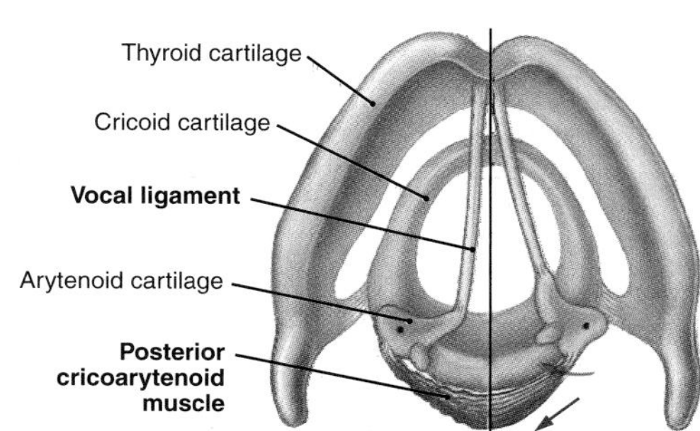
Thyroid cartilage
Cricoid cartilage
Vocal ligament
Arytenoid cartilage
Posterior cricoarytenoid muscle

Figure 597.2 **Action of Posterior Cricoarytenoid:** See NOTE 3 below.

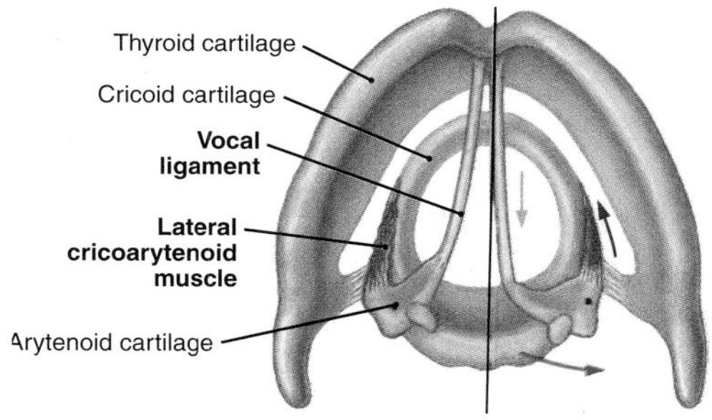
Thyroid cartilage
Cricoid cartilage
Vocal ligament
Lateral cricoarytenoid muscle
Arytenoid cartilage

Figure 597.3 **Action of Lateral Cricoarytenoid:** See NOTE 3 below.

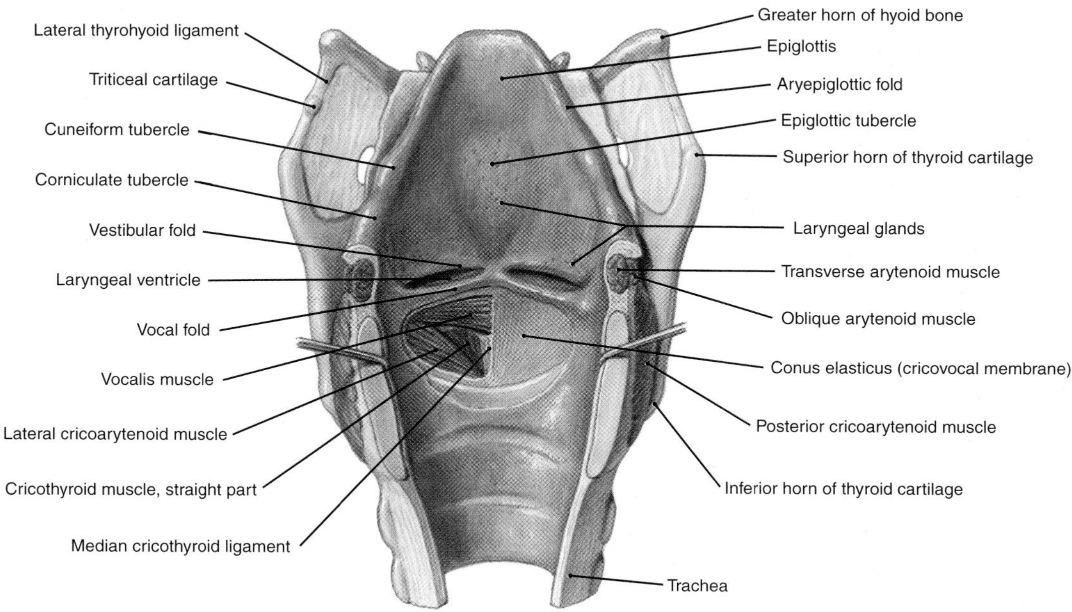
Lateral thyrohyoid ligament
Triticeal cartilage
Cuneiform tubercle
Corniculate tubercle
Vestibular fold
Laryngeal ventricle
Vocal fold
Vocalis muscle
Lateral cricoarytenoid muscle
Cricothyroid muscle, straight part
Median cricothyroid ligament
Greater horn of hyoid bone
Epiglottis
Aryepiglottic fold
Epiglottic tubercle
Superior horn of thyroid cartilage
Laryngeal glands
Transverse arytenoid muscle
Oblique arytenoid muscle
Conus elasticus (cricovocal membrane)
Posterior cricoarytenoid muscle
Inferior horn of thyroid cartilage
Trachea

Figure 597.4 **Larynx Opened from Behind (Posterior View)**

NOTE: The lateral walls of the larynx have been opened widely, and the left part of the conus elasticus has been removed.

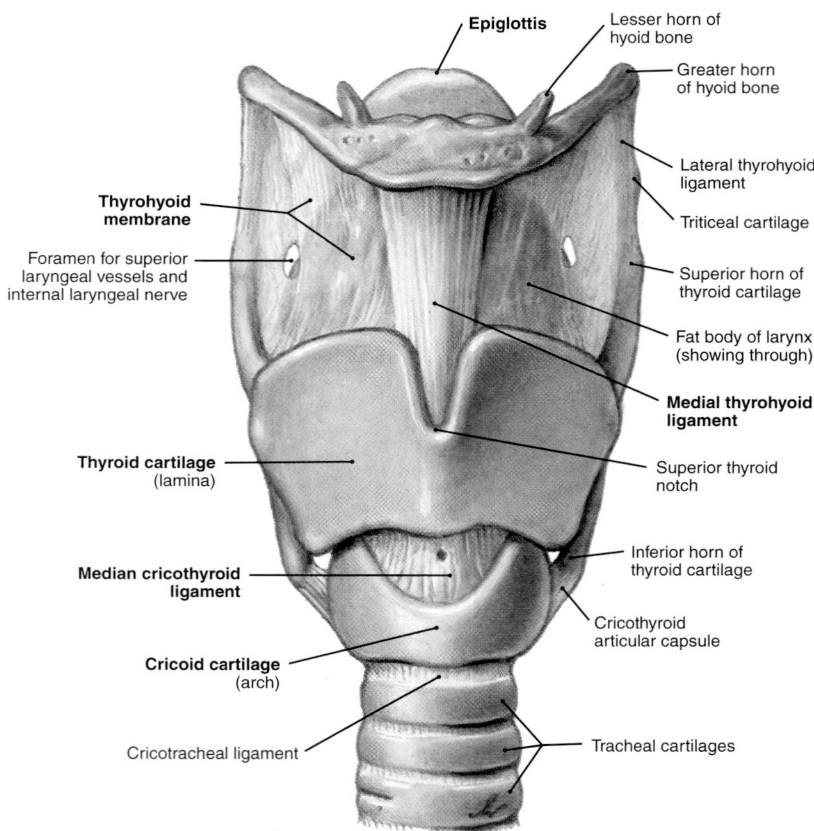
Epiglottis
Lesser horn of hyoid bone
Greater horn of hyoid bone
Lateral thyrohyoid ligament
Thyrohyoid membrane
Triticeal cartilage
Foramen for superior laryngeal vessels and internal laryngeal nerve
Superior horn of thyroid cartilage
Fat body of larynx (showing through)
Medial thyrohyoid ligament
Thyroid cartilage (lamina)
Superior thyroid notch
Inferior horn of thyroid cartilage
Median cricothyroid ligament
Cricothyroid articular capsule
Cricoid cartilage (arch)
Cricotracheal ligament
Tracheal cartilages

Figure 598.1 Cartilages and Ligaments of the Larynx (Ventral View)

NOTE: (1) The laryngeal cartilages form the skeleton of the larynx, and they are interconnected by ligaments and membranes. There are three larger **unpaired** cartilages (**cricoid, thyroid,** and **epiglottis**) and three sets of **paired** cartilages (**arytenoid, corniculate,** and **cuneiform**). In this anterior view, the unpaired cricoid, thyroid, and epiglottis are all visible.

(2) The **thyrohyoid membrane** and the centrally located thyrohyoid ligament. Attached to the upper border of the thyroid cartilage, this membrane stretches across the posterior surfaces of the greater horns of the hyoid bone. The medial thyrohyoid ligament extends from the thyroid notch to the body of the hyoid bone. The membrane is pierced by the **superior laryngeal vessels** and the **internal laryngeal branch of the superior laryngeal nerve.**

(3) The **cricothyroid ligament** attaches the apposing margins of the cricoid and thyroid cartilages. This ligament underlies the cricothyroid muscles.

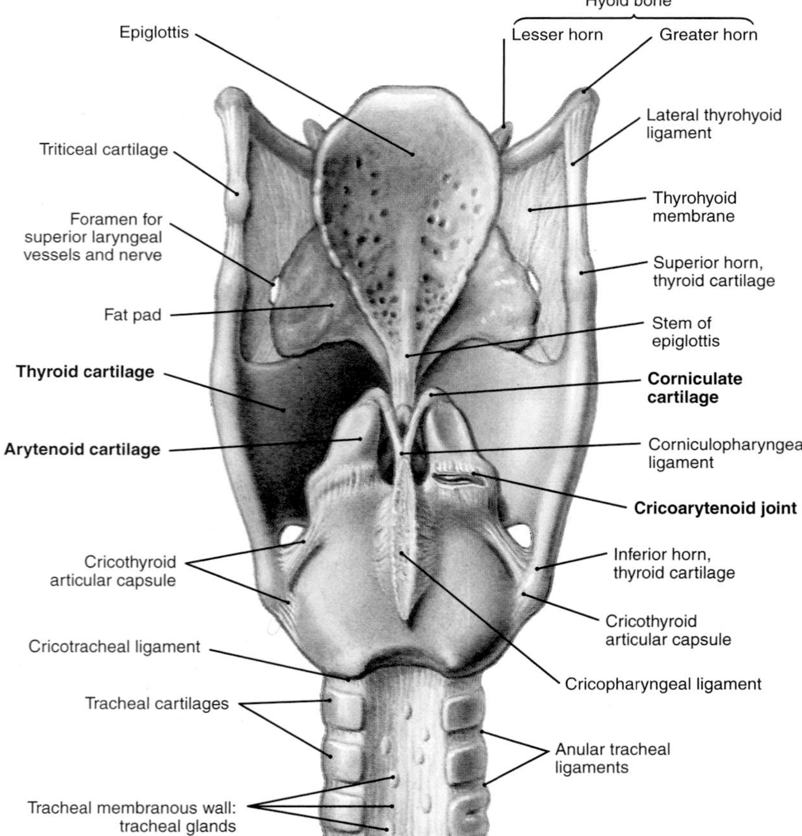
Hyoid bone
Lesser horn
Greater horn
Epiglottis
Lateral thyrohyoid ligament
Triticeal cartilage
Thyrohyoid membrane
Foramen for superior laryngeal vessels and nerve
Superior horn, thyroid cartilage
Fat pad
Stem of epiglottis
Thyroid cartilage
Corniculate cartilage
Arytenoid cartilage
Corniculopharyngeal ligament
Cricoarytenoid joint
Inferior horn, thyroid cartilage
Cricothyroid articular capsule
Cricothyroid articular capsule
Cricotracheal ligament
Cricopharyngeal ligament
Tracheal cartilages
Anular tracheal ligaments
Tracheal membranous wall: tracheal glands

Figure 598.2 Cartilages and Ligaments of the Larynx (Dorsal View)

NOTE: (1) The articulation of the paired arytenoid cartilages with the cricoid cartilage below. These synovial cricoarytenoid joints are surrounded by articular capsules and strengthened by the posterior cricoarytenoid ligaments.

(2) The cricoarytenoid joints allow for: (a) **rotation of the arytenoid cartilage** on an axis that is nearly vertical and (b) the **horizontal gliding movement** of the arytenoid cartilages.

(3) Rotation of the arytenoid cartilages results in medial or lateral displacement of the vocal folds, thereby increasing or decreasing the size of the opening between the folds, the **rima glottis.**

(4) Horizontal gliding of the arytenoid cartilages permits the bases of these cartilages to be approximated or moved apart. Medial rotation and medial gliding of the arytenoid cartilages occur simultaneously, as do the two lateral movements.

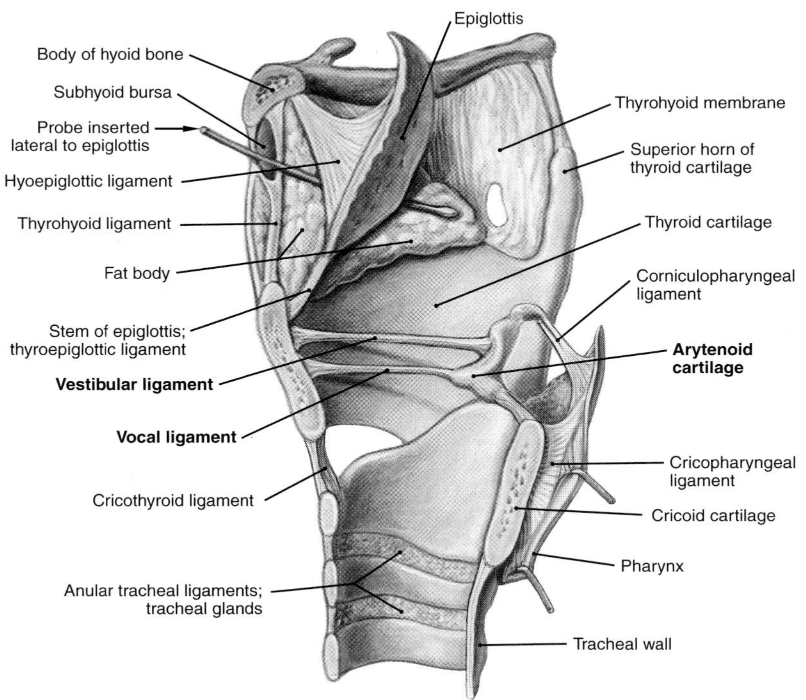

Epiglottis
Body of hyoid bone
Subhyoid bursa
Probe inserted lateral to epiglottis
Hyoepiglottic ligament
Thyrohyoid ligament
Fat body
Stem of epiglottis; thyroepiglottic ligament
Vestibular ligament
Vocal ligament
Cricothyroid ligament
Anular tracheal ligaments; tracheal glands
Thyrohyoid membrane
Superior horn of thyroid cartilage
Thyroid cartilage
Corniculopharyngeal ligament
Arytenoid cartilage
Cricopharyngeal ligament
Cricoid cartilage
Pharynx
Tracheal wall

Figure 599.1 Right Half of the Larynx Showing the Cartilages and Vestibular and Vocal Ligaments

NOTE: (1) The **vestibular ligament** is a compact band of fibrous tissue attached anteriorly to the thyroid cartilage and posteriorly to the anterior and lateral surface of the arytenoid cartilage. It is enclosed by mucous membrane to form the vestibular fold (or false vocal fold).

(2) The **vocal ligament** consists of elastic tissue and is attached anteriorly to the thyroid cartilage and posteriorly to the vocal process of the arytenoid cartilage. It, too, is covered by mucous membrane, which, along with the vocalis muscle forms the vocal fold. Laryngeal sounds are produced by oscillations of the vocal folds initiated by puffs of air.

Figure 599.2 Vocal Ligaments and Conus Elasticus (Seen from Above)

NOTE: (1) The **conus elasticus** is a membrane consisting principally of yellow elastic fibers; it interconnects the thyroid, cricoid, and arytenoid cartilages. It underlies the mucous membrane below the vocal folds and is overlaid to some extent by the thyroarytenoid and cricothyroid muscles on the exterior of the larynx.

(2) The symmetry of the arytenoid cartilages and their related vocal ligaments.

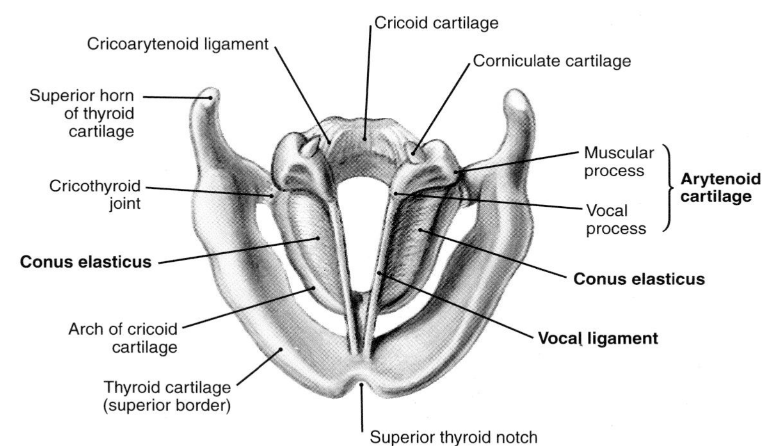

Cricoid cartilage
Cricoarytenoid ligament
Corniculate cartilage
Superior horn of thyroid cartilage
Cricothyroid joint
Conus elasticus
Arch of cricoid cartilage
Thyroid cartilage (superior border)
Superior thyroid notch
Muscular process
Vocal process
Arytenoid cartilage
Conus elasticus
Vocal ligament

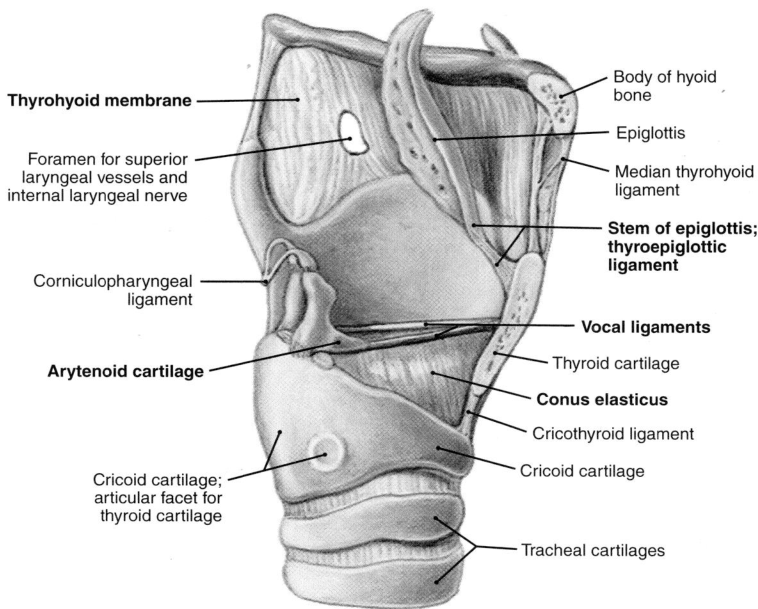

Thyrohyoid membrane
Foramen for superior laryngeal vessels and internal laryngeal nerve
Corniculopharyngeal ligament
Arytenoid cartilage
Cricoid cartilage; articular facet for thyroid cartilage
Body of hyoid bone
Epiglottis
Median thyrohyoid ligament
Stem of epiglottis; thyroepiglottic ligament
Vocal ligaments
Thyroid cartilage
Conus elasticus
Cricothyroid ligament
Cricoid cartilage
Tracheal cartilages

Figure 599.3 Upper Left Part of the Larynx

NOTE: (1) The right halves of the hyoid bone, epiglottis, and thyroid cartilage have been removed to open the upper left portion of the larynx. The two vocal ligaments, the arytenoid cartilages, and the conus elasticus are also displayed.

(2) The attachment of the stem of the epiglottis to the thyroid cartilage by means of the thyroepiglottic ligament.

(3) The conus elasticus as it forms the vocal ligament and attaches to the arytenoid, thyroid, and cricoid cartilages.

(4) Although sounds are initiated at the vocal folds, the pitch, range, quality, volume, tone, and overtones of the human voice also incorporate structures in the mouth (tongue, teeth, and palate), nasal sinuses, pharynx, rest of the larynx, lungs, diaphragm, and abdominal muscles.

Larynx (Frontal and Midsagittal Sections)

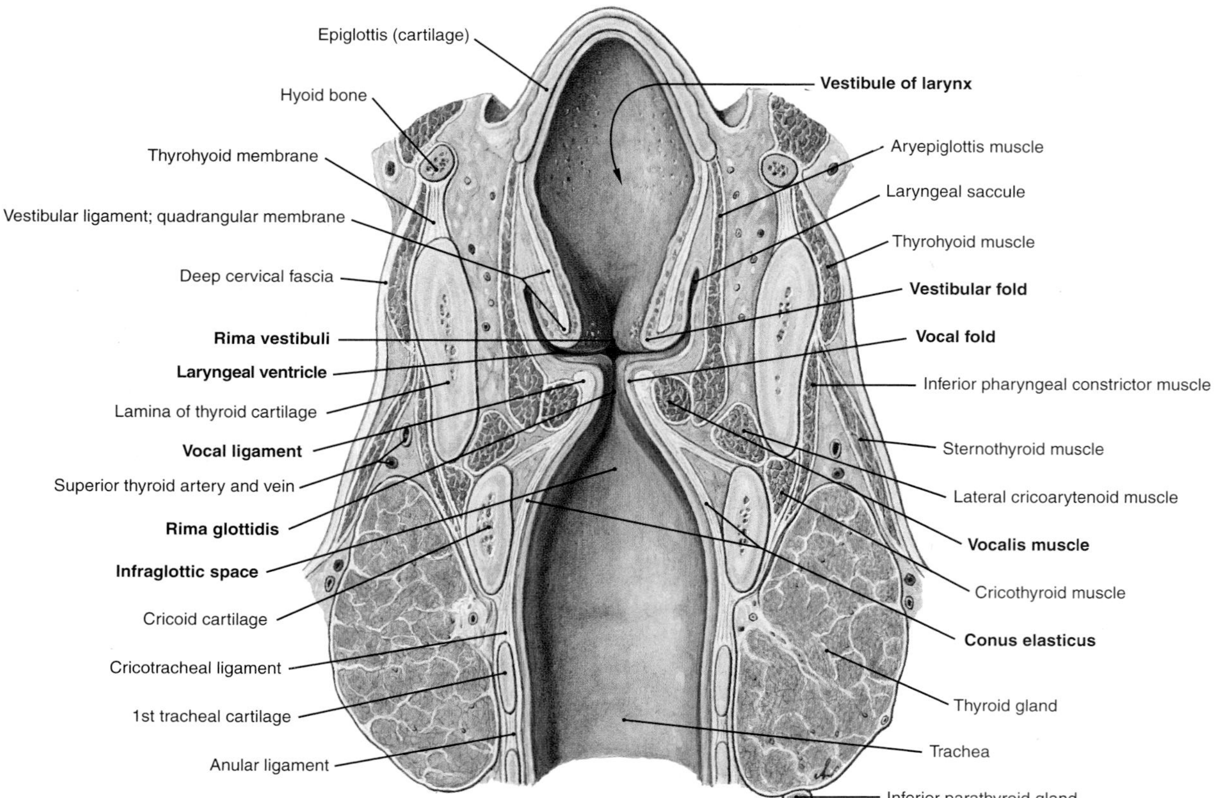

Epiglottis (cartilage)
Hyoid bone
Thyrohyoid membrane
Vestibular ligament; quadrangular membrane
Deep cervical fascia
Rima vestibuli
Laryngeal ventricle
Lamina of thyroid cartilage
Vocal ligament
Superior thyroid artery and vein
Rima glottidis
Infraglottic space
Cricoid cartilage
Cricotracheal ligament
1st tracheal cartilage
Anular ligament
Vestibule of larynx
Aryepiglottis muscle
Laryngeal saccule
Thyrohyoid muscle
Vestibular fold
Vocal fold
Inferior pharyngeal constrictor muscle
Sternothyroid muscle
Lateral cricoarytenoid muscle
Vocalis muscle
Cricothyroid muscle
Conus elasticus
Thyroid gland
Trachea
Inferior parathyroid gland

Figure 600.1 **Frontal Section through the Larynx Showing the Laryngeal Folds and Cavities in Its Anterior Half**

NOTE: (1) The paired **vocal folds** consist of mucous membrane overlying the **vocal ligaments** and **vocalis muscles.** Just superior to the vocal folds observe the **vestibular folds,** which are separated from the vocal folds by a recess called the **laryngeal ventricle** (or sinus).

(2) Above the vestibular folds is the **vestibule** of the larynx, which lies just below the laryngeal inlet. Below the vocal folds is the **infraglottic space,** which communicates with the trachea below and is limited above by the **rima glottis** between the two vocal folds.

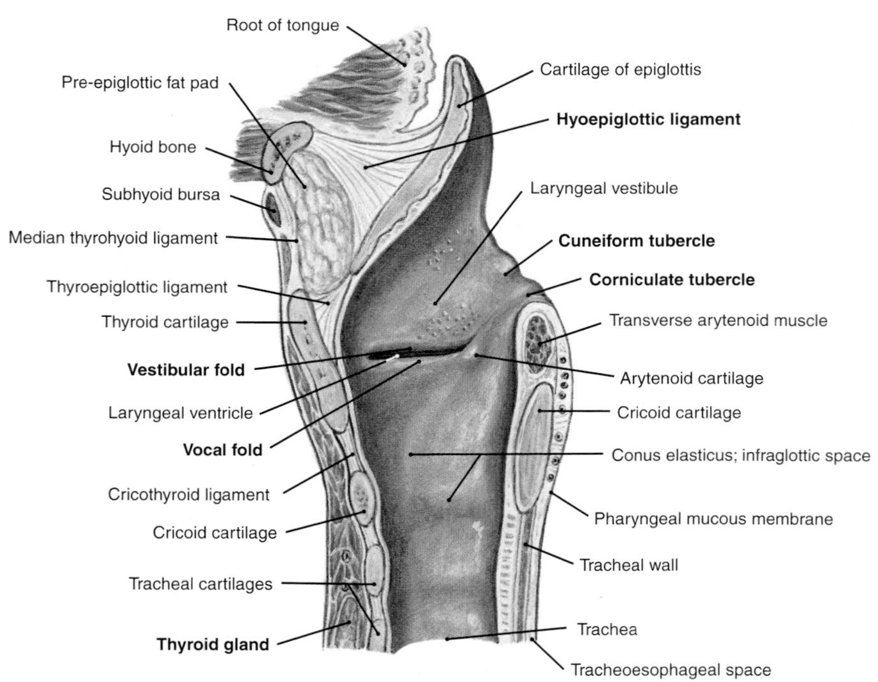

Root of tongue
Pre-epiglottic fat pad
Hyoid bone
Subhyoid bursa
Median thyrohyoid ligament
Thyroepiglottic ligament
Thyroid cartilage
Vestibular fold
Laryngeal ventricle
Vocal fold
Cricothyroid ligament
Cricoid cartilage
Tracheal cartilages
Thyroid gland
Cartilage of epiglottis
Hyoepiglottic ligament
Laryngeal vestibule
Cuneiform tubercle
Corniculate tubercle
Transverse arytenoid muscle
Arytenoid cartilage
Cricoid cartilage
Conus elasticus; infraglottic space
Pharyngeal mucous membrane
Tracheal wall
Trachea
Tracheoesophageal space

Figure 600.2 **Midsagittal Section of Larynx**

NOTE: (1) The laryngeal inlet leads to the laryngeal vestibule, the anterior border of which is the epiglottis. The **aryepiglottic folds,** marked by oval elevations (cuneiform and corniculate cartilages), define the borders of the laryngeal inlet.

(2) The epiglottis attaches **superiorly** to the hyoid bone (by the hyoepiglottic ligament); **inferiorly** to the thyroid cartilage (by the thyroepiglottic ligament); and **laterally** to the arytenoid cartilages (by the aryepiglottic folds).

Figure 601.1 Cross Section of Larynx at the Vocal Folds

NOTE: (1) The orientation of the arytenoid cartilages and their articulations with the cricoid cartilage.

(2) The vocal folds consist of mucous membrane over the vocal ligaments, lateral to which extend the deeper part of the thyroarytenoid muscle.

(3) By drawing the arytenoid cartilages forward, the thyroarytenoids shorten and relax the vocal folds. At the same time, they medially rotate the arytenoid cartilages and, thus, approximate the vocal folds.

(4) The intercartilaginous part of the rima glottidis is bounded by the arytenoid and cricoid cartilages, while the intermembranous part is bounded by the vocal fold mucous membrane.

I = intermembranous part of the rima glottidis
II = intercartilaginous part of the rima glottidis

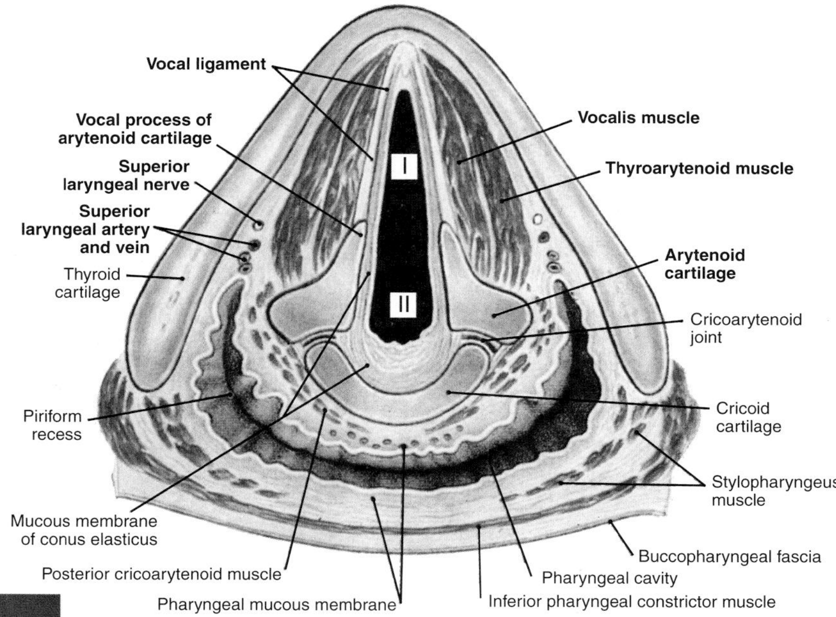
Vocal ligament
Vocal process of arytenoid cartilage
Superior laryngeal nerve
Superior laryngeal artery and vein
Thyroid cartilage
Piriform recess
Mucous membrane of conus elasticus
Posterior cricoarytenoid muscle
Pharyngeal mucous membrane
I
II
Vocalis muscle
Thyroarytenoid muscle
Arytenoid cartilage
Cricoarytenoid joint
Cricoid cartilage
Stylopharyngeus muscle
Buccopharyngeal fascia
Pharyngeal cavity
Inferior pharyngeal constrictor muscle

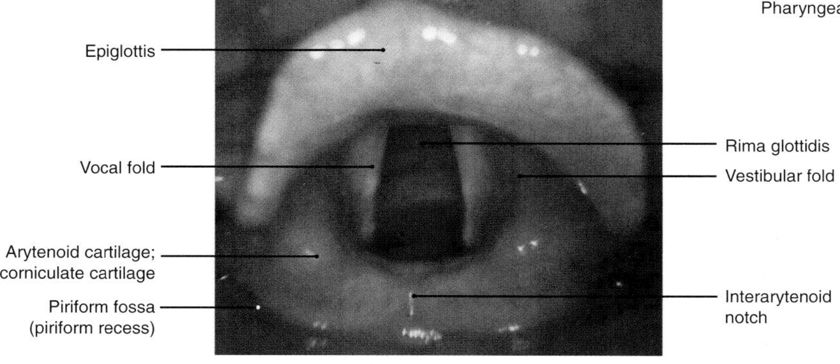
Epiglottis
Vocal fold
Arytenoid cartilage; corniculate cartilage
Piriform fossa (piriform recess)
Rima glottidis
Vestibular fold
Interarytenoid notch

Figure 601.2 Rima Glottidis in Forced or Deep Inspiration (Direct Laryngoscopy)

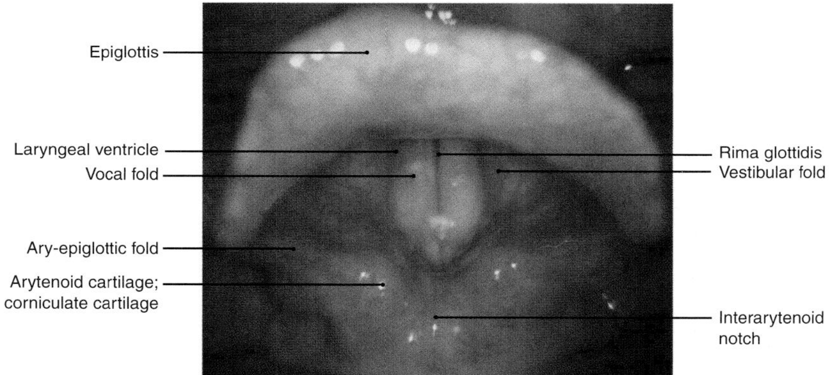
Epiglottis
Laryngeal ventricle
Vocal fold
Ary-epiglottic fold
Arytenoid cartilage; corniculate cartilage
Rima glottidis
Vestibular fold
Interarytenoid notch

Figure 601.3 Rima Glottidis during Shrill Tone Phonation (Direct Laryngoscopy)

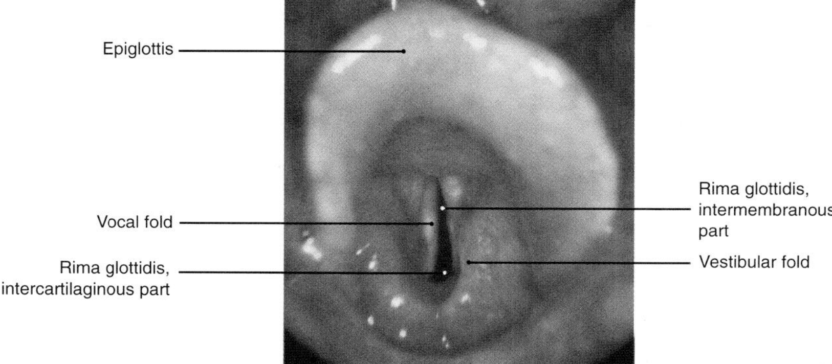
Epiglottis
Vocal fold
Rima glottidis, intercartilaginous part
Rima glottidis, intermembranous part
Vestibular fold

Figure 601.4 Rima Glottidis during Whispering: Intercartilaginous Part Open (Direct Laryngoscopy)

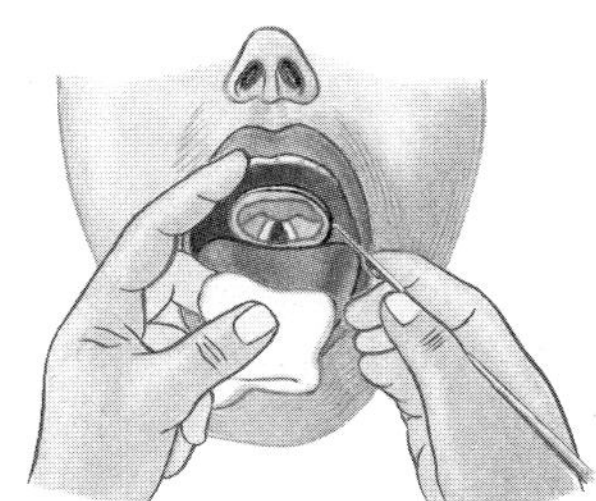

▲ **Figure 601.5 Indirect Laryngoscopy**

NOTE: Protraction of the tongue creates space for a laryngoscopic mirror so that the vocal folds can be visualized indirectly by their reflection in the mirror.

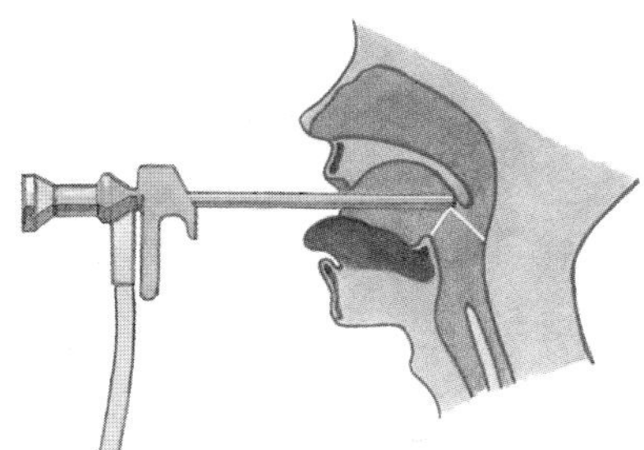

▲ **Figure 601.6 Direct Laryngoscopy**

NOTE: The use of an endoscope allows visualization of the vocal folds directly.

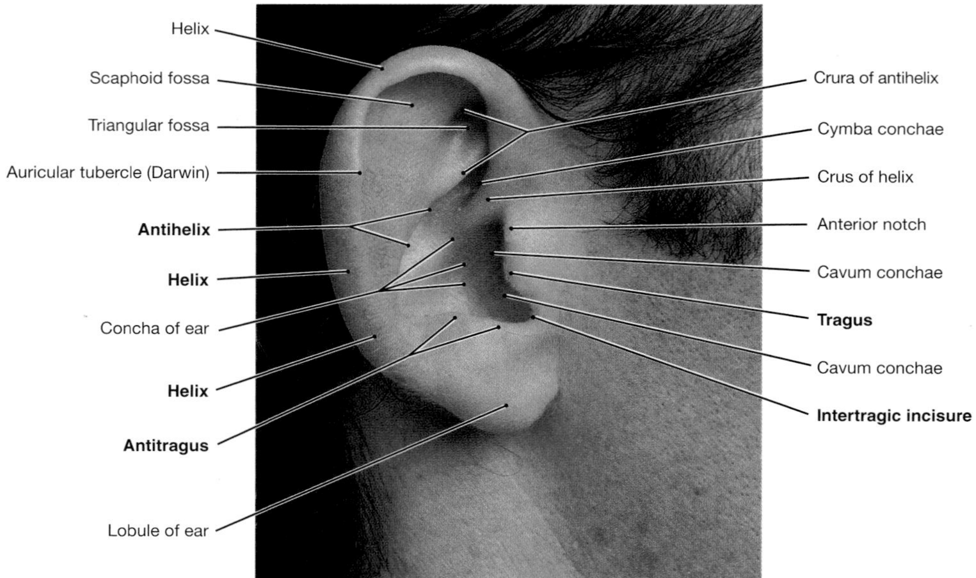
Helix
Scaphoid fossa
Triangular fossa
Auricular tubercle (Darwin)
Antihelix
Helix
Concha of ear
Helix
Antitragus
Lobule of ear
Crura of antihelix
Cymba conchae
Crus of helix
Anterior notch
Cavum conchae
Tragus
Cavum conchae
Intertragic incisure

Figure 602.1 Right External Ear (Lateral View)

NOTE: (1) The external ear (or auricle) consists of skin overlying an irregularly shaped elastic fibrocartilage. The ear lobe, or lobule, does not contain cartilage, but is soft and contains connective tissue and fat.

(2) The **external acoustic meatus** courses through the auricle to the tympanic membrane. It is an oval canal that extends for about 2.5 cm in an S-shaped curve to the tympanic membrane. It consists of an outer cartilaginous part (1 cm) and a narrower more medial part that is osseous (1.5 cm).

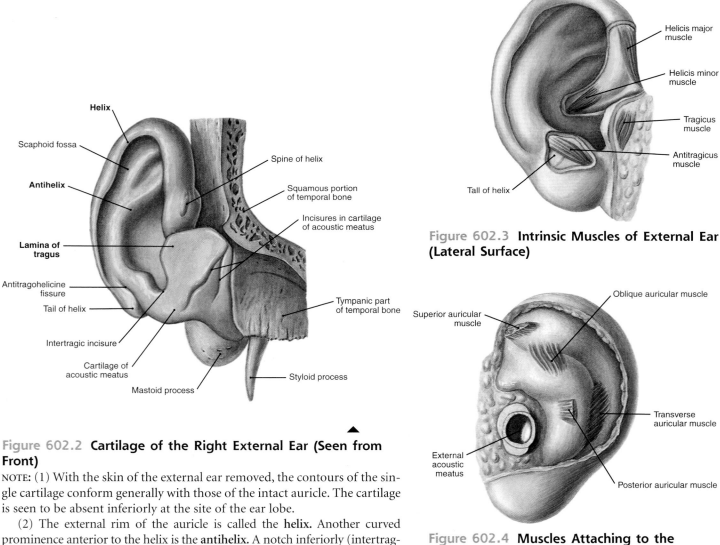

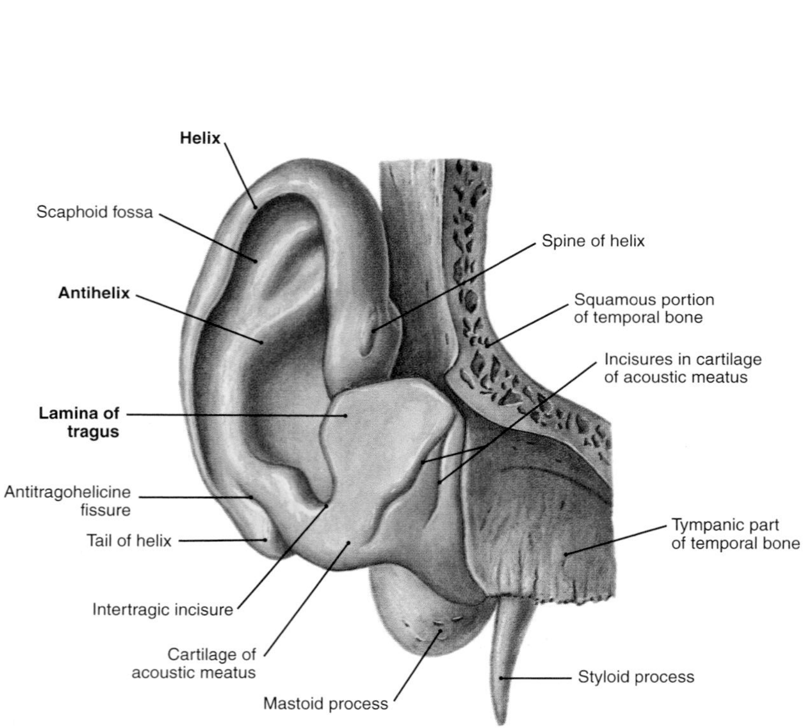
Helix
Scaphoid fossa
Antihelix
Lamina of tragus
Antitragohelicine fissure
Tail of helix
Intertragic incisure
Cartilage of acoustic meatus
Mastoid process
Spine of helix
Squamous portion of temporal bone
Incisures in cartilage of acoustic meatus
Tympanic part of temporal bone
Styloid process

Figure 602.2 Cartilage of the Right External Ear (Seen from Front)

NOTE: (1) With the skin of the external ear removed, the contours of the single cartilage conform generally with those of the intact auricle. The cartilage is seen to be absent inferiorly at the site of the ear lobe.

(2) The external rim of the auricle is called the **helix.** Another curved prominence anterior to the helix is the **antihelix.** A notch inferiorly (intertragic incisure) separates the **tragus** anteriorly from the **antitragus** posteriorly.

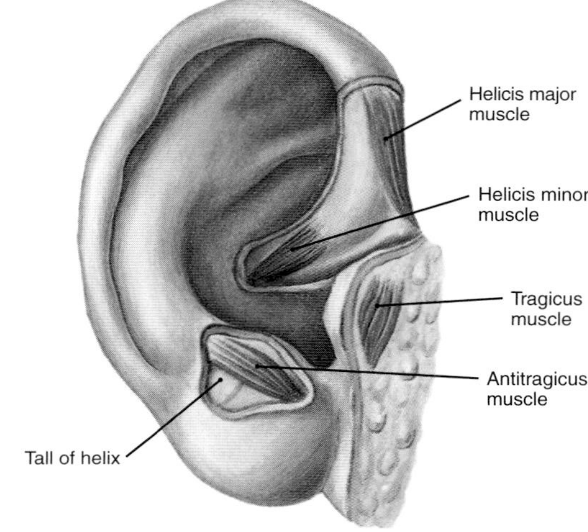
Helicis major muscle
Helicis minor muscle
Tragicus muscle
Antitragicus muscle
Tail of helix

Figure 602.3 Intrinsic Muscles of External Ear (Lateral Surface)

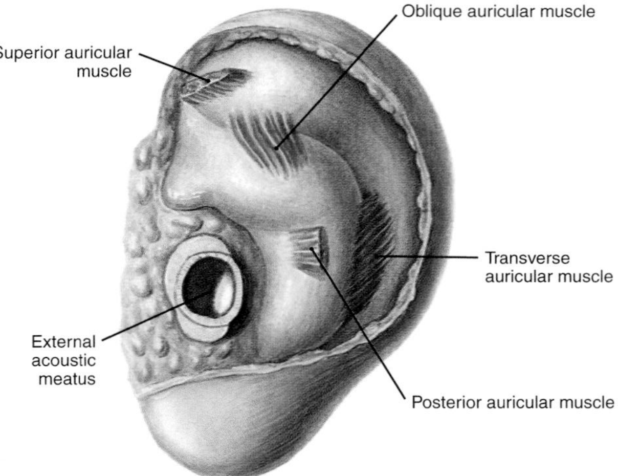
Oblique auricular muscle
Superior auricular muscle
Transverse auricular muscle
External acoustic meatus
Posterior auricular muscle

Figure 602.4 Muscles Attaching to the Medial Surface of External Ear

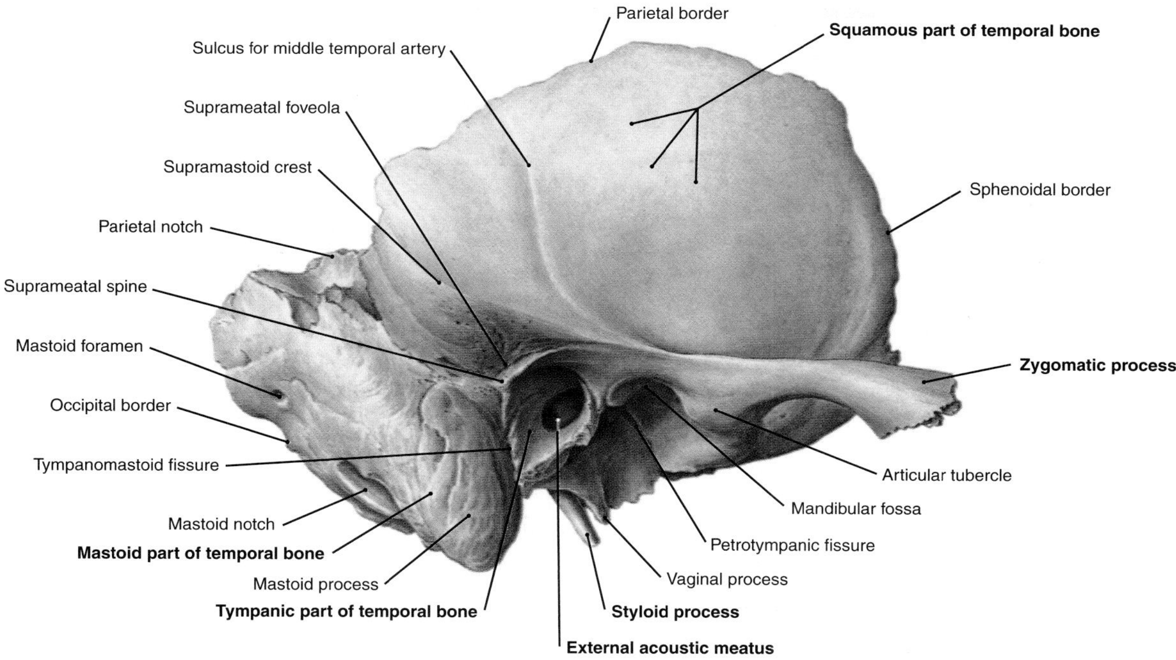
Parietal border
Squamous part of temporal bone
Sulcus for middle temporal artery
Suprameatal foveola
Supramastoid crest
Sphenoidal border
Parietal notch
Suprameatal spine
Mastoid foramen
Zygomatic process
Occipital border
Tympanomastoid fissure
Articular tubercle
Mandibular fossa
Mastoid notch
Mastoid part of temporal bone
Petrotympanic fissure
Mastoid process
Vaginal process
Tympanic part of temporal bone
Styloid process
External acoustic meatus

Figure 603.1 Right Temporal Bone (Lateral View)

NOTE: (1) The temporal bone forms the osseous encasement for the middle and internal ear and consists of three parts: **squamous, tympanic,** and **petrous.**

(2) The **squamous part** is broad in shape, and it is thin and flat. From it extends the zygomatic process. The **tympanic part** is interposed below the squamous and anterior to the petrous parts. The external acoustic meatus, which leads to the tympanic membrane, is surrounded by the tympanic part of the temporal bone.

(3) The hard **petrous part** contains the organ of hearing and the vestibular canals. Its mastoid process is not solid but contains many air cells, and its external surface affords attachment to several muscles.

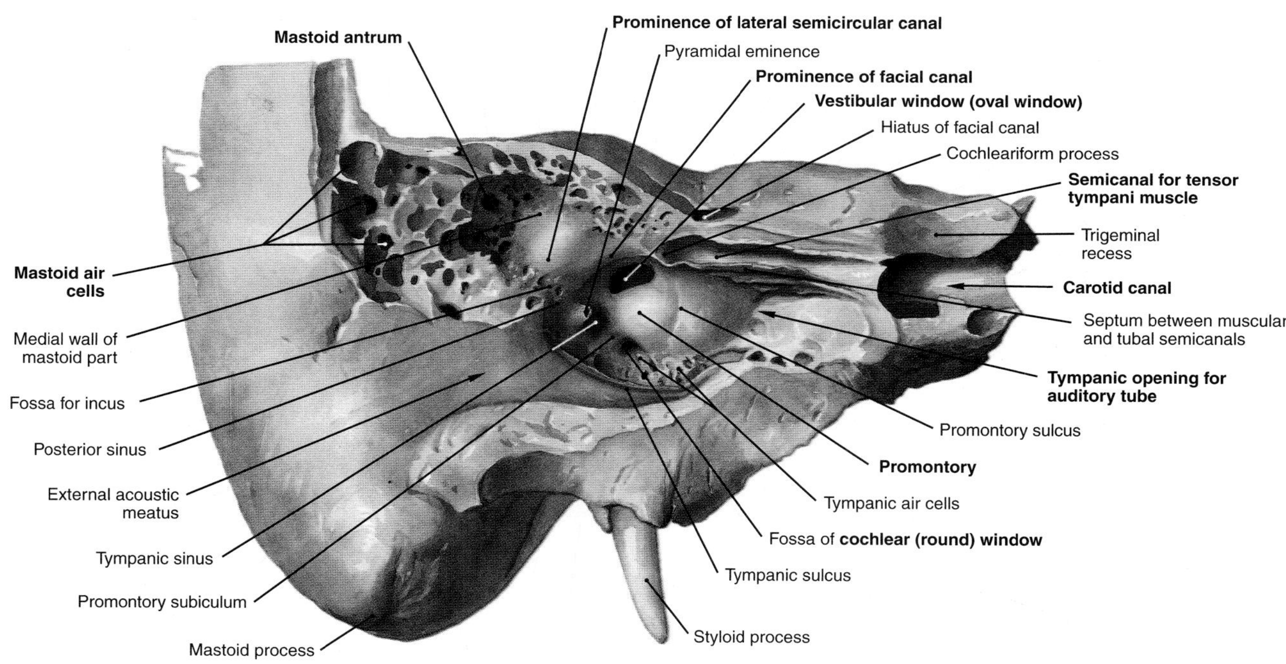
Prominence of lateral semicircular canal
Mastoid antrum
Pyramidal eminence
Prominence of facial canal
Vestibular window (oval window)
Hiatus of facial canal
Cochleariform process
Semicanal for tensor tympani muscle
Trigeminal recess
Mastoid air cells
Carotid canal
Septum between muscular and tubal semicanals
Medial wall of mastoid part
Tympanic opening for auditory tube
Fossa for incus
Promontory sulcus
Posterior sinus
Promontory
External acoustic meatus
Tympanic air cells
Fossa of cochlear (round) window
Tympanic sinus
Tympanic sulcus
Promontory subiculum
Styloid process
Mastoid process

Figure 603.2 Lateral Dissection of the Right Temporal Bone Showing the Tympanic Cavity

NOTE: (1) The tympanic cavity (middle ear) communicates posteriorly with the mastoid antrum and, in turn, with the mastoid air cells. It also is in communication with the nasopharynx by way of the auditory tube.

(2) The **lateral wall** of the tympanic cavity is formed by the tympanic membrane (not shown), while the **medial wall** (or labyrinthine wall) presents the following important structures: the **promontory** (projection of the first turn of the cochlea); the **vestibular window** (oval window); the **cochlear window** (round window); the bony prominence of the **facial canal;** and posteriorly, the prominence of the **lateral semicircular canal** and the **pyramidal eminence.**

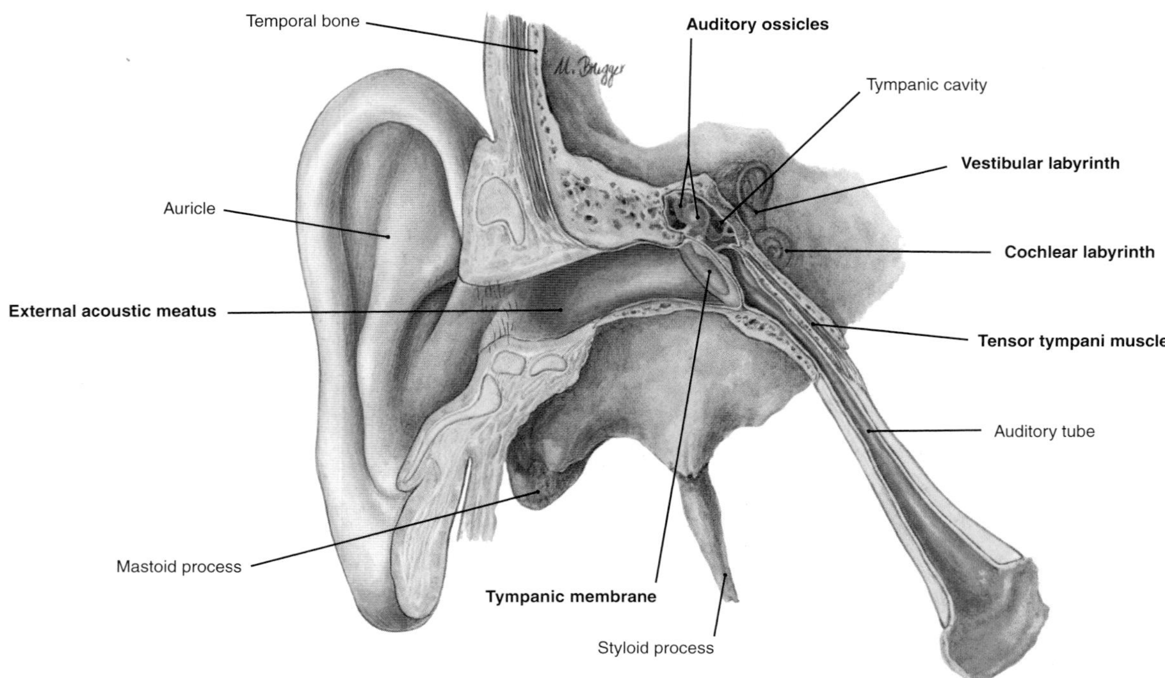
Temporal bone
Auditory ossicles
Tympanic cavity
Vestibular labyrinth
Auricle
Cochlear labyrinth
External acoustic meatus
Tensor tympani muscle
Auditory tube
Mastoid process
Tympanic membrane
Styloid process

Figure 604.1 **Frontal Section through the Right External, Middle, and Internal Ear**

NOTE: (1) The external acoustic meatus commences at the auricle and leads to the external surface of the tympanic membrane. Through the meatus course the sound waves that cause vibration of the tympanum.

(2) The **middle ear** (or tympanic cavity) contains three ossicles (malleus, incus, and stapes) and two muscles (tensor tympani and stapedius; the latter is not shown).

(3) The cavity of the middle ear communicates with the **mastoid antrum** and **mastoid air cells** posteriorly, and the nasopharynx by way of the **auditory tube**. This tube courses downward, forward, and medially from the middle ear.

(4) The ossicles interconnect the tympanic membrane with the inner ear. The inner ear contains the coiled **cochlea** (or organ of hearing) and the three **semicircular canals** (the vestibular organ) and their associated vessels and nerves.

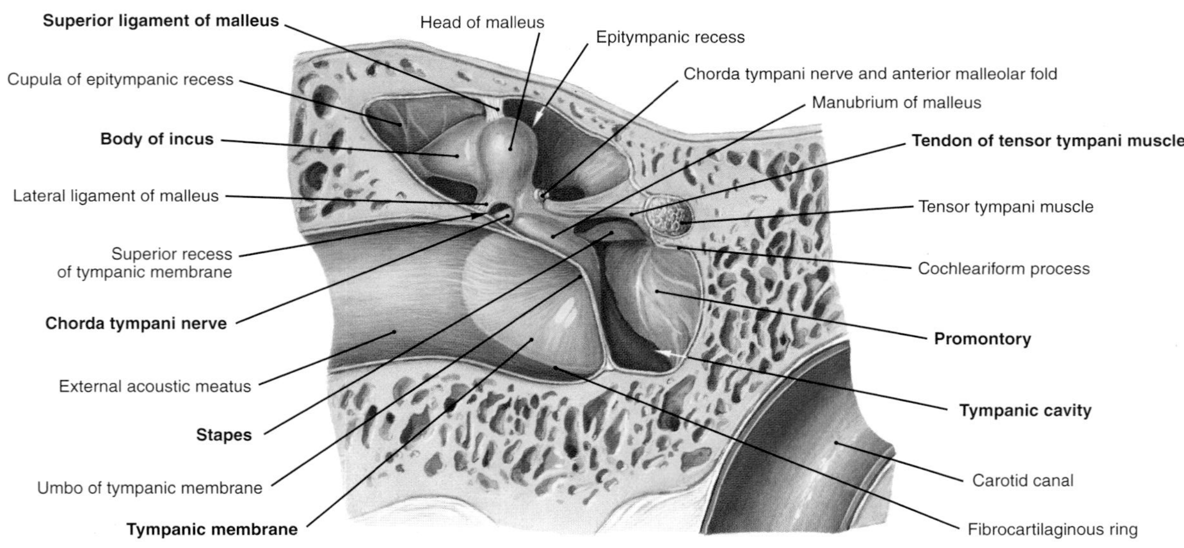
Superior ligament of malleus
Head of malleus
Epitympanic recess
Cupula of epitympanic recess
Chorda tympani nerve and anterior malleolar fold
Manubrium of malleus
Body of incus
Tendon of tensor tympani muscle
Lateral ligament of malleus
Tensor tympani muscle
Superior recess of tympanic membrane
Cochleariform process
Chorda tympani nerve
Promontory
External acoustic meatus
Tympanic cavity
Stapes
Carotid canal
Umbo of tympanic membrane
Tympanic membrane
Fibrocartilaginous ring

Figure 604.2 **Frontal Section through the Right External and Middle Ear**

NOTE: (1) The slender tendon of the *tensor tympani muscle* turns sharply upon reaching the tympanic cavity to terminate on the manubrium of the malleus.

(2) The tympanic cavity is extended superiorly by the epitympanic recess located above the level of the tympanic membrane. On the medial wall of the middle ear observe the promontory that protrudes into the tympanic cavity. This bony prominence is formed by the spiral cochlea of the internal ear.

(3) The lateral and superior ligaments attaching to the head of the malleus. The anterior ligament of the malleus, which interconnects the neck of the malleus to the anterior wall of the tympanic cavity, is not shown.

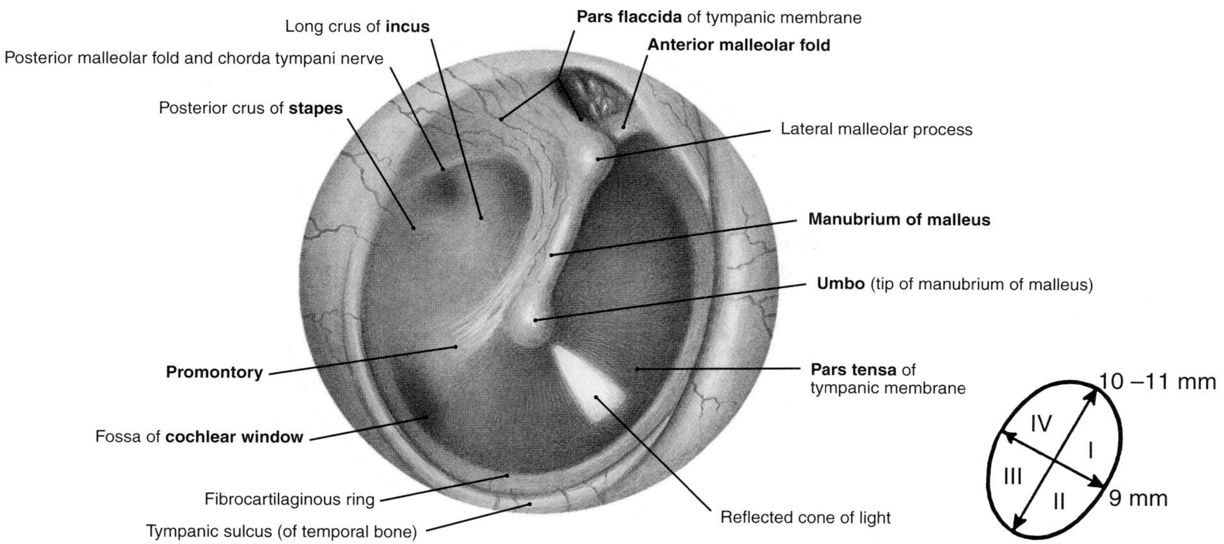
Long crus of incus
Posterior malleolar fold and chorda tympani nerve
Posterior crus of stapes
Pars flaccida of tympanic membrane
Anterior malleolar fold
Lateral malleolar process
Manubrium of malleus
Umbo (tip of manubrium of malleus)
Promontory
Pars tensa of tympanic membrane
Fossa of cochlear window
Fibrocartilaginous ring
Tympanic sulcus (of temporal bone)
Reflected cone of light
10 –11 mm
IV
I
III
II
9 mm

Figure 605.1 Right Tympanic Membrane as Seen with an Otoscope in a Living Person

NOTE: (1) The tympanic membrane is oval and measures about 9 mm across and from 10 to 11 mm vertically; it often is described as consisting of four quadrants (see lower inset diagram).

(2) The **anterior** and **posterior malleolar folds.** The more lax part (pars flaccida) of the tympanic membrane lies above and between these folds, while the rest is more tightly stretched (pars tensa).

(3) The blood supply of the membrane is derived from the **deep auricular** and **anterior tympanic branches** of the maxillary artery and the **stylomastoid branch** of the posterior auricular artery.

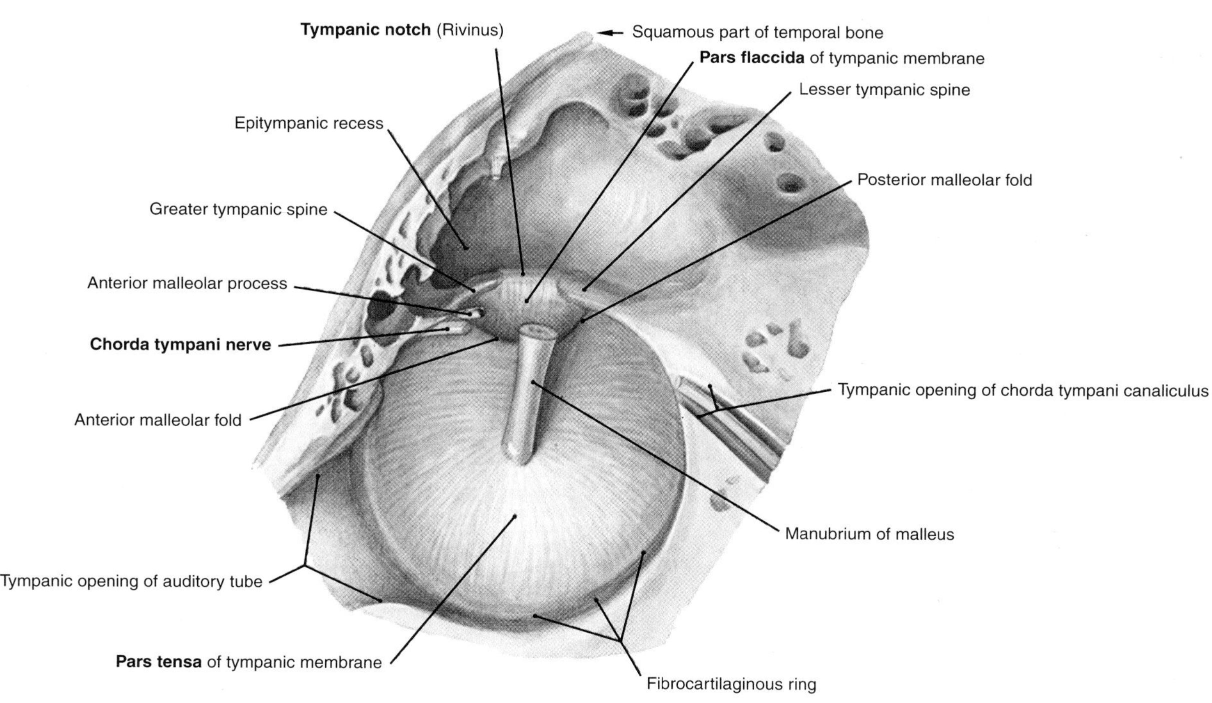
Tympanic notch (Rivinus)
Squamous part of temporal bone
Pars flaccida of tympanic membrane
Lesser tympanic spine
Epitympanic recess
Posterior malleolar fold
Greater tympanic spine
Anterior malleolar process
Chorda tympani nerve
Tympanic opening of chorda tympani canaliculus
Anterior malleolar fold
Manubrium of malleus
Tympanic opening of auditory tube
Pars tensa of tympanic membrane
Fibrocartilaginous ring

Figure 605.2 Lateral Wall of the Right Middle Ear (Tympanic Membrane Viewed from within the Tympanic Cavity)

NOTE: (1) The **manubrium** of the **malleus** has been severed from the remainder of the ossicle and left attached to the tympanic membrane. The fibrocartilaginous tympanic ring is deficient superiorly, forming the **tympanic notch** (of Rivinus). The looser portion of the tympanic membrane (**pars flaccida**) covers this zone.

(2) The tympanic membrane below the malleolar folds is the **pars tensa.** This portion is made taut by the **tensor tympani muscle,** which attaches to the manubrium of the malleus.

(3) The external surface of the tympanic membrane is innervated by the **auriculotemporal branch** of the mandibular nerve (V) and the **auricular branch** of the vagus nerve (X). The internal surface of the membrane is supplied by the **tympanic branch** of the glossopharyngeal nerve (IX).

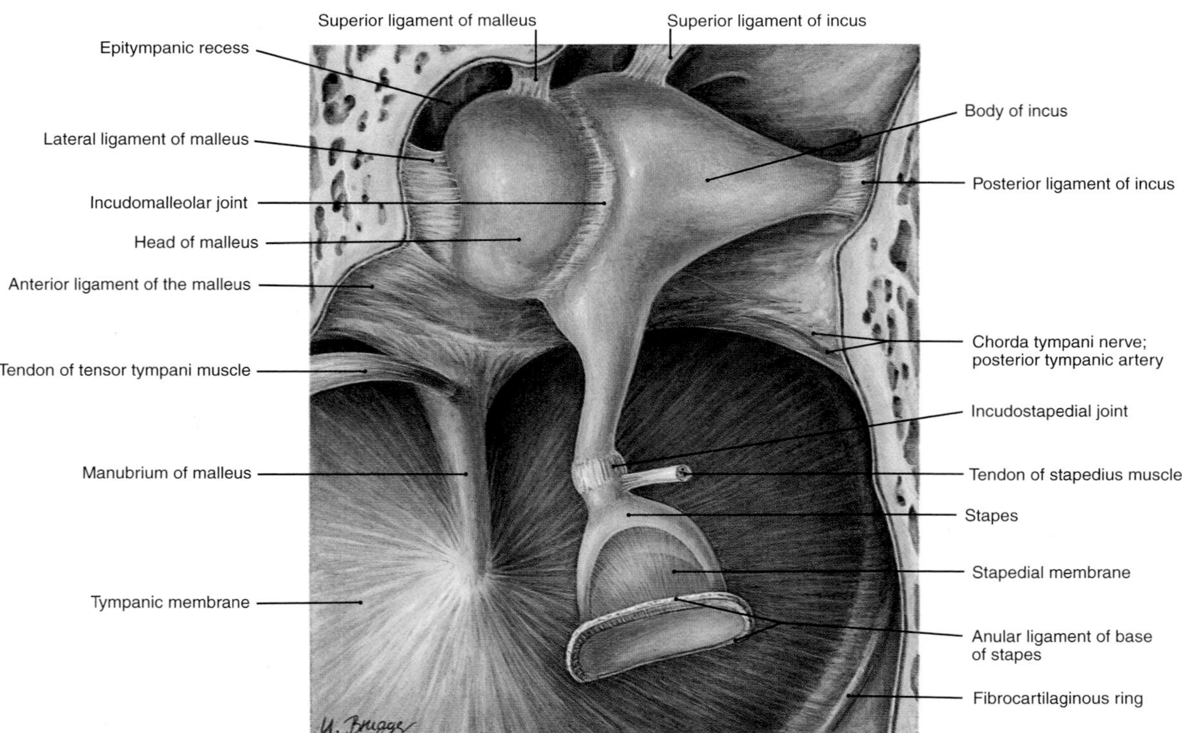
Superior ligament of malleus
Superior ligament of incus
Epitympanic recess
Body of incus
Lateral ligament of malleus
Posterior ligament of incus
Incudomalleolar joint
Head of malleus
Anterior ligament of the malleus
Chorda tympani nerve; posterior tympanic artery
Tendon of tensor tympani muscle
Incudostapedial joint
Manubrium of malleus
Tendon of stapedius muscle
Stapes
Stapedial membrane
Tympanic membrane
Anular ligament of base of stapes
Fibrocartilaginous ring
U. Brugger

Figure 606.1 Middle Ear Ossicles and Attachment of Muscle Tendons (Right Side)

NOTE: (1) The tendon of the **tensor tympani muscle** inserts on the manubrium of the malleus and the short tendon of the **stapedius muscle** inserts onto the neck of the stapes close to its articulation with the incus.

(2) The tensor tympani draws the manubrium medially, thereby making the tympanic membrane taut. At the same time its action pushes the base of the stapes more securely into the vestibular window. The tensor is innervated by the mandibular division of the **trigeminal nerve.**

(3) The stapedius opposes the action of the tensor at the vestibular window, tilting the head of the stapes away from the window. Its denervation results in hyperacusis, a condition in which sounds are perceived as unduly loud. The stapedius is supplied by the **facial nerve.**

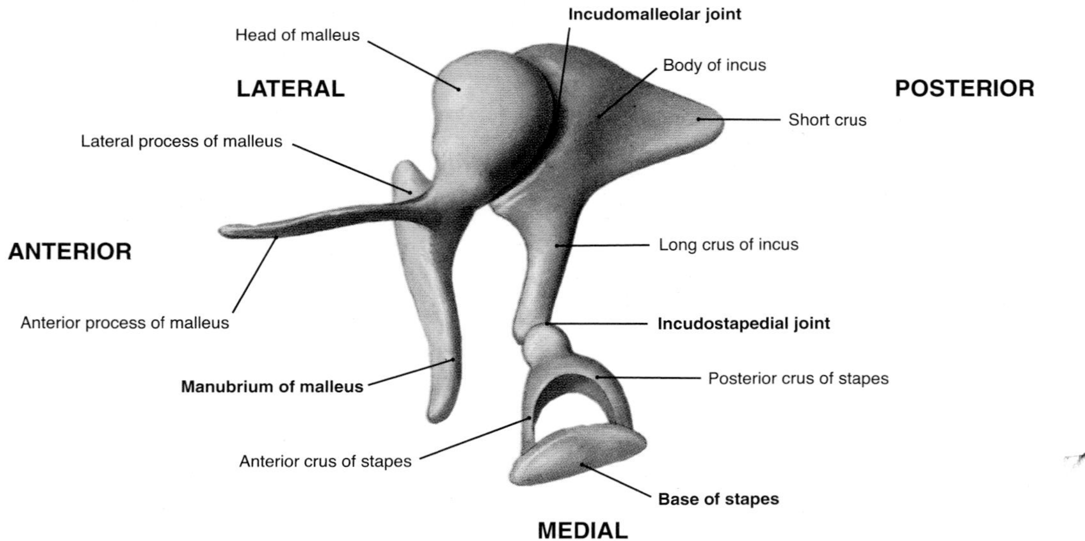
Incudomalleolar joint
Head of malleus
Body of incus
LATERAL
POSTERIOR
Short crus
Lateral process of malleus
ANTERIOR
Long crus of incus
Anterior process of malleus
Incudostapedial joint
Posterior crus of stapes
Manubrium of malleus
Anterior crus of stapes
Base of stapes
MEDIAL

Figure 606.2 Right Auditory Ossicles

NOTE: (1) When sound waves are received at the tympanic membrane, they cause a **medial** displacement of the manubrium of the malleus. The head of the malleus is then tilted **laterally,** pulling with it the body of the incus. At the same time the long process of the incus is displaced **medially,** as is the articulation between the incus and stapes.

(2) The base of the stapes rocks as if it were on a fulcrum at the vestibular window, thereby establishing waves in the perilymph. These waves stimulate the auditory receptors and become dissipated at the secondary tympanic membrane covering the cochlear window.

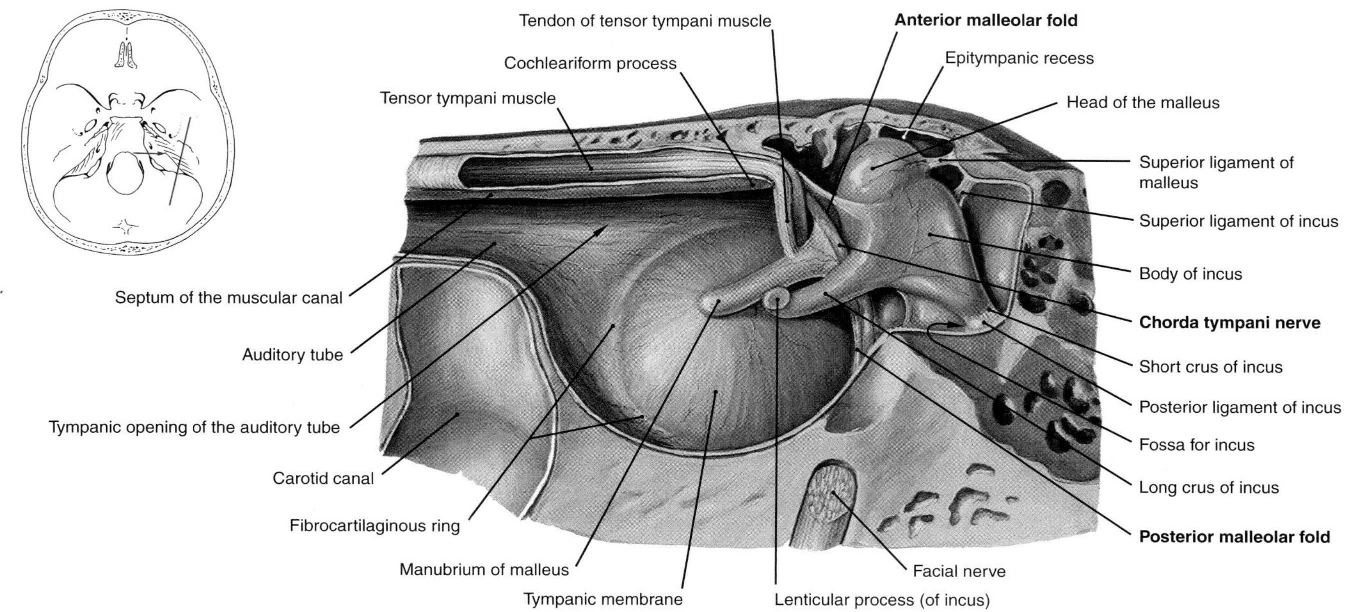
Tendon of tensor tympani muscle
Anterior malleolar fold
Epitympanic recess
Cochleariform process
Tensor tympani muscle
Head of the malleus
Superior ligament of malleus
Superior ligament of incus
Body of incus
Chorda tympani nerve
Short crus of incus
Posterior ligament of incus
Fossa for incus
Long crus of incus
Posterior malleolar fold
Septum of the muscular canal
Auditory tube
Tympanic opening of the auditory tube
Carotid canal
Fibrocartilaginous ring
Manubrium of malleus
Tympanic membrane
Lenticular process (of incus)
Facial nerve

Figure 607.1 Lateral Wall of the Right Tympanic Cavity (Viewed from the Medial Aspect)

NOTE: (1) The tympanic cavity is completely lined with a mucous membrane that attaches onto the surface of all the structures of the middle ear. This tympanic mucosa is continuous with that lining the mastoid air cells posteriorly and the auditory tube anteriorly.

(2) Reflections of the tympanic mucous membrane form the **anterior** and **posterior malleolar folds.** These are also reflected around the **chorda tympani nerve** as it curves along the medial side of the manubrium of the malleus.

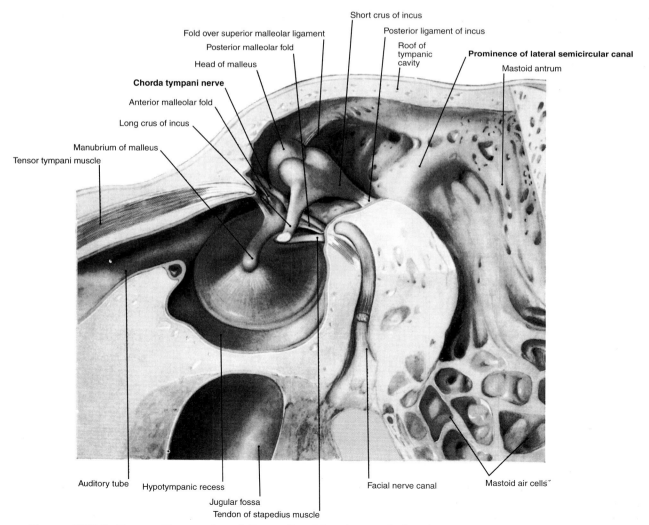

Short crus of incus
Fold over superior malleolar ligament
Posterior ligament of incus
Posterior malleolar fold
Roof of tympanic cavity
Prominence of lateral semicircular canal
Head of malleus
Mastoid antrum
Chorda tympani nerve
Anterior malleolar fold
Long crus of incus
Manubrium of malleus
Tensor tympani muscle
Auditory tube
Hypotympanic recess
Jugular fossa
Tendon of stapedius muscle
Facial nerve canal
Mastoid air cells

Figure 607.2 Tensor Tympani and Stapedius Muscles and Chorda Tympani Nerve (Right Side)

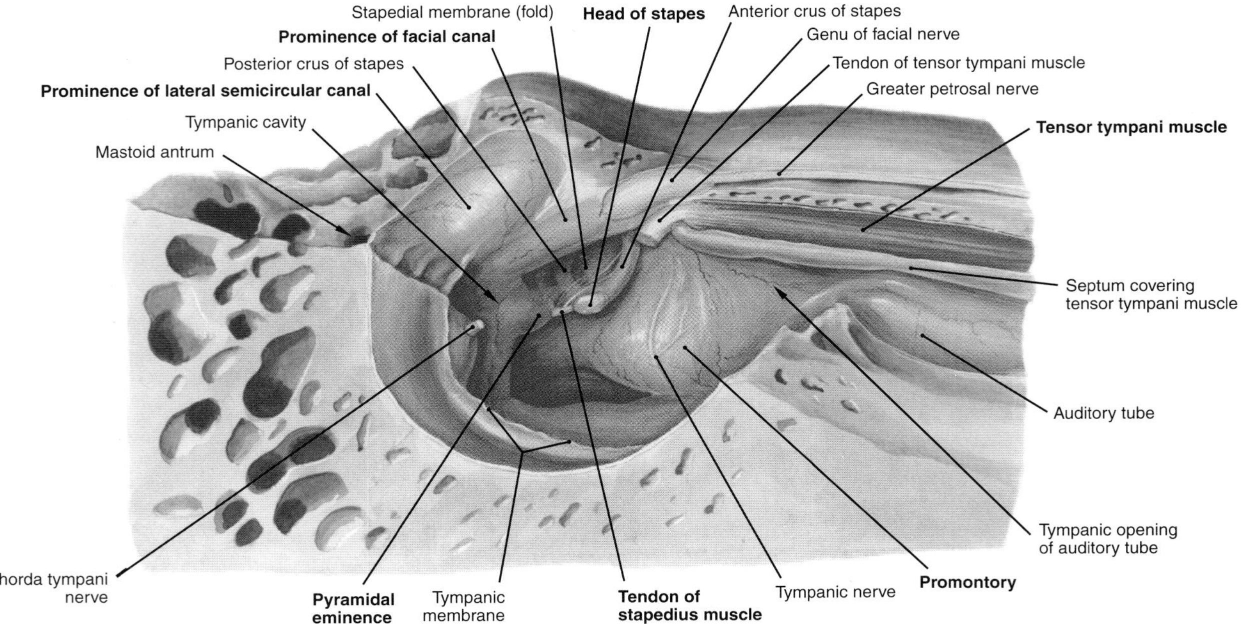

Stapedial membrane (fold)
Head of stapes
Anterior crus of stapes
Prominence of facial canal
Genu of facial nerve
Posterior crus of stapes
Tendon of tensor tympani muscle
Prominence of lateral semicircular canal
Greater petrosal nerve
Tympanic cavity
Tensor tympani muscle
Mastoid antrum
Septum covering tensor tympani muscle
Auditory tube
Tympanic opening of auditory tube
Chorda tympani nerve
Pyramidal eminence
Tympanic membrane
Tendon of stapedius muscle
Tympanic nerve
Promontory

Figure 608.1 Medial Wall of the Right Tympanic Cavity (Viewed from Lateral Aspect)

NOTE: (1) The tympanic membrane has been removed, along with the bony roof of the tympanic cavity. The malleus and incus have also been removed and the tendon of the tensor tympani severed. Observe the **stapes** with its base directed toward the vestibular window and the **stapedius muscle** still attached to its neck.

(2) Several bony markings: (a) the prominence containing the **lateral semicircular canal**, (b) the curved prominence of the **facial canal** with its facial nerve, (c) the **promontory**, which is a rounded thin bony covering over the **cochlea**, and (d) the hollow **pyramidal eminence,** from which arises the **stapedius muscle.**

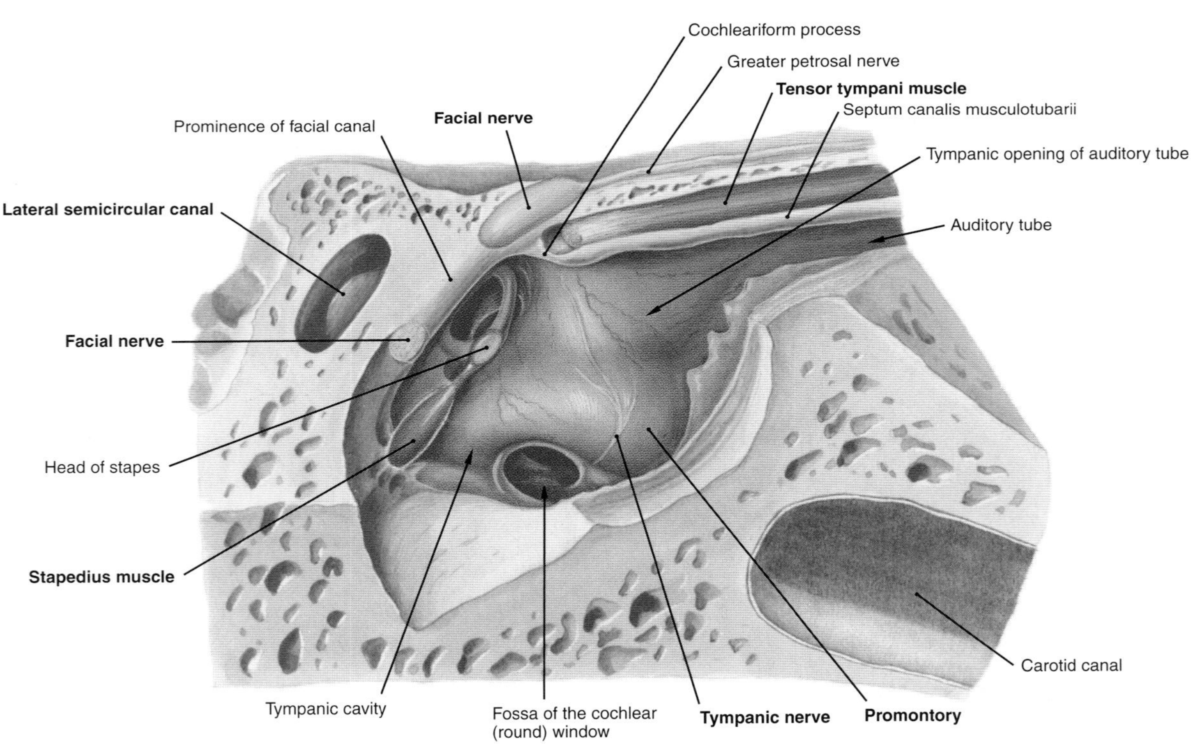

Cochleariform process
Greater petrosal nerve
Tensor tympani muscle
Septum canalis musculotubarii
Prominence of facial canal
Facial nerve
Tympanic opening of auditory tube
Lateral semicircular canal
Auditory tube
Facial nerve
Head of stapes
Stapedius muscle
Carotid canal
Tympanic cavity
Fossa of the cochlear (round) window
Tympanic nerve
Promontory

Figure 608.2 Medial Wall of the Right Tympanic Cavity Showing the Stapedius Muscle

NOTE: (1) The stapedius muscle emerges through the apex of the pyramidal eminence and it is about 4 mm in length. It pulls the base of the stapes laterally and protects the inner ear from damage caused by loud sounds.

(2) The **tympanic** branch of the **glossopharyngeal nerve** (IX) coursing along the promontory. This nerve is sensory to the mucous membrane of the middle ear, and is also known as the nerve of Jacobson. Its fibers are joined by sympathetic fibers to form the **tympanic plexus.**

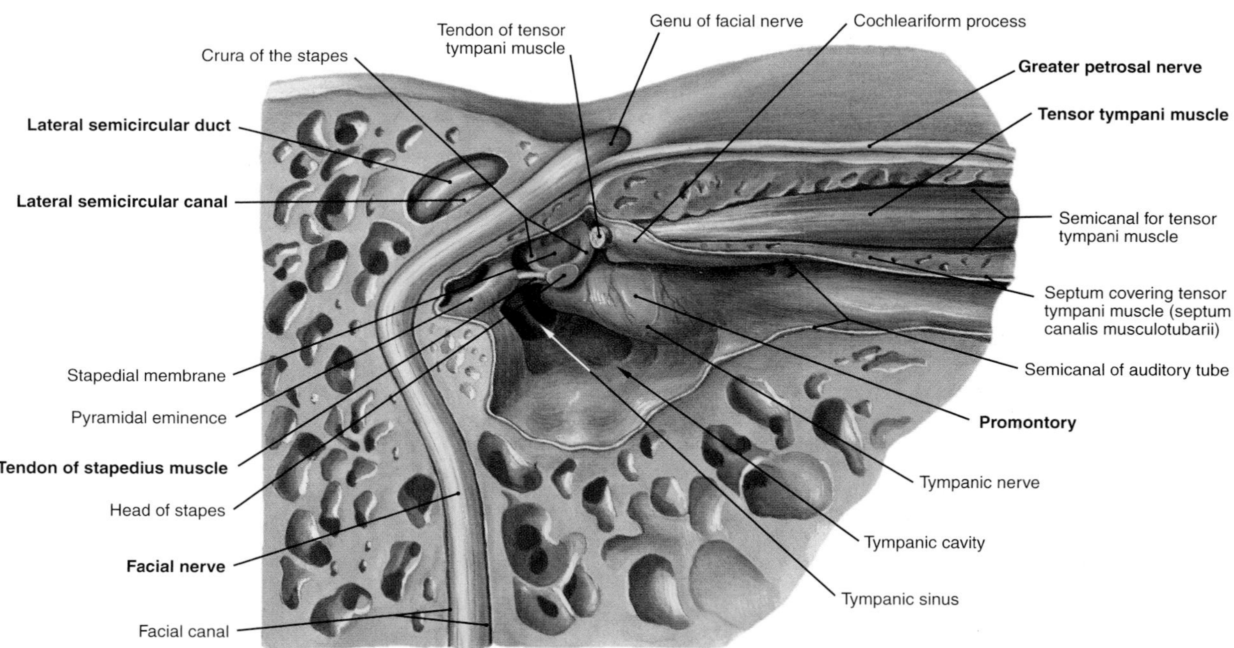
Crura of the stapes
Tendon of tensor tympani muscle
Genu of facial nerve
Cochleariform process
Greater petrosal nerve
Tensor tympani muscle
Lateral semicircular duct
Lateral semicircular canal
Semicanal for tensor tympani muscle
Septum covering tensor tympani muscle (septum canalis musculotubarii)
Semicanal of auditory tube
Stapedial membrane
Pyramidal eminence
Promontory
Tendon of stapedius muscle
Tympanic nerve
Head of stapes
Tympanic cavity
Facial nerve
Tympanic sinus
Facial canal

Figure 609.1 Medial Wall of Right Tympanic Cavity (Lateral View)

NOTE: (1) The bone forming the prominences of the **lateral semicircular canal** and the **facial canal** has been removed to reveal their internal structures.

(2) The **greater petrosal nerve** carries preganglionic parasympathetic fibers from the facial nerve to the pterygopalatine ganglion as well as many taste fibers from the soft palate.

(3) Coursing along the surface of the promontory can be seen the **tympanic branch** of the **glossopharyngeal nerve** and the tympanic vessels along with sympathetic fibers from the carotid plexus (caroticotympanic nerves).

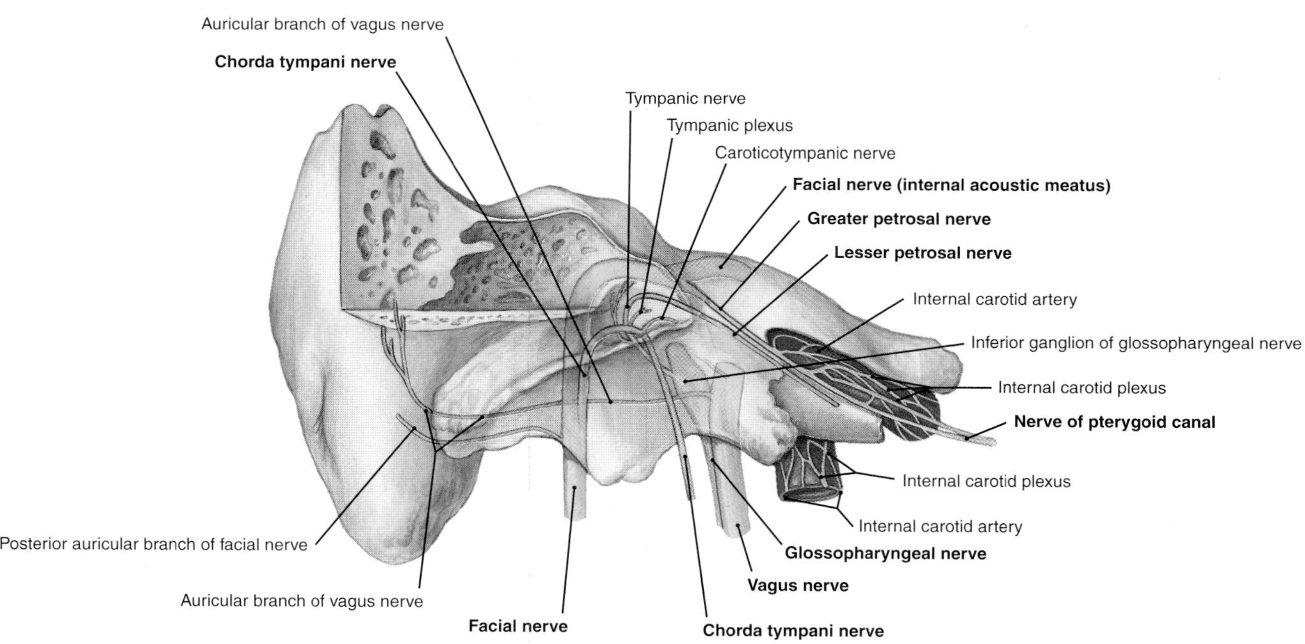
Auricular branch of vagus nerve
Chorda tympani nerve
Tympanic nerve
Tympanic plexus
Caroticotympanic nerve
Facial nerve (internal acoustic meatus)
Greater petrosal nerve
Lesser petrosal nerve
Internal carotid artery
Inferior ganglion of glossopharyngeal nerve
Internal carotid plexus
Nerve of pterygoid canal
Internal carotid plexus
Internal carotid artery
Posterior auricular branch of facial nerve
Glossopharyngeal nerve
Vagus nerve
Auricular branch of vagus nerve
Facial nerve
Chorda tympani nerve

Figure 609.2 Facial, Glossopharyngeal and Vagus Nerves Projected on Temporal Bone

NOTE: (1) From the tympanic plexus (see NOTE 3, Fig. 609.1) emerges the **lesser petrosal nerve**, which courses to the **otic ganglion.**

(2) The **greater petrosal nerve** joins with sympathetic branches of the internal carotid plexus (actually the **deep petrosal nerve**) to form the nerve of the **pterygoid canal.**

(3) The **auricular branch** of the **vagus nerve** is distributed to the upper surface of the external auricle, to the posterior wall and floor of the external acoustic meatus, and to part of the lateral (outer) surface of the tympanic membrane.

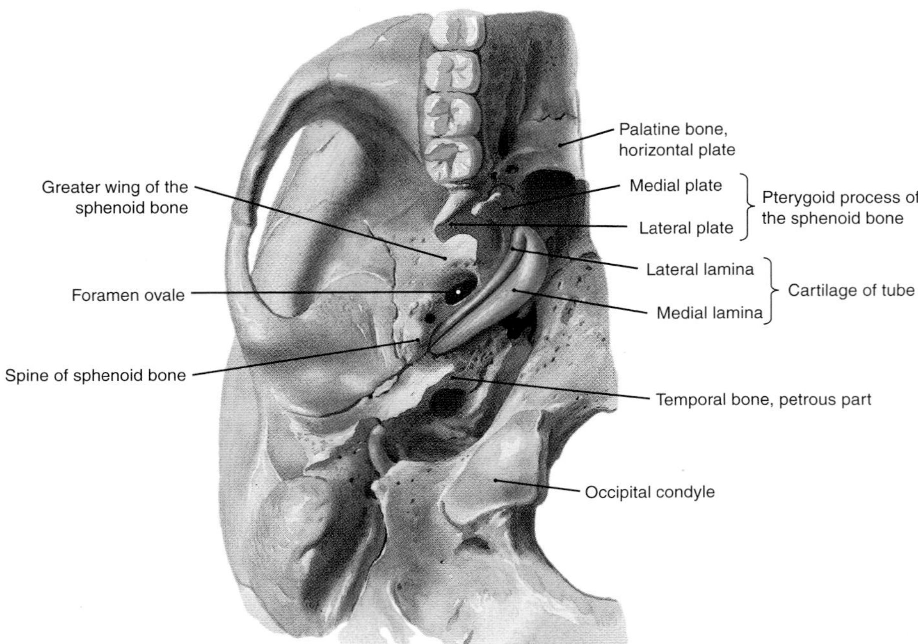

Palatine bone, horizontal plate
Greater wing of the sphenoid bone
Medial plate
Lateral plate
Pterygoid process of the sphenoid bone
Lateral lamina
Medial lamina
Cartilage of tube
Foramen ovale
Spine of sphenoid bone
Temporal bone, petrous part
Occipital condyle

Figure 610.1 Cartilaginous Part of the Auditory Tube at the Base of the Skull

NOTE: (1) The auditory tube is an air channel between the tympanic cavity of the middle ear and the nasopharynx. Air passes through the tube and thereby equalizes the air pressure on both sides of the tympanic membrane.

(2) The auditory tube has a bony or osseous part (about 12 mm long; not seen in this figure) and a cartilaginous part (about 24 mm long; shown in this figure). The osseous part is an extension of the bony walls of the middle ear (see Plate 608), while the cartilaginous part (continuous with the bony part) extends to and opens into the nasopharynx.

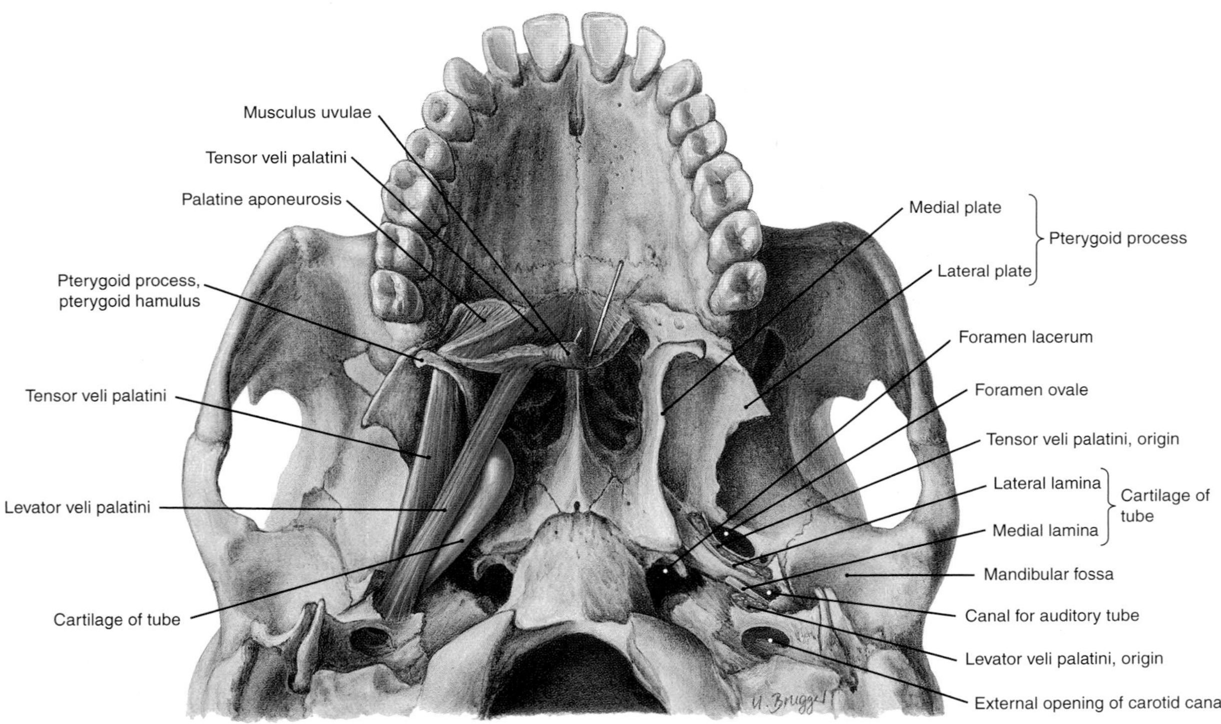

Musculus uvulae
Tensor veli palatini
Palatine aponeurosis
Pterygoid process, pterygoid hamulus
Tensor veli palatini
Levator veli palatini
Cartilage of tube
Medial plate
Lateral plate
Pterygoid process
Foramen lacerum
Foramen ovale
Tensor veli palatini, origin
Lateral lamina
Medial lamina
Cartilage of tube
Mandibular fossa
Canal for auditory tube
Levator veli palatini, origin
External opening of carotid canal

Figure 610.2 Auditory Tube and the Tensor and Levator Veli Palatini Muscles

NOTE: (1) The close relationship of the tensor and levator veli palatini muscles at their origins on the base of the skull with the auditory tube. Some muscle fibers of the tensor arise from the lateral lamina of the cartilaginous part of the auditory tube and may act as a dilator of the tube.

(2) The manner by which the tensor and levator insert into the soft palate. The tendon of the tensor courses around the hamulus of the pterygoid process before inserting into the soft palate, while the levator inserts directly into the soft palate.

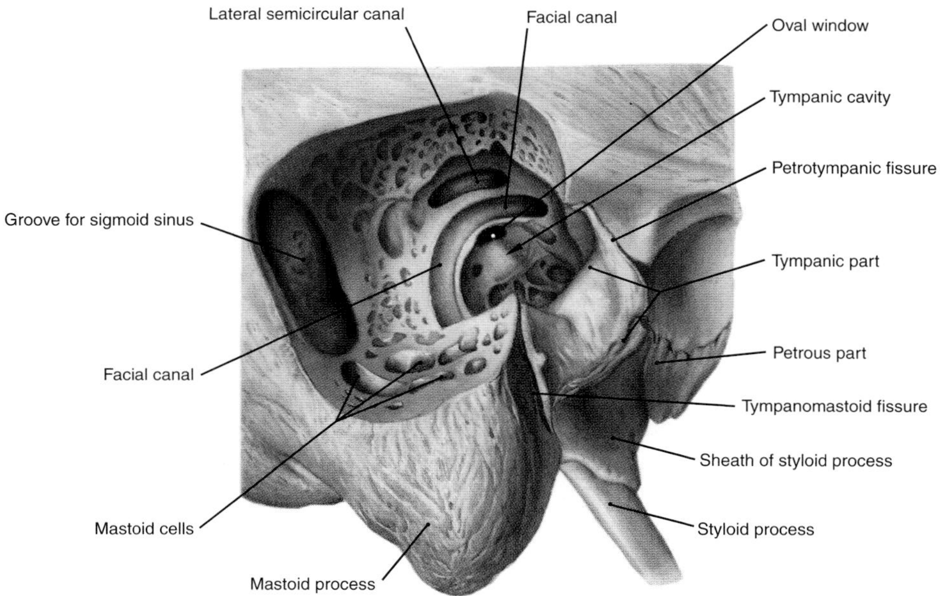
Lateral semicircular canal
Facial canal
Oval window
Tympanic cavity
Petrotympanic fissure
Groove for sigmoid sinus
Tympanic part
Petrous part
Facial canal
Tympanomastoid fissure
Sheath of styloid process
Mastoid cells
Styloid process
Mastoid process

Figure 611.1 Dissected Right Temporal Bone

NOTE: (1) Through the facial canal courses the **facial nerve.** The canal commences at the internal auditory meatus and continues through the petrous part of the temporal bone to its exit at the stylomastoid foramen (see Figure 611.2).

(2) In its descent, the facial canal courses posterior to the cavity of the middle ear (tympanic cavity), where the facial nerve gives off the nerve to the stapedius muscle and the chorda tympani branch.

(3) The location of the lateral semicircular canal superiorly and the groove for the sigmoid sinus posteriorly.

(4) Within the tympanic cavity is located the oval window adjacent to which would be found the base of the stapes.

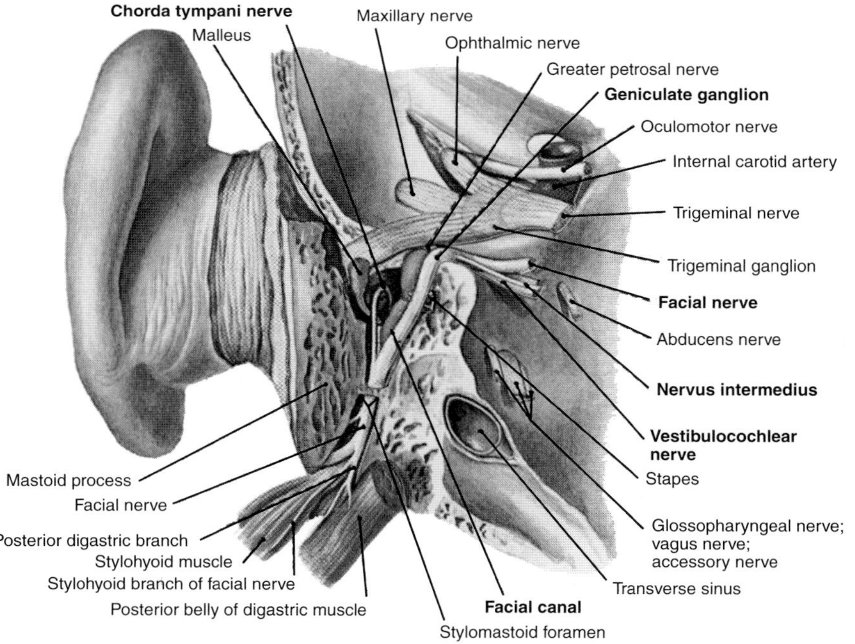
Chorda tympani nerve
Malleus
Maxillary nerve
Ophthalmic nerve
Greater petrosal nerve
Geniculate ganglion
Oculomotor nerve
Internal carotid artery
Trigeminal nerve
Trigeminal ganglion
Facial nerve
Abducens nerve
Nervus intermedius
Vestibulocochlear nerve
Stapes
Mastoid process
Facial nerve
Posterior digastric branch
Stylohyoid muscle
Stylohyoid branch of facial nerve
Posterior belly of digastric muscle
Glossopharyngeal nerve; vagus nerve; accessory nerve
Transverse sinus
Facial canal
Stylomastoid foramen

Figure 611.2 Intracranial Course of the Facial Nerve Viewed Posteriorly

NOTE: (1) This is a frontal section of the temporal bone that opens the facial canal from behind. Observe the **chorda tympani nerve** coursing from the **facial nerve** across (from posterior to anterior) the tympanic cavity along the inner surface of the tympanic membrane.

(2) The internal acoustic meatus in the floor of the skull transmits the facial nerve (and **nervous intermedius**) and the **vestibulocochlear nerve.**

(3) Distal to the **geniculate ganglion** (the sensory ganglion of the facial nerve) the facial nerve enters the facial canal where it first courses laterally and then turns sharply backward and inferiorly (see Figure 609.1).

(4) Beyond the chorda tympani branch, the trunk of the facial nerve descends in the temporal bone to emerge on the side of the face through the stylomastoid foramen posterior to the ear lobe.

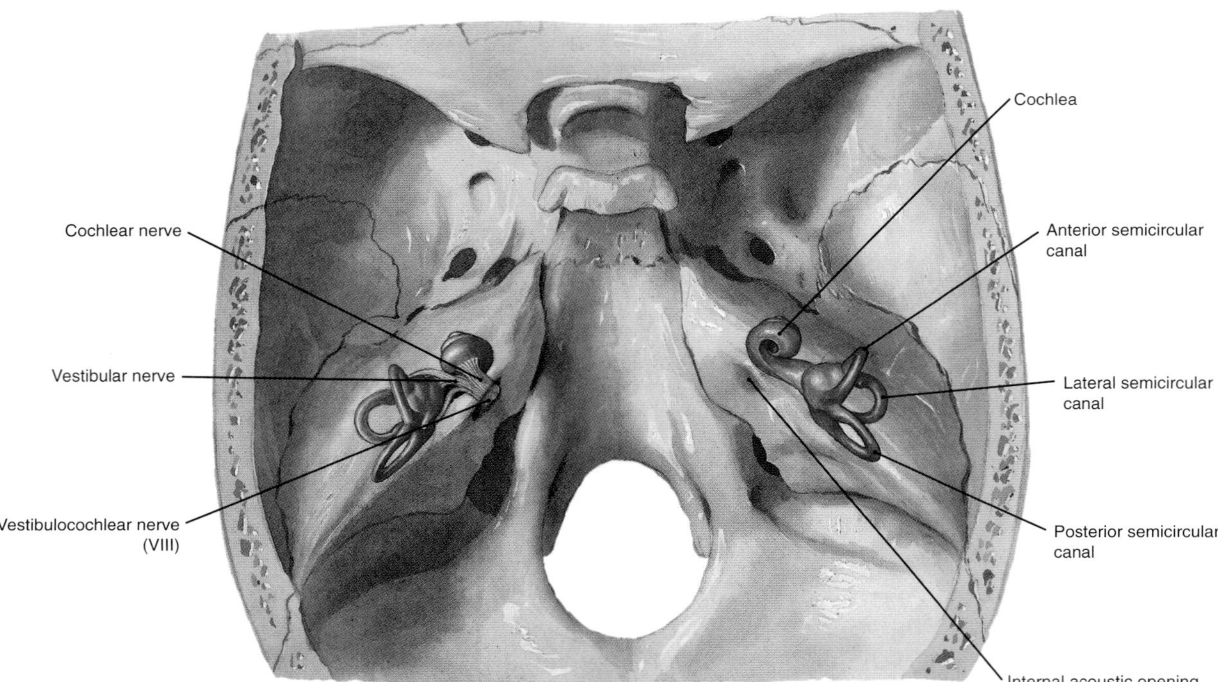
Cochlea
Cochlear nerve
Anterior semicircular canal
Vestibular nerve
Lateral semicircular canal
Vestibulocochlear nerve (VIII)
Posterior semicircular canal
Internal acoustic opening

Figure 612.1 Cochlea and Semicircular Canals Projected onto the Petrous Part of the Temporal Bone

NOTE: (1) The internal ear lies in the petrous part of the temporal bone just deep to the crest of that bone (called the arcuate eminence [not labeled]) that separates the middle cranial fossa from the posterior cranial fossa. Observe also the internal acoustic (auditory) meatus on the posterior aspect of the arcuate eminence through which pass the facial and vestibulocochlear nerves.

(2) The orientation of the anterior, lateral, and posterior semicircular canals, and the cochlea is positioned slightly medial and anterior to the canals. Note also (on the reader's left) the vestibular and cochlear divisions of the vestibulocochlear nerve that carries impulses from the vestibular receptors in the semicircular canals that inform the brain of the position of the head in space and the receptors in the cochlea that transmit the special sense of hearing.

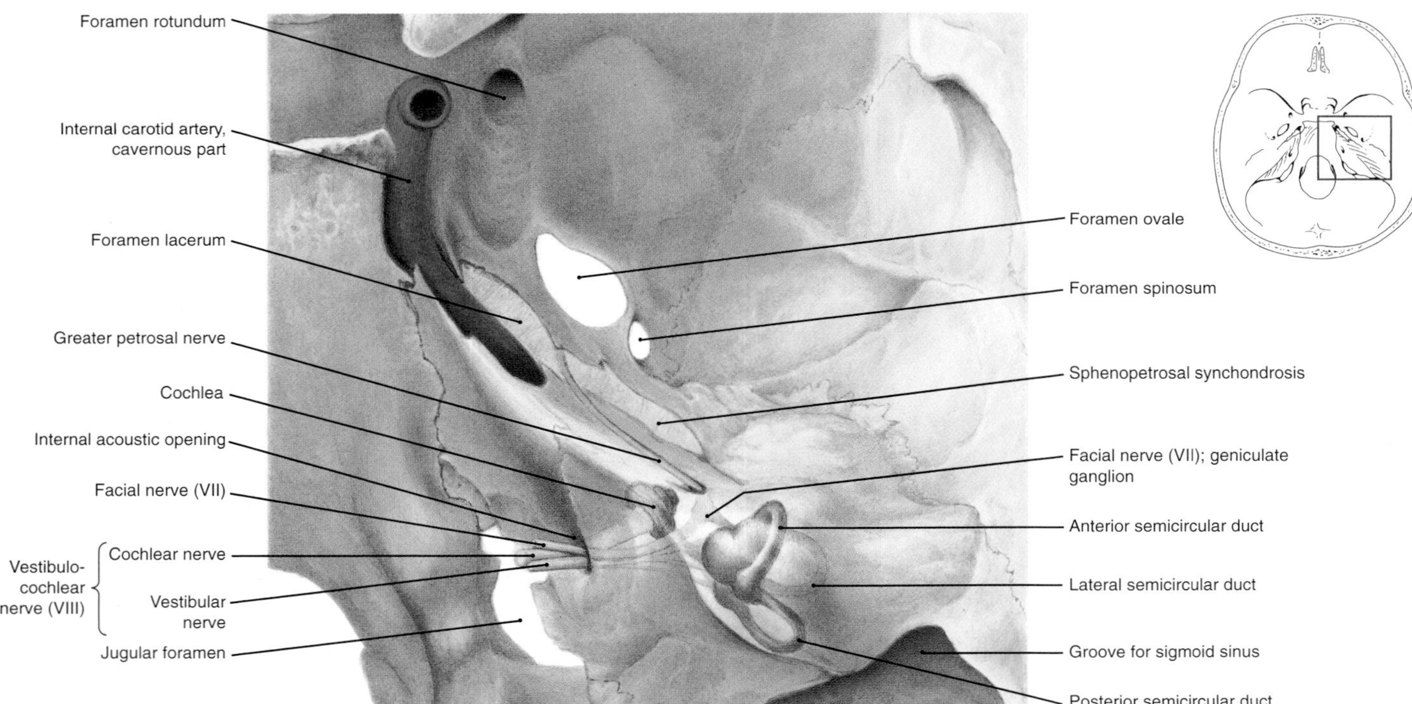
Foramen rotundum
Internal carotid artery, cavernous part
Foramen lacerum
Greater petrosal nerve
Cochlea
Internal acoustic opening
Facial nerve (VII)
Vestibulocochlear nerve (VIII)
Cochlear nerve
Vestibular nerve
Jugular foramen
Foramen ovale
Foramen spinosum
Sphenopetrosal synchondrosis
Facial nerve (VII); geniculate ganglion
Anterior semicircular duct
Lateral semicircular duct
Groove for sigmoid sinus
Posterior semicircular duct

Figure 612.2 Structures of the Right Inner Ear and the Vestibulocochlear and Facial Nerves Visualized from Above

NOTE: (1) The semicircular canals and the cochlea of the inner ear are projected onto the superior surface of the petrous portion of the temporal bone. Observe also the **facial nerve** and **the vestibular and cochlear divisions** of the **vestibulocochlear nerve** traversing the internal acoustic (auditory) meatus.

(2) The orientation of the cochlea is similar to that in Fig. 612.1. Note also the **geniculate ganglion** through which course the fibers that form the greater petrosal nerve. This ganglion contains the cell bodies for the taste fibers in the chorda tympani nerve for the anterior two-thirds of the tongue.

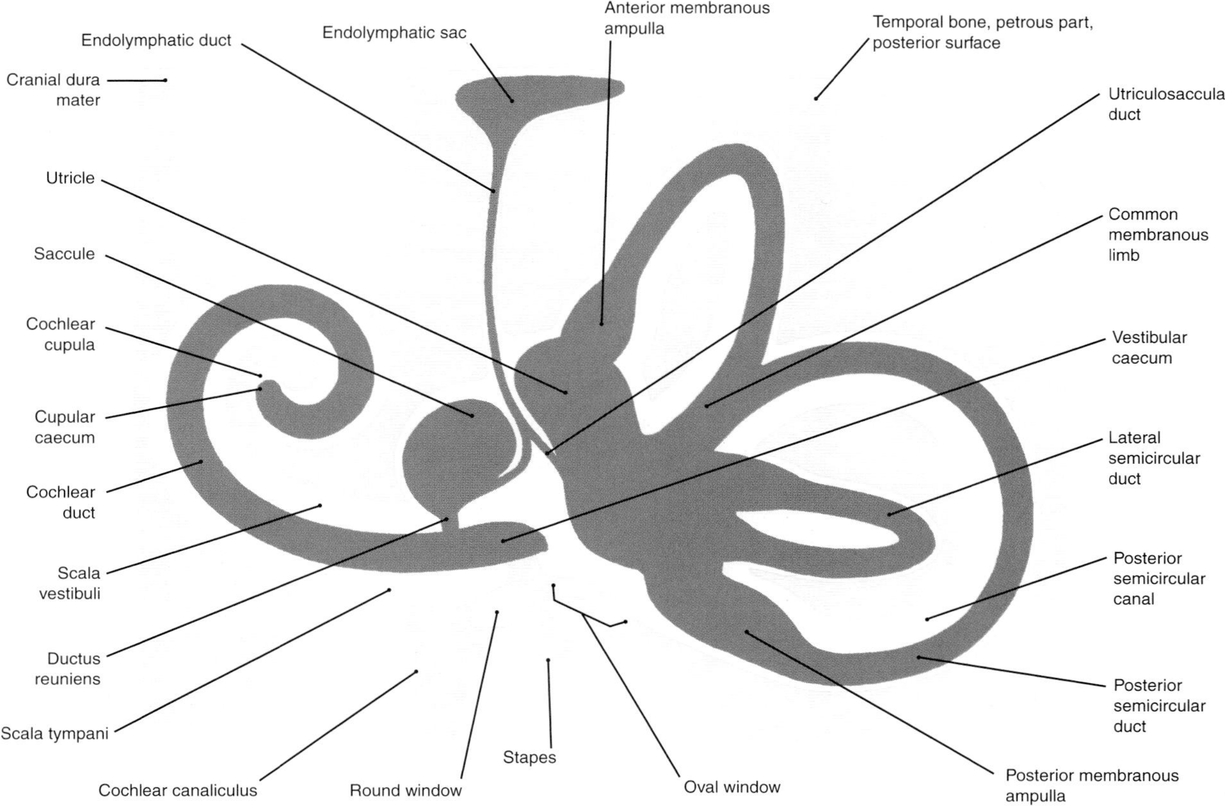
Endolymphatic duct
Endolymphatic sac
Anterior membranous ampulla
Temporal bone, petrous part, posterior surface
Cranial dura mater
Utriculosaccular duct
Utricle
Common membranous limb
Saccule
Vestibular caecum
Cochlear cupula
Cupular caecum
Lateral semicircular duct
Cochlear duct
Scala vestibuli
Posterior semicircular canal
Ductus reuniens
Posterior semicircular duct
Scala tympani
Stapes
Posterior membranous ampulla
Cochlear canaliculus
Round window
Oval window

Figure 613.1 Membranous Labyrinth of the Inner Ear

NOTE: The membranous labyrinth is a closed system of ducts and sacs surrounded by the bony labyrinth of the inner ear. It contains endolymph surrounded by perilymph and consists of the ducts of the semicircular canals, the utricle, the saccule, the endolymphatic duct, and the duct of the cochlea.

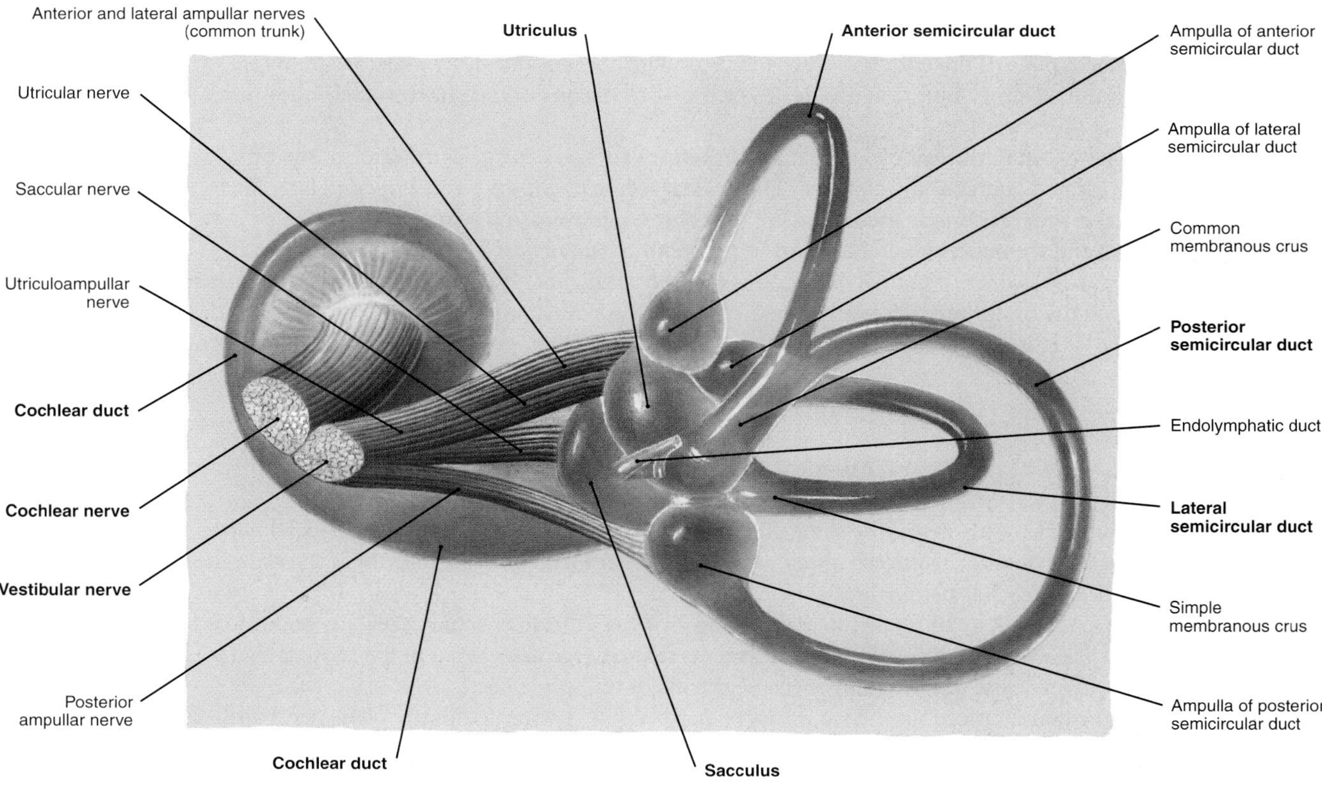
Anterior and lateral ampullar nerves (common trunk)
Utriculus
Anterior semicircular duct
Ampulla of anterior semicircular duct
Utricular nerve
Ampulla of lateral semicircular duct
Saccular nerve
Common membranous crus
Utriculoampullar nerve
Posterior semicircular duct
Cochlear duct
Endolymphatic duct
Cochlear nerve
Lateral semicircular duct
Vestibular nerve
Simple membranous crus
Posterior ampullar nerve
Ampulla of posterior semicircular duct
Cochlear duct
Sacculus

Figure 613.2 Right Membranous Labyrinth (Medial View)

NOTE: The ampullae of the three semicircular ducts, the sacculus, the utriculus, and the cochlear duct, and the connections of the endolymphatic duct to the utriculus and sacculus.

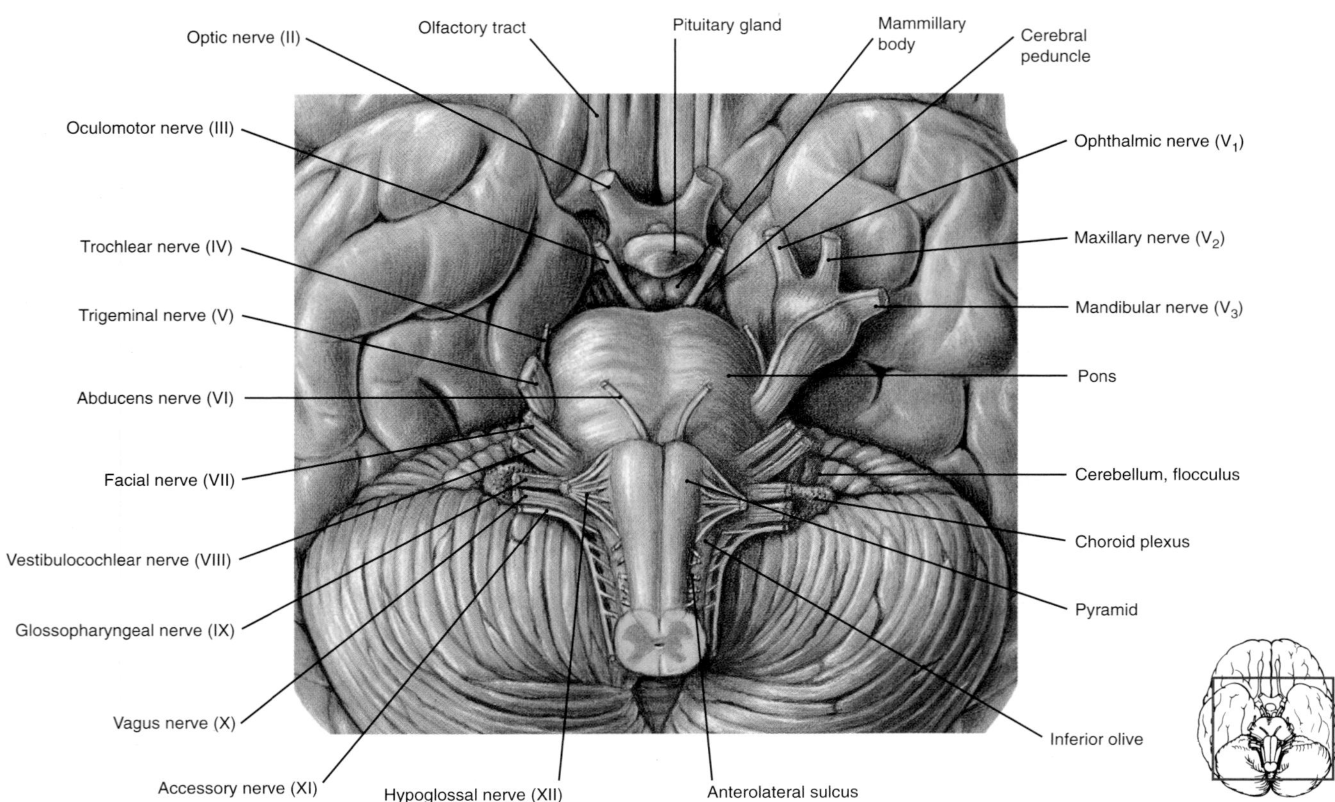
Optic nerve (II)
Olfactory tract
Pituitary gland
Mammillary body
Cerebral peduncle
Oculomotor nerve (III)
Ophthalmic nerve (V_1)
Trochlear nerve (IV)
Maxillary nerve (V_2)
Trigeminal nerve (V)
Mandibular nerve (V_3)
Pons
Abducens nerve (VI)
Facial nerve (VII)
Cerebellum, flocculus
Vestibulocochlear nerve (VIII)
Choroid plexus
Glossopharyngeal nerve (IX)
Pyramid
Vagus nerve (X)
Inferior olive
Accessory nerve (XI)
Hypoglossal nerve (XII)
Anterolateral sulcus

Figure 614 Ventral View of the Brain and the Sites of Attachment of the Cranial Nerves

NOTE: (1) The cranial nerves supply motor and sensory innervation to the head and, in some instances, to other region of the body. There are 12 pairs of cranial nerves, and these are attached to the brain from the basal forebrain to the medulla oblongata.

(2) The cranial nerves pass through openings in the skull to (or from) extracranial structures, and they are subject to damage along their paths due to vascular or traumatic incidents or from infections or neoplasms.

SITES OF ATTACHMENT OF THE CRANIAL NERVES TO THE BRAIN

I **Olfactory Nerves:** These are neurons from receptors for the special sense of smell in the nasal cavity that pierce through foramina in the cribriform plate of the ethmoid bone and terminate on neurons of the olfactory bulb (about 20 bundles). The axons from neurons in the olfactory bulbs (which are second-order neurons in the olfactory pathway) form the **olfactory tracts** that attach to the basal forebrain.

II **Optic Nerves:** These join at the optic chiasma. The **anterior cerebral artery** lies anterior to the optic chiasma and the **internal carotid artery** is located lateral to the chiasma. The optic tracts then course posteriorly and laterally to enter the diencephalon.

III **Oculomotor Nerve:** Emerges on the medial side of the ventral midbrain and passes between the posterior cerebral artery (superior to the nerve) and the superior cerebellar artery (inferior to the nerve).

IV **Trochlear Nerve:** Most slender of cranial nerves. It is the only cranial nerve that emerges from the posterior aspect of the brainstem. It attaches to the brain immediately below the inferior colliculus in the upper pons.

V **Trigeminal Nerve:** It is attached to the anterior surface of the pons near its upper border. The smaller motor root is covered by the large sensory root.

VI **Abducens Nerve:** Emerges at the lower border of the pons, in a furrow between the pons and pyramid of the medulla oblongata (the pontomedullary junction).

VII **Facial Nerve:** Also attaches at the lower border of the pons (at the cerebellopontine angle) medial and slightly anterior to the vestibulocochlear nerve.

VIII **Vestibulocochlear Nerve:** Attaches in the same groove as the facial nerve but lateral to the facial nerve.

IX **Glossopharyngeal Nerve:** Attached to the upper aspect of the medulla oblongata in front of the vagus nerve in a groove between the medulla and the cerebellar peduncle.

X **Vagus Nerve:** Attached by 8 to 10 filaments in the same groove as the glossopharyngeal nerve but just posterior to it.

XI **Accessory Nerve:** The **cranial root** is formed by filaments that emerge just caudal to the rootlets that form the vagus nerve. The **spinal root** arises from fibers from the upper five segments of the spinal cord.
The fibers from the cranial root join the **vagus nerve** and become distributed in the pharyngeal and laryngeal branches of the vagus. The fibers of the spinal root leave the cranial fibers and descend from the jugular foramen to supply the sternocleidomastoid and trapezius muscles.

XII **Hypoglossal Nerve:** Fibers emerge from the ventrolateral aspect of the caudal medulla in line with the ventral roots spinal cord. They represent the four fused precervical nerves.

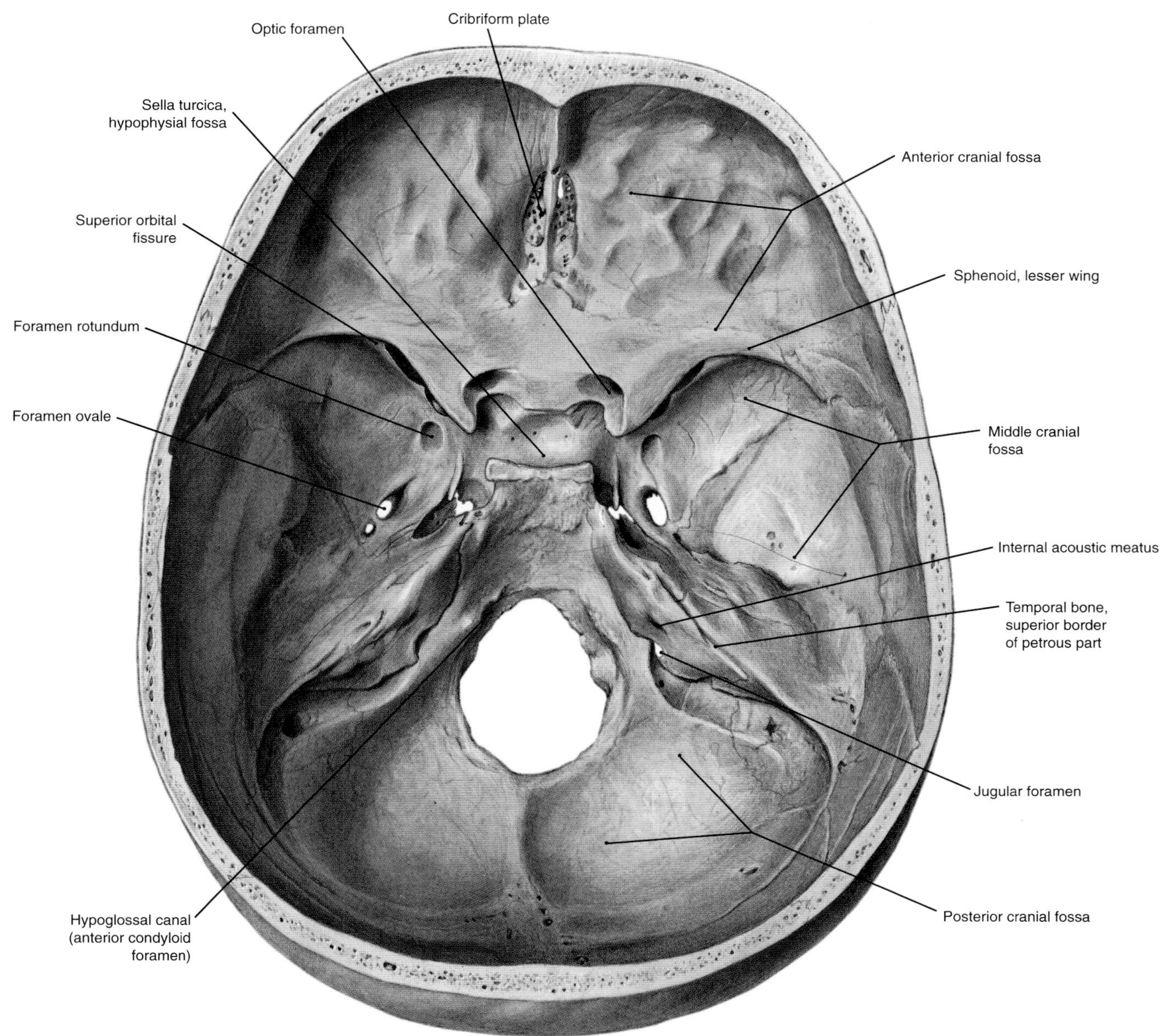
Optic foramen
Cribriform plate
Sella turcica, hypophysial fossa
Anterior cranial fossa
Superior orbital fissure
Sphenoid, lesser wing
Foramen rotundum
Foramen ovale
Middle cranial fossa
Internal acoustic meatus
Temporal bone, superior border of petrous part
Jugular foramen
Posterior cranial fossa
Hypoglossal canal (anterior condyloid foramen)

Figure 615 **Base of the Skull Showing Foramina through Which Traverse the Cranial Nerves**

I. Olfactory Nerve: **Cribriform plate** of the ethmoid bone
II. Optic Nerve: **Optic foramen** of sphenoid bone (with the ophthalmic artery)

III. Oculomotor Nerve:
IV. Trochlear Nerve:
V_1. Ophthalmic division, Trigeminal Nerve:
} **Superior orbital fissure** of sphenoid bone

V_2. Maxillary division, Trigeminal Nerve **Foramen rotundum** of sphenoid bone
V_3. Mandibular division, Trigeminal Nerve **Foramen ovale** of sphenoid bone

VI. Abducens Nerve **Superior orbital fissure of sphenoid bone**

VII. Facial Nerve:
VIII. Vestibulocochlear Nerve:
} **Internal acoustic meatus** of temporal bone (petrous part)

IX. Glossopharyngeal Nerve:
X. Vagus Nerve:
XI. Accessory Nerve:
} **Jugular foramen**, between the occipital bone and petrous portion of temporal bone

XII. Hypoglossal Nerve: **Hypoglossal Canal** (anterior condylar foramen)

Figure 616.1 **Lateral Wall of the Nasal Cavity and Olfactory Receptors (Olfactory Nerves) Cranial Nerve I**

Figure 616.2 **Nasal Septum and Olfactory Receptors (Olfactory Nerves) Cranial Nerve I**

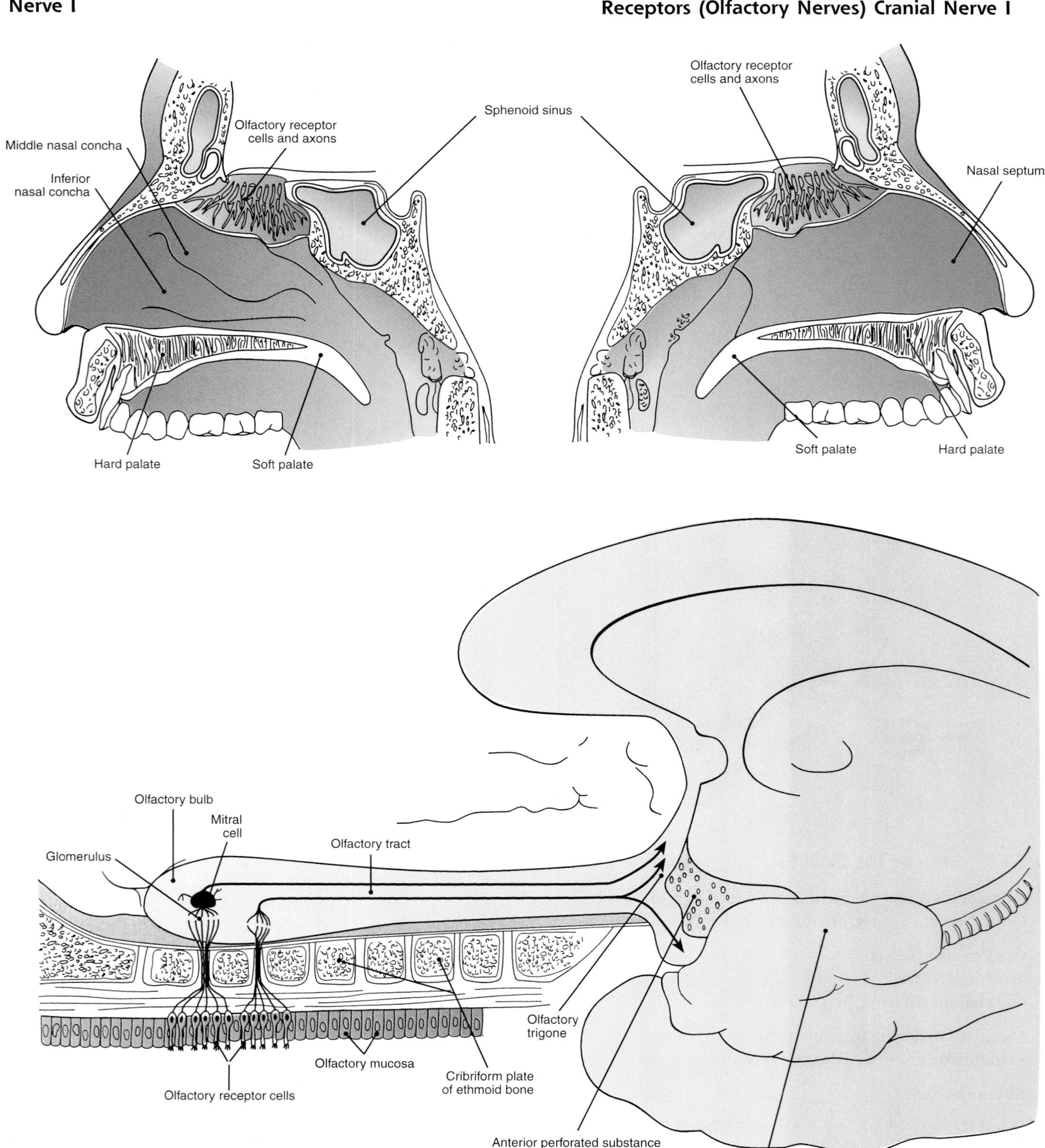

Middle nasal concha
Inferior nasal concha
Olfactory receptor cells and axons
Sphenoid sinus
Hard palate
Soft palate
Olfactory receptor cells and axons
Nasal septum
Soft palate
Hard palate
Olfactory bulb
Mitral cell
Glomerulus
Olfactory tract
Olfactory trigone
Olfactory mucosa
Cribriform plate of ethmoid bone
Olfactory receptor cells
Anterior perforated substance
Piriform lobe

Figure 616.3 **Olfactory Mucosa, Receptors, and Nerves (Cranial Nerve I) and Olfactory Bulb and Tract of the Central Nervous System (CNS)**

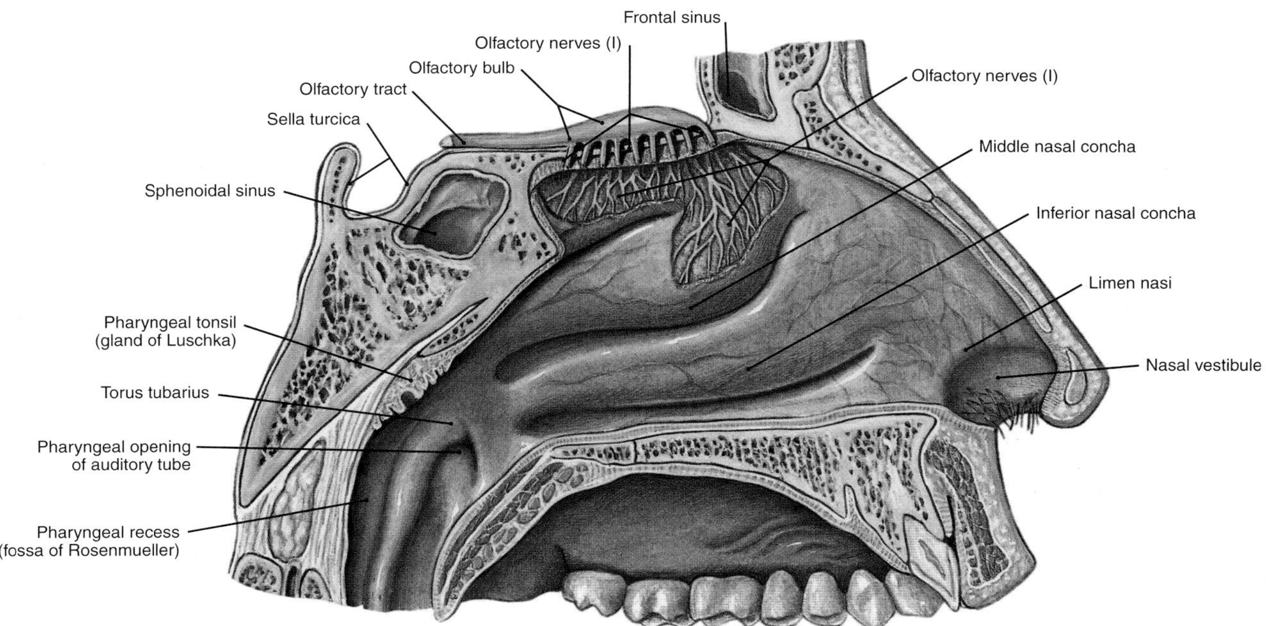
Frontal sinus
Olfactory nerves (I)
Olfactory bulb
Olfactory tract
Sella turcica
Sphenoidal sinus
Pharyngeal tonsil
(gland of Luschka)
Torus tubarius
Pharyngeal opening
of auditory tube
Pharyngeal recess
(fossa of Rosenmueller)
Olfactory nerves (I)
Middle nasal concha
Inferior nasal concha
Limen nasi
Nasal vestibule

Figure 617.1 **Lateral Wall of the Nasal Cavity: Olfactory Nerves (Cranial Nerve I) and Olfactory Bulb and Tract**

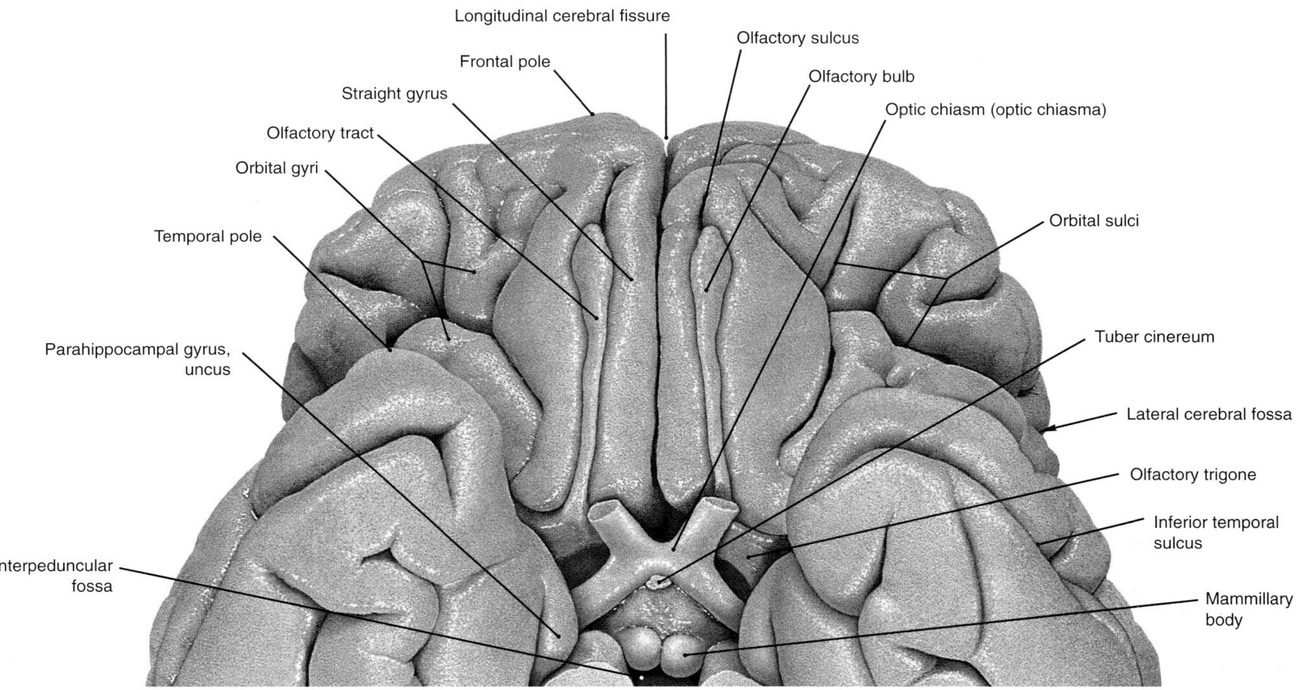
Longitudinal cerebral fissure
Frontal pole
Straight gyrus
Olfactory tract
Orbital gyri
Temporal pole
Parahippocampal gyrus,
uncus
Interpeduncular
fossa
Olfactory sulcus
Olfactory bulb
Optic chiasm (optic chiasma)
Orbital sulci
Tuber cinereum
Lateral cerebral fossa
Olfactory trigone
Inferior temporal
sulcus
Mammillary
body

Figure 617.2 **Basal Forebrain Showing the Olfactory Bulb, Olfactory Tract, and Olfactory Trigone (CNS)**

Figure 617.1 and Figure 617.2

NOTE: (1) The olfactory receptor cells and their axons that enter the olfactory bulb constitute the first cranial nerve. These are peripheral nerves (PNS), while the olfactory bulb and olfactory tract are brain (CNS) structures;.

(2) The olfactory receptors are located in the **olfactory epithelium** that overlies the superior concha in the lateral wall of the nasal cavity and the adjoining mucosa that covers the superior aspect of the nasal septum (see Fig. 616.1 and 616.2);

(3) About 20 small bundles of nerve fibers from the receptor cells enter the olfactory bulbs on each side by passing through the foramina of the cribriform plate of the ethmoid bone (see Fig. 616.3).

(4) The receptor neuron fibers synapse with tufted and mitral cells in the olfactory bulb and project their axons centrally to form the olfactory tracts (see Figs. 616.3 and 617.2). These tracts are often mistakenly considered the first pair of cranial nerves. The receptor cells and their axons form the first cranial nerve. Second-order neurons (such as the tufted cells and mitral cells in the olfactory bulb) send their axons posteriorly to form the olfactory tract, which is completely a CNS tract.

(5) Damage to the olfactory filaments or the olfactory tracts may occur following fractures of the skull in the anterior cranial fossa or by tumors or inflammation in this fossa. This can result in **anosmia** (loss of the sense of smell).

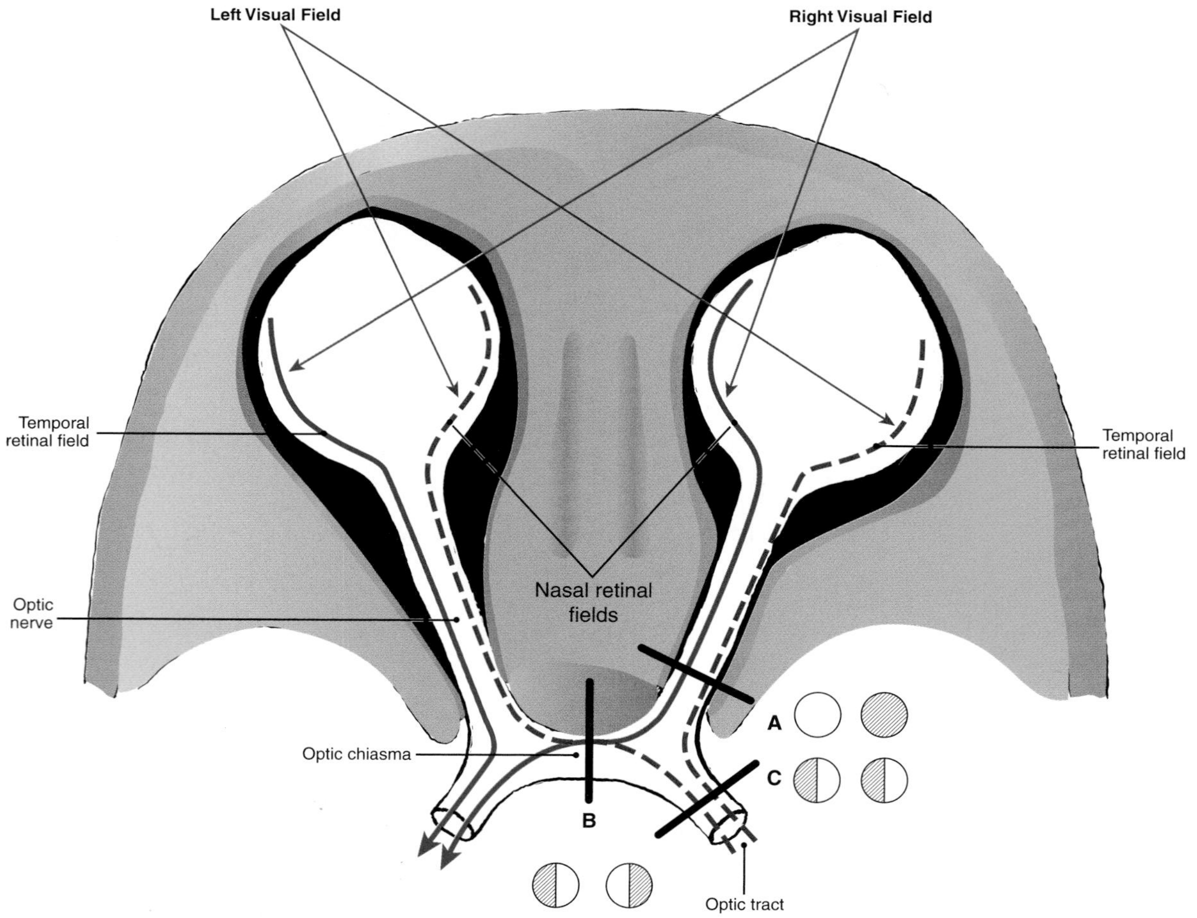
Left Visual Field
Right Visual Field
Temporal retinal field
Temporal retinal field
Optic nerve
Nasal retinal fields
A
C
B
Optic chiasma
Optic tract

Figure 618 Visual Fields; Retinal Fields; Retina; Optic Nerve; Optic Chiasma (Diagram)

NOTE: (1) The **optic nerves** transmit visual impulses from the retina posteriorly to the brainstem. The fibers that form the optic nerves are axons from the ganglion cells if the retina. These cells form the innermost layer of the retina and emerge from the bulb of the eye at the optic disk (see Plates 554–556).

(2) A **visual field** is the area in space that is visible to an eye at a given position. A visual field is also called a field of vision. The **nasal retina** is the nasal half of the retina medial to the optic disk (sometimes called the **nasal retinal field**); the **temporal retina** is the outer half of the retina lateral to the optic disk (sometimes called the **temporal retinal field**).

(3) As the optic nerves course posteriorly from the eyeball, half of its fibers cross to the opposite side of the brain at the **optic chiasma.** Fibers from the temporal retina of both eyes DO NOT cross at the optic chiasma, while fibers from the nasal retinas of the two eyes CROSS at the optic chiasma.

(4) Posterior to the optic chiasma the optic fibers form the **optic tracts** that carry the fibers to the midbrain, where they synapse with neurons in the lateral geniculate body. These latter neurons send their fibers to the cerebral cortex.

(5) Because of the crossed and uncrossed fibers in the optic chiasma, different lesions in the visual pathway will result in varying losses of vision:

(a) An **optic nerve** lesion results in a loss of vision in that eye, thus, there is a loss of both nasal and temporal field vision in that one eye (**A**).

(b) An **optic chiasma** (**B**) lesion that cuts though the middle of the optic chiasma results in a loss of vision from the nasal half of the retina of the right eye (right temporal visual field) and the nasal half of the retina of the left eye (left temporal visual field). This condition is called **bitemporal hemianopia** because both temporal visual fields are lost and indicates that the crossed fibers at the optic chiasma are cut, while the uncrossed fibers are intact.

(c) A lesion in the **optic tract** (**C**) on one side (e.g., in the right optic tract) will eliminate vision from the temporal half of the retina of the right eye and the nasal half of the retina of the left eye. This means that there is a loss of input from the contralateral visual fields to both eyes, resulting in a loss of input to the left nasal retinal field and to the right temporal retinal field. This is called **homonymous hemianopia.**

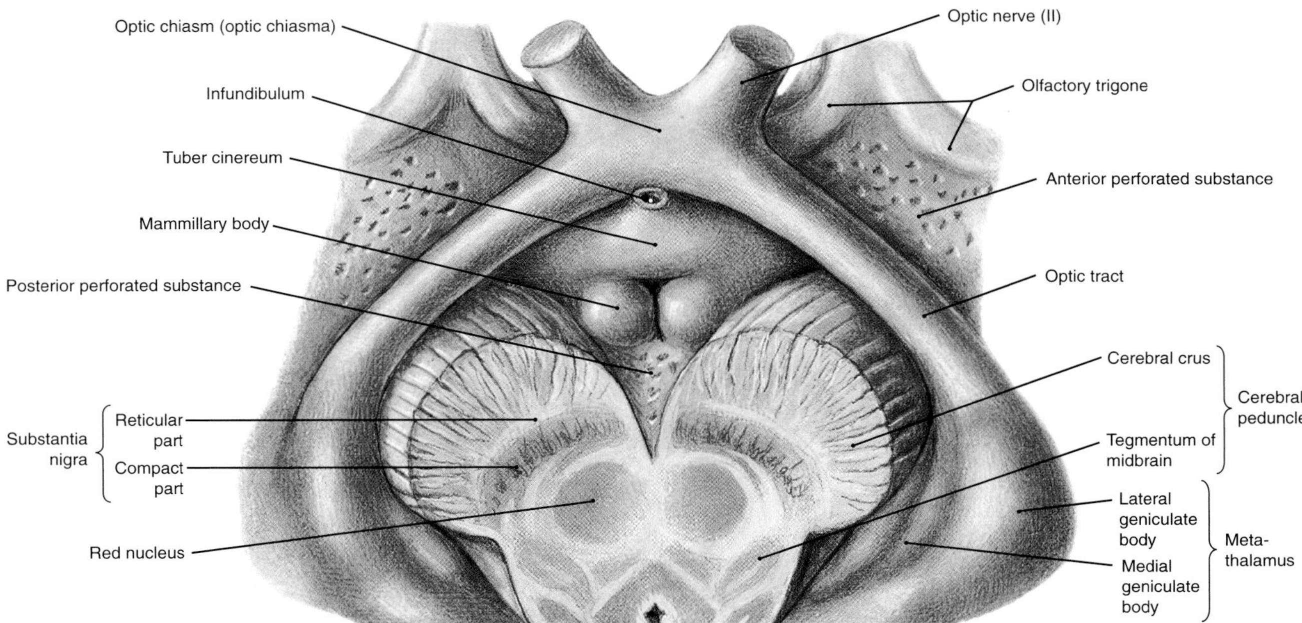
Optic chiasm (optic chiasma)
Infundibulum
Tuber cinereum
Mammillary body
Posterior perforated substance
Substantia nigra
Reticular part
Compact part
Red nucleus
Optic nerve (II)
Olfactory trigone
Anterior perforated substance
Optic tract
Cerebral crus
Tegmentum of midbrain
Cerebral peduncle
Lateral geniculate body
Medial geniculate body
Meta-thalamus

Figure 619.1 **Optic Chiasma, Optic Tract, and Lateral Geniculate Body; Severed Midbrain (Caudal View)**

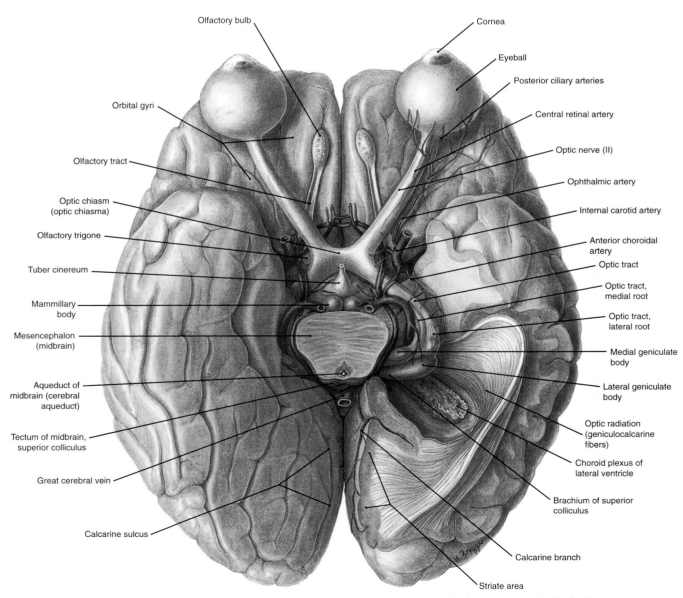

Olfactory bulb
Orbital gyri
Olfactory tract
Optic chiasm (optic chiasma)
Olfactory trigone
Tuber cinereum
Mammillary body
Mesencephalon (midbrain)
Aqueduct of midbrain (cerebral aqueduct)
Tectum of midbrain, superior colliculus
Great cerebral vein
Calcarine sulcus
Cornea
Eyeball
Posterior ciliary arteries
Central retinal artery
Optic nerve (II)
Ophthalmic artery
Internal carotid artery
Anterior choroidal artery
Optic tract
Optic tract, medial root
Optic tract, lateral root
Medial geniculate body
Lateral geniculate body
Optic radiation (geniculocalcarine fibers)
Choroid plexus of lateral ventricle
Brachium of superior colliculus
Calcarine branch
Striate area

Figure 619.2 **Visual Pathway from the Optic Nerve to the Cerebral Cortex; Ophthalmic Artery**

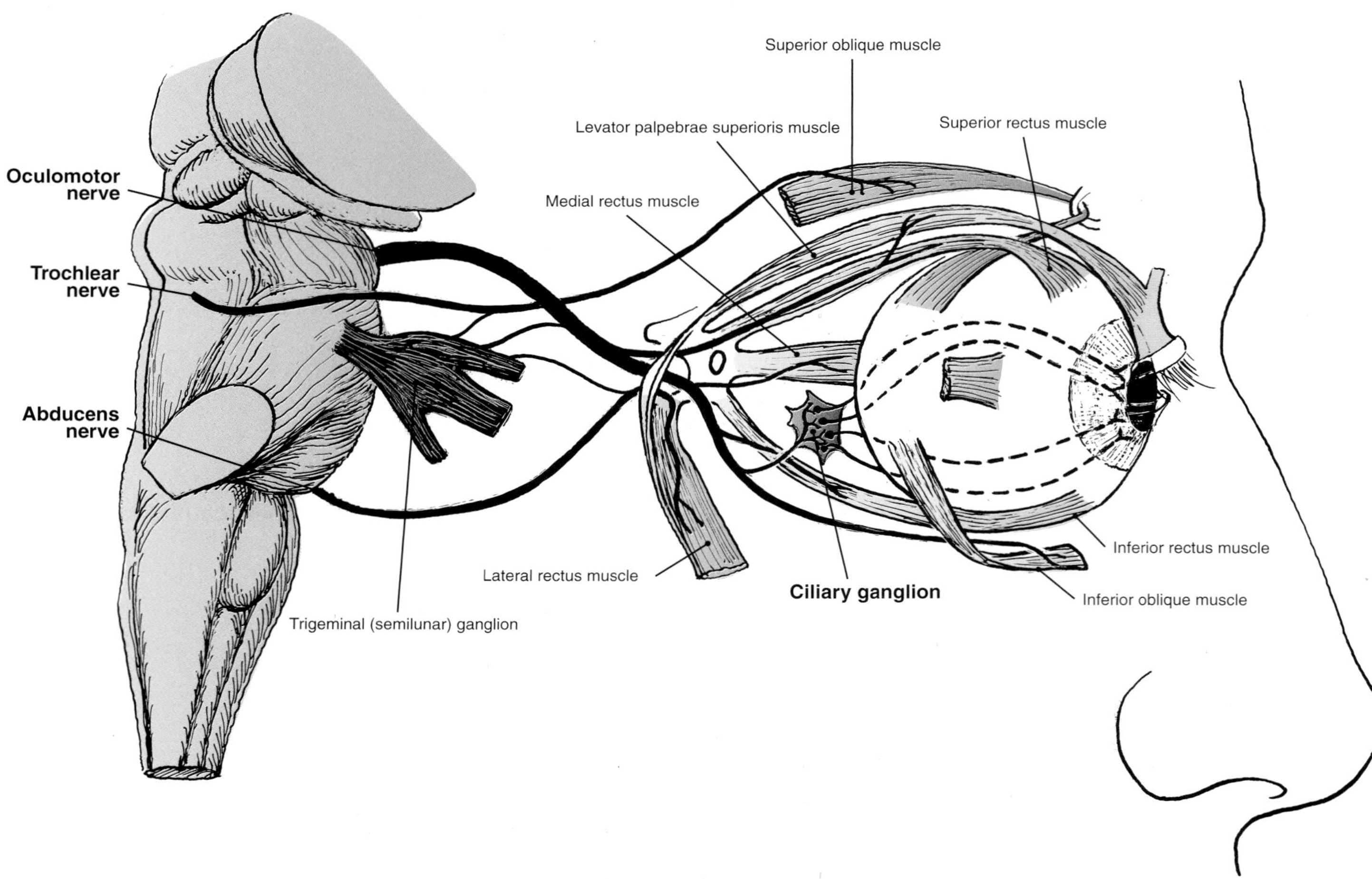
Superior oblique muscle
Levator palpebrae superioris muscle
Superior rectus muscle
Oculomotor nerve
Medial rectus muscle
Trochlear nerve
Abducens nerve
Inferior rectus muscle
Lateral rectus muscle
Ciliary ganglion
Inferior oblique muscle
Trigeminal (semilunar) ganglion

Figure 620 **Oculomotor (III), Trochlear (IV), and Abducens (VI) Nerves: Lateral View (Diagram)**

OCULOMOTOR NERVE (III)

NOTE: (1) The **oculomotor nerve** principally carries **somatomotor fibers** to five extraocular muscles and **preganglionic parasympathetic fibers** to the **ciliary ganglion.** These fibers have their cell bodies in the midbrain: those to the extraocular muscles in the **main oculomotor nucleus,** while the preganglionic parasympathetic fibers have their cell bodies in the **accessory** or **autonomic nucleus** (of Edinger–Westphal).

(2) The oculomotor nerve emerges from the midbrain between the posterior cerebral artery (superior to the nerve) and the superior cerebellar artery (just caudal to the nerve). Hardening of these pulsating arteries and plaques within them can injure the nerve.

(3) The oculomotor nerve courses through the cavernous sinus and enters the orbit by way of the superior orbital fissure and within the annulus tendinous; the nerve then divides into **superior and inferior divisions** and within the orbit supplies five extraocular muscles.

(4) The **superior division** is the smaller of the two and ascends lateral to the optic nerve to supply the **levator palpebrae superioris** and the **superior rectus muscles;** the **inferior division** divides into three branches to supply the **medial rectus,** the **inferior rectus,** and the **inferior oblique muscles.**

(5) The **preganglionic parasympathetic fibers** emerge from the midbrain with the somatomotor fibers and course in the inferior division of the oculomotor nerve in the branch to the inferior oblique muscle. The parasympathetic fibers then leave the nerve to the inferior oblique and pass directly to the **ciliary ganglion,** where they synapse with postganglionic parasympathetic cell bodies.

(6) The postganglionic parasympathetic fibers emerge from the ganglion and course along the **short ciliary nerves** to supply the **ciliary muscle** and the **constrictor of the pupil.** The ciliary muscle controls the shape of the lens, while the constrictor of the pupil controls the size of the pupil by reducing its diameter.

(7) Lesions of the oculomotor nerve result in a condition called **ophthalmoplegia.** Its symptoms include: (a) **strabismus,** which is the inability to direct both eyes to the same object, this effect results in a downward and abducted eyeball, (b) **a dilated pupil,** (c) **a droopy eyelid** because the levator muscle is denervated, and (d) **a loss of accommodation.**

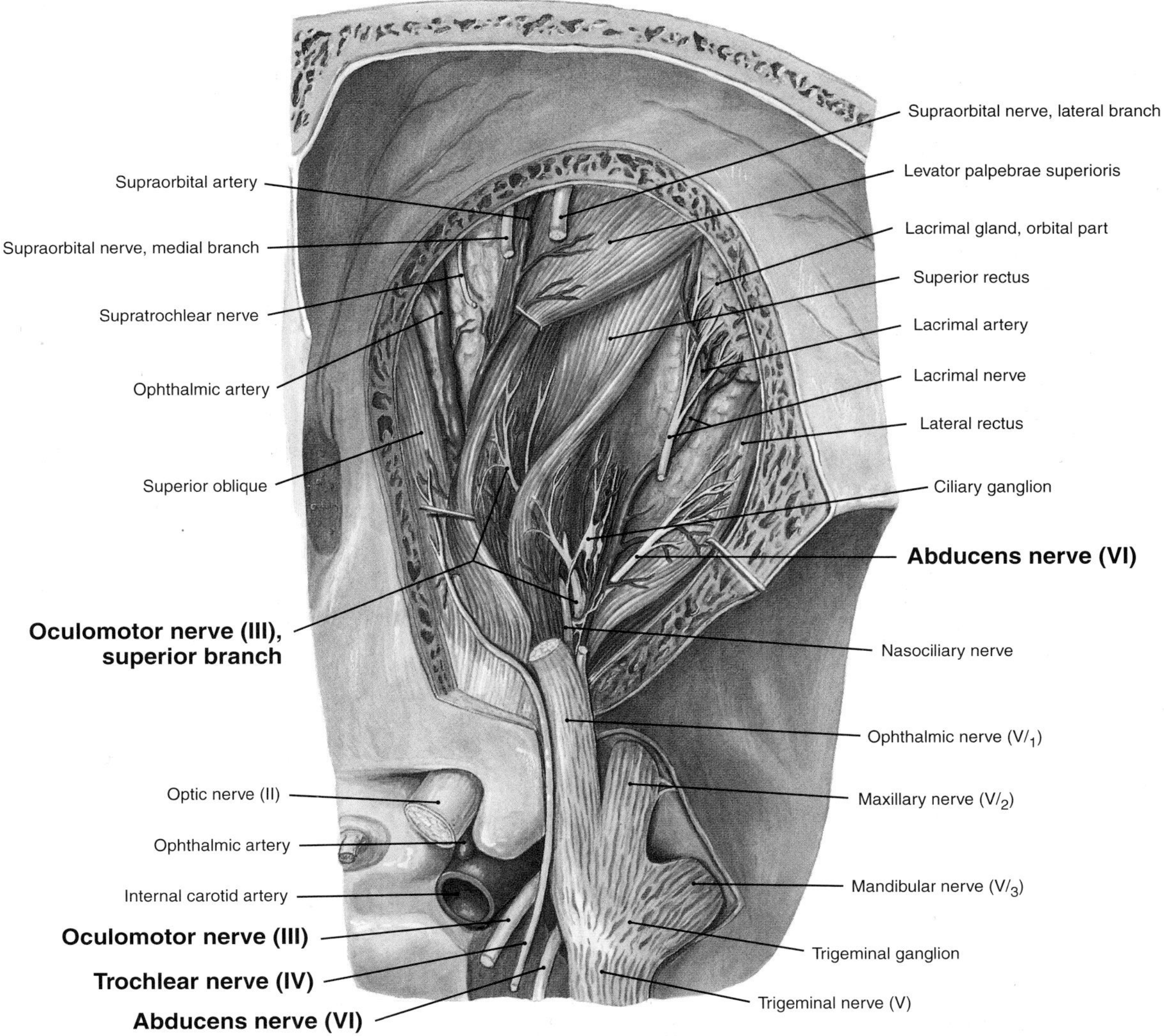
Supraorbital nerve, lateral branch
Levator palpebrae superioris
Lacrimal gland, orbital part
Superior rectus
Lacrimal artery
Lacrimal nerve
Lateral rectus
Ciliary ganglion
Abducens nerve (VI)
Nasociliary nerve
Ophthalmic nerve (V/1)
Maxillary nerve (V/2)
Mandibular nerve (V/3)
Trigeminal ganglion
Trigeminal nerve (V)
Supraorbital artery
Supraorbital nerve, medial branch
Supratrochlear nerve
Ophthalmic artery
Superior oblique
Oculomotor nerve (III), superior branch
Optic nerve (II)
Ophthalmic artery
Internal carotid artery
Oculomotor nerve (III)
Trochlear nerve (IV)
Abducens nerve (VI)

Figure 621 **Oculomotor, Trochlear, and Abducens Nerves as They Enter the Orbital Cavity (Superior View)**

TROCHLEAR NERVE (IV)

NOTE: (1) The **trochlear nerve** is the smallest of all the cranial nerves and it supplies only the **superior oblique muscle** in the orbit. It is the only cranial nerve to emerge from the central nervous system on the dorsal aspect of the brain.

(2) The fibers of the trochlear nerve cross to the contralateral side before leaving the dorsal midbrain; after emerging, the nerve is directed laterally around the brainstem immediately above the pons between the posterior cerebral and superior cerebellar arteries.

(3) The nerve then passes rostrally in the lateral wall of the **cavernous sinus** below the oculomotor nerve and superior to the ophthalmic division of the trigeminal nerve (see Fig. 525.1). Anteriorly, it crosses the oculomotor nerve from lateral to medial and it enters the orbit through the **superior orbital fissure** outside the annulus tendineus. In the orbit, the nerve lies superior to the extraocular muscles and it pierces the superior surface of the superior oblique muscle.

(4) **If the oculomotor nerve is injured,** the superior oblique muscle is denervated and it causes an impairment in turning the eye downward and outward. The eye is extorted (outward rotation) because the inferior oblique muscle is acting unopposed.

ABDUCENS NERVE (VI)

NOTE: (1) The **abducens nerve** supplies only the **lateral rectus muscle** within the orbit. Its fibers descend from the abducens nucleus located in the caudal pons, just deep to the fourth ventricle.

(2) The abducens fibers emerge from the ventral surface of the brainstem in the sulcus between the anterior medulla and the posterior border of the pons.

(3) The nerve then courses superiorly, anteriorly, and laterally through the pontine cistern. It then bends acutely forward to traverse the cavernous sinus and it enters the orbital cavity through the **superior orbital fissure** and within the annulus tendineus. It pierces the lateral rectus along the medial surface of the muscle.

(4) The nerve travels a long course from the lower pons to the orbit and is subject to damage due to skull fractures or in cases involving increased intracranial pressure.

(5) If the lateral rectus muscle is denervated, the medial rectus acts unopposed (**internal strabismus**).

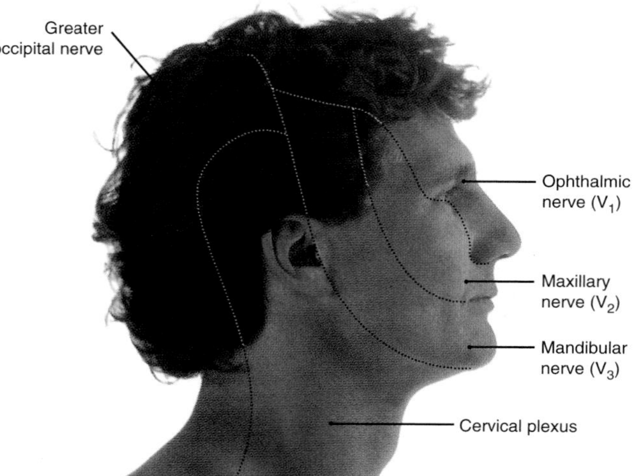
Greater occipital nerve
Ophthalmic nerve (V_1)
Maxillary nerve (V_2)
Mandibular nerve (V_3)
Cervical plexus

Figure 622.1 Lateral View of the Face: Surface Areas Supplied by the Three Divisions of the Trigeminal Nerve

NOTE: (1) The **ophthalmic nerve** supplies the skin of nose, upper eyelid, and the scalp from the eyebrow posteriorly to the vertex or top of the skull cap.

(2) The **maxillary nerve** supplies the region between the eyelid and the upper lip, including the skin over the cheek bone.

(3) The **mandibular nerve** supplies the skin of the lower jaw, the lateral part of the face anterior to the ear, and the skin of the temple region on the lateral side of the head.

Supratrochlear nerve
Supraorbital nerve
Ciliary ganglion
Nasociliary nerve
Meningeal branch
Frontal nerve
Infratrochlear nerve
Auriculotemporal nerve
External nasal nerve
Temporal nerve
V_1
V_2
V_3
Pterygopalatine ganglion
Tensor tympani nerve
Medial pterygoid nerve
Tensor veli palatini nerve
Buccal nerve
Lingual nerve
Lateral pterygoid nerve
Masseter nerve
Buccinator muscle
Inferior alveolar nerve
Parotid gland
Sublingual gland
Submandibular gland
Geniohyoid muscle
Nerve to mylohyoid muscle
Mylohyoid muscle

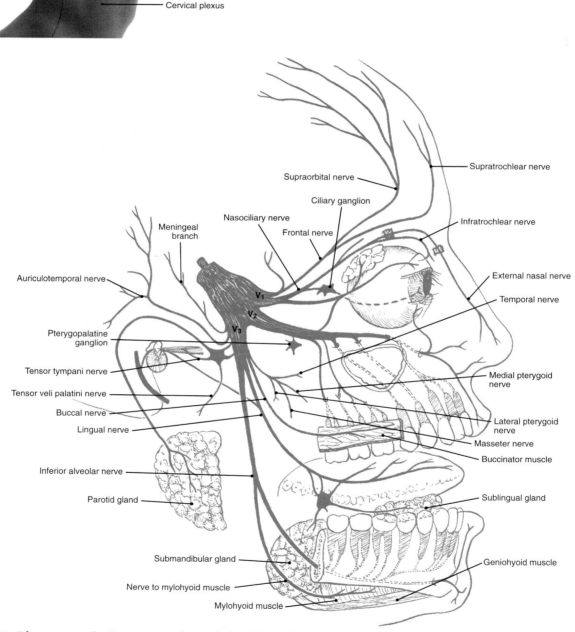

Figure 622.2 Diagrammatic Representation of the Trigeminal Nerve and Its Branches

NOTE: (1) The trigeminal nerve is the largest of the cranial nerves, and it is the great sensory nerve of the face and of the orbital, oral and nasal cavities; it also supplies much of the anterior scalp and all of the teeth.

(2) In addition to its sensory functions the trigeminal nerve, through its mandibular division, supplies the **four muscles of mastication**, the **mylohyoid muscle**, the **anterior belly of the digastric muscle,** and two tensors: the **tensor veli palatini** and the **tensor tympani** muscles.

(3) The cell bodies of the sensory fibers in the **ophthalmic, maxillary,** and **mandibular divisions** of the trigeminal nerve and located within the **trigeminal** (or semilunar) **ganglion.** The ganglion is located in a cleft or recess covered by dura mater, called the **trigeminal cave,** on the anterior aspect of the petrous portion of the temporal bone in the middle cranial fossa of the bony base of the skull.

Ophthalmic Division of the Trigeminal Nerve

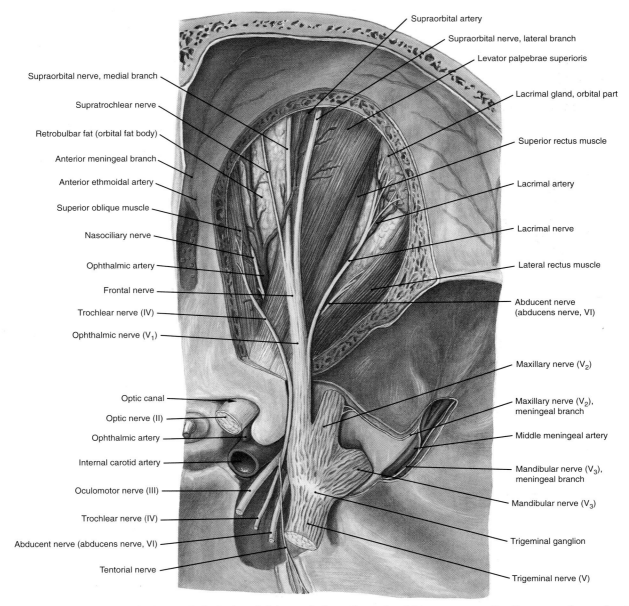

Supraorbital artery
Supraorbital nerve, lateral branch
Levator palpebrae superioris
Supraorbital nerve, medial branch
Lacrimal gland, orbital part
Supratrochlear nerve
Retrobulbar fat (orbital fat body)
Superior rectus muscle
Anterior meningeal branch
Anterior ethmoidal artery
Lacrimal artery
Superior oblique muscle
Lacrimal nerve
Nasociliary nerve
Ophthalmic artery
Lateral rectus muscle
Frontal nerve
Abducent nerve (abducens nerve, VI)
Trochlear nerve (IV)
Ophthalmic nerve (V_1)
Maxillary nerve (V_2)
Optic canal
Maxillary nerve (V_2), meningeal branch
Optic nerve (II)
Ophthalmic artery
Middle meningeal artery
Internal carotid artery
Mandibular nerve (V_3), meningeal branch
Oculomotor nerve (III)
Mandibular nerve (V_3)
Trochlear nerve (IV)
Abducent nerve (abducens nerve, VI)
Trigeminal ganglion
Tentorial nerve
Trigeminal nerve (V)

Figure 623.1 **Branches of the Ophthalmic Division of the Trigeminal Nerve upon Its Entrance into the Orbit**

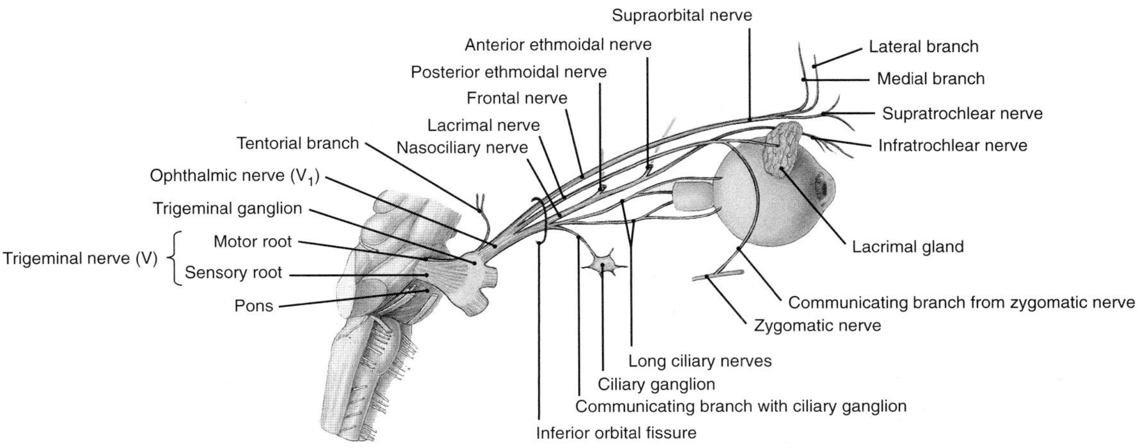
Supraorbital nerve
Anterior ethmoidal nerve
Lateral branch
Posterior ethmoidal nerve
Medial branch
Frontal nerve
Supratrochlear nerve
Lacrimal nerve
Tentorial branch
Nasociliary nerve
Infratrochlear nerve
Ophthalmic nerve (V_1)
Trigeminal ganglion
Motor root
Lacrimal gland
Trigeminal nerve (V)
Sensory root
Pons
Communicating branch from zygomatic nerve
Zygomatic nerve
Long ciliary nerves
Ciliary ganglion
Communicating branch with ciliary ganglion
Inferior orbital fissure

Figure 623.2 **Ophthalmic Division of the Trigeminal Nerve**

NOTE: (1) The **frontal, lacrimal,** and **nasociliary nerves** along with the small tentorial (dural) branch are the nerves that stem from the trunk of the ophthalmic nerve.

(2) The frontal nerve gives rise to the **supraorbital** (medial and lateral branches) and the **supratrochlear** branches.

(3) The lacrimal nerve courses to the lacrimal gland and then pierces the skin over the lateral orbit. It receives a communicating branch from the maxillary nerve carrying postganglionic parasympathetic fibers to the lacrimal gland.

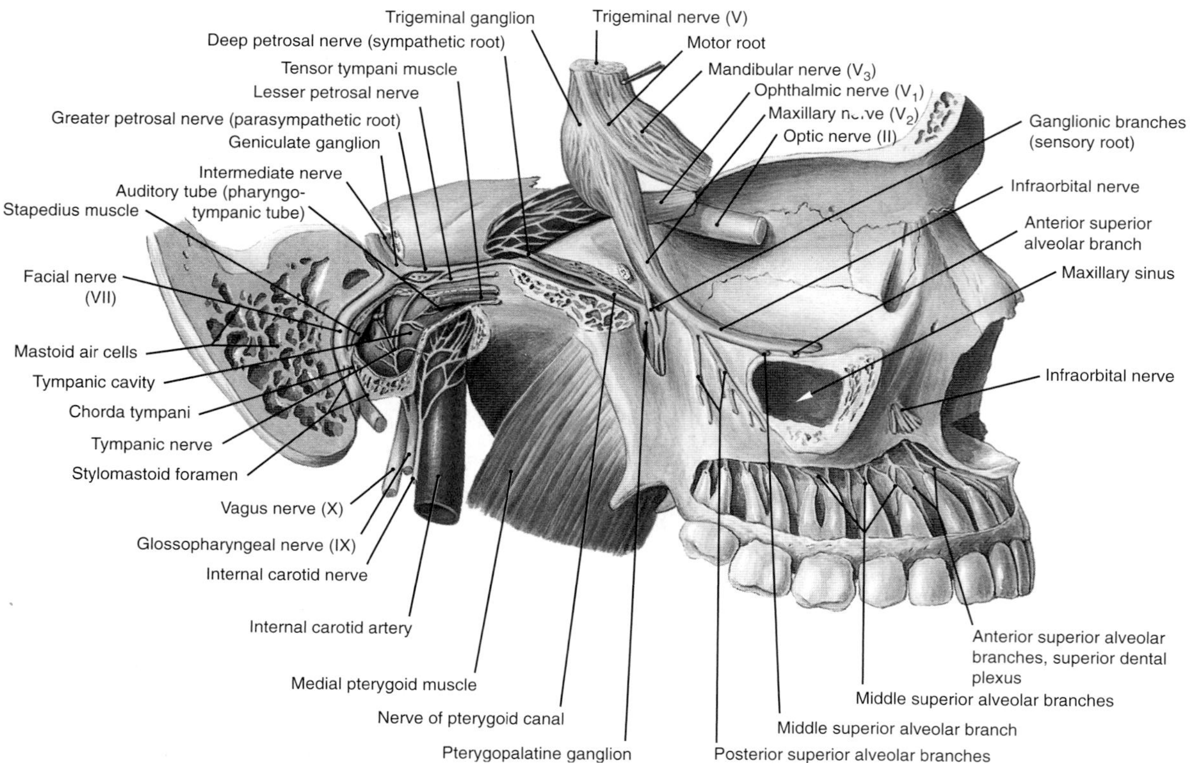
Trigeminal ganglion
Trigeminal nerve (V)
Deep petrosal nerve (sympathetic root)
Motor root
Tensor tympani muscle
Mandibular nerve (V_3)
Lesser petrosal nerve
Ophthalmic nerve (V_1)
Greater petrosal nerve (parasympathetic root)
Maxillary nerve (V_2)
Geniculate ganglion
Optic nerve (II)
Ganglionic branches (sensory root)
Intermediate nerve
Auditory tube (pharyngo-tympanic tube)
Stapedius muscle
Infraorbital nerve
Anterior superior alveolar branch
Facial nerve (VII)
Maxillary sinus
Mastoid air cells
Tympanic cavity
Infraorbital nerve
Chorda tympani
Tympanic nerve
Stylomastoid foramen
Vagus nerve (X)
Glossopharyngeal nerve (IX)
Internal carotid nerve
Internal carotid artery
Anterior superior alveolar branches, superior dental plexus
Medial pterygoid muscle
Middle superior alveolar branches
Nerve of pterygoid canal
Middle superior alveolar branch
Pterygopalatine ganglion
Posterior superior alveolar branches

Figure 624.1 **Maxillary Nerve and Its Infraorbital and Superior Alveolar Branches**

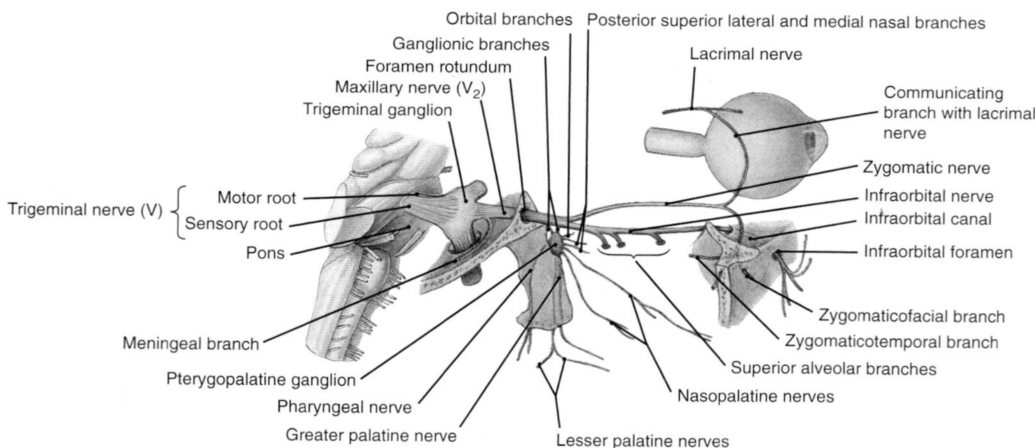
Orbital branches
Posterior superior lateral and medial nasal branches
Ganglionic branches
Lacrimal nerve
Foramen rotundum
Maxillary nerve (V_2)
Communicating branch with lacrimal nerve
Trigeminal ganglion
Zygomatic nerve
Motor root
Trigeminal nerve (V)
Sensory root
Infraorbital nerve
Infraorbital canal
Pons
Infraorbital foramen
Zygomaticofacial branch
Meningeal branch
Zygomaticotemporal branch
Superior alveolar branches
Pterygopalatine ganglion
Nasopalatine nerves
Pharyngeal nerve
Greater palatine nerve
Lesser palatine nerves

Figure 624.2 **Maxillary Division of the Trigeminal Nerve**

NOTE: (1) The **zygomatic, infraorbital, nasopalatine, greater** and **lesser palatine, lateral** and **medial nasal,** and **pharyngeal** branches derive from the trunk of the maxillary nerve. These are all sensory nerves.

(2) This nerve supplies all of the upper teeth through the superior alveolar branches that come off of the infraorbital nerve. After emerging on the face, the infraorbital nerve supplies the skin from the upper lip to the lower eyelid.

(3) The nasopalatine and greater and lesser palatine branches supply the nasal septum and the hard and soft palates, while the pharyngeal nerve supplies the mucosa of the nasopharynx.

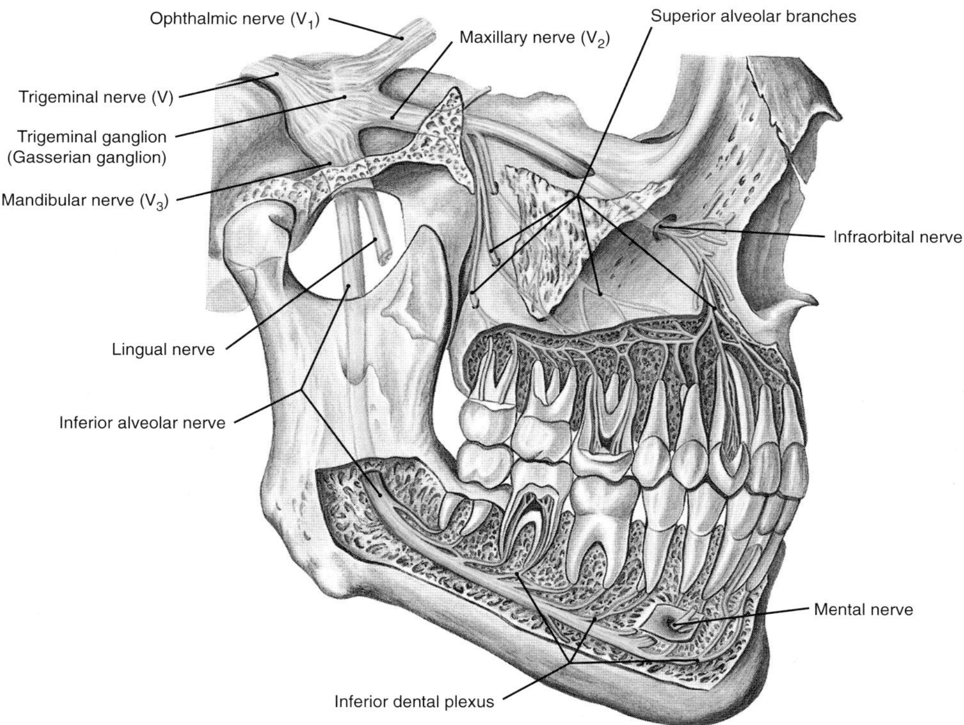
Ophthalmic nerve (V_1)
Maxillary nerve (V_2)
Superior alveolar branches
Trigeminal nerve (V)
Trigeminal ganglion
(Gasserian ganglion)
Mandibular nerve (V_3)
Infraorbital nerve
Lingual nerve
Inferior alveolar nerve
Mental nerve
Inferior dental plexus

Figure 625.1 Maxillary and Mandibular Nerves

NOTE: (1) In this figure, only the **inferior alveolar nerve** and the proximal stump of the cut **lingual nerve** from the mandibular nerve are shown.

(2) The infraorbital and superior alveolar branches of the maxillary nerve are seen supplying structures in the maxillary region.

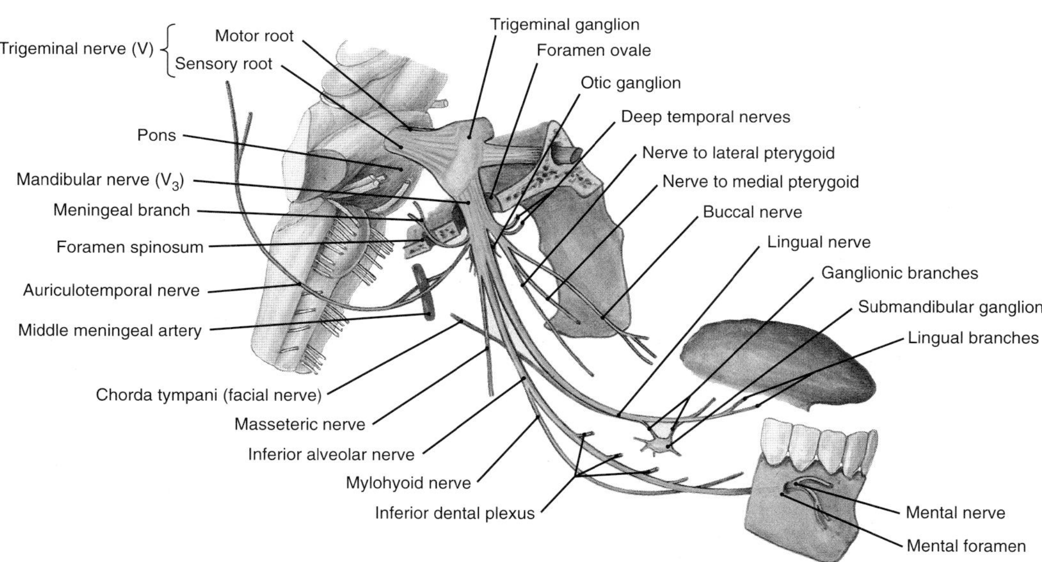
Trigeminal nerve (V)
Motor root
Sensory root
Trigeminal ganglion
Foramen ovale
Otic ganglion
Deep temporal nerves
Pons
Nerve to lateral pterygoid
Nerve to medial pterygoid
Mandibular nerve (V_3)
Meningeal branch
Buccal nerve
Foramen spinosum
Lingual nerve
Ganglionic branches
Auriculotemporal nerve
Submandibular ganglion
Middle meningeal artery
Lingual branches
Chorda tympani (facial nerve)
Masseteric nerve
Inferior alveolar nerve
Mylohyoid nerve
Inferior dental plexus
Mental nerve
Mental foramen

Figure 625.2 Mandibular Division of the Trigeminal Nerve

NOTE: (1) The **auriculotemporal, inferior alveolar,** and **lingual nerves** and the branches that supply the muscles of mastication: the **masseteric** and **deep temporal nerves** and the **nerves to the lateral and medial pterygoid muscles.**

(2) The mylohyoid branch of the inferior alveolar nerve that supplies the mylohyoid muscle and the anterior belly of the digastric muscle.

(3) Not shown in this figure but shown in Figure 624.1, are the small, delicate branches that supply two tensor muscles: the **tensor veli palatini** that tenses the soft palate and the **tensor tympani muscle** that tenses the tympanic membrane in the middle ear.

(4) The mandibular nerve supplies sensory innervation to all of the lower teeth, the skin of the chin, lower lip, and the side of the face and head anterior to the external ear.

Figure 626.1 Facial Nerve Descending in the Facial Canal

NOTE: (1) The facial nerve emerges from the brainstem by motor and sensory roots. The cells bodies of the fibers in the sensory root are located in the **geniculate ganglion.**

(2) The sensory fibers of the facial nerve are of two types: **general sensation** and **special sense** of **taste** from the anterior two-thirds of the tongue that course centrally in chorda tympani nerve.

(3) The motor fibers of the facial nerve also are of two types: **somatomotor** to the muscles of facial expression, the stapedius muscle, and to the posterior belly of the digastric muscle and stylohyoid muscle and **visceromotor** (preganglionic parasympathetic) that go to the pterygopalatine and submandibular ganglia.

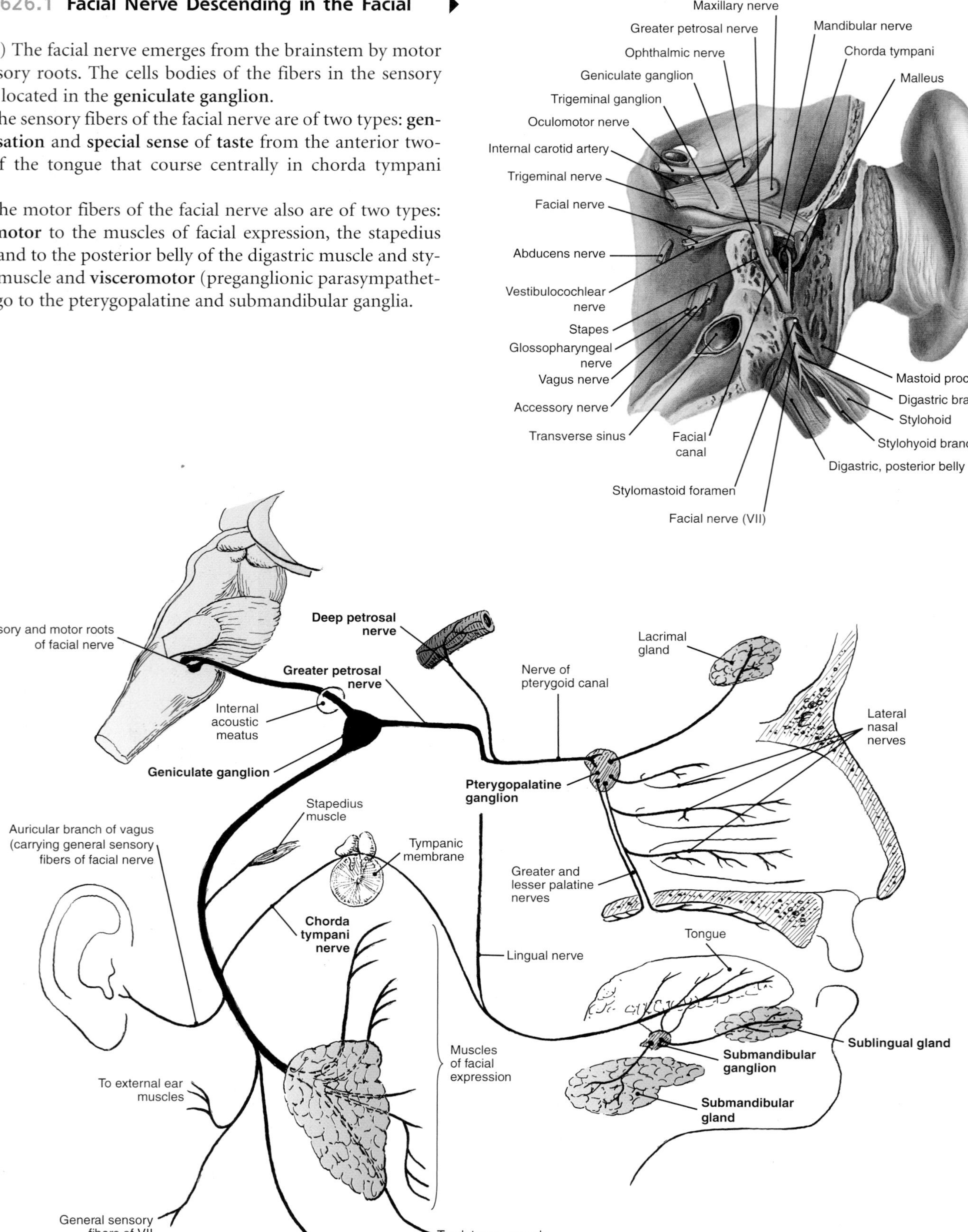
Maxillary nerve
Greater petrosal nerve
Mandibular nerve
Ophthalmic nerve
Chorda tympani
Geniculate ganglion
Malleus
Trigeminal ganglion
Oculomotor nerve
Internal carotid artery
Trigeminal nerve
Facial nerve
Abducens nerve
Vestibulocochlear nerve
Stapes
Glossopharyngeal nerve
Vagus nerve
Accessory nerve
Transverse sinus
Facial canal
Mastoid process
Digastric branch
Stylohoid
Stylohyoid branch
Digastric, posterior belly
Stylomastoid foramen
Facial nerve (VII)
Sensory and motor roots of facial nerve
Deep petrosal nerve
Greater petrosal nerve
Internal acoustic meatus
Geniculate ganglion
Nerve of pterygoid canal
Lacrimal gland
Lateral nasal nerves
Pterygopalatine ganglion
Stapedius muscle
Tympanic membrane
Auricular branch of vagus (carrying general sensory fibers of facial nerve
Greater and lesser palatine nerves
Chorda tympani nerve
Tongue
Lingual nerve
Sublingual gland
Submandibular ganglion
Muscles of facial expression
To external ear muscles
Submandibular gland
General sensory fibers of VII
To platysma muscle
To posterior belly of digastric muscle
To stylohyoid muscle

Figure 626.2 Diagrammatic View of the Facial Nerve

NOTE: (1) The **greater petrosal nerve** branches from the main stem of the facial nerve at the genu of the facial nerve (i.e., where the nerve turns about 90 degrees inferiorly from its horizontal course through the internal acoustic meatus).

(2) The **chorda tympani nerve** branches along the facial canal posterior to the middle ear. It then enters the middle ear cavity courses across the tympanic membrane and emerges in the deep face. It joins the **lingual nerve** (a branch of the trigeminal nerve) and descends to the submandibular ganglion.

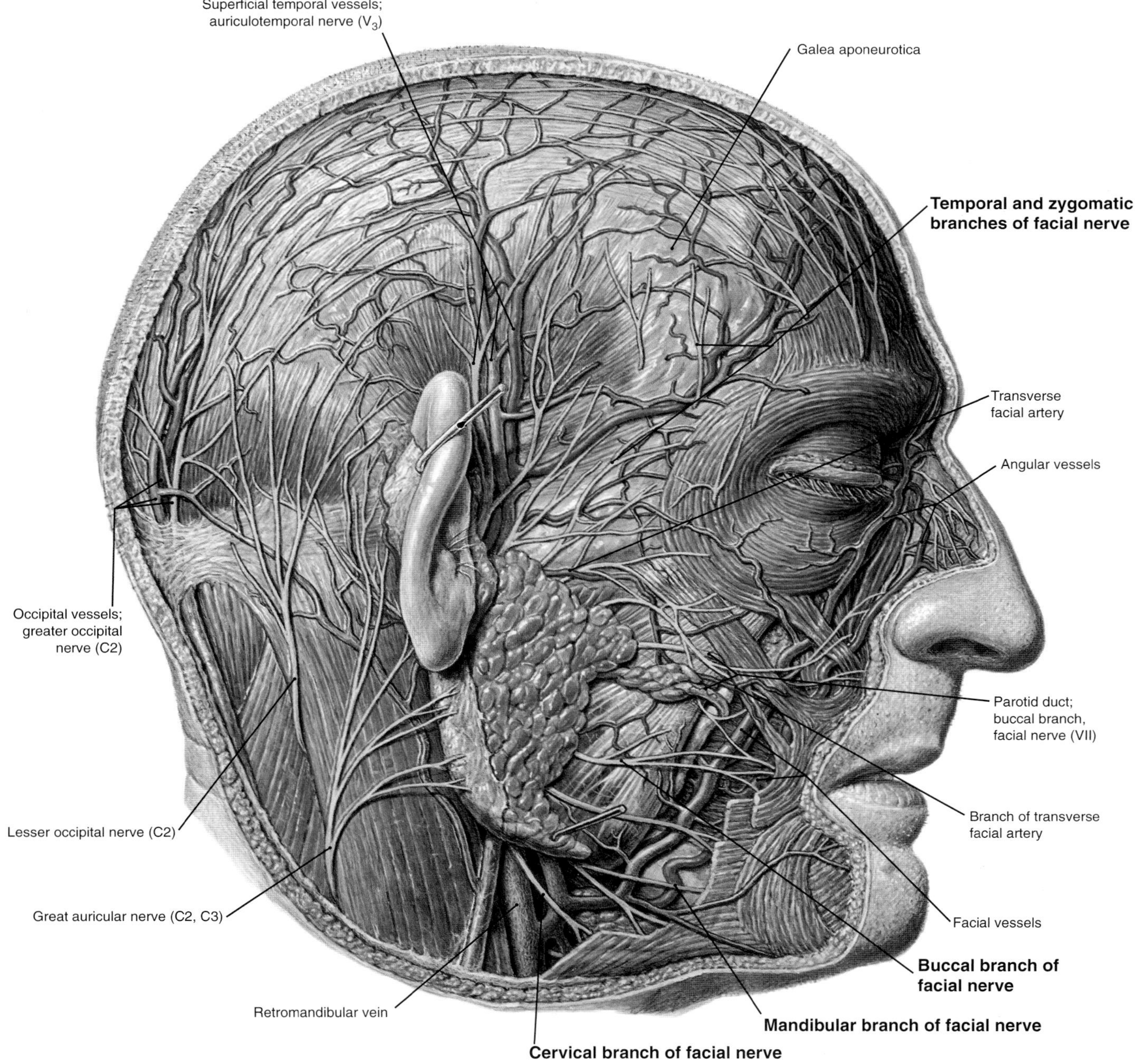

Superficial temporal vessels; auriculotemporal nerve (V_3)
Galea aponeurotica
Temporal and zygomatic branches of facial nerve
Transverse facial artery
Angular vessels
Occipital vessels; greater occipital nerve (C2)
Parotid duct; buccal branch, facial nerve (VII)
Branch of transverse facial artery
Lesser occipital nerve (C2)
Great auricular nerve (C2, C3)
Facial vessels
Buccal branch of facial nerve
Retromandibular vein
Mandibular branch of facial nerve
Cervical branch of facial nerve

Figure 627 Facial Nerve on the Side of the Face

NOTE: (1) The facial nerve emerges from the facial canal at the stylomastoid foramen behind the ear lobe, courses through the parotid gland, and divides into muscular branches for the muscles of facial expression.

(2) The following branches of the facial nerve supply the muscles of facial expression: **temporal, zygomatic, buccal, mandibular,** and **cervical** branches. These nerves contain somatomotor fibers that are under voluntary control.

(3) Injury to the facial nerve or dysfunction of the facial nerve on one side because of paralysis (Bell's palsy) leaves that side of the face expressionless and results in a loss of tone of the superficial facial muscles. This is usually recognizable because of a loss of firmness and a sagging of the face on the afflicted side compared with the normal side.

(4) Because the branches of the facial nerve cross the face horizontally, any incision that might be necessary should be a horizontal one and NOT VERTICAL.

(5) The parotid gland overlies the facial nerve anterior and inferior to the external ear.

(6) The posterior aspect of the scalp is supplied by sensory fibers from the greater occipital nerve (posterior primary ramus of C2), and the skin posterior to the ear and on the lateral side of the upper neck is supplied with sensory fibers from lesser occipital nerve and the great auricular nerve from the cervical plexus and not from either the facial or trigeminal nerves.

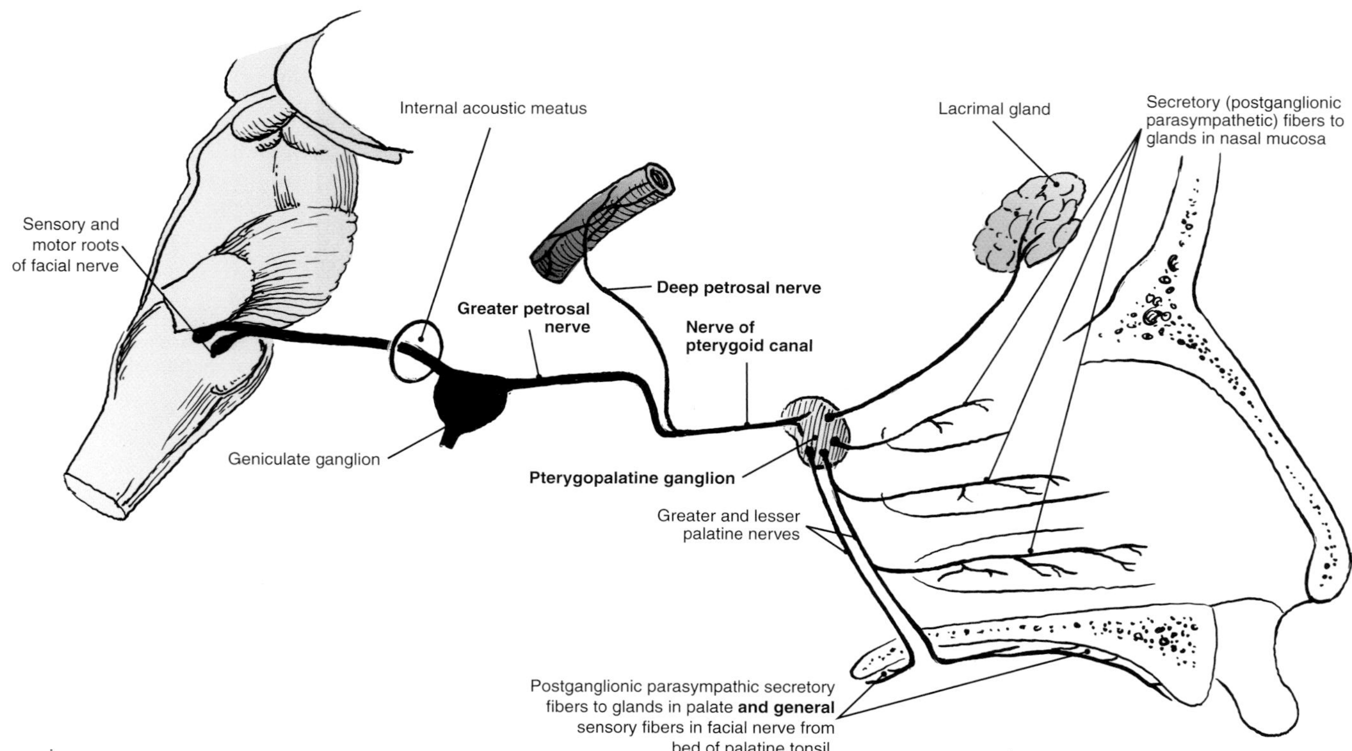
Internal acoustic meatus
Lacrimal gland
Secretory (postganglionic parasympathetic) fibers to glands in nasal mucosa
Sensory and motor roots of facial nerve
Deep petrosal nerve
Greater petrosal nerve
Nerve of pterygoid canal
Geniculate ganglion
Pterygopalatine ganglion
Greater and lesser palatine nerves
Postganglionic parasympathetic secretory fibers to glands in palate and general sensory fibers in facial nerve from bed of palatine tonsil

Figure 628.1 **Diagrammatic Representation of the Facial Nerve and Its Connections**

NOTE: (1) The **greater petrosal nerve** commences at the **geniculate ganglion** and is joined by the **deep petrosal nerve** to form the nerve of the pterygoid canal. The greater petrosal nerve is carrying preganglionic parasympathetic fibers to the pterygopalatine ganglion and taste fibers from the palate. It receives postganglionic sympathetic fibers from the **deep petrosal nerve,** and together these various fibers form the **nerve of the pterygoid canal.**

(2) From the pterygopalatine ganglion postganglionic parasympathetic fibers course: (a) to the lacrimal gland by way of the zygomatic branch of the maxillary nerve and then the lacrimal branch of the ophthalmic nerve, (b) to mucous glands in the lining of the lateral wall of the nasal cavity and septum, and (c) to mucous glands in the lining of the soft and hard palate by way of the greater and lesser palatine nerves. It is also thought that these nerves carry taste fiber from the palate as well.

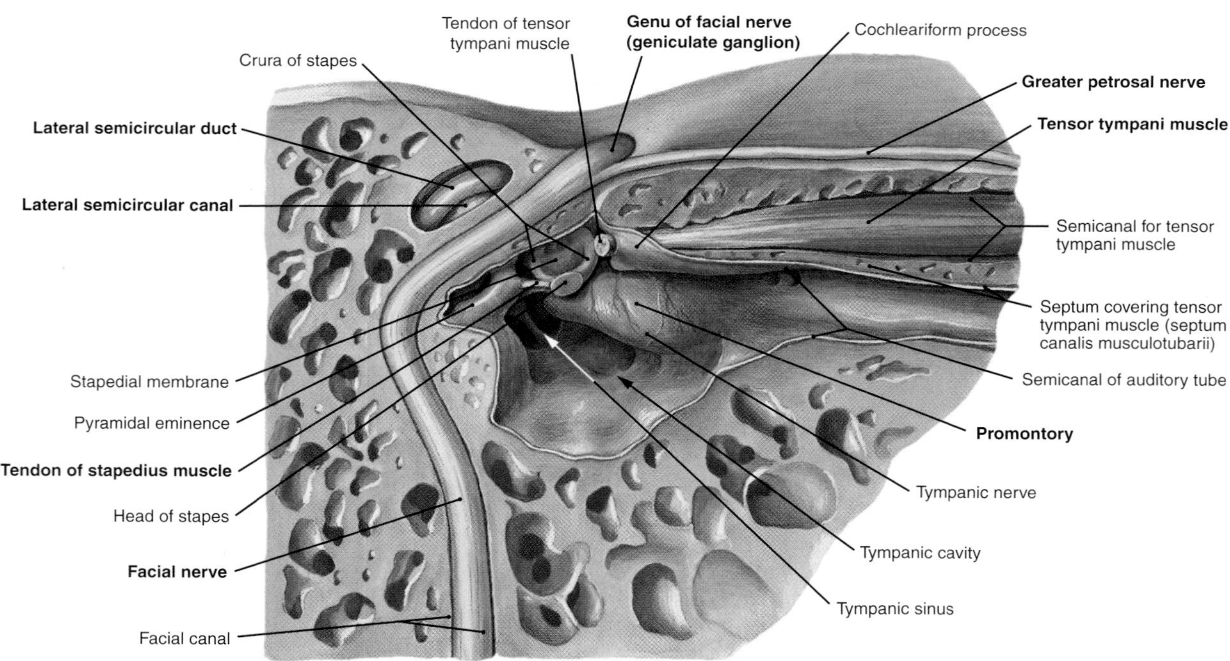
Tendon of tensor tympani muscle
Genu of facial nerve (geniculate ganglion)
Cochleariform process
Crura of stapes
Greater petrosal nerve
Lateral semicircular duct
Tensor tympani muscle
Lateral semicircular canal
Semicanal for tensor tympani muscle
Septum covering tensor tympani muscle (septum canalis musculotubarii)
Stapedial membrane
Semicanal of auditory tube
Pyramidal eminence
Promontory
Tendon of stapedius muscle
Tympanic nerve
Head of stapes
Tympanic cavity
Facial nerve
Tympanic sinus
Facial canal

Figure 628.2 **Facial Nerve in the Facial Canal and Its Greater Petrosal Branch**

NOTE: The greater petrosal nerve branches from the facial nerve at the genu (90-degree turn). It carries preganglionic parasympathetic fibers and taste fibers from the palate.

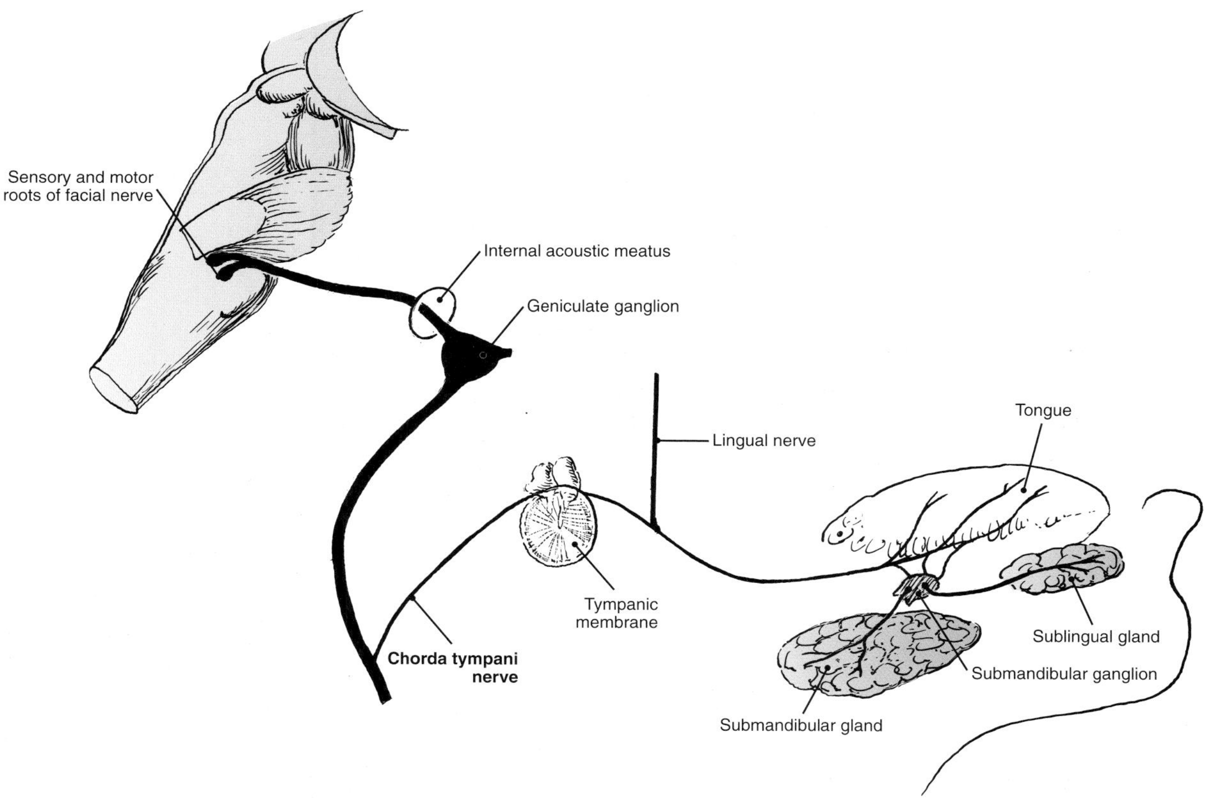
Sensory and motor roots of facial nerve
Internal acoustic meatus
Geniculate ganglion
Lingual nerve
Tongue
Tympanic membrane
Chorda tympani nerve
Sublingual gland
Submandibular ganglion
Submandibular gland

Figure 629.1 **Diagrammatic Representation of the Facial Nerve and Its Chorda Tympani Branch**

NOTE: (1) The facial nerve descends in the facial canal and at the level of the tympanic cavity it gives off the chorda tympani nerve that pierces the bone to enter the tympanic cavity.

(2) This nerve carries visceromotor (preganglionic parasympathetic) nerve fibers that synapse in the submandibular ganglion to supply the submandibular and sublingual glands. It also carries special sensory taste fibers from the anterior two-thirds of the tongue.

(3) Within the tympanic cavity the nerve courses over the medial surface of the tympanic membrane adjacent to the superior border of the membrane.

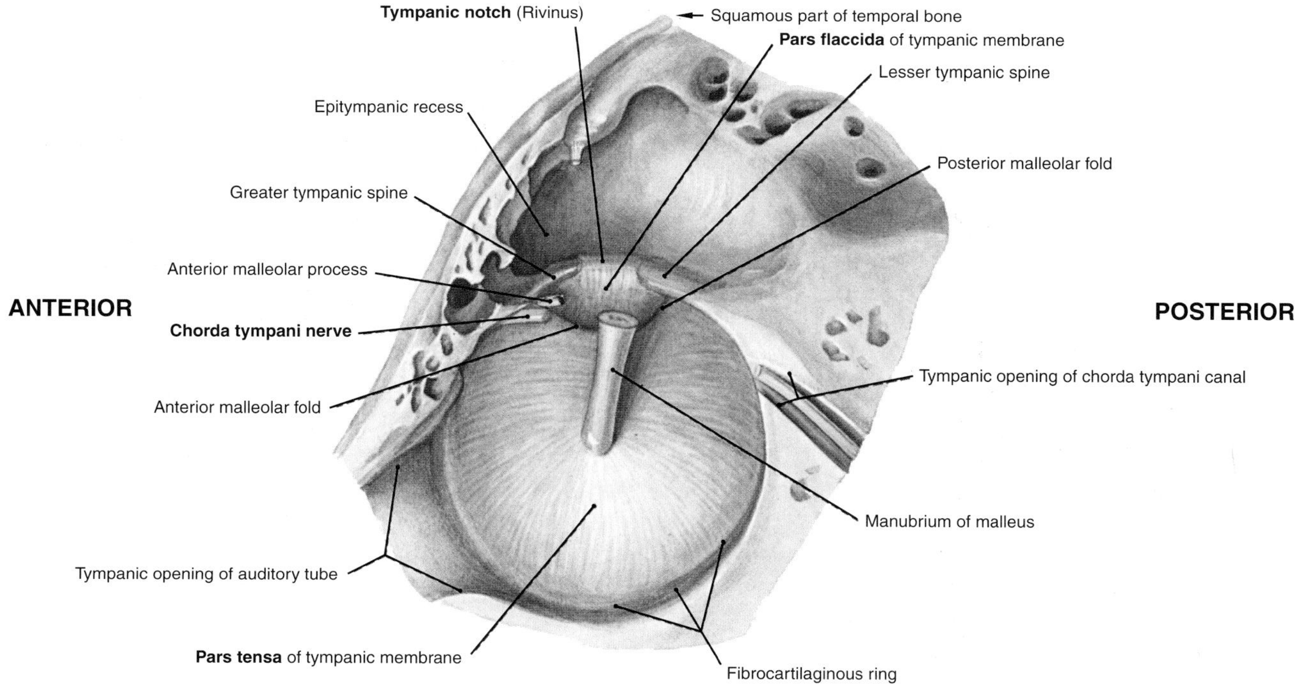
Tympanic notch (Rivinus)
Squamous part of temporal bone
Pars flaccida of tympanic membrane
Lesser tympanic spine
Epitympanic recess
Posterior malleolar fold
Greater tympanic spine
Anterior malleolar process
ANTERIOR
Chorda tympani nerve
POSTERIOR
Tympanic opening of chorda tympani canal
Anterior malleolar fold
Manubrium of malleus
Tympanic opening of auditory tube
Pars tensa of tympanic membrane
Fibrocartilaginous ring

Figure 629.2 **Medial View of the Tympanic Membrane in the Middle Ear Cavity**

NOTE: The chorda tympani nerve enters the posterior aspect of the tympanic cavity and after crossing the tympanic membrane, it leaves the cavity anteriorly to enter the superior aspect of the deep face (see Fig. 513).

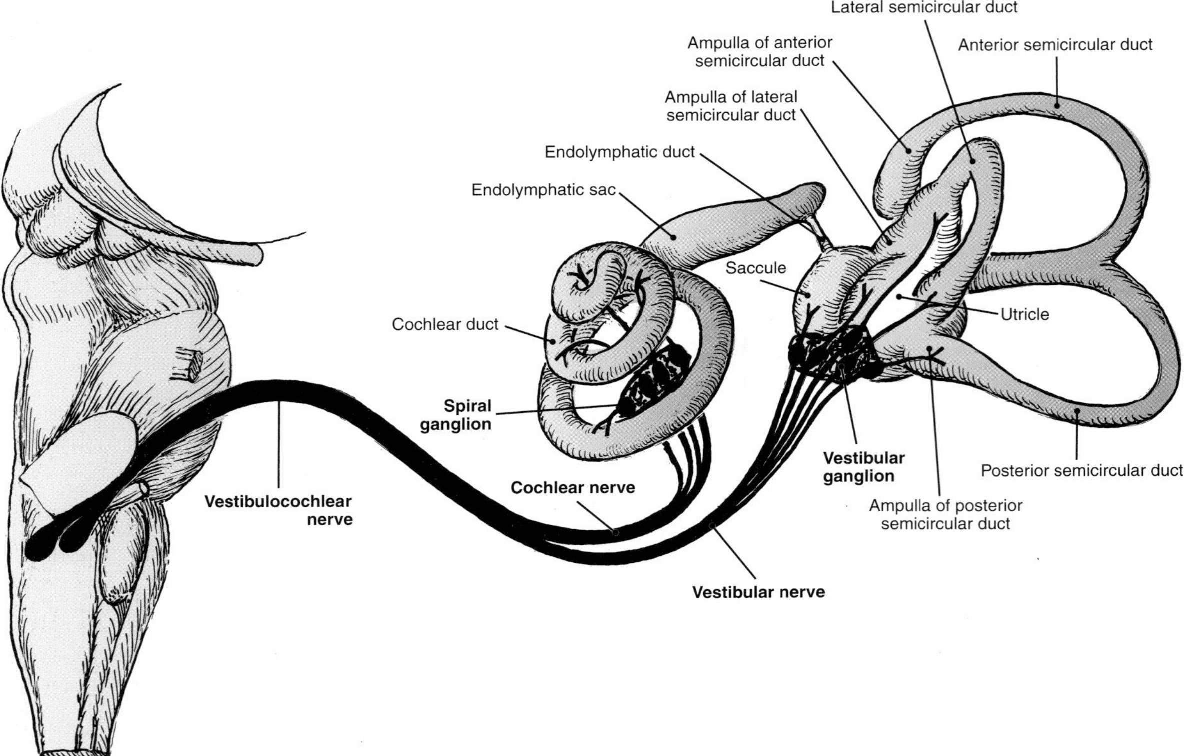
Lateral semicircular duct
Ampulla of anterior semicircular duct
Anterior semicircular duct
Ampulla of lateral semicircular duct
Endolymphatic duct
Endolymphatic sac
Saccule
Cochlear duct
Utricle
Spiral ganglion
Vestibular ganglion
Posterior semicircular duct
Cochlear nerve
Vestibulocochlear nerve
Ampulla of posterior semicircular duct
Vestibular nerve

Figure 630.1 Eighth Cranial Nerve (VIII): Vestibulocochlear Nerve

NOTE: (1) The **spiral organ of Corti** within the internal ear contains the receptor cells for the special sense of hearing. These receptors, called **hair cells,** are in the **cochlear duct,** and they are innervated by the peripheral processes of sensory neurons whose cell bodies are in the **spiral ganglion.** The central processes of these neurons form the **cochlear nerve.**

(2) The **vestibular apparatus** of the eighth cranial nerve consists of three semicircular canals, the utricle, the saccule, receptors within these structures and the neurons in the **vestibular ganglion.** These neurons send peripheral processes to these receptor cells and their central processes to the brain by way of the **vestibular nerve.**

(3) The cochlear and vestibular nerves join to form the **vestibulocochlear** or **eighth cranial nerve.**

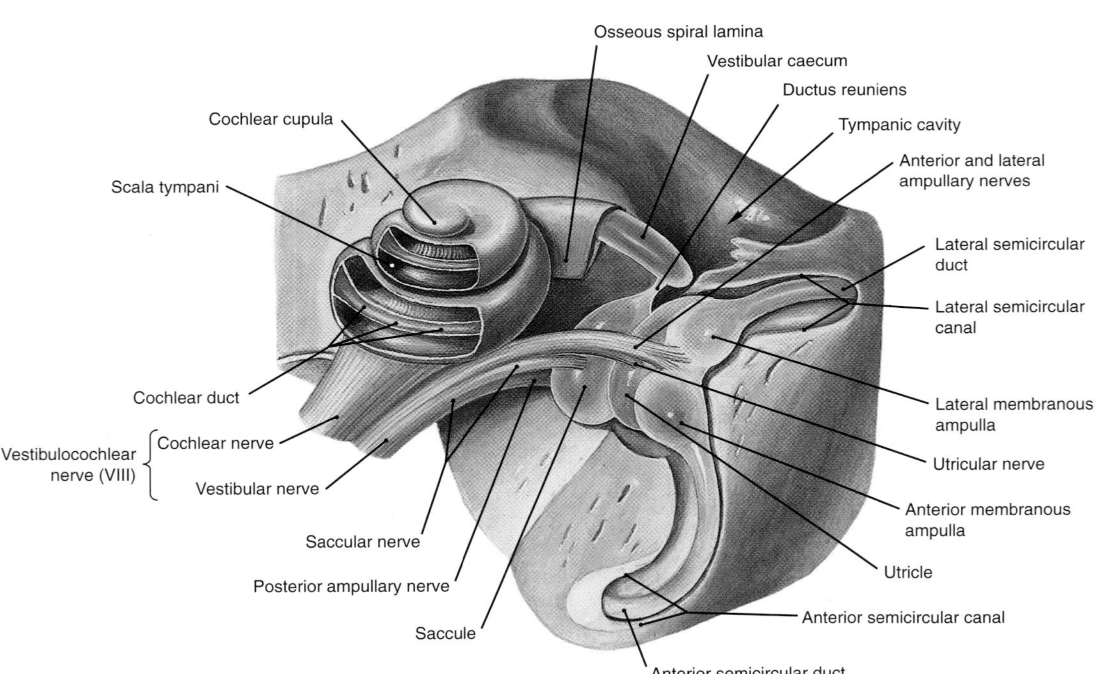
Osseous spiral lamina
Vestibular caecum
Ductus reuniens
Cochlear cupula
Tympanic cavity
Anterior and lateral ampullary nerves
Scala tympani
Lateral semicircular duct
Lateral semicircular canal
Cochlear duct
Lateral membranous ampulla
Vestibulocochlear nerve (VIII)
Cochlear nerve
Vestibular nerve
Utricular nerve
Anterior membranous ampulla
Saccular nerve
Utricle
Posterior ampullary nerve
Anterior semicircular canal
Saccule
Anterior semicircular duct

Figure 630.2 Right Vestibulocochlear Nerve, the Cochlea, and the Membranous Labyrinth of the Internal Ear

NOTE: (1) The anterior, lateral, and posterior **ampullary nerves** of the semicircular canals and the delicate **saccular** and **utricular nerves** all join to form the **vestibular nerve.**

(2) The fibers of the cochlear nerve receive input from the cochlear receptor cells in the **spiral organ of Corti.**

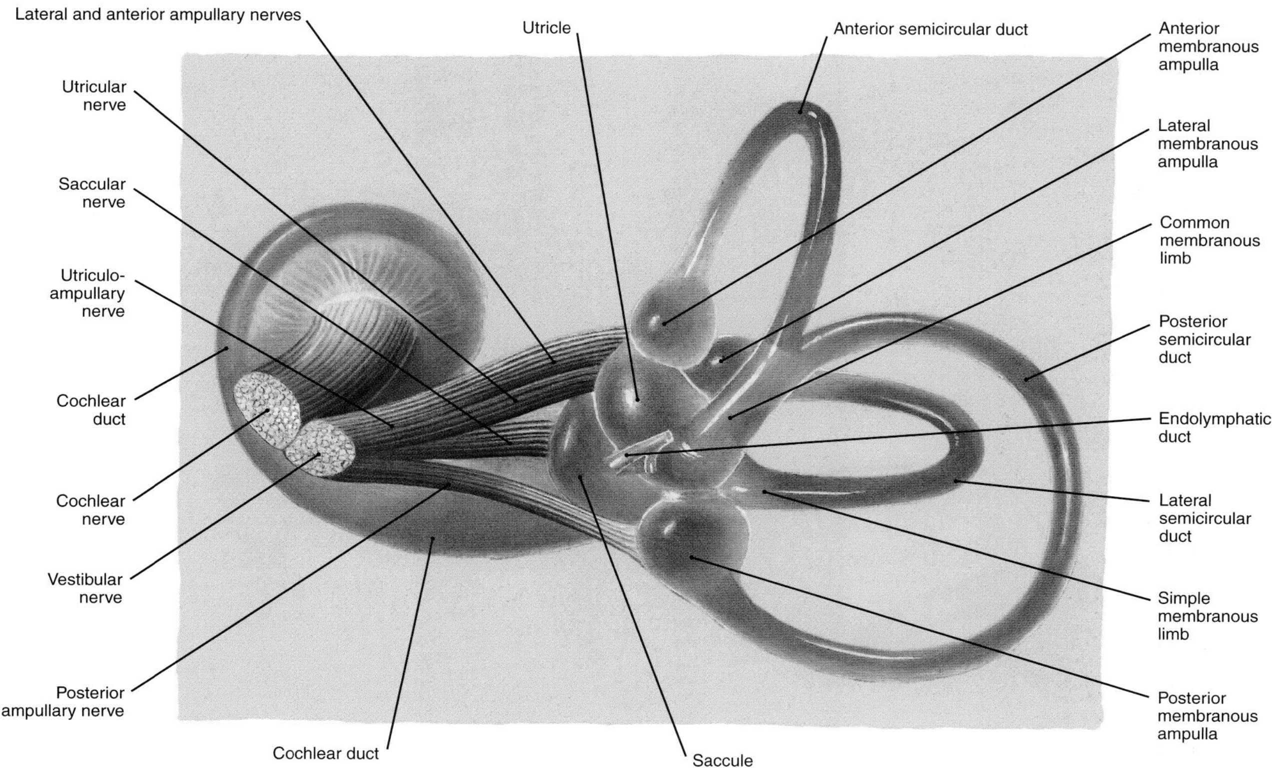
Lateral and anterior ampullary nerves
Utricle
Anterior semicircular duct
Anterior membranous ampulla
Utricular nerve
Lateral membranous ampulla
Saccular nerve
Common membranous limb
Utriculo-ampullary nerve
Posterior semicircular duct
Cochlear duct
Endolymphatic duct
Cochlear nerve
Lateral semicircular duct
Vestibular nerve
Simple membranous limb
Posterior ampullary nerve
Posterior membranous ampulla
Cochlear duct
Saccule

Figure 631.1 **Membranous Labyrinth, the Organ of Corti, and the Vestibular and Cochlear Nerves**

NOTE: (1) The vestibular nerve is the nerve of equilibrium, and because of its connections in the brain, sensory input from this nerve is able to alter eye movements and movements of the head and body that might counteract a loss of balance in an attempt to prevent a fall and thereby maintain equilibrium.

(2) The membranous labyrinth lies within the walls of the bony or osseous labyrinth.

(3) The receptors within the saccule and utricle are able to sense the position of the head with respect to gravity and are sometimes called the **static labyrinthine receptors.** These receptors (**maculae**) contain ciliated hair cells with a gelatinous substance over them and small crystals (**otoliths**) within the gel; since they react to head position in relationship to gravity, they are considered the organ of **static balance.**

(4) The receptors on the ampullae of the semicircular canals are related to kinetic balance and are stimulated by angular acceleration of the head. These are referred to as organs of **kinetic balance.**

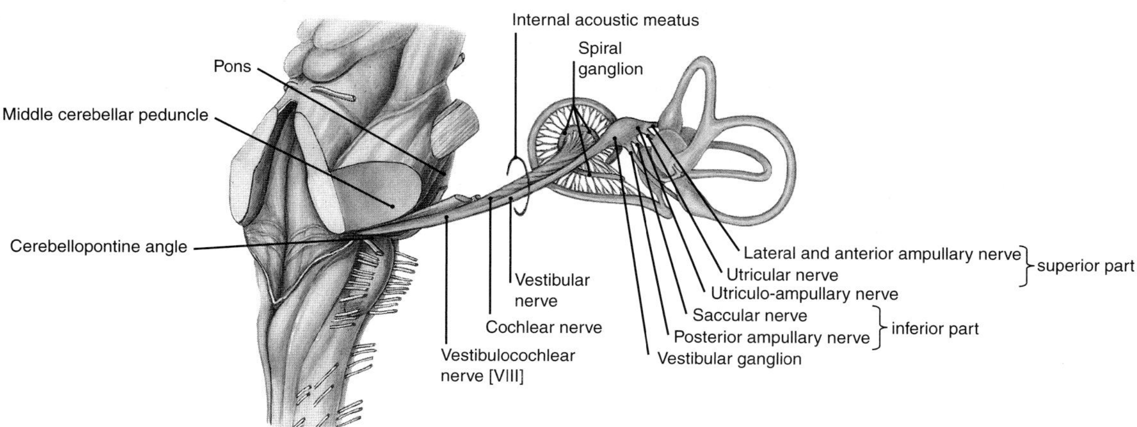
Internal acoustic meatus
Spiral ganglion
Pons
Middle cerebellar peduncle
Cerebellopontine angle
Lateral and anterior ampullary nerve
Utricular nerve
superior part
Utriculo-ampullary nerve
Saccular nerve
Posterior ampullary nerve
inferior part
Vestibular ganglion
Vestibular nerve
Cochlear nerve
Vestibulocochlear nerve [VIII]

Figure 631.2 **Diagrammatic Schema of the Vestibulocochlear Nerve**

NOTE: The vestibulocochlear and facial nerves attach to the brain at the cerebellopontine angle just posterior to the middle cerebellar peduncle.

Figure 632.1 Sensory Innervation of the Pharynx

NOTE: The glossopharyngeal nerve supplies the oral pharynx with sensory innervation and is the afferent limb of the gag reflex.

Maxillary nerve (V_2)

Glossopharyngeal nerve (IX)

Vagus nerve (X)

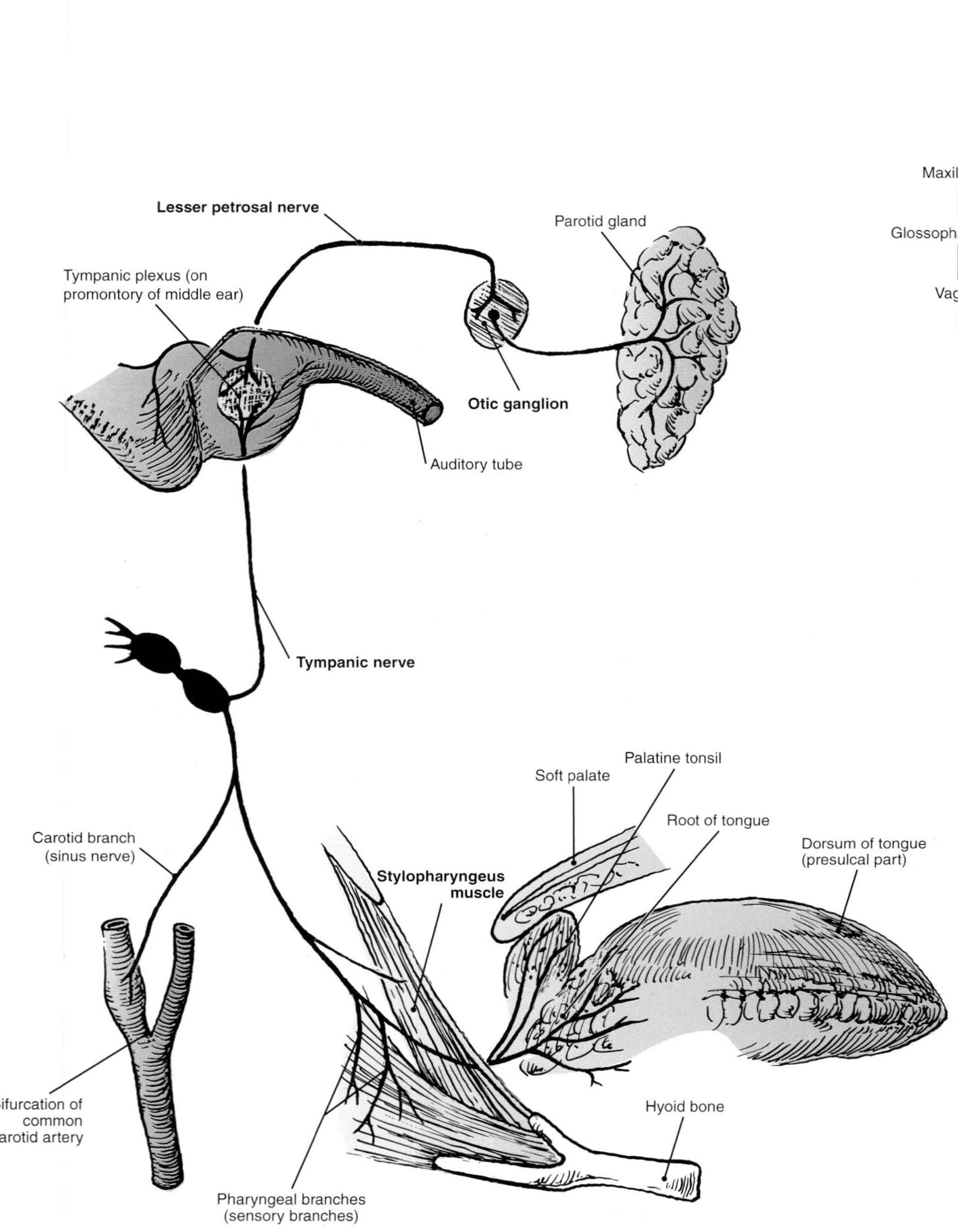
Lesser petrosal nerve
Tympanic plexus (on promontory of middle ear)
Parotid gland
Otic ganglion
Auditory tube
Tympanic nerve
Palatine tonsil
Soft palate
Root of tongue
Carotid branch (sinus nerve)
Dorsum of tongue (presulcal part)
Stylopharyngeus muscle
Bifurcation of common carotid artery
Hyoid bone
Pharyngeal branches (sensory branches)

Figure 632.2 Diagrammatic Representation of the Glossopharyngeal Nerve (after J.C.B. Grant)

NOTE: (1) The glossopharyngeal nerve supplies one voluntary muscle, the **stylopharyngeus.** This muscle (on both sides) elevates the pharynx during the act of swallowing. After supplying this muscle, the nerve supplies the posterior third of the tongue with both general sensory fibers and fibers of the special sense of **taste.**

(2) The glossopharyngeal nerve also has preganglionic parasympathetic nerve fibers that ascend in the **tympanic branch** to the middle ear and divides to form the **tympanic plexus** over the surface of the promontory.

(3) From this plexus, the fibers reassemble to form the **lesser petrosal nerve,** which enters the base of the skull on the superior surface of the temporal bone. It leaves the skull base through a small foramen adjacent the greater petrosal nerve and passes through the foramen ovale to join the **otic ganglion.**

(4) From the otic ganglion, postganglionic parasympathetic fibers join the **auriculotemporal nerve** and innervate the parotid gland.

(5) The **pharyngeal branches** of the glossopharyngeal nerve supply sensory innervation to the mucosa of the oropharynx and participate in the **gag reflex** (see Fig. 632.1).

(6) The **carotid branch** contains visceral afferent fibers and with the vagus nerve supplies the carotid body.

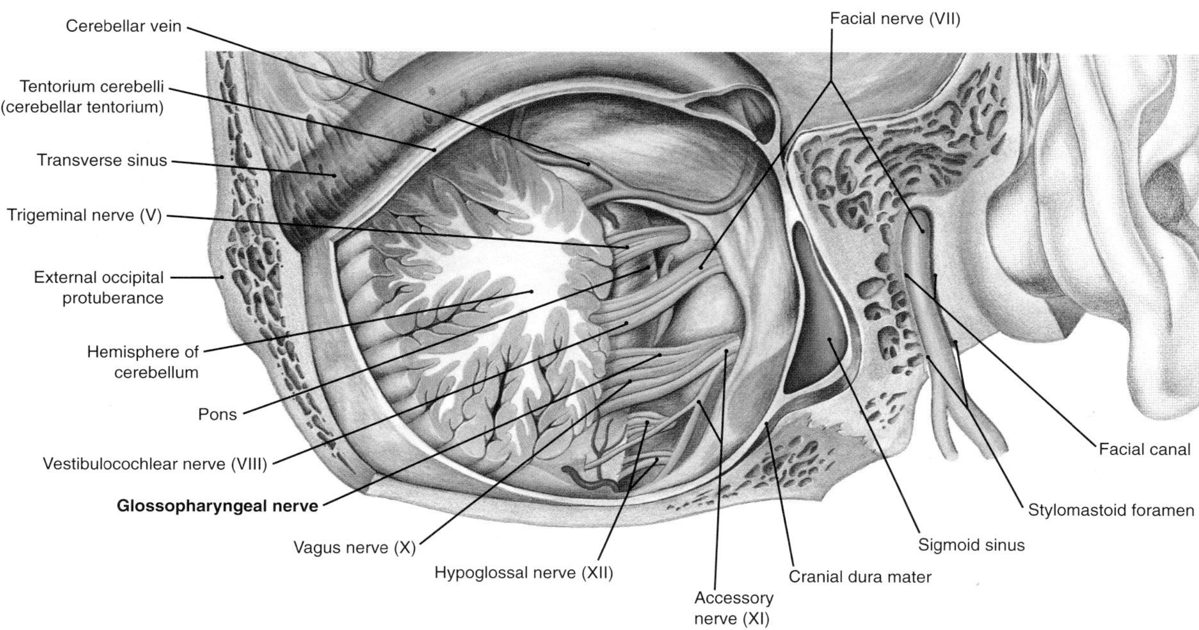
Cerebellar vein
Tentorium cerebelli (cerebellar tentorium)
Transverse sinus
Trigeminal nerve (V)
External occipital protuberance
Hemisphere of cerebellum
Pons
Vestibulocochlear nerve (VIII)
Glossopharyngeal nerve
Vagus nerve (X)
Hypoglossal nerve (XII)
Accessory nerve (XI)
Cranial dura mater
Sigmoid sinus
Stylomastoid foramen
Facial canal
Facial nerve (VII)

Figure 633.1 **Glossopharyngeal Nerve Coursing from the Skull Base through the Jugular Foramen**

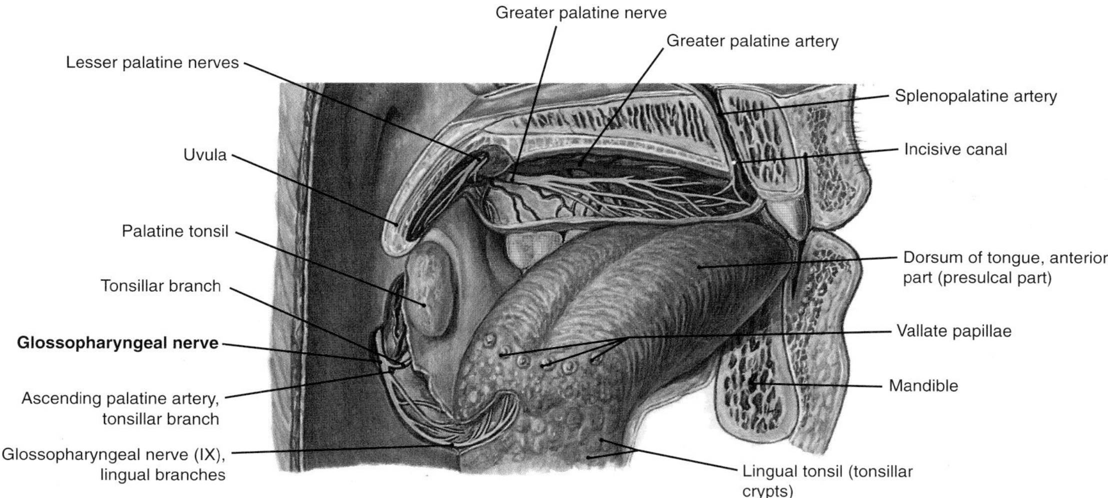
Greater palatine nerve
Greater palatine artery
Lesser palatine nerves
Splenopalatine artery
Incisive canal
Uvula
Palatine tonsil
Tonsillar branch
Glossopharyngeal nerve
Ascending palatine artery, tonsillar branch
Glossopharyngeal nerve (IX), lingual branches
Dorsum of tongue, anterior part (presulcal part)
Vallate papillae
Mandible
Lingual tonsil (tonsillar crypts)

Figure 633.2 **Glossopharyngeal Nerve in the Oropharynx and Penetrating the Posterior Third of the Tongue**
NOTE: At this site the glossopharyngeal nerve is sensory and carries general sensory and special sensory fibers (taste) to the posterior third of the tongue.

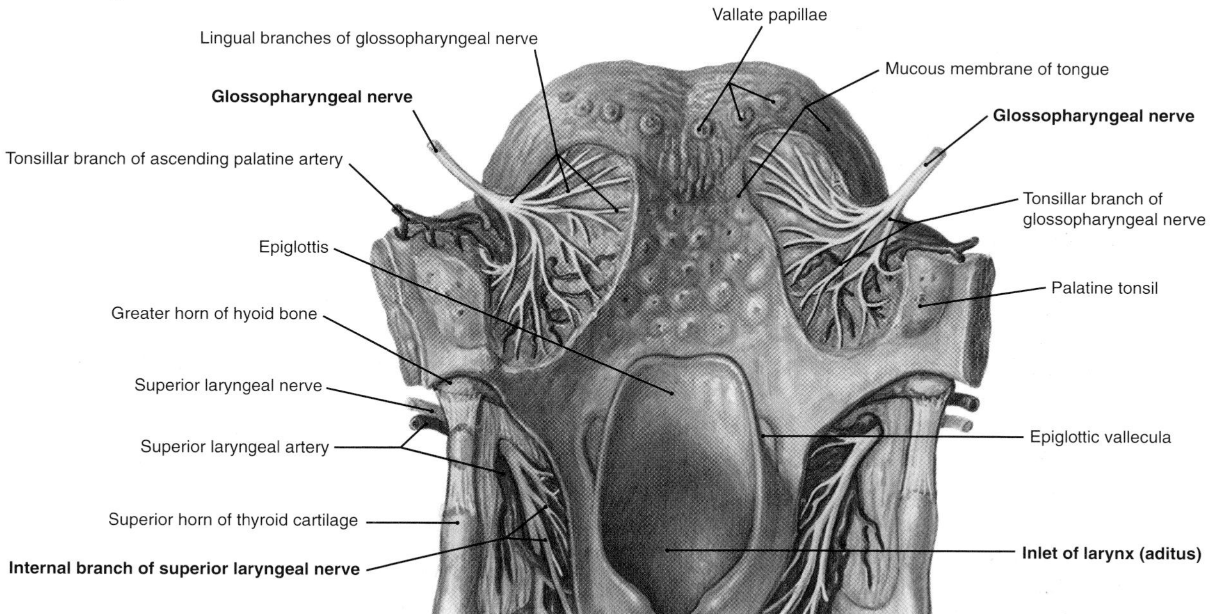
Vallate papillae
Lingual branches of glossopharyngeal nerve
Mucous membrane of tongue
Glossopharyngeal nerve
Glossopharyngeal nerve
Tonsillar branch of ascending palatine artery
Tonsillar branch of glossopharyngeal nerve
Epiglottis
Palatine tonsil
Greater horn of hyoid bone
Superior laryngeal nerve
Superior laryngeal artery
Epiglottic vallecula
Superior horn of thyroid cartilage
Internal branch of superior laryngeal nerve
Inlet of larynx (aditus)

Figure 633.3 **Glossopharyngeal Nerve and Its Lingual Branches to the Posterior Tongue and to the Vallate Papillae**

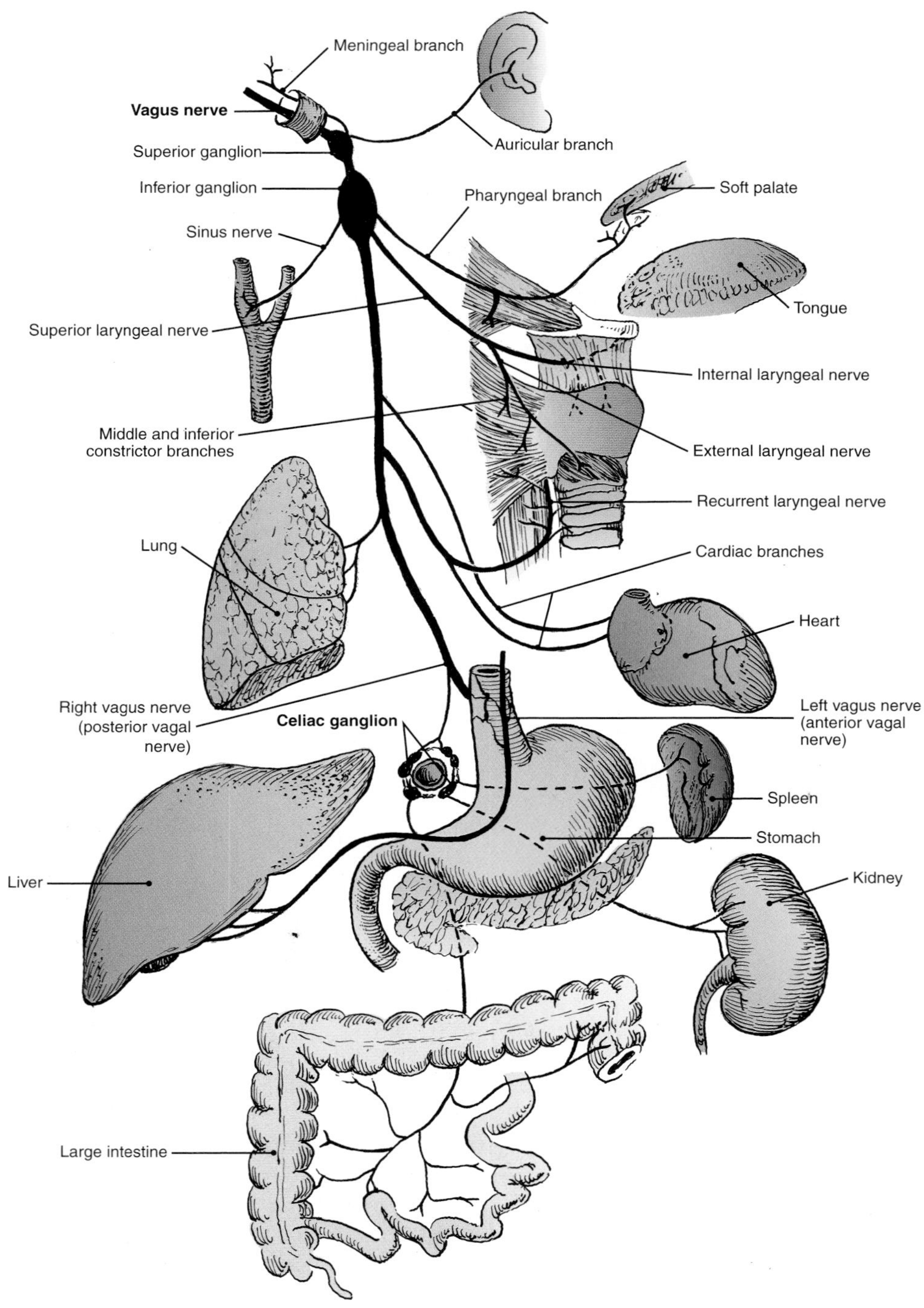
Meningeal branch
Vagus nerve
Superior ganglion
Inferior ganglion
Auricular branch
Pharyngeal branch
Soft palate
Sinus nerve
Tongue
Superior laryngeal nerve
Internal laryngeal nerve
Middle and inferior constrictor branches
External laryngeal nerve
Recurrent laryngeal nerve
Lung
Cardiac branches
Heart
Right vagus nerve (posterior vagal nerve)
Celiac ganglion
Left vagus nerve (anterior vagal nerve)
Spleen
Stomach
Kidney
Liver
Large intestine

Figure 634 Diagrammatic Representation of the Vagus Nerve

NOTE: (1) The vagus nerve contains both visceromotor and viscerosensory fibers as well as somatomotor fibers. The latter come from the medullary part of the accessory nerve, and they supply voluntary muscles in the larynx, pharynx, and soft palate.

(2) The visceromotor fibers are preganglionic parasympathetic fibers that innervate the organs in the neck, thorax, and the abdomen as far as the splenic flexure of the transverse colon.

(3) The vagus also contains a few somatosensory fibers in its **auricular branch** that supply some skin of the external ear; other sensory fibers are in the **superior laryngeal** and **recurrent laryngeal** branches that supply the internal mucosa of the larynx. In addition, the vagus contains visceral afferent fibers from organs in the neck, thorax, and abdomen. All of these sensory fibers have their cell bodies in the **superior and inferior ganglia** of the vagus.

(4) Visceral afferent fibers in the **carotid sinus** nerve are from pressoreceptor cells that respond to blood pressure changes.

(5) The **pharyngeal branch** of the vagus supplies motor fibers to the pharyngeal constrictor muscles as well as to the muscles of the soft palate (except the tensor veli palatini muscle). These motor fibers in the vagus are from the accessory nerve and are often described as 11 via 10 (i.e., accessory via the vagus).

(6) The **superior laryngeal branch** has an **external branch** supplying the cricothyroid muscle and an **internal branch** to the mucosa of the upper larynx. All other muscles of the larynx are supplied by the recurrent laryngeal branch.

Vagus Nerve (Continued)

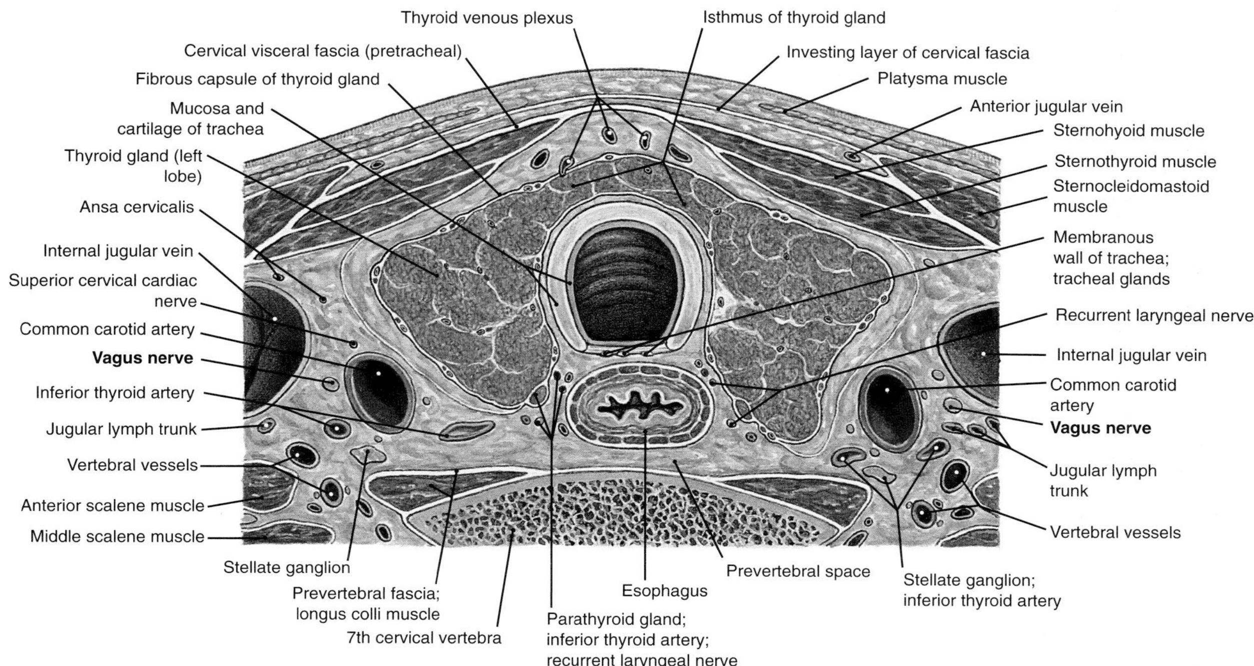
Thyroid venous plexus
Isthmus of thyroid gland
Cervical visceral fascia (pretracheal)
Investing layer of cervical fascia
Fibrous capsule of thyroid gland
Platysma muscle
Mucosa and cartilage of trachea
Anterior jugular vein
Sternohyoid muscle
Thyroid gland (left lobe)
Sternothyroid muscle
Sternocleidomastoid muscle
Ansa cervicalis
Membranous wall of trachea; tracheal glands
Internal jugular vein
Superior cervical cardiac nerve
Recurrent laryngeal nerve
Common carotid artery
Internal jugular vein
Vagus nerve
Common carotid artery
Inferior thyroid artery
Vagus nerve
Jugular lymph trunk
Vertebral vessels
Jugular lymph trunk
Anterior scalene muscle
Middle scalene muscle
Vertebral vessels
Stellate ganglion
Prevertebral space
Prevertebral fascia; longus colli muscle
Esophagus
Stellate ganglion; inferior thyroid artery
7th cervical vertebra
Parathyroid gland; inferior thyroid artery; recurrent laryngeal nerve

Figure 635.1 **Vagus Nerve in the Neck at the Level of the Second Tracheal Cartilage**

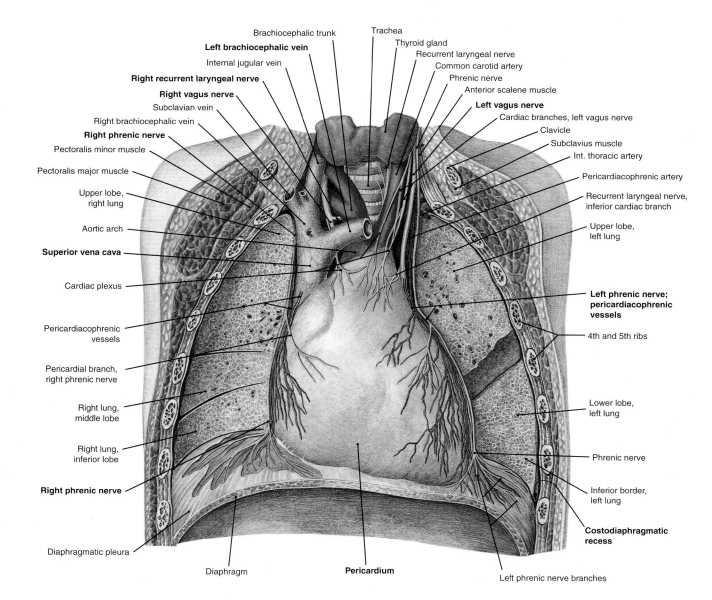

Brachiocephalic trunk
Trachea
Left brachiocephalic vein
Thyroid gland
Recurrent laryngeal nerve
Internal jugular vein
Common carotid artery
Right recurrent laryngeal nerve
Phrenic nerve
Anterior scalene muscle
Right vagus nerve
Left vagus nerve
Subclavian vein
Cardiac branches, left vagus nerve
Right brachiocephalic vein
Clavicle
Right phrenic nerve
Subclavius muscle
Pectoralis minor muscle
Int. thoracic artery
Pectoralis major muscle
Pericardiacophrenic artery
Upper lobe, right lung
Recurrent laryngeal nerve, inferior cardiac branch
Upper lobe, left lung
Aortic arch
Superior vena cava
Cardiac plexus
Left phrenic nerve; pericardiacophrenic vessels
Pericardiacophrenic vessels
4th and 5th ribs
Pericardial branch, right phrenic nerve
Lower lobe, left lung
Right lung, middle lobe
Right lung, inferior lobe
Phrenic nerve
Right phrenic nerve
Inferior border, left lung
Costodiaphragmatic recess
Diaphragmatic pleura
Diaphragm
Pericardium
Left phrenic nerve branches

Figure 635.2 **Vagus Nerves in the Upper Thorax**

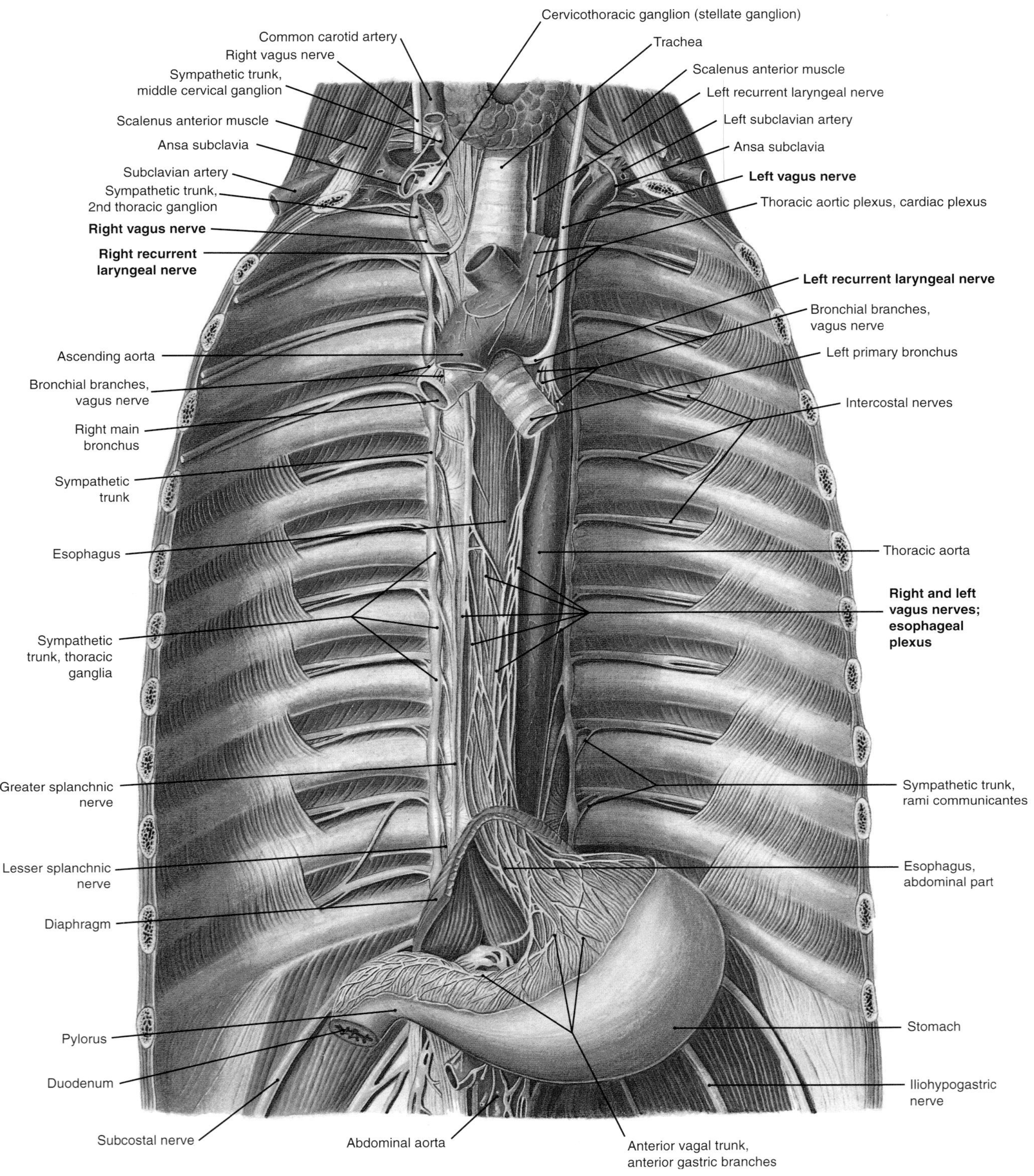
Cervicothoracic ganglion (stellate ganglion)
Common carotid artery
Trachea
Right vagus nerve
Scalenus anterior muscle
Sympathetic trunk,
middle cervical ganglion
Left recurrent laryngeal nerve
Scalenus anterior muscle
Left subclavian artery
Ansa subclavia
Ansa subclavia
Subclavian artery
Left vagus nerve
Sympathetic trunk,
2nd thoracic ganglion
Thoracic aortic plexus, cardiac plexus
Right vagus nerve
Right recurrent
laryngeal nerve
Left recurrent laryngeal nerve
Bronchial branches,
vagus nerve
Left primary bronchus
Ascending aorta
Bronchial branches,
vagus nerve
Intercostal nerves
Right main
bronchus
Sympathetic
trunk
Esophagus
Thoracic aorta
Right and left
vagus nerves;
esophageal
plexus
Sympathetic
trunk, thoracic
ganglia
Greater splanchnic
nerve
Sympathetic trunk,
rami communicantes
Lesser splanchnic
nerve
Esophagus,
abdominal part
Diaphragm
Pylorus
Stomach
Duodenum
Iliohypogastric
nerve
Subcostal nerve
Abdominal aorta
Anterior vagal trunk,
anterior gastric branches

Figure 636 Vagus Nerve in the Thorax

NOTE: (1) The vagus nerves enter the superior mediastinum, give off the recurrent laryngeal nerves, and then course medially toward the bronchi, where they form bronchial plexuses, and then toward the esophagus.

(2) The **left vagus nerve** splits into branches and forms the **anterior** esophageal plexus, while the **right vagus nerve** forms the **posterior** esophageal plexus.

(3) The fibers of these plexuses enter the abdomen through the esophageal hiatus. The left vagal fibers become the **anterior gastric branches** and the right vagal fibers become the **posterior gastric branches.** The anterior branches supply the anterosuperior aspect of the stomach, while the posterior branches supply the posteroinferior aspect of the stomach.

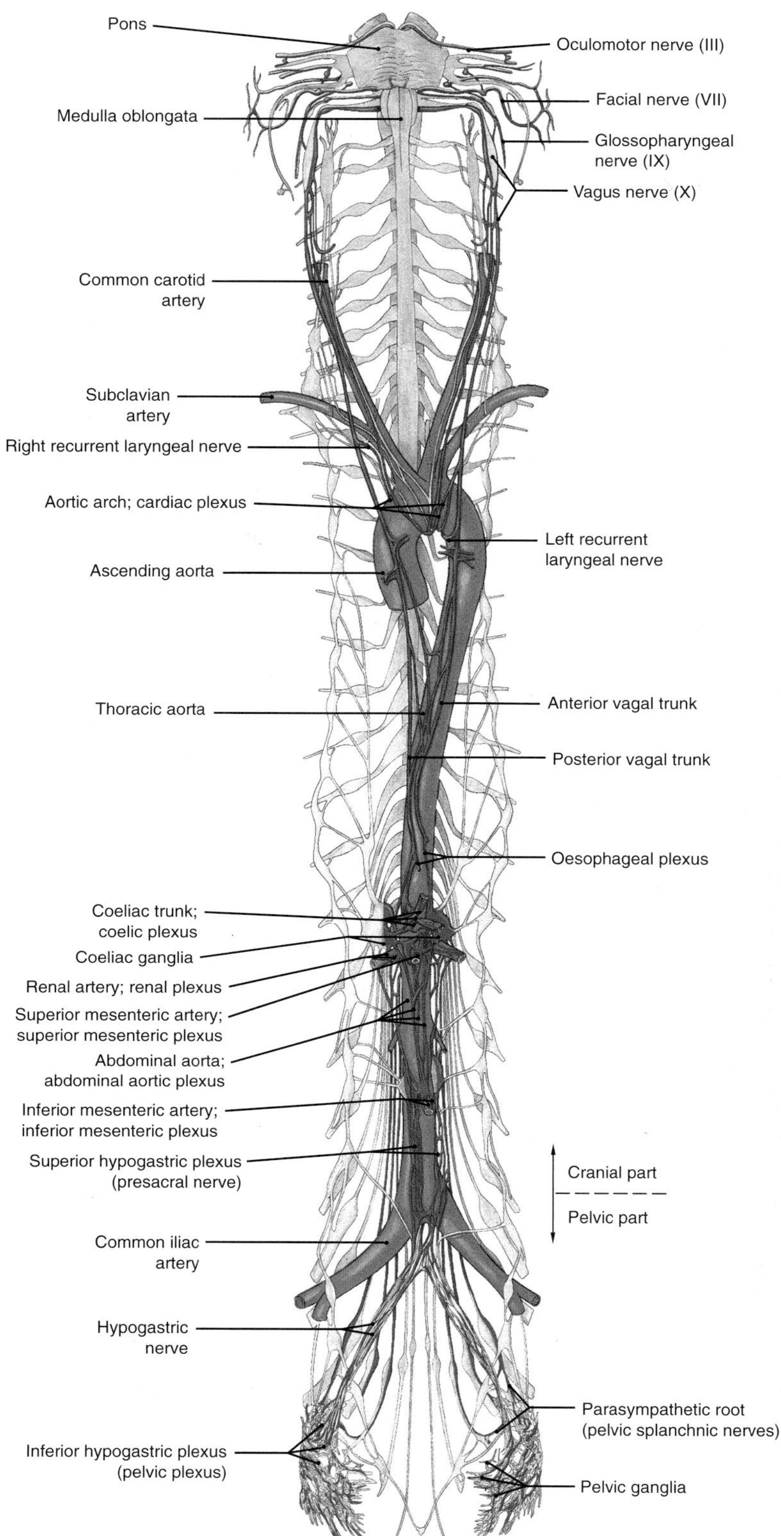
Pons
Oculomotor nerve (III)
Medulla oblongata
Facial nerve (VII)
Glossopharyngeal nerve (IX)
Vagus nerve (X)
Common carotid artery
Subclavian artery
Right recurrent laryngeal nerve
Aortic arch; cardiac plexus
Left recurrent laryngeal nerve
Ascending aorta
Thoracic aorta
Anterior vagal trunk
Posterior vagal trunk
Oesophageal plexus
Coeliac trunk; coelic plexus
Coeliac ganglia
Renal artery; renal plexus
Superior mesenteric artery; superior mesenteric plexus
Abdominal aorta; abdominal aortic plexus
Inferior mesenteric artery; inferior mesenteric plexus
Superior hypogastric plexus (presacral nerve)
Cranial part
Pelvic part
Common iliac artery
Hypogastric nerve
Parasympathetic root (pelvic splanchnic nerves)
Inferior hypogastric plexus (pelvic plexus)
Pelvic ganglia

Figure 637 **Parasympathetic Division of the Autonomic Nervous System**

NOTE: (1) Four cranial nerves carry preganglionic parasympathetic nerve fibers: the 3rd, or **oculomotor;** the 7th, or **facial;** the 9th, or **glossopharyngeal;** and the 10th, or **vagus.**

(2) The preganglionic parasympathetic fibers in the third, seventh, and ninth nerves course to ganglia in the head, but the vagus nerve does not send parasympathetic fibers to the head. Vagal fibers seek postganglionic parasympathetic neuron in the walls of viscera in the neck thorax and abdomen.

(3) Below the splenic flexure of the transverse colon, preganglionic parasympathetic fibers come from the second, third, and fourth sacral spinal nerves. The descending colon, sigmoid colon, and rectum, and all other organs in the pelvis are supplied with parasympathetic fibers from these sacral nerves (also called pelvic splanchnic nerves).

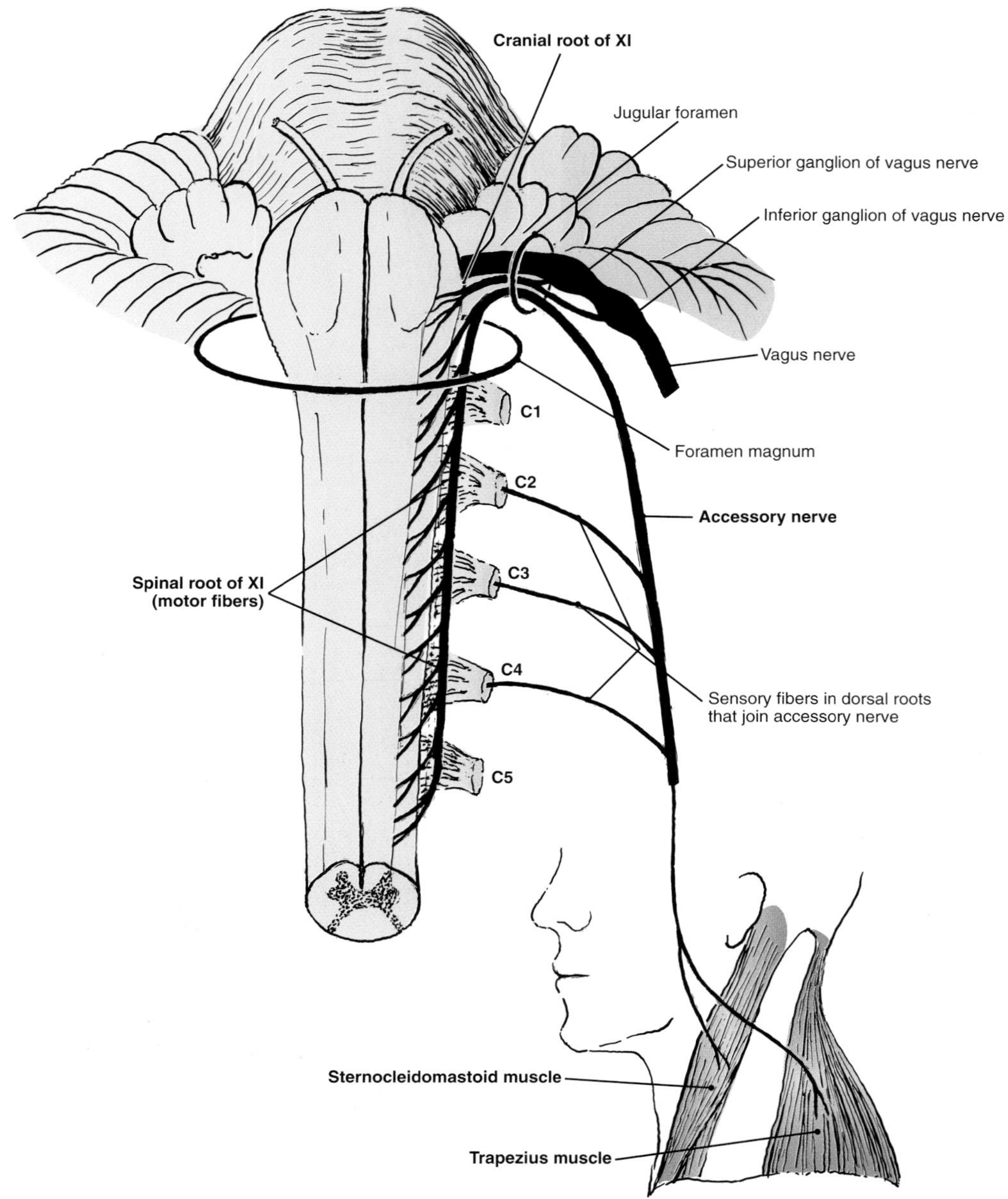

Cranial root of XI
Jugular foramen
Superior ganglion of vagus nerve
Inferior ganglion of vagus nerve
Vagus nerve
C1
Foramen magnum
C2
Accessory nerve
Spinal root of XI
(motor fibers)
C3
C4
Sensory fibers in dorsal roots
that join accessory nerve
C5
Sternocleidomastoid muscle
Trapezius muscle

Figure 638 Diagrammatic Representation of the Accessory Nerve (XI Cranial Nerve)

NOTE: (1) The **accessory nerve** (sometimes called the spinal accessory nerve) is formed by the brief union of fibers that originate in the spinal cord and others that emerge from the medulla oblongata.

(2) Motor nerve fibers leave the spinal cord from cervical segmental levels down as far as C5. The fibers from these upper cervical segments join to form a single trunk that ascends in the spinal canal and enters the cranial cavity through the foramen magnum. This constitutes the **spinal root**.

(3) Within the cranial cavity the spinal root is joined by the smaller **cranial root,** which consists of five or six delicate rootlets that leave the medulla oblongata just inferior to the rootlets of the vagus nerve.

(4) The cranial root briefly joins the spinal root and then **separates from it and merges with the rootlets of the vagus nerve,** with which it descends through the jugular foramen.

(5) The spinal root (now consisting of the original spinal motor fibers) turns inferiorly and also leaves the cranial cavity through the jugular foramen to enter the neck, where it supplies the **sternocleidomastoid muscle**, and crosses the posterior triangle to innervate the **trapezius muscle.**

(6) The medullary fibers that join the vagus nerve become distributed in its pharyngeal and recurrent laryngeal branches to supply striated fibers of the pharyngeal and laryngeal muscles and the muscles of the soft palate (except for the tensor veli palatini muscle).

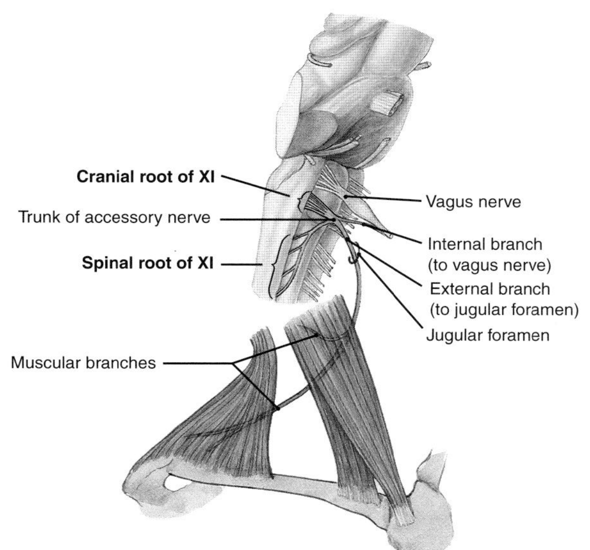
Cranial root of XI
Trunk of accessory nerve
Spinal root of XI
Muscular branches
Vagus nerve
Internal branch
(to vagus nerve)
External branch
(to jugular foramen)
Jugular foramen

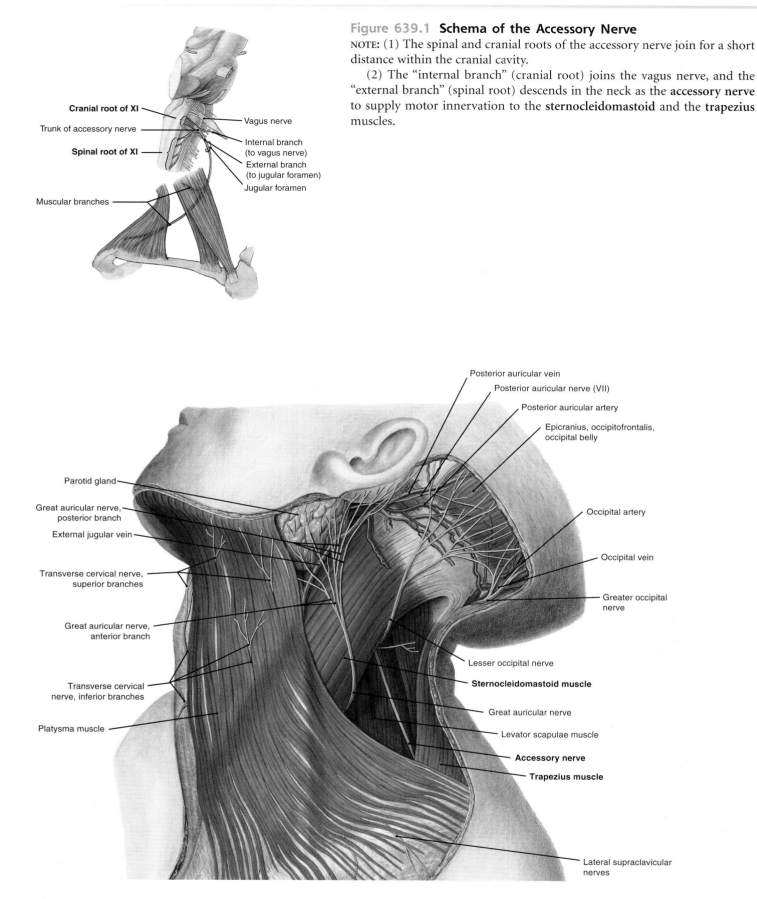

Figure 639.1 Schema of the Accessory Nerve

NOTE: (1) The spinal and cranial roots of the accessory nerve join for a short distance within the cranial cavity.

(2) The "internal branch" (cranial root) joins the vagus nerve, and the "external branch" (spinal root) descends in the neck as the **accessory nerve** to supply motor innervation to the **sternocleidomastoid** and the **trapezius** muscles.

Posterior auricular vein
Posterior auricular nerve (VII)
Posterior auricular artery
Epicranius, occipitofrontalis, occipital belly
Parotid gland
Great auricular nerve, posterior branch
External jugular vein
Transverse cervical nerve, superior branches
Great auricular nerve, anterior branch
Transverse cervical nerve, inferior branches
Platysma muscle
Occipital artery
Occipital vein
Greater occipital nerve
Lesser occipital nerve
Sternocleidomastoid muscle
Great auricular nerve
Levator scapulae muscle
Accessory nerve
Trapezius muscle
Lateral supraclavicular nerves

Figure 639.2 Accessory Nerve Traversing the Posterior Triangle of the Neck

NOTE: (1) Distal to the jugular foramen, the accessory nerve descends in the neck deep to the **sternocleidomastoid muscle** as it innervates it. Then it crosses the posterior triangle of the neck to the deep surface of the **trapezius muscle,** which it also supplies.

(2) Sensory fibers from the **C3, C4,** and **C5** segments also join the nerve. Some of these supply proprioceptors that allow the individual to know the positions of the head and shoulder as the muscles act.

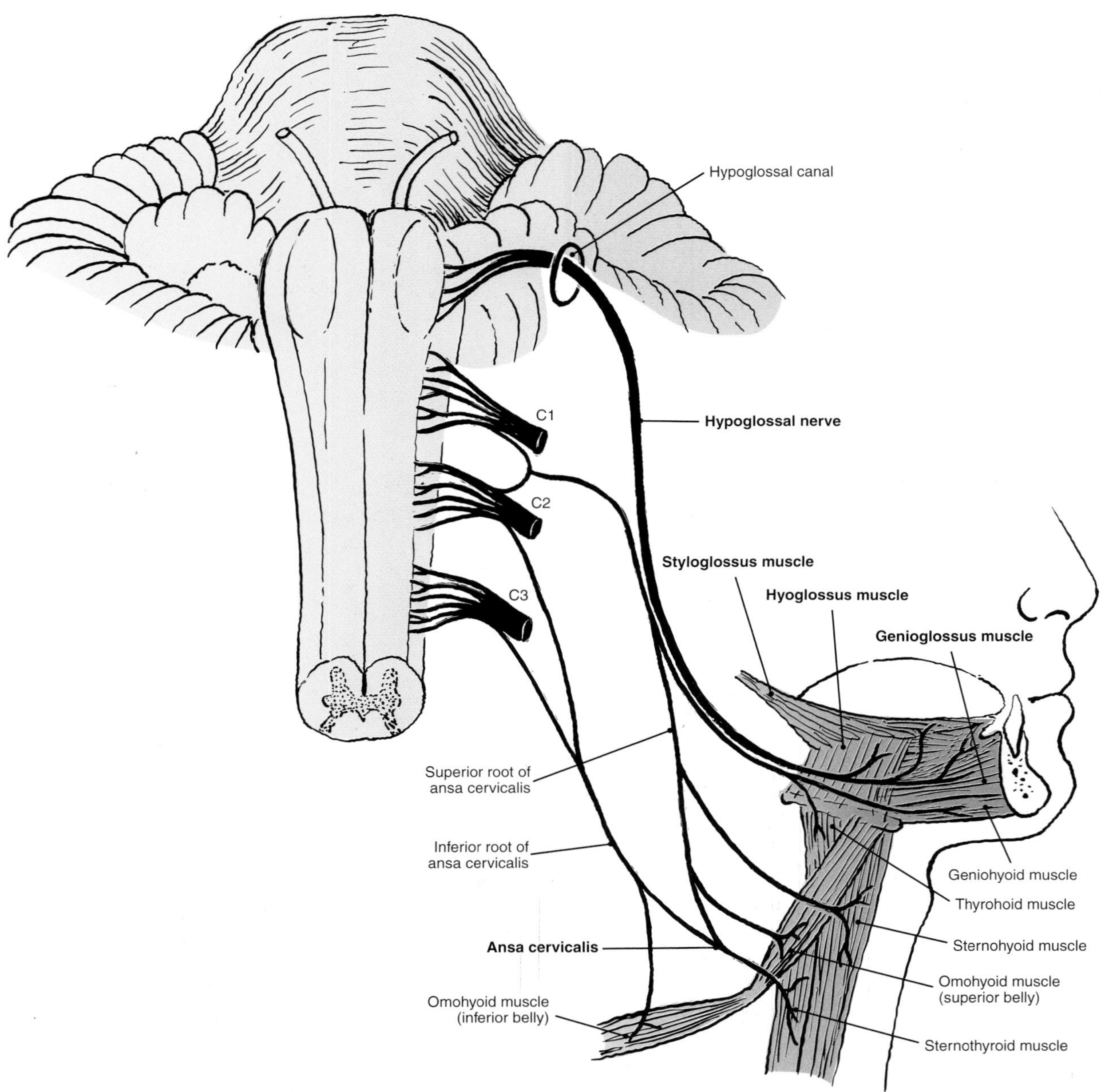
Hypoglossal canal
C1
Hypoglossal nerve
C2
Styloglossus muscle
C3
Hyoglossus muscle
Genioglossus muscle
Superior root of ansa cervicalis
Inferior root of ansa cervicalis
Geniohyoid muscle
Thyrohoid muscle
Sternohyoid muscle
Ansa cervicalis
Omohyoid muscle (superior belly)
Omohyoid muscle (inferior belly)
Sternothyroid muscle

Figure 640 **Hypoglossal Nerve (Diagrammatic Representation)**

NOTE: (1) The hypoglossal nerve is the motor nerve of the tongue. Its fibers emerge from the medulla oblongata in a line with the oculomotor, trochlear, and abducens nerves and the anterior roots (motor) of the spinal cord.

(2) This nerve supplies all the **intrinsic muscles** (longitudinal, transverse, and vertical) of the tongue and all of the **extrinsic muscles** (except the palatoglossus) that move the tongue (i.e., the **styloglossus, hyoglossus,** and **genioglossus**).

(3) The palatoglossus muscle is innervated by the pharyngeal branch of the vagus and forms the anterior pillar of the fauces in the oral cavity. It is the only muscle with the term "glossus" in its name not supplied by the hypoglossal nerve.

(4) In the upper neck, the hypoglossal nerve takes a 270-degree turn deep to the posterior belly of the digastric muscle and enters the oral cavity between the hyoglossus and mylohyoid muscles (see Fig. 641.2).

(5) The C1, C2, and C3 nerves emerge from the spinal cord and form two descending nerve trunks: the **superior** and **inferior roots** of the **ansa cervicalis.** The superior root (C1 and C2 fibers) courses with the hypoglossal nerve for a short distance, *but they are NOT hypoglossal fibers.*

(6) The superior root (C1 and C2) joins the inferior root (C2 and C3) and together they join as a loop called the **ansa cervicalis.** From this cervical nerve formation the strap muscles of the neck are innervated.

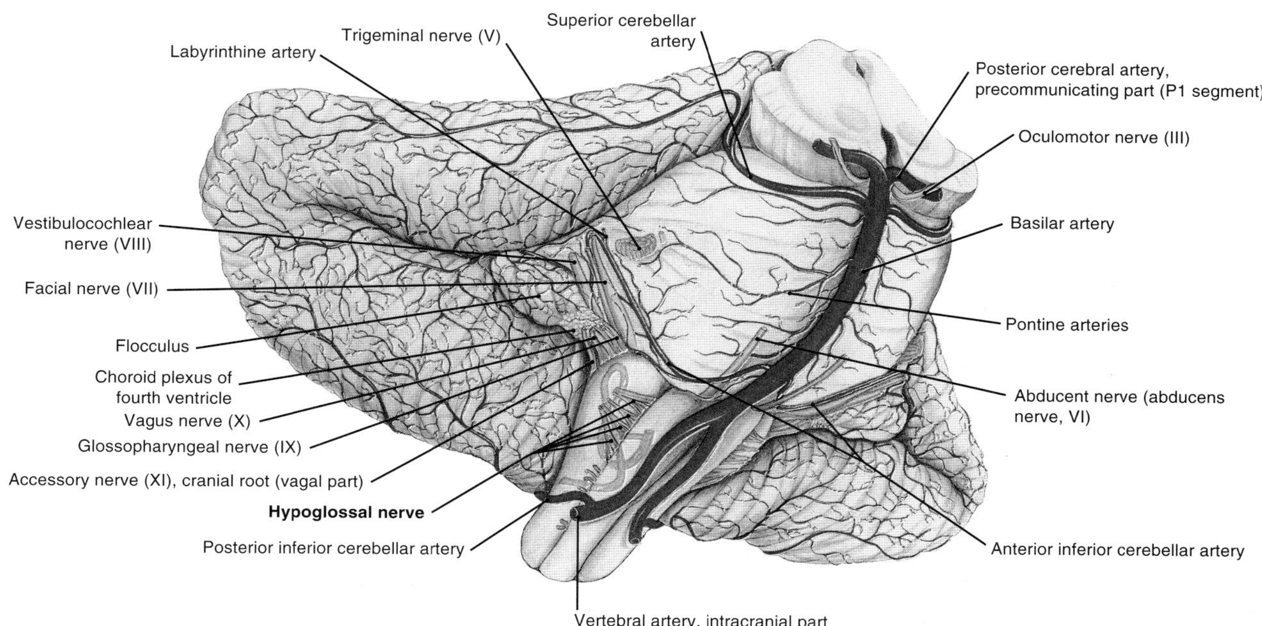
Labyrinthine artery
Trigeminal nerve (V)
Superior cerebellar artery
Posterior cerebral artery, precommunicating part (P1 segment)
Oculomotor nerve (III)
Vestibulocochlear nerve (VIII)
Basilar artery
Facial nerve (VII)
Pontine arteries
Flocculus
Choroid plexus of fourth ventricle
Abducent nerve (abducens nerve, VI)
Vagus nerve (X)
Glossopharyngeal nerve (IX)
Accessory nerve (XI), cranial root (vagal part)
Hypoglossal nerve
Posterior inferior cerebellar artery
Anterior inferior cerebellar artery
Vertebral artery, intracranial part

Figure 641.1 **Medulla Oblongata and the Pons of the Brainstem Showing the Exit of the Hypoglossal Nerve**

NOTE: (1) The hypoglossal nerve emerges from the anterolateral sulcus of the medulla oblongata by a series of 24 to 16 rootlets that form two bundles before traversing the occipital bone by way of the hypoglossal canal (condylar canal).

(2) From the cervical end of the hypoglossal canal, the hypoglossal nerve descends in the neck somewhat posterior to the internal jugular vein and internal carotid artery (see Fig. 641.2).

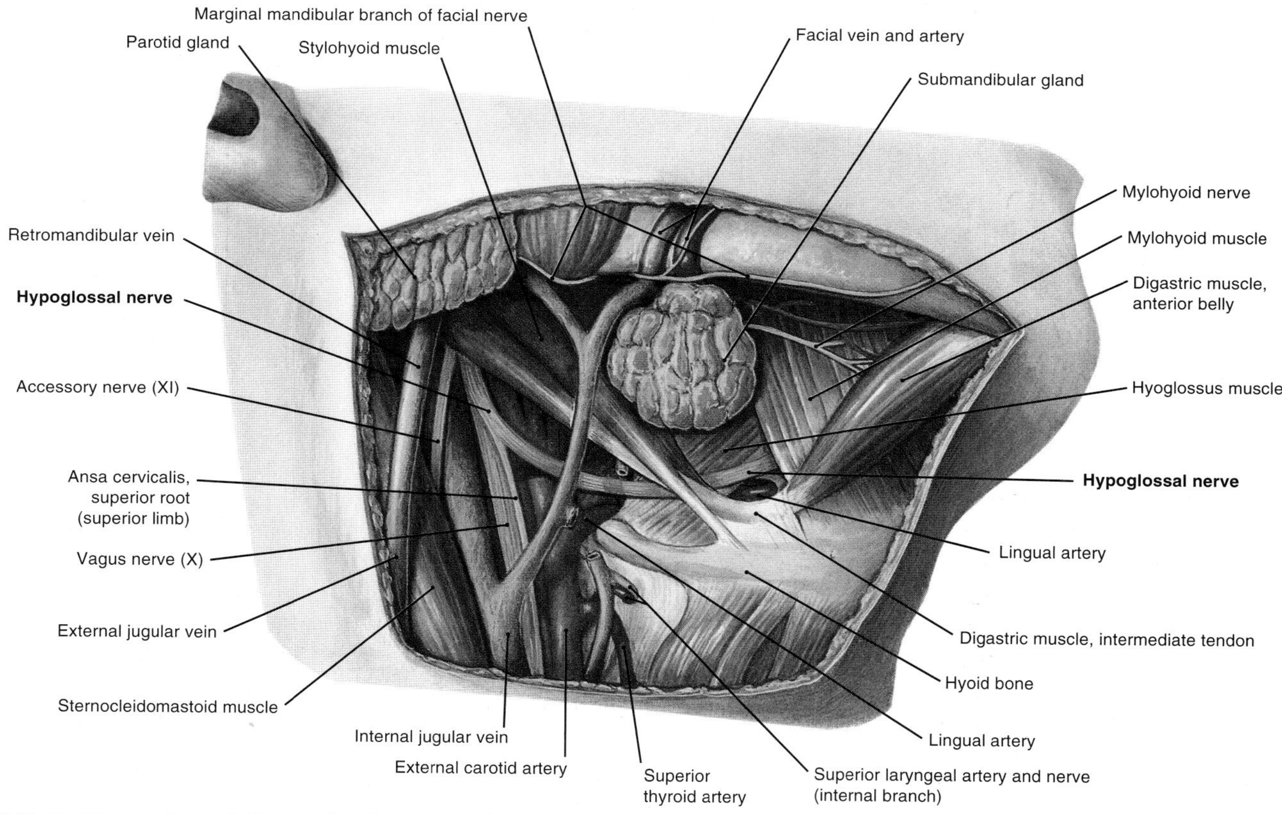
Marginal mandibular branch of facial nerve
Parotid gland
Stylohyoid muscle
Facial vein and artery
Submandibular gland
Mylohyoid nerve
Retromandibular vein
Mylohyoid muscle
Digastric muscle, anterior belly
Hypoglossal nerve
Accessory nerve (XI)
Hyoglossus muscle
Ansa cervicalis, superior root (superior limb)
Hypoglossal nerve
Vagus nerve (X)
Lingual artery
External jugular vein
Digastric muscle, intermediate tendon
Hyoid bone
Sternocleidomastoid muscle
Internal jugular vein
Lingual artery
External carotid artery
Superior thyroid artery
Superior laryngeal artery and nerve (internal branch)

Figure 641.2 **Hypoglossal Nerve in the Superior Neck Region**

NOTE: (1) In the upper neck region, the hypoglossal nerve (in addition to passing deep to the internal jugular vein and the internal carotid artery) descends posterior to the glossopharyngeal, vagus and accessory nerves.

(2) At the lower end of the posterior belly of the digastric muscle and below the angle of the mandible, the hypoglossal nerve **turns medially and superiorly** deep to the tendon of the posterior belly of the digastric muscle and the stylohyoid muscle to enter the submandibular triangle.

(3) Lying lateral (or superficial) to the hyoglossus muscle, the hypoglossal nerve passes between that muscle and the mylohyoid muscle to enter the oral cavity.

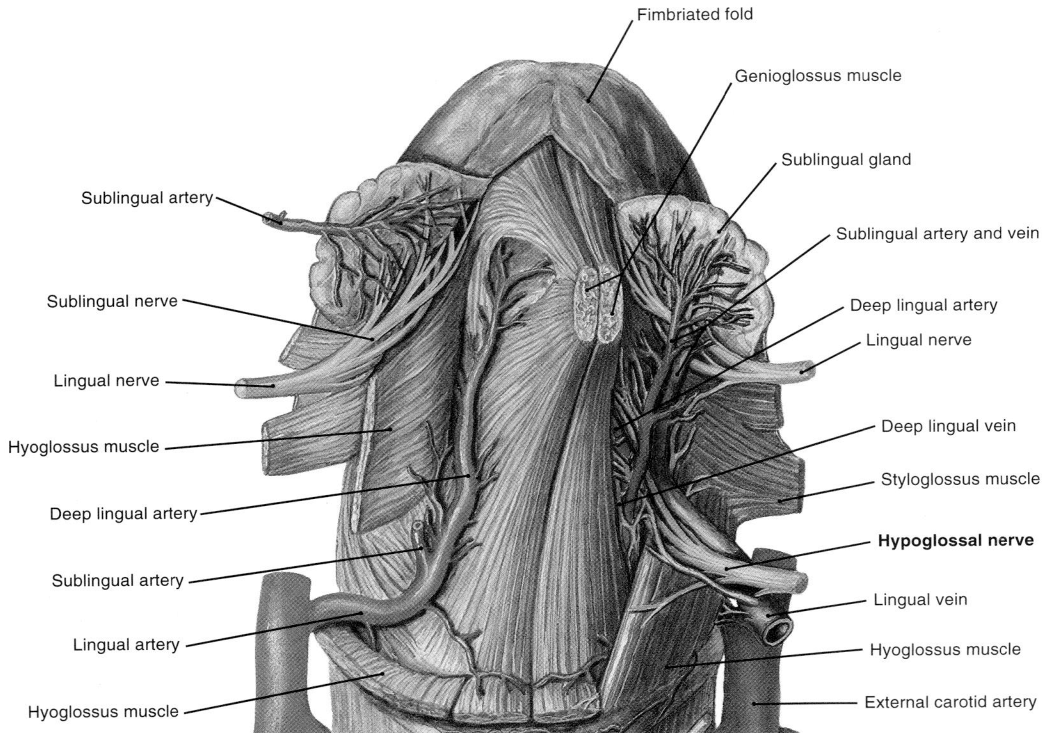

Fimbriated fold
Genioglossus muscle
Sublingual gland
Sublingual artery and vein
Deep lingual artery
Lingual nerve
Deep lingual vein
Styloglossus muscle
Hypoglossal nerve
Lingual vein
Hyoglossus muscle
External carotid artery
Sublingual artery
Sublingual nerve
Lingual nerve
Hyoglossus muscle
Deep lingual artery
Sublingual artery
Lingual artery
Hyoglossus muscle

Figure 642.1 **Hypoglossal Nerve as It Enters the Tongue (Inferior View)**

NOTE: (1) The hypoglossal nerve enters the oral cavity deep to the mylohyoid muscle and superficial (shown here) to the hyoglossus muscle. The nerve often courses with a pair of accompanying veins (called **vena comitans nervi hypoglossi**); which drain either into the facial vein or the lingual vein.

(2) When the hypoglossal nerve is cut or injured, the muscles on that side of the tongue are denervated. Upon physical examination when the patient is asked to protrude the tongue, it is directed toward the paralyzed side because the innervated muscles on the normal side are acting unopposed.

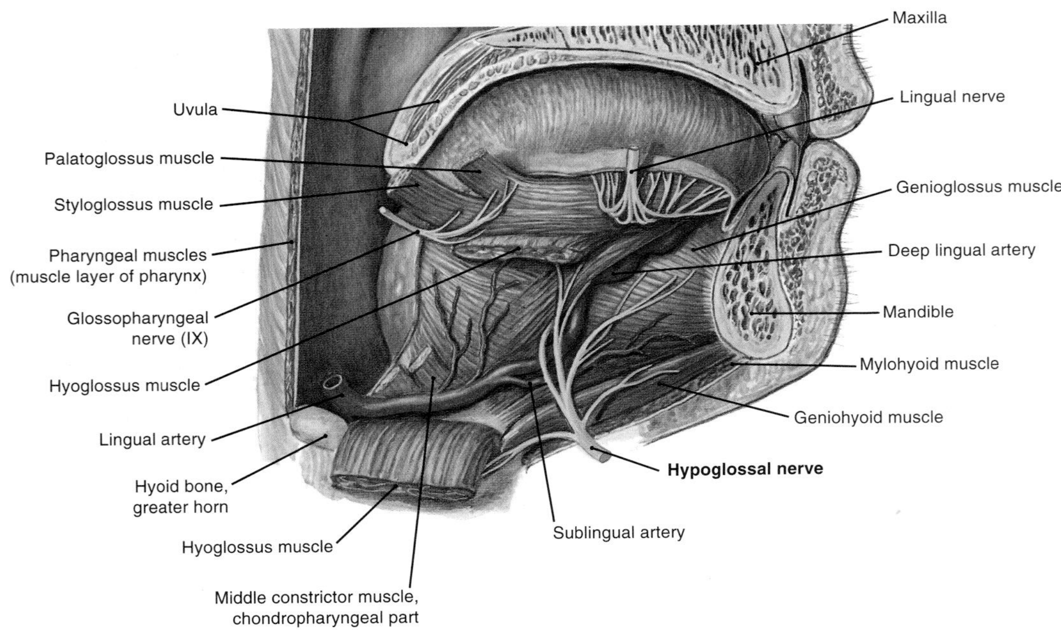

Maxilla
Lingual nerve
Genioglossus muscle
Deep lingual artery
Mandible
Mylohyoid muscle
Geniohyoid muscle
Hypoglossal nerve
Sublingual artery
Uvula
Palatoglossus muscle
Styloglossus muscle
Pharyngeal muscles (muscle layer of pharynx)
Glossopharyngeal nerve (IX)
Hyoglossus muscle
Lingual artery
Hyoid bone, greater horn
Hyoglossus muscle
Middle constrictor muscle, chondropharyngeal part

Figure 642.2 **Hypoglossal Nerve in the Oral Cavity**

NOTE: (1) As the hypoglossal nerve approaches the tongue from its inferolateral aspect, it gives off branches to the hyoglossus, genioglossus, styloglossus, and geniohyoid. The fibers to the geniohyoid, however, are not true hypoglossal fibers in origin, but come from the C1 nerve.

(2) From the lateral aspect of the genioglossus muscle, the hypoglossal nerve continues forward within the muscular substance of the tongue as far as the tip.

Index

Numbers refer to **Plates**
Numbers in **boldface** type indicate main references.

* Muscle chart describes action, innervation, insertion, and origin.

* Muscle chart describes action, innervation, insertion, and origin.

* Muscle chart describes action, innervation, insertion, and origin.

* Muscle chart describes action, innervation, insertion, and origin.